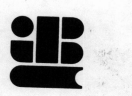

Issues
in the Care of Children
with Chronic Illness

A Sourcebook
on Problems, Services,
and Policies

Nicholas Hobbs
James M. Perrin
General Editors

with the assistance of
Henry T. Ireys
May W. Shayne
Linda C. Moynihan

Issues
in the Care of Children
with Chronic Illness

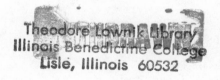
 Jossey-Bass Publishers
San Francisco • London • 1985

ISSUES IN THE CARE OF CHILDREN WITH CHRONIC ILLNESS
A Sourcebook on Problems, Services, and Policies
  by Nicholas Hobbs and James M. Perrin, General Editors

Copyright © 1985 by: Jossey-Bass Inc., Publishers
                     433 California Street
                     San Francisco, California 94104

&

Jossey-Bass Limited
28 Banner Street
London EC1Y 8QE

Library of Congress Cataloging in Publication Data
Main entry under title:

Issues in the care of children with chronic illness.

   Jossey-Bass social and behavioral science series)
(Jossey-Bass health series)
   Includes bibliographies and indexes.
   1. Chronic diseases in children—United States.
2. Chronically ill children—Services for—United
States.   3. Chronically ill children—Education.
4. Chronically ill children—Government policy—
United States.   I. Hobbs, Nicholas.   II. Perrin,
James M. (James Marc)   III. Series.   IV. Series:
Jossey-Bass Health series. [DNLM: 1. Chronic Disease—
in infancy & childhood.   2. Chronic Disease—
rehabilitation.   3. Health Policy—United States.
WS 200 I86]
RJ380.I87   1985   362.1′9892   85-45056
ISBN 0-87589-650-2 (alk. paper)

Manufactured in the United States of America

The paper in this book meets the guidelines for
permanence and durability of the Committee on
Production Guidelines for Book Longevity of the
Council on Library Resources.

JACKET DESIGN BY WILLI BAUM

FIRST EDITION

Code 8523

A joint publication in
The Jossey-Bass
Social and Behavioral Science Series
and
The Jossey-Bass Health Series

Preface

Childhood chronic illness in America has changed dramatically in the last two decades. Major advances in medical treatments and in the organization of health services have led to the survival of many children who in years past would have succumbed to their illness. Today, most children with severe chronic illnesses survive to adulthood. The task now is to enhance their lives and those of their families and to enable them to participate fully in American society.

It was the changing nature of illness in childhood that led us to a careful review of public policies for families with children with chronic illnesses. Most of the infectious diseases that claimed the lives of children earlier in the century have been eradicated or brought under control. Chronic and continuing afflictions have largely replaced earlier severe acute conditions as a central problem in child health care in America. Ten to 15 percent of children in America have a chronic health condition. Of this group, about 10 percent—or 1 to 2 percent of all children—have a condition severe enough to interfere with their daily activities.

Our intent has been to define and examine the opportunities available to families who are trying to meet their own needs in raising a child with the special burden of a chronic illness. As we began the task of gathering information about childhood chronic illness and making it available to interested citizens and those in policy making positions, the lack of literature available, outside technical and disciplinary journals, became clear. There was no place for interested people to turn for information on the broad array of topics reflecting the changes in care and service for children with chronic illnesses and their families. Thus the genesis of this book, the chapters of which were commissioned from leaders in their respective fields, representing a wide variety of perspectives, including those of

ix

specialists in specific chronic illnesses, in the training of health providers, in the needs of special populations, and in the education of children with chronic illnesses. These chapters will provide guidance to anyone wishing to explore in depth the policy issues and options brought about by the fact of larger numbers of children with chronic illness in the United States.

Government officials—in state departments and legislatures, in the Congress and federal agencies responsible for public programs or for the allocation of public resources—will find here the evidence and experience that can strengthen policy making and implementation. Parents will recognize the similarity of their experiences to those of many other families with chronically ill children, and child advocates will gain greater insight into the problems affecting a group of children neglected in recent public attention. Physicians, social workers, nurses, and mental health professionals, who all work closely with families with chronically ill children, will learn more about the programs that work for children, the range of family and social needs engendered by chronic illness in a child, and the complex matters of costs and financing of services. Other health workers—among them, nutritionists, occupational and physical therapists, and respiratory care workers—can gain understanding of the broad array of problems affecting the children with whom they work, and the prospects for meeting those children's needs. Teachers and educational administrators can find information here to help them provide children with chronic illnesses the best possible education and integrate them into schools and communities.

This book is organized into seven topical parts comprised of several chapters each, plus an Overview and Epilogue by the editors. The Overview depicts with a broad brush the topics that are analyzed in detail in subsequent chapters. It provides a definition of the population of children with severe chronic illnesses and summarizes issues in the organization and financing of services, school policies, professional training, and research. Part One introduces basic concepts about childhood chronic illness and its impact on the child and family. The nature of chronic illness as a constant shadow is graphically portrayed by Robert Massie. Next follows consideration of the common elements among diverse chronic illnesses, the special ethical problems raised by childhood chronic illness, developments in genetics and their implications, and the important nature of research in the field of chronic illness. Current efforts in genetics hold great promise for the prevention of disease and some of its consequences. Complex ethical questions and other issues in the implementation of effective genetic programs accompany these developments.

Part Two begins with a discussion of the epidemiology and demography of childhood chronic illness, addressing such questions as How many children are currently affected, and what are the prospects for the size of the population with childhood illnesses? What are the prevalence rates of representative conditions? Which conditions carry most promise of long-term survival? Part Two continues with up-to-date reviews of eleven groups of severe childhood chronic health conditions. These descriptions, while hardly exhaustive of the vast variety of chronic illnesses in childhood, are representative of the larger group. The chapters review current knowledge of cause, treatment, and outcome for each of the groups of diseases, as well as the family, developmental, and financial and social impacts of the illness. The authors provide recommendations, some specific to these illnesses, but most generalizable to policies affecting children with a wider variety of chronic conditions.

Part Three describes populations at special risk of long-term illness, particularly rural and inner-city groups. Residents of these areas also face difficult problems of access to needed general and specialty medical services. The chapters in Part Four examine professional activities on behalf of children with chronic illnesses as well as issues in training various providers to work with children. Recent changes in education of physicians, nurses, social workers, and mental health professionals are considered in the context of current training efforts and recommendations for closing key gaps in professional education. The chapter examining interprofessional issues clarifies problems inherent in the overlap of professional responsibilities and suggests opportunities for greater professional teamwork in supporting families.

The interface of children with chronic illnesses and the educational system is often complex, both because illness creates special problems in the school setting and because illness and its treatment interfere with the educational process. The authors of chapters in Part Five discuss chronically ill children in schools, the impact of chronic illness on cognitive functioning, the developmental aspects of chronic illnesses, and opportunities in vocational training for chronically ill children. These chapters offer a framework from which to encourage the better development of children with chronic illnesses. The strengths and limitations of Public Law 94–142 are described, and recommendations for federal, state, and local policies to integrate children effectively into school settings are provided.

Part Six discusses organizational issues, with chapters on the history of public support for the care of chronically ill children and on the need for and benefits of integrating services, especially at the state level. Families may benefit through the integration of limited public resources at the state and local level, where most families receive services. Self-help groups, voluntary associations, and professional organizations have all contributed greatly to the lives of chronically ill children, and these chapters provide recommendations to heighten this impact further.

Part Seven describes economic issues. How costly is the care of chronically ill children, and how is it currently financed? How does health insurance serve families with chronically ill children? Children with chronic illnesses consume a share of health resources that is much larger on a per-child basis than that used by able-bodied children. The presence of chronic illness in the child creates major economic hardship for many families and affects the work patterns of parents. Private health insurance currently provides a large amount of the support for needed health services for children with chronic illnesses, yet major gaps in coverage remain. These chapters define the gaps and provide recommendations that may lead to better coverage.

The book concludes with an Epilogue that summarizes important recent developments in the care of chronically ill children and their families. It outlines opportunities for further policy and program development and suggests a set of principles that may guide policy makers, families, health providers, teachers, and others as they collaborate to strengthen the lives of children with chronic illnesses.

What becomes apparent from this book is that much is known that can help to inform the nation of the special burdens carried by families with a wide range of rare and severe childhood chronic illnesses. The severity of these burdens and the variability with which they have been addressed in the public response become clear from multiple discussions with parents and from reading the poignant, compelling, at times angry ideas reflected in the chapters in this volume. That most families cope as well as they do is a measure of the strength of families in American society. This book should deepen understanding of the relative neglect of the problem of childhood chronic illness in America and of the rich opportunities to help families nurture their children, with or without illness, most effectively.

Nashville, Tennessee   James M. Perrin, M.D.
September 1985

Acknowledgments

In the preparation of this volume, we have been aided by a number of colleagues. The authors of the chapters have been exceptional, bearing through numerous revisions and our efforts to condense much important material into a manageable length. Our three main colleagues, Henry T. Ireys, May W. Shayne, and Linda C. Moynihan, contributed greatly to the editing of this volume, helping to clarify structure and language and to make key points apparent. They worked diligently to check references, to communicate with authors, and to keep the drafts in order. And Mary Dane Wadkins has worked valiantly throughout this effort, keeping track marvelously of each chapter and its revisions.

To carry out our study of public policies affecting chronically ill children and their families, we had the support and help of several other colleagues on the staff at the Vanderbilt Institute for Public Policy Studies. Each took responsibility early on for certain chapters, exploring with the authors the types of issues that might be addressed. Samuel Ashcroft, Susie Baird, and Eng-Bee Dy, all experienced in matters of childhood education, were key in the development and consideration of programs and policies for children with chronic illnesses in schools. Mark Merkens, pediatrician, and Carolyn Burr, pediatric nurse clinician, both seasoned clinicians experienced in the ongoing care of chronically ill children and their families, provided leadership and support in the area of health services. Karen Weeks, Robert Hauck, and John Harkey worked on varied issues, including the costs and financing of care for children with chronic illnesses, the political science considerations, and the changing demography of chronic illness in childhood. Alice Christensen and Lisa Reichenbach provided important staff support, exploring such areas as the ethical nature of policy for children, the difficulties in defining costs of care, and models of care in other countries.

Several groups aided us in planning this book. Most important were the National Advisory Committee to the project and the members of the Research Consortium on Chronic Illness in Children, several of whom also contributed chapters to the volume. The National Advisory Committee met frequently during the course of the study, and their advice has been invaluable in every phase. They reviewed the initial selection of chapter titles, recommended authors, and reviewed the outcomes, offering a great breadth of experience in their commitment. The consortium, a group of scholars actively involved in research on the epidemiological, developmental, and family impact of childhood chronic illness, was organized early in the history of the Vanderbilt study to provide advice and consultation as research findings became available in important areas affecting families. This group continues, after the conclusion of the study of public policies, working on joint research efforts and helping together to define basic concepts in this field of research. In addition, a group of parents in Nashville whose children have a variety of severe chronic illnesses provided an invaluable perspective, by generously sharing with the project staff their experiences and views.

The research effort was supported by grants (MCR-470444-02-1 and MCJ-473306-01-0) from the Division of Maternal and Child Health of the Department of Health and Human Services and the Office of Special Education and Rehabilitative Services of the Department of Education. Colleagues in these offices, and most especially Vince Hutchins and Merle McPherson, helped with advice in all phases of this research. With their aid, we convened groups representing several federal agencies and child health charities. These groups in turn shared with us their achievements, plans, and problems and directed our attention to new issues in the organization and financing of health services and in medical research. These representatives helped also in the choice of topics and authors for this book. The National Association of Maternal and Child Health and Crippled Children's Services Directors, through a group ably directed by William Hollingshead III, discussed with us the special issues of organizing services at the state level.

Many other groups and individuals helped in the development of this book and we are grateful to them all. The responsibility for any errors of omission or commission rests entirely with the editors.

Contents

Contents

The Editors

Nicholas Hobbs was professor emeritus of psychology at Vanderbilt University and senior research associate at the Vanderbilt Institute for Public Policy Studies prior to his death in January 1983. He was awarded the B.A. degree from The Citadel, the M.A. and Ph.D. degrees from Ohio State University, and honorary degrees from the University of Louisville, The Citadel, and Université Paul Valéry in Montpellier, France.

Hobbs taught at the Teachers College of Columbia University, Louisiana State University, and George Peabody College for Teachers. At George Peabody College for Teachers, he was the first director of the John F. Kennedy Center for Research on Education and Human Development. He was provost of Vanderbilt University from 1967 to 1975, then joined the Vanderbilt Institute for Public Policy Studies, where he was director of the Center for the Study of Families and Children for five years. He served on a number of regional and national bodies concerned with children, health, and education; was the first director of selection and research for the Peace Corps; was a member of the advisory committee on child development of the National Research Council; and was a member of the Select Panel for the Promotion of Child Health established by Congress in 1979. For the American Psychological Association, Hobbs chaired the committee that first developed the *Ethical Standards of Psychologists* and, in 1966, served as the association's president. In 1980, he received the American Psychological Association's Award for Distinguished Professional Contributions and the award for Distinguished Contributions to Psychology in the Public Interest.

Hobbs's previously published books include *The Futures of Children* (1975), *Issues in the Classification of Children* (1975), *The Troubled and Troubling Child* (1982), and *Strengthening Families* (1984).

James M. Perrin is senior research associate at the Institute for Public Policy Studies and assistant professor of pediatrics at Vanderbilt University. He received his B.A. degree (1964) from Harvard College in chemistry and his M.D. degree (1968) from Case Western Reserve University. Perrin did his pediatric residency and fellowship training at the University of Rochester. He then became medical director of the Oak Orchard Community Health Center in Brockport, New York, while continuing teaching and research at Rochester. Since coming to Vanderbilt University in 1977, he has headed the Division of General Pediatrics and directed the Vanderbilt Primary Care Center, a multidisciplinary teaching and research program of the School of Medicine.

Perrin's research interests are in child health, behavioral medicine, and health policy. His publications include work on middle ear disease in childhood, problems of lead in the environment, policies relating to high-cost illness in childhood, and distribution of health manpower.

Contributors

Louis Aledort, M.D., is professor and vice-chairman, Department of Medicine, Mount Sinai Medical Center, New York City.

Virginia Andrews, M.S.W., is assistant professor, School of Social Work, Syracuse University, New York.

Samuel C. Ashcroft, Ed.D., is professor of special education, George Peabody College, Vanderbilt University, Nashville, Tennessee.

Susie M. Baird, M.Ed., is assistant coordinator, Healthy Children Initiative, Tennessee Department of Health and Environment, Nashville.

Kathleen Bajo, M.S., is consultant, Ross Planning Associates, Ross Laboratories, Columbus, Ohio.

Corinne M. Barnes, Ph.D., R.N., F.A.A.N., is professor and director, Graduate Program, Nursing Care of Children, School of Nursing, University of Pittsburgh, Pennsylvania.

Nina Berlin is executive director, Pennsylvania Diabetes Task Force, Philadelphia.

Leonard D. Borman, Ph.D., is founder and president of the Self-Help Center and adjunct professor of anthropology and lecturer at the College of Arts and Sciences, Northwestern University, Evanston, Illinois.

Peter Budetti, M.D., J.D., is counsel, Subcommittee on Health and the Environment, U.S. House of Representatives, Washington, D.C.

Carolyn Keith Burr, R.N., M.S., is assistant professor of nursing, Florida Atlantic University, Boca Raton.

Marcy Bush, M.A., is research assistant, Department of Psychology, Case Western Reserve University, Cleveland, Ohio.

John A. Butler, Ed.D., is assistant professor of health policy, Community Services Program, The Children's Hospital Medical Center, Boston, Massachusetts.

Mary C. Cerreto, Ph.D., is chief psychologist and associate professor of pediatrics, University of Texas Medical Branch, Galveston.

Ronald L. Chard, Jr., M.D., is associate head, Division of Hematology/Oncology, Department of Pediatrics, University of Washington, Seattle.

C. William Daeschner, Jr., M.D., is John Sealy Professor and chairman, Department of Pediatrics, University of Texas Medical Branch, Galveston.

Donald W. Day, M.D., is assistant professor of pediatrics and genetics and director of the Center for Craniofacial Anomalies, University of Illinois College of Medicine, Chicago.

Shelby L. Dietrich, M.D., is assistant vice-president of medical affairs and director, Pediatrics, Orthopedic Hospital, Los Angeles, California.

Dorothy A. Downes, R.N., M.S.W., M.P.A., is policy research associate, Office of the Assistant Secretary for Planning and Evaluation, U.S. Department of Health and Human Services, Washington, D.C.

Allan Lee Drash, M.D., is professor of pediatrics, University of Pittsburgh School of Medicine, and director, Division of Pediatric Endocrinology, Children's Hospital of Pittsburgh, Pennsylvania.

Dennis Drotar, Ph.D., is associate professor of pediatrics, Departments of Psychiatry and Pediatrics, Case Western Reserve School of Medicine, Cleveland, Ohio.

Antoinette Parisi Eaton, M.D., is professor of pediatrics and preventive medicine, Ohio State University, and associate medical director, Children's Hospital, Columbus.

Julie T. Elworth, M.A., is research specialist, Batelle Human Affairs Research Center, Seattle, Washington.

Richard Fine, M.D., is professor of pediatrics and head, Division of Pediatric Nephrology, University of California at Los Angeles Center for the Health Sciences.

Donald C. Fyler, M.D., is associate chief of cardiology, Children's Hospital, Boston, Massachusetts.

Patricia J. V. Giardina, M.D., is assistant professor, Department of Pediatrics, New York Hospital/Cornell University Medical College, New York.

Irene S. Gilgoff, M.D., is staff pediatrician, Rancho Los Amigos Hospital, Downey, California.

Stephen L. Gortmaker, Ph.D., is associate professor, Department of Behavioral Sciences, Harvard School of Public Health, Boston, Massachusetts.

Morris Green, M.D., is Perry W. Lesh Professor and chairman, Department of Pediatrics, Indiana University School of Medicine, and physician-in-chief, James Whitcomb Riley Hospital for Children, Indianapolis.

John R. Hartmann, M.D., is head, Division of Hematology/Oncology, Department of Pediatrics, University of Washington, Seattle.

Margaret W. Hilgartner, M.D., is professor of pediatrics and director, Division of Pediatric Hematology/Oncology, Department of Pediatrics, New York Hospital/Cornell University Medical College, New York.

Paul Hippolitus, M.A., is employment advisor, President's Committee on Employment of the Handicapped, Washington, D.C.

Neil A. Holtzman, M.D., M.P.H., is professor of pediatrics, Johns Hopkins University School of Medicine, Baltimore, Maryland.

Debra P. Hymovich, Ph.D., R.N., F.A.A.N., is lecturer and consultant, Gulph Mills, Pennsylvania.

Henry T. Ireys, Ph.D., is assistant professor of pediatrics and psychiatry, Albert Einstein College of Medicine, Bronx, New York.

Francine H. Jacobs, Ed.D., is research associate, Harvard Graduate School of Education, Cambridge, Massachusetts.

Susan M. Jay., Ph.D., is assistant professor of pediatrics, University of Southern California School of Medicine, Los Angeles.

Dorothy Jones Jessop, Ph.D., is assistant professor of pediatrics, Albert Einstein College of Medicine, Bronx, New York.

Tom Joe, M.A., is director, Center for the Study of Social Policy, Washington, D.C.

Lorraine V. Klerman, Dr. P.H., is professor of public health, head of Health Services Administration, Department of Epidemiology and Public Health, School of Medicine, Yale University, New Haven, Connecticut.

Loretta Kopelman, Ph.D., is associate professor of humanities and director of the Humanities Program, East Carolina University School of Medicine, Greenville, North Carolina.

Barbara Korsch, M.D., is professor of pediatrics, Children's Hospital of Los Angeles, California.

Fred Leffert, M.D., is clinical associate professor of pediatrics, Medical University of South Carolina, Greenville.

Arthur J. Lesser, M.D., is former director, Maternal and Child Health Service, U.S. Public Health Service, Washington, D.C.

Norman J. Lewiston, M.D., is associate professor of pediatrics, Stanford University, and chief, Pediatric Allergy and Pulmonary Diseases, Children's Hospital at Stanford, Palo Alto, California.

Margaret A. McManus, M.H.S., is health policy consultant, Washington, D.C.

Phyllis R. Magrab, Ph.D., is professor of pediatrics, Georgetown University Medical School, Washington, D.C.

Robert K. Massie, Jr., M. Div., is chaplain and assistant minister, Grace Church, New York City.

Judith S. Mearig, Ph.D., is professor of educational psychology and coordinator of the School of Psychology Graduate Studies Program, St. Lawrence University, Canton, New York.

Margaret Millsap, R.N., Ed.D., is professor and chairperson, Nursing Division, Birmingham-Southern College, Alabama.

Carl Milofsky, Ph.D., is associate professor, Department of Sociology, Bucknell University, and research associate, Program on Nonprofit Organizations, Yale University, New Haven, Connecticut.

Linda C. Moynihan is research associate, Institute for Public Policy Studies, Vanderbilt University, Nashville, Tennessee.

Gary J. Myers, M.D., is professor of pediatrics and director, Sparks Center, University of Alabama, Birmingham.

Paul W. Newacheck, M.P.P., is assistant professor of health policy, Institute for Health Policy Studies, School of Medicine, University of California, San Francisco.

Eleanor N. Nishiura, Ph.D., is assistant professor, Department of Community Medicine, College of Medicine, Wayne State University, Detroit, Michigan.

Thomas W. Pendergrass, M.D., M.S.P.H., is assistant professor of pediatrics and adjunct associate professor of epidemiology, University of Washington and Children's Orthopedic Hospital and Medical Center, Seattle.

Kathryn K. Peppe, R.N., M.S., is core staff nursing consultant, Division of Maternal and Child Health, Ohio Department of Health, Columbus.

I. Barry Pless, M.D., F.R.C.P.(C), is professor of pediatrics and epidemiology, McGill University, Montreal, Canada.

Kathryn Strother Ratcliff, Ph.D., is assistant professor, Department of Sociology, University of Connecticut, Storrs.

Julius B. Richmond, M.D., is director of the Harvard University Division of Health Policy Research and Education and John D. MacArthur Professor of Health Policy and Management, Harvard University, Boston, Massachusetts.

Cheryl Rogers, M.Ed., is research associate, Center for the Study of Social Policy, Washington, D.C.

Claire Rudolph, Ph.D., M.S.W., is professor, School of Social Work, and associate director, Maxwell School Health Studies Program, Syracuse University, New York.

David S. Salkever, Ph.D., is professor, Department of Health Policy and Management, and director, Interdepartmental Program in Public Health Economics, School of Hygiene and Public Health, Johns Hopkins University, Baltimore, Maryland.

May W. Shayne, M.S.S.W., is research associate, Institute for Public Policy Studies, Vanderbilt University, Nashville, Tennessee.

Barbara Starfield, M.D., M.P.H., is professor and head, Division of Health Policy, School of Hygiene and Public Health, Johns Hopkins University, Baltimore, Maryland.

Ruth E. K. Stein, M.D., is professor of pediatrics, Albert Einstein College of Medicine, Bronx, New York.

Suzanne Stenmark, M.S., is associate, Browne, Bortz, and Coddington, Inc., Denver, Colorado.

Deborah Klein Walker, Ed.D., is assistant professor, Department of Behavioral Sciences, Harvard School of Public Health, Boston, Massachusetts.

Karen H. Weeks, M.A., is research associate, Vanderbilt Institute for Public Policy Studies, Nashville, Tennessee.

Michael Weitzman, M.D., is associate professor of pediatrics and public health, Boston City Hospital, Boston University School of Medicine, Massachusetts.

Charles F. Whitten, M.D., is professor of pediatrics, associate dean for curricular affairs, and director, Comprehensive Sickle Cell Center, Wayne State University, School of Medicine, Detroit, Michigan.

Logan Wright, Ph.D., is director, Institute of Health Psychology for Children, Oklahoma City, Oklahoma.

Issues
in the Care of Children
with Chronic Illness

A Sourcebook
on Problems, Services,
and Policies

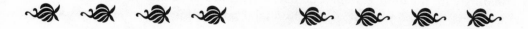

Introduction
James M. Perrin, M.D.

Significance of the Problem

Children who suffer from severe chronic illness are a neglected group in our society. A growing segment of the childhood population, chronically ill children have lacked serious public attention to their needs and to the heavy burdens their families bear. Major advances in medical and surgical technologies have allowed many children who would have died in years past to survive to adulthood, although often with great psychological or physical disability. Marked improvement in survival has brought new problems for greater numbers of children with chronic illnesses and their families and new opportunities for the larger community. Essential efforts in disease prevention and treatment will continue (Nyhan, 1983), yet a central task for the coming decades is to diminish handicap arising from chronic illness in children and to help these children grow into accomplished and vital members of society (Pless and Pinkerton, 1975).

This volume provides much of the information that the shapers and makers of policy need to address effectively one of the nation's least known but most urgent problems. The book examines closely eleven diseases representative of the severe chronic illnesses of childhood: juvenile-onset diabetes, muscular dystrophy, cystic fibrosis, spina bifida, sickle cell anemia, congenital heart disease, chronic kidney diseases, hemophilia, leukemia, cleft palate, and severe asthma. The eleven conditions serve as marker diseases—that is, they have characteristics that make them representative of the total range of such illnesses. Considered separately, each disease is relatively rare and occurs in a small percentage of the childhood population. Taken altogether, however, perhaps a million children are severely involved and another ten million have less severe chronic illnesses (Gortmaker and Sappenfield, 1984). In considering a million

1

children with severe chronic illnesses, we also refer indirectly to at least three million family members burdened with caring responsibilities, affected by anxiety and sometimes by guilt, strapped by unpredicted expenses and possible economic ruin, and facing an uncertain future that may include the premature death of the child. Thus the emphasis on families in our work. Our concern is mainly with the more extreme end of the distribution of chronically ill children, with less than 1.5 percent of the childhood population whose problems are so special that the health system falters and extraordinary efforts are required to make it work even moderately well. The directions charted here are primarily concerned with public policies—that is, with policies of governments (federal, state, and local) and of large organizations such as professional associations and insurance companies.

Chronicity and Severity: Definitions

A chronic illness is one that lasts for a substantial period of time or that has sequelae that are debilitating for a long period of time. The common diseases of childhood provide a convenient reference point for defining chronicity. Most illnesses of childhood are self-limiting and run their course in a period of hours, days, or weeks. Even the acute and serious illnesses of childhood, with proper treatment, require a month or so for complete convalescence. By contrast, most of the severe, chronic illnesses of childhood persist for a few to a number of years after onset and have a variable course with some improving, some remaining stable, and some becoming progressively worse. A general definition of *chronic illness* is a condition that interferes with daily functioning for more than three months in a year, causes hospitalization of more than one month in a year, or (at time of diagnosis) is likely to do either of these.

Although the meaning of *chronicity* can be rather readily agreed upon, defining *severity* is a much more complex matter. There are simply no good reference points that find ready acceptance. For some of the chronic illnesses here considered, there is a strong inclination among physicians to refuse to assess severity at all, at least on a physiological basis. For example, a child either has cystic fibrosis or has not, and how well that child may be getting along at any particular time is as much a reflection of the quality of care and compliance as of severity.

For the purposes of this inquiry into public policies affecting chronically ill children and their families, we advance five criteria with which to assess the severity of impact of an illness. These are in addition to available criteria of physiological severity.

1. The illness places a large financial burden on the family. For the diseases considered here, out-of-pocket medical costs may exceed 10 percent of family income after taxes.
2. The illness restricts significantly the child's physical development. Many of the children here considered will be well below normal height and weight as the result of the illness.

3. The illness impairs significantly the ability of the child to engage in accustomed and expected activities.
4. The illness contributes significantly to emotional problems for the child as expressed in maladaptive coping strategies.
5. The illness contributes significantly to the disruption of family life as evidenced, for example, in increased marital friction and sibling behavior disorders.

Defining chronicity and severity on a generic basis to serve public policy purposes is hazardous. The definitions we propose emphasize the social impacts of the diseases in an effort to broaden the conventional disease-oriented definitions. Perhaps most important in considering severity is the recognition that these criteria identify very different groups of children and families. Children with the most physically debilitating arthritis, for example, may have far fewer emotional problems from the illness than children with milder disease (McAnarney and others, 1974).

The Epidemiology of Childhood Chronic Illness

The dramatic medical advances of the past few decades have meant that many children who previously would have died of their chronic illnesses now survive to young adulthood. For almost all childhood illnesses, there is little evidence of changing incidence—that is, the number of new cases appearing in the population. Furthermore, there is evidence that most potential gains in longevity have already occurred (see Chapter Seven). The number of children with chronic illnesses presently depends, in large measure, on the number of new children in the population, and with a stable (rather than growing) child population, the numbers of children with chronic illnesses will also be stable.

About 10 to 15 percent of the childhood population have a chronic illness. Among chronically ill children, about 10 percent (or 1 to 2 percent of the total childhood population) have *severe* chronic illnesses. With the marked decline in morbidity and mortality from infectious diseases among children and with the increasing survival of children with severe chronic illnesses, that 1 to 2 percent has become a much larger part of child health practice. Among adults, chronic illnesses tend to be few in number and fairly common: arthritis, hypertension, diabetes, coronary artery diseases, and so on. In contrast, the chronic illnesses of children are relatively rare, and there is a tremendous variety of conditions.

The etiologies of childhood chronic illness vary greatly. Most known etiologies incorporate both genetic and environmental factors, with different prospects for prevention and intervention. Methods of intervention include avoidance of procreation by parents at risk for having a child with chronic illness; detection in utero of a chronic disorder, followed by termination of pregnancy or by medical treatment of the fetus; treatment of genetic diseases through genetic engineering; screening of newborns to detect chronic illnesses before they are expressed symptomatically, followed by early treatment; and control of environmental causes, such as toxic chemicals, drugs, tobacco, and viruses (Harkey, 1983). All of the strategies for intervention have associated technical uncertainties and raise perplexing ethical questions.

Tremendous advances in understanding the mechanisms of diseases and the possibilities of prevention have occurred during the last decade. There remain, nevertheless, real barriers (some ethical and some technological) to preventing many or most chronic childhood illnesses. A key problem results from the large number of specific conditions because preventive approaches usually develop on a disease-by-disease basis. Thus, chances appear high that children with severe chronic illnesses will remain part of the nation's population for the foreseeable future. A balanced appraisal encourages basic research on prevention coupled with recognition of the need for continued attention to ameliorating the secondary physiological, social, and psychological effects of childhood chronic illnesses.

Chronically Ill Children as a Class

For the purpose of organizing services and allocating resources, chronically ill children can be considered as a class. The special needs of severely and chronically ill children and their families cannot be met efficiently and effectively simply by extending to this group policies that are efficient for children with routine illnesses, with acute or even fatal illnesses, with stable handicapping conditions (such as mental retardation), or with mild chronic illnesses such as allergies, transient asthma, and minor gastrointestinal problems.

For several reasons, there has been a tendency to regard each chronic illness separately. Among the reasons are the physiological diversity of the diseases, the diversity of treatments, and the variation in the expected length of life. The many chronic illnesses of childhood can be classified in many ways, such as by age of onset, whether the illness affects the child's cognitive or motor skills, or whether its course is stable or unpredictable. Each disease has its corps of specialists, its affiliation with specialty clinical centers, its advocacy group, and its champions in the Congress and in the state legislatures, each disease's advocates competing with the others for scarce funds.

From the many reports of parents and from a policy perspective, however, the diseases have more in common with each other than they do with other illnesses of childhood. In general, severe chronic illnesses of childhood share the following characteristics. Most of the diseases are costly to treat. Direct medical treatment costs, including hospitalization, are often high. Long-term care may be costly, too, involving expenses for blood and blood products, insulin, syringes, special diets, drugs, orthopedic devices, transportation, wheelchairs, long-distance telephone calls, occupational or physical therapy, oxygen, control of environmental temperature, glasses, hearing aids, special schooling, and nursing care provided professionally or by family members and friends. Most of the diseases require care over an extended period of time; thus costs mount steadily. In acute diseases, costs may be high but for a short period. By contrast, severe chronic illnesses have both high costs for brief periods and continuing costs (never low) for a long period of time. The costs of these diseases may be so great that a family can be made bankrupt, insurance may be impossible to obtain, and employment opportunities for parents and family members may be severely curtailed.

Most of the diseases require medical services intermittently—at the time of diagnosis and the establishment of a treatment regimen, at subsequent routine checks, and in periods of crisis. The daily burden of care, day after day, week after week, year after year, falls on the family. Means exist to provide care for many kinds of handicapped people, young and old, but not the chronically ill child. Formal resources for the daily out-of-hospital care of such children are almost nonexistent.

Many of the diseases entail a slow degeneration and premature death. The course of all the diseases is highly unpredictable. The uncertainty generated creates great psychological problems for the child and the child's family.

Most of the diseases are accompanied by pain and discomfort, sometimes beyond appreciation by the normal individual. Furthermore, most of the diseases require treatments that in themselves are arduous, often painful, sometimes embarrassing, to the point that the afflicted family may wonder whether a prolonged life is worth it after all.

The integration of medical care, not normally a problem, takes on serious proportions when severe, chronic illness of children is involved. The integration of general and specialty health services is essentially nonexistent (Palfrey, Levy, and Gilbert, 1980). Primary care physicians rarely see one child with each of the marker diseases, and there may be difficulties in early identification and referral, in allocation of responsibility for continuing care, and in coordination among health providers and schools.

As a further link among these disparate physiological states, policy itself creates ties among the chronically ill. It is policy for some states to provide treatment for sickle cell disease; for others it is not. Some provide treatment for the complications of diabetes; others do not. Parents who are fortunate enough to be informed may move to communities where there are specialty care centers or to states that have policies providing assistance to children with their particular disease. The nation as a whole simply does not provide, at a cost manageable by most parents, the resources it takes to treat a child with a severe, chronic illness. Perhaps there is no stronger bond among children with severe and chronic illnesses (and among their families as well) than the absence of an examined public policy pertaining to them.

Many children without chronic illnesses but with other potentially handicapping conditions face similar problems. A main distinction is the need of families with chronically ill children for access to specialty medical and surgical services of high quality, services not required by other children. Recognition that families face similar problems and challenges regardless of the specific illness of their child allows the pursuit of policy and the development of programs that provide for these families jointly rather than on a disease-by-disease basis. Other families can benefit as well from better policies and programs. The definition of a class of children with chronic illnesses is meant to encourage joint efforts rather than to exclude other children also deserving of similar services and public attention.

Advances in Health Care and in Public Programs

Dramatic progress has been made in preventing some diseases, in bringing others under at least a measure of control, and in actually curing some children with certain diseases that were formerly incapacitating or lethal. Much of the progress has resulted from research leading to new knowledge and from technological developments leading to improved treatment techniques. Progress has also been made in shaping public and private health care programs so that afflicted children and their families can benefit from scientific and clinical advances. As a consequence, the prospects today for the child seriously ill with a chronic disease or disorder are considerably better than they were in years past.

Examples of twentieth-century achievements in acquiring knowledge and then in putting that knowledge to work through enlightened public policies are the discovery of insulin, enabling the control of juvenile diabetes; research leading almost to the elimination of three major disabling conditions of childhood: poliomyelitis, tuberculosis, and rheumatic heart disease; progress in treating renal disease through transplants and home dialysis; development of surgical techniques to alleviate several heart conditions; advances in the treatment of leukemia with chemical and radiation therapies and by bone marrow transplants; better prevention of pulmonary complications in cystic fibrosis; development of means to detect various fetal anomalies in utero, making early intervention possible; and genetic typing and counseling that can improve family planning and reduce the incidence of some illnesses.

The scientific and clinical achievements have been paralleled in many instances by the development of social structures. They include the establishment of the Crippled Children's Services in 1935; mandatory immunization against poliomyelitis and other childhood illnesses including public expenditures to ensure availability; reimbursement for health care for children through Medicaid, the Supplemental Security Income/Disabled Children's Program, and Medicare (for treatment of end-stage renal disease); the Developmental Disabilities Program, extended in the late 1970s to allow inclusion of children with severe and chronic illnesses; Public Law 94-142, (the Education for All Handicapped Children Act), which includes some chronically ill children in its definition of handicapped children; and registers to determine correlations between environmental hazards and birth defects and chronic illnesses.

Challenge: The Tasks Ahead

Although much has been accomplished, there is much to be done in the acquisition of knowledge and its application through organizational and financial mechanisms. Certain basic issues have lacked public attention in the last two decades; among them are inequities in access to services, incentives emphasizing high-cost and high-technology services to the neglect of other needed services, insensitivity on the part of many providers, and lack of attention from schools.

Diversity and fragmentation characterize the organization of health services for chronically ill children. Because it is based on such characteristics as the interest of specialists in an academic center, the urban or rural nature of a community, and the organization of governmental services, especially Crippled Children's Services, there is tremendous variation in the care families receive. In some areas, a broad variety of family support services is available; in others, services to families are limited to medical and surgical interventions.

Fragmentation of services often causes families to experience great frustration. One or more of the specialists they see may be a distance from their home, and among their specialists, there may be disagreement about plans for the child. Granted, the availability of needed medical and surgical services, notably for specialty care, has improved dramatically during the past fifteen or twenty years. Among health care providers, there has also been a great improvement in the distribution of general physicians and nurse practitioners in the past ten to twenty years, such that far more small communities have adequate general health services available. However, despite greater availability of general health services, access to adequate specialty medical services is a problem in many communities. Most chronic conditions of childhood are rare, and community pediatricians and other general providers may have little experience with an unusual malignancy, severe renal disease, or hemophilia. Similarly, regardless of the quality of its nursing staff, the hospital with just a few hundred deliveries per year will have very little experience with conditions that occur in one in ten thousand live births. Not only may identification be a complex issue; referral may be a problem as well.

Access to nonmedical services is highly variable. Some communities may have excellent comprehensive programs for children with specific health problems. An example is the comprehensive hemophilia centers in some areas (Smith and others, 1984). In other locales, general health care providers offer coordination that assures availability of a broad range of nonmedical services to families of children with chronic illnesses. The emphasis on families can have a great impact on a child's development and functional abilities. A child undergoing corrective cardiovascular surgery needs attention not only to necessary medical and surgical care but also to schooling. What can be done to diminish the degree to which that child falls behind classmates? What plans should be made for the child's activity upon return to school? Are homebound teachers appropriate for a period of time?

Nonmedical services can be provided in many ways. Yet the fundamental problem in providing many of them is the lack of reimbursement for such services. Payment in almost all circumstances is skewed to a narrow range of services, mainly medical and surgical. Genetic counseling, for example, is often dependent on federal research or service support, and with the cyclical variations inherent in such support, genetic services may come and go in a relatively brief period of time.

Children with chronic conditions require much greater than average use of hospital and ambulatory care. In 1977, for example, less than 5 percent of children with chronic conditions accounted for 36 percent of total hospital days for all children less than fifteen years of age in the United States (see Chapter Forty). In 1980, expenditures for physician visits and hospitalization of children with activity limitations totaled more than $1.6 billion; 65 percent of these costs were for hospitalization.

The typical pattern of a high-cost childhood chronic illness involves a series of outpatient treatments and hospitalizations over many years, together with routine daily home-care or self-care procedures (Perrin and Ireys, 1984). This pattern generates many obvious medical costs—for hospitals and physicians, medications, laboratory and x-ray services, and often for such services as physical therapy or social work. Many costs less easily categorized or assessed are also generated; these include transportation costs, extra telephone costs, costs associated with time lost from work or school, costs for special diets, and emotional costs associated with increased worry and stress within the family. For each illness, the specific medical, social, and emotional costs will differ, but for almost every family, both types of cost will be major factors in the financial picture.

The system for financing health care in this country for chronically ill children is a complex interaction of federal programs, state programs, and private insurance arrangements. Although most chronically ill children have a large portion of their medical care supported by some third-party arrangement, there are major gaps in coverage. There is great variability of financial coverage by income, condition, severity, type of services, and geography. Sizable sectors of the population remain uncovered. Ten percent of all children with functional limitations have no insurance, public or private; 20 percent of low-income children with functional limitations are uninsured. Among specific public programs, Medicaid covers only 25 percent of the disabled child population and only about 60 percent of disabled children below poverty.

These challenges in the organization and financing of health services for chronically ill children are accompanied by similar issues in other realms. School policies have not kept pace with the greater opportunity for chronically ill children to receive schooling (see Chapter Thirty). Schools often lack arrangements for giving medicines or for handling special diets needed by some children. Physical barriers may hinder access for other children. The presence of a nurse at school only once a week may keep away the child who needs daily nursing care. In years past, it was assumed that, for many of these children, schooling was good but relatively unimportant insofar as they often did not survive to graduate. The changing nature of childhood chronic illness no longer supports this assumption.

Instructional programs for children who are absent from school are usually available only for those who are absent for long and continuous periods of time. Yet exacerbations of chronic illnesses often cause frequent, brief absences for which schools rarely make provisions. Health providers and schools communicate infrequently about families with chronically ill children. Often physicians make educational recommendations with only limited knowledge of the skills and resources of the school system. And schools similarly may make judgments about the health status of a chronically ill child based on misinformation or on a total lack of understanding of the child's condition and its consequences. Yet there are few incentives to encourage health and education people to work together with families to aid the educational functioning of children.

Basic biomedical research has greatly enhanced the lives of children by increasing understanding of the causes and mechanisms of diseases and potential medical and surgical therapies. This research has been highly focused and effective in bringing about the major advances described earlier. Much less attention has been paid in new areas of concern that arise partly because of the success in keeping many children alive. Why is it that some children at risk develop a certain disease and others do not? What are the social and environmental factors at work? Many families cope very effectively with the tremendous demands placed by a chronic childhood illness on their resources and activities. What are the mechanisms by which they do so, and what interventions are available and effective for those families coping less well? What services are most effective in helping families raise their children? What role and importance have various services for families, and how should they be organized? The opportunities for new research are wide and now encompass far more than the basic biomedical research that has brought our understanding of chronic childhood illness to its present high level.

Professional training too has not kept pace with the changing needs of families with chronically ill children. Although chronicity obviously connotes persistence over long periods of time, professionals in training—especially physicians—usually work with children over only brief periods. They become knowledgeable about the episodes of illness but not about the illness over time or about the development of the child and family as they grow with the illness. Other professionals in training may have even less direct exposure to the longitudinal care of children with chronic illnesses, and for most professionals, the concepts presented throughout this book are rarely available to those in training. Although many training institutions have a multitude of specialists in specific groups of diseases, few have faculty that considers directly the problems of chronic childhood illness in general. In adult medicine, the varied medical problems of older people are increasingly considered together under the terms *gerontology* or *geriatric medicine*. Similar models have not gained widespread acceptance within the child health community.

Summary

The successes of the past foretell the very real achievements that lie ahead in the alleviation of the adverse effects of severe chronic childhood illnesses. It is the purpose of this volume to lay a groundwork for understanding the problems of childhood chronic illnesses in America and for exploring solutions that may lighten the burdens families carry.

References

Gortmaker, S. L., and Sappenfield, W. "Chronic Childhood Disorders: Prevalence and Impact." *Pediatric Clinics of North America,* 1984, *31,* 3-18.

Harkey, J. "The Epidemiology of Selected Chronic Childhood Health Conditions." *Children's Health Care,* 1983, *12*(2), 62-71.

McAnarney, E., and others. "Psychological Problems of Children with Chronic Juvenile Arthritis." *Pediatrics,* 1974, *53,* 523-528.

Nyhan, W. L. "Promising Directions in Pediatric Research." *Advances in Pediatrics,* 1983, *30,* 1-12.

Palfrey, J., Levy, J., and Gilbert, K. L. "Use of Primary Care Facilities by Patients Attending Specialty Clinics." *Pediatrics,* 1980, *65,* 567-572.

Perrin, J. M., and Ireys, H. T. "The Organization of Services for Chronically Ill Children and Their Families." *Pediatric Clinics of North America,* 1984, *31,* 235-257.

Pless, I. B., and Pinkerton, P. *Chronic Childhood Disorders: Promoting Patterns of Adjustment.* Chicago: Yearbook Medical Publishers, 1975.

Smith, P. S., and others. "The Benefits of Comprehensive Care of Hemophilia: A Five-Year Study of Outcomes." *American Journal of Public Health,* 1984, *74,* 616-617.

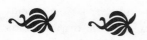 # Part I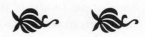

Basic Concepts

What is life like for children with chronic illnesses, and how do their families manage to meet these children's special needs? In spite of the distinct characteristics of specific illnesses, chronically ill children have much in common in terms of their family experiences, psychological adjustment, and social development. The chapters in Part One focus on the role of the family in the life of a child with a chronic illness and the impact of the child's condition on the family.

Chapter One is an account of chronic illness by a young man, Robert K. Massie, Jr., who has struggled with severe classical hemophilia all his life. Although Massie observes that each afflicted person and family is unique, he recounts experiences, feelings, and observations that are common strands weaving chronically ill children and their families together. Massie describes chronic illness as a constant and at times overwhelming companion, a shadow—inseparable and persistent. The strengths of family members, and the importance of support for the family while it nurtures the chronically ill child, are major emphases in this chapter. The caring, or lack of it, on the part of the medical community and the community-at-large shapes significantly the future of these children and their families. Massie concludes that compassion must be the responsibility of all rather than simply a response of the few.

In Chapter Two, Carolyn Keith Burr examines a variety of issues for families with chronically ill children. Burr analyzes the effects of a child's illness on the family's ability to carry out its developmental tasks and on family adaptation. She presents eight family developmental tasks and discusses them in depth. Burr then addresses the relationship between family functioning and the psychosocial adjustment of the chronically ill child. Finally, she looks at policy implications from the perspectives of financing the services that families need, making health care resources and social services available, and improving communication within the family and between the family and the community.

I. Barry Pless and James M. Perrin, in Chapter Three, discuss the increasing evidence that children and families of children with chronic illnesses face many of the same social and psychological issues, regardless of the children's specific conditions. In fact, they point out, the nature of the family is more likely to determine the frequency with which certain problems are experienced than is the distinct nature of the disorder or chronic illness. Pless and Perrin give special attention to the needs of families, the delivery of services, and the implications for public policy, and conclude that for purposes of program development and policy recommendation, chronically ill children should be considered as a broad class of children with special common needs.

Paternalism and autonomy in the care of chronically ill children, as defined by Loretta Kopelman in Chapter Four, are compatible approaches. Both include creating opportunities for children to develop independence and take on responsibilities—and are comparable to encouraging autonomy for children who are not ill. Kopelman states that the degree of control exercised in presenting such opportunities to minors should, perhaps, be greater for chronically ill children than for other children. In reviewing moral and legal policies concerning the care of children, Kopelman includes discussions of children's rights, the achievement of autonomy, and the need for truthfulness and informed consent. Kopelman links each policy to three basic and binding moral principles—justice, utility, and benevolence—which she analyzes in depth.

In Chapter Five, Neil A. Holtzman and Julius Richmond present what is currently known about prevention of several major chronic diseases and consider the controversies that have been generated by new scientific discoveries. They explicate the conflicts and dilemmas that attend the newly expanded capacities for prenatal diagnosis, intrauterine therapy, preconceptional control of reproduction, and genetic engineering. They also address the need to effectively disseminate information about the genetic bases of disease in order to increase public awareness, especially among young adults. In the realm of genetic screening and counseling policy, the authors point out essential safeguards, such as public participation, education and consent, counseling, and testing and follow-up. Policy issues affecting the future of preventive services in genetics are also discussed.

The last chapter in Part One concentrates on the research needed to inform policymaking. Reminding the reader that a research agenda should consider feasibility, or the current state of knowledge, Barbara Starfield describes various types of research and general research strategies and identifies nine general areas in which specific research on chronically ill children is needed. She defines principles to guide theoretical and population-based studies, emphasizing the importance of new theoretical frameworks to understand illness causation and health behavior. Starfield offers suggestions for the development of information systems and standardized nomenclature for problems and their functional impact, in order to enhance the comparability of diverse research efforts. She concludes by recommending that research be incorporated into the training of practitioners and that new models be developed and funded to provide research across diseases and categorical lines.

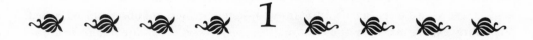

The Constant Shadow:
Reflections on the Life
of a Chronically Ill Child

Robert K. Massie, Jr., M.Div.

When first asked to write on what it is like to be a chronically ill child, I failed to realize how much of a challenge this would be. Although I have struggled all my life with severe classical hemophilia and its frequent internal joint bleedings and constant arthritis, I am now twenty-five years old and have some difficulty recalling my view of things at the age of, say, nine. Perhaps more perplexing was the question that immediately posed itself: Although I have lived with hemophilia, how can I speak for the millions of chronically ill children whose diagnoses range from Down's syndrome to blindness to leukemia? Hemophilia, sometimes a brutal and excruciating illness, has its merciful moments of respite when I am left to breathe, think, and go about my life almost as if it were not there. Is there a common denominator between my experiences and those of a child who has muscular dystrophy or is dying of cancer?

I sought to answer this question by reflecting on my own experiences, both as a child and as a former chaplain at Yale New Haven Hospital, where my assignments included a pediatric floor, and by rereading some of the hundreds of letters my family received when my parents' book, *Journey*, which describes our life with hemophilia, appeared in 1975. I also read a dozen books by chronically ill people and their families in my search for the common strands that weave us together.

I found a strange and marvelous paradox: although each story is different and every afflicted person and family unique, there are certain experiences and feelings that seem to be common. One woman wrote that "though the names and

13

the faces are different, I feel as if you were telling my story," and she was echoed by dozens of others. Each of the books I read, although different in style, content, and outcome, contained many of the same emotions and observations. Each parent and child I worked with in the hospital was strikingly different, yet the looks of anguish, uncertainty, and relief were often the same.

So what I offer here is quite limited—a few stories and observations culled from my experience with one chronic illness—yet I set them down here with the conviction that there are thousands, perhaps millions, of children and their families who share these feelings but who are not as fortunate as I have been to have the freedom, the ability, and the opportunity to record them.

The most important thing to remember about a chronic illness is that it is exactly that: chronic. Most chronically ill children face the presence of a relentless illness, sometimes from the moment they are born to the moment they die. I have never known a moment when I did not have hemophilia, and that fact has pervaded my family life, my education, my experiences with medicine, and my spiritual growth. Every morning of every day I wake up with my corroded leg joints painfully stiff from arthritis that has set in during the night, and I must hobble to the bathroom and sit in a hot tub for ten or fifteen minutes before I can walk. Two or three times a week I must administer an intravenous injection of a specially prepared plasma protein—factor VIII—to compensate for the absence of that protein in my blood. And there is no end in sight for me, unless something dramatically changes in hematological research. There is no hope for improvement of my damaged knee and ankle joints, only the attempt to slow the deterioration. One day, replacement with an artificial joint might be possible, but currently there are no artificial ankles, which are my most painful joints.

I do not offer this as an example of a particularly great burden, for I have known children who have struggled to take a few steps, who battle against decaying motor control, who endure radiation, chemotherapy, and other treatments far more frequent, painful, and intrusive than those I experience. Yet, for me and for them, a chronic illness is a constant and sometimes overwhelming companion, a shadow both inseparable and eternal. I think this is a hard thing for most people to imagine, particularly medical professionals who are trained in a broad array of diseases and disciplines and who routinely treat dozens of different people with different problems.

"Having a chronic illness" is sometimes an elusive concept because one's illness becomes melded into one's identity. To ask what I would be like without hemophilia is an impossible question to answer, like asking who Abraham Lincoln would have been if he had been a midget. Clearly, there *is* a me distinct from hemophilia, but it is hard to say sometimes where the boundaries to that me are. Who would Helen Keller have been if she had been a sighted and hearing little girl?

The quality of relentlessness inherent in all chronic illness creates a tremendous need in the patient—child or adult—for a group of supportive and caring human beings who show by their words and actions that they will stay with the patient through the physical and emotional roller-coaster ride of disease.

Thus, the single most important factor in the life of chronically ill children—other than the medical care they receive—is their relationship with their parents and family.

Children sense parental moods and attitudes and from them take the cue for their own emotional response. If the parents are fearful, despairing, or angry at the doctor (or each other), the child will feel the pressure. If the parents are supportive, patient, and caring, the child draws tremendous comfort. This is not to say that parents should be falsely cheerful or dishonest with a child because children can almost always detect the true emotion lurking beneath a nervous smile. It is to point out what may seem to be a truism: that the health of any child is inextricably bound to the quality of emotional support provided by the parents.

Chronic illness does not strike individuals; it strikes the whole living unit of the family. The presence of a chronic illness creates such enormous financial and emotional demands that every family member is affected—the parents and the brothers and sisters as well. The ability of the family to respond and the manner in which its members choose to do so can be the decisive element in how a child learns to work with and overcome the effects of a chronic illness.

This has unquestionably been true for me. The story of how my parents responded to my hemophilia is told in their own words in *Journey*, and I think that entire book stands as a testimony to their courage and love. With a marvelous combination of sympathy and challenge, my mother helped me fight off the occasional bouts of depression that would seize me when I was confined to my bed. She brought me books and games, helped me learn to cook, and refused to let me belittle or pity myself. During the storm of crisis, she was an anchor. During the long, boring stretches of convalescence, she constantly looked for ways to make little, demonstrable improvements. Instinctively, she knew ways to cheer me up, by straightening up the pillows to support my swollen knee, by organizing my papers so they would readily accessible, or by bringing me a surprise pizza. During those interminable nights when pain banished sleep, she spent hours holding my hand and telling me stories of faraway places.

My father also supported me, but in a different way. He never once made me feel he was disappointed not to have a son who could play football, ski, or be a Boy Scout (when I was young, the Scouts did not make the effort to include handicapped children that they do today). I can remember distinctly a conversation I had with him when I was about six, in which he told me that since he had gotten thirty-six good years out of his legs, he wished that he could give them to me in exchange for mine.

"After all," he said, "I'm a writer, and I could sit and do my writing while you dashed around."

My first reaction was that he was *crazy:* Why would he want to trade a pair of perfectly good legs for my rigid and (at that time) braced ones? Then it hit me: He was willing to sacrifice them *for me,* and the seriousness and awesomeness of such a love sank in deeply.

In later years, when it became possible for parents to administer the factor VIII concentrate at home rather than having it done in a hospital or a doctor's office, my father became more personally involved in my medical care. He and I would discuss the mechanics of transfusions: where this or that bubble had come from, why the fluid was not flowing down a tube when it should, and so on. His continuous involvement and patience gradually enabled me to begin administering the injections myself, giving me new freedom to live and travel on my own.

My sisters, Susanna and Elizabeth, were affected in many ways by my hemophilia. They had to contend with the unusual amount of attention my parents were required to devote to my care. They had to deal with the unwitting comments and inquisitive looks of their friends. They have always treated me "normally," maintaining a careful balance between respect for the problems I faced and a refusal to grant me special status. We fought over who had to do the dishes; we teased each other; we shared games and secrets. By doing so, they taught me how to be with people my own age. Now that they are adults, hemophilia continues to affect their lives through its silent genetic grip.

The importance of the family to the well-being and medical improvement of a child may seem obvious, but it is shocking how often this is forgotten by medical institutions. Throughout my childhood, my parents were frequently treated like useless—even counterproductive!—appendages by doctors and nurses who banished them to waiting rooms. Many hospitals still do not allow parents to remain overnight with their children, even though a hospital stay may be the single most terrifying experience the child has yet had.

Mercifully, this widespread attitude seems to be diminishing, but there are still hospitals across the country where inflexibility and arrogance are rife. Even on the pediatric ward where I worked as chaplain, with its excellent nursing care and unusually attentive staff, some parents were labeled "difficult," although in reality they were more scared or frustrated than anything else. A few minutes of listening, a small gesture of concern offered at the right time can change a parent's and a child's world.

Even assuming that the home is a supportive and stable environment (which for many chronically ill children, it tragically is not), the child must eventually face the challenge of emerging into a world of peers. For those whose medical conditions permit, this excursion is usually into a schoolroom filled with gawking children and a nervous teacher. Here the protective shield of the parents melts, and the child is exposed to the full impact of insensitive comments, blunt questions, and occasional ostracism.

I spent my first years in a public school in suburban New York, and I can remember how difficult it was to be part of the group when I had full-length leg braces. A delicate balance had to be struck by the teacher responsible for informing the children of my condition (to explain unexpected absences) without emphasizing it so much that the children accused me of being a teacher's pet. When I was in sixth grade, I went to a small private boys' school near my house and used to join my classmates in the wrestle and tussle matches that sometimes followed lunch, with very few resulting physical problems. One day I returned to class after a few days at home (with a cold!) and was informed by a friend that the headmaster of the school had announced at the previous day's assembly that no one was to touch Bobby Massie under pain of Saturday detention. My sudden transformation into an untouchable—for whatever well-intentioned reasons— filled me with a sense of powerlessness and stinging humiliation.

Fortunately, I was able to benefit from the duality that rules American education: the simultaneous emphasis on intellect and on athletic achievement. In grade school, there were those who dominated the classroom with their brains, others who dominated the playgrounds with their bodies. Because I was barred from most team sports (except kickball, where a heavy metal brace proved an asset in driving the ball great distances), I used my mind. I read, I talked, I wrote. I also learned to play jacks, a game that required coordination and could be played sitting. Because in the early 1960s jacks was (at least in my town) strictly a girls' game, I inadvertently broke a sex barrier by becoming quite proficient.

For children whose medical problems affect their motor control, their reading, and their speaking, life with peers—with siblings or classmates—is all the more difficult. People who speak in a slow or garbled manner or who cannot talk at all are often deemed stupid, although the stupidity in fact lies in our inability to be patient enough to listen. A child whose head lolls to one side or who must wear protective devices must endure the frightened looks that mark every initial encounter.

I am strongly encouraged by the developments that have taken place in the United States in recent years. Mainstreaming of children into public schools, although sometimes presenting some great challenges, is to everyone's advantage. Handicapped children must eventually learn to live in a world where acceptance takes time, and normally functioning children must learn how to act with those who do not enjoy all of the same physical gifts.

Apart from the worlds of family and friends, chronically ill children must also learn to survive in the world of medicine. This strange land of machinery, white coats, frequent medication, and alternating states of anxiety, boredom, and suffering is a challenge to any person, but for the chronically ill child, it is part of daily life. For those chronically ill children who commute between a normal school and occasional hospitalizations, there is a constant challenge to reconcile the two worlds, to explain to one's friends about medicines and procedures, and to retain in the midst of the medical world an active hope to return to a more normal life. For the chronically ill child who is hospitalized most or all of the time, there is the struggle of learning to live in a world of which most people are not even aware or, if they are, of which they are afraid.

A child quickly learns that the medical world portrayed in our literature and on our television screens is not an accurate mirror of reality. Doctors, no matter how good they are, are not able to cause quick healing. Hospitals, by virtue of their size and complexity, are slow-moving leviathans, whose speed, even in the emergency rooms, is a rarity unless the matter is one of life and death. The result is that most chronically ill children spend the bulk of their time waiting: waiting for tests, waiting for doctor's appointments, waiting for physical therapy, waiting for meals, waiting to get better. I can remember spending hours sitting in the same orange plastic chair, flipping through the same old magazine, swinging my legs and fidgeting as I waited for my fifteen-minute audience with a physician.

Children in the hospital must contend not only with the siege of boredom but also with innumerable intrusions. Doctors and medical students enter in flocks, pull down sheets and examine sometimes painful limbs, then discuss the case in a strange language as though the child weren't there. Nurses enter to check vital signs, and technicians come in to draw blood. In short, an array of unfamiliar people parades through, most of them intent on doing something that hurts. Small wonder that many of the children I met as a chaplain would cry at the sight of me, fearful that I was a doctor. Only after three or four visits would they calm down, trusting gradually that I would not touch them.

Clearly, the procedures and examinations are a necessary component of good medical care. Some of the treatments are unavoidable, and even the most thoughtful doctor or nurse cannot lessen the physical pain. Yet my concern is not so much the physical pain—for that is something most children can learn to face—as it is the attitude with which some medical professionals go about their work and the stupidity of some hospital regulations that make the problems worse. For example, as a child, whenever I was admitted to the hospital, the diagnosis of hemophilia dictated that a hematologist had to be called to give me my transfusion. The hematologist, however, was inexperienced at getting into a child's veins, so I would have to endure five or six failed venipuncture attempts before the doctor would request a pediatrician. My parents soon learned to ask for a pediatrician as soon as I reached the hospital, but hospital rules would not permit it! Fortunately, my parents also learned to insist. Today, many hospitals have *pediatric* hematologists and more flexible rules, although less than two years ago, I was in a hospital in Kentucky speaking to a group of parents when a mother asked me, "Why does my son have to be stuck five or six times by a hematologist before the hospital will allow the pediatrician to be called?"

Some doctors and medical students apparently think that when they are brisk in manner they are being professional. In fact, they are being bad doctors. The art of medicine involves a commitment to the patient as a *person,* and that person is often scared and uncertain, desperate to ask questions but intimidated by the doctor's demeanor and obvious impatience. This is especially true for patients who are children and for their young parents. In my life, I have had many different doctors, doctors who were ice cold and doctors who were warmly concerned, young doctors and older doctors, male and female. Those who have taken the time, even a few minutes, to answer my questions and to listen to my worries have my strongest respect, trust, and affection.

Healing is a mysterious process of which medical science is only a part. If the environment in which a child lives at home is a decisive element in that child's health, this is no less true at the hospital. And this, I think, is the key point that is still missed by most of American medicine today: We heal not only with our machines, but also with ourselves, when we reach out to each other as human beings.

Although this may sound like a vaguely mystical assertion, it is based on a simple and basic human need, the need not to feel abandoned. Doctors and nurses are trained to do everything they can to bring their patient back to health, but sometimes the situation is complex or so grave that there remains little that can be done *medically*. At this point—the point of inefficacy of further treatment—doctors and nurses are faced with their own limitations, and in one sense, with their professional failure. It is also at this point that most doctors—out of fear, or frustration, or demands from elsewhere—withdraw, emotionally if not physically.

Yet, for the patient, particularly for the patient who is a child, the very moment that medical techniques are proving inadequate is the moment when the patient most needs to sense that he or she is not being abandoned. Here, at the point when the doctor is in a unique position to offer human care, perhaps even to trigger unexpected healing, is the crucial moment of encounter between physician and patient. And it is this moment for which many physicians are tragically unprepared.

When I was twelve years old, I was vacationing in Maine when my left knee began to bleed internally in a very serious manner. My left knee has always been my most precarious joint, and when I saw it swelling rapidly, I knew that this incident was going to be far worse than most. My father, after telephone conversations with several doctors, decided to drive me to Boston, some five hours away, so my knee could be surgically aspirated. We drove all evening, stopping for a quick roadside meal, and arrived around 11 p.m. The doctors were ready to take me into the operating room but were dismayed to find that I had eaten before the procedure, thus ruling out normal anesthesia. Instead, they gave me a narcotic that knocked me cold.

Some hours later, the aspiration successfully performed and my knee bandaged up, I was taken to a hospital room to recover. As I began to emerge from my stupor, I began to hallucinate, experiencing wild sights, bizarre sounds, hideous nightmares. Every time I turned, I felt I was falling into a bottomless crevice; every time I opened my eyes, I felt like an explosion had been ignited in my face. I was terrified, and I was certain I was going to die.

Somewhere in the midst of all that, I heard a calm voice talking to me, repeating soothing words over and over. Through the kaleidoscope of frightening images, I felt a hand take mine and I held on to it tightly. As I twisted and babbled, these words and that hand became a lifeline to reality, to safety. "I'm not going to die," I said to myself, "there's someone there; there's someone whose face I cannot see, but that person is there." And so gradually, after several hours of unforgettable torment, the narcotic wore off, and I was able to open my eyes and see the face of the nurse who had stayed at my bedside. I never saw her again, but her compassion earned my eternal gratitude.

Indeed, if there is one word that embodies what I feel is too often lacking in the world of medicine and should be nurtured in nursing and medical schools, it would be this: *compassion.* The word *compassion* comes from the Latin roots *cum pati,* meaning "to suffer with." When we are compassionate, even though there may be nothing more we can do, we stay with a person, and "suffer with" him or her. To be compassionate also means to be patient (another derivative of *pati*), to wait with the person as they struggle. This does not mean that highly trained physicians and hard-pressed nurses must always spend hours sitting by someone's bedside; compassion is a *quality* of care rather than a technical achievement or a certain quantity of time. Compassion exists in hospitals today— I have seen it as a patient and as a chaplain—but it is still too rare and struggles against too many pressures and entanglements. For me, compassion is manifested in the little gestures and statements, like the nurse who carefully washed a dying girl who had already sunk into a coma, and after drying her forehead, kissed her lightly and tenderly. Or the answer I received to a question I asked my hematologist when I was riding in a car with her one day. "Why did you become a hematologist?" I had asked, expecting her to respond that it was an interesting field or that she had a particularly inspiring teacher in medical school. She looked at me quietly and steadily and then answered, "Because I wanted to help people like you."

It would seem that the challenges faced by chronically ill children as they learn to walk, talk, and live in a world still too insensitive to their needs would be enough for one person to be obliged to face. Unfortunately, in America virtually every child and family who struggle with chronic illness must also battle against the enormity and insanity of the American health insurance system. Anyone who has had contact with the gargantuan costs a chronic illness can engender knows that health care in the United States is an empire of inequity, a system that provides extraordinary care to some while largely neglecting others. Insurance companies routinely bar the chronically ill because of their preexisting conditions. Parents have been thrown out of their jobs when their employer's insurer complained that their child was going to provide a rate hike for the company. One man whose chronically ill son was born while he was in the Marine Corps reluctantly decided to stay in the Marines because it was the only place he could be sure of adequate medical coverage.

Some governmental authorities have recognized this problem and tried to deal with it, either disease by disease, state by state, or group by group. The result is a crazy patchwork of assistance and exclusion. Some states have programs that provide for most of the care of the hemophiliacs in their states; others have nothing at all. The federal government funds renal dialysis (after several senators were jolted by a dialysis performed in a Senate hearing room) but will not assist other illnesses.

Thus, parents and children must fight not only the disease but sometimes also insurance companies, employers, government agencies, and hospital financial screening offices that create whirlpools of worry that often contribute to the destruction of the family structure so important to the child's health. A further result is that many diseases end up competing with each other for the attention of the public, using talkathons, walkathons, turkey raffles, barbecues, and other events to raise research and operating funds. Admittedly, such activities can sometimes be a positive and necessary source of funds and educational outreach, although all too often, I have seen them deteriorate into maudlin and humiliating events, with the diseased child brought into the television lights in the hope that the sympathetic stares will translate into dollars and cents. Is this a dignified way for the United States of America, which prides itself on its fairness and its generosity, to provide for its least advantaged citizens?

The problem results from a deeply ingrained and illogical principle lying at the base of the system of health insurance in the United States: Those who least need the coverage (who have the lowest risk) receive the highest benefits at the lowest costs, whereas those who most need the coverage (such high-risk groups as the elderly, the chronically ill, and the poor) receive the lowest benefits at the highest cost. This is a horrendous way to organize health insurance. The federal and state governments have erratically tried to pick up those categories of people who would simply be left uninsured if left to private industry—the elderly, the poor, and the handicapped. In doing so, the government is providing a huge subsidy to the private health insurance industry.

Does this need to be the case? No. Since 1948, most of the nations of Europe have had broad-based national health insurance systems that combine public and private institutions into a network of easily accessible, high-quality care. Most opponents of health insurance in the United States have pointed accusatory fingers at the system in Great Britain, with its high emphasis on governmentally run institutions. Although England has its problems, I doubt that many of its citizens would wish to switch to a system such as ours. Moreover, how often do we hear about the systems in Holland, in Germany, or in Japan, where partnerships between government and private companies have resulted in even, high-quality care?

I lived in France for four years and, during my stay, received some of the best medical care I have ever had. Although I was a foreign resident, I was given factor VIII concentrate free of charge, and because of this, I owe my ability to walk to French medicine. The French system is one of national *health insurance* (not "socialized medicine," a spurious term coined by an advertising firm hired by the AMA in the early 1950s). Employers and employees make contributions to the system, then pay for medical services that are automatically reimbursed along a scale of fixed percentages. The system works so well that few people even think about it, let alone debate its merits.

Society possesses no magic wand to wave over the heads of chronically ill children to make their medical conditions evaporate, but it does have a responsibility to alleviate the huge financial and psychological burdens imposed by decades of uninterrupted confusion.

For the first two decades of my life, my struggle was with hemophilia, and although hundreds of people gave me assistance, such an illness always has a dimension that remains solitary. In recent years, my health has improved and my vocation has led me to spend time with many children struggling with other illnesses. I have watched the face of a child who knows that the next morning her leg must be amputated. I have seen the tenacity with which a young boy fought to recover from repeated open-heart operations. I have known a young man who did not reach his sixteenth birthday before being struck down by muscular dystrophy, and a two-year-old victim of brain cancer who left this life knowing as little about it as it knew about her.

Through my life and through such experiences, I have come to believe that the true test of greatness for any group of people—be they a family, a community, or a nation—is the manner in which they care for those suffering in their midst. Just as we judge parents on the way they educate and care for their children, and friends on their constancy and sensitivity, so should we judge society by the way it assists those who bear life's greatest burdens: the chronically ill, the poor, and the elderly. Our goal should be a society made up of people who are both individually and collectively compassionate.

The United States has far to go along these lines. For one thing, we have fallen into the trap of professionalizing compassion, making it a job for the few rather than a responsibility for all. The result is that someone might work with handicapped children all day and ignore the elderly woman who lives alone next door. We might dedicate our lives to medicine, to social work, or to ministry and find that our caring is still somehow abstract. Although chronic illness touches every family in America in some way, we still prefer the idols of health, youth, and omnipotence nurtured by our industry and our own fears.

Indeed, fear is what most keeps us from compassion. Illness reminds us of our limitations, of our own inability to affect much of what happens in life. Ultimately, illness reminds us of our own death. Illness in children is somehow even more frightening because we look to children to bring us new life, purer life, and not the tragedy and disfiguration of disease.

Yet, I believe such fear causes most of us to miss a great opportunity to learn from chronically ill children. When we care for them, we are not only giving but also receiving. When I see children straining to pronounce a single word or sweating to walk the first step, my occasional frustration at my slow-moving arthritic legs is transformed into a wondrous appreciation for the many gifts I have been given. When I watch a child fight back against physical pain, loneliness, and depression, I begin to see the meaning and power of courage. So often when I told people that I was working in a hospital as a chaplain, they would respond, "Oh, but isn't that awfully depressing?" I have been joyful and I have wept; I have been exhausted and I have been drained; but I have never felt the kind of depression that would cause me to want to flee from those who were struggling there. This is because I have come to believe that somehow, enclosed in those hospital rooms and homes, in the privacy of a child's attempt to live as well as possible against the most difficult of circumstances, is a vision that taps into the very substance of life.

So when we ask how we can help chronically ill children and launch into an examination of policies and programs, medical and educational techniques, institutional and financial resources, we must not forget to explore the one place that is often overlooked: our own hearts. The greatest burden for a chronically ill child is not the pain, the anguish, or the disappointment; it is the wall of emotional isolation with which we have encircled that child because of our own fears. We must look inside ourselves, face those fears, and despite them, reach out. Only the power of a warm heart can alleviate the deep chill of a child's constant shadow.

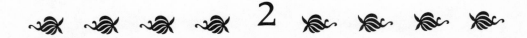

2

Impact on the Family
of a Chronically Ill Child

Carolyn Keith Burr, R.N., M.S.

Families provide for the growth and well-being as well as the physical and emotional support of their members. Families who have a child with a chronic illness carry out these functions in the face of additional stresses and needs brought about by that illness.

Recent research has taken an increasingly broad view of childhood chronic illness, examining not only the effect of illness on the child's physical and emotional health, but also the dynamic relationship between the child, the illness, and the health of the family. Families are viewed not only as contributors to the child's physical and psychosocial health but also as potential victims of the effects of the illness. This broader perspective emphasizes both the negative influences of a chronic illness on a child and family and the positive strengths and resources that affect coping by children and families.

Three main issues regarding the families of chronically ill children are addressed here. First, what is the impact on a family of having a child with a chronic illness? Specifically, does the child's illness interfere with the family's ability to carry out its developmental tasks? Is that ability, in some cases, enhanced? What factors (of family, illness, or community) play a role in family adaptation and in the family's accomplishment of developmental tasks?

The second issue is the relationship of family functioning to the psychosocial adjustment of the chronically ill child. Do children do better in families that function well? Does illness in a child greatly influence family stability or communication? Third, is the issue of how public policy can be more responsive to the needs of families with chronically ill children in order to promote healthier families and children.

Theories of Family Development

Family developmental theory offers a framework for organizing and analyzing the findings of many studies of a broad range of chronic physical illnesses in children. It provides a structure for looking at the impact on children and families across disease entities and for describing commonalities and differences in impact.

Within family developmental theory, the family is viewed as a semiclosed system of interacting personalities (Hill and Rodgers, 1964). It is composed of dynamic people who are seen as family members and individuals at the same time. Because the nature of the interactions within a family changes over time, the concept of a family life cycle was added to "focus attention on the longitudinal career of the family system" (Rowe, 1966, p. 199).

The stages in the family life cycle are determined by the degree of transition the family experiences as the result of a particular family event—for example, marriage, birth of first child, last child leaving home. The two major divisions in the family life cycle—expansion and contraction of the family—are based on children entering and leaving the family. Theorists have formulated from eight (Duvall, 1977) to twenty-four (Hill and Rodgers, 1964) developmental stages in a family life cycle.

As a family moves through the life cycle, certain role expectations or developmental tasks must be met (Rowe, 1966). The concept of family developmental tasks is an expansion of Havighurst's (1948) work on individual developmental tasks from birth to old age. A family developmental task is "a growth responsibility that arises at a certain stage in the life of a family, the successful achievement of which leads to present satisfaction, approval, and success with later tasks—whereas, failure leads to unhappiness in the family, disapproval by society and difficulty with later family developmental tasks" (Duvall, 1977, p. 167). The central importance of the accomplishment of developmental tasks is well stated by Rowe (1966, p. 199): "The better equipped a family is for each of its members to meet his developmental tasks and the more closely the family accomplishes its group tasks, the more successful is the development of the family." For the purposes of this chapter the term *family* encompasses a variety of models including single-earner nuclear families, dual-career families, single-parent households, blended families, and multigenerational families in one household.

Most studies of chronically ill children and their families are disease-specific, and with some exceptions, families in various developmental stages are grouped together in a study. Therefore, our discussion is organized not according to family developmental stages but rather according to family developmental tasks common to each stage. The potential impact of having a chronically ill child on a family's ability to accomplish its developmental tasks is examined utilizing Duvall's (1977) eight categories of family developmental tasks:

1. physical maintenance
2. allocation of resources

3. division of labor
4. socialization of family members
5. maintenance of order and establishment of communication
6. reproduction, release, and recruitment of members
7. placement of members in the larger society
8. maintenance of motivation and morale

Physical Maintenance. The first developmental task—physical mainte-nance—includes providing food, clothing, shelter, and health care for family members. Families with a chronically ill child especially need access to special-ized health care. Pless and Satterwhite (1975a), in a community-based study of families with chronically ill children, found that 55 percent of the children had seen a physician for the chronic illness in the year prior to the study and 25 percent of those had seen more than one physician. Especially indicative of the burden on families is the finding that 11 percent of parents estimated more than ten doctor visits in the year.

Family decisions regarding other aspects of life may be based, in part, on continued access to specialized health care. Notable among these decisions are those surrounding travel (Vance and others, 1980) and career mobility of parents (Meyerowitz and Kaplan, 1967; Salk, Hilgartner, and Granich, 1972). Other aspects of physical maintenance of a family may be directly affected by having a chronically ill child—for example, the need of a family with hemophilia for a grassy play area (Salk, Hilgartner, and Granich, 1972) and the special dietary needs of children with cystic fibrosis (Crozier, 1974). More broadly, the ability to provide for the physical maintenance of the family is often seriously impaired by the financial burden of having a chronically ill child.

Allocation of Resources. In an optimally functioning family, financial, space, and time resources are allocated according to family members' needs. A child who has a chronic illness may have a disproportionate need for family resources leaving fewer resources available for other family members.

Financial concerns are frequently expressed by parents of children with various chronic illnesses (Turk, 1964; Salk, Hilgartner, and Granich, 1972). When families of children with nephrosis were compared with families with healthy children, finances were one of only two areas of difference between the groups, and affected families related their financial problems specifically to the disease (Vance and others, 1980). Sixty-six percent of families with a variety of chronic illnesses mentioned significant financial difficulties as a concern (Pless and Satterwhite, 1975b).

For chronic illnesses requiring medical and nursing tasks on a daily basis (such as cystic fibrosis) or causing the child to become increasingly dependent in activities of daily living (such as muscular dystrophy), a disproportionate amount of time must be spent with the ill child to maintain that child's health and function. Parents of children with cystic fibrosis felt the time demanded by the illness deprived them of leisure time, time for activity with the family, time to be with spouse and engage in adult activities, and time for self (Turk, 1964).

For some families, the difficulties of allocating resources are made more difficult by other circumstances in the family. Even before the additional burden of a chronic illness, single-parent families may already have major constraints on parent-child time together and often have fewer financial resources than do two-parent families. Similarly, in low-income families, resources are often stretched thin even before a child's illness. Families living in areas where medical and support services are scarce, such as rural or inner-city areas, find that much time is spent seeking out and traveling to the services the chronically ill child needs.

Appropriate and equitable allocation of family resources is a difficult task for many families with chronically ill children. Scarcity and maldistribution of resources available to these families adds to their burdens.

Division of Labor in the Family. Determining individual roles in support, management, and care of the home and of family members is the third family developmental task. The increased burden of care for the chronically ill child may fall to one parent, usually the mother. Five of twelve mothers of children with cystic fibrosis stated that their husbands were unable to assist in the child's care at all. However, families who did share the work and worry with each other found sharing to be an important source of personal and family strength (Mikkelsen, Waechter, and Crittenden, 1978). For families with children with diabetes (Simpson and Smith, 1979) and with cystic fibrosis (Turk, 1964), the need to foster communication in the family, to facilitate task-sharing between parents, and to involve the children in their own care has been stressed. Community resources such as visiting nurses or homemaker services can provide parents relief from the constant burden of care. The broader impact on families of the burden of a child with a chronic illness is demonstrated in the finding of fatigue cited as a concern by 55 percent of parents whose child had a severe chronic illness (Pless and Satterwhite, 1975b). The burden may be shared less well in families on whom the disease makes daily demands than in those in which there are episodic crises caused by the disease.

In some families, the burden of care is shared by the parents. Mattson and Gross (1966) found that, from the time of diagnosis, the majority of fathers took an active part in caring for their sons with hemophilia. Active involvement with the child was seen as a way of accepting mutual responsibility for bearing and rearing the child and as an attempt to relieve the mother's guilt as the carrier of the disease.

Another aspect of the division of labor tasks in a family relates to parental employment. Half of mothers employed at the time of diagnosis of cystic fibrosis left their jobs to stay home with the child (Meyerowitz and Kaplan, 1967). In contrast, in a small controlled study of families with hemophilia, mothers of children with hemophilia worked solely for financial reasons in comparison with the control mothers who worked for personal satisfaction as well as financial reward (Markova, MacDonald, and Forbes, 1979). A recent survey of parents of children with hemophilia revealed that one third of the mothers worked to meet expenses, one fifth of the fathers held a second job, and 11 percent of the fathers had been influenced in their selection of their present job by the child's illness (see Hilgartner, Aledort, and Giardina's discussion in Chapter Fifteen). Thus, the nature of the illness may put pressure on the parent to enter or leave the work force and may limit employment mobility.

Shifts in the division of labor within a family have an impact on both the well siblings and the ill child. Lavigne and Ryan (1979), in a study of adjustment of siblings of hematology, cardiology, and plastic surgery patients compared with adjustment of children with healthy siblings, found the relationship between the age and sex of the sibling and the sibling's adjustment to be a complex one. Younger female siblings appeared to have more adjustment problems than younger male siblings while older female siblings had slightly fewer adjustment problems than older male siblings. The authors speculate that sex roles in the family may account for these differences. Younger sisters may feel more displaced by an older ill sibling in a dependent role than do younger brothers from whom less dependence is tolerated. Older sisters, in contrast, may be better prepared to accept the additional responsibilities brought about by an ill sibling than are older brothers, who have had fewer responsibilities initially. The authors note that, if these interpretations are correct, they would be most noticeable in families with acquired rather than congenital disease.

In a family with a chronically ill child, decisions regarding division of labor seem to be influenced by several factors, including the nature of the illness, the financial and task burdens it causes, the ability of parents to communicate and to share tasks, and the age and sex of the affected child and the siblings. How these issues of division of labor are resolved has important implications for overall family functioning. According to Hansen and Hill (1964, p. 806), "Stress causes change in [family] role patterns; expectations shift, and the family is forced to work out different patterns. In the process, the family is slowed up in its affectional and emotion-satisfying performances until new patterns are worked out and avenues for expressing affection are open once more."

Socialization of Family Members. Families assure each member's socialization through internalization of increasingly mature roles (Duvall, 1977). The first step is development of an affectional bond or attachment to a newborn. The development of parental attachment to a newborn can be negatively influenced by circumstances surrounding an infant's birth—for example, illness, prematurity, or congenital defect (Leifer and others, 1972; Rose, Boggs, and Alderstein, 1960; Green and Solnit, 1964). Within the psychoanalytic literature, the birth of an infant with a defect is viewed as causing parents to experience a sense of loss. The birth of a child with a defect brings about a grief reaction in the mother caused by the loss of the expected perfect child (Solnit and Stark, 1961). Attachment to the imperfect child is impeded until the mourning process allows for a gradual reduction of the wished-for normal child.

Drotar and his colleagues (1975) identify five stages that parents of children with congenital defects experience. The stages include initial shock, followed by a period of denial, and then a stage marked by sadness, anger, and anxiety. The fourth stage is marked by decreased anxiety and less intense emotional reaction. Finally, in the fifth stage—reorganization—parents are able to develop a more rewarding level of interaction with the infant. The ability of parents to regain equilibrium is affected by their ability to be mutually supportive of each other.

Other important variables influence the attachment process. Separation of mother and newborn because of illness or prematurity of the infant has been shown to have a profound effect on attachment (Leifer and others, 1972; Klaus and Kennell, 1976). Availability of treatment also affects the mother's response. In a study comparing seventy-five mothers of infants with cleft lip and a control group of mothers of healthy infants, the birth of a baby with a defect caused a crisis for the mothers in this sample. However, the resolution of the crisis was more cohesive than divisive. Clifford and Crocker (1971) note that the timing of showing the baby to the mother and the availability of treatment may lessen the impact of the defect.

In another study of maternal attachment to infants with visible defects, no significant differences in attachment behavior were noted between five mothers of infants with defects and five matched control mothers at three observation times between birth and ten weeks of age (Burr, 1978). Mothers of infants with defects cited seeing and holding the baby soon after birth, the support of their families, and easy access to health care providers caring for the infant as the important factors in resolving the crisis around the birth of the child.

Many studies have discussed the socialization of a child with a chronic illness in terms of the risks of parental overprotection or neglect (Waechter, 1975; Apley, Barbour, and Westmacott, 1967; MacKeith, 1973). Mourning the loss of the healthy child and feelings of self-blame are aspects of parental reaction (Mattson, 1972). Parents who are aware of their self-accusatory feelings and are able to verbalize and master them are more able to accept the reality of the disease and its impact on child and family. Guilt-ridden parents are more likely to overprotect the child and limit activities with other children. Overprotection seems not to be related to the actual severity of the defect but rather to the parent's perception of the defect (Offord and Aponte, 1967).

Socialization of the healthy sibling can be affected by a chronically ill child in the family. Earlier studies report that parents noted the attention-seeking behavior of healthy siblings but failed to deal with it (Turk, 1964). A recent study compared the adjustment of siblings of cardiology, hematology, and plastic surgery patients to that of children with healthy siblings (Lavigne and Ryan, 1979). Siblings of patients were more withdrawn and irritable than the healthy controls, and siblings of children with visible handicaps were more severely affected on measures of emotional and behavioral problems than were siblings of children with nonvisible handicaps. The severity of the illness was not found to be significantly related to the siblings' adjustment. The psychological adjustment of siblings of children with one of four types of chronic conditions did not differ significantly from that of the control group in overall symptomatology (Breslau, Weitzman, and Messenger, 1981). However, they did score significantly higher on two scales measuring interpersonal aggression with peers and in school.

A controlled study of the siblings of children with spina bifida found that four times more siblings of children with spina bifida scored in the maladjustment range than siblings of control children (Tew and Laurence, 1973). When severity was controlled for, a bimodal distribution was found in which siblings of mildly and severely handicapped children had the highest maladjustment while siblings of moderately handicapped children had the least.

In a well-controlled study of children with nephrotic syndrome and their families, serious problems among parents and siblings were less common than expected (Vance and others, 1980). However, the physical and emotional health of the siblings of the sick children was significantly worse than that of the healthy controls, as rated by parents. Similarly, brothers and sisters of the children with kidney disease had significantly lower academic performance, self-acceptance, and social confidence than did the control group. There was less fighting among siblings in families with a child with kidney disease but more embarrassment concerning the ill child. The authors suggest that from the findings, "a picture of a sheltered, protected family environment emerges in the descriptions by parents [which] may be interpreted as suggesting preoccupation with the sick child" (p. 954).

Maintenance and Order. The fifth family developmental task involves establishment of ways of interacting, communicating, and expressing affection, aggression, and sexuality in the family within limits acceptable to society (Duvall, 1977). Communication breakdown within families who have a chronically ill child is discussed frequently in the literature. Turk (1964) found that parents of children with cystic fibrosis were able to discuss day-to-day issues of the child's management with each other but did not discuss the child's illness with their other children, family, or friends. Significantly, 60 percent never discussed the diagnosis with the child. A more recent study found that all parents discussed the nature of the disease and the reasons for treatment with the child and one third of the families were able to discuss the prognosis (Mikkelsen, Waechter, and Crittenden, 1978). Another study of families of children with cystic fibrosis concluded that the less communicative and the less emotionally supportive the family was, the greater the likelihood of adjustment difficulties (Tropauer, Franz, and Dilgard, 1970). Parents of children in long-term remission of leukemia (more than four years) reported that they had difficulty talking with each other about the illness or discussing it with the child (Obetz and others, 1980).

In contrast, findings from a controlled study of families of mildly and severely affected boys with hemophilia indicate that parents of mildly affected boys cooperated more, trained the child to be more independent, and had more clearly formulated views on childrearing than the parents of severely affected sons or healthy controls. Parents of mildly affected boys may profit from the experience by mobilizing emotional strengths, which results in increased parental cooperation and more attention to childrearing (Markova, MacDonald, and Forbes, 1979). These studies seem to indicate that parents' ability to communicate with each other about the child and the disease may be affected by the long-term prognosis of the disease. Parents of children with cystic fibrosis and leukemia, whose life spans are considerably shortened, seem less able to communicate about the illness than parents of children with mild hemophilia whose disease causes life-threatening episodes but who generally have a more favorable prognosis.

Anecdotal reports often suggest increased rates of marital breakdown among families with a chronically ill child (Lavigne and Ryan, 1979). Although the proportion of actual divorce may be overstated, the stress on marital relationships as reported by parents in studies is clear (Salk, Hilgartner, and Granich, 1972; Simpson and Smith, 1979). In families who have marginal family functioning, the stress of a child with a chronic illness may further impair functioning. Inability of parents to communicate with each other about the child's disease isolates them from each other, their children, and their social support systems.

Reproduction, Recruitment, and Release of Family Members. Having a child with a chronic illness has a marked impact on parents' decisions to have more children. Fifty-three percent of families felt that already having a son with hemophilia affected their decision regarding having more children—usually not to have more (Salk, Hilgartner, and Granich, 1972). Similarly, parents of children with spina bifida and cystic fibrosis (Turk, 1964) have shown reluctance to have further children who might be affected. Advancing techniques in prenatal diagnosis and genetic counseling give some families hope of having unaffected children.

Later in the family life cycle, releasing the chronically ill late adolescent into the community may present logistical as well as emotional difficulties. The continuing need for medical support services and the assistance of another person in diseases such as cystic fibrosis (McCollum and Gibson, 1970) and spina bifida (Hayden, Davenport, and Campbell, 1979) makes the child's achievement of independence appropriate for this age very difficult. For other illnesses, such as diabetes (Mattson, 1972)) and kidney disease (Kaplan De-Nour, 1979), issues around compliance with medical regimens can become the arena in which the adolescent's struggle for independence is waged.

The foundation for accomplishment of adolescent tasks can be laid in a family as the child is growing up. In a study of adolescents with cystic fibrosis, 70 percent of those judged to be competent and functioning well had grown up in families where the mothers worked outside the home or were active in community affairs and where the child had daily responsibility for self-care in the home (Boyle and others, 1976). Similarly, among children aged seven through seventeen who had diabetes, adequate self-concept and an appropriate balance of dependence and independence were closely and significantly associated with acceptance of the disease by the child, adjustment at home, and the emotional tone of the home (Swift, Seidman, and Stein, 1967). An emotional climate within a family that fosters acceptance of the illness and promotes the development of a healthy self-concept in the child facilitates achievement of developmentally appropriate tasks in adolescence.

Improved treatment has dramatically lengthened the life expectancy for many with childhood chronic diseases. As increasing numbers of chronically ill children live into adolescence and adulthood, more concern must be directed toward helping these children and families achieve the complex developmental tasks of transition to adulthood. Some available guidance examines adolescent concerns about sexuality, career choices, and independence in the context of a childhood chronic illness. However, more work is needed, particularly in such areas as career counseling in high schools, insurance coverage, and medical care for young adults with childhood chronic illnesses.

In some situations, parents' experience of having a child with a chronic illness may prepare them emotionally for the child's increasing independence later. Parents of children with leukemia in long-term remission (Obetz and others, 1980) stated they had learned to appreciate their children for what they are and to appreciate each day with them.

Family Members in the Larger Society. The seventh family developmental task involves the relationship of family members to the larger society including work, school, church, friends, and extended family. For some families, the volume of care associated with the child's illness (as in cystic fibrosis) may limit the family's time for other activities (Turk, 1964). For other illnesses such as muscular dystrophy and spina bifida, difficulties surrounding mobility of the child may keep parents at home and isolated (Holroyd and Guthrie, 1979). In one study, three fourths of mothers of children with spina bifida felt isolated (Walker, Thomas, and Russell, 1971), while in another study of adolescents with spina bifida, 42 percent of families had to make special arrangements or found social life difficult or impossible (Dorner, 1975). The fear of the child's contracting an infection (for families of children with cystic fibrosis or leukemia) will also limit the families' involvement with the larger community (Meyerowitz and Kaplan, 1967; Klopovich, 1979). Parents may feel a lack of caring support as a result of diligently maintaining low social visibility by keeping the obvious manifestations of the disease in good control (Simpson and Smith, 1979). Whatever the causes, the lack of social support systems limit parents' mechanisms for sharing the burden of the ill child beyond the family.

For all children, school provides a long-term relationship with the larger society. Responsibility of schools for meeting the special needs of the chronically ill child remains an area of controversy beyond the scope of this chapter. The effect of chronic illness on the child's participation in school, however, is noted clearly in the literature. Pless and Satterwhite (1975a) found that the number of school days missed was directly related to the severity of the chronic illness. Also, severity, as perceived by the mother, is directly related to days absent (Parcel and others, 1979). Children with asthma have a significantly higher absentee rate from school (8.4 percent of days) than that of nonasthmatic controls (5.9 percent) regardless of sex or ethnicity and for most socioeconomic groups. Absences decrease as children grow older, but the relationship is the same.

For some chronic illnesses, school performance, adjustment, and the presence of illness are significantly interrelated. Among forty-two children with chronic juvenile rheumatoid arthritis, three times as many children with arthritis had low achievement scores and twice as many were referred to the school psychologist as healthy children (McAnarney and others, 1974). One third of children with arthritis (compared with 9 percent of healthy children) had low overall school adjustment ratings. A number of measures indicated that the relationship between severity of arthritis and maladjustment was curvilinear, with children with severe disability and those with no disability having the greatest adjustment problems. For twelve of sixteen measures, nondisabled children with arthritis had poorer adjustment than moderately or severely disabled.

The stage of the disease and the required treatment may have a serious impact on the child's participation in school and vocational training. Adolescents on chronic hemodialysis had a significantly decreased level of functioning in the area of vocational rehabilitation when compared with adult patients (Kaplan De-Nour, 1979). In contrast, among children one to five years post-kidney-transplant, all but two of nineteen older children were in appropriate jobs or colleges and all but five of sixteen younger children were attending school (Korsch and others, 1973). Although the initial disruption caused by kidney disease is great, it appears that equilibrium is reestablished in the child and the family within about a year after the transplant procedure. For children with other chronic diseases, such as cystic fibrosis, academic achievement may provide an opportunity for success denied them in other areas (Mikkelsen, Waechter, and Crittenden, 1978).

Parental career aspirations are affected by having a child with a chronic illness. Career mobility is seen by parents as being negatively affected (Meyerowitz and Kaplan, 1967; Salk, Hilgartner, and Granich, 1972). The need for access to specialized health care and the need to maintain adequate health insurance coverage with job changes are two of many factors limiting parents' career choices.

Mobilizing support systems for families, fostering school adjustment in ill children, and removing barriers to parental career mobility are all areas where intervention could improve families' abilities to meet this developmental task.

Maintenance of Morale and Motivation. This final family developmental task includes rewarding achievement, meeting personal and family crises, setting attainable goals, and developing family loyalties and values (Duvall, 1977). Morale may be lower in families of children with chronic illnesses. For example, a controlled study of families of children with juvenile diabetes found the emotional tone to be poorer in these homes, with turmoil and conflict more strongly present (Swift, Seidman, and Stein, 1967). In one study, three fourths of parents of children with spina bifida reported that they felt worried or depressed (Walker, Thomas, and Russell, 1971), while, in another study, mothers of adolescents with spina bifida had significantly more moderate to marked depression than had mothers of healthy adolescents (Dorner, 1975). When asked the most difficult part of caring for a chronically ill child, 43 percent of parents in a large community-based study said worry (Pless and Satterwhite, 1975b).

The presence of a chronic illness in a child may provide the stimulus to mobilize untapped family resources and strengthen the family. Parents in one study noted that the chronic illness had been a unifying force in the family and had increased family members' sensitivity to others (Pless and Satterwhite, 1975b). Eight of sixteen parent couples in a study of hemophilia felt their child's illness had brought them closer together (Markova, MacDonald, and Forbes, 1979). Parents of children with leukemia in long-term remission felt the experience had altered their values and priorities in life and that they had experienced personal growth as a result of the illness (Obetz and others, 1980).

A family's ability to deal with day-to-day situations as part of their maintenance of morale can be positively or negatively affected by a chronic illness in their child. Parents of children with diabetes had less agreement on how to handle the child and more marital conflict than parents of healthy children (Crain, Sussman, and Weil, 1966). However, among families of boys with and without hemophilia aged three to five years, no differences were found in parental agreement and consistency in childrearing practices, in mothers' attentiveness or amount of time spent with the child, or in parents' planning for the child's future (Markova, MacDonald, and Forbes, 1979). Differences attributable to the disease or differences in families' abilities to cope with chronic illness could account for these conflicting findings.

Families may be unaware of the dynamics underlying their difficulties in managing day-to-day problems. Parents of children with diabetes expressed fear of finding the child's urine sugar to be high (Simpson and Smith, 1979). They felt helpless and angry when an elevated urine sugar occurred, and the child became angry as well. When parents were able to recognize that this reaction stemmed from their own and the child's sense of failure, they were able to develop new approaches to the problem including acknowledging the child's feelings as normal and "reinforcing the nature of the urine test [as] measuring percentage of glucose, not self-worth" (p. 294). Open communication in the family encouraged a sense of self-worth in the child and moved the family toward maintenance of morale and motivation.

The tasks of maintaining morale and motivation, of setting and attaining goals, and of establishing values are difficult and complex for any family. In families with a chronically ill child where emotional and physical resources may be strained, these tasks may prove particularly difficult.

Family Functioning

A dynamic relationship exists between family functioning and the functioning of family members. How is the psychosocial adjustment of the chronically ill child affected by family functioning? According to family developmental theory, the ability of the family to accomplish its developmental tasks fosters both the growth of the family unit and the growth of individual family members. Thus, the family's capability in accomplishing developmental tasks is reflected in the development of individual family members. Within the large body of literature examining the psychological adjustment of chronically ill children, several studies have investigated the specific influence of the family on child adjustment.

Grey, Genel, and Tamborlane (1980), in a study of twenty children aged seven to thirteen, all of whom had diabetes, examined the relationship between the children's psychosocial adjustment, their self-esteem, the parents' self-esteem, and family functioning. Fifty-five percent of the children had moderate to severe maladjustment. In the group of well-adjusted children, the authors found that "better adjustment was associated with higher parental and child self-esteem and optimal family functioning" (p. 70). A partial correlation analysis of these four variables revealed high parental self-esteem to be the key to the child's self-esteem and psychosocial adjustment and to family functioning.

Swift, Seidman, and Stein (1967) found similar results in a controlled study of fifty children with juvenile diabetes. They found adequate self-concept and an appropriate dependence-independence balance in the child with diabetes to be closely and significantly associated with disease acceptance by the patient, adjustment of the home, and emotional tone of the home. A positive emotional tone in the home and a parental attitude of acceptance of the disease contribute not only to the child's psychosocial adjustment but also to consistent regulation of the disease process.

The influence of the family on the child's psychosocial adjustment may, in some instances, be stronger than the impact of the disease itself. Among children with asthma, a positive correlation between the level of family disturbance and the child's psychosocial adjustment has been determined, but no correlation has been found between the severity of the disease and adjustment (McLean and Ching, 1973). Minuchin, Rosman, and Baker (1978) studied families of children with diabetes and asthma who manifested emotional conflicts in the family with somatic symptoms of the disease. They found that the functioning of the "psychosomatic families" differed both from the functioning of healthy families and of other families that had children with diabetes in five characteristics: enmeshment of family interactions, overprotectiveness, rigidity, lack of conflict resolution, and the child's involvement in parental conflict. With intensive family therapy, some families were able to establish healthier patterns of interaction and conflict resolution, and the child's disease control improved markedly.

How a family interacts with a child with a chronic illness regarding individual and family responsibilities may have long-term consequences for the child's adjustment. Adolescents with cystic fibrosis whose families had given them daily responsibility for their own care were found to be functioning better and to be more competent than their peers with cystic fibrosis whose mothers had assumed responsibility for their care (Boyle and others, 1976).

Implications for Policy

A review of studies of chronically ill children and their families reveals methodological limitations that must be considered when evaluating variations in the studies for policy implications. Results of the studies, even those of the same disease, are at times contradictory or inconclusive. For example, the low incidence of many chronic illnesses has resulted in studies with small sample sizes, which limits the validity and generalizability of the studies. Collaborative studies among institutions have more recently been conducted to increase the number of children with a particular chronic illness in a study and thus improve the applicability of the findings.

Studies of chronically ill children and their families have often lacked control groups of healthy children and families, and this limits the generalizability of the conclusions. Some studies have also failed to differentiate among children by disease severity or extent of disability, an important variable in adjustment of children and families according to recent research (McAnarney and others, 1974; Pless and Satterwhite, 1975a).

Finally, an overriding concern in the literature of chronically ill children and their families is how well conclusions reached about the impact of one illness can be generalized to other illnesses. Newer studies are looking at groups of children with different illnesses within the same study and using the same measures of family function and child adjustment for all (Lavigne and Ryan, 1979; Stein, Jessop, and Riessman, 1983). Measures are also being developed to provide an objective measure of the burden of the illness and the impact on the family regardless of the specific disease (Stein and Riessman, 1979, 1980). This noncategorical approach to the study of chronically ill children and their families highlights the commonalities of their concerns across disease conditions and should guide future research (Stein and Jessop, 1982).

Although many questions remain unanswered, important trends in the literature re-emerge and provide the basis for discussing how society, through public policy, can begin to address better the needs of families with chronically ill children. A number of areas in which public policy response needs to be examined are apparent. One important area of concern for these families is the availability of financial resources for meeting the direct and indirect health care expenses for the ill child. The financial burden of childhood chronic illness on a family is pervasive through most studies and affects families' accomplishment of developmental tasks. Public policies limiting program access to children with certain illnesses or to families who meet particular income guidelines must be re-examined. Similarly, the availability and distribution of health care resources should be examined, both in terms of the quality of services available and in terms of the effects, both financial and psychosocial, on families for whom resources are unavailable or distant.

Families' needs for services beyond the traditional biomedical services are also apparent (Kanthor and others, 1974; Palfrey, Levy, and Gilbert, 1980; Pless, Satterwhite, and Van Vechten, 1978; Ireys, 1981). Families need to be provided with more information and a better understanding of the disease, its cause, and its treatment, and particularly, with advice regarding daily management of the disease at home (Stein, Jessop, and Riessman, 1983).

In addition, access of families to social services and health resources such as homemaker services, visiting nurses, and respite care, needs to be improved through policy changes and increased provider awareness of families' needs.

A number of other services can also assist families with chronically ill children as they progress through the family life cycle. Availability of services such as genetic screening and genetic counseling, which allow families to make more informed decisions about future childbearing, needs to be assured. Community-based services, which can increase families' sense of social support, need to be encouraged. Barriers that limit parents' career mobility, such as insurance gaps, inequities in program availability, and unequal access to services, require careful consideration in policy analysis. Public policy review should also examine the availability to families of support groups and mental health services that promote better communication in families and better sharing of tasks and can improve a family's ability to carry out its developmental tasks.

The end result of public policies more responsive to the needs of families with chronically ill children will be improved resources that enable families to decrease their burden, to improve communication within the family, and to increase their involvement in the community. The goal of such public policy is the promotion of healthier, more functional families and children who are contributing, vital members of the community despite the presence of a chronic illness.

References

Apley, J., Barbour, R. F., and Westmacott, I. "Impact of Congenital Heart Disease on the Family: Preliminary Report." *British Medical Journal*, 1967, *1*, 103–105.

Boyle, I. R., and others. "Emotional Adjustment of Adolescents and Young Adults with Cystic Fibrosis." *Journal of Pediatrics*, 1976, *88*, 318–326.

Breslau, N., Weitzman, M., and Messenger, K. "Psychological Functioning of Siblings of Disabled Children." *Pediatrics*, 1981, *67*, 344–353.

Burr, C. K. *The Effect of an Infant's Congenital Defect on Maternal Infant Attachment.* Unpublished master's thesis, School of Nursing, University of Rochester, 1978.

Clifford, E., and Crocker, E. C. "Maternal Responses: The Birth of a Normal Child as Compared to the Birth of a Child with a Cleft." *Cleft Palate Journal*, 1971, *8*, 298–304.

Crain, A., Sussman, M. B., and Weil, W. B. "Effects of a Diabetic Child on Marital Integration and Family Function." *Journal of Health and Human Behavior*, 1966, *7*, 122–127.

Crozier, D. N. "Cystic Fibrosis: A Not-So-Fatal Disease." *Pediatric Clinics of North America*, 1974, *21*, 935–950.

Dorner, S. "The Relationship of Physical Handicap to Stress in Families with an Adolescent with Spina Bifida." *Developmental Medicine and Child Neurology*, 1975, *17*, 765–776.

Drotar, D., and others. "The Adaptation of Parents to the Birth of an Infant with a Congenital Malformation: A Hypothetical Model." *Pediatrics*, 1975, *56*, 710–717.

Duvall, E. M. *Marriage and Family Development*. Philadelphia: Lippincott, 1977.

Erikson, E. *Childhood and Society* (2d ed.). New York: Norton, 1963.

Green, M., and Solnit, A. J. "Reactions to a Threatened Loss of a Child: A Vulnerable Child Syndrome." *Pediatrics*, 1964, *34*, 58–66.

Grey, M. J., Genel, M., and Tamborlane, W. V. "Psychosocial Adjustment of Latency Aged Diabetics: Determinants and Relationships to Control." *Pediatrics*, 1980, *65*, 69–72.

Hansen, D. A., and Hill, R. "Families Under Stress." In H. T. Christensen (Ed.), *Handbook of Marriage and the Family*. Chicago: Rand McNally, 1964.

Havighurst, R. *Developmental Tasks and Education*. Chicago: University of Chicago Press, 1948.

Hayden, P. W., Davenport, S. L., and Campbell, M. M. "Adolescents with Myelodysplasia: Impact of Physical Disability on Emotional Maturation." *Pediatrics*, 1979, *64*, 53–59.

Hill, R., and Rodgers, R. H. "The Developmental Approach." In H. T. Christensen (Ed.), *Handbook of Marriage and the Family*. Chicago: Rand McNally, 1964.

Holroyd, J., and Guthrie, D. "Stress in Families with Neuromuscular Disease." *Journal of Clinical Psychology*, 1979, *35*, 735–739.

Ireys, H. T. "Health Care for Chronically Disabled Children and Their Families." In U.S. Department of Health and Human Services, *Better Health for Our Children: A National Strategy*. Vol 4: *Background Papers*. Publication 79-55071. Washington, D.C.: U.S. Government Printing Office, 1981.

Kanthor, H., and others. "Areas of Responsibility in the Health Care of Multiply Handicapped Children." *Pediatrics*, 1974, *54*, 779–785.

Kaplan-De-Nour, A. "Adolescents' Adjustment to Chronic Hemodialysis." *American Journal of Psychiatry*, 1979, *136*, 430–433.

Klaus, M. H., and Kennell, J. H. *Maternal Infant Bonding*. St. Louis, Mo.: Mosby, 1976.

Klopovich, P. "Immunosuppression of the Child Who Has Cancer." *MCN: The American Journal of Maternal Child Nursing*, 1979, *4*, 288–292.

Korsch, B. M., and others. "Kidney Transplantation in Children: Psycho-Social Follow-up Study on Child and Family." *Journal of Pediatrics*, 1973, *83*, 399–408.

Lavigne, J. V., and Ryan, M. "Psychologic Adjustment of Siblings of Children with Chronic Illness." *Pediatrics*, 1979, *63*, 616–627.

Leifer, A., and others. "Effects of Mother-Infant Separation on Maternal Attachment Behavior." *Child Development*, 1972, *43*, 1203–1218.

McAnarney, E., and others. "Psychological Problems of Children with Chronic Juvenile Arthritis." *Pediatrics*, 1974, *53*, 523–528.

McCollum, A. T., and Gibson, L. E. "Family Adaptation to the Child with Cystic Fibrosis." *Journal of Pediatrics*, 1970, *77*, 571–578.

MacKeith, R. "The Feelings and Behavior of Parents of Handicapped Children." *Developmental Medicine and Child Neurology*, 1973, *15*, 524–530.

McLean, J. A., and Ching, A. Y. "Follow-Up Study of Relationships Between Family Situation and Bronchial Asthma in Children." *Journal of the American Academy of Child Psychiatry*, 1973, *12*, 142-161.

Markova, I., MacDonald, K., and Forbes, C. "Impact of Haemophilia on Child-Rearing Practices and Parental Cooperation." *Journal of Child Psychology/Psychiatry*, 1979, *21*, 153-161.

Mattsson, A. "Long-Term Physical Illness in Childhood: A Challenge to Psycho-Social Adaptation." *Pediatrics*, 1972, *50*, 801-811.

Mattsson, A., and Gross, S. "Social and Behavioral Studies on Hemophilic Children and Their Families." *Journal of Pediatrics*, 1966, *68*, 952-964.

Meyerowitz, J. H., and Kaplan, H. B. "Familial Responses to Stress: The Case of Cystic Fibrosis." *Social Science and Medicine*, 1967, *1*, 249-266.

Mikkelsen, C., Waechter, E., and Crittenden, M. "Cystic Fibrosis: A Family Challenge." *Children Today*, July/August 1978, pp. 22-26.

Minuchin, S. *Families and Family Therapy*. Cambridge, Mass.: Harvard University Press, 1974.

Minuchin, S., Rosman, B. L., and Baker, L. *Psychosomatic Families: Anorexia Nervosa in Context*. Cambridge, Mass.: Harvard University Press, 1978.

Obetz, W. S., and others. "Children Who Survive Malignant Disease: Emotional Adaptation of the Children and Families." In J. L. Schulman and M. J. Kupst (Eds.), *The Child with Cancer*. Springfield, Ill.: Thomas, 1980.

Offord, D. R., and Aponte, J. F. "Distortion of Disability and Effect on Family Life." *Journal of the American Academy of Child Psychiatry*, 1967, *6*, 499-511.

Palfrey, J. S., Levy, J., and Gilbert, K. L. "Use of Primary Care Facilities by Patients Attending Specialty Clinics." *Pediatrics*, 1980, *65*, 567-572.

Parcel, G. S., and others. "A Comparison of Absentee Rates of Elementary School Children with Asthma and Non-Asthmatic Schoolmates." *Pediatrics*, 1979, *64*, 878-881.

Pless, I. B., and Satterwhite, B. B. "Chronic Illness." In R. Haggerty, K. Roghmann, and I. B. Pless (Eds.), *Child Health and the Community*. New York: Wiley, 1975a.

Pless, I. B., and Satterwhite, B. B. "Family Functioning and Family Problems." In R. Haggerty, K. Roghmann, and I. B. Pless (Eds.), *Child Health and the Community*. New York: Wiley, 1975b.

Pless, I. B., Satterwhite, B. B., and VanVechten, D. "Division, Duplication and Neglect: Patterns of Care for Children with Chronic Disorders." *Child Care, Health and Development*, 1978, *4*, 9-19.

Rose, J., Boggs, T., and Alderstein, A. "The Evidence for a Syndrome of 'Mothering Disability' Consequent to Threats to the Survival of Neonates: A Design for Hypothesis Testing Including Prevention in a Prospective Study." *American Journal of Diseases of Children*, 1960, *100*, 776-777.

Rowe, G. P. "The Developmental Conceptual Framework to the Study of the Family." In F. I. Nye and F. M. Berardo (Eds.), *Emerging Conceptual Frameworks in Family Analysis*. New York: Macmillan, 1966.

Salk, L., Hilgartner, M., and Granich, B. "The Psychosocial Impact of Hemophilia on the Patient and His Family." *Social Science and Medicine*, 1972, *6*, 491-505.

Simpson, O. W., and Smith, M. A. "Lightening the Load for Parents of Children with Diabetes." *MCN: The American Journal of Maternal Child Nursing*, 1979, *4*, 293-296.

Solnit, A. J., and Stark, M. H. "Mourning and the Birth of a Defective Child." *The Psychoanalytic Study of the Child*, 1961, *16*, 523-537.

Stein, R.E.K., and Jessop, D. J. "What Diagnosis Does Not Tell: The Case for a Noncategorical Approach to Chronic Physical Illness." Paper presented at the meetings of the Society for Pediatric Research/Ambulatory Pediatric Association, Washington, D.C., May 1982.

Stein, R.E.K., Jessop, D. J., and Riessman, C. K. "Health Care Services Received by Children with Chronic Illness." *American Journal of Diseases of Children*, 1983, *137*, 225-230.

Stein, R.E.K., and Riessman, C. K. "Development of an Objective Burden Index for Chronic Illness in Childhood." Ambulatory Pediatric Association, 1979.

Stein, R.E.K., and Riessman, C. K. "Impact on Family Scale." *Medical Care*, 1980, *18*, 465-472.

Swift, C., Seidman, F., and Stein, H. "Adjustment Problems in Juvenile Diabetics." *Psychosomatic Medicine*, 1967, *29*, 555-571.

Tew, B., and Laurence, K. M. "Mothers, Brothers and Sisters of Patients with Spina Bifida." *Developmental Medicine and Child Neurology*, 1973, *15*(29), 69-76.

Tropauer, A., Franz, M. N., and Dilgard, V. W. "Psychological Aspects of the Care of Children with Cystic Fibrosis." *American Journal of Diseases of Children*, 1970, *119*, 424-432.

Turk, J. "Impact of Cystic Fibrosis on Family Functioning." *Pediatrics*, 1964, *34*, 67-71.

Vance, J. C., and others. "Effects of Nephrotic Syndrome on the Family: A Controlled Study." *Pediatrics*, 1980, *65*, 948-955.

Waechter, E. H. "Developmental Consequences of Congenital Abnormalities." *Nursing Forum*, 1975, *14*, 108-129.

Walker, J. H., Thomas, M., and Russell, I. T. "Spina Bifida and the Parents." *Developmental Medicine and Child Neurology*, 1971, *13*, 462-476.

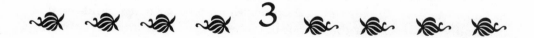

Issues Common
to a Variety of Illnesses

I. Barry Pless, M.D., F.R.C.P.[C]
James M. Perrin, M.D.

The chronic illnesses of childhood are, individually, usually rare, but as a group, they affect from 10 to 15 percent of the population under eighteen years of age. Of children with chronic illnesses, about 10 percent (1 percent of the total childhood population) have disabilities severe enough to interfere with the ability to carry out ordinary tasks appropriate for their age (Pless and Roghmann, 1971; Ireys, 1981). The remainder have disabilities of lesser degrees, and indeed some with well-established disorders are not disabled in any detectable way. Nonetheless, the needs and problems of chronically ill children cannot be predicted from the severity or type of disability alone.

As a group, chronically ill children and their families merit public attention for several reasons. First, chronically ill children are the recipients of sizable public investment, especially for medical services, and consume a large proportion of total dollars spent on child health. Second, as a class, they present special needs not likely to be met through any existing or proposed programs for general child health care. Third, because of tremendous technological and health care advances of the past quarter century, many children who would have succumbed to an early death are surviving into adulthood, perhaps with a relatively greater frequency of handicaps.

We wish not only to review some of the specific issues that distinguish one chronic illness from another but also to look at their similarities, especially from the perspective of the needs of families, the delivery of services, and the implications for public policy.

Continuity and Commonality

The use of the term *continuities* in connection with the care of children with chronic illnesses is a deliberately ambiguous way of describing two distinct but related concepts. The first sense in which the term is used refers to consistency or lack thereof in the pattern of care provided for any particular child—that is, continuity of care. Care is continuous in the sense that the medical needs of most of these children are long lasting and require frequent, if not constant, attention. It is discontinuous, however, in that these needs are usually divided among several practitioners or involve a variety of health providers. One very common example is the break in care between the primary care provider and those at the secondary or more specialized levels. Discontinuity may also occur within secondary care when many specialists are involved—the extent to which these doctors and their colleagues provide services that are in any sense continuous and coordinated is highly problematic. This concept describes much of the pattern and work of people who deal at every level with chronically ill children and their families.

The second sense reflects the notion of continuity of condition—that there are found, across a wide range of disorders, some dissimilar but many other important similar elements affecting chronically ill children and their families. *Commonalities* is a more satisfactory term to describe this concept than *continuities*. From the point of view of either service or research, a strong case can be made for viewing all chronic conditions, regardless of their individual characteristics, as one group having many problems in common, although it is true that, in some disorders, the elements shared with other conditions are heavily outweighed by those that are unique to that condition. This chapter focuses on this second use of the term, considering both the categorical and common issues in chronic childhood illness, as they are seen by the family, and then developing a synthesis between the two seemingly opposing views. It is hoped that such a synthesis will provide a rational and realistic guide in the development of future health policy.

Families with children who have chronic illnesses face complex problems in obtaining support for the various special needs brought about as a result of such illness. These needs vary from very specialized diagnostic and therapeutic medical care of a highly technical sort through less specialized nursing care and family care of common complications. Families with a chronically ill child often require educational, psychological, financial, and social support. Family tasks range from seeking skilled, specialized medical care (likely to provide quality and up-to-date technological services) through the search for optimal school placement, counseling, and advice to meeting the general need for respite from the complex parenting demands of many of these children.

Background: History and Epidemiology

Historically, most research and service programs for children with chronic illnesses have developed from a categorical or disease-by-disease approach, emphasizing the unique characteristics of individual disease entities. In large part, the way medical knowledge is organized—by organ systems—has been the principle around which specialized diagnostic and treatment skills have evolved. Thus, those with special knowledge of the cardiovascular system become cardiologists and provide care in cardiology clinics, and a cardiology clinic will be held at a time and place different from a neurology clinic. The philosophy of care prevailing in each clinic may, however, differ markedly, and the differing philosophies can create problems especially for the many children who have two or more major disabilities.

These structural constraints make less likely any consideration of the commonalities among sick children with different diseases. Similarly, public policies relating to these children have generally developed from a narrow, categorical base. To some degree, this background results from the relative ease of mobilizing and continuing support for one condition rather than many. Initially, federal investment in children with chronic conditions via the Crippled Children's Services (CCS) represented an effort to provide specific orthopedic services. The growth of CCS programs, especially in earlier years, generally reflected a disease-by-disease addition to the list of those eligible for coverage (Select Panel for the Promotion of Child Health, 1981). In many states, however, CCS still covers few categories of chronic conditions, and the criteria for inclusion are generally arbitrary. The disarray among CCS programs is further reflected in the wide variety of poorly coordinated efforts—such as those of Developmental Disabilities Councils, university-affiliated facilities (for developmentally handicapped children), and state Medicaid programs—directed toward children with special needs.

Only relatively recently has there been much recognition of issues such as impact on family, psychological adjustment, and social development that are common to children with different chronic diseases. Increasing evidence of these commonalities has indicated the need for a more coordinated public response. This need is reflected in the organization of health services, the response of schools and other community institutions, and the further extension of research into untoward consequences of the illness for child and family and the most effective means of intervention.

The epidemiology of chronic illness in childhood is different from that of chronic illness in adults. Most importantly, where adult chronic illness consists mainly of a relatively large number of fairly common illnesses (such as hypertension, diabetes, and osteoarthritis) and a few rare diseases, chronic illness in childhood is characterized by very few disorders that are common and by many that are quite rare. Of the group of serious illnesses considered in this policy study, only asthma has a prevalence greater than one in a thousand in a childhood population. The average pediatrician usually has fewer than two thousand children actively enrolled in his or her practice. Unless there is a means of concentrating children with specific chronic illnesses in a particular practice, it is unlikely that a pediatrician will see many children with any single specific chronic illness during his or her practice lifetime. Similarly, community schools encounter children with specific illnesses only sporadically. This special issue of prevalence is, on the one hand, a contributing factor in the historical focus on specific categories and, on the other hand, a primary argument in favor of the new movement toward a more generic approach.

In order to develop expertise in such rare conditions as cystic fibrosis, leukemia, and myelomeningocele, it has been necessary to organize centralized referral programs that attract families referred from a fairly wide population base. Such expertise has generally developed within tertiary-care academic medical centers. The development of specific disease programs has evolved with increasing specialization in medical care, which has, in turn, led to the presence in some centers not only of specialists in such areas as hematology (diseases of the blood and blood-forming organs), but also of specialists in diseases of specific blood parts (for example, white cells, red cells, and serum components). Indeed, because of the history of the past quarter century, most academic centers have organized their services around increasingly narrow organ- or disease-specific clinics, even to the extent of separating children with relatively related organ disorders—into, for example, a thyroid disorder clinic and a growth clinic.

This intense specialization has accounted for a significant number of the important developments in the therapy of childhood disorders over the past few decades. However, academic institutions have only rarely developed a comparable intellectual pursuit of the generic issues of chronic childhood illness. Although most academic health centers will have staff with experience with most specific forms of chronic childhood illness, only rare pediatric departments or schools of nursing have faculty members with a focus on the generic problems of chronic childhood illness. Because there are few medical experts in childhood chronic illness who serve as generalists with a focus on management as opposed to treatment, academic researchers often find it difficult to gather together from their multitude of disease-specific clinics children with a variety of chronic illnesses. Moreover, medical leadership for community agencies and for illness interest groups often rests with the local specialists.

Finally, federal funding policies have generally supported specialization within academic health centers. Funding for academic institutions has become increasingly dependent on disease-specific programs within the National Institutes of Health (NIH). Only relatively recently has the NIH supported significant amounts of behavioral research in chronic illness, and this support still represents only a very small percent of total NIH commitments to childhood chronic illness. The large majority of NIH-supported behavioral research has had a disease-specific focus.

As indicated in other chapters of this book, it is clear that the emphasis on special biological problems of specific diseases has led to important developments improving the longevity and quality of life of many. Such activities, which will continue to foster basic technological advances, need ongoing support. But with the increase in our understanding of the problems faced by families of chronically ill children, there is also a growing need for advances in understanding the more generic issues. There should be an expansion of the intellectual base for the development of new preventive and therapeutic programs as well as research into basic mechanisms regarding the generic issues.

Categorizing Chronic Childhood Illnesses

The categorical approach, bringing together numbers of children with a specific illness, encourages more in-depth attention to the health, developmental, and research questions associated with that disease. Only by review of sizable numbers of children with, say, cystic fibrosis can the spectrum of symptoms, severity, and response to treatment be well understood. There are potential benefits as well in developing a *partial* categorical approach; that is, one that takes into account some of the common physiological and therapeutic character- istics of groups of disorders. For example, although lymphoma and leukemia are clearly different diseases, there are some important similarities in manifestations, in therapy, and in complications that make it appropriate to consider them together. We will consider some of the ways of categorizing and distinguishing classes of chronic illnesses that may have implications for the delivery of services and for related public policies.

Prevalence. As stated, only a few of the chronic disorders in childhood are common. These are mainly allergic diseases (especially asthma), neurologic disorders (seizures and forms of cerebral palsy), and behavioral problems. Others are all increasingly rare, varying from diabetes or sickle-cell anemia (with a prevalence of about one in a thousand in the childhood population) to disorders like phenylketonuria and other metabolic disorders or immunologic diseases that have prevalence rates of less than one in thirty thousand. The more common disorders are likely to be found in most communities, schools, and medical practices and should therefore lend themselves to primary care management. Given the relatively greater prevalence of the more common disorders, general physicians should be able to maintain the technical ability to provide ongoing services for uncomplicated cases. Similarly, schools and other child-related institutions should have the flexibility to respond appropriately to these children.

The rare disorders, however, raise more complex issues in appropriate early identification, referral, and long-term management. In general, it must be assumed that general physicians will have had little experience with a rare disorder during their training and essentially no experience since entering practice. Consequently, they may have difficulty recognizing the disorder and little knowledge of where to refer it or how best to advise the family. As an example, spina bifida occurs approximately once in three thousand births. There are major disagreements about the best technological approach to early manage- ment of these children, varying from advocating early surgical intervention for all such children to advocating restriction of surgical intervention to those meeting certain prognostic criteria. The general physician has limited experience with the disorder and is not usually familiar with the specialist groups techni- cally prepared to care for children with spina bifida. Referrals may, therefore, be made on the basis of acquaintance. And parents, who cannot be expected to know the different philosophies of the available doctors, will be unable to participate in important decisions involving their child. Yet both steps are crucial determinants of the care that will follow.

Primary care providers have a key responsibility in early identification and referral of children with rare disorders. Their responsibility for long-term medical management also needs clarity. It can be argued that rare disorders are best managed by specialists in centers. The primary provider can remain up to date in the technological advances for rare diseases only with difficulty and is unlikely to have enough clinical experience to understand the subtle but important issues associated with complications of the disease or its treatment or in the usual course of the disorders. On the other hand, to the degree that concern is more focused on the broader issues involving the management of the child and the child's family in the community, it may be the primary provider who is more knowledgeable about the general issues than the specialist.

Mobility-Activity. A second issue in the categorization of chronic illness is whether the disorder has significant (real or perceived) impact on mobility. Many disorders that affect mobility require major orthopedic surgery as well as costly appliances and physical therapy for habilitation. Decreased mobility hinders access to public institutions (including schools) and job opportunities. Diseases that directly affect mobility may prevent children from participating in sports and other activities with their peers and separate them from siblings at home as well.

For diseases affecting mobility, children at the margin (boundary between health and illness—those with mild or moderate rather than severe disease) may have greater problems in psychological adjustment. Paradoxically, for some children with a chronic disorder, psychological adjustment may be worse when the physiologic severity of the disease is relatively minimal in comparison with children coping with greater physiologic severity (McAnarney and others, 1974). This finding may be more common with disorders affecting mobility or when children perceive that their ability to participate in usual childhood activities is diminished. Children at the margin may become easily frustrated by their attempts to compete with their able-bodied peers, whereas children with more significant interference with mobility may feel less compelled to compete (Pless and Pinkerton, 1975).

Course of Illness. A third issue in the categorization of chronic illness is the course of the illness, which can be described, among other ways, as static or dynamic. Static disorders include those with a fixed deficit (although that deficit may likely manifest itself in varied ways at different developmental stages). Dynamic disorders are those in which there is a change over time in the effects of the illness. The dynamic disorders may be further categorized as to whether the course is predictably toward improvement or decline or whether it is marked by exacerbations, with times when the child may be relatively healthy and others when she or he may be quite ill. Among the dynamic disorders, muscular dystrophy is one with a persistent downhill course. In contrast, asthma is one with frequent exacerbations but with not infrequent general improvement and alleviation of the disease. Others, like diabetes, are usually quite stable over time. Additionally, the likelihood that a disease will lead to death in childhood distinguishes it from conditions in which most children survive to adulthood.

These differences in the course of illness may be reflected in important variations in children's adjustment to illness. Diseases with frequent exacerbations are characterized by frequent, brief absences from school and by problems of mobilizing needed support services, such as homebound educational programs, for short periods. Children with asthma, for example, account for a substantial proportion of school absenteeism due to chronic illness (Parcel and others, 1979); yet, each episode of school absence tends to be relatively short. Many community resources require a certain minimum length of disability before support services can be obtained.

Age of Onset. Age of onset may be important in predicting child and family adjustment to chronic illness. Children with early (usually birth) onset problems (such as spina bifida or congenital heart disease) have different developmental and service needs from those with later onset (diabetes, asthma). Children with congenital heart disease usually need extensive care, including one or more complex surgical procedures, early in life, and for most families, once this intense early period is over, children can lead active lives with little impact on their condition. Children born with a condition affecting their functioning appear to adjust to it more readily or to develop in the context of their illness in different ways from those able-bodied children who, having gone through typical developmental phases, develop permanent conditions later in childhood. Children with spina bifida, as an example, have different patterns of adjustment from children rendered paraplegic from injury in adolescence. Children who have once had an ability react to its loss differently from those who never had it.

Cognitive and Sensory Functioning. A fourth issue in categorization is the impact of the disorder on cognitive ability. Problems directly impairing cognitive functioning will have different implications for child development and for such concomitants of disease as psychological adjustment. Such problems also lead to service needs different from those of children without cognitive impairment.

Similarly, children who have major sensory impairments (for example, in their ability to communicate with their environment due to speech, hearing, or vision impairment or some combination of these), have special service needs and are likely to have a different pattern of psychological adjustment from that of children without sensory impairment.

Visibility. Childhood chronic illness can be categorized, as well, according to whether or not the disorder is visible. For example, congenital heart diseases are usually invisible, whereas spina bifida usually has visible aspects. Visibility has the greatest effect in areas of peer relations, where the response of other children often varies according to the extent to which the condition can be seen. As documented in Gliedman and Roth (1980), the social and developmental consequences of being seen as handicapped can be pervasive.

Additional Categorical Considerations. A final issue that may be considered in categorizing chronic illness is the amount of time necessary for diagnosis

of the problem. In most cases, a diagnosis can be made relatively soon after the
family or the clinician first becomes aware of the symptoms. For some, however,
there may be a lengthy and often anxiety-provoking time between the onset of
symptoms and the formal confirmation of the diagnosis. Additionally, some
chronic illnesses have a significant genetic component. Where the genetics are
understood and where they are important in the disease, careful investigation and
counseling must be provided. Conditions such as diabetes require more ongoing
medical supervision than do others, such as stable cerebral palsy.

Commonality of Chronic Conditions

The case for commonality, that is, for viewing all chronic conditions as
having common elements, is based heavily on the results of a variety of research
studies. From a clinical point of view, however, the opposite impression
undoubtedly prevails: all physicians are trained to make diagnoses by recognizing
features specific to a particular disease and distinct from others. Furthermore,
within individual disease categories, good clinicians recognize individual characteristics that represent the uniqueness of each patient as a person. These
clinicians value "clinical judgment" and personalized decision making, and
many constantly move between trying to identify common elements on the one
hand and unique elements on the other. The best of clinical medicine represents
a delicate balance between these dynamics. Thus, it is likely that if specialist
physicians were asked whether children with diabetes have much or little in
common with those with asthma or epilepsy, their first reaction is likely to be
"little." On further reflection, however, it is likely that many would agree that
the element of chronicity alone is one feature shared equally by all such children
that has widespread implications.

From a sociopsychological point of view, the element of chronicity is
thought to have a very powerful effect on the child's development and on the
family's functioning. In particular, a considerable body of empirical data
supports the belief that the presence of a disorder that renders children "different"
from their peers and persists for a significant period of time poses a potential risk
for normal psychosocial adjustment. We return to this point later because it is
central to several of the main arguments in support of the notion of
commonalities.

The persuasive evidence for this position derived equally from studies of
individual disorders and from those in which chronic conditions are considered
as a group (Pless and Pinkerton, 1975). What emerges from these studies is a body
of data pointing to several important and recurring themes that must be
considered in the planning of appropriate health services at a clinical level, at
a policy level, or both. For example, the typical pattern of medical care for
children with a chronic disorder begins with a primary physician who suspects
or makes a diagnosis of the disorder. This physician, a general practitioner,
family physician, or general pediatrician will, more often than not, seek

confirmation of the diagnosis from a specialist or subspecialist with training pertinent to that disorder.

Once the diagnosis is confirmed, the pattern varies somewhat depending on local custom (Pless, Satterwhite, and VanVechten, 1976). This custom, in turn, may be strongly influenced by geographic considerations. Children who live in an urban area where a university medical center is located and where subspecialist physicians are plentiful, will likely find that the bulk of their care is provided in that center by a specialist. The process of handing over responsibility from primary physician to specialist may be done deliberately and explicitly after thorough discussion with the primary physician, or it may simply come about in a more passive, gradual, and informal fashion with the passage of time. What happens, in effect, is that primary physicians are eventually removed (or remove themselves) from the picture through what may be regarded as a process of attrition.

In the case of many chronic conditions, a second, third, and possibly fourth or fifth specialist may become involved following the initial referral. This is especially likely when children have disorders such as spina bifida for which, at various stages of the illness, there are different technical needs. Each stage requires medical or surgical attention of a specialized kind, and the extent to which they are provided in a continuous or discontinuous fashion depends entirely on the organization of the particular services involved. In cases of complex handicapping conditions, then, the ideal of continuity applies not only to the interaction between primary and tertiary care settings but also to the interaction among the involved specialists.

Even in circumstances in which a number of specialists are involved in the care of a single child or a single category of chronic disorder, it is unlikely that they will view this condition as similar to other chronic conditions (that is, from a noncategorical perspective). In general, it is unusual for specialist physicians as a group to appreciate the common elements between and among chronic disorders, nor is there much incentive for them to do so.

The best evidence for commonalities among conditions arises from studies in which the views of parents (or the children themselves), as well as others outside the medical system, are obtained systematically. When these views are analyzed, it becomes clear that there are a limited number of difficulties frequently experienced by many, if not most, families who have a child with a chronic disorder. These analyses suggest that the difficulties vary only slightly from disorder to disorder or from family to family. If anything, the nature of the family, more than the nature of the disorder, is likely to determine the frequency with which certain problems are experienced.

Certainly, one of the most common and most extensively studied problems is that of secondary psychosocial difficulties. For a long while, it was argued that personality and behavioral disorders were specific to individual conditions. The literature purported to describe characteristic constellations of traits of, for example, children with diabetes (Swift, Seidman, and Stein, 1967), asthma (Purcell and others, 1969), or rheumatoid arthritis (Grokoest, Snyder, and

Schleger, 1962). It was only after many years of more systematic and better-designed research that this myth was laid to rest. Eventually, it became clear that there is no such thing as a typical personality profile or behavioral problem that applies to a specific disorder. Rather, where there are apparent patterns, factors related to the family and other social circumstances of the child have been shown to be the important determinants of who is troubled and who is not. There remains little evidence that the nature of a child's psychosocial difficulties is related in any way to a specific medical condition.

A second example of commonalities is found in the literature describing the impact of the disease on the family. Here again, older studies, often focusing on a specific disease (usually one with catastrophic qualities such as spina bifida, cerebral palsy, or a terminal illness), documented in an uncontrolled fashion the frequency with which certain problems are reported by a representative of the family, usually the mother (Pless and Pinkerton, 1975). It is striking, however, that even an examination of this older literature, which must be viewed as simply descriptive, suggests the existence of a common pattern that applies to most conditions. Thus, although the studies frequently dealt with only a single condition, the nature of the problems documented (financial, transportation, social disruption, or the effects on marriage or siblings) were similar across different conditions.

In order to strengthen the conclusion that they are truly attributable to the child's condition, the more recent literature in the area of family impact attempts to look at such problems in comparison with those of nonaffected populations. In some areas, the results suggest that the previous conclusions may be somewhat overstated. For example, the older literature stated, almost without exception, that the presence of a chronic disorder resulted in serious marital difficulties. Almost as consistent were reports of disturbances experienced by siblings of a disabled child. It is only in recent years that studies have been sufficiently well controlled so that comparisons are made with families of similar social composition (for example, Vance and others [1980]). From recent studies, it appears that the impact on families is extremely variable.

A variety of methodological problems makes it difficult to reach more definite conclusions about the impact of the child's illness on the family. Most parents with a disabled or chronically ill child are interviewed years after onset of the event, at a point far removed in time from that when problems may have been most severe. Over time, most families learn to adapt and may do so by suppressing or denying the nature of the difficulties they have experienced. Others may, consciously or otherwise, exaggerate difficulties in order to earn the sympathy of the interviewer. Furthermore, in the case of healthy families being interviewed for purposes of comparison, it is extremely difficult to conceive of meaningful questions that would be similar in content to those asked of the family of a disabled child. Notwithstanding these methodologic problems, several current studies reveal potentially important common problems among families of children with diverse conditions. Not one, however, suggests that the impact is universal or that it is invariably negative. There is reasonable evidence for the belief that, in many instances, families are unified or otherwise strengthened by the shared experience. Clearly the effects are selective and complex, and much remains for researchers to untangle.

The extent to which problems are noncategorical is well illustrated by several early studies of handicapped children. These generally community-based projects had the broad aim of defining the plight of handicapped children and their families systematically and in detail. For example, the study undertaken by the Carnegie United Kingdom Trust (1964) includes children with a wide variety of neurologic and orthopedic disorders as well as some with certain sensory problems. The list of conditions included in these early studies (and in the early American studies) is shown in Table 1. The composition of the sample varied somewhat from substudy to substudy, but in general, the conclusions about the child and family needs generated by illness were remarkably similar, regardless of the specific health conditions. A later review of a wide variety of studies headed by Kellmer-Pringle, (1964a, 1964b) reached similar conclusions. In these important landmark British reports, no essential distinctions are made among different types of disabilities with regard to the nonmedical needs of children.

Using a more systematic and rigorous approach, several early American studies—Wishik in Georgia (1956), Richardson and Higgins in Alamance County (1965), and Sultz and others in Erie County (1972), among others—show a similarity of conclusions about needs, both medical and nonmedical, that is striking. More recent community-based surveys in Monroe County, New York (Haggerty, Roghmann and Pless, 1975) and in Genesee County, Michigan (Walker, Gortmaker, and Weitzman, 1981) also sound the same note. In these instances, children with various chronic disorders were identified based on reports obtained from parents in a random sample of households whereas, in the earlier studies (Alamance, Erie), cases were identified through hospital and agency records or by clinic examinations. In both sets of findings, parents and officials alike describe many problems—in everyday living, in the organization of health care, and in the provision of educational services—that cut across diagnostic lines. If there are any significant variations in the conclusions of these reports, they are related more to the time and place in which the studies were carried out than to the composition of the sample.

One important finding of the Alamance study (Richardson and Higgins, 1965), particularly in view of the time when it was conducted, was that many sociodemographic factors (among them, social class, economic status, education, age, race, and sex) appeared to be related to the need for medical care. The study drew attention to what the authors describe as "the social folkways and values of the community, the organization, goals and specific interests and interrelationships of the community agencies, and the legal and policy restrictions of services and programs" (p. 123). The authors noted that these factors are as important as the availability of services in determining whether handicapped children really receive the care they need, and this conclusion applies as well now as it did twenty years ago.

Three general family needs that were identified then (Richardson and Higgins, 1965, p. 126) have been repeatedly identified by other investigators. The

Table 1. Chronic Disorders Represented in Various Studies of Handicapped Children.

Categories and Entities of Chronic Disorders Represented	Younghusband and others	Anderson	Carnegie United Kingdom Trust	Richardson and Higgins	Wishik	Sultz and others	Haggerty, Roghmann, and Pless	Walker, Gortmaker, and Weitzman	Rutter, Tizard, and Whitmore
Blind/partially sighted	X		X	X	X		X	X	
Deaf/partially hearing	X		X	X	X		X	X	X
Speech	X		X	X	X		X	X	
Physical handicaps									
Orthopedic	X		X	X	X				X
Nonorthopedic			X						
Cerebral palsy	X	X	X	X	X		X	X	X
Spina bifida	X	X							
Spinal injury/polio	X	X	X						
Achondroplasia		X				X			
Congenital absence of limbs								X	
Thalidomide		X							
Rheumatoid arthritis, etc.		X				X	X	X	
Muscular dystrophy						X			
Epilepsy	X		X	X	X	X	X	X	X
Delicate	X		X	X		X			
Asthma/hay fever						X	X	X	X
Heart disease					X	X	X	X	X
Kidney						X	X	X	
Diabetes						X	X	X	X
Gastrointestinal		X				X	X		
Cystic fibrosis						X			
Anemia/other blood						X	X		
Hemophilia	X								
Cleft lip/palate				X	X				
Skin/cosmetic				X	X	X	X		X

first was "for free or part-pay clinics and/or financial assistance for services needed." It is a sad commentary that, so many years later, this problem persists, albeit to a somewhat lesser degree. The second need was for "social and counseling services" aimed at diminishing the strain on intrafamilial relationships and on the emotional problems generated among siblings. It was evident that public health nurses and medical social workers were insufficient to overcome this deficiency. Finally, a third general problem identified was for "a broadly based, soundly conceived, energetically pursued community educational program to overcome the fear, prejudice, and ignorance of available sources of health and care."

Perhaps most important historically was the recognition by Richardson and Higgins (1965) of the fact that services for the handicapped were characterized by specialization and fragmentation; by a lack of systematic, continuous communication and referral between health agents and the agencies; and by the fact that there was "no agency which was in a position to provide a measure of coordination among the diverse agencies and services involved" (p. 127). They stated, "It is our considered judgment that the greatest need in the whole field of childhood handicapping is for a program which can provide for the coordination of all the interested services in the community, facilitate the needed communication and referral, and ensure that the focus of service will be the child and his total needs and not just a specific handicapping condition" (p. 128).

Very much the same sort of conclusion was reached by the Working Party on Children with Special Needs, which reported to the National Bureau for Cooperation in Child Care in Britain (Younghusband, Birchall, Davie, and Kellmer-Pringle, 1970). The basic objective of the working party was "to examine a wide range of handicapping conditions from mild to severe and to focus on the health, educational, family and social needs of these children" (p. 5). (The use of the term *handicap*, at least by British workers of that time, is quite nonspecific and derives from institutional origins, thus differing from the more sophisticated interpretation that is more consistent with present-day usage.) A brief summary of the principal conclusions clearly underscores the noncategorical nature of the working party's recommendations: the focus is on the child's family; the care provided must be interdisciplinary and comprehensive; it should draw upon voluntary organizations and local communities. Although priority is placed on preschool children, it is stressed that care must extend through to late adolescence. The conclusions also draw attention to the need for more efficient translation into practice of our knowledge about prevention of handicap. Much emphasis is placed on the value of initial detection (including screening), on the role of comprehensive assessment teams, and on the need for local authorities to compile and maintain comprehensive registers of handicapped children. It is suggested that social service departments should have a coordinating function to ensure continuity of care.

Above all, the report stresses the need for more and better supporting services for families—services that include information, advice, and counseling and see the role of parents as participants in the team. A long list of specific services is discussed; these include sitting in, home help, laundry, housing, aids to living, and daycare facilities. The report also draws attention to the need for improved design and adaptation of buildings and to the need for hostels, special education boarding schools, and long-stay hospitals. The importance of preparation for leaving school, for employment, and for the special needs of handicapped adolescents is underscored.

The studies by the Carnegie United Kingdom Trust (1964) of the problems of 600 handicapped children and their families identified common needs parallel to those just noted; these needs include: (1) adequate counseling services to give systematically offered advice to parents on the nature, prospect, and consequence of their child's handicaps; on their doubts and anxieties; and on the daily problems of caring for their children; (2) services in the home, especially for cases involving serious problems of behavior or care; (3) more and better aftercare services designed to meet the needs of children leaving school and concerned not only with employment, but also with emotional and social problems; (4) better coordination of and guidance for home teachers of handicapped children; and (5) services to provide relief to parents, particularly for leisure time and holidays.

Recently, Stein and Jessop (1982a, 1982b) reported the findings of an important study of children with varied chronic illnesses who attended the clinics of the Bronx Municipal Hospital Center. They examined a number of important child and family factors, including mother's psychiatric symptoms, child's psychological adjustment, impact of illness on the family, social support of mother, satisfaction with care, and general health status of the child. No difference in any of these child or family indicators could be accounted for by different diagnoses. The only exception was in physician's estimates of the burden involved in the care of the child. In other words, in the areas studied, chronic illness has a basically similar impact regardless of the specific diagnostic group.

In the preceding paragraphs we have provided a general description of the results of surveys of health needs that apply to groups of children with varied chronic disorders. In the large majority of cases there are more features that are held in common among different diagnostic groups than there are features that distinguish them. It must be clearly understood however that these data do not negate the obvious and important biological differences that distinguish one disease from another. As a result of these differences, the treatment of a child with cystic fibrosis is, in a medical sense, a very different matter from that provided for a child with diabetes. Similarly, the treatment for seizures, essentially medicinal, is entirely different from treatment for spina bifida, where a combination of surgical interventions is often indicated.

These distinctions are clear and important; they are easily recognized and generally appreciated; indeed they form the foundation of the organization of our health care system for most children with chronic disorders. Nonetheless, we have tried to demonstrate that there are many other aspects of care where the differences in the needs between children in specific diagnostic groups are usually unimportant. This seeming paradox may be most easily understood when one shifts gears mentally from thinking about the *treatment* of the disease to thinking about *management* of the child and family.

Management is a concept that encompasses therapies of a variety of specific kinds, medicinal as well as surgical. The term also carries with it clear connotations about other skills of equal importance. These skills have to do with the development and coordination of personal and social resources to provide support for the child and family as well as with the direct use by the health care profession of whatever personal skills may be available to address the social and psychologic needs of the child and family.

As has been illustrated through a variety of examples, it is in these broad areas that needs are remarkably similar. These needs range from simple coordination of a wide number of technical services to the coordination and integration of the technical with the supportive services provided by different members of the health team, of community agencies, or both. The actual number of helpers (persons involved in the care of the child and family with a particular illness) is often very large. In the absence of a unifying link, it is conceivable and indeed probable that, in spite of the good intentions of all concerned, more problems may be created than are resolved by the many actors involved. Even in the simplest clinical situations, there is a need for better coordination between the health care provided by a specialist physician and that provided by the primary physician.

Beyond coordination, there is the demand for the provision of counseling and advice about matters that are strictly speaking nonmedical. Again, these matters are often independent of the specific disease in question. Whether a child has diabetes, asthma, or epilepsy, all parents want advice about how to deal with certain common situations. For example, they need to discuss with someone how much a child should tell friends about the illness and whether, when, and how teachers should be told. They need guidance about special education. Most parents require some idea of what lies ahead for the child. If a child with any chronic disease has a behavioral problem, parents will want advice about whether, because of the disease, they should be lenient or strict or at least as strict as they would be if the child were healthy. They need advice about how to deal with the child's siblings, whose need for attention may, at some stages, reflect a sense of competition with the attention being devoted to the ill child. Parents often need advice about very practical matters, such as the availability of financial aid, the extent of insurance coverage, and help available through community agencies. They may also need help with such practical matters as when and where to secure appliances, wheelchairs, or other devices to aid the disabled.

The examples are almost endless, for every facet of life poses special questions when one is living with a disability. All that the nondisabled take for granted becomes potentially problematic. The task of the physician is to be able to respond to those problems with skill, wisdom, and judgment. Clearly the broader the experience with handicapped children, the better the response is likely to be.

In summary, chronically ill children have much in common. As Ireys (1981) notes, they all have the potential for severe disruption of psychological well-being and of the life of the family. The latter is a result of the endless, repetitive, and demanding routines of medical care as well as the more subtle emotional strain on the parents. Travis (1976) puts it well: "Chronic illness is not an entity but an umbrella" and although "each illness is unique," the limitations on child and family are truly widespread.

Summary and Policy Implications

In a very general sense, a principal conclusion that can be drawn from this review for policymakers is that categorical versus noncategorical, or generic, approaches are not dichotomous but rather represent a spectrum. Emphasis at either extreme is not helpful because families with chronically ill children have a variety of both specific and common needs. The great biological and medical variation among diseases mandates distinct treatments (medical and surgical) for each disease (and for each child with a certain disease). Yet the strikingly similar problems (of family financial burden, development and psychologic impact, and the many other areas noted earlier in this chapter) faced by chronically ill children and their families strongly support the notion that for program development and public policy consideration, chronically ill children can be considered as a broad class of children with special needs.

Based on the preceding review, the following recommendations can be made:

1. Chronically ill children and their families should have access both to very specific services dependent on the specific disease and to generic services needed by essentially all children with chronic illness.

   Children with chronic illness can be considered as a category in themselves because of the many similarities of demands placed on them and their families despite the important distinctions among specific disease entities. These relatively common demands include increased financial burdens, a need for specialized services, and a need for access to appropriate technology. In addition, there are clearly increased risks of significant psychological maladjustment and developmental problems. For all, there is an increased need for family support. Children with chronic illnesses also often face special problems as they become adolescents, and many have special needs in school health areas. Finally, chronically ill children have a greater need for better coordination in their primary care and, indeed, for *having* primary care services available to them. It does, therefore, make sense to develop policies of a public nature that reflect the common elements and needs of families with varied chronic conditions.

   At the same time, the consideration of individual diseases, from the viewpoint of patients and families, focuses special attention on technological issues. Although complications of chronic illness are generally rare, it is necessary to ensure access to important new therapeutic measures. Attention to individual diseases leads in turn to development of experts (especially clinicians) with special knowledge of specific diseases, who offer an expertise not otherwise available. Optimally, services should reflect both specific and generic needs.

Despite these common elements, access to the array of needed services is generally more dependent upon geographic considerations and the activities of the medical community and disease-oriented voluntary associations than it is upon the needs of families. Uniformity of need does not guarantee uniformity of access. Families will be offered counseling and social support services only if the clinician concerned with their child's illness is also concerned with having such services available or if the local chapter of the disease-specific association accepts as part of its mission the provision of such services. Not infrequently, a child with a related condition will not receive support services because that condition does not fall within the interests of the association's primary disease. We believe not only that services should be coordinated but also that access to both specialized and generic services should be uniform across disease entities.

2. Services should be provided in a coordinated and efficient way. Health care services are better when they are appropriately coordinated and efficiently organized. Being faced with the need to receive medical care on an ongoing basis from a variety of providers is, in and of itself, bad enough. When such care is so poorly organized that some services are duplicated and others neglected, the burden on the family and child is unnecessarily increased. That problems of duplication and neglect arising from the fundamental division of medical services into categorical blocks continue to exist in spite of general recognition of their implications is well demonstrated in recent studies by Kanthor and others (1974), Pless, Satterwhite, and VanVechten (1978), and Stein and Jessop (1982a, 1982b). In each instance, regardless of the fundamental manner in which the services were organized (through a birth defects clinic, a traditional disease-focused specialty clinic, or a home care program, respectively), many services were provided by several doctors while many other services were offered by none.

To foster integration of services, each family should have a case coordinator responsible for identifying needs and assuring adequate and appropriate communication among service providers and the family to ensure that the full range of needed services has been made available to the family. The coordinator could be any of a number of different people within the service system (nurse, social worker, lay community worker, physician); in some families, the coordinator could be a family member. It is less important who carries out these functions than that they be carried out routinely and well.

3. Services for chronically ill children and their families should be regionalized. Regionalization of child health services in North America has developed so far only for high-risk newborn infants. Central referral (tertiary care) units now exist along with secondary-level centers in small communities. Together they emphasize outreach to nurse and physician providers in smaller communities and hospitals. Regionalization, emphasizing easy access to appropriate specialized care, attention to generic common family needs, and support of services at the community level will go a long way to filling present gaps.

Some key elements of an effective regionalization program include the identification of community resources (hospitals, physicians, teachers, and the like) capable of providing ongoing services to the families of children with chronic conditions and the development of communication systems ensuring easy referral to services in a specialty center and transfer of information back to the local community. Community educational programs, utilizing the skills of the tertiary center staff, should improve the quality of care available on the local level. Care plans should be developed emphasizing the broad range of services needed by families, and clear agreement should be obtained on responsibility for carrying out plan components between the referral center and the local providers. A regional system is an important step in ensuring that families have access to both specific and generic services.

4.   Preparation of providers should include skills in identifying and managing common problems of childhood chronic illness. Although chronic illnesses may be rare in *specific* forms in childhood, it is important to recognize that they are not rare in *general*. Thus, service providers, especially in health and education areas, need to have the training and skills with which to work effectively with the sizable proportion of their population that have chronic conditions. Service providers, too, need access to quality special advice for specific conditions, but they should be equipped to respond to the generic needs of these families.

5.   Research efforts, both in areas common to all chronic illnesses and in the very special problems of specific diseases, must continue. Excellent research in specific diseases has led to new devices, such as the insulin pump, and to the significantly improved care and outcome of childhood leukemia. This emphasis on high-quality research in specific diseases should be extended to similar research in the generic issues of chronic illness—in the more detailed description of the common problems of psychological adjustment, the need for special education programs, and in intervention programs with the aim of improving such areas as physiological functioning, family functioning, and psychological adjustment.

6.   Systematic collaboration among the disease-oriented voluntary associations would be an important step toward improving the lives of all chronically ill children. Policies and constituencies will develop best with combinations of generic and specific approaches to children with chronic handicapping conditions. Among federal programs, the Medicaid program has the largest dollar investment in chronic childhood illness.

This represents a relatively noncategorical program, insofar as it emphasizes delivery of health services regardless of disease category. On the other hand, as a generic program, it does not actively take into account any of the special, coordinated, team- or multidisciplinary-based problems of children with chronic illnesses. In contrast, the Crippled Children's Services, which began as a very categorical program emphasizing one or two specific groups of diseases, especially (initially) orthopedic ones, has become significantly less disease-specific and has, mainly by adding on numerous specific diseases, become a more generically oriented childhood chronic illness program. Similarly, the development of a constituency for chronically ill children and their families seems sometimes to need a very specific disease approach and other times to need collaboration among several disease-specific groups. In developing some support for, say, muscular dystrophy, it makes good sense to gather together interested relatives of children with dystrophy. However, in developing public support for transportation services for handicapped children, it seems logical to encourage the muscular dystrophy groups to work with groups concerned with other handicapping disorders.

7.   Children with chronic illnesses will continue to need special public policy attention. It seems to us that, even with relatively broad entitlement to health

services and/or health insurance, there will continue to be a need for public programs that focus special attention on chronically ill children. They face medical and health risks quite different from those faced by able-bodied children, and they have special needs for comprehensive and coordinated health, psychological, developmental, and social services different from those required by able-bodied children and their families. Although other programs will generally improve the base of services available to these families, it is unlikely that any general program will provide adequate incentives for a careful response to these special needs.

References

Anderson, E. M. *The Disabled Schoolchild: A Study of Integration in Primary Schools.* London: Methuen, 1973.

Carnegie United Kingdom Trust. *Handicapped Children and Their Families: Reports to the Carnegie United Kingdom Trust on the Problems of 600 Handicapped Children and Their Families.* Dumferline, Scotland: Carnegie United Kingdom Trust, 1964.

Gliedman, J., and Roth, W. *The Unexpected Minority.* New York: Harcourt Brace Jovanovich, 1980.

Grokoest, A., Snyder, A., and Schleger, R. *Juvenile Rheumatoid Arthritis.* Boston: Little, Brown, 1962.

Haggerty, R. J., Roghmann, K. J., and Pless, I. B. *Child Health and the Community.* New York: Wiley, 1975.

Ireys, H. T. "Chronic Illness in Childhood." In *Better Health for Our Children: A National Strategy,* vol. 4. Publication 79-55071. Washington, D.C.: U.S. Department of Health and Human Services, 1981.

Kanthor, H., and others. "Areas of Responsibility in the Health Care of Multiply Handicapped Children." *Pediatrics,* 1974, *54,* 779–785.

Kellmer-Pringle, M. L. *The Emotional and Social Adjustment of Blind Children.* London: National Foundation for Educational Research in England and Wales, 1964a.

Kellmer-Pringle, M. L. *The Emotional and Social Adjustment of Physically Handicapped Children.* London: National Foundation for Educational Research in England and Wales, 1964b.

McAnarney, E., and others. "Psychological Problems of Children with Chronic Juvenile Arthritis." *Pediatrics,* 1974, *53,* 523–528.

Parcel, G. S., and others. "A Comparison of Absentee Rates of Elementary School Children with Asthma and Non-Asthmatic Schoolmates." *Pediatrics,* 1979, *64,* 878–881.

Pless, I. B., and Pinkerton, P. *Chronic Childhood Disorders—Promoting Patterns of Adjustment.* London: Henry Kimpton, 1975.

Pless, I. B., and Roghmann, K. "Chronic Illness and Its Consequences: Some Observations Based on Three Epidemiological Surveys." *Journal of Pediatrics,* 1971, *79,* 351–359.

Pless, I. B., Satterwhite, B., and VanVechten, D. "Chronic Illness in Childhood: A Regional Survey of Care." *Pediatrics*, 1976, *58*, 37–46.

Pless, I. B., Satterwhite, B., and VanVechten, D. "Division, Duplication and Neglect: Patterns of Care for Children with Chronic Disorder." *Child Care: Health and Development*, 1978, *4*, 9–19.

Purcell, K., and others. "A Comparison of Psychologic Findings in Variously Defined Asthmatic Subgroups." *Journal of Psychosomatic Research*, 1969, *13*, 67–75.

Richardson, W. P., and Higgins, A. C. *The Handicapped Children of Alamance County, North Carolina: A Medical and Sociological Study*. Wilmington, Del.: Nemours Foundation, 1965.

Rutter, M., Tizard, J., and Whitmore, K. *Education, Health and Behavior: Psychological and Medical Study of Childhood Development*. New York: Wiley, 1970.

Select Panel for the Promotion of Child Health. *Better Health for Our Children: A National Strategy*, vol. 2. Publication 79-55071. Washington, D.C.: U.S. Department of Health and Human Services, 1981.

Stein, R.E.K., and Jessop, D. J. "A Noncategorical Approach to Chronic Childhood Illness." *Public Health Records*, 1982a, *97*, 354–362.

Stein, R.E.K., and Jessop, D. J. "What Diagnosis Does *Not* Tell: The Case for a Noncategorical Approach to Chronic Physical Illness." Paper presented at the annual meeting of the Society for Pediatric Research, Washington, D.C., 1982b.

Sultz, H. A., and others. *Long-Term Childhood Illnesses*. Pittsburgh, Pa.: University of Pittsburgh Press, 1972.

Swift, C., Seidman, F., and Stein, H. "Adjustment Problems in Juvenile Diabetes." *Psychosomatic Medicine*, 1967, *29*, 555–571.

Travis, G. *Chronic Illness in Children: Its Impact on Child and Family*. Stanford, Calif.: Stanford University Press, 1976.

Vance, J., and others. "Effects of Nephrotic Syndrome on the Family: A Controlled Study." *Pediatrics*, 1980, *65*, 948–955.

Walker, D. K., Gortmaker, S. L., and Weitzman, M. *Chronic Illness and Psychosocial Problems Among Children in Genesee County*. Boston: Community Child Health Studies, Harvard School of Public Health, 1981.

Wishik, S. M. "Handicapped Children in Georgia: A Study of Prevalence, Disability, Needs and Resources." *American Journal of Public Health*, 1956, *46*(2), 195–203.

Younghusband, E., Birchall, D., Davie, R., and Kellmer-Pringle, M. L. (Eds.) *Living with Handicap: The Report of a Working Party on Children with Special Needs*. London: The National Bureau for Co-operation in Child Care, 1970.

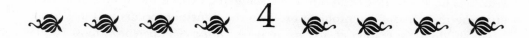

4

Paternalism and Autonomy in the Care of Chronically Ill Children

Loretta Kopelman, Ph.D.

Children with catastrophic or major chronic diseases have all the rights of other children, but they also have special and important needs. Faced with the greater likelihood of crises, momentous decisions, or restricted opportunities, clarification of these rights and evaluation of minors' abilities to make decisions on their own behalf can be crucial for these children. The purpose of this chapter is to examine some of the policies that directly affect them—to determine what constitutes proper consent for diagnostic or therapeutic procedures, how best to study their conditions, and when it is appropriate to seek assent from older children. Viewed in one way, this discussion is about encouraging warranted paternalism for chronically ill children. We act paternalistically when our goal is to protect another from harm or to act for that person's benefit. Children whose potential is developing and who cannot act for themselves have a right to paternalism. It is necessary for adults to make decisions for them based on estimates of what is in their best interest, given the circumstances. However, viewed in another way, this discussion is also about encouraging autonomy for children. That is, it is about how best to foster purposeful and responsible actions under conditions that allow expression of their nature (Kant [1790] 1949; Rawls, 1971; Murphy, 1978).

Insofar as paternalism seeks to create opportunities for development, independence, and responsibility for children, it is not incompatible with fostering autonomy. Rather, autonomy presupposes paternalism. Most children mature and develop autonomy under protection and encouragement. Accord-

61

ingly, the goals of paternalism require its gradual elimination and demise in favor of autonomy.

Obviously, the transition from dependence to independence is gradual in childhood. Infants have a right to full paternalism, and well-adjusted seventeen-year-olds have a justified claim to understand and express themselves in actions affecting their lives. The problem of when the transition occurs becomes acute when children are neither clearly incompetent nor as competent as most adults and when, due to their catastrophic or major chronic illness, we want to know how much they can comprehend and whether they should participate in important care decisions. In the acute phase of a catastrophic illness, there may be too little time to assess individual maturity; however, in protracted illness, estimates of intellectual and emotional development are important enough to be kept current. With major illness, then, assessment of the degree of paternalism appropriate for minors can be more important than it ordinarily is. An arbitrary chronological age for recognition of maturity and full civil rights works well enough in most circumstances. However, it seems an inadequate policy from our point of view, which is that of caring for and about children with catastrophic or chronic diseases.

What we call a catastrophic or chronic disease or illness depends on the prognosis, given available treatment. Actual or imminent departure from normal function inclines us to call something an illness or disease, but its permanence, seriousness, or lack of treatability, or the irreversibility of its effects lead us to call it catastrophic or chronic. In part, this may depend on the services or technology that happen to be available. For example, if no reliable treatment is available, acute pneumonia may be a catastrophic illness.

Whatever recalcitrant moral or legal problems arise in the care of adults with catastrophic and chronic illnesses (and there are many), they are even harder to deal with and more stubbornly resistant to solution when children are involved. Although the law presumes, until proven otherwise, that adults are able to decide their own destinies, such issues as informing, consent for therapy or research, competence, undue pressure, voluntariness, and the limits of paternalism are nonetheless troublesome. In part, this is because the law generally maintains the fiction (important for some reasons) that people are either wholly competent or they are not. That is, there are legally no intervening categories between competence and incompetence that take into account confusion, depression, misassessment of the prognosis, inability to sort out what is in one's best interest, ignorance about medical matters, or fear (Jackson and Younger, 1979). Where there are important consequences riding on these decisions, staff sometimes have difficulty accepting what they perceive to be poor choices by legally competent adults for themselves or their wards.

Personal and policy choices are made more complicated for minors by the great range of developmental and intellectual ability encompassed by the category of *minor*. In addition, difficulties arise from disagreements about ends and goals, such as the proper role and limitation of paternalism or third-party consent. Still, health care policies are necessary to foster the care, respect, and protection of children. For in caring for catastrophically ill children, the goals adopted and policies enforced and funded have a profound effect on the lives of these children.

This review of some moral and legal policies concerning the care of children with catastrophic and chronic illness will focus on children's rights, fostering autonomy, truthfulness, informed consent, research involving children, and problems of reconciling theory and practice. The policies and the controversies surrounding these issues will be related to three basic and binding moral principles, which may show that the policies are less fragmented or situational than they might seem. These are (1) the principle of *justice*—treat similarly those who are situated similarly and extend to others the measure of liberty and control rational for ourselves as self-governing beings, (2) the principle of utility—follow a policy that maximizes the total amount of good in the world, and (3) the principle of beneficence—do good and prevent harm (Frankena, 1963; Donagan, 1977). Paternalistic justifications appeal to the precepts of utility and benevolence; justifications using autonomy, to that of justice.

As we discuss some of these policies, the role of one or more of these precepts should be apparent. Moreover, the perplexities and lingering dissatisfaction inherent in the most difficult of these choices can frequently be traced to conflicts relating to these principles. For example, we value freedom of choice and religion, yet most of us would view the decision of an older teenager, who as a Jehovah's Witness rejects a life-saving transfusion, as a needless tragedy. Although we may agree it would be unjust to interfere with that teenager's free choice, it seems to most of us that such a death is a great and avoidable harm. At other times, the source of the problem involves not conflicts between principles as discussed above but conflicts arising from different applications of the same principle. For example, two parents, with equal claim to decide, may have important and sustained disagreement about what therapy is best for their child.

Children's Rights

People must achieve a certain degree of maturity before they attain full civil rights. As a matter of administrative convenience, an arbitrary age, such as eighteen or twenty-one years, is selected as the age at which the person is assumed to be sufficiently mature to be granted full civil rights. Until minors reach the age of majority, adults are generally authorized to make decisions for them. As a rule, guardians are suited to protect, identify, and act in children's best interests: they want to foster development to the point that children take responsibility for themselves. Such paternalism, in general, is quite justified and necessary (Dworkin, 1971; Dworkin, 1979; Gutmann, 1981; Bok, 1978).

In the past, it was assumed that guardians had an unqualified right to control their children's destiny until adulthood. Reasons commonly given for this policy were (1) children were their property, (2) children, until they reached a particular birthday, were always incompetent to make rational decisions, (3) guardians and parents had the right to the labor of their children, or (4) thoroughgoing direction was necessary to help children properly develop their potential (Worsfold, 1974; Rodham, 1974; Locke [1690], 1937). Gradually, and only in the past century, have minors been recognized as individuals with their own rights (Pilpel, 1971; Raitt, 1974-1975; Hofmann and Pilpel, 1974; Pilpel, 1972).

The increasing restriction of guardians' authority through laws and courts during the last century represents a major policy shift (Worsfold, 1974; Rodham, 1974; Raitt, 1974-1975). In accordance with the goals of justified paternalism, the rationale for extending many specific legal rights to children was to protect them from harm (laws on abuse and neglect, for example) and to promote their interests (such as physical examinations for school children). Some practices intended to protect minors in the courts, however, have had untoward effects by denying them due process (Rothman and Rothman, 1980). Minors recently have gained rights to due process, rights to counsel, and protection from self-incrimination (Pilpel, 1972; Raitt, 1974-1975). In the area of medical care, many rights have recently been guaranteed to minors under the right of privacy (Raitt, 1974-1975; Pilpel, 1972). These include the right to contraceptive information and devices, abortion, and treatment for venereal disease, alcoholism, and drug-related problems (*Planned Parenthood of Central Missouri* v. *Danforth*, 1976; Pilpel, 1971; Paul, 1974-1975). Minors may obtain such information or services without parental consent, and health professionals are, by law, immune from prosecution by parents or guardians for providing such care or information. Too often, minors in need went without treatment rather than face disapproving parents. More extensive rights are sometimes recognized for older minors who are in the category of emancipated minors, which acknowledges that minors who earn their own living, are married, or are otherwise independent should be free to control their own persons (although not necessarily all of their property) (Hofmann and Pilpel, 1974).

Different views about how to apply the precepts of utility, justice, and beneficence are apparent in these shifting policies. In the past, before children were granted rights independent of their parents, it was assumed the best care and protection of children was simply to let guardians make the decisions. The authority of guardians, however, was limited when this reasoning seemed untenable in light of abuse, neglect, conflicting interests, and exploitation of some children by their parents or guardians. The overall importance of fostering the development of minors, looking out for their well-being, and preventing harm to them by limiting parental authority in such instances was recognized (Baker, 1969; Pilpel, 1972; Worsfold, 1974; Rodham, 1974; Rothman and Rothman, 1980).

Rights language can be used to mark out two sorts of justified claims (there is also a *slogan use of rights*, which does not concern us), and both are illustrated by the laws guaranteeing children's rights that were just discussed. On the one hand, rights language is used to mark out liberties with which others may or may not interfere. These freedoms concern the decisions and choices not harming others but affecting our lives and destinies. Rarely can one justify interfering with the liberties of competent people "for their own good." But interference because someone harms another (as in child abuse) or because the choice is impaired (as by ignorance) may be justified. But this does not mean one can always intervene for someone's "own good"—such paternalistic interference would be an affront to one's dignity as a fully qualified person capable of acting in one's best interest. Such rights may be called *autonomy rights* (Murphy, 1978; Kant [1790], 1949). As we have seen, some of the rights granted to older minors are liberties of this sort.

A second kind of right or justified claim is used to distinguish what we believe ought to be guaranteed to people, no matter what their level of functioning. These entitlements are unlike autonomy rights because they do not require people to have special capacities to make decisions for themselves. Many of this second type of right are paternalistic in character because they protect people (such as laws that protect children from abuse, neglect, or incompetent caretakers); others try to give equal opportunities to people or are paternalistic in character because they provide basic things for the development of persons (such as laws that require schooling, innoculations, eye tests, screening, and physical examinations for school children). To have these rights, one does not have to have special status or ability as a moral agent capable of free choice. Rather, these are rights we believe to be morally reasonable for society to guarantee to people. Some call them "social contract rights" (Murphy, 1978), others, "rights to well-being" (Peffer, 1978).

Liberties and entitlements are different. Many liberties are legally guaranteed. For example, the right of competent adults to refuse treatment and not be interfered with is guaranteed by law (Byrn, 1978), but not all autonomy rights can be guaranteed by law. For example, suppose that, in order to make a patient (child or adult) hold still, a nurse promises a procedure will not be painful, knowing it is likely to be painful. This is morally wrong, even if we do not make it illegal. Such behavior to a child or adult shows lack of respect for the individual, and harms by eroding trust. Any child old enough to understand is old enough not to be manipulated in this way. Another example will show that entitlements are sometimes set aside at the request of the person and from respect for their liberties. For example, a seventeen-year-old minor with kidney disease was uncooperative and frequently violent in refusing dialysis treatment. He insisted and finally won his right not to be interfered with, setting aside what others took to be his own good.

As to which claims society ought to enforce, we need to consider our priorities and resources and what each of us would want for ourselves or our families if we were in a disadvantaged position. If rational people would want to be protected from abuse and from certain major losses, then we ought to extend a welfare net or a minimum floor for those who, through no fault of their own, have the bad luck to be sick or poor. For example, rational persons, even selfish ones who care primarily about themselves and their families, might want hospitals to have enough intensive care beds for children and adults to serve each region, just in case they need one. None of us are immune from tragedy, so prudence, if not compassion, suggests we protect ourselves.

To summarize, these two kinds of rights are important in making children be and become responsible. To help children become responsible, it is often as important to treat them as if they were responsible as it is to protect them. Frequently they show us that they want and are prepared for more responsibility than we thought they should have. Phasing out paternalism and phasing in autonomy is an art of great importance in the care of children with chronic and catastrophic illness.

Fostering Autonomy

Children with catastrophic or chronic illnesses have conditions that single them out. Their disease may cause temporary or permanent disability or handicap. It is difficult for anyone to cope with major acute or long-term illness; for the child, whose self-image is developing and who longs to be like other children, the emotional stress may be especially great. In addition, there is a tendency, called the spread effect, for negative appraisals to dominate in our estimation of people. Thus, people with disabilities tend to be perceived by themselves and others as more disabled than they are (Wright, 1979). Open communication with children about their illness and its effects may help foster their personal development and prevent or correct misconceptions (Turk, 1964; Mattsson, 1972). Still, sometimes holding back or at least careful planning about discussions is indicated. One sad incident involved a dying teenager who locked herself in the bathroom, refusing to come out until people promised to stop talking about dying. Denial or agreement on silence is, for some, an effective means of dealing with crisis. Some people clearly indicate they do not want to be informed, make decisions, or talk to certain persons; and this desire, especially for children, deserves to be honored as well.

Because of the great intellectual and developmental variation in children, it is difficult to specify the chronological age at which a minor can understand and participate in treatment choices. But, a child's expressed desire to be informed and to participate in decisions affecting his or her life should be respected. "If they are old enough to ask, they are old enough to be told" expresses only part of this principle because some children who want to know have difficulty asking.

One can object, however, that our encouragement of as much communication and autonomy as possible is an ineffective policy because it allows for such wide interpretation. After all, it is hard enough to make decisions about adults' competency and to estimate what information adults do or do not want; when children are involved, it is much harder. Although this objection is important and practical, too much emphasis on the difficulties can cause one to miss the point. What we recommend is a certain way of looking at the treatment of children and use of a conceptual framework that *seeks to include, rather than exclude, children as much as possible*. In deciding how to act, I believe it can be as potent (but in a more worthwhile way) as an earlier policy that, in general, patients (children as well as adults) ought to be excluded from serious decisions (Percival [1803], 1977; American Medical Association, 1977). The value of our policy is to dispose us toward informing and seeking assent.

There are interesting parallels between this position and that in the federal rules on Research Involving Children (U.S. Department of Health and Human Services, 1983). These rules recommend seeking the assent of the child if possible, and no specific age is mentioned. Presumably, the term *assent* rather than *consent* is used to distinguish it from the more legalistic notion. The document states that assent should be based on the sort of information appropriate to the child's level of understanding. In determining when assent should be sought, the Institutional Review Board (IRB) plays a crucial role: Assent should be sought "when in the judgment of the IRB the children are capable of providing assent. In determining whether children are capable of assenting, the IRB shall take into account the ages, maturity, and psychological state of the children involved in research under a particular protocol, or for each child, as the IRB deems appropriate" (U.S. Department of Health and Human Services, 1983). Like the policy we recommend—of trying to inform and seek assent—no reference is made to age in this Department of Health and Human Services recommendation. Rather, it too relies on judgments about the appropriateness of informing and seeking permission.

Obviously, these judgments about who to inform and when and how to do it should be affected by studies about the likely effects of informing and seeking assent from children at certain ages. For example, there is evidence that children under twelve have great difficulty understanding what it means to be research subjects (Schwartz, 1972). But if we agree first that children have a justified claim to information about themselves and to control over their lives, if possible and if they want it, and second that we ought to try to seek the assent of children, then this agreement should encourage systematic examination of when, what, and how information should be given to children of different ages and maturity, or of what verbal or nonverbal clues are reliable markers that children want or do not want to be informed.

If this is correct, then although consent from the child's guardian is typically needed for certain therapy or research, the understanding and assent of the child is also desired. This seems to be justified on the basis of all three moral precepts. For to disregard a child's need to know, control, or assent seems neither fair nor kind nor useful. Anyone, child or adult, who wants to know and be part of decisions about himself or herself and is excluded, feels frustration, isolation, and loss of control. Seeking the child's assent, when possible, respects and recognizes the child's important and independent perspective. This is small restitution for children who, by virtue of catastrophic and chronic illnesses, have been restricted in the ways they can express and assert themselves.

Truthfulness

Due to the nature of diseases we call catastrophic or chronic, information about the patient will sometimes be sad. If a case can be made for routinely withholding depressing news from adults, then our position that as much candor as possible should be used with children is weakened. And odd though it may seem, not too long ago a prevailing view was that physicians were exempt from the usual moral requirements about truthfulness (Sedgwick [1907], 1966; Cabot [1903], 1977; Percival [1803], 1977; American Medical Association [1847], 1977). Paternalistic arguments about what was for the patients' own good or to prevent their harm were used to defend withholding information, deceiving, manipulating, and even lying. A frequently used but erroneous argument was that one need not be truthful because it is hard to know for sure what the truth really is. However, in asking for truthfulness, we ask for a statement about what the other person sincerely believes and not for absolute truth, whatever that may be (Chisholm and Feehan, 1977; Kalin, 1976; Morano, 1975). Further, we are asking not only that the professional not perform an act of commission but also that the professional not intentionally withhold information it is believed will have important consequences (that is, not perform an act of omission). An influential source of the recommendation to withhold depressing news is found in Percival's *Medical Ethics* (1803, p. 22). The following passage from this work is repeated verbatim in the "Code of Medical Ethics" adopted by the American Medical Association [1847], 1977, p. 29):

> A physician should not be forward to make gloomy prognostications, because they savor of empiricism, by magnifying the importance of his services in the treatment or cure of the disease. But he should not fail, on proper occasions, to give to the friends of the patient, timely notice of danger, when it really occurs, and even to the patient himself, if absolutely necessary. This office however is so peculiarly alarming, when executed by him, that it ought to be declined whenever it can be assigned to any other person of sufficient judgment and delicacy. For the physician should be the minister of hope and comfort to the sick; that by such cordials to the drooping spirit, he may smooth the bed of death, revive expiring life, and counteract the depressing influence of those maladies.

Writing decades apart, both Cabot ([1803] 1979) and Fletcher (1954) criticized this view, arguing that, in spite of the good intentions, the position had bad consequences. It reduces the physicians' credibility, undermines trust, and insults patients by assuming that they are not capable of handling bad news about themselves. These effects can apply to children as well as adults. For adults, the position also holds that such an exercise of power and control by one private citizen over another steals something that belongs to the latter, namely, information that will affect how that person will conduct his or her life—and even has an untoward effect on the person who is not candid (Kant [1790], 1949; Beck, 1975; Veatch, 1976; Bok, 1978).

Research done about twenty years ago, when this paternalistic view was more frequently defended, showed that whereas physicians thought it was a good idea not to inform patients of sad news, most patients (80 percent or more) did want the information (Oken, 1961; Bok, 1978; Veatch, 1976). Some physicians objected that these surveys were unreliable, arguing that, although patients may *say* that they want to be told, they *really* do not. It is not difficult to imagine an example of this, but it is just as easy to imagine that, for one reason or another, the physician, in spite of what he or she *says*, does not *really* want to tell the patient. We are all subject to self-deception or rationalization. The difficulty with this view, then, is the assumption that the parties are on a different footing as persons who know their own minds (Beck, 1975; Kant [1790], 1949).

Investigators further suggested that, rather than make patients feel better, withholding or manipulating information had the opposite result, often isolating them from discussions, decisions, and support; giving free reign to destructive imaginings; and causing them to feel a loss of control over their lives (Kubler-Ross, 1967; Bok, 1978; Veatch, 1976).

These studies and candid discussions with adult patients changed prevailing attitudes and had an effect on pediatric care as well (Mnookin, 1978). Instead of treating adult patients like children, it appeared that older children could sometimes be treated more like adults. Still, a good case can occasionally be made for withholding information, for force, or even for deception. For example, were I a physician, I would not go out of my way to inform the father (or "father") of a child with sickle cell disease that he did not have sickle cell trait. Or, imagine situations where life or limb are at stake: a child will not take urgently needed medicine because it is nauseating and will cause loss of hair; a disfiguring operation is life-saving but the child does not want it; if no one can think of any methods to save a child other than by force, it might be justifiable to use it. Deception would rarely seem justified because of the lasting damage it would do to someone's ability to trust others. However, suppose a child is in urgent need of life-saving surgery; although in general, force is preferable to deception, either one would be better than allowing the child to die, especially as there would be time enough later to set things straight about why deception or force was used.

It is interesting that appeals have been made to likely utility, benefits, or harms (that is, to the principles of utility and beneficence) to try to justify very different policies—namely, routinely informing and also not informing (Sedgwick [1907], 1966; Percival [1803], 1977; American Medical Association [1847], 1977). This process shows a problem with the use of very general principles that seek to vindicate complex actions now by what will occur in the future. For in using the principles, we presuppose that we know well enough the likely consequences. Do we? Often this requires doing studies or appraising data in relation to scientific theories in order to explain and predict—as opposed to following the well-intentioned hunch that too often takes the place of studies. The results can surprise us. Studies indicate that routine withholding of information does not usually lead to good results. Furthermore, some of the important arguments favoring candor focus on liberties and not utility or beneficence. These arguments are used to stress the justice of giving information that affects how people will control their lives, information we would want for ourselves in similar circumstances. According to these arguments, we have a prima facie right to this information (Veatch, 1976; Engelhardt, 1975; Beck, 1975).

Informed Consent

During this century, legal decisions have increasingly supported the right of adults to certain information and the corresponding duty of physicians to inform them (*Natanson* v. *Kline,* 1960; Katz, 1978; Holder, 1976; *Canterbury* v. *Spence,* 1972). Examination of the law does not settle moral questions. For one thing, as we shall see, the law is rarely unambiguous. Even more important, if we ever want to say some laws are wrong, we must separately evaluate what is legal and moral. Although it attempts to recognize the importance of different values, current informed consent policy is not a model of clarity or consistency.

Consent, whether given for oneself or one's ward, has three necessary features: it must be given by someone who is competent, it must be given voluntarily, and it must be based on information a reasonable person would consider adequate (Katz, 1978; Holder, 1976; Curran, 1979; *Canterbury* v. *Spence,* 1972). Thus, consent policy as it relates to children almost always concerns obtaining consent from adults (Raitt, 1974–1975). In gaining consent, physicians have the obligation not only to provide enough information but also to do so in a way most people would find understandable. The goals of giving enough information and doing so in a comprehensible way can lead to somewhat different (although not mutually exclusive) professional behaviors. Those interested in getting the information across to most people may have to spend many sessions reviewing the same material. Those concerned principally about the legal implications may concentrate on what courts, colleagues, and lawyers would view as adequate information, especially on written consent forms. The latter tendency may account for why consent forms are all too often unnecessarily difficult to read or are viewed as protection for the hospital and/or physician rather than as information for the patient (Cassileth and others, 1980; Grundner, 1980).

In most cases, the third-party consent for therapy that guardians give for minors works well, for there is usually a consensus between the family and health professionals about the child's best interest. Difficulties arise when there are important and irresolvable disagreements among the staff, the parents, and/or the child (especially the older minor). Sometimes parents refuse to give consent for treatment the staff regards as essential. The refusal may be stated or may take the form of deliberate noncompliance. In other cases, parents seek to withdraw prescribed medication in favor of inadequate or discredited care (such as laetrile to treat cancer). If other means are exhausted to resolve such disputes, it may be appropriate for staff or others to bring in the courts as fact finder and decision maker. Although the law supports the right of competent adults to refuse treatment, even life-saving treatment, for themselves (Byrn, 1978), such a decision is not binding when giving third-party consent. In such a case, the staff may be obligated to challenge the guardian's decision. The Supreme Court has made this clear, for example, in cases involving children in great need of blood transfusions whose parents are Jehovah's Witnesses (*In re Simpson,* 1972). If the child is endangered, parental directives prohibiting essential therapy should not be followed automatically. A court can take temporary or even permanent custody of the child and grant consent as the child's guardian. Some courts have ordered nonvital care over a guardian's objection; others are reluctant to do so unless the child's life is in peril (Raitt, 1974–1975). Where the threat is real but distant (surgery should be done now, for in ten years the risk will be great), the courts are less inclined to overrule parents (Baker, 1969).

One source of the doctrine of informed consent is the *fiduciary relationship* between the professional and the client, which presumes that professionals, by the codes of their professions, are in a position of special trust to look out for the interests of their clients. This source invites a kind of paternalism. But a second source of the doctrine of informed consent does not. It is the principle that a person of sound mind has a right to determine what shall be done with his or her own body. This *right of self-determination* has been an important part of recent litigation on informed consent. Judge Schroeder, in *Natanson* v. *Kline* (1960, p. 1104), stressed that people do not lose their civil rights when they enter a medical setting: "Anglo-American law starts with the premise of thoroughgoing self-determination. It follows that each man is considered to be master of his own body, and he may, if he be found of sound mind, expressly prohibit the performance of life-saving surgery, or other medical treatment. A doctor may well believe that an operation or form of treatment is desirable or necessary but the law doesn't permit him to substitute his own judgment for that of the patient by any form of artifice or deception."

However, as if to show that the doctrine of informed consent is shaped by both the right of self-determination and reliance on professional trust, Judge Shroeder almost immediately modifies his strongly libertarian position: "The duty of the physician to disclose, however, is limited to those disclosures which a reasonable medical practitioner would make under the same or similar circumstances. . . . So long as the disclosure is sufficient to assure an informed consent, the physician's choice of plausible courses should not be called into question if it appears, all circumstances considered, that the physician was motivated only by the patient's best therapeutic interest and he proceeded as a competent medical man would have done in a similar situation" (p. 1106).

Different courts and states have given different weight to these two sources (Katz, 1978). Some states stress the fiduciary relationship and adopt a standard requiring the physician or professional to reveal what most would be inclined to reveal in similar situations. Excessive reliance on this as a standard, however, has been increasingly criticized and rejected by many courts that maintain it gives insufficient recognition to the right of self-determination (Holder, 1976; Katz, 1978). According to recent rulings, the right of persons to exercise free choice and take responsibility for decisions affecting their bodies shapes the boundaries of the disclosure rule. The *Canterbury* v. *Spence* court stressed the right of self-determination, adopting a standard that enough information must be provided to patients or their representatives to enable them to make an intelligent treatment choice based on their needs. Many others also hold that patients or their representatives, if circumstances permit, should be told in an understandable way about diagnoses, procedures, risks, prognosis with and without treatment, and alternative treatments, if any (Holder, 1976; American Hospital Association, 1978).

.   The right of self-determination, however, is modified even in *Canterbury* v. *Spence* (1972) where two exceptions are cited that reintroduce the importance of the fiduciary relationship. The first is in an emergency in which neither the patient nor the family is able to consent and "harm from a failure to treat is imminent and outweighs any harm threatened by the proposed treatment" (p. 788). The second is "when risk-disclosure poses such a threat of detriment to the patient as to become unfeasible or contraindicated from a medical point of view" (p. 789). Here, as in *Natanson* v. *Kline*, the libertarian tone is tempered.

These two different sources of the doctrine of informed consent acknowledge each of the three moral principles of justice, utility, and benevolence. The doctrine recognizes liberties—for competent persons, giving enforcement of the right to privacy and self-determination and autonomy in framing the informed consent doctrine. This acknowledges the importance of the moral principle of justice. Also, the doctrine recognizes the need to protect: In acknowledging the prudence of relying on professionals to act in the best interests of their clients, it also recognizes the importance of the principles of utility and beneficence. For patients not competent to decide for themselves, choices about them are to be made by the family with the advice of physicians about the patient's prognosis and best interests (*In re Quinlan*, 1976). In this case, the fiduciary relationship can offer special protection to minors because the primary obligation of the professional is to the incompetent patient, not the guardian. Physicians and others are obligated to seek court action if the child is endangered. These same three precepts have had at least as obvious a role in shaping policy about research involving children as they did about consent doctrine.

Research Involving Children

It is not unusual to exhaust standard therapies in the care of patients with chronic and catastrophic illness, and experimental therapies may then be used to try to stay ahead of the ravages of the illness. Therapeutic research combines therapy and gaining new information. The primary goal, however, should be to provide each patient with the best available care; gaining new information should be a secondary goal. The "Declaration of Helsinki" states this forcefully: "The doctor can combine medical research with professional care, the object being the acquisition of new medical knowledge only to the extent that medical research is justified by its potential diagnostic or therapeutic value for the patient" (World Medical Association, 1978, p. 407).

Of course, one would want children to get the therapy they need, even if they are unable to give consent for it. Therapy as such is intended to benefit, so it fits the paternalistic role to have guardians seek it and consent for them. Third-party consent for therapy and for therapeutic studies, then, is not considered problematic. Consent for therapeutic research is also noncontroversial if the information is collected and used in a way that maintains confidentiality and respect.

What is controversial is whether, or when, third-party consent is appropriate for nontherapeutic research involving children. The primary goal of such studies is to gain new information, not to provide direct therapeutic benefit to the patient. It may be, of course, that a nontherapeutic study could generate information that might eventually benefit those studied. Unknown future benefits, however, do not transform research into therapy. The controversy is not about whether such research is important. It centers on the propriety of using persons for studies without their consent if there is no direct benefit to them.

Some have argued for forbidding nontherapeutic research on subjects who cannot consent for themselves (Jonas, 1970; Ramsey, 1970). If this policy were adopted, then children, retarded persons, and many people who are mentally ill could not be subjects in any research study that did not have therapeutic or diagnostic goals. Those who defend this view hold that enough progress could be made using consenting adults and animal models or in conjunction with needed diagnostic or therapeutic procedures. According to this position, people used in nontherapeutic studies without their consent are abused, even if they are not otherwise harmed (Ramsey, 1970; Jonas, 1970).

The position that children and others who do not give consent should never be subjects in nontherapeutic studies might seem humane and reasonable. For it seems to advocate not exploiting those who are unable to give consent. Although well intentioned, this view fails on several counts. Not all nontherapeutic studies on subjects who do not consent for themselves necessarily involve rights violations. Many important studies that are virtually without physical or psychosocial risk do not seem to violate their subjects' rights or dignity. For example, in order to understand the extent of a three-year-old's motor handicap, it is necessary to compare that child's performance to what most three-year-olds do. Thus, it is necessary to find out how quickly most three-year-olds can do certain tasks, such as stacking blocks. But for all but one of these children, who are not patients in need of diagnosis or therapy, this is a nontherapeutic research project. One could not call stacking blocks therapeutic just because the three-year-olds had a good time. To forbid this important kind of low-risk study on the grounds that the three-year-olds are being exploited because someone observes how they stack blocks seems counterproductive.

Many nontherapeutic studies involve little or no risk to the subject and are extremely important in gaining new information. These include techniques that can sometimes be used without being risky, such as follow-up or retrospective studies, questionnaires, testing of perceptual discrimination, analysis of growth and development data obtained during routine examination, or observational studies. A ban on all nontherapeutic studies involving dependent subjects would mean abandoning even such safe, noninvasive studies.

Moreover, defenders of this position may fail to appreciate the medical uniqueness of persons of different ages or conditions. For example, premature infants are functionally different from older children and adults. They suffer from different diseases and react to drugs, immunization, and therapy differently. Two well-known tragic examples concern the uses of the antibiotics sulfisoxazole (gantrisin) and chloramphenicol (chloromycetin), which are effective in treating older persons but resulted in illness and deaths when they were inappropriately administered to premature infants. Thus, there is a limit to what can be inferred from studies done on other groups. Studies should, of course, be done first on animals and then on adults if possible.

In short, although doing research is an ethical issue, not doing research is one as well. Not supporting research for minors' catastrophic and chronic illnesses would be paramount to denying advances in care for them. But some of these studies would have components that are nontherapeutic—for example, those studies conducted in order to establish norms.

The charge that children would be denied the benefits of improved therapy if nontherapeutic research on children were halted is supported by consideration of the number of drugs available to children as a consequence of restrictions on drug usage adopted by the Food and Drug Administration (FDA) since 1962. The Kefauver-Harris Law (a response to the thalidomide tragedy) requires labels on drugs identifying safe dosage for all groups on which they are being used. Such labeling requires research, testing, and evaluation of drugs before their release for general therapeutic use. Currently 75 percent of all therapeutic agents are not FDA approved for children because insufficient evidence is available about their efficacy and safety (American Academy of Pediatrics, 1974). As a result, children are either denied the opportunity to have such drugs in their treatment or the drugs must be used on them without adequate testing. Moreover, as older drugs and procedures become discredited and fewer can be used to replace them, Shirkey's argument that children are becoming "therapeutic orphans" seems more compelling (Shirkey, 1972).

If utility justifies some nontherapeutic studies with children as subjects, then which studies should be permitted? It hardly seems just to do the same studies on children as on adults, for adults can assess risks or benefits and decide for themselves. Besides, it is not at all clear that guardians have the right to volunteer dependents under their care for procedures that not only do not benefit them but also may be risky. The guardians' role is to protect their dependents— to act in their interest, and to safeguard their well-being. It violates that role to intentionally volunteer a dependent person for a procedure involving risk when there is no prospect of compensatory benefit. Important ends such as the goals of scientific advance and improving therapy for other members of the community do not justify such means to achieve those ends. One is not justified in jeopardizing another, even for a good cause. Utility could also cause further harm by having a brutalizing effect upon a society that would condone using helpless individuals in situations involving risk. Volunteering others for procedures involving risks, then, sets a dangerous precedent and violates the guardian's protective role (Kopelman, 1978b).

A more defensible position is to allow nontherapeutic research if there is appropriate third-party consent and if a competent Institutional Review Board

(IRB) judges that the physical and psychosocial risk is minimal (Kopelman, 1981). This is the position generally taken in the federal regulations (U.S. Department of Health and Human Services, 1981, 1983; U.S. Department of Health, Education, and Welfare, 1978). Strictly speaking, these regulations apply only to studies seeking funds from the federal government. However, they have had an important role in setting general standards for acceptable research on subjects and in confirming the importance of some nontherapeutic studies. This position does so by restricting nontherapeutic research on children to that which is virtually without risk to them.

The federal guidelines propose additional safeguards for children (U.S. Department of Health and Human Services, 1983). The guidelines recommend adequate attention to the worthiness of the study, to its scientific soundness and significance, to preceding the study by appropriate animal studies. Risks should be minimized and adequate provision made for confidentiality and fairness in the selection of subjects. Therapeutic studies involving more than minimal risk are justified by their probable direct benefit to the child. Some provision is made to allow IRB approval of some studies that do not hold out direct benefit to the child and have a minor increase over minimal risk. What constitutes a minor increase over minimal risk remains unclarified; it seems to fall into an area the Office for Protection from Research Risks refers to as "judgment calls" by IRBs.

The Department of Health and Human Services has exempted some studies on adults from consent requirements (U.S. Department of Health and Human Services, 1981; Kopelman, 1981) and exempts some research involving children under similar conditions. These are studies that, in the opinion of the IRB, do not present risk or confidentiality problems and would include certain surveys, observational research, or research designed to study large-scale social, economic, or health service trends.

Thus, several distinct categories emerge:

1. Research that is exempt from the Department of Health and Human Services requirements, including research related to normal educational practices, observation of public behavior, educational testing, and collection or study of existing data.
2. Research not involving greater than minimal risk (46.404).
3. Research involving greater than a minimal risk but presenting the prospect of direct benefit to the individual subjects (46.405).

The following two categories are controversial (McCartney, 1978). They were included out of the sincere belief that some such research would be rational and justifiable, and that enough safeguards exist to keep them from being misused:

4. Research involving minor increase over minimal risk and holding out no prospect of direct benefit to individual subjects may be approved by an IRB if it is likely to yield generalizable knowledge. Adequate provisions for the child's assent and the parent's or guardian's permission is made (46.406).
5. Research not otherwise approvable by the IRB but that presents an oppor-

tunity to understand, prevent, or alleviate a serious problem affecting the health or welfare of children. In this case the secretary, in consultation with a panel of experts, may approve the study. Adequate provisions for the child's assent and the parent's or guardian's permission are made.

Consequently, assessment of risk is a necessary step for the IRB when determining whether research should be permitted. Most of us would agree that, except in extraordinary circumstances, it is unethical to do risky studies with children as subjects unless the studies or the risky component of studies can be justified as diagnostically or therapeutically beneficial to them. Their vulnerability and inability to consent places special responsibilities on us to protect them. Most now agree it is justifiable to approve some nontherapeutic studies with acceptably low risks. But the consensus over this position is chimerical if there is not also substantial agreement about how to assess risks. The category of minimal risk, therefore, could become the new procrustean bed of research involving children.

The key issue, then, is where to draw the line between risks that are and are not acceptably low. The U.S. Department of Health and Human Services (1981, 46.102[g]) has adopted a general definition of *minimal risk* that is in use as a standard: "'Minimal risk' means that the risks or harm anticipated in the proposed research are not greater, considering probability and magnitude, than those ordinarily encountered in daily life or during performance of routine physical or psychological examinations or tests."

Although it is important to offer such a standard, this definition is troublesome (Kopelman, 1981). First, studies can be risky because they violate confidentiality, create self-fulfilling prophesies, or cause anxiety. This definition fails to adequately address problems of such psychosocial risks. After all, a great deal of confidential information can come to light in routine physical or psychological examinations. Second, it presupposes what is by no means obvious, that we know what the risks in daily life are, both in their probability and magnitude. The risks all or some of us encounter are not only difficult to ascertain but may not be minimal at all. The ordinary risks of daily life, then, are a poor base from which to judge whether or not there is a low enough risk to justify studies on special nonconsenting groups.

The second part of the definition, however, is helpful for judging what is or is not physically risky. It offers a relatively well-defined basis for judging whether the physical risk is of a kind that is too great to be called minimal. One need only ask, is this the kind of thing done in a routine examination? Still, by this definition, a project with a low physical risk but a high psychosocial risk (such as the XYY screening of infants) could be argued to have minimal risk. That study was discontinued, however, on the grounds that the psychosocial risks were inappropriately high (Kopelman, 1978a).

After seeing the inadequacies of this definition of minimal risk, it should not come as a surprise that there is great difference in how different IRBs assess risk. A survey by Janofsky and Starfield (1981) of pediatric department chairmen and pediatric clinical research center directors found considerable differences on estimates about whether some procedures, such as arterial puncture and gastric and intestinal intubation, had less than minimal risk, minor increase over minimal risk, or a more-than-minor increase over minimal risk.

The standard for judging risk and the definition of minimal risk, thus, could be improved. This might be accomplished by identifying the considerations, all things being equal, that need to be applied fairly and impartially by a conscientious IRB; for example, if with adequate information, they judge that (1) the kind of physical harm or risk, both in its probability and magnitude, is no greater than ought reasonably to be expected in a routine physical examination of a healthy individual and (2) the study would not reasonably be expected to cause harm from overtesting (minor annoyance when repeated can be unkind, painful, or terrifying), inconvenience, invasion of privacy, stigmatization, loss of self-esteem, labeling, or other psychosocial problems. Furthermore, disagreement within the IRB over approval of a study, and the reason for that disagreement, should be recorded permanently and made available for review, especially to prospective subjects or their guardians (Kopelman, 1981).

Some disagreements over risk assessment and whether certain tests are indicated diagnostically are common. The final decisions usually fall to the IRB. In practical terms, the board's conscientious action may offer more protection to most minors than the guardian's well-intentioned consent.

Reconciling Theory and Practice

The courts have affirmed repeatedly that the primary decision maker, acting with information and advice from the physician, is the competent patient and, if the patient is incompetent, the patient's representative (*In re Quinlan,* 1976; Katz, 1978; Glantz and Swazey, 1979). The guidelines on research maintain this as well. This is the theory; practice is another matter. Privately, physicians and physician-investigators admit they think they could get most people to agree to almost anything.

Consider some difficulties of legally competent adults. How can staff determine whether patients who are very ill, perhaps heavily medicated or even on a ventilator, are adequately informed or competent to make a momentous decision? Even if patients are informed and express strong preferences, it is sometimes difficult to know how to interpret them. Despair, pain, depression, anxiety, fear, and misconception distort the judgment of otherwise competent persons. It seems wrong simply to abandon people to what most of us view as a bad choice because it is their right to decide (Jackson and Younger, 1979; Engelhardt, 1975). A compassionate and caring staff may try to reach and convince them that another decision is better. One might argue that this is paternalism, for it is an unwarranted interference with adults who are not legally incompetent. What is troubling about this argument, however, is that it fails to appreciate that autonomy is not any particular behavior but rather responsible or purposeful choices that express one's nature. For some, the desire to be uninformed, to escape important choices, or to make decisions most of us regard as tragic may express their nature. If so, these choices deserve to be respected. However, when we believe a "bad" choice is the expression of situational fear, anxiety, depression, pain, or misconception, then we suspect that the choice is not autonomous. (This condition is captured by such common expressions as "She is not herself today" or "It is not like him to do that.") In such circumstances, the staff's so-called paternalistic actions can make autonomy possible for these people.

After the patient, the patient's representative, which is typically the family, is the primary decision maker. Theory aside again, some families cannot or will not exercise such responsibility. Some show by their actions that they want to escape the choice, and they withdraw physically or psychologically. It is not uncommon for patients or families to seek to transfer responsibility, using such expressions as "I'm in your hands" or "Do what you would do for a member of your own family." If we focus on this sort of example, it is easy to become cynical about informing and consent.

Some physicians are willing to accept responsibility for decision making. Others take the time and trouble to encourage those reluctant to exercise responsibility to do so. Good results have been reported by some who encourage patients or families to understand what is at stake and to decide for themselves. For example, Imbus and Zawacki (1977, p. 308) seek to preserve autonomy for patients so severely burned that they are not expected to survive. During the first few hours of hospitalization consent for therapy is sought: "While still lucid, and with sufficient information, the patient is asked if he wishes to choose between a full therapeutic regime or ordinary care, reassured that with either choice, the burn team will provide the constant presence of human caring and full use of its professional skills. This approach has not changed the mortality rate of such patients, but has increased both the self-determination that they exercise and the empathy that they receive."

Duff and Campbell (1973) also report success in including parents of infants with severe birth defects in decisions to terminate or continue treatment. They reject arguments that these parents are too upset to understand. They state that parents can act responsibly but they need the support and understanding of the hospital personnel. Subsequent studies support this (Benfield, Leib, and Vollman, 1978). They argue that the entire staff and family should discuss the situation, and they even urge including someone such as a minister, who might be of special help to the family. Duff and Campbell argue for adoption of a social policy flexible enough to allow some tolerance of different choices made by different persons in rather similar circumstances.

There is a serious objection to the view that, in practice, the patient or the patient's family should be the primary decision maker. Even if we agree these are not purely medical decisions, they normally require knowledge of the prognosis and treatment options. Such information is often complicated and presented at a time the patient and family are upset, so patients or families are likely to be swayed by the way the situation is described, what information is presented, and how it is presented. One can wonder, for example, how Imbus and Zawacki conveyed the suffering of the severely burned person when they gave "sufficient information." The physician, or whoever informs, cannot be entirely free from the attitudes he or she brings to the informing sessions. Thus, the argument continues, it is better to acknowledge that consent from patients and families is usually a subterfuge. Either they respond automatically, "Do what you think best" or "Do what you can," or they are unduly swayed by the professional staff's judgment. Therefore, they say, it is better not to deceive ourselves and simply to acknowledge that the burden of the decision is going to fall on the professional staff. It is all very well to talk about patient rights and justice in the medical setting, but the best and most useful policy is for professionals to recognize that they are largely in charge.

The extreme version of this view is that physicians, by virtue of their knowledge, know what is best for patients; thus, they ought to disclose only the information they judge to be beneficial. This extreme view is easy to dispose of. First, knowledgeable physicians certainly disagree, so there is uncertainty about what is best for some patients. Second, it presumes that physicians always know what is best for patients, and that is not so. Third, people have special beliefs, ways of living, or ways of evaluating ends and goals that are different. Physicians, who are after all private citizens, cannot restrict the liberties of other citizens just because it seems best to them. Moreover, many of these decisions, although made in a medical setting and with medical consequences, are moral or religious choices. Physicians can claim expertise only in the medical aspects of the decisions (Veatch, 1976).

The less extreme version of this view is that physicians and other professionals really make the decision, whether they want to or not, because they control the information. What they choose to say or stress, and their preferences or biases, generally determine what patients or their families will do. This objection points up the importance of revealing differences of opinion between the professionals to the decision maker. The law also stresses this (Holder, 1976; Katz, 1978). But the objection may mean that, because such choices are affected by the information given, patients or families never really choose. If so, it is mistaken. First, sometimes they do disagree and seek consultations, switch physicians, and so on. Second, and more generally, all of our choices are influenced by the information we receive. (Indeed, one way of intentionally manipulating or restricting the liberty of another is to control the information received.) To single out one group—patients—for special treatment because of what is generally true is unfair and assumes they are on a different level of freedom and responsibility. Moreover, professionals are also patients or families of patients. So, the manner in which they treat others helps create the policy for how they will be treated. If each of us would want to be consulted about ourselves or our family then we ought to extend this right of self-determination to others. This willingness to treat others the way we want to be treated is a necessary feature of morally justified judgments. It shows the social dimension of these judgments. The moral point of view has, as its ideal, judgments based on adequate information, impartiality of application, and the use of reasons that have been stated and defended.

It seems ironic that the health care team, sometimes (justly) criticized by the patients' rights movement for paternalism and encouragement of dependence, is also typically necessary for patient-family autonomy in important medical decisions. As a rule, if the condition is serious, then unless the professionals are prepared to be very supportive when informing patients or families, they will probably have no genuine role in the decisions. Being adequately informed has two components: provision of enough information to the patient or family and comprehension of that information by the patient or family. Many times they will be too troubled to hear the information when they are initially informed. The physician or others determined to inform a family facing a serious chronic or life-threatening illness may have to spend a lot of time with them. Yet, one could fulfill one's legal obligations to them simply by providing sufficient information in a way that a reasonable person would understand (Curran, 1979; *Canterbury* v. *Spence*, 1972), and a signed consent form is some legal protection for the staff. But the staff who goes through complex or upsetting material repeatedly until the family understands it, goes beyond legal obligations; by acting beyond what is required of them, they may make autonomy a possibility for many patients or families.

Conclusion

This review of some moral and legal policies affecting children with chronic or catastrophic illness has been related to three fundamental moral precepts. For in addition to considering particular experiences, it is also important to think of our actions and policies in terms of general principles. As Hare (1972-1973, pp. 7-8) has written, "We learn from experience, in morality as in other matters; and we also learn by precept. The two kinds of learning are not so different in practice as might be supposed; for the precepts very often relate to experiences, and the point of the experiences is that they lead to the adoption of certain precepts. Learning from experience is not just empirical observation; it is the adoption of precepts or principles as a result of our reflection on what has happened to us."

Let us briefly consider the role of the three moral principles of justice, utility, and beneficence in this discussion about autonomy and paternalism. One strength of using justice and rights to guide actions is to set limits. Defining a base that is not ordinarily negotiable by conditions of expediency or of what others perceive as kindness is an important social safeguard. Liberties and entitlements state what is or ought to be the minimum for just treatment of persons in a society. For example, Massachusetts and California have passed laws enforcing the legal right of females with stage 1 breast cancer to be informed of treatment options and the corresponding obligations of physicians to inform them that there are choices (Curran, 1979). Apparently, such a specific law about rights to know and decide seemed necessary because too few physicians told women about these treatment options or refused to separate initial screening from subsequent surgery. Clarifying patients' or subjects' rights correlatively clarifies the obligations of the professionals. It defines their basic responsibilities and what counts as discharging them in an imperfect world.

Consideration of justice alone, although important in clarifying rights and duties, seems inadequate to illuminate fully the nature of compassion, caring, or beneficence. A principle of justice may show why some are entitled to certain rights but not why we ought to help our fellow human beings or why we should do good rather than harm. It fails to account for why, for example, staff who have fulfilled all specific legal requirements believe they ought to take more time to inform or to support a family after the death of a patient (Duff and Campbell, 1973). Yet beneficence unrestrained by what can be offered to all as a matter of justice can foster wishful thinking and false hopes. Moreover, it can give insufficient recognition to the requirements of fair and respectful treatment of persons. The importance of these principles and the tensions between them are apparent in informing and consent policies in the law where the right to self-determination and the fiduciary relationship are both stressed.

Concerning the ranking of these three principles, Frankena (1963, p. 37) writes:

> Now, I wish to contend, as has already been suggested, that we not have any moral obligations, prima facie or actual, to do anything which does not, directly or indirectly, have some connection with what makes someone's life good or bad, better or worse. If not our particular actions, then at least our rules must have some bearing on the increase of good or the decrease of evil. Morality was made for man, not man for morality. Even justice is concerned about the distribution *of good and evil*. In other words, all our duties, even that of justice, *presuppose* the principle of benevolence, though they do not all *follow from* it. To this extent, and only to this extent, is the old dictum that love is what underlines and unifies the rules of morality correct. It is the failure to recognize the importance of the principle of benevolence that makes so many deontological systems unsatisfactory.

Frankena's general comments seem especially relevant when considering how to exercise enough paternalism for children while encouraging their autonomy. The policies we adopt should presuppose kindness and love, but it does not follow that kindness and love alone will get us to the best policies.

Of course, not everyone agrees with Frankena about how to rank these principles. But serious and sustained disagreements in policy between informed persons of good will can often be traced to different assessments of either the relative importance or the nature of the application of one of these principles. An example is the controversy over research involving children. Employing the principle of utility, different positions result from different views about the likely effects. In one view, many stress the need to do research in order to advance knowledge and keep children from becoming "therapeutic orphans" (Shirkey,

1972). In another view and using the same principle, others argue it would have a damaging effect on children and society to *use* them in this way. There are also controversies about how to apply the principle of justice; there is some disagree-ment, for example, about whether doing nontherapeutic research on children violates their rights. These principles are so general that they can be used to generate different positions (Hare, 1972–1973). The upshot is that sorting out what policies are useful requires data and principles. We did conclude that arguments using the principle of justice to disallow all nontherapeutic research on children were unconvincing. Rather, it was argued that children's rights could be protected and important studies could continue if carefully restricted. Criti-cism of the Department of Health and Human Services' definition and use of "minimal risk" was stated and an alternative standard offered.

Truthfulness was also discussed in relation to these principles and the need for further studies. In contrast to a position that was influential for many decades, the practice of being as candid as possible seems justified for children as well as adults. Although it had been presumed that (paternalistically) withholding bad news was a useful and kindly policy, studies have suggested otherwise. This earlier but mistaken assumption that deception was comforting once again reveals a difficulty with using general principles such as those of utility and beneficence: They can rely on predictions of future events to justify complex actions, and these predictions may not be reliable. It was argued that a more justifiable policy in terms of recent studies and of the three principles of justice, utility, and beneficence is, whenever possible, to be candid with and include persons of any age in decisions that affect their lives. Because of the develop-mental and intellectual differences in minors, the procedure for implementa-tion of such a policy cannot be stated as unequivocally for children as for adults. Still its benefit could be in gaining predisposition to or a perspective that favors autonomy and including, rather than excluding, children.

This discussion has focused on policies regarding children who are under care. But many children are doubly unlucky in that they need medical care and do not get it. Children with catastrophic and chronic illnesses have special needs that are important, often apparent, and too frequently unmet. Where they could be met but are not, the result can be a further restriction of opportunities and happiness in their lives. Still, no society has unlimited resources, so the problem is how to relate the special needs of these children to what is owed to them in a just society with its own certain resources, technology, and heritage (Peffer, 1978; Daniels, 1981). Although it would seem reasonable to provide at least as much funding for children's programs as for adults', because children have a lifetime of benefit ahead of them, too often it is their programs that get the least funding.

The principles of justice, utility, and beneficence suggest the same policy as moral, given the resources, in allocation of sufficient funds for study and prevention of and screening for catastrophic and chronic childhood illness. In the long run, such policy has generally been shown to be cost-effective, contributing to the well-being of individuals and society by increasing the opportunities for development of individual potential. As the chronically ill are people with rights as well as special needs, the policy acknowledges their right to equality of consideration. When kindness, utility, and fairness suggest the *same* policy, as they do here, the justification for action seems complete.

References

American Academy of Pediatrics. "General Guidelines for the Evaluation of Drugs to Be Approved for Use During Pregnancy and Treatment of Infants and Children." A Report of the Committee on Drugs, American Academy of Pediatrics, to the Food and Drug Administration, U.S. Department of Health, Education, and Welfare, July 1974.

American Hospital Association. "Statement on a Patient's Bill of Rights." In T. L. Beauchamp and L. Walters (Eds.), *Contemporary Issues in Bioethics.* Belmont, Calif.: Dickensen, 1978.

American Medical Association. "Code of Medical Ethics." (Adopted May 1847). In S. R. Reiser, A. J. Dyck, and W. J. Curran (Eds.), *Ethics in Medicine: Historical Perspectives and Contemporary Concerns.* Cambridge, Mass.: M.I.T. Press, 1977.

Baker, J. A. "Court Ordered Non-Emergency Medical Care for Infants." *Cleveland-Marshall Law Review,* 1969, *18*(2), 296–307.

Beck, L. W. *The Actor and the Spectator.* New Haven, Conn.: Yale University Press, 1975.

Benfield, D. G., Leib, S. A., and Vollman, J. H. "Grief Response of Parents to Neonatal Death and Parent Participation in Deciding Care." *Pediatrics,* 1978, *62*(2), 171–177.

Bok, S. O. *Lying: Moral Choice in Public and Private Life.* New York: Pantheon Books, 1978.

Byrn, R. M. "Compulsory Lifesaving Treatment for the Competent Adult." In T. L. Beauchamp and L. Walters (Eds.), *Contemporary Issues in Bioethics.* Belmont, Calif.: Dickensen, 1978.

Cabot, R. C. "The Use of Truth and Falsehood in Medicine." In S. R. Reiser, A. J. Dyck, and W. J. Curran (Eds.), *Ethics in Medicine: Historical Perspectives and Contemporary Concerns.* Cambridge, Mass.: M.I.T. Press, 1977. (Originally published 1903.)

Canterbury v. *Spence.* 464 F.2d 772, 791 (D.C. Cir., 1972) (conclusion only). In T. L. Beauchamp and L. Walters (Eds.), *Contemporary Issues in Bioethics.* Belmont, Calif.: Dickensen, 1978.

Cassileth, B. R., and others. "Informed Consent—Why Are Its Goals Imperfectly Realized?" *New England Journal of Medicine,* 1980, *32*, 896–900.

Chisholm, R. M., and Feehan, T. D. "The Intent to Deceive." *Journal of Philosophy,* March 1977, *74*, 143–159.

Curran, W. J. "Informed Consent, Texas Style: Disclosure and Nondisclosure by Regulation." *New England Journal of Medicine,* 1979, *300*(9), 482–483.

Daniels, N. "Health-Care Needs and Distributive Justice." *Philosophy and Public Affairs,* 1981, *10*(2), 146–179.

Donagan, A. *The Theory of Morality.* Chicago, Ill.: University of Chicago Press, 1977.

Duff, R. S., and Campbell, A.G.M. "Moral and Ethical Dilemmas in the Special-Care Nursery." *New England Journal of Medicine,* 1973, *289,* 890–894.

Dworkin, G. "Paternalism." In R. A. Wasserstrom (Ed.), *Morality and the Law.* Belmont, Calif.: Dickensen, 1971.

Dworkin, R. "Liberalism." In S. Hampshire (Ed.), *Public and Private Morality.* New York: Cambridge University Press, 1979.

Engelhardt, H. T., Jr. "A Demand to Die." *Hastings Report,* 1975, *5,* 9–10.

Fletcher, J. *Morals and Medicine.* Boston: Beacon Press, 1954.

Frankena, W. *Ethics.* Engelwood Cliffs, N.J.: Prentice-Hall, 1963.

Glantz, L.H.G., and Swazey, J. B. "Decisions Not to Treat: The Saikewicz Case and Its Aftermath." *Forum on Medicine,* 1979, *2,* 22–32.

Grundner, T. M. "On the Readability of Surgical Consent Forms." *New England Journal of Medicine,* 1980, *302,* 900–902.

Gutmann, A. "Children, Paternalism, and Education." *Philosophy and Public Affairs,* 1981, *10*(1), 27–46.

Hare, R. N. "Principles." *Proceedings of the Aristotelean Society,* 1972–1973, *73,* 1–18.

Hofmann, A. D., and Pilpel, J. D. "The Legal Rights of Minors." *Pediatric Clinics of North America,* 1974, *20,* 989–1004.

Holder, A. "Informed Consent." *Journal of the American Medical Association,* 1976, *214,* 1181–1182.

Imbus, S. H., and Zawacki, B. E. "Autonomy for Burn Patients When Survival Is Unprecedented." *New England Journal of Medicine,* 1977, *297,* 308–334.

In re Quinlan, New Jersey Supreme Court, 70 N.J. 10, 355 A.2d 647, 1976.

In re Simpson, 278, N.E. 2d 918, 328 N.Y./S. 2d 686, 1972.

Jackson, D. L., and Younger, S. "Patient Autonomy and 'Death with Dignity.'" *New England Journal of Medicine,* 1979, *301*(8), 404–408.

Janofsky, B. A., and Starfield, B. "Assessment of Risk in Research on Children." *Journal of Pediatrics,* 1981, *98*(5), 842–846.

Jonas, H. "Philosophical Reflections on Experimentation with Human Subjects." In P. A. Freud (Ed.), *Experimentation with Human Subjects.* New York: George Braziller, 1970.

Kalin, J. "Lies, Secrets, and Love: The Inadequacy of Contemporary Moral Philosophy." *Journal of Value Inquiry,* 1976, *10,* 253–265.

Kant, I. "On the Supposed Right to Lie from Altruistic Motives." In L. W. Beck (Ed. and trans.), *Critique of Practical Reason.* Chicago: University of Chicago Press, 1949. (Originally published 1790.)

Katz, J. "Informed Consent in Therapeutic Relationships: Legal and Ethical Aspects." In W. T. Reich (Ed. in Chief), *Encyclopedia of Bioethics,* Vol. 2. New York: Free Press, 1978.

Kopelman, L. "Ethical Controversies in Medical Research: The Case of XYY Screening." *Perspectives in Biology and Medicine,* 1978a, *21*(1), 196–204.

Kopelman, L. "On the Use of Children and Retarded Persons as Subjects in Non-Therapeutic Research." In L. Kopelman and F. G. Coisman (Eds.), *The Rights of Children and Retarded Persons*. Rochester, N.Y.: Rock Printing Company, 1978b.

Kopelman, L. "Estimating Risk in Human Research." *Clinical Research*, 1981, *29* (1), 1–8.

Kubler-Ross, E. *On Death and Dying*. New York: Macmillan, 1967.

Locke, J. *Treatise of Civil Government*. (C. L. Sherman, Ed.) New York: Appleton-Century-Crofts, 1937. (Originally published 1690.)

McCartney, J. J. "Research on Children: National Commission Says 'Yes, If . . . '" *Hastings Report*, 1978, *8* (5), 26–31.

Mattsson, A. "Long-Term Physical Illness in Childhood: A Challenge to Psychosocial Adaptation." *Pediatrics*, 1972, *50*, 801–811.

Mnookin, R. H. "Children's Rights: Legal and Ethical Dilemmas." *Pharos*, 1978, *41*, 2–7.

Morano, D. V. "Truth as a Moral Category." *Journal of Value Inquiry*, 1975, *9*, 243–259.

Murphy, J. G. "Rights and Borderline Cases." In L. Kopelman and F. G. Coisman (Eds.), *The Rights of Children and Retarded Persons*. Rochester, N.Y.: Rock Printing Company, 1978. (Also in *Arizona Law Review*, 1978, *19*.)

Natanson v. *Kline*, 186 Kansas 393, 350 P. 2d 1092 (1960). 187 Kansas 186. 354 P. 2d 670 (1960).

Oken, D. "What to Tell Cancer Patients: A Study of Medical Attitudes." *Journal of the American Medical Association*, 1961, *175*, 1120–1128.

Paul, E. W. "Legal Rights of Minors to Sex-Related Medical Care." *Columbia Human Rights Law Review*, 1974–1975, *6*, 357–377.

Peffer, R. "A Defense of Rights to Well-Being." *Philosophy and Public Affairs*, 1978, *8* (1), 65–87.

Percival, T. *Medical Ethics*. In S. R. Reiser, A. J. Dyck, and W. J. Curran (Eds.), *Ethics in Medicine: Historical Perspectives and Contemporary Concerns*. Cambridge, Mass.: M.I.T. Press, 1977. (Originally published 1803.)

Pilpel, H. F. "Teenage Patients." *Medical World News*, 1971, *12* (19), 48–57.

Pilpel, H. F. "Minors' Rights to Medical Care." *Albany Law Review*, 1972, *36*, 462–487.

Planned Parenthood of Central Missouri v. *Danforth*, 428 U.S. 52 (1976).

Raitt, G. E., Jr. "The Minor's Right to Consent to Medical Treatment: A Corollary of the Constitutional Right to Privacy." *Southern California Law Review*, 1974–1975, *48*, 1417–1456.

Ramsey, P. *The Patient as Person*. New Haven, Conn.: Yale University Press, 1970.

Rawls, J. *A Theory of Justice*. Cambridge, Mass.: Harvard University Press, 1971.

Rodham, H. "Children under the Law." In *The Rights of Children, Harvard Educational Review*, 1974, *9*, 1–28.

Rothman, D. J., and Rothman, S. M. "The Conflict Over Children's Rights." *Hastings Report*, 1980, *10* (3), 7–10.

Schwartz, A. H. "Children's Concept of Research Hospitalization." *New England Journal of Medicine,* 1972, *287* (12), 589-592.

Sedgwick, H. *The Methods of Ethics.* New York: Dover, 1966. (Originally published 1907.)

Shirkey, H. C. "Therapeutic Orphans—Who Speaks for Children?" In H. C. Shirkey (Ed.), *Pediatric Therapy.* (4th ed.) St. Louis, Mo.: Mosby, 1972.

Turk, J. "Impact of Cystic Fibrosis on Family Functioning." *Pediatrics,* 1964, *34,* 67-71.

U.S. Department of Health and Human Services, Office of the Secretary. "Final Regulations Amending HHS Policy for the Protection of Human Research Subjects." Public Law 45, CFR 46, *Federal Register,* 1981, *46* (16), 8366-8392.

U.S. Department of Health and Human Services, Office of the Secretary. "Additional Protection for Children Involved as Subjects in Research." Public Law 45, CFR 46, *Federal Register,* 1983, *48* (46), 9814-9820.

U.S. Department of Health, Education, and Welfare, Office of the Secretary. "Report and Recommendations of the National Commission for the Protection of Human Subjects: Research Involving Children." *Federal Register,* 1978, *43* (9), 2085-2114.

Veatch, R. M. *Death, Dying, and the Biological Revolution.* New Haven, Conn.: Yale University Press, 1976.

World Medical Association. "Declaration of Helsinki, 1964." (Rev. ed.) In T. L. Beauchamp and L. Walters (Eds.), *Contemporary Issues in Bioethics.* Belmont, Calif.: Dickensen, 1978.

Worsfold, V. L. "A Philosophical Justification of Children's Rights." *The Rights of Children, Harvard Educational Review,* 1974, 29-40.

Wright, B. A. "Atypical Physique and the Appraisal of Persons." *Connecticut Medicine,* 1979, *43,* 19-24.

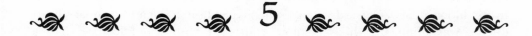

5

Genetic Strategies
for Preventing Chronic Illnesses

Neil A. Holtzman, M.D., M.P.H.
Julius B. Richmond, M.D.

The prospect for preventing many chronic diseases of children, or the disabilities resulting from them, is much greater today than even ten years ago. In contrast to earlier periods, new discoveries have been rapidly communicated to the public, increasing expectations of further progress and benefits, on the one hand, and fear of misuse, on the other. Nowhere has this occurred more rapidly than in genetics. During the last thirty years the molecular basis of inheritance and the genetic origin of many diseases have been discovered. Innovative diagnostic and therapeutic techniques followed. Mutation, the basis of inherited disease, has been incriminated in the pathogenesis of some birth defects and cancer. In this chapter, we consider first the knowledge base for the prevention of several major chronic diseases of children and then the controversies generated by new discoveries. We next examine the means by which the resources for the dissemination of technologies have been generated and conclude with a discussion of strategies for assuring their appropriate use.

Knowledge Base for Prevention

Single-Gene Conditions. Five of the conditions reviewed in the Vanderbilt project result from the inheritance of a mutant gene either from both parents (these are autosomal recessive conditions: cystic fibrosis, sickle cell anemia, thalassemia, some forms of muscular dystrophy) or from the mother (X-linked conditions: hemophilia, other forms of muscular dystrophy) or from either parent (dominant conditions: still other forms of muscular dystrophy). Many other disorders causing chronic impairment are inherited by similar mechanisms.

For other disorders that have been thought to have a complex etiology, epidemiological surveys have suggested a simple mode of inheritance. The discovery, for instance, that the distribution of serum cholesterol concentrations in the blood relatives of individuals with hypercholesterolemic coronary heart disease was bimodal, which is more consistent with a single-gene than a multigene etiology, encouraged a search for a genetically determined molecular defect. The entire process, from the epidemiological study to the discovery of the molecular defect, occurred within ten years! A survey of all individuals with mental retardation born during a ten-year period suggested that X-linked disorders might account for much of the male excess in populations with mental retardation. This suggestion was shortly borne out by the discovery of the X-linked fragile X syndrome. After Down syndrome, it is the leading cause of retardation in males.

In conditions due to the presence of a single mutant gene (in either single or double dose) the base sequence of the DNA of the gene in question is altered. The change will be present in the DNA of every cell developing from the fertilized egg, not only those in which the gene is expressed. In those cells in which the gene is expressed, a protein—usually an enzyme—whose synthesis is determined by the gene will be quantitatively or qualitatively altered, frequently resulting in an alteration in the concentration of certain metabolites not only in the cell but in other tissues such as blood and urine as well. These features have major implications for detection, treatment, and prevention.

By the use of recombinant DNA technology, the DNA coding for single human genes can be purified and used to identify DNA fragments of the gene in cell extracts from subjects suspected of having the mutant gene. The size of the fragments, obtained by digestion of the DNA with specific restriction endonucleases, indicates whether the mutant gene is present, either alone (homozygote) or together with the "wild-type" gene (heterozygote). DNA analysis of amniotic fluid cells from fetuses suspected of being homozygotes can be used for prenatal diagnosis, for example, in pregnancies in which both parents are carriers of the sickle cell or thalassemia genes. The extension of the technique to virtually any other single-gene condition is theoretically possible because the DNA of the gene will be altered in every cell, not only those in which the gene is expressed. The limitation lies in identifying and purifying the DNA of the specific gene.

If the gene in question is expressed in amniotic fluid cells, protein or enzyme assays can be performed on amniotic fluid cell preparations obtained from amniocentesis. More than fifty inherited disorders have been diagnosed by this approach. Through fetoscopy, fetal blood can be collected and analyzed for substances that are not found in amniotic fluid cells but that are present in fetal blood. This technique, as well as the DNA analysis described above, can be used for diagnosis of hemoglobinopathies and the thalassemias. It also has been used to assay for factor VIII, which is deficient in hemophilia. Although not without risk, the assay provides an advance over the earlier method of prenatal diagnosis of hemophilia (one that must be still used for the X-linked form of muscular dystrophy): fetal sex determination. If a male pattern is observed on chromosome analysis, there is a 50 percent chance that the fetus will have the condition, whereas if a female pattern is observed, the fetus will not be affected. If the parents choose to terminate male pregnancies, half of the time an unaffected fetus will be aborted.

Amniocentesis and fetoscopy are relatively expensive and not completely without risk. (The chance of fetal death as a result of amniocentesis in the hands of experienced physicians is less than 1 percent, of fetoscopy, probably less than 5 percent.) Consequently, they are used for single-gene conditions only when both parents are carriers for autosomal recessive conditions or when the mother is a carrier for an X-linked condition.

Knowledge of the parents' carrier status is obtained in two ways: by the birth of a previously affected child or by screening for the carrier state. Screening of entire populations is possible when the product of the mutant gene is detectable in readily accessible tissues (such as blood or urine) by inexpensive techniques. Screening for carriers of the Tay-Sachs, sickle cell, and thalassemia genes is possible and in wide use in many populations in which these genes occur with relatively high frequency.

There remain a number of single-gene conditions that cannot be detected prenatally because the DNA for the gene has not yet been isolated, the gene defect is not known, or the gene is not active in utero or in any accessible fetal tissue. Cystic fibrosis, muscular dystrophy, and phenylketonuria (PKU) fall in this category, although a probe for the human PKU gene has recently been reported. Such conditions can be detected postnatally; screening of newborns for PKU is widespread in the United States and other developed countries and has resulted in a marked reduction in disability due to the disorder. Although screening is also possible for cystic fibrosis and muscular dystrophy, the tests yield many false positives, and no definitive treatments are currently available. Newborn screening for sickle cell anemia is being carried out in a number of states; no definitive treatment is available.

The deleterious consequences of single-gene defects can sometimes be overcome. Substitutes for the defective protein have been effective in hemophilia, growth-hormone deficiency, and diabetes. The availability of human factor VIII, growth hormone, and insulin will be increased by the use of recombinant DNA technology for synthesizing human proteins. Organ or tissue transplantation sometimes provides missing proteins, as in Fabry's disease and some immunodeficiency states. In other disorders, damage can be prevented by lowering the concentration of the material acted on by the defective enzyme, as in phenylketonuria. In some disorders, the enzyme in question normally begins to function in utero, and irreversible damage may already be sustained in affected infants by the time of birth. Intrauterine therapy has been successful in at least two inborn errors of metabolism in which high doses of vitamin cofactor are needed: methylmalonic acidemia and multiple carboxylase deficiency.

Disability from several single-gene defects can be prevented by the initiation of therapy before irreversible damage occurs. In some cases, this requires laboratory diagnosis; irreversible damage will be present by the time the first symptoms and signs appear. When screening is available, as for PKU, there is no need to wait for the birth of one affected child in a family; all infants can be screened and the burden of the disease in the entire population markedly reduced.

For most single-gene conditions, definitive therapy is not yet available. For those for which prenatal diagnosis is available, the parents can be provided with sufficient information to consider the option of terminating the pregnancy, another means of avoiding the burden of disabling genetic conditions. If prenatal diagnosis is not possible, genetic counseling can provide couples with precise prediction of recurrence risks. Alternatives to taking the chance of bearing an affected child include avoiding reproduction and adoption. In the case of autosomal recessive conditions (or of dominant conditions in which the male is the carrier) artificial insemination by donor provides another alternative. In the case of X-linked conditions, some couples may opt for using a noncarrier, surrogate mother inseminated by the husband's semen, or in the future, in vitro fertilization of a surrogate mother's ovum with the husband's semen, with subsequent implantation into the wife's uterus.

Genetic engineering may be another means of preventing disability from single-gene disorders. Technology is at hand to introduce DNA that contains the wild-type gene into cells whose function is impaired by the presence of the mutant gene. Thus far, attempts to improve hemoglobin synthesis by introduction of normal globin genes into bone marrow cells of patients with thalassemia have failed.

Three criteria must be satisfied in animal experiments before genetic engineering can be used in humans: (1) Enough product must be made to be effective (this was the problem in the thalassemia experiment). (2) The transplanted gene must continue to function for a period of time long enough to be helpful. (3) The harm from the process must not exceed the benefit. Harm might result if the amount of protein produced by the new gene were not regulated in the same way as protein synthesized under the instructions of the subject's own genes, if the new gene interfered with other regulatory or surveillance processes, or if malignant transformation or deleterious immunological reactions occurred.

Another approach involves insertion of the wild-type gene into a just-fertilized egg (zygote) that is at risk of developing into an infant with genetic disease because, for instance, both parents are carriers of the same mutant gene. The modified zygote would then be reimplanted into the mother's uterus. Recently, mice developed from zygotes into which rabbit hemoglobin gene was injected contained rabbit hemoglobin in their red blood cells. The outcome of preliminary animal experiments would have to assure that viable offspring with other severe derangements would virtually never occur before such engineering could be undertaken in humans.

The prospect for effective treatment or prevention appears much greater for single-gene disorders than for polygenic conditions. In a small proportion of patients with conditions that are usually polygenic, or due to environmental as well as genetic factors (such as spina bifida, congenital heart disease, or cleft palate), the defect results from the presence of a mutant gene. Determining whether a single-gene defect is present, beginning with a detailed family history, may be important for the future reproductive decisions of the family. At the very least, knowledge that a single gene is responsible can provide the parents, through genetic counseling, with precise predictions of recurrence risks.

Genetic-Environmental Interactions. Mutation of the genetic material in germ cells and somatic cells can occur as spontaneous errors in DNA replication or as a result of exposure to environmental agents such as ionizing radiation and chemicals. New mutations in germ cells are responsible for a significant proportion of X-linked and dominant conditions that cause impairment in the young. Although birth defects in which the chromosomes are abnormal, such as Down syndrome, may be inherited, most occur either spontaneously or as a result of mutagenic effects of environmental factors. Associations between radiation exposure and Down syndrome have been reported. Certain mutations in somatic cells lead to malignant changes, sometimes heralded (as in several forms of leukemia) by characteristic chromosome changes.

In order to correlate trends and clusters of cases with exposures to environmental agents some of which may be mutagens, birth defect and cancer registries have been established in a number of countries. Bacteria and animal test systems are also used to identify mutagenic and carcinogenic substances. Some of these systems have been used to assay body fluids from subjects who work with potentially mutagenic substances.

The reduction of exposure to harmful substances, which could result from monitoring, constitutes a primary form of prevention of birth defects and cancer. Awareness of the carcinogenic effects of x-ray exposure led to the reduction of the use of fluoroscopy and radiotherapy for benign disorders such as enlarged thymus. This probably contributed to the lower incidence of childhood leukemia in the 1960s compared to the 1950s. It should contribute to a reduction of thyroid carcinomas in the coming decades.

Until primary prevention becomes possible for more conditions, prenatal diagnosis of chromosome abnormalities offers a way of avoiding the birth of individuals with environmentally induced serious handicaps. Prenatal diagnosis is being offered with increasing frequency to older pregnant women who are at much higher risk of having infants with Down syndrome and other chromosome defects. If, as is currently the trend, a greater proportion of women delay childbearing, prenatal diagnosis followed by pregnancy termination could significantly reduce the frequency of Down syndrome. Despite their much greater risk, women over age thirty-five constitute fewer than 5 percent of pregnancies in the United States. Consequently, most Down syndrome infants are born to younger women despite their lower risks. Because of limited resources and the risk (even though small), current techniques of prenatal diagnosis probably will never be available to all women.

Epidemiological studies, frequently triggered by astute observations of practicing physicians, have also incriminated certain drugs (thalidomide), tobacco, alcohol, and infectious agents (rubella, cytomegalovirus) in the occurrence of specific birth defects or retarded fetal growth. The mechanism of action of these agents is poorly understood. Postnatal lead poisoning, infection, and accidents are beyond the scope of this paper, but they are pernicious environmental causes of acute (sometimes fatal) and chronic impairment in children. It has also become evident that familial factors can operate nongenetically. Parents' habits, such as smoking, can contribute to disease in their children, and agents brought home from the workplace can also have deleterious effects.

The susceptibility of somatic cells to malignant transformation from exposure to carcinogens may be enhanced by the presence of certain mutant genes. Two childhood cancers, retinoblastoma and Wilms tumor, can occur as the result of inheritance of particular autosomal dominant genes, but in addition, a somatic cell mutation—possibly resulting from an environmental insult—may have to occur before the tumors develop. Specific chromosome translocations and deletions, some of which are inherited, also predispose to cancer. If these changes prove to be highly associated with the development of malignancy, prenatal diagnosis followed by pregnancy termination could eliminate them from pedigrees in which cancer abounds. Avoiding excessive exposure to environmental mutagens in combination with periodic examinations to detect neoplasia might reduce, if not prevent, the burden of malignancy in people with genetic predispositions.

The mechanism by which the genes discussed above predispose to cancer is unknown. In some recessive conditions (Bloom's syndrome, ataxia-telangiectasia, Fanconi anemia, and xeroderma pigmentosum), defects of DNA-repair mechanisms probably increase the chance of malignancy. Inherited immune deficiencies may also predispose to cancer, partly by increasing the propensity of certain viruses to cause cancer.

Attention has been given recently to the possibility of screening workers for genotypes that increase their susceptibility to harm from substances in the workplace. Few such predispositions have been established, and available screening procedures are not highly predictive.

Some diseases that usually do not become manifest until adulthood may arise from genetic susceptibilities to harmful effects of environmental agents. Approximately one in five hundred individuals who are heterozygotes for defective low-density lipoprotein receptor genes are sensitive to cholesterol and have a high chance of developing coronary heart disease. Screening for this genotype is not yet feasible but would be far more specific in identifying individuals at risk for coronary heart disease than screening for high cholesterol levels.

Specific alleles at the histocompatibility (HLA) gene loci occur in higher frequency in patients with ankylosing spondylitis, psoriasis, juvenile diabetes mellitus, celiac disease, acute lymphocytic leukemia, renal and testicular carcinomas, and several other chronic conditions. The HLA allele occurring with high frequency in one condition—juvenile diabetes, for instance—is not the same as in other conditions. Except for hemochromatosis and one form of adrenal hyperplasia (21 hydroxylase deficiency), in both of which closely linked genes are responsible, it is not yet clear whether the HLA alleles themselves, or closely linked ones, increase the chance that the specific disease will develop. Because only a fraction of individuals with a specific allele develop the condition in question, an environmental exposure is needed before the disease develops. For instance, an abnormal response (dependent on the presence of a specific HLA allele) to certain viral infections has been proposed to account for the formation of insulin antibodies in juvenile diabetes mellitus. Further knowledge of these genetic-environmental interactions offers the possibility of prevention. The administration of a vaccine to prevent the viral infection (if one is incriminated) in children with the predisposing allele might be effective in preventing juvenile diabetes mellitus. Until more specific associations with genes in the HLA region are established and the nature of the environmental interactions determined, screening for specific alleles will identify individuals who will never suffer from the disorder whose prevention is being sought.

The environment of the fetus is also influenced by the mother's genotype. The presence of anti-Rh antibodies in Rh-negative women results in hemolytic disease if the fetus is Rh-positive. Prevention of sensitization by the administration of anti-Rh immunoglobulin to Rh-negative women following pregnancy has greatly reduced the frequency of hearing impairment and cerebral palsy due to Rh incompatibility.

The fetus of a mother with untreated PKU will almost certainly sustain brain damage as a result of intrauterine exposure to high levels of phenylalanine. It is not yet clear whether dietary restriction of phenylalanine during pregnancy will prevent damage to the fetus. An alternative is in vitro fertilization: ova are removed from the PKU woman, fertilized in vitro by sperm from her spouse; the fertilized egg is then implanted in a surrogate mother.

Disorders of Unknown Etiology. Knowledge of etiology is not always needed to develop diagnostic or therapeutic interventions. Although we remain ignorant of the causes of neural tube defects, the discovery that alpha-fetoprotein (AFP) is usually elevated in the blood of pregnant women carrying fetuses with open defects of the tube (anencephaly, spina bifida) provides women with the option of terminating the pregnancy of affected infants. Very recent work incriminates vitamin deficiency, particularly folic acid, in some cases of neural tube defects; if proven, this opens up the possibility of primary prevention.

Visualization of the fetus by ultrasound, or directly by fetoscopy, can be used for the prenatal diagnosis of gross skeletal or organ deformities. Until recently, termination of pregnancy was the only option. Successful fetal surgery for bladder obstruction and for correction of hydrocephalus may open a new era of surgical intervention with the fetus. Yet the likelihood of substantially improving the outcome of fetuses with visible defects, which may represent only one manifestation of much more extensive malformations, seems small at the moment and very expensive. Fetal surgery and therapy must still be viewed as experimental techniques.

Conflicts, Controversies, and Dilemmas

The gains in knowledge outlined in the previous sections expand the opportunities for early detection of those at risk of developing childhood chronic diseases or of giving birth to children who would develop them. For relatively few conditions have advances in conventional modes of therapy matched advances in early detection. Advances in four unconventional areas offer new options: (1) prenatal diagnosis—offering abortion of affected fetuses or, if possible, intrauterine treatment, (2) intrauterine therapy or surgery, (3) preconceptional control of reproduction—artificial insemination by donor, surrogate motherhood, in vitro fertilization, and (4) postconceptional alterations of the genetic material—genetic engineering. A fifth option (for which there is precedent) is primary prevention—reducing exposures to environmental agents involved in etiology. Although the unconventional technologies could lower the prevalence of seriously handicapping conditions, they raise problems, generate controversies, and pose dilemmas that will be difficult for society to resolve. Primary prevention also poses problems, to which we will turn after considering the unconventional technologies.

Unconventional Technologies. Three problems are common to all of the unconventional technologies. The first is how to avoid outcomes that all would agree are undesirable. No one would want to see a pregnancy terminated when a healthy fetus has been mistakenly diagnosed as having a disorder. Nor could the appearance of major disabilities that occur as a result of preconceptional control or of genetic engineering be tolerated. The rules governing research on human subjects in the United States make it unlikely that harmful outcomes will result during the development of new technologies. Whether the same careful scrutiny will be given to the safety and effectiveness of these technologies once they become routinely available is more problematic. (The issue of quality assurance is dealt with later in this chapter.) Certain consequences of new technologies may be unknowable until the technology receives fairly extensive use in humans. We do not know, for instance, and probably cannot find out from animal studies, the effect of in vitro fertilization or surrogate motherhood on maternal-child interactions. Ongoing, systematic evaluation will be needed.

The second problem relates to the distribution of new technologies. Should costly interventions be made available to all who are at risk, regardless of ability to pay? If because of high costs this is not possible, should the technology be made available to the wealthy? These questions should be considered before large sums are allocated to the development of new technologies. Investing in the development of a costly technology not all could afford often forecloses development in other areas in which the benefits could be more widely distributed.

The third and most overriding problem is the effect that the opportunities for reducing handicaps will have on society's and parents' tolerance for handicaps. Society would most likely (but not assuredly) accept parents' refusal of interventions that are intended to avoid the birth of children with handicaps, but it might not continue to pay for the care of such children, placing the burden on the parents and the children. With greater expectations of prevention, resources for caring for all types of handicaps might be reduced. But because it will remain impossible to prevent all (or even most handicaps, including some of the most severe), the result could be poorer care and poorer acceptance of those with major disabilities.

In addition to parents who refuse prenatal diagnosis and abortion of affected fetuses for religious or moral reasons, parents who already have had children with serious conditions, for which prenatal diagnosis became available subsequent to the birth of the affected child, might be likely to refuse. For instance, parents of children with spina bifida often feel caught between not wanting to repeat their (and their child's) ordeal, on the one hand, and on the other, fear of conveying to their living affected children that they would not be alive had prenatal diagnosis been available before they were born.

As we gain the knowledge and skill to detect prenatally a broader range of defects, prospective parents may be less and less willing to accept even minor defects in their offspring. How this will affect the rearing of children who do not satisfy their parents' expectations remains unknown; obviously parents will differ. In our quest to eliminate a broader range of defects we may unwittingly be searching for a greater degree of conformity. But the notion that there is an "ideal human genotype which it is desirable to bestow upon everybody is not only unappealing, but is almost certainly wrong—it is human diversity that acted as a leaven of creative effort in the past and will so act in the future" (Dobzhansky, cited in Milunsky and Annas, 1980). Despite the most strenuous efforts, diversity will persist; because of the continued and unavoidable occurrence of mutations as well as the inevitable inability to predict which genes from the mother and the father will combine in the zygote, we will never be able to assure the qualities of offspring (even when preconceptional control or genetic engineering is used).

Having dealt with some general issues of unconventional technologies, let us briefly examine some conflicts that pertain to specific technologies. The first of these is prenatal diagnosis and termination of pregnancy. If anti-abortion forces triumph, a major option made possible by prenatal diagnosis will be removed. Prenatal diagnosis itself, which carries a small chance of harm to the fetus, would seldom be undertaken. Couples at risk of conceiving offspring with serious defects might decide not to have any children, a point frequently ignored by prolife groups. On the other hand, if such couples decide to take their chances, the incidence of chronically handicapping conditions would increase.

While the right to life of the fetus has received considerable publicity, the question of whether a fetus who will become seriously impaired has the right not to be born has also been raised. So-called wrongful life cases have been brought to the courts, with the parents acting on behalf of the fetus against physicians who did not provide adequate prenatal diagnosis. With few exceptions, the courts have not awarded damages to the infants wrongfully born, although they have awarded damages to the parents, primarily for economic suffering.

One problem with the wrongful life doctrine lies in determining how severe a condition must be for the life to be wrong. When a relatively mild, possibly repairable defect (for example, cleft palate) or a finding of unknown significance is discovered by prenatal diagnosis, do parents have the right to terminate the pregnancy? Cytogenetic techniques, which are most frequently used in prenatal diagnosis, can reveal chromosome changes other than the one being sought; some are associated with conditions whose severity is unknown or known to be relatively mild. These techniques also reveal the sex of the fetus. It is doubtful from a legal point of view that physicians could withhold information from the parents about the sex of the fetus or about findings whose consequences are unknown or mild.

At the present time, because resources for providing prenatal diagnosis are scarce, women at lower risk can be turned away. If and when resources become abundant, it is unclear whether providers could (or would) refuse prenatal diagnosis for what they perceive to be frivolous reasons (either because the risk is low, or the defect sought is not, in their view, serious).

Let us turn now to a second unconventional technology, preconceptional reproductive control. The use of artificial insemination by donor, in vitro fertilization, and surrogate motherhood to allow conception using the germ cells of one but not both of the parents to reduce the risk of a single-gene disorder in their offspring avoids the abortion issue but raises problems of parental rights and responsibilities that have not been completely resolved. A sperm or ovum donor might also carry the same gene that a couple sought to avoid by artificial mating. Whenever possible, donors should be screened for the defect. This is seldom done today. Infants with Tay-Sachs disease and PKU have resulted from artificial insemination. Sperm donors have been held not to be responsible for support of their progeny by artificial insemination and not to have any claim on the offspring. One would expect the same to be true for a woman who donated her ova for in vitro fertilization by another woman's husband with subsequent implantation in the wife's uterus. (This could be done to avoid an X-linked disorder.) A conflict more difficult to resolve will arise when a woman serves as a surrogate with either her ova, or the wife's ova, fertilized by the husband's sperm in vivo or in vitro respectively. In both of these cases the issue is whether carrying the fetus and giving birth establishes a right to motherhood. In the case where the wife's ova is used, does it establish a compelling competing right?

The sperm donor's identity is not usually made available to the child. However, just as adopted children frequently demand to know the identity of their biological parents, so might those conceived by artificial insemination or in vitro fertilization. This information would help them understand their genetic heritage as they plan their own families. This is particularly important with artificial insemination by donor because of the risk of consanguinity; sperm from a single donor may be used to inseminate many women in the same community, and it is conceivable that the offspring of those inseminations—who are half siblings—will subsequently mate. The chance of handicapping autosomal recessive conditions in their offspring would be increased.

It is questionable whether artificial reproduction techniques will ever become widespread or whether prenatal diagnosis will often be accepted without remorse by parents who feel they must choose abortion. The more feasible and satisfying means of prevention will be the elimination of the causes of the defects themselves. But here, too, problems arise.

Primary Prevention. Most environmental substances that have been, or will be, incriminated as mutagens, carcinogens, or teratogens are also likely to have some beneficial function. Society must determine, then, whether the benefits exceed the risks. In some situations, a reduction of ambient levels of toxic substances will lower the chance of harmful reactions sufficiently to yield a favorable benefit:risk ratio. Alternatively, efforts may be sought to reduce exposure only of those at excessive risk.

Harmful substances frequently find their way into the environment as a result of industrial use. Not only those who work with harmful substances are exposed; inadequate storage of industrial wastes exposes those beyond the factory as well. Without governmental regulation, industry is unlikely to pay for changes to reduce exposures. Thus the question of how much government regulation of industry is appropriate is germane to the prevention of disease. The extent to which federal, state, or local governments and the industry doing the dumping are responsible for removal of toxic wastes, relocation of exposed families, and reimbursement for damages has not yet been determined.

All individuals will not be at equal risk of harm from industrial exposures. Efforts to identify unusually susceptible workers and exclude them from exposure to substances especially harmful to them or their offspring (for instance, by denying them employment) might replace efforts to lower exposure of all workers. Rather than risk suits for damage to children as a result of intrauterine exposure, several corporations have excluded fertile women from jobs that could expose the fetus to harmful agents; such policies have not stood up in the courts.

Genetic screening could be used to identify and exclude workers who are unusually susceptible to the toxic effects of industrial chemicals. At the present time, few such susceptibilities are known, and even fewer are amenable to screening. Nor is it clear that among human populations there is a discontinuity in susceptibility. Workers who pass genetic screening tests for susceptibility may be at less risk than those who fail. Nevertheless, they may suffer harm from exposure. Screening tests could provide a false sense of security and reduce efforts to lower ambient levels of toxic substances.

Although seldom used by private industry, the United States government itself has used genetic screening to exclude sickle cell carriers from the U.S. Air Force Academy on the belief that they are at increased risk of harmful consequences from high-altitude flying. Challenge to its scientific basis has led to reconsideration of this policy.

The health professions themselves may be responsible for harmful exposures. The largest exposure of the public to ionizing radiation comes from dental and medical sources. Some radiation is unnecessary or excessive due to poor equipment. Any exposure to radiation carries with it a risk of mutation. At low levels, the risk is small but still present.

In addition to environmental exposures over which they have no control, people may choose to expose themselves to potentially harmful substances, such as cigarettes and alcohol, often induced to do so by advertising and social pressures. Should society reduce consumption of these substances to reduce the unhealthful consequences? Here, too, there is the possibility of detecting individuals who are unusually susceptible on a genetic basis. Such individuals may be more receptive to altering their behavior than those less susceptible, who could continue to indulge. The usefulness of this selective screening approach remains to be demonstrated.

Strategies to Disseminate New Technologies

Although some of the controversies and dilemmas posed in the previous section will never be resolved, ignorance and distorted notions of the nature and objectives of new technologies may hinder the diffusion of preventive strategies. Recent efforts to undermine the teaching of evolution in the name of scientific creationism contribute to the persistence of ignorance. Mutations—the same events that account for evolution—account for genetic and gene-influenced diseases. A greater appreciation of how mutations occur will help remove the stigmatization that frequently surrounds genetic diseases and increase understanding of their detection.

Increasing Awareness. There is little need to increase public awareness of those genetic conditions whose prevention is possible only after they occur once within a family. These are diseases for which screening is not possible or not cost-beneficial (usually because the diseases are extremely rare). With their firsthand contact, family members are likely to ask about recurrence and what can be done to prevent it. In some instances, however, physicians will not appreciate the genetic aspects of the disease and will not offer services to other family members. Thus, there is a need to increase providers' knowledge of genetics and assure adequate resources for diagnosis and counseling. Out of fear of stigmatization, family members may not want to inform other relatives who are at risk of having an affected child. Failure to inform does not pose a threat to the public health or even (very often) a high probability of harm to other family members. Nevertheless, a client's refusal to have others informed places providers in a difficult position; maintaining confidentiality may jeopardize others.

The situation is far different for those conditions amenable to population-based screening through which individuals at risk of disease or of conceiving infants with a disease can be detected before any affected relative suffers the consequence of late diagnosis. Most people will not have had contact with the illness; increasing their appreciation of the importance of screening poses a major challenge.

Little has been taught in schools about the scientific discoveries, particularly in human genetics, on which early detection and prevention are based. Surveys of high school students in the United States and Canada, of adults coming to screening programs, and of those who have children with genetic diseases all reveal poor knowledge of heredity and its biological basis. Human genetic diseases have been mentioned in classrooms, either as rare oddities (such as PKU) or as the plight of minority groups. Neither approach is likely to foster recognition that everybody is likely to carry deleterious genes. Starting in the elementary grades, greater emphasis on the genetic as well as environmental basis of human variability should be taught, and in high school, students should be confronted with the controversies we have enumerated.

Increasingly, books, magazines, newspaper articles, and television have conveyed information about new discoveries to the adult public. Organizations concerned about specific diseases, or diseases in specific ethnic groups, have disseminated information. Surprisingly, physicians are not so important a source of information about new genetic services to people who come for screening as are friends, relatives, and the media. Physicians may be unaware or unaccepting of new technologies: recent surveys, including scores on questions about genetics on the National Board examinations, showed significant deficiencies of physicians' knowledge of human genetics. A few medical schools in the United States still do not have genetics courses, and genetics is infrequently a topic of continuing education programs. (The deficiencies are even more marked in nurses' training.) Even in the late 1970s, only a minority of obstetricians were making referrals for prenatal diagnosis, although not apparently because of the opposition of pregnant women. An intensive effort to inform low-income, primarily black, high-risk pregnant women about prenatal diagnosis, providing a full explanation of risks and procedures, resulted in 60 percent accepting amniocentesis. Among middle-income white women, the proportion who say they would accept termination of pregnancy of an infant with a serious mental or physical defect is higher. The anti-abortion campaign may have had a more profound effect on providers than on consumers. As a result, women with some college education, who are more likely to be aware of prenatal diagnosis, obtain a disproportionate share of prenatal diagnostic services.

Dissemination Strategies. The slowness with which new approaches were incorporated into routine medical practice led organizations and professions concerned about specific diseases to seek help outside the medical profession. When hospitals and physicians were slow to screen newborns for PKU, chapters of the National Association of Retarded Children (consisting largely of parents) advocated, often successfully, state laws and regulations to make screening mandatory. In the early 1970s, several states passed laws requiring sickle cell screening of newborns, school-age children, or applicants for marriage licenses. The early legislation mandated screening, with little concern for education, counseling, or effectiveness. With much political fanfare, the federal government entered the picture in 1972, when Congress passed the National Sickle Cell Anemia Control Act. Later that year, it passed the National Cooley's Anemia Control Act. Although specific appropriations did not accompany either act, federal funds were awarded to local sickle cell programs. To correct deficiencies of many existing programs, the guidelines stipulated that testing had to be voluntary, that education and counseling had to be provided, and that laboratories had to participate in a national proficiency testing program. Further efforts in genetic services resulted, in 1975, in passage of a program to develop Hemophilia Diagnostic and Treatment Centers and Blood Separation Centers.

By the late 1970s, Congress was growing wary of single-disease legislation and in 1976 it combined the sickle cell and Cooley's anemia legislation into the National Sickle Cell Anemia, Cooley's Anemia, Tay-Sachs, and Genetic Diseases Act, which named eleven genetic conditions. In 1978 (the first year of appropriations for the act), Congress clarified, through amendments, that it listed these only as examples. Concerns about compulsory testing and confidentiality of results, particularly in carrier-screening programs, were expressed frequently by the time the act was drafted. Consequently, the requirement for voluntary testing in the original sickle cell act was carried over into the Genetic Diseases Act, and requirements for confidentiality of individual data and community representation in the development and operation of genetic services were included as well. By 1981, funds appropriated under the Genetic Diseases Act supported genetics and sickle cell programs in forty states, the District of Columbia, and Puerto Rico. As a result, education, diagnostic, and counseling services became available to populations remote from tertiary genetics centers. Treatment was omitted from the act, precluding the criticism that federal funds would be used to pay for abortion.

The courts have also been used, albeit sporadically, to speed dissemination. Recent rulings hold physicians liable if they do not tell pregnant women who are at high risk of having an infant with a serious defect of the likelihood of its occurrence or if they fail to inform those women for whom prenatal diagnosis is indicated of its availability.

In the early 1970s, ethnic groups interested in Tay-Sachs, sickle cell anemia, and thalassemia, frequently led by parents of affected individuals, arranged detection programs for carriers in schools, churches, synagogues, and other community centers, using private donations and voluntary contributions for support. The programs were often aimed at people entering their reproductive years, who frequently do not have a regular source of medical care.

Local health departments serving predominantly black populations also provide sickle cell screening, sometimes with federal or state support. Hospitals sometimes screen black patients for hemoglobinopathies, particularly when anesthesia is scheduled.

By advertising to physicians or the public, manufacturers of screening tests, or commercial laboratories who perform them, increase awareness of new technologies and speed the dissemination of screening through their marketing. At least one commercial laboratory advertised neonatal hypothyroid screening tests directly to the public, and may have accelerated the incorporation of thyroid testing into statewide newborn screening programs.

Although the unit costs of screening are low, the potential volume is enormous, making screening a lucrative enterprise. As a result of commercial availability and pressure, screening tests could be widely adopted before sufficient provider and consumer understanding have developed and before adequate resources for follow-up and counseling are available. These problems are discussed further in the next section.

Improving Public Policy for Genetic Screening and Counseling

The history of dissemination of genetic-screening technologies indicates that programs rarely emerge from broad public consensus. Two problems have interfered with rational public policy making. First, policy makers often lack an objective analysis of the benefits, risks, and costs of new technologies before establishing policy. Nor have they had an opportunity to place each new discovery into perspective with other parallel or future discoveries. Second, pressure groups interested in specific diseases have capitalized on this lack of perspective and have been the dominant force in establishment of public policy on both state and federal levels. Often well intentioned, these groups stress benefits more than costs and risks and ignore competing demands for the investment of public funds.

Steps are being taken to overcome these problems. Congress has established the Office of Technology Assessment, which has begun to examine policy implications of new discoveries including those in genetics. It also created a National Center of Health Care Technology (which has now been merged with the National Center for Health Services Research) to foster studies regarding the use of new as well as existing technologies that influence health care. One of the earliest priorities of the center was for studies relating to maternal serum alpha fetoprotein (MSAFP) testing for fetal neural tube defects.

Public Participation in Policy Making. In its epochal report, "Genetic Screening," a committee of the National Academy of Sciences proposed formation of state commissions, composed of health professionals, legislators, lawyers, educators, and the general public, to review and approve screening projects receiving public support, set standards for routine operations of these programs, and assist educational efforts in genetics. In that report, the Committee for the Study of Inborn Errors of Metabolism (1975, p. 3) also stated, "Broad public representation among members of the commission could also protect the community from the pressure of special-interest groups who, in their preoccupation with their own concerns, may obtain official or even legislative sanctions for programs that are not in the general interest."

Among the states, Maryland has gone farthest with this approach by creating a Commission on Hereditary Disorders that has authority to regulate the detection and management of hereditary disorders provided it holds public hearings before doing so. Composed of five lay members, two legislators, and four health professionals, the commission has promulgated regulations for assuring the quality of newborn and hemoglobinopathy screening as well as consent and confidentiality. It has proceeded cautiously in approving new screening programs, insisting on pilot phases before giving approval for routine use. Such pilot programs can pinpoint deficiencies before they become ingrained.

Both public participation in deciding whether a screening program should be launched and the use of pilot programs help assure the adoption of enlightened policies for prevention of genetic diseases. Additional safeguards are needed, especially in three areas we examine in this section: education and consent, counseling, and testing and follow-up.

Education and Consent. It has been suggested that "it is more important for society to follow a conscious policy of protecting individual autonomy in assessing the social implications of one's individual genotype than to mobilize social resources behind a coercive model of genetic 'normality' " (Committee for the Study of Inborn Errors of Metabolism, 1975, p. 188). In some screening programs, written informed consent is not obtained, and education is minimal or nonexistent. Subtle pressures can coerce individuals who do not understand the objectives of screening or what being a carrier means into being screened. More intensive education prior to screening might alleviate some of these problems. There has been concern, however, that informing potential screenees about innocuous tests might do more harm than good. In Maryland, 55 percent of obstetricians opposed informed consent for MSAFP testing, primarily because they believed it would heighten women's anxiety about having an infant with a severe birth defect. Thirty-five percent of pregnant women were also opposed to consent for MSAFP screening. A study of the pilot MSAFP screening in Maryland showed that providing women with information about screening for neural tube defects did not generate anxiety.

The law establishing the Maryland Commission on Hereditary Disorders required that all genetic screening be voluntary. The commission interpreted this to incude newborn screening, and the legislature subsequently agreed when it repealed the mandatory requirement. A study of the informed consent policy for newborn screening in Maryland showed that fewer than 0.05 percent of parents refused consent and that considerable knowledge about screening and the disorders for which it was being performed was gained by the parents as a result of the disclosure-consent process. Nevertheless, in situations such as PKU screening, in which the benefits to every affected child are enormous and the risks negligible, it is arguable whether parents should have the right to refuse.

The documented inability of physicians to interpret screening test results correctly, as well as their lack of knowledge about how positive test results should be interpreted, indicates the need for intense provider education before screening becomes routine and for regulating the use of new methods for screening to assure appropriate patient management. Invoking its power to regulate when there is a potential for harm, the Food and Drug Administration under the Carter administration proposed restrictions in the distribution of MSAFP screening kits. They require patient education prior to testing, and coordination between laboratories and physicians as well as documentation of high laboratory quality.

Pressure for the restrictions came from public interest groups as well as the Spina Bifida Association of America, whose members (many of them parents of children with neural tube defects or patients themselves) feared the spread of inaccurate information about the condition. Organizations representing obstetricians and pediatricians also favored the restrictions while the American Medical Association and organizations representing clinical pathologists vehemently opposed them as an unnecessary intrusion into the practice of medicine. In June 1983, the FDA withdrew these proposed restrictions.

Counseling. Feelings of stigmatization and diminished self-esteem sometimes follow the identification of individuals as carriers, pointing up the need for counseling as well as for confidentiality. Those discovered to be noncarriers sometimes have a heightened self-image, pointing up the inadequacy of their prescreening education; they too carry genes for serious disorders. There are often deficiencies in counseling following screening and also deficiencies in counseling provided to families who already have a child with a genetic disorder. Recent reviews indicate poor retention or comprehension of counseling information.

The measurement of attitudes toward altering reproduction is more complex and could pose difficult policy issues. For if it is discovered that, after counseling, families are inclined to take greater risks than before, modification of counseling to "correct" this problem implies a eugenic intention and not really a desire to present parents with sufficient information to allow them to make a rational, independent decision. A careful assessment might reveal, however, that information about probabilities has not been conveyed in a manner that allows the counselee to make a rational decision.

Testing and Follow-Up. When screening procedures are initiated on a broad scale, attention must be given to the reliability and validity of the tests under conditions of routine use and to the availability of adequate resources for follow-up. In the early days of sickle cell screening, 14 percent of federally supported laboratories engaged in routine testing could not correctly identify a specimen of SA hemoglobin. Deficiencies of PKU and hypothyroid testing in large-scale programs have also been uncovered. A few states (most notably New York) have developed proficiency-testing programs for cytogenetic laboratories and require participation for licensing. Unfortunately, many providers, particularly commercial laboratories, do not participate in proficiency testing. State licensure requirements are frequently weak or nonexistent.

Screening tests are not an end in themselves. When New York City was required under state law to start newborn screening for sickle cell anemia, it did not have adequate resources to ensure follow-up, and 48 percent of infants presumed to have sickle cell anemia were never located. A number of the professional and consumer organizations that urged the Food and Drug Administration to restrict the release of reagents for MSAFP screening feared that, with inadequate resources for confirmatory diagnostic procedures and for counseling of women with positive tests, unaffected fetuses could be aborted. No more than one in thirty women with a positive MSAFP screening test will be carrying a fetus with a neural tube defect.

Sometimes mass screening uncovers previously unknown variants whose prognosis is uncertain and for which, consequently, the appropriate intervention is unknown. In the early days of PKU screening, infants with persistent but moderate phenylalanine levels were placed on restricted diets and sometimes developed phenylalanine deficiency. It is now known that these infants would have developed normally without any treatment. At the present time, some infants identified through newborn screening as having congenital hypothyroidism may be treated unnecessarily; the information is not yet available to predict with complete accuracy which infants will benefit from treatment. In such situations, systematic efforts to establish criteria for treatment and to monitor the effects of treatment are needed.

The Future of Preventive Services in Genetics

Programmatic Support. In 1981, the Genetic Diseases Act was absorbed into the Maternal and Child Health Services Block Grant Act. The appropriation was substantially reduced, and states whose programs were largely based on federal support found the existence of their programs threatened. If the trend continues, there will be even less federal support in the future. With state governments now responsible for deciding whether to allocate block grant or other funds to genetic services, disparities among states in the availability and quality of services are likely to increase. Unless the states assume support, or Medicaid and other third-party insurers adequately reimburse for preventive services, the overall level of services will fall. In fiscal year 1983, states whose federal funding for genetics and sickle cell services was cut off were unable to replace this support with funds from other sources.

The cutback in funds also increases the likelihood that fees will be charged for newborn screening and for carrier screening. Fees pose the greatest problem for the poor, who if they are unable to pay for screening can expect to be burdened most by birth of affected infants. Once states with efficient centralized screening programs begin to charge, hospitals and commercial laboratories are likely to set up their own competing screening programs, which will result in fragmentation of screening and a likely decline in quality.

With this bleak outlook and the growing competition for funds, the danger of reverting to single-disease programs in response to the pressures of special issues groups looms unless coalitions are formed to fight for continuation of all existing, effective programs. A further blow to genetic services programs will result from anti-abortion legislation and the exclusion of abortion from Medicaid reimbursement.

Quality Assurance. Despite the gloomy outlook for publicly supported services, as technologies for early detection and intervention continue to expand, additional resources eventually will be attracted to preventing childhood chronic diseases. As an example, the current scarcity of resources, which requires setting priorities among women for amniocentesis, may be replaced by a surplus. Services that have been delivered almost exclusively through university-affiliated programs will be offered by other providers. Although university affiliation is no assurance of quality, there is even less assurance that newcomers to the field will have competence in diagnosis and counseling. A more serious situation may develop in the provision of laboratory services. Cytogenetics testing, in particular, depends on the judgment of individual technicians, and there is plenty of room for error.

The newly created American Board of Medical Genetics offers certifying examinations in clinical and laboratory aspects of genetics. The Association of Cytogenetic Technologists certifies cytogenetic technicians. Although there is little evidence to suggest that consumers use certification in selecting providers, third-party insurers, both public and private, could reimburse only for services provided by a certified clinician or laboratory. State agencies that license laboratories could also require that key personnel be competent in medical genetic laboratory techniques, as judged by their having passed one of the national exams in genetics.

Integration of Services. The establishment of genetics as a specialty may have unwanted consequences. Primary care providers may be less inclined to offer testing and counseling and instead refer individuals or families at risk to genetic specialists. With limited reimbursement for genetic services, some people will not obtain the consultation and will receive no counseling instead of some. Genetic specialists may also be less inclined to educate primary care providers in genetic counseling. Yet, repeated counseling, which can be given by a primary care provider, seems far more effective than one-shot consultation.

Although many genetic conditions become evident during the perinatal period, providers of neonatal care often do not count them among the diagnostic possibilities, and when they do, do not offer counseling to parents of affected infants. Infants dying from inborn errors of metabolism may often be thought to have primary respiratory distress or idiopathic conditions. An excellent mechanism to reduce this problem has been undertaken at the Ben Gurion Medical Center in Israel. A team of an obstetrician, a pediatrician, and a geneticist reviews all perinatal deaths and, within two months, meets with the parents to discuss the likely causes of the problem and chances of recurrence.

Reimbursement. Counseling constitutes a major component of genetic services. Yet, third-party insurers are often reluctant to reimburse for it. Part of their reluctance stems from provision of counseling by nonphysicians. A more fundamental reason is their unwillingness to reimburse for preventive services. The cost-saving benefits of genetic counseling are seldom immediate and tangible, yet without counseling, families have little accurate basis on which to gauge their risks for bearing children with major disabilities.

Greater third-party coverage of screening and counseling, and reimbursement for counseling provided by nonphysicians is needed. Although insurance companies have been slow to respond, Blue Cross, in cooperation with the March of Dimes and the Health Services Administration of the U.S. Department of Health and Human Services, will soon field-test an expanded package of counseling services. Eventually, legislation requiring expanded coverage as a condition of state licensure of insurance companies may be needed.

Primary Prevention. Lack of systematic observation has hampered progress in elucidating environmental agents that may play an etiological role in chronic handicapping conditions. Greater attention has recently been given to investigating the effects of exposure to potentially toxic substances and to the association of illness with environmental agents. Data on the incidence of congenital malformations or specific cancers in defined populations are frequently lacking. Consequently, there is no baseline against which suspected changes can be measured. In the area of congenital malformations, surveillance of birth defects (such as that carried out by the Centers for Disease Control in Atlanta) or required reporting of birth defects (as required in a handful of states) could provide the needed information. In Maryland, beginning in 1983, reports of birth defects will be linked to a registry of toxic substances, facilitating discovery of associations between birth defects and release of substances into the environment.

Conclusion—Benefit:Cost Analysis

Economic analyses of newborn screening for PKU and hypothyroidism, prenatal screening for neural tube defects, prenatal diagnosis of Down syndrome in older women, and carrier screening for Tay-Sachs all demonstrate that benefits exceed costs. Screening for other conditions, which if performed alone would not be cost beneficial, can be economically added to existing programs because start-up and collection and transportation of the specimens comprise a significant proportion of all costs. For some disorders, technologies for early detection may be available, but their use can be questioned.

An interesting case is neonatal screening for branched-chain ketoaciduria (BCK). In contrast to PKU, in which untreated infants usually survive and incur significant costs for management of their severe retardation, infants with BCK who are not detected early in life and treated usually die. Thus, averted economic costs are small although the family's grief may be enormous. Moreover, dietary treatment, which must be maintained for life, is relatively expensive (compared to PKU), and the prevention of retardation or death is far less certain. It costs very little to add BCK screening to existing programs, and by so doing, early death will probably be prevented. Whether there are long-term monetary savings is doubtful.

Newborn screening is also possible for sickle cell anemia and cystic fibrosis. As mentioned earlier, no definitive treatment is available for either condition. Newborn screening would result in much earlier diagnosis for both conditions, but the evidence is not yet in that early diagnosis will improve outcomes. If early administration of antibiotics prophylactically reduces morbidity for either of these conditions, or if parental or physician awareness leads to more appropriate and prompt medical care, then early detection would be of benefit. If, as a result of newborn screening, parents become aware of the risks of recurrence before they conceive another child, then screening could result in avoidance of the birth of additional children with these conditions. With small family size and most affected children being the first born, the reduction in births of affected infants as a result of newborn screening is not likely to be great. Even with the most recent procedure for newborn screening for cystic fibrosis (serum immuno-reactive trypsin assay), there will be false positives and false negatives, thus reducing the benefit:cost ratio of screening.

The maximum benefit:cost ratio from screening will occur when all subjects at risk are screened and when those identified through screening choose the pathway that will lead to the lowest increment in costs. Few economic analyses consider the proportion of people who will avail themselves of screening. This is not surprising in the studies of newborn screening because it is compulsory in most states. In prenatal detection, in which abortion may be the least costly option, it is far from clear what proportion of women will choose screening or abortion. This proportion appears to be high for Tay-Sachs disease. No evidence has been collected in the United States to indicate the extent to which screening for sickle cell carriers reduces the incidence of sickle cell anemia. In Greece, a sickle cell screening program failed to reduce matings between carriers. At the time of the study, the only means of avoiding the birth of an affected infant was for a carrier to avoid mating with another carrier. Fear of both stigmatization and failure to find a mate by announcing one's carrier status may have contributed to carriers' failure to act on screening-test results. Now that prenatal diagnosis of both sickle cell anemia and the thalassemias are possible, carrier screening may lead to a reduction in the number of affected offspring born. In several Mediterranean countries, prenatal diagnosis of thalassemia is being used by carrier couples (detected either by screening or by previous birth of an affected infant). When affected fetuses are diagnosed, couples are electing abortion. (In the Mediterranean countries, fetoscopy is used to collect blood for prenatal diagnosis. This procedure carries with it a risk of fetal death of about 5 percent. In the United States, recombinant DNA techniques for prenatal diagnosis of both thalassemia and sickle cell anemia, which are much safer, are just starting to be used. For sickle cell anemia, most, but not all, couples in whom an affected fetus is discovered are electing to terminate the pregnancy.)

Thus the use of benefit:cost analysis points up the conflict between individual freedom and societal benefits. To maximize benefit:cost ratios, new technologies must be imposed on everyone. However, out of fear of intrusion or of pressure from groups morally opposed to interfering with the reproductive process, new technologies may be denied those who want to use them. If the middle ground is struck and the technologies are made available on a voluntary basis, and if the number who use them is small, the continued investment of public funds in development or support of these technologies will be questioned. Increasing public and provider understanding and development of mechanisms that allow all points of view to be heard and new proposals to be pilot-tested before public policies are promulgated will provide the best guarantee for preventing chronic illness of children in accord with the values of a democratic society.

References

Anderson, W. F. "Gene Therapy." *Journal of the American Medical Association,* 1981, *246,* 2737–2739.

Antonarakis, S. E., Phillips, J. A., and Kazazian, H. H., Jr. "Genetic Disease: Diagnosis by Restriction Endonuclease Analysis." *Journal of Pediatrics*, 1982, *100*, 845–856.

Bloom, A. D. (Ed.) *Guidelines for Studies of Human Populations Exposed to Mutagenic and Reproductive Hazards.* White Plains, N.Y.: March of Dimes Birth Defects Foundation, 1981.

Cohen, B. A., Lilienfeld, A. M., and Huang, P. C. (Eds.) *Genetic Issues in Public Health and Medicine.* Springfield, Ill.: Charles C. Thomas, 1978.

Committee for the Study of Inborn Errors of Metabolism. *Genetic Screening: Programs, Principles and Research.* Washington, D.C.: National Academy of Sciences, 1975.

Gerald, P. S. "X-Linked Mental Retardation and the Fragile-X Syndrome." *Pediatrics*, 1981, *68*, 594–595.

Harrison, M. R., and others. "Fetal Treatment." *New England Journal of Medicine*, 1982, *307*, 1651–1652.

Holtzman, N. A., Leonard, C. O., and Farfel, M. R. "Issues in Antenatal and Neonatal Screening and Surveillance for Hereditary and Congenital Disorders." *Annual Review of Public Health*, 1981, *2*, 219–251.

Milunsky, A., and Annas, G. J. (Eds.) *Genetics and the Law II.* New York: Plenum, 1980.

Office of Technology Assessment. *The Role of Genetic Testing in the Prevention of Occupational Disease.* Washington, D.C.: U.S. Government Printing Office, 1983.

President's Commission for the Study of Ethical Problems in Medicine and Biomedical and Behavioral Research. *Splicing Life.* Washington, D.C.: U.S. Government Printing Office, 1983.

Sorenson, J. R., Swazey, J. P., and Scotch, N. A. *Reproductive Pasts, Reproductive Futures: Genetic Counseling and Its Effectiveness.* New York: Alan R. Liss, 1981.

Stanbury, J. B., and others (Eds.) *The Metabolic Basis of Inherited Disease.* New York: McGraw-Hill, 1983.

van Eys, J., and Sullivan, M. P. (Eds.) *Status of Curability of Childhood Cancers.* New York: Raven Press, 1980.

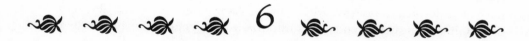

6

The State of Research on Chronically Ill Children

Barbara Starfield, M.D., M.P.H.

This chapter addresses the need for research, particularly research that helps inform policy concerning children who are chronically ill.

Although the focus is on chronically ill children and their families, a broader view of the problem is necessary because all children are relatively vulnerable as compared with adults. Most adults have some control over their environment, or at least they have potential for such control. In contrast, children are dependent upon adults. If those adults fail to appreciate the role the environment plays in shaping responses to health-threatening events or if they fail to pursue measures to reduce these threats, children are at risk of both acute and long-lasting problems. Moreover, the terms *chronic illness, impairment,* and *handicap* lack precise definition. A chronic illness or a handicap or an impairment in one child is not necessarily a similar phenomenon in another child. Conditions of unknown etiology or with unclear pathogenesis are likely to be even more variable than diseases with clearly elucidated causes and manifestations.

In the development of a research agenda, it is necessary to be aware not only of needs for research but also of the possibilities. Research takes place within social, economic, and epistemological constraints. In some societies, particular types of research are proscribed, severely restricted, or discouraged. In the United States, some types of research are effectively prevented by constraints on funding, and unless social priorities dictate the transfer of funds from other things, such research becomes impossible. Social research is particularly vulnerable to shifts with changes in public policy. The state of knowledge may also affect the feasibility of research—some answers cannot be obtained because there is insufficient knowledge with which to frame precise questions. Even when questions can be precisely framed, answers may be unobtainable because there are inadequate tools for measuring the phenomena of interest. The most unjustifiable research is research undertaken too early thus consuming resources that could have been devoted to research with some probability of succeeding. Therefore, in developing a research agenda, it is important to be cognizant of the state of the art.

In general, research proceeds in stages from the exploratory to the descriptive to the analytical to the experimental. In the first stage, the aim is to develop insights that allow a potentially unlimited range of characteristics to be narrowed sufficiently to make it possible to observe them. At this stage, researchers seek ideas from literature, personal contacts, or other encounters and attempt to integrate diverse pieces of information. In contrast to other types of studies, the researcher's subjective impressions are often helpful in formulating strategies and approaches. In this stage, there are no data; there are only intuitive knowledge and conventional wisdom. Life experiences are required for mastery of a subject in this phase of knowledge. In the second (descriptive) phase of research, unplanned events are systematically observed. Although there are no hypotheses, the variables of interest are specified. In this stage of knowledge, there are isolated, disparate data, but only in small areas, and the findings are not generalizable. Case studies are examples of research in this stage. In the third (analytical) stage, research focuses on unplanned events, but there are specific hypotheses about interrelationships among observed events or characteristics. Experience can be validated by data, and data supplement experience in informing decisions. The fourth (experimental) phase is based on knowledge gained in the prior stages to provide a theoretical framework. Events are manipulated to test their effects, and specific hypotheses guide the search for knowledge about the interrelationships among variables. When there is a theory and when events can be tested within this theory, education and learning can occur without direct experience.

So little is known about the subject of chronic illness in childhood that much research is of the descriptive or analytic type. But as is the case in any field of endeavor, accumulation of knowledge is uneven, and in some areas, there is more than in others. In this chapter, only certain types of research are discussed. In health care, biomedical research provides knowledge about biological, physiological, biochemical, biophysical, and pathophysiological phenomena. Although much remains to be learned about the biomedical facets of chronic illness, this chapter focuses on the other two types of health care research: clinical and health services. The longer an illness persists and the more complex the etiology, the greater the likelihood that it will involve variables outside the biomedical model. Therefore, clinical and health services research needs are even more pressing for chronic illness than they are for acute illness. Clinical research deals with individual patients, whereas health services research deals with populations. A further distinction is in the nature of the variables. In clinical research, the variables derive primarily from biomedical phenomena, whereas in health services research, at least one variable must be other than a biomedical one (Institute of Medicine, 1979). The framework that guides health services research is presented in Figure 1. The health care system comprises a structure, a process, and an outcome. Impinging on all three are the social and physical environments, and there are interactions among all components. These interactions occur within constraints imposed by the genetic composition of the patient or population (Starfield, 1973). Although this framework specifies the general classes of variables involved in health services research, it does not specify the wide variety of components subsumed under each class. Definitions of most of the classes and of their components are available in the medical care literature, which is too extensive to summarize here. Also, the issue of costs of care, although not specified in the model, is understood to be superimposable on all aspects of the structure, process, and outcome of the health care system.

Figure 1. The Health Services System.

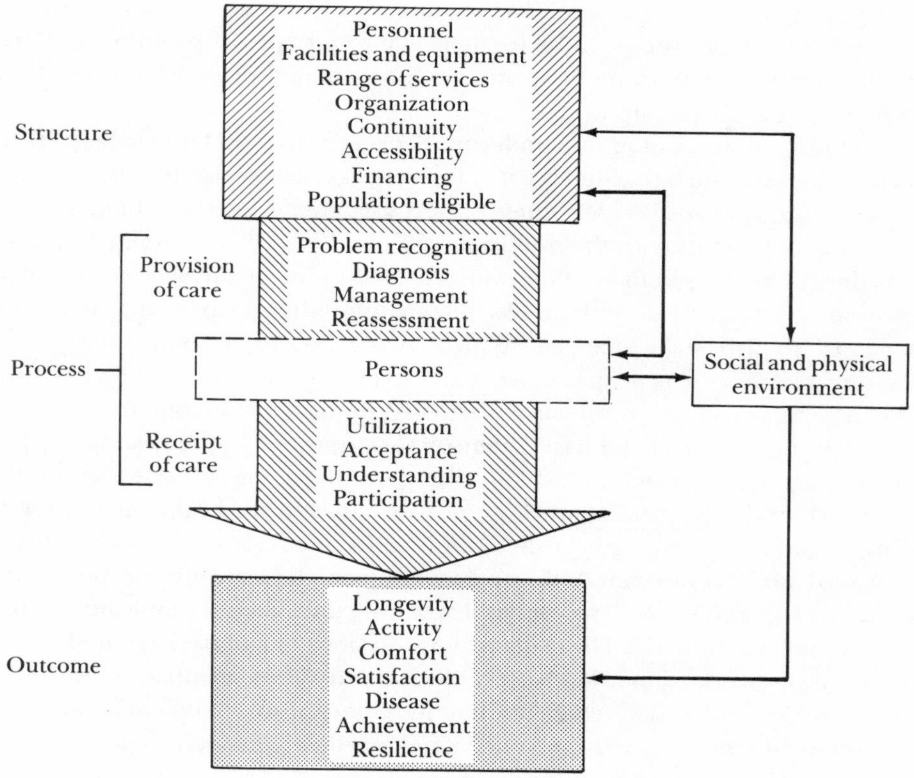

Source: Starfield, 1973.

Needed Research

Distribution and Etiology of Illness. Knowledge of the distribution, incidence, and prevalence of most chronic illnesses in childhood is limited. In fact, only one publication systematically examines the issue (Sultz and others, 1972). Except for the class of conditions with a known genetic defect, most of the problems have no precise definition. Therefore, estimation of their frequency in the population depends on application of criteria for which there is consensus as to their appropriateness. For example, the prevalence of asthma can be determined by the application of a set of questions derived from the "Question-naire on Respiratory Symptoms" developed and approved by the British Medical Research Council's Committee on the Etiology of Chronic Bronchitis (Medical Research Council, 1960). There are, however, no standard criteria for many conditions, even such common ones as otitis media (acute or chronic), enuresis, and (most notably) psychosocial problems in childhood.

Therefore, efforts to describe the nature of chronic problems and to use these descriptions to derive a consensus about ways to measure their prevalence in the population are high in priority. Without such efforts, there will continue to be erroneous perceptions of the frequency of occurrence of common and rare conditions alike, and failure to appreciate their magnitude as health problems to which children are subject.

Studies of the etiology of conditions depend in part on knowledge of their distribution. Most such research is generated in large medical centers, but because of their nature as referral centers, these centers see patients unrepresentative of the population of patients with the conditions (White, 1961). In addition, researchers in medical centers are more likely to see conditions relatively late in their evolution and to see those with more severe manifestations. Conditions that have progressed to this stage may be atypical of conditions as they exist in the community, and there is no assurance that the etiology of this subset of problems is the same as that of the problems as they exist in the wider community.

Although clinical and basic biomedical techniques are now being applied to determine etiology of almost all illnesses, limitation of research to the biomedical model is insufficient. Yet, most research in medical centers is done by investigators trained only in the biomedical model. Exclusive focus on the biomedical model compromises the understanding of disease causation and limits the range of therapies that can be employed to reduce diseases and their effects (Mishler and others, 1981). The classical formulations of Dubos (1961) and Cassel (1974) and the work of many other physicians and social scientists attest to the social causes of illness; their elucidation requires an approach, research tools, and techniques different from those suited to biomedical research. The effects of phenomena such as poverty (Black, 1980; Egbuonu and Starfield, 1982), stress, social isolation—for example, the effect of widowhood—(Susser, 1981), and conditions of work (American Public Health Association, 1975) are often so profound as to dwarf biological defects, yet research into these as concomitants of disease is generally neglected. A more consistent policy to include demographic and social factors in studies of disease is essential in providing an adequate base of knowledge about the etiology, natural history, and prognosis of chronic conditions in children.

Natural History and Prognosis of Illness in Childhood. As is the case with regard to distribution and etiology of illnesses in childhood, little is known about their natural history and prognosis. Most available information derives from experience in tertiary medical centers. Notable in this regard are the long-term studies of children with diabetes who received their care from the Joslin Clinic. Although data gained from such studies can provide the very important descriptive information necessary for the formulation of hypotheses for research, experience in tertiary centers is limited by virtue of its focus on individuals who choose to be cared for in those facilities and who are likely to be unrepresentative of all patients with the condition. A typical child receives care from many different sources (Levy and others, 1979), and each place deals with only a portion of the child's health problems. Moreover, physicians vastly overestimate the extent to which they are central in the patient's health care: With the exception of those in public clinics, physicians in Washington, D.C., claimed that most of their patients were regular users of care at their facility; in three of the facilities, the doctors thought all patients were regular patients (Dutton, 1981). Yet, in some facilities, more than two of five visits children made were to sources of care other than the one identified as the regular source.

Physicians are frequently unaware of the fact that patients under their care are receiving care elsewhere. In a study in three different facilities (a teaching hospital, an urban prepaid group, and a suburban prepaid group), a large proportion of child patients made a visit elsewhere during a period in which they were under care of a particular physician for a particular problem (Starfield and others, 1976). The primary care practitioner scheduled a visit to another clinic or physician for one in nine children sometime during the interval between two regular follow-up visits. In addition, at least one in ten children made an unanticipated visit elsewhere during this intervening period. The physicians who were caring for the patient sometimes followed up on the occurrence of the visits they themselves scheduled, but they infrequently followed up on (or knew about) visits the patients made on their own. At most, only about a quarter of these visits were recognized. Moreover, the content of these visits and their diagnoses and therapies were rarely integrated into the care given these patients even though, in some proportion of cases, it must have had a bearing on the management of the problem being followed. It is clear that physicians seeing children generally do not know the full burden of the children's illnesses. Most children are seen sporadically or not at all, whether their care is provided in offices, outpatient departments, or specialty clinics. And even if some children are seen regularly in general or specialty clinics it is for only a subset of their problems.

Although evidence is scant, a review of the literature regarding the relative constancy and change of physical health in childhood suggests that many childhood conditions generally considered to be acute and self-limited may not be so (Starfield and Pless, 1980). Rather, they may be associated with persistent or recurrent dysfunction manifested years later. Although the conclusions for specific health conditions are tentative because of relatively limited data, it appears that children who experience otitis media, mild respiratory illnesses, and such problems as frequent school absences, misuse of medication, and restricted activity are at relatively high risk of having those or related problems later on. Moreover, it appears that children having certain conditions later on in childhood were much more likely than children without these problems to have had antecedents early in life; that is, conditions such as enuresis, teenage respiratory problems, and urinary tract infection when present later on are found often to have been present earlier. There is also evidence that illnesses—acute, chronic, and both together—cluster in the population rather than being distributed randomly (Hinkle and Wolff, 1957; Starfield and others, 1984). Some people have much more than their share of illnesses of all types than others, and some have very little.

Despite the historical attention given to the concept of the vulnerable child (Levy, 1980), little is known about the distribution and characteristics of such children or the likelihood of reversing the ominous prognosis conveyed by the term *vulnerability*. Poor children, children from certain minority groups, children with physical and mental handicaps, children with chronic illness, and children born prematurely are all thought to be at increased risk of subsequent problems and therefore vulnerable. However, it is increasingly clear that other children may also be vulnerable, including those with recurrent acute illnesses (Starfield and Pless, 1980) and psychosocial problems (Starfield, 1982). Although much is known about the characteristics that predispose chronically ill children to poor adaptation (Pless, 1981), most of the research is descriptive and based on studies of limited numbers of children with specific health problems in individual clinics. So far, there has been little attempt to develop a theory of vulnerability that could guide research of a more sophisticated, analytical form. Focus on specific conditions in disparate facilities also impedes generalizability and retards the development of the conceptual framework that would facilitate hypothesis testing. Therefore, conduct of studies that involve different types of populations and that do not limit the number of specific conditions or handicaps is of the greatest priority in this area.

This is also the case for use of health services. The median and modal number of visits in a population of children is below the mean, and a relatively small percentage of children accounts for a relatively large proportion of visits (Starfield, 1981a). Moreover, children who are high users in one year are much more likely to continue to be high users than would be the case if utilization were distributed by chance alone. In two facilities separated by three thousand miles and ten years, the proportion of children who are consistently high users is more than three times (13 percent) greater than could be accounted for by chance distribution of high use (4 percent). The reason for this uneven distribution is unclear; it is unlikely to be a reflection of the presence of chronic illness in relatively few children because the proportion of children who are high users is greater than the prevalence of serious chronic illness in the population (Starfield, van den Berg, and Katz, 1979).

Children who are persistently high users are much more likely than other children to have multiple types of morbidity, only one of which is a typical chronic illness (Starfield and others, manuscript in preparation). That is, chronic illness by itself does not produce high use of services; it does so only in combination with other types of illness. Illness, like utilization, does not distribute randomly in the population. What makes some children prone to a variety of types of ailments and some children relatively free of any? What factors ameliorate risk? Current clinical and epidemiological research focuses on the detection of factors predisposing to disease. In contrast, little effort is expended in identifying protective factors (Orchard, 1980). Attention to both risk factors and protective factors should provide an understanding of why all vulnerable children do not suffer problems and why some children ostensibly not at risk do. As is the case with risk factors, protective factors may be social as well as biological, and both types must be considered (Starfield, 1983a). Children vulnerable to illness and its sequelae as a result of poverty are an especially challenging group. Not all poor children are destined to experience health problems, and some are notably free of the physical and psychological morbidity that is of relatively high prevalence among the group as a whole. To what extent is there a protective effect, and what is its nature? Research is needed on the independent effects of the various dimensions of social stratification (income, education, parental occupation, housing) (Black, 1980) as well as on genetic factors and familial aggregation, individual and group health behaviors, and access to and receipt of medical care. Carefully planned and longitudinal studies of the development of illness in childhood should help elucidate the social and biological concomitants of this phenomenon.

Impact of Illness. Between 10 and 20 percent of children have an illness that can be considered chronic in the sense that it persists longer than a few days or a few weeks (Mahoney, 1979; Pless and Pinkerton, 1975). According to the definition used by the National Center for Health Statistics, a chronic illness is one that lasts three months or more or is a diagnosis that is widely considered to be chronic. Examples of the latter are asthma, allergies, diabetes, epilepsy, "mental or nervous trouble," and rheumatic fever. Impairments are conditions such as deafness, vision problems, congenital defects such as cleft palate, stammering, cerebral palsy, and skeletal deformities. These conditions have little in common except for their tendency to persist. As a class, chronic illness is heterogeneous in type of etiology, severity, and prognosis. Although physicians and other medical practitioners rely heavily on the diagnostic rubric to guide them in management of care of patients, the significant feature for patients and families is not the name of the illness but rather its outcome including its prognosis and impact on function. Studying children with a variety of chronic illnesses, Stein and colleagues examined functional status, impact on family, child and mother's psychological adjustment, satisfaction with care, unmet health needs, burden of illness, and social resources for coping (Stein and Jessop,

1982). These investigators demonstrated that the variability within diseases was much greater than the variability among them, a finding that supports the legitimacy of a noncategorical approach to assessing the impact of illness on children.

Measurement of outcome is even more a challenge in children than in adults. In adults, the impact of illness and its alleviation by medical care are usually reflected in changes in limitation of physical activities and ability to carry on the tasks necessary to daily life and to earn a livelihood. In contrast to children, the lives of adults are relatively routine over long periods of time. In children, the rapidity of the processes of development and learning presents the individual with opportunities to meet ever new challenges. Adaptability, a desirable trait at all ages, is imperative for the optimum growth of children. Therefore, any approach to the measurement of health status in children must include not only the well-accepted measures of physical function but also physical and psychological characteristics that reflect adaptability.

It has been customary to divide health status into three components: physical, psychological, and social. Impact of illness on the child's family is an additional dimension that has received wide currency. The state of the art of measures of health status has been summarized by Ware and others (1981). There are also summaries relating specifically to children (Eisen and others, 1979) and relating to impact of children's ill health on the family (Pless, 1981).

Research on the development of measures of outcome is still in its infancy, although there are signs of progress in conceptualization and instrumentation. A conceptual model consisting of a profile categorizes outcome along seven dimensions: longevity, activity, comfort, satisfaction, disease, achievement, and resilience (Starfield, 1974). In contrast to most other measures of health, this model does not divide health into separate physical, psychological, and social components; rather, it reflects their inseparability in real life. The development of a valid system of scoring along each of the dimensions requires a collaborative effort involving individuals with expertise in clinical medicine, psychology, and sociology as well as experts in measurement. Such teams would identify all existing methods of measuring the dimensions and identify a series of positions along each dimension. Each existing instrument would have to be examined to determine both its applicability to the general population of children (not only to those with particular illnesses or from particular sociodemographic strata) and its sensitivity to changes in function as a result of normal development and the illness remissions or regressions that occur naturally or as a result of the receipt of medical care. Of particularly high priority are the development of measures that are more appropriate to the child's world than the measures currently in existence. Adults unconsciously bring their own preconceptions to bear in the instruments they develop. Very few investigators have consulted children for their concepts of normal and abnormal behavior. Because children's self-images are in large measure determined by their perceptions of how their peers regard them, any adequate functional status measure must incorporate the expectations that children have of each other.

The pressing need for methodological research on development of a measure of health status that also reflects the impact of illness need not preclude the application of measures already in existence. The pioneering efforts of the staff of the National Health Survey have already provided policy makers with benchmarks to measure the impact of important public programs (Starfield, 1981b; Newacheck and others, 1981). Although these measures are not sensitive enough for use on an individual level, others have used additional measures to refine or supplement the concepts of "restricted activity due to acute illness" and "limitation of activity due to chronic illness" (Clouser, Culver, and Gert, 1981; Schach and Starfield, 1973).

Pressures to hold down the costs of health care and to increase benefits are already requiring demonstrations of the effectiveness and efficiency of various clinical modalities and interventions. Demands of accountability to the public and for public participation in decision making are also putting stress on the medical care system. Pless (1981, p. 205) cogently stated this imperative as follows: "Another broad issue which must be addressed more directly in the future is that related to trade-offs in outcomes. Parents, children, and physicians may place different values on the many possible outcomes which may pertain to a particular intervention. The choice of a single or several closely related measures reveals some of the investigators' values and biases. There are, however, many other values implicit in such studies, and it is essential that these be identified and weighted appropriately."

There is a critical need for studies of the impact on health status of a variety of interventions. What type of practitioner does best, given certain types of populations and problems? What are the relative advantages of drug therapy, behavioral therapy, and social therapy? Under what circumstances do practitioner and patient suffice to bring about problem resolution, and what circumstances require other community and environmental alteration? How applicable is the time-honored professional dominance of the patient-physician relationship to the needs of modern medicine? Exploration of all of these important concerns requires a concentrated effort to transform the fragmented approaches to health status measurement into a system that can be applied in comparable fashion (with appropriate adaptations) to populations of children in different facilities and systems.

Recognition, Diagnosis, and Management of Illness. Efforts at assessing the quality of health care have traditionally addressed the processes of diagnosis and management. Medical curricula focus almost exclusively on training practitioners to make diagnoses; to support these diagnoses with appropriate information from the history, physical examination, and laboratory; and to institute therapy appropriate to the diagnoses. The focus is largely on the biochemical and biophysical basis of disease, and relatively little attention is devoted to the social and psychological causes of ill health. The emphasis is on assigning single causes for disease and on arriving at a single diagnosis. Students are taught how diseases typically manifest themselves and what therapies are typically appropriate, but they have little exposure to the concept of variability (the range of expression of illness and response to therapy in the population). Students learn about illness through experience with it rather than by any inferences or deductions from theory. Because the patients to whom students are exposed are not a representative sample of all patients with the illness (patients in teaching institutions are generally sicker and of different sociodemographic characteristics than patients in the wider population), what students learn may be appropriate only to a subset of patients. Moreover, students' exposure to patients is short-term. The educational process ill prepares them to assume responsibility for patients over long periods of time because it precludes their getting to know patients well enough to understand the dynamics of their illnesses. Yet, such understanding is critical to the success of medical care interventions.

A summary of the process by which physicians develop ways of understanding their patients has been adapted from Barnlund (1976) as follows: (1) individuals have their own frame of reference, which provides meaning out of the chaos of life events; (2) language plays a critical role in the construction of the frames of reference (although the research of others also indicates the important role of other means of expression); (3) every individual problem is in part a symbolic one; neither physicians nor patients are free of the influence of the way they define their situation. Therefore, there is no patient who does not present the medical problem with, at least in part, a symbolic problem that has a semantic dimension.

This formulation makes it clear that emphasis solely on diagnosis and management is inadequate in assuring the quality of health care. Although necessary, they are by themselves insufficient without attention to the critical first step of problem recognition. Elstein and colleagues (1978) have shown that physicians formulate a limited number of hypotheses about the patient's diagnosis early in their interaction with the patient. Once formed, these hypotheses are very difficult to discard, and positive evidence in support of them easily outweighs negative evidence against them.

If the process of medical education emphasizes certain aspects of the etiology and pathogenesis of illness, the mind-set of physicians makes it difficult for them to assimilate cues about other aspects of etiology and pathogenesis in their hypothesis generation and confirmation. Despite its critical importance, this process of problem recognition has not received the attention it merits in research. At least the following are known with some assurance:

1. Satisfaction with medical care is related to the degree to which patients believe their physician understands their concerns (Roter, 1977; Svarstad, 1976).
2. Adequate recognition of patients' problems is associated with better compliance (Hulka and others, 1976; Korsch, Freeman, and Negrete, 1971).
3. Professional dominance of the practitioner-patient interaction can be reduced by encouraging patients to express their problems more forcefully (Roter, 1977).
4. The outcome of care is associated with accurate recognition of patients' problems (Starfield and Scheff, 1972; Stewart, McWhinney, and Buck, 1979)

and with the degree to which the patient and practitioner agree on what the problem is (Starfield and others, 1979, 1981).

5. Physicians and nonphysician practitioners differ in the extent to which they identify and follow up on certain types of problems, and their skills are potentially complementary. The data also indicate that this potential is not fully exploited, particularly by physicians (Simborg, Starfield, and Horn, 1978).

6. Continuity of practitioner facilitates the follow-up of patients' problems from one visit to another (Starfield and others, 1976). It is associated with fewer total visits to health care facilities, probably due to increased use of the telephone as a result of increased familiarity of the practitioner with the patient (Breslau and Haug, 1976). Continuity of practitioner also increases parents' satisfaction with a wide variety of aspects of care (Breslau and Mortimer, 1981). Continuity of a practitioner team also enhances the disclosure of behavior problems by parents (Becker, Drachman, and Kirscht, 1974). However, a change in practitioner increases the extent to which there is follow-up of patients' problems if the initial practitioner failed to recognize the problem at a prior visit.

7. Certain medical record formats facilitate the follow-up of patients' problems (Simborg and others, 1976; Starfield and others, 1977).

These findings indicate directions for new research as follows:

1. Under what conditions and for what types of patients does continuity of practitioner improve recognition of patients' problems?

2. What types of personnel are best at recognizing what types of problems, and how can complementarity of skills be maximized in organization and provision of services?

3. What role does explicit conflict play in recognition of patients' problems? Medical education generally assumes a relatively passive, compliant role for patients with the doctor's role being one of educator. Roter's (1977) findings suggest that intentional precipitation of conflict may be a useful strategy for achievement of problem resolution, but the circumstances in which this is the case need exploration.

4. How can the role of patients themselves be maximized? Practitioners and patients could discuss problems and concerns and arrive at a consensus regarding their mutual expectations. Patients could maintain copies of records, generated by themselves or by their practitioners, that would contain a list of their problems and strategies used by both to alleviate them. Patients could also be given tape recordings of their interactions with practitioners or copies of encounter notes and be permitted to amend them.

5. Research regarding the characteristics of the practitioner-patient interaction, the practitioner's recognition of the variety of concerns of patients with different types of illnesses, and the impact of changes in these phenomena on the health of children is relatively sparse and much needed.

The Effects of Medical Care. Although the medical profession continues to enjoy a generally high image in the minds of the public, there is increasing skepticism about the benefits of individual medical interventions. In response to popular demand, access to care was improved in the 1960s and 1970s primarily by providing financing of care for those with low incomes and by taking steps to increase the supply of health manpower by training more physicians, nurses, and physician assistants. Although there is evidence that this resulted in greater (and undoubtedly needed) use of services, particularly among the poor, anticipated great improvements in health status as a result of increased access have not been evident. In particular, the prevalence of chronic illness has increased and continues to increase over the most recent two decades, even among children (Starfield, 1981b; Wilson, 1981; Colvez and Blanchet, 1981). Declining death rates cannot, alone, account for these increases, at least part of which may be a result of better access to care and, hence, increased diagnosis of chronic ailments. The increase may also be a result either of enhanced risk of chronic disease or of a declining ability of the health profession to deal adequately with problems of this nature.

Attempts to improve effectiveness and reduce costs of medical care have taken various forms, but little is known either about the usefulness of the approaches or their differential effects on individuals with various types of problems. Outstanding questions for research include the following:

1. To what extent does comprehensiveness facilitate the recognition, diagnosis, and management of children with various types of problems? The findings of early research were ambiguous about the usefulness of comprehensiveness, but in no case was the concept of comprehensiveness translated into any operational measure. More recent studies, which are more precise in specifying comprehensiveness as a full range of services, suggest that it is probably less important than related but distinguishable features of care such as continuity of physician (Breslau and Mortimer, 1981). There is also the possibility that comprehensiveness may be disadvantageous, particularly to the extent that responsibility for routine preventive care is in the same hands as care for illness (Silver, 1979). Researchers who address comprehensiveness should be aware of the importance of defining the concept in designing their study. Comprehensiveness requires specification of the range of services that a health facility agrees to provide as well as ascertainment of the extent to which its practitioners recognize the need to provide appropriate services (Starfield, 1979).

2. To what extent does the development of a relationship over time, regardless of the presence or absence of particular types of problems, facilitate recognition, diagnosis, and management of health problems, and especially, to what extent does it prevent the emergence of health problems? There are those who believe that preventive care in childhood is best achieved by separating it from the other functions of the health care system (Silver, 1979). In the United States, prevention is considered a function to be performed by the primary care practitioner. Evidence on this issue would be useful in designing better systems to achieve health and prevent illness.

3. What kinds of problems are best managed by the general pediatrician (or other primary care practitioner) and which are best referred to subspecialists? When problems do require referral, what mechanisms are required to achieve coordination of care so that conflicting recommendations and duplication of procedures are avoided?

4. What is the proper balance between primary care (general) pediatricians, general and family physicians, nonphysician practitioners, and pediatric

subspecialists? In the United States, generalist and family physicians are as likely as pediatricians to be identified as a child's regular source of care (Starfield, 1983a). Pediatricians contribute a slightly greater proportion of visits than family-oriented physicians primarily because they are more likely to see younger children who visit more frequently. But more than 20 percent of all visits made by children are to other types of physicians, and the proportion of these visits that are for primary care problems (as distinct from problems requiring expertise in a particular type of problem) is unknown. What training is required for generalists (pediatricians or family physicians) to enable them to achieve these essentials of primary care: accessibility, coordination, comprehensiveness, and longitudinality (Starfield, 1979)? How can the training of practitioners stress mechanisms of referral to specialists and assure that primary care physicians learn how to provide adequate information to consultants as well as how to receive adequate information back from them?

5. What effect do the vagaries of public policy have on receipt of medical care and on response to it? Cutbacks in federal funding of programs for the poor, without assurances that other agencies will assume responsibility, can be expected to reduce access for the poor, and especially for poor children. Maintenance of data systems and monitoring for these effects, as well as for effects on health status, are essential. At the very least, trends in neonatal mortality, postneonatal mortality, childhood mortality, disability days (including school absences), and limitations of activity due to health conditions in each of several subgroups of children (those in different income groups especially) require ongoing assessment to observe for signs that progress is not being maintained or is reversing.

   Planning More Adequate Health Services. In contrast to many other industrialized nations, the United States does not have a regionalized system of health care. Historically, regionalization has been attempted in certain areas since the 1930s. But recent attempts at formalizing relationships among various levels of care (for example, the Regional Medical Programs of the 1960s) have not met with success. The only current example of attempted regionalization in child health care concerns perinatal care, and evaluations of experiments on regionalization for high-risk perinatal care are just becoming available (Shapiro and others, 1981).

   Rising health care costs and attempts to reduce them dictate a more rational deployment of resources. Practitioner's offices and community hospitals cannot maintain expensive technology unless it can be used justifiably and with sufficient frequency and accuracy to make it practical.

   Priorities of research are the following:

1. What technologies are appropriate at what levels of care? To what extent can procedures such as tympanometry be justified in primary care practice? What are its benefits in terms of patients' convenience, satisfaction, and maintenance of health; and what are its costs and unintended effects? To what extent can rehabilitative therapy for chronic illness and impairments be carried out in primary care practice, and to what extent should it be a responsibility of referral and consultative centers? To what extent can diagnostic procedures be decentralized into small laboratories, and what is the impact of decentralization on quality of testing and on costs?

The impact on costs of frequently performed technology, such as that carried out in office laboratories, is only recently being recognized (Moloney and Rogers, 1979). Should the performance of screening procedures, such as those employed in the newborn period, be at the discretion of the primary care physician, or does the maintenance of quality and penetration of the population demand that such procedures be organized at the secondary or tertiary level of care? Under what circumstances is screening justified, and when do the benefits cease to outweigh the costs? Unfortunately, no test is completely sensitive or specific; that is, there are always false negative results and false positive results (Griner and others, 1981). False negative tests give an unwarranted sense of security to both the physician and the patient, but false positive tests have equally undesirable effects. Patients with false positive results are destined to experience additional examinations that require expenditure of time, funds, and inconvenience. Most seriously, the possibility of iatrogenic complications increases with the number of procedures performed. The degree of likelihood of unintended psychological, economical, or physical trauma needs to be evaluated for existing and new technologies and screening procedures. Public concern mandates that the profession provide data that will help society make rational decisions about which procedures are warranted and which facilities should be reimbursed for performing them.

2. Rational planning for health services demands much more data about children's needs than has been the case up to now. A low occupancy rate in many hospitals results in demands for the closing of beds, particularly beds for children. Efforts to reduce inflation in the health care sector are causing many states to impose new methods of paying hospitals for care.

In the past, hospitals and physicians have been reimbursed according to their fee for every service rendered, a process thought to encourage performance of many nonessential procedures. As states increasingly adopt reimbursement schemes based on cases rather than services and on prepayment rather than fee-for-service, it is imperative that research provide the data that make the process rational. Different practitioners and different facilities are likely to differ in their case-mix (the diversity of problems seen and their severity); thus it is illogical to devise schemes that reimburse each facility equally because their expenses will differ. At present, no method for specifying case-mix has been developed for widespread use. Several approaches to case-mix definition in adults are under development (Horn, 1982), and the method of staging specific illnesses (Gonella and others, 1977) includes some conditions occurring in childhood. Both efforts are limited to inpatient care. Researchers involved in concerns of children with ambulatory care problems have not yet become involved in this area, which promises to be an increasingly important one in public policy and organization of child health facilities and services.

Alternative Strategies for Dealing with Chronic Illness and Its Effects. Preeminence of the medical model in medical education and practice is responsible for primary emphasis on pharmaceutical management in medical care. Alternative strategies are frequently not even considered. The problem of enuresis is a case in point. In a recent survey of physicians' and parents' attitudes toward enuresis carried out in nine different facilities, 28 percent of physicians usually suggested medication for the management of enuresis, even though only 6.6

percent of parents felt that medication was a very good way of dealing with the problem (Shelov and others, 1981). Research on management of enuresis in Great Britain and Australia largely focuses on methods involving conditioning therapy. In contrast, most research carried out by physicians in the United States involves the testing of various drugs. Although several groups of psychologists have developed and assessed the effectiveness of behavioral approaches to enuresis (Azrin and Thienes, 1978), their work fails to reach pediatricians because their reports are published in journals not generally read by physicians. Another example concerns iron-deficiency anemia. The standard therapy for this type of anemia is iron-containing medication. Yet a study of the effectiveness of care for children with low hemoglobin revealed that maternal awareness of the problem was the factor most related to increases in the hemoglobin level. On the other hand, prescription of iron medication by itself was not highly related to outcome (Starfield and Scheff, 1972). Health professionals (such as nurses), whose training is based less on the medical model and more on social support models, prescribe more nondrug therapies than physicians (Simborg, Starfield, and Horn, 1978).

The predictable and relatively frequent adverse effects of drugs and their relatively high cost as compared with nondrug therapy suggest a pressing need for controlled trials of alternative modes of therapy. Behavioral therapy, particularly that involving individual patients in an active rather than passive role, is one type of alternative. Other types involve interventions that are more social in nature. An example of a social intervention is provided by the multicenter hypertension detection and follow-up program, which in addition to facilitating drug therapy, involved patients in group social activities during the course of the study (Hypertension Detection and Follow-Up Program Cooperative Group, 1979).

The development and testing of mechanisms for social support received particular attention in a recent report of the National Research Council (1981, p. x) in which the preface states that, largely because children "are hardly ever viewed as entire human beings in their homes, families, and community environments . . . services for children are falling short of the expectations of parents, program administrators, and legislators." Focusing on services for children with particular categories of problems (such as particular diseases or handicaps) detracts from attention to children as entire human beings who live, work, and play in communities. The report recommended enlarging the frame of reference for children's services and chose three areas to illustrate how to do this: (1) Research should take into account that it is no longer atypical for children, even preschoolers, to be cared for outside the home for at least part of the average day. How can this time away from home be used to provide the social support so necessary for the proper development of every person? (2) For adolescents, the report recommended research on the "social context and incidence of specific behaviors," on "patterns of family care," on the "effectiveness of community-based services," and on "adolescent emancipation" (pp. 60–65). (3) Research "should include measures of the costs to parents, communities, and society of providing or not providing particular services, [including] both direct benefits to children and indirect benefits to their families and other institutions participating in their care" (p. 74).

The Effects of Research Itself. The National Commission for the Protection of Human Subjects of Biomedical and Behavioral Research took much longer to produce its recommendations regarding research on children than it did for adults (U.S. Department of Health, Education, and Welfare, 1978). Even at the date of this writing, federal regulations for research on children had not yet been adopted. Procedures to be followed under the proposed regulations depend on decisions about the degree of risk to which children are subjected by the research. Institutional Review Board (IRB) members need not address issues of benefit or assent if a project is of minimal risk or less. The proposed regulations state that whether a procedure involves more than minimal risk should be determined by comparing it to procedures normally encountered in the daily lives or in the routine medical, dental, or psychological examination of healthy children. Despite this definition, a substantial proportion of respondents to a survey rated procedures such as intestinal intubations, placebo injections, bone scans, and placement on a metabolic bed for twenty-four hours as of no more than minimal risk (Janofsky and Starfield, 1981). Evidence derived from clinical or epidemiological studies is lacking, and at present, the only alternatives (which are not mutually exclusive) are to rely on judgments of individual IRB members, to take into account the judgments of a population of pediatric research experts, or to seek the input of individuals such as community representatives, the clergy, and lawyers. None of these types of individuals should have the same vested interest in the conduct of research as researchers themselves. Support of the collection of data from multiple research units employing comparable techniques of observation to determine the difficulties and complications of research procedures is required if important decisions are to be based on fact rather than on opinion.

Principles for obtaining the assent of children involved in research are also unclear. Although the involvement of parents in providing informed consent is required by the regulations, there are few data that examine the risks and benefits of informed consent and no data dealing with the risks and benefits of the child's assent or the conditions under which risks are minimized and benefits maximized. Characteristics of particular interest are the child's developmental and chronological age, degree and type of illness, social supports, and psychological characteristics. Work under way to examine the effects of informed consent for newborn screening provides a model for the kinds of efforts that are required for all research on children (Holtzman and others, 1980). Research designed to determine the nature and degree of risk of research itself and ways to alter these is of great priority in order to maximize safeguards to health.

Research on Illness Paradigms. A long-term agenda for research would be incomplete without mention of the need for research to explore new ways of viewing illness. The current paradigm of illness, which derives primarily from anatomical-physiological models, is reflected in existing methods for classifying illness. Although this classification of illness is consistent with the disease-by-disease approach taken in clinical education and therefore with the nature of current medical practice, it may become dysfunctional as the nature of illnesses changes. Advances in medical care have led to improved survival of individuals with illnesses that used to be rapidly fatal, and this places individuals at risk of having multiple diagnoses. The effects of multiple diagnoses on physiological function, on physical function, on need for medical care or requirements for therapy, and on prognosis for length of productive life are largely unknown. Continued classification by individual diseases may increasingly impede understanding of these phenomena because the impact of a multiplicity of diagnoses is certainly different from the sum of the impacts of the individual components. Also, the immensely greater exposure to new types of environmental and social pathogens consequent to technological advances creates new risks, the manifestations of which have not even begun to be catalogued. It is virtually certain that these will lead to biological and psychological derangements that will be more or less symptomatic but certainly not classifiable using standard nomenclature of disease. More population-based research will be necessary to point to directions that can be exploited by clinical and basic research.

The nature of the new paradigms is not yet clear, but several alternatives come to mind. Systems based on type of etiology rather than anatomical site may be useful, as might systems based on prognosis for duration of normal activity, reduced activity, or life itself. The paradigm under which we now operate has served well for several hundred years, but rapidity of technological development makes demands on the imagination of scientists and clinicians for new ones.

Principles to Guide Research

A Theoretical Model. Research is a systematic process designed to produce generalizable knowledge. If the process is to be systematic and if knowledge is to be generalizable, research ultimately must be conducted within a theoretical framework or model that guides the testing of postulated relationships between characteristics or events. Earlier in this chapter, a model was described that can serve as a theoretical framework for both clinical and health services research and is based on the assumption that health is a function of genetic factors, personal behavior, medical care interventions, and the social and physical environment. Clinical research stresses the relationships between components of the process and outcome of the health care system. Health services research involves the investigation of two or more of the variables in the model, but at least one of the variables is derived from a conceptual framework other than that of contemporary biomedical science (Institute of Medicine, 1979). (Biomedical science views the human organism in terms of its anatomical structure and physiological processes and identifies, classifies, and explains diseases, which are usually defined as structural malformations, chemical lesions, or behavioral abnormalities.) The ability to draw inferences from a myriad of separate research activities conducted by a variety of types of researchers at diverse institutions will depend on the extent to which their research is guided by a common theoretical framework. Therefore, the first step in planning new research should be an attempt to specify precisely where in the common framework the research fits. The appropriate literature can then be reviewed to determine the state of the art on the subject and to provide clues to guide the development of hypotheses, definition of variables, and tools of measurement.

Population-Based Approaches. There are at least five reasons why population-based approaches should be part of investigations on determinants of health and effects of medical care (Starfield, 1981a). First, the distribution of health problems in the community cannot be understood by concentrating only on patients appearing in teaching centers or tertiary care hospitals. Second, knowledge of how problems initially present cannot be derived without research based in the community where problems initially arise. Third, the results of care cannot be understood without efforts to follow up on the effects of management strategies in the communities where people live and work. Controlled clinical trials of therapeutic interventions can provide information on the efficacy of these interventions (that is, on their effects under controlled conditions), but the effectiveness of the interventions (their impact when used under usual life circumstances) can be understood only by examining their effect when they are carried out by ordinary people under everyday conditions of living. Fourth, certain types of problems cannot be recognized without a broader view than is customary in clinical facilities catering to referred patients or organized by types of medical specialties. Most patients have a diversity of problems whose interactions can be understood only by viewing patients in the context of their community. Fifth, a population-based approach is necessary to understand the interrelationships between the existence of health problems, the use of health services, and the effect of these on subsequent health. Singular focus on particular clinical manifestations of illness without adequate attention to children as they grow and develop over long periods of time will produce gaps in knowledge about the dynamics of illnesses, their causes, and their prognoses.

Development of Information Systems and Standardized Nomenclature for Problems and Their Functional Impact. Because the health problems, particularly the traditional chronic illnesses, of children are relatively uncommon as compared with adults, research to elucidate their nature, impact, and prognosis frequently requires that comparable research be conducted in several different sites to produce a sufficient number of children for stable estimates of results. Research may be done collaboratively, with joint planning and analysis, or it may be done separately. In either case, comparability of concept, of definition of variables, and of methods of analysis is essential. The basic system for collecting data on children seen in the various facilities should be similar. Advances in instrumentation that enable office-based practitioners to have their own mini-computers provide an opportunity that was previously impossible. Although most commercially available systems are devised for administrative purposes, including billing, several can be adapted for research purposes. An adequate data system should have the capability of providing data on the characteristics of individual children as well as on the characteristics of visits.

Use of coding schemes more appropriate to ambulatory care problems than the International Classification of Diseases (ICD) should be encouraged. The International Classification of Health Problems in Primary Care (ICHPPC) provides one example of a system based on the ICD but supplementing it to make it more suited to health problems experienced by children in communities (World Organization of National Colleges, 1979). Other new and better systems are under development. Where different facilities use different schemes for classifying problems, an early step in planning research involves the translation of one classification scheme into the other. As this is generally a tedious process, forethought in the development of schemes so they are comparable at the outset will provide for much greater consistency and efficiency. Encouragement of research on children should be accompanied by efforts to explore the potential of adapting existing data systems and for developing additional ones where they are needed.

Incorporating Research into Training of Practitioners. During their medical training, students and house officers have little exposure to the type of research addressed in this chapter. As a result, interest in these areas is not generated during the years when career ideas are formed, and opportunities to learn the skills required to address these areas are missed. All trainees should be required to keep records of all inpatients and outpatients for whom they provide any care. Periodically, the patients' medical charts should be reviewed by a preceptor and the trainee to determine the patients' patterns of care and their responses to therapy. At least once during the training, all trainees as a group should review their experiences to determine sociodemographical and clinical characteristics of patients seen, approaches taken toward understanding and managing their problems, and results of interventions. The primary aim of this exercise is to provide trainees with skills in looking at populations of patients, to recognize evidence of variability among patients and among physicians, to explore reasons for that variability, and to consider its implications for future patient care and research. Trainees who become interested in particular aspects of this exercise should be encouraged to develop specific questions that lend themselves to research and to design and conduct a small research project under appropriate guidance.

The generation of issues requiring investigation is a fruitless task if there are too few trained individuals to translate them into research. Development of a research agenda requires parallel consideration of the development of needed resources. Although this section has considered only the preliminary stages involving the stimulation of interest in research, the formal training of researchers and the requirements of that training also must be addressed.

Broadened Focus of Research. Previous sections of this chapter have stressed the need to view illness from the perspective of the individual rather than from the perspective of the disease. For research of this type to develop and flourish, new organizational and financial arrangements for the conduct of research are required. Models of research that focus on diseases or organ systems are not appropriate for research of the type described in this chapter. Parenthetically, we should note that the research program of the National Institutes of Health is categorical in the sense that it is addressed toward particular diseases, conditions, or organ systems. Although it has been eminently successful in producing knowledge about the biomedical correlates of disease, it has not adequately addressed concerns that transcend individual diseases, types of diseases, functional impact of illness, or etiologies other than biomedical. The new imperatives require approaches that cross diseases and categorical agencies. New mechanisms of organization and funding may have to be developed to support this endeavor to provide knowledge to prevent illness and maximize the healthy development of children.

References

American Public Health Association. *Health and Work in America: A Chart Book*. Washington, D.C.: American Public Health Association, 1975.

Azrin, N., and Thienes, P. "Rapid Elimination of Enuresis by Intensive Learning Without a Conditioning Apparatus." *Behavior Therapy*, 1978, *9*, 342–354.

Barnlund, D. "The Mystification of Meaning: Doctor-Patient Encounters." *Journal of Medical Education*, 1976, *51*, 716–725.

Becker, M., Drachman, R., and Kirscht, J. "A Field Experiment to Evaluate Various Outcomes of Continuity of Physician Care." *American Journal of Public Health*, 1974, *64*, 1062–1070.

Black, D. *Inequalities in Health: Report of a Research Working Group*. London: Department of Health and Social Security of Great Britain, 1980.

Breslau, N., and Haug, M. "Service Delivery Structure and Continuity of Care: A Case Study of a Pediatric Practice in Process of Reorganization." *Journal of Health and Social Behavior*, 1976, *17*, 339–352.

Breslau, N., and Mortimer, E. "Seeing the Same Doctor: Determinants of Satisfaction with 'Specialty Care' for Disabled Children." *Medical Care*, 1981, *19*, 741–758.

Cassel, J. C. "Psychosocial Processes and Stress: Theoretical Formulation." *International Journal of Health Services*, 1974, *4* (3), 471–482.

Clouser, K., Culver, C., and Gert, B. "Malady: A New Treatment of Disease." *The Hastings Center Report*, 1981, *11*, 29–37.

Colvez, A., and Blanchet, M. "Disability Trends in the United States Population, 1966–76: Analysis of Reported Causes." *American Journal of Public Health*, 1981, *71*, 464–471.

Dubos, R. *Mirage of Health: Utopias, Progress and Biological Change*. New York: Anchor Books, 1961.

Dutton, D. "Children's Health Care: The Myth of Equal Access." In Select Panel for the Promotion of Child Health, *Better Health for Our Children: A National Strategy*. Vol. 4. Washington, D.C.: U.S. Government Printing Office, 1981.

Egbuonu, L., and Starfield, B. "Child Health and Social Status." *Pediatrics*, 1982, *69*, 550–555.

Eisen, M., and others. "Measuring Components of Children's Health Status." *Medical Care,* 1979, *17,* 902-921.

Elstein, A., Shulman, L. and Sprafka, S. *Medical Problem-Solving: An Analysis of Clinical Reasoning.* Cambridge, Mass.: Harvard University Press, 1978.

Gonella, J., and others. "Use of Outcome Measures in Ambulatory Care Evaluation." In G. Giebink, N. White, and E. Short (Eds.), *Ambulatory Medical Care—Quality Assurance, 1977: Proceedings of a Conference.* La Jolla, Calif.: La Jolla Science Publications, 1977.

Griner, P., and others. "Selection and Interpretation of Diagnostic Tests and Procedures: Principles and Applications." *Annals of Internal Medicine,* 1981, *94* (4), 553-600.

Hinkle, L., and Wolff, H. "The Nature of Man's Adaptation to His Total Environment and the Relation of This to Illness." *Archives of Internal Medicine,* 1957, *99,* 442.

Holtzman, N., and others. "Informed Consent Improves Knowledge of Neonatal Screening, Abstracted." *Pediatric Research,* 1980, *14,* 489.

Horn, S. "Severity Index Applied to DRGs Accounts for Sicker Patients." *Hospitals,* 1982, *56* (24), 37.

Hulka, B., and others. "Communication, Compliance, and Concordance Between Physicians and Patients with Prescribed Medication." *American Journal of Public Health,* 1976, *66,* 847-853.

Hypertension Detection and Follow-Up Program Cooperative Group. "Five-Year Findings of the Hypertension Detection and Follow-Up Program." *Journal of the American Medical Association,* 1979, *242,* 2562-2576.

Institute of Medicine. *Health Services Research.* Washington, D.C.: National Academy of Sciences, 1979.

Janofsky, J., and Starfield, B. "Assessment of Risk in Research on Children." *Journal of Pediatrics,* 1981, *98,* 842-846.

Korsch, B., Freeman, B., and Negrete, V. "Practical Implications of Doctor-Patient Interaction Analyses for Pediatric Practice." *American Journal of Diseases of Children,* 1971, *121,* 110-114.

Levy, J. "Vulnerable Children: Parents, Perspectives, and the Use of Medical Care." *Pediatrics,* 1980, *65,* 956-963.

Levy, J., and others. "Primary Care: Patterns of Use of Pediatric Medical Facilities." *Medical Care,* 1979, *17,* 881-893.

Mahoney, M. "A Perspective on Child Care Needs in the 1980s." Address to the Institute of Medicine, National Academy of Sciences, October 25, 1979.

Medical Research Council. "Standardized Questionnaire on Respiratory Symptoms." *British Medical Journal,* 1960, *2,* 1665.

Mishler, E., and others. *Social Contexts of Health, Illness, and Patient Care.* Cambridge, England: Cambridge University Press, 1981.

Moloney, T., and Rogers, D. "Medical Technology—A Different View of the Contentious Debate over Costs." *New England Journal of Medicine,* 1979, *301,* 1413-1419.

National Research Council. *Services for Children: An Agenda for Research.* Study Project on Children's Services, Committee on Child Development Research and Public Policy, Assembly of Behavioral and Social Sciences. Washington, D.C.: National Academy Press, 1981.

Newacheck, P., and others. "Income and Illness." *Medical Care*, 1981, *18*, 1165–1176.

Orchard, T. "Epidemiology in the 1980s—Need for a Change." *Lancet*, 1980, *2*, 845–846.

Pless, I. B. "Children with Special Needs: State of the Field, 1981." Manuscript prepared for the Conference on Research Priorities in Maternal and Child Health, Brandeis University, Waltham, Mass., June 1981.

Pless, I. B., and Pinkerton, P. *Chronic Childhood Disorders: Promoting Patterns of Adjustment.* London: Henry Kimpton, 1975.

Roter, D. "Patient Participation in the Patient-Provider Interaction: The Effects of Patient Question-asking on the Quality of Interaction, Satisfaction, and Compliance." *Health Education Monographs*, 1977, *5* (4), 281–315.

Schach, E., and Starfield, B. "Acute Disability in Childhood: Examination of the Agreement Between Various Measures." *Medical Care*, 1973, *11*, 297–309.

Shapiro, S., and others. "Effectiveness of Regionalization for Perinatal Care." Paper presented at the Annual Meeting, American Public Health Association, Los Angeles, Calif., November 3, 1981.

Shelov, S., and others. "Enuresis: A Contrast of Attitudes of Parents and Physicians." *Pediatrics*, 1981, *67*, 707–710.

Silver, G. *Child Health: America's Future.* Germantown, Md.: Aspen Publications, 1979.

Simborg, D., Starfield, B., and Horn, S. "Physicians and Non-Physician Health Practitioners: The Characteristics of Their Practices and Their Relationships." *American Journal of Public Health*, 1978, *68*, 44–48.

Simborg, D., and others. "Information Factors Affecting Problem Follow-Up on Ambulatory Care." *Medical Care*, 1976, *14*, 848–856.

Starfield, B. "Health Services Research: A Working Model." *New England Journal of Medicine*, 1973, *289*, 132–136.

Starfield, B. "Measurement of Outcome: A Proposed Scheme." *Milbank Memorial Fund Quarterly*, 1974, *52*, 39–50.

Starfield, B. "Measuring the Attainment of Primary Care." *Journal of Medical Education*, 1979, *54*, 361–369.

Starfield, B. "Patients and Populations: Necessary Links Between the Two Approaches to Pediatric Research." *Pediatric Research*, 1981a, *15*, 1–5.

Starfield, B. "Poverty, Ill Health, and Medical Care." Presidential address to the Ambulatory Pediatric Association, San Francisco, May 1, 1981b.

Starfield, B. *Behavioral Pediatrics and Primary Health Care.* Philadelphia: Saunders, 1982.

Starfield, B. "Social Factors and Child Health." In M. Green and R. Haggerty (Eds.), *Ambulatory Pediatrics III.* Philadelphia: Saunders, 1983a.

Starfield, B. "Special Responsibilities: The Role of the Pediatrician." *Pediatrics*, 1983b, *71* (3), 433–440.

Starfield, B., and Pless, I. B. "Constancy and Change in Physical Health." In O.

Brim and J. Kagan (Eds.), *Constancy and Change in Human Development.* Cambridge, Mass.: Harvard University Press, 1980.

Starfield, B., and Scheff, D. "Effectiveness of Pediatric Care: The Relationship Between Process and Outcome." *Pediatrics,* 1972, *49,* 547–552.

Starfield, B., van den Berg, G., and Katz, H. "Variations in Utilization of Health Services by Children." *Pediatrics,* 1979, *63,* 633–641.

Starfield, B., and others. "Continuity and Coordination in Primary Care: Their Achievement and Utility." *Medical Care,* 1976, *14,* 625–636.

Starfield, B., and others. "Coordination of Care and Its Relationship to Continuity and Medical Records." *Medical Care,* 1977, *15,* 929–938.

Starfield, B., and others. "Patient-Provider Agreement About Problems: Influence on Outcome of Care." *Journal of the American Medical Association,* 1979, *242,* 344–346.

Starfield, B., and others. "The Influence of Patient-Practitioner Agreement on Outcome of Care." *American Journal of Public Health,* 1981, *71,* 127–131.

Starfield, B., and others. "Morbidity in Childhood: A Longitudinal View." *New England Journal of Medicine,* 1984, *310* (13), 824–829.

Starfield, B., and others. "Utilization and Morbidity: Random or Tandem?" *Pediatrics,* 1985, *75* (2), 241–247.

Stein, R. K., and Jessop D. "What Diagnosis Does *Not* Tell: The Case for a Non-Categorical Approach to Chronic Physical Illness." *Pediatric Research,* 1982, *16* (Part 2), 188A.

Stewart, M., McWhinney, I., and Buck, C. "The Doctor-Patient Relationship and Its Effect on Outcome." *Journal of the Royal College of General Practice,* 1979, *29,* 77–82.

Sultz, H., and others. *Long-term Childhood Illness.* Pittsburgh, Pa.: University of Pittsburgh Press, 1972.

Susser, M. "Widowhood: A Situational Life Stress or a Stressful Life Event?" *American Journal of Public Health,* 1981, *71,* 793–795.

Svarstad, B. "Physician-Patient Communication and Patient Conformity with Medical Advice." In D. Mechanic (Ed.), *The Growth of Bureaucratic Medicine.* New York: Wiley-Interscience, 1976.

U.S. Department of Health, Education, and Welfare. "Protection of Human Subjects: Proposed Regulations on Research Involving Children." 45 CFR 46.6., *Federal Register,* 1978, *43,* 31786.

Ware, J., and others. "Choosing Measures of Health Status for Individuals in General Populations." *American Journal of Public Health,* 1981, *71,* 620–625.

White, K. L. "The Ecology of Medical Care." *New England Journal of Medicine,* 1961, *265,* 885–892.

Wilson, R. "Do Health Indicators Indicate Health?" *American Journal of Public Health,* 1981, *71,* 461–463.

World Organization of National Colleges, Academies, and Academic Associations of General Practitioners/Family Physicians. *International Classification of Health Problems in Primary Care.* (2d ed.) Oxford, England: Oxford University Press, 1979.

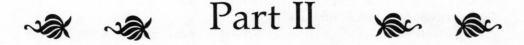

Part II

Chronic Childhood Illnesses: Epidemiology, Demography, and Representative Conditions

Part Two focuses initially on the prevalence of chronic conditions in the United States, the increased survival rates among chronically ill children, and the considerable impact these illnesses have had on expenditures for childhood chronic diseases.

Noting the lack of reliable population data as a major constraint on the development of sound demographic knowledge about chronically ill children, Steven L. Gortmaker, the author of Chapter Seven, reviews what is known about the demography of childhood chronic illnesses. Gortmaker focuses on patterns of population dynamics in his description of the relationships among the birthrate and the incidence, survival, and prevalence rates of childhood chronic illnesses. Gortmaker discusses these demographic trends in relation to geographic variation and migration. He indicates that, although the prevalence rate of childhood conditions should continue to increase, the numbers of chronically ill children are probably leveling off due to the lower birthrate and other factors. He discusses the implications of increased survival rates of chronically ill children and the impact on current and future expenditures for childhood chronic diseases.

The authors of Chapters Eight through Eighteen provide readers with perspectives on the more prevalent severe chronic illnesses of childhood: juvenile-onset diabetes is discussed by Allen Lee Drash and Nina Berlin; muscular dystrophy, by Irene S. Gilgoff and Shelby L. Dietrich; cystic fibrosis, by Norman J. Lewiston; spina bifida, by Gary J. Myers and Margaret Millsap; sickle cell anemia, by Charles F. Whitten and Eleanor N. Nishiura; congenital heart disease,

133

by Donald C. Fyler; chronic kidney diseases, by Barbara Korsch and Richard Fine; thalassemia and hemophilia, by Margaret W. Hilgartner, Louis Aledort, and Patricia J. V. Giardina; leukemia, by Thomas W. Pendergrass, Ronald L. Chard, Jr., and John R. Hartmann; craniofacial birth defects, by Donald W. Day; and asthma, by Fred Leffert. These eleven "marker diseases" represent the larger class of severe childhood chronic illnesses.

Each chapter provides a clinical description of the "marker disease" in lay terms, documents to the extent possible the costs of the disease, and discusses the impacts of the disease on children and their families. The authors raise policy questions related to each disease and offer recommendations that address those questions.

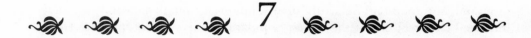

7

Demography
of Chronic Childhood Diseases

Steven L. Gortmaker, Ph.D.

Demographic data concerning children with rare chronic diseases are not widely available. Some extremely important questions concerning populations of chronically ill children, however, require consideration of key demographic issues, including questions of population size, distribution, socioeconomic status, and dynamic change. Recent medical advances, for example, have substantially increased the survival chances of children with a number of chronic diseases; children with cystic fibrosis (Dynesen and Flensborg, 1978), spina bifida (Elwood and Elwood, 1980), acute lymphocytic leukemia (Simone, 1979), congenital heart disease (Roberts and Cretin, 1980), and chronic kidney diseases (Vaughan, McKay, and Nelson, 1975) have experienced significantly improved chances of living into adulthood. These increases in survival also imply, however, increasing numbers of children needing often expensive treatment and services. Some key demographic questions include the following: How have the sizes of these populations changed? Are the incidence and survival of chronically ill children changing rapidly? How are populations of chronically ill children distributed throughout the United States?

A major constraint on the development of sound demographic knowledge of these populations lies in the lack of reliable and valid population data. All of

Note: This research was supported by funds provided by the Charles Stewart Mott Foundation and the Maternal and Child Health and Crippled Children's Services Research Grants Program, Bureau of Community Health Services, Department of Health and Human Services (MC-R-250437).

James Perrin, M.D., and Michael Weitzman, M.D., provided helpful comments on earlier drafts.

the childhood chronic illnesses discussed in this book, with the exception of asthma, are relatively rare. Prevalence estimates of many of these illnesses are on the order of one per thousand children, or less. Asthma constitutes the most common of the chronic conditions, and estimates of the prevalence of moderate and severe asthma in children often are on the order of ten to twenty per thousand. Most population health surveys, however, contain data on less than ten thousand children; one of the largest populations surveys, the National Health Interview Survey in the United States, contains data on perhaps forty-three thousand children, ages birth through seventeen (National Center for Health Statistics, 1973). Because few children with any one of these specific chronic illnesses are likely to be found in this sample, no adequate population data exist for many of these illnesses in the United States; the same is true for most other countries. The formation of surveillance systems for monitoring congenital malformations constitutes one relatively recent improvement in the available data. Because of the paucity of data in the United States, we examine data from both North American and European countries—the Scandinavian countries, for example, have perhaps the most complete data on some chronically ill populations (Kallen and Winberg, 1979; Bjerkedel and Bakketeig, 1975).

This chapter reviews what is known about the demography of childhood chronic illnesses, with a focus on patterns of population dynamics. Because population projections often prove incorrect, some assumptions that may be subject to change and the illnesses for which change is likely in the future are pointed out.

A general theme that emerges from the analyses is that drastic changes in the numbers of children with these chronic illnesses are not expected in the United States in the coming decades. A variety of forces will both encourage and discourage the growth of these populations of children. In general, increasing survival of a variety of groups of chronically ill children will be offset by the decreasing absolute numbers of children with chronic diseases because the "baby boom" cohorts of the 1950s have given way to smaller numbers of births. For some illnesses, the current population of children may well be the largest in the United States for many years to come.

Demographic Concepts and Rare Chronic Illnesses

Perhaps the most important concept in demography is a quite simple one: the demographic equation (Population^{t1} – Population^{t2}) = (Births) – (Deaths) + (Inmigration – Outmigration)(1). This equation states that the population of a given age range in a defined geographic area as it changes from time 1 to time 2 can be precisely predicted if the births, deaths, and net migration for this area can be estimated. This rather simple equation can be extended into more complex series of equations that trace the future course of the population in the area (Keyfitz, 1977). Application of this equation to the present problem tells us that, even though good quality population data concerning chronically ill children are not available, we can obtain useful projections of chronically ill populations knowing the likely trends in components of the demographic-change equation. For example, we can look for data concerning the changing incidence of illnesses, changing survival, and migration patterns. For some illnesses, good data concerning these components may be available. At the least, we will construct order-of-magnitude estimates of the population dynamics of groups of children with these chronic conditions.

Relationships Among Numbers of Births, Incidence, Survival, and Prevalence

Several concepts are used in describing populations of children with chronic illnesses. One concept refers to the absolute number of children of a given age that exhibit a chronic condition. A second concept refers to the proportion of children with a given condition. The two concepts are related, but they may differ considerably in their variation over time. For example, although the proportion of all births in any given year that results in a child with a chronic illness may remain relatively stable from year to year, the numbers of these children born may change dramatically if the sizes of birth cohorts change. The number of children born with a given disease in a particular year is calculated as the product of the corresponding proportion and the size of the birth cohort. Thus, changing proportions and changing numbers of total births can influence the number of chronically ill children.

There are various ways to refer to these proportions of children. One is the incidence rate—that is, the number of new occurrences of disease per unit of population during a specified period of time (MacMahon and Pugh, 1970). Incidence of some childhood chronic diseases is difficult to estimate because occurrence can vary from before birth (for example, spina bifida) to a range of times following (for example, leukemia). For application to the demographic equation given earlier, we thus must recognize that births into the population of interest can occur either at birth (here the incidence may have taken place either at conception or at any time up to the time of birth—spina bifida, for example, is thought to occur at approximately four weeks gestation [Elwood and Elwood, 1980, p. 31]) or at the onset of disease symptoms (as in juvenile-onset diabetes), which can occur throughout the years one through twenty.

Prevalence, the number of cases of a disease per thousand children from birth to twenty years, is another useful measure. The prevalence of a chronic disease varies as the product of the incidence rate of the disease multiplied by the average duration of the disease from onset to termination (MacMahon and Pugh, 1970). We can adjust for the later onset of certain diseases by noting how it affects prevalence estimates. Our estimation process assumes that the age of onset of these diseases is not changing significantly over time and uses incidence rates at birth because the onset of most of these diseases occurs within a few years of birth.

The preceding facts make techniques used for projecting trends in the population of children with chronic illnesses slightly different from the projection techniques conventionally used in mathematical demography. Central to conventional techniques are fertility rates (which specify the extent to which a given population group produces offspring) as well as survival rates. For example, given fixed schedules of fertility and survival by age and a beginning population distribution by age, matrix techniques can be used to project the size of a population over time (Keyfitz, 1977).

The situation with chronically ill children is a little different because the vast majority are not born to parents with a similar chronic illness. Although there is a genetic component to many of these illnesses, most of the dynamics of these populations are contingent upon growth of the total population and on their reproductive behavior, which includes, for example, all of those individuals who carry a particular recessive gene but who do not exhibit the associated chronic illness. Thus, for the children being discussed here, the numbers of births entering the population in a given year will be for the most part a function of the incidence of these children in the population of all births, as well as the number of children born in a given year.

Trends in the Size of Birth Cohorts. The most precise data and accurate projections are of the current total numbers of births in the United States and the likely trends in these births in the future. In contrast, data on the past and future incidence of the diseases and on the past and future survival of these children are more speculative.

The number of births in the United States each year is recorded quite accurately; there were three significant periods of change in the size of these cohorts during the past fifty years. The first period occurred prior to the end of World War II (1930–1945); generally, the birth cohorts during this period were between 2.3 and 3.1 million births per year. From 1946 to 1961, there was a steady rise in the size of birth cohorts, beginning with 3.4 million and ending with 4.4 million in 1960. Between 1962 and the present, the sizes of birth cohorts decreased to a low of 3.1 million, which was in 1975.

Projections concerning the sizes of birth cohorts are constantly reevaluated. The U.S. Census mid-range projections indicate that these cohorts could increase to about 4.0 million in 1990, then decrease to about 3.7 million in the year 2000. Then the numbers are projected to rise slowly and finally again to reach 4.3 million in 2040 (U.S. Bureau of the Census, 1977). Such projections are, of course, fraught with uncertainty, mainly regarding assumptions about the average number of lifetime births per woman. The projections noted above assume a value of 2.1 and assume that this value will persist throughout the period projected.

This level of completed cohort fertility is larger than current experience. The experience of the past, however, is that completed fertility rates have changed repeatedly, and thus the assumption of unchanged completed fertility rates throughout this entire projection period must be considered unrealistic. Even if there are some changes, however, the previous high levels probably will not occur again: improvements in fertility control and the increasing participation of women in the labor force should keep rates at or below replacement (Bumpass, 1973). The Census Bureau projections cited earlier thus appear to be reasonable estimates of the future size of birth cohorts in the United States.

Trends in the Incidence of Childhood Chronic Diseases. Trend data on the incidence of childhood chronic diseases are scattered throughout the literature. The data vary widely across disease categories, and the quality of the data varies as well. An exact accounting of new cases of a disease in a geographical area is rarely available. For that reason, emphasis in this section is upon making order-of-magnitude estimates rather than precise inferences concerning trends in incidence.

As we noted earlier, the estimation of incidence rates is particularly difficult because, although most chronic conditions appear at birth or soon after, some appear at varying ages up to adulthood. Thus, it is important that, when incidence rates are compared, similar age ranges are assumed. A related caveat is that improved casefinding and diagnosis can result in the apparent increased incidence of a disease when, in fact, the disease is merely being detected earlier.

There are various reasons for changes in the incidence of chronic diseases. A change in the age distribution of pregnant women, for example, can influence the incidence of some birth defects, notably Down's syndrome (Apgar, 1970). The teratogenic effects of drugs can influence incidence—for example, amphetamines and congenital heart disease (Vaughan, McKay, and Nelson, 1975). Environmental influences and social and political decisions can affect the incidence of diseases—for example, the ability to detect spina bifida with alpha-fetoprotein screening and amniocentesis offers the possibility of lowering the incidence of these births (Sunderland and Emery, 1979). However, if abortion laws deny the opportunity to terminate pregnancy, a lowered incidence may not be possible. Also, many women may not have access to prenatal diagnostic services for reasons of cost, availability, and knowledge.

Table 1 summarizes data on incidence, age of onset, and evidence for changes in incidence among eleven representative childhood chronic diseases. In general, there is little evidence for significant changes in incidence, although some differences are noted among different population groups, and there is evidence for substantial rises and decreases in the incidence of spina bifida over time. A reason for the relatively minor changes may be a lack of substantial time-series data; good quality population data on the incidence of most illnesses are relatively recent, and the evidence for lack of change must be tempered with this caveat. Nonetheless, changes in incidence during the past two to three decades, as shown in the table, are much smaller in magnitude than the changes in the sizes of birth cohorts. The data thus indicate that changes in incidence of chronic illnesses are not currently a major factor leading to changes in the number of affected children in the population. If significant changes do occur, these could very well involve decreases in incidence as improved genetic counseling and improved detection techniques during pregnancy lead to more avoidance of births of affected children.

Trends in Survival. Estimates of the survival of children with chronic diseases are difficult to compare precisely among disease categories. Some survival data come from studies of birth cohorts, some from studies of children identified at different ages of onset, some from mathematical models fitted to

Table 1. Incidence Data: Eleven Childhood Chronic Diseases.

Disease	Typical age of onset	Typical incidence per 1,000 live births (or young children)	Evidence for change (or possibility of change) in incidence and magnitude of that change
Cystic fibrosis	Variable: Most in first year (Dynesen and Flensborg, 1978)	.50 (Frydman, 1979)	No evidence for change, although some variation related to genetics to be expected (Ten Kate, 1977). Limited effects of genetic counseling; usually only after child has been born with cystic fibrosis are parents identified as carriers.
Spina bifida	Birth	1.00 (Elwood and Elwood, 1980)	Evidence for threefold rise in 1930s in North America, rise in 1960s in Ireland. Alpha-fetoprotein testing can lead to reduction in incidence; questions of cost, ethics, and efficacy limit applicability (Elwood and Elwood, 1980). Further evidence for continuing decrease to 1978 (Windham and Edmonds, 1982).
Leukemia	Maximum onset at 3–4 years (Vaughan, McKay, and Nelson, 1975)	.03 (Birch and others, 1981; Moe, 1976)	Little evidence for change.
Congenital heart disease	88% by first year (Hoffman and Christianson, 1978)	8.00 (Vaughan, McKay, and Nelson, 1975; Hoffman and Christianson, 1978; Roberts and Cretin, 1980)	No change recently observed in England (Bound and Logan, 1975); evidence for twofold rise in ventricular septal defects from U.S. (Layde and others, 1980). These defects comprise about 35% of total (Hoffman and Christianson, 1978).
Asthma	First year or two of life is typical (Vaughan, McKay, and Nelson, 1975)	10.00 (Haggerty, Roghmann, and Pless, 1975) 20.00 (Rutter, Tizard, and Whitmore, 1970) (moderate and severe cases only)	Little evidence for change.

Condition	Onset	Incidence rate	Evidence for change
Sickle cell anemia	Latter part of first year (Vaughan, McKay, and Nelson, 1975; Goldenson, Dunham, and Dunham, 1978)	.36* (Goldenson, Dunham, and Dunham, 1978)	No evidence for change noted. Genetic counseling can lead to reduced incidence, but probably quite limited effects.
Chronic kidney disease	Varies substantially 1–15 years (Vaughan, McKay, and Nelson, 1975)	Imprecise estimate due to varied conditions. 2.00 (among 0–18-year-olds) (Haggerty, Roghmann, and Pless, 1975)	No significant evidence for change overall; some prevention is possible (Vaughan, McKay, and Nelson, 1975, p. 1234) but of limited magnitude.
Juvenile diabetes	Onset increases and peaks at about age 12. Half of cases appear after age 9 (Deckert, Poulsen, and Larsen, 1979)	.40 (among all 0–15-year-olds) (Vaughan, McKay, and Nelson, 1975)	Little evidence for change.
Muscular dystrophy	After age 3 (Vaughan, McKay, and Nelson, 1975)	.14 (Duchenne's form; Vaughan, McKay, and Nelson, 1975) .13**	No evidence for change.
Hemophilia	90% of patients with severe disease have clinical evidence of increased bleeding by age 3–4 (Vaughan, McKay, and Nelson, 1975)		No evidence for change. Genetic counseling, amniocentesis can reduce some incidence (male carriers can be identified) (Goldenson, Dunham, and Dunham, 1978).
Cleft palate	Birth	.40 (Vaughan, McKay, and Nelson, 1975)	Evidence for 20% increase in Denmark (1939–1961), but no recent change in Norway (1967–1974) (Abyholm, 1978). Evidence for a rise then a decrease in Australia, with a peak in 1969, coincides with these data and fertility patterns (Brogan and Murphy, 1978).

* Assumes 1/500 incidence in blacks in the United States (Goldenson, Dunham, and Dunham, 1978) and that 18 percent of births in the U.S. are black.

** Assumes a rate of .25 per 1,000 among male children (Goldenson, Dunham, and Dunham, 1978) and that 50 percent of births are male.

Table 2. Survival Data (to age eighteen): Eleven Childhood Chronic Diseases.

Disease	Recent survival estimate by age and year	Evidence for changes in survival and magnitude of that change
Cystic fibrosis	70% to 21 (1965–1969); projected from data in Dynesen and Flensborg (1978). Life expectancy at birth of 15–20 years (Vaughan, McKay, and Nelson, 1975).	Sevenfold increase noted in Denmark 1950–1970; 5% survival to age 21 in 1945–1959; 70% estimate for 1965–1969.
Spina bifida	45% to ages 4–8 (1968) (Elwood and Elwood, 1980).	Twofold increase noted from 21% to ages 4–8 (cases untreated) to 45% for treated cases (Elwood and Elwood, 1980). Evidence that physical and mental handicaps also increase.
Leukemia	50% to age 2 (1970–1975) (Szklo and others, 1978). More recent estimates indicate 50% remain in initial complete remission for 3 years. If therapy stopped, hazard of relapse drops to virtually zero after fourth year (Simone, 1979). Thus, 40% survival to age 20 is a current estimate.	Greater than twofold increase in survival to age 2. 30% (1960–1964) to 80% (1970–1975). Five-year survival increased to perhaps 40% (Simone, 1979).
Congenital heart disease	74% survival to ages 5–13 (1959–1960) (Hoffman and Christianson, 1978); 52% at 15 years (1963–1973) (Laursen, 1980).	Recent increases in survival of two- to sevenfold noted for certain defects (British Medical Journal, 1971; Roberts and Cretin, 1980).
Asthma	Similar to normal. Rackemann and Edwards (1952) found 1% died of asthma after being followed for 20 years.	Some increased risks noted at times for certain treatments (for example, aerosols) but no substantial change.

Sickle cell anemia	93% to age 20 (1960–1980) (Murthy and Haywood, 1981).	Dramatic increases in survival as a result of early diagnosis, patient education, and therapeutic intervention (Lukens, 1981).
Chronic kidney disease	If treatment provided, few children die now as consequence of renal failure (Vaughan, McKay, and Nelson, 1975).	Significant improvement in therapy, 1965–1975 (Vaughan, McKay, and Nelson, 1975).
Juvenile diabetes	85% survive to age 20 (onset before 1953) if onset age is 0–10 (Deckert, Poulsen, and Larsen, 1979). Life expectancy of two thirds of general population at time of onset (Vaughan, McKay, and Nelson, 1975). Currently expect somewhat higher survival to age 20, perhaps 95% (James M. Perrin, M.D., personal communication with the author, 1983).	No recent change noted, but increased supervision is related to reduced mortality (Deckert, Poulsen, and Larsen, 1979).
Muscular dystrophy	25% survival to age 20 (Vaughan, McKay, and Nelson, 1957) (Duchenne's form most common).	No change noted; no effective treatments.
Hemophilia	Relatively normal survival to age 20.	No changes noted.
Cleft palate	Normal survival, except with associated chromosomal abnormalities (Vaughan, McKay, and Nelson, 1975). Mortality within first year of life was 6.5% in Norway, 1967–1974. In majority of these deaths, multiple malformations was the main cause of death (Abyholm, 1978).	No recent changes noted. Earlier increases in survival due to improved operative results (Abyholm, 1978).

samples of affected children classified by age, and some from samples of affected children being given particular treatments. Another distinction that should be made is that the estimates of incidence discussed generally refer to the incidence of a particular disease among children at birth. However, as already noted, it is more precise to speak of incidence taking place at many points before birth for some diseases; thus, from this point of view, survival could in fact be altered before birth through techniques such as abortion. To simplify discussions in the present situation, this chapter refers to incidence at birth, incidence among young children, and subsequent survival among these affected children.

In spite of differences in definition, a significant percentage of children with the eleven representative diseases survive into adulthood (Table 2). In addition, recent improvements in survival have been noted for children with six of the diseases. There is evidence for a sevenfold increase in survival to age twenty-one among children with cystic fibrosis in Denmark (1945–1973) and increases of twofold or greater for children with spina bifida, leukemia, and congenital heart disease.

Changes in survival have direct implications for changes in the total chronically ill childhood population. If one assumes there have been no significant changes in incidence, then it should be obvious that changes in survival will produce higher prevalence estimates of these children (aged birth through twenty). There is an upper bound to the increase in prevalence that increased survival can produce: When incidence is constant and duration and survival to adulthood are 100 percent, the childhood prevalence rate equals the incidence rate. The only factor that complicates this simple approach to estimating prevalence is the varying age of onset among the different diseases.

Table 3 combines data on incidence, age of onset, duration, and survival to produce current prevalence estimates. It also includes maximum prevalence estimates that can be expected under the same conditions of age of onset, duration, and incidence, assuming 100 percent survival to age twenty. If one assumes no overlap among diseases, the prevalence estimates can be added up; overall figures are provided at the bottom of Table 3.

Overall estimates of prevalence indicate that more than 80 percent of the maximum prevalence of these diseases among children aged birth to twenty years has been reached. The estimates, of course, are heavily weighted by the fact that asthma has the greatest prevalence. If asthma is excluded, 86 percent of the maximum prevalence estimate has been obtained (again, assuming constant incidence in the future). The implications of these analyses should be fairly clear: There is little room to expand the numbers of chronically ill children via improved survival. Overall, only a 16 percent increase could be expected if survival among *all* of these children were increased to 100 percent—and such an event is not likely, at least in the near future. Substantial increases, however, could occur among a couple of disease categories, for example, leukemia and muscular dystrophy. Both conditions, however, are among the rarer chronic illnesses of childhood.

Table 3. Estimated Prevalence and Maximum Prevalence Estimates for Eleven Childhood Chronic Diseases, Ages 0–20, United States, 1980.

Disease	Estimated proportion surviving to age 20* (percent)	1980 prevalence estimate per 1,000**	Estimated maximum prevalence, assuming 100% survival to age 20, constant incidence and age of onset***
Asthma (moderate and severe)	98	10.00	10.20
Congenital heart disease	65	7.00	9.33
Diabetes mellitus	95	1.80	1.89
Cleft lip/palate	92	1.50	1.62
Spina bifida	50	.40	.67
Sickle cell anemia	90	.28	.29
Cystic fibrosis	60	.20	.26
Hemophilia	90	.15	.16
Acute lymphocytic leukemia	40	.11	.22
Chronic renal failure	25	.08	.19
Muscular dystrophy	25	.06	.14
Estimated total (assuming no overlap)		21.58	24.97

Source: Gortmaker and Sappenfield, 1984.

  * Estimate refers to the survival expected of a birth cohort to age 20 given current treatments. For more detailed estimates, see Gortmaker and Sappenfield, 1984.

  ** Estimates are from population prevalence data or are derived from estimates of incidence (or prevalence at birth) and survival data. For details, see Gortmaker and Sappenfield, 1984.

  *** Most of the rates used in our calculations are not true incidence rates, but rather prevalence estimates at birth.

Although survival may be extended through childhood for many children, they may still experience a shortened life span. However, significant changes in population size will occur among older age groups as changes in survival continue. Increasing numbers of adults with what are often defined as childhood diseases constitute an area of significant policy research.

Geographic Variation and Migration. There are significant geographic variations in the incidence and prevalence of various chronic diseases. Spina bifida, for example, has greater than fourfold differences in estimated incidence rates among different geographic areas (Elwood and Elwood, 1980); cystic fibrosis has fourfold variations among Caucasian populations and even greater variation when Caucasian populations are compared to non-Caucasian populations (Ten Kate, 1977). Although much variation in these estimates is due to different methods of data collection and analysis, some differences are too large to be explained on this basis alone. Furthermore, biological variation in gene frequency exists in autosomal recessive disorders, and thus variation in the observed incidence rates for cystic fibrosis should be expected (Ten Kate, 1977). In addition, given the known relationships between certain birth defects and intrauterine infections and environmental teratogens, variations in the incidence of some of the other diseases should be expected in different social, economic, and physical environments.

Secular variations in the incidence of childhood diseases should be interpreted with these comments in mind. The trend data discussed here usually refer to studies confined to a single geographic area, and the periods of time under observation are, at most, a few decades. Thus, the variations in population genetics and the physical and social environment observed in most of these data are quite limited. If larger variations were observed in the environment, for example, larger variations in incidence could be expected. Studies of ethnic groups who have migrated provide data to use in estimating the influence of such large changes in environment. Naggan and MacMahon (1967), for example, compared rates of spina bifida and anencephalus among women who either migrated from Ireland or were first-generation Irish with rates among other mothers; substantial differences were observed.

Massive migrations that would rapidly alter the genetic makeup of a population or rapid and massive changes in the social, economic, and physical environment of the United States are, however, unlikely in the near future. Migration has typically been a small component of population growth of the United States; net immigration has been about four hundred thousand per year in the United States in the recent past (U.S. Bureau of the Census, 1977). Although net levels of illegal migration to the United States are larger, perhaps one million per year, the total population genetics can be expected to change very slowly. Changes in the social, economic, and physical environment also occur relatively slowly over time, although natural or manmade disasters could have significant effects on the incidence of chronic diseases.

Evidence concerning geographical variation in the incidence and prevalence of diseases throughout the United States does not indicate large differences.

There is evidence for up to a 1.5-fold difference in reported rates of congenital anomalies in different regions of the United States, although this is due partly to differences in reporting practices (National Center for Health Statistics, 1978). Asthma is a childhood chronic disease that is significantly influenced by the environment, and thus variations in incidence and prevalence (due to variations in the environment and migration) can be expected. National data indicate 1.5-fold differences in the prevalence of asthma among regions of the United States (National Center for Health Statistics, 1973).

Differences in the prevalence of asthma are also reported in a comparison of data from population surveys in two different parts of the United States when compared with national data (Walker, Gortmaker, and Weitzman, 1981). In this study, differences among geographic areas for a variety of other childhood chronic conditions, however, were not statistically significant. These findings imply that childhood chronic diseases likely have slightly varying incidence rates in different parts of the United States. However, it is likely that the variations are relatively random with respect to one another and that the aggregate incidence and prevalence of childhood chronic diseases do not vary substantially across the United States.

Data on migration patterns of families of children with chronic diseases are sparse; however, this factor may not be large. A study of 369 children enrolled in specialty clinics in the Cleveland metropolitan area, for example, shows that 82 percent of the families indicated that they had never moved to meet the child's needs (Breslau and others, n.d.).

In summation, one finds little evidence for significant migration either of new populations into the United States or of families with these diseases throughout the United States; migration is not of a magnitude to greatly alter the population genetics of the United States in the foreseeable future. Similarly, significant changes in genetics or in the environment in particular geographic areas of the United States are not expected. This analysis should apply to most geographic areas of the United States, although diseases that occur mainly among certain populations (such as cystic fibrosis among Caucasians) will have less relevance to areas with mostly minority populations, and vice versa.

Demographic Trends: A Case Example. Cystic fibrosis provides an example of the implication of these trends. One may assume for this analysis that the incidence of cystic fibrosis remains constant at .5 per thousand live births (with a simplifying assumption of diagnosis soon after birth) (Frydman, 1979). One also assumes little migration of families of children with cystic fibrosis. If survival data from Denmark approximate those in the United States, one can estimate the numbers of children born in a given year with cystic fibrosis who would survive to their twenty-first birthday. For children born in 1946, a 10 percent survival rate to age twenty-one is assumed. By 1959, this survival rate would have increased to an estimated 30 percent (projected from data in Dynesen and Flensborg, 1978). During the same period of time, the numbers of births in the United States increased from about 3.1 million in 1946 to 4.4 million in 1959.

Even with significant errors in survival and incidence estimates, the implications of these assumptions are instructive. If survival rates had remained unchanged from the 1946 to the 1959 cohorts, the total number of children surviving to age twenty-one would increase from an estimated 155 to 220 in the United States simply because of increasing cohort size. The change in survival from 10 percent to 30 percent at age twenty-one would change the latter number to an estimated 660. Furthermore, if we extrapolate from the early survival data of more recent cohorts, survival rates are probably currently 60 percent or higher (projected from data in Dynesen and Flensborg, 1978). A 60 percent survival rate to age twenty-one among the 1969 birth cohort of 3.6 million would imply 1,080 of the cohort surviving to age twenty-one.

These data clearly indicate how both changing cohort size and changing survival during recent decades could lead to a sevenfold increase in the numbers of children with cystic fibrosis who survive to adulthood. Because even larger proportions survive at earlier ages, the increases in early childhood prevalence are even greater. In this case, increasing survival was the dominant factor in the predicted demographic change. Many chronic diseases, however, are not accompanied by significantly lower survival during childhood. Thus, the numbers of children with function-impairing asthma would have increased in large part during this same period because of the growing size of birth cohorts. If we assume a constant incidence of function-impairing asthma of ten per thousand and almost complete survival to school age, the numbers of school-age children with asthma in 1952 in the United States would have been about 31,000. By 1965, this estimate would have increased to 44,000.

These examples provide an illustration of recent effects of both changing birth cohort size and changing survival of children with chronic diseases upon the numbers of these children in the United States.

National Estimates of Activity Limiting Chronic Conditions: 1967–1980

The preceding demographic analysis has identified two major forces currently determining the population size and percentage distribution of children with childhood chronic diseases in the United States. The increasing survival into adulthood of many of these children should lead to increased prevalence of these childhood chronic diseases, although the "maximum" attainable prevalence (under the assumption of constant age of onset, duration, and incidence rates) for these diseases is now close to being realized. Survival to age twenty of most chronically ill children is now quite high, and little room for improvement in survival remains.

Although the *prevalence* of childhood conditions should still be increasing, the *numbers* of chronically ill children in the United States population has probably been leveling off recently, and may decline in the near future (particularly for some conditions) because the cohort sizes will remain relatively stable into the next century. Some tests of these hypothesized trends are provided using a time-series analysis of data from the National Health Interview Survey. Data concerning children with limitation of activity due to chronic conditions have been collected using comparable questions and definitions since 1967 (National Center for Health Statistics, 1970).

Prevalence estimates obtained via these data are not strictly comparable with the estimates derived earlier for the individual childhood diseases via demographic analysis. The national estimates include children with many childhood conditions and illnesses not discussed here (children with cerebral palsy and Down's syndrome, to name two of the most prevalent). In addition, a substantial number of children with childhood conditions and illnesses do not experience activity limitation as defined in the national estimates (for example, children with cystic fibrosis and juvenile diabetes function normally in school). Differences between the two sets of data appear to roughly offset each other when prevalence estimates are made. The prevalence estimate from Table 3 (2.2 percent) is not far from the most recent estimate of children under 17 with limitation in major activity due to chronic conditions (2.0 percent in 1980). Thus, national data provide a useful test of the trends predicted via our disaggregated demographic analysis.

Table 4 summarizes data from the National Health Interview Survey, 1967–1980. Figure 1 displays estimates of the prevalence of children with limitation in major activity due to chronic conditions. It confirms a substantial increase in estimated prevalence (of more than 70 percent) during the years 1967 to 1973 and evidence for a smaller increase during the period 1973 to 1980. In general, the hypothesized trends are supported by the data from the National Health Interview Survey.

Implications and Conclusions

During recent decades, the numbers of children with a variety of childhood chronic diseases have increased substantially. As noted in the section on demographic concepts, changes in a specified population in a given geographic area can come about only via net migration, the entrance of new births, or changes in survival. Migration patterns into the United States have had little impact on these recent increases. In addition, few data indicate significant changes in the incidence of these diseases during this period. In contrast, there is substantial evidence for changes in the survival into adulthood of children with many childhood chronic diseases. Furthermore, although there is little evidence for change in incidence, there have been large increases in the numbers of children born and hence in the number of children born with or who develop chronic diseases.

The analyses and data indicate that significant changes in the size of the population of children with childhood chronic diseases have occurred in the past. However, the estimated population has plateaued beginning in 1973, and our demographic analysis finds little evidence for a significant increase in the future. Our analysis implies that the prevalence of children with childhood chronic diseases can increase only a limited amount in the future, the main determinant

Table 4. Persons Aged 0–16 with Limitation of Activity Due to
Chronic Conditions in the United States, 1967–1980.

	Estimated Number in Thousands		Percentage Distribution	
Year	With Activity Limitation	With Limitation in Major Activity	With Activity Limitation (percent)	With Limitation in Major Activity (percent)
1967	1,418	712	2.1	1.1
1968	1,427	825	2.1	1.2
1969	1,760	810	2.6	1.2
1970	1,820	873	2.7	1.3
1971	1,942	972	2.9	1.5
1972	1,921	1,037	3.0	1.6
1973	2,149	1,191	3.4	1.9
1974	2,305	1,199	3.7	1.9
1975	2,283	1,165	3.7	1.9
1976	2,267	1,179	3.7	1.9
1977	2,012	1,104	3.4	1.8
1978	2,309	1,178	3.9	2.0
1979	2,291	1,232	3.9	2.1
1980	2,223	1,180	3.8	2.0

Source: National Center for Health Statistics, Current Estimates from the National
Health Interview Survey, Series 10, Annual Reports 1967–1980, Nos. 52, 60, 63, 72, 79, 85,
95, 100, 115, 119, 126, 130, 136, 139.

Figure 1. Estimated Percentage of U.S. Children, Aged Birth Through
Sixteen, with Limitation of Activity Due to Chronic Conditions, 1967–1980.

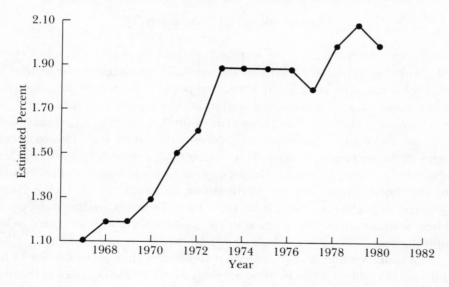

Source: National Center for Health Statistics, Current Estimates from the National
Health Interview Survey, Series 10, Annual Reports 1967–1980.

being that the majority of chronically ill children survive into adulthood. Overall, if survival to age twenty increased to 100 percent among all the different disease categories, we could only expect an increase in numbers surviving to adulthood of 16 percent. In addition, current population projections indicate that the maximum birth cohort sizes achieved during the late 1950s and 1960s will likely not be replicated for many years. We will not again achieve larger numbers of children with childhood chronic diseases until the next century.

Some qualifications need to be added to this projection. Children with some diseases could experience substantially increased survival if new medical treatments are discovered. Thus, there could still be significant increases in the numbers of children with leukemia, muscular dystrophy, congenital heart disease, spina bifida, or cystic fibrosis. The "ceiling effect" described earlier refers to the aggregation of all of the eleven representative disease categories and most particularly to those diseases where little reduction in life during childhood is currently experienced.

Large increases in absolute numbers could have a variety of influences on public policies. Just as the baby boom resulted in the construction of new schools and new medical and social service facilities and personnel, the increasing number of children with chronic diseases has resulted in the need for more facilities and personnel to serve their special needs. In the case of diseases where survival through childhood has been relatively complete (asthma, hemophilia, cleft palate), increases in numbers have paralleled the general growth of the baby boom generation. For others, where significant changes in survival have occurred (cystic fibrosis, spina bifida, leukemia, congenital heart disease, chronic kidney disease), increases have been much more dramatic.

It is interesting to speculate upon the extent to which the demographic changes in the absolute sizes of chronically ill populations have influenced public policy. It is an oversimplification to say that the Education for All Handicapped Children Act of 1975, P.L. 94-142, was due to increased demands generated by the largest cohorts of handicapped children in United States history. However, the increase in numbers was undoubtedly implicated in countless decisions concerning construction of new facilities and hiring of specialized personnel. The underlying demographic trends thus laid the groundwork for establishment of a legal framework to protect the rights of chronically ill children to education.

It is not difficult to imagine how increased numbers could lead to organization for change. In 1950, a community of 500,000 could expect to have perhaps fifteen children with cystic fibrosis, aged birth to twenty-one (assuming the figures cited earlier). By the 1960s, this number would have increased to about seventy and could lead to an increased consciousness among families and providers concerning the children's needs. The increases can also provide the economic base (sufficient numbers) necessary for development of specialty clinics and educational programs. As more children survive into adulthood, larger numbers of adults will require treatment and services.

The pattern predicted via the analysis of this chapter is for little change of the numbers of children with childhood chronic diseases. One significant implication of this projection is that expenditures for services to children with chronic diseases should not be driven up significantly in the future by increasing numbers of chronically ill children. In fact, reductions in service levels for certain disease categories may be seen. Precise estimates of future resource requirements as well as their optimal allocation require detailed research by disease category. These questions should provide important topics of future research.

References

Abyholm, F. "Cleft Lip and Palate in Norway." *Scandinavian Journal of Plastic and Reconstructive Surgery*, 1978, *12*, 29-34.

Apgar, V. "Down's Syndrome (Mongolism)." *Annals of the New York Academy of Sciences*, 1970, *171*, 303-688.

Birch, J. M., and others. "Childhood Leukemia in North West England, 1954-1977: Epidemiology, Incidence and Survival." *British Journal of Cancer*, 1981, *43*, 321-329.

Bjerkedel, T., and Bakketeig, L. S. "Surveillance of Congenital Malformations and Other Conditions of the Newborn." *International Journal of Epidemiology*, 1975, *4* (1), 31-36.

Bound, J. P., and Logan, W. E. F. "Incidence of Congenital Heart Disease in Blackpool, 1957-1971." *British Heart Journal*, 1977, *39*, 445-450.

Breslau, N., and others. "Children with Disabilities and Their Families: 1978-1981." Unpublished study, Case Western Reserve School of Medicine, Cleveland, Ohio, no date.

British Medical Journal. "Survival in Severe Congenital Heart Disease." 1971, *5764*, 723-724.

Brogan, W. F., and Murphy, B. P. "The Effects of Zero Population Growth on the Incidence of Cleft Lip and Palate in Western Australia." *Medical Journal of Australia*, 1978, *1*, 126-131.

Bumpass, L. "Is Low Fertility Here to Stay?" *Family Planning Perspectives*, 1973, *5* (2), 67-69.

Deckert, T., Poulsen, J. E., and Larsen, M. "The Prognosis of Insulin Dependent Diabetes Mellitus and the Importance of Supervision." *Acta Medica Scandinavica, Supplement*, 1979, *624*, 48-53.

Dynesen, A. H., and Flensborg, E. W. "Prognosen for Cystisk Fibrose i Danmark 1945-1974. Betydning af Centraliseret Kontrol og Behandling." *Ugeskrift Laeger*, 1978, *140*, 463-470.

Elwood, J. M., and Elwood, J. H. *Epidemiology of Anencephalus and Spina Bifida*. New York: Oxford University Press, 1980.

Frydman, M. I. "Epidemiology of Cystic Fibrosis: A Review." *Journal of Chronic Diseases*, 1979, *32*, 211-219.

Goldenson, R. M., Dunham, J. R., and Dunham, C. S. *Disability and Rehabilitation Handbook*. New York: McGraw-Hill, 1978.

Gortmaker, S., and Sappenfield, W. "Chronic Childhood Disorders: Prevalence and Impact." *Pediatric Clinics of North America,* 1984, *31* (1), 3–18.

Haggerty, R. J., Roghmann, K. J., and Pless, I. B. *Child Health and the Community.* New York: Wiley, 1975.

Hoffman, J.I.E., and Christianson, R. "Congenital Heart Disease in a Cohort of 19,502 Births with Long-term Follow-up." *American Journal of Cardiology,* 1978, *42,* 641–647.

Kallen, B., and Winberg, J. "Dealing with Suspicions of Malformation Frequency Increase. Experience with the Swedish Register of Congenital Malformations." *Acta Paediatrica Scandinavica,* 1979, *275,* 66–74.

Keyfitz, N. *Introduction to the Mathematics of Population with Revisions.* Reading, Mass.: Addison-Wesley, 1977.

Laursen, H. B. "Some Epidemiological Aspects of Congenital Heart Disease in Denmark." *Acta Paediatrica Scandinavica,* 1980, *69,* 619–624.

Layde, P. M., and others. "Is There an Epidemic of Ventricular Septal Defects in the U.S.A.?" *Lancet,* 1980, February 23, pp. 407–408.

Lukens, J. N., "Sickle Cell Disease." *Disease-a-Month,* 1981, *27* (5), 1–56.

MacMahon, B., and Pugh, T. *Epidemiological Methods,* Boston: Little, Brown, 1970.

Moe, P. J. "Childhood Leukemia in Norway from 1963–1974 with Special Emphasis on Own Material." *Acta Paediatrica Scandinavica,* 1976, *65,* 529–533.

Murthy, V. K., and Haywood, L. J. "Survival Analysis by Sex, Age Group and Hemotype in Sickle Cell Disease." *Journal of Chronic Diseases,* 1981, *34,* 313–319.

Naggan, L., and MacMahon, B. "Ethnic Differences in the Prevalance of Anencephaly and Spina Bifida in Boston, Massachusetts." *New England Journal of Medicine,* 1967, *227,* 1119–1123.

National Center for Health Statistics. "Current Estimates, 1967." Series 10, No. 52. Washington, D.C.: U.S. Department of Health, Education, and Welfare, 1970.

National Center for Health Statistics. "Prevalence of Selected Chronic Respiratory Conditions, United States, 1970." Series 10, No. 84. Washington, D.C.: U.S. Department of Health, Education, and Welfare, 1973.

National Center for Health Statistics. "Congenital Anomalies and Birth Injuries Among Live Births: United States, 1973–74." Washington, D.C.: U.S. Department of Health, Education, and Welfare, 1978.

Rackemann, F. M., and Edwards, M. D. "Asthma in Children: A Follow-Up Study of Six Hundred Eighty-Eight Patients After an Interval of Twenty Years." *New England Journal of Medicine,* 1952, *246,* 815–858.

Roberts, N. K., and Cretin, S. "The Changing Face of Congenital Heart Disease." *Medical Care,* 1980, *18* (9), 930–939.

Rutter, M., Tizard, J., and Whitmore, K. *Education, Health and Behavior.* London, England: Longman, 1970.

Simone, J. "Childhood Leukemia as a Model for Cancer Research: The Richard and Linda Rosenthal Foundation Award Lecture." *Cancer Research*, 1979, *39*, 4301–4306.

Sunderland, R., and Emery, J. L. "The Mortality and Birth Rates of Spina Bifida During a Period of Treatment, Selection and Antenatal Screening in Sheffield, 1963–1978." *Zeitschrift für Kinderchirurgie und Grenzgebiete*, 1979, *28* (4), 294–301.

Szklo, M., and others. "The Changing Survivorship of White and Black Children with Leukemia." *Cancer*, 1978, *42*, 59–66.

Ten Kate, L. P. "Cystic Fibrosis in the Netherlands." *International Journal of Epidemiology*, 1977, *6* (1), 23–34.

U.S. Department of Health and Human Services, Bureau of the Census. "Projections of the Population of the U.S.: 1977 to 2050." *Current Population Reports*, Series P-25, No. 104. Washington, D.C.: U.S. Government Printing Office, 1977.

Vaughan, V. C., McKay, R. J., and Nelson, W. E. *Textbook of Pediatrics.* Philadelphia: Saunders, 1975.

Walker, D., Gortmaker, S., and Weitzman, M. "Chronic Illness and Psychosocial Problems Among Children in Genesee County." Harvard School of Public Health, August 1981.

Windham, G., and Edmonds, L. "Current Trends in the Incidence of Neural Tube Defects," *Pediatrics*, 1982, *70* (3), 333–337.

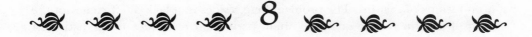

8

Juvenile Diabetes

Allen Lee Drash, M.D.
Nina Berlin

Clinical Description

Diabetes mellitus is a systemic disease resulting from either an absolute or a relative deficiency of insulin, the polypeptide hormone produced by the beta cells of the pancreas. Insulin is the primary regulator of energy homeostasis, having important effects on the uptake and utilization of energy from glucose, amino acids, and fat. In a state of partial or complete insulin deficiency, significant alterations in metabolism occur leading to the clinical symptomatology of diabetes mellitus.

Classification of Diabetes Mellitus. Until recently, diabetes mellitus was felt to be a single homogeneous disease. This, now, is clearly not the case. If carbohydrate intolerance (blood glucose concentration in excess of the upper limits of normal) is to be the basis for diagnosis of diabetes, then there are a large number of genetic and acquired conditions that may lead to this diagnosis. From a practical point of view, however, diabetes may be thought of broadly as two distinct diseases, insulin-dependent diabetes mellitus (IDDM) and non-insulin-dependent diabetes mellitus (NIDDM).

For many years, the form of diabetes that is characteristically seen in the child has been referred to as juvenile diabetes mellitus, or juvenile-onset diabetes (JOD). The condition has also been referred to as ketosis-prone diabetes. A recent reclassification of diabetes (National Diabetes Data Group, 1979) classifies this condition as insulin-dependent diabetes mellitus (IDDM). The condition is also called Type I in the new English nomenclature. This condition is a result of essentially complete destruction of the beta cells resulting in eventual complete insulin deficiency.

The other major form of diabetes mellitus has traditionally been referred to as maturity-onset diabetes, or obesity-related or ketosis-resistant diabetes. The recent reclassification refers to this condition as non-insulin-dependent diabetes (NIDDM)—Type II in the new English nomenclature. Unlike IDDM, this condition is not a result of beta-cell failure or a deficiency of circulating concentrations of insulin. The problem here resides in a lack of efficiency of the timing of insulin release or, more often, peripheral resistance to the action of insulin. NIDDM is characteristically associated with excessive body weight and is usually detected in midlife or beyond. The primary therapeutic approach to NIDDM patients is dietary restriction and weight loss, although insulin administration or treatment with one of the oral hypoglycemic agents may be of value.

Diabetes Mellitus in Our Society. Diabetes is very common in the Western world. Approximately 2 percent of the American public have diabetes mellitus; that is, they have been diagnosed and are under some form of therapy. Epidemiological studies indicate that approximately another 2 percent of the American public have diabetes and have not yet been diagnosed. It is estimated that at least 85 percent of diabetics, diagnosed and undiagnosed, have the non-insulin-dependent form of the disease. Thus, something less than 15 percent of the total diabetic population in the United States require insulin on a daily basis to sustain life. Although insulin dependency is characteristic of diabetes in childhood, it may occur at any age. Insulin-dependent patients are particularly susceptible to the ravages of small-blood-vessel disease, leading to retinopathy (eye damage), neuropathy (peripheral nerve damage), and nephropathy (kidney damage), but they experience increased mortality from accelerated atherosclerosis (hardening of the arteries) as well. Kimmelstiel-Wilson disease is a progressive damage to the glomeruli of the kidney resulting directly from diabetes mellitus. It frequently leads to terminal renal failure and is the major cause of death in patients with insulin-dependent diabetes mellitus. Myocardial infarction (heart attack) is the second most common cause of death in these patients.

Diabetes is the third major cause of death in the United States, the number one cause of acquired blindness in adults, and one of the most frequent causes of terminal renal failure. The loss of time from school and work, the impairment of the ability to perform optimally in personal and public situations, the necessary alteration in life style, and the impact on the family all lead to an enormous toll in time, dollars, and human suffering. Many of these losses can be significantly moderated, if not eliminated, by general application of currently known information on improved management techniques and specialized procedures.

Epidemiology of IDDM in the Child. Probably more than 98 percent of children with diabetes mellitus have the classical disorder resulting from beta-cell damage and loss of ability to synthesize and release insulin. However, a small percentage of patients have other forms of diabetes, including maturity-onset (non-insulin-dependent) diabetes (NIDDM). In our experience, most of these latter patients are grossly overweight, black, adolescent females. In addition a small number of patients have a condition referred to as maturity-onset diabetes of youth (MODY), a specific genetic disease that is autosomal dominant in transmission, usually identifiable in at least three generations, and not necessarily associated with obesity, and that usually requires low doses of insulin for management. The remainder of this discussion focuses on insulin-dependent diabetic children.

The incidence of IDDM is approximately fifteen per hundred thousand normal children and adolescents under twenty years of age per year (Drash and others, 1981; La Porte and others, 1981a, 1981b; Wagener and others, 1982). It is uncommonly diagnosed in the younger child, increasing gradually with increasing age, reaching a peak during the early adolescent years, and then declining with the completion of growth. The peak incidence occurs approximately one and a half years earlier in girls than in boys, consistent with their earlier onset of adolescence. The disease occurs equally in boys and girls, although a few studies have suggested a slight excess of males. Diabetes occurs slightly less often in black children than in white, comparable incidence figures being fifteen per hundred thousand per year in whites and ten per hundred thousand per year in blacks. Other investigators have suggested that the incidence in blacks is approximately one fifth of that in whites. There is an increased risk of NIDDM in individuals from lower socioeconomic groups; however, this is probably not the case in insulin-dependent diabetes in children. Our own recent studies have documented no evidence of a socioeconomic effect in either black or white children over a period of approximately twenty years.

Many investigators have documented a clear seasonality to the diagnosis of diabetes mellitus in adolescents. The disease is more commonly diagnosed in winter than in summer, strongly suggesting a link to infectious diseases. A number of specific viral agents have been implicated as either provocative triggers or direct causative factors. The identified viruses include coxsackie viruses, rubella, mumps, cytomegalovirus, Epstein-Barr virus, and others (Drash, 1979). There have been several reports suggesting that IDDM is increasing in our society. Our own studies in Allegheny County, Pennsylvania, do not confirm this observation. In an analysis of incidence of diabetes initially diagnosed in individuals under twenty years of age, we find no statistically significant increases when the past twenty years' experience is analyzed in four-year intervals. It is our interpretation that the suggestion of increasing secular trend is a reflection of improved statistics in recent years.

Etiology of IDDM. Insulin-deficient diabetes occurs as a result of inflammatory destruction to the beta cells of the pancreas leading eventually to complete or almost complete loss of the capacity to synthesize and release insulin. The mechanism of this inflammatory damage has been the object of intense investigation by many investigators over a period of several years. This work is in an accelerating stage, and we have increasing insights into the underlying mechanisms, although no final explanation for the etiology of IDDM can be elucidated at this time. The recent excellent review by Cahill and McDevitt (1981) places into perspective all current relevant information.

It has been known for many years that diabetes mellitus is a genetic disease. However, the disease is not inherited. A certain genetic predisposition increases the likelihood of beta-cell damage under certain environmental conditions. Many recent studies have identified the unique relationship between human lymphocyte antigen (HLA) and IDDM. From literally several thousand possible blood-typing combinations, a very few specific types are seen in approximately 85 percent of patients with IDDM. Patients with NIDDM have the same distribution of HLA types as the general population, further evidence of the genetic distinction between these two metabolic disorders. The HLAs are located on human chromosome number 6, which is also the genetic locus of much of the immunological machinery of the body. Immunological response to injury, infection, or inflammation is a very complex, coordinated integration of both cellular and humoral responses. Circulating antibodies to foreign or offending agents are regularly and swiftly produced by certain specialized cells. In addition, specialized lymphocytes are involved in attacking infectious or noxious agents and eliminating them from the body. Pathologic alterations in this integrated defense mechanism may result in the direction of this process to one's self.

Autoimmunity is the term applied to that process involving humoral or cellular damage of a highly specific or generalized nature. The process is the aberration of the normal host-defense mechanisms and is destructive rather than healing in nature. IDDM is now known to be a classical autoimmune disease in many cases. Genetic alterations in the host-defense mechanism may increase the risk of viremia and viral infection of the pancreas. In rare instances, this viral infectious process may be the complete cause of eventual beta-cell destruction in diabetes mellitus. More often, the viral infection or, in other cases, environmental poisons such as Vacor simply initiate an inflammatory response that leads to beta-cell destruction. The clinical documentation of this destructive process is the identification of circulating islet-cell antibodies. There are a number of different antibodies that have been identified in blood samples of newly diagnosed diabetic patients. There is considerable controversy as to whether the islet-cell antibodies actively participate in destruction of the beta cells or whether they are a secondary effect of the inflammation and not specifically toxic to the beta cells.

Pathophysiology of IDDM. The small polypeptide hormone, insulin, has pervasive effects on energy homeostasis. Insulin is released promptly from the beta cells into the blood stream in response to the ingestion of foodstuffs. The stimulants for insulin release include not only glucose but also several amino acids and possibly fat and ketone bodies. Insulin affects glucose metabolism by promoting the uptake of glucose in such peripheral tissues as muscle and organ and by controlling the rate of glucose release from liver, the major storage depot. Insulin promotes protein synthesis and growth by working synergistically with growth hormone to promote an increased rate of amino acid uptake into cells. Insulin controls fat metabolism by stimulating conversion of excess dietary carbohydrate into fat stores, thus promoting circulating fat uptake to adipose tissue and preventing the excessive outflow of free fatty acids and glycerol (the breakdown products of stored triglyceride) from adipose tissue. In a very real sense, insulin can be considered an anabolic (body-building) hormone, promoting glucose utilization for energy needs and for synthesis and storage of protein and fat. In the absence of insulin, these metabolic processes are reversed. Glucose metabolism is impaired secondary to decreased peripheral glucose uptake and increasing glucose production by the liver, both of which events lead to increased blood sugar (hypoglycemia) and, subsequently, sugar in the urine. Protein synthesis is stopped and replaced by protein breakdown (proteolysis) and an increased rate of gluconeogenesis, leading to further hyperglycemia. Lipid (fat) synthesis stops, and lipid mobilization greatly increases; this results in hyperlipidemia and eventually in diabetic ketoacidosis.

Presentation and Initial Clinical Course. The clinical features of IDDM are clearly understandable in terms of the pathophysiological events: With the decline in insulin production, hyperglycemia results leading to sugar in the urine and excessive urination (Drash and Becker, 1978; Drash, 1980). The body's natural defense against continuing excessive losses of water through the urine is an increase in fluid intake, polydipsia. When this response is found to be inadequate to meet energy losses, increased caloric ingestion (polyphagia) follows. The overall result of increasing fluid intake is to increase further the concentration of circulating nutrients, particularly glucose, leading to further urinary glucose losses. These classical symptoms (polyuria, polydipsia, and polyphagia), referred to as the triad of diabetes, usually result in clinical diagnosis of this disorder within two to three weeks of onset. Medical help is usually sought because of concern about kidney disease. If a diagnosis is not established during this initial phase of energy wasting, it will occur as the metabolic status further deteriorates with excessive mobilization of body fat leading to ketone body accumulation and the potentially fatal complication of diabetic ketoacidosis, a presenting finding in slightly less than half of newly diagnosed children and adolescents. Characteristically, at the time of diagnosis, patients have had a significant weight loss and have additional complaints including extreme muscle weakness, visual disturbance, and abdominal pain. Not infrequently, infections may have triggered the process that leads to diagnosis of the disease.

IDDM is an incurable lifelong disease. Management requires daily injections of insulin and adherence to a regularized life-style including a specialized diet and integration of exercise into daily activities. It is a very demanding disease for both patient and family because they must be integrally involved in therapeutic decisions and medication administration from the very beginning.

Initial evaluation and confirmation of the diagnosis usually occurs in the hospital. Therapy with insulin is promptly initiated, administered several times per day by injection as rapid-acting insulin or continuously by intravenous administration if the patient has diabetic ketoacidosis. Initial stabilization occurs within a period of a few days, allowing the child to be switched to one of the intermediate-acting insulins (such as NPH or Lente) that has a time duration of approximately twenty-four hours. Most patients are treated with a combination such as NPH plus regular given once or, in many cases, twice daily. Characteristically, there is a fairly dramatic decrease in insulin requirement occurring in the initial weeks after diagnosis. This period is referred to as a remission or the honeymoon phase and is a period of increasing good health, good metabolic control, and decreasing insulin requirement. In a very small number of patients, probably less than 3 percent, total remission occurs, and the patient may be removed from insulin injections completely for a variable period of time from a few weeks to as long as one or two years. Invariably, however, the remission is lost and increasing insulin requirements result leading to an average insulin dose of approximately 1.0 units/kg/day within two years after diagnosis (Drash and others, 1980).

Therapeutic Objectives. The obvious objective of therapy for the patient with IDDM would be to manage the patient in such a way that all of the metabolic alterations are returned to normal. This is currently not possible because our techniques for insulin administration do not approach the highly sophisticated and sensitive insulin release mechanisms of the normal healthy beta cell as it responds to food ingestion, stress, exercise, and the like. Consequently, the physician and patient must accept a therapeutic compromise from what is highly desirable to what is practically achievable, keeping in mind that therapeutic improvements should be incorporated into the patient's program as they become available. The primary concern about therapy is the increasing evidence that there is some direct relationship between the frequency and severity of such serious small-blood-vessel complications of diabetes as retinopathy, neuropathy, and nephropathy and the characteristic metabolic disturbances of diabetes, particularly hyperglycemia but probably also amino acid, protein, and lipid derangement.

The therapeutic objectives of the clinic at Children's Hospital of Pittsburgh include the following:

1. Complete elimination of the acute symptoms of diabetes mellitus including polyuria, polydipsia, and polyphagia
2. Prevention of ketonuria, ketonemia, and ketoacidosis (although ketonuria can be expected to occur transiently in association with intercurrent infections, the development of ketoacidosis in the child with previously diagnosed diabetes should not occur. It is a treatment failure, the responsibility for which should be borne by the physician as well as the patient and the family.)
3. Prevention of hypoglycemia
4. Control of hyperglycemia and glycosuria to the extent that caloric losses are minimized (a twenty-four-hour urine glucose loss of less than 7 percent of the ingested carbohydrate (twenty to twenty-five grams of glucose per day) is a reasonable goal that can be achieved in a high percentage of patients)
5. Maintenance of blood-lipid concentrations within the limits of normal for age
6. Achievement of normal growth and development including the normal timing of secondary sexual development
7. Maintenance of a high level of physical fitness
8. Avoidance of obesity
9. Full participation in activities appropriate to age and interest
10. Acceptance of a diet that helps minimize postprandial hyperglycemia and prevent hyperlipidemia

11. Education of the patient and family regarding diabetes and its treatment so they can effectively participate in all management decisions
12. Assumption by the patient of progressively more responsibility for insulin administration, urine testing, and dietary and other daily management activities
13. Development on the part of the patient of sound psychological acceptance of the problems of diabetes including a positive outlook for the future
14. Eventual achievement of full intellectual, physical, and emotional potential as a contributing member of society
15. Prevention of cardiovascular complications of diabetes including atherosclerosis and microvascular disease

The physician should help the patient achieve the best level of metabolic control possible but must at the same time be acutely aware of the psychological hazards that may accompany a highly regimented, restrictive management approach. Daily maintenance of a normoglycemic state is not achievable in the great majority of children with diabetes. In a few children, near normality can and indeed should be reached. However, a therapeutic approach that places a high premium on achievement of biochemical normality invariably carries with it increasing danger of recurrent hypoglycemia (low blood sugar) and psychological sequelae. The rules of the clinic or physician may come to be unconsciously viewed as ethical commandments by the patient and family. A reward and punishment system develops, and guilt feelings rise when the rules are transgressed. If, in reality or in the eyes of the patient, the objectives of the clinic or physician cannot be achieved, the patient will become discouraged and will be progressively less cooperative.

A number of recent methodological advances have improved our abilities to assess the level of metabolic control in the diabetic patient accurately and thus improve management. In the face of persistent hyperglycemia, glucose attaches to a number of body proteins by a chemical bond referred to as glycosylation. This process, involving the hemoglobin molecules of the red blood cells, has turned out to be a highly sensitive index of blood-glucose control over a period of three to four months. The optimal therapeutic objective would be to achieve normal glycosylated hemoglobin levels in IDDM patients. This has been possible in only 3 to 5 percent of our patients. A more achievable goal is to keep glycosylated hemoglobin levels no more than two or three percentage points above the upper limit of normal. The other recent technical advance has been development of accurate, safe, and relatively painless methods for home blood-glucose monitoring. This involves the patient obtaining a drop of blood by a small lancet and analyzing this blood specimen for glucose content by using impregnated glucose oxidase strips that are read either visually or with a small colorimeter. Many physicians now request their patients carry out such tests from two to seven times per day and to adjust their insulin, diet, and exercise according to their observations. Fasting blood-glucose values below 120 mg/percent and values below 180 mg/percent after a meal are generally accepted as reasonable therapeutic objectives. Although, technically, older children and adolescents are capable of carrying out home blood-glucose monitoring, the long-term value of this approach, particularly as it relates to emotional well-being, has not yet been established.

The Therapy of IDDM. Daily insulin administration is essential to the patient with IDDM. If the patient should miss the usual daily insulin injection for even two or three days, the development of diabetic ketoacidosis can be expected to occur, with death inevitable unless active therapy is reinstated. Insulin is regularly administered by injection into the subcutaneous tissue where it is absorbed into the circulation. However, insulin may be given intramuscularly or intravenously, both of which result in more rapid onset of action. The commercially available insulin preparations are all extracted from pancreas obtained from beef or pork sources. The insulins are chemically slightly different from the chemical formulation of human insulin. Consequently, antibodies to commercial insulin invariably develop in insulin-treated diabetic patients. Allergic problems may also result. Current research is directed toward development of human insulin by recombinant-DNA methods. It is probable that insulin produced by this method will become the primary source of insulin for patient use in the near future. This development should result in diminishing problems due to insulin allergy or immunologic reaction.

Daily insulin injections are given to IDDM patients either by themselves or by a family member. The dose of insulin is carefully worked out on a trial-and-error basis, utilizing the patient's observations on urine glucose concentration and blood glucose concentration as well as clinical symptoms to determine dosage needs. Increasingly, multiple-dose insulin injection therapy is being advocated and accepted. Many patients receive insulin injections prior to breakfast and the evening meal, and some patients now take injections of regular insulin before each meal and a long-acting insulin preparation in the evening to cover the period of sleep. There is increasing research to improve the mode of insulin delivery and mimic as closely as possible the insulin release methods of the normal healthy beta cell. The open-loop insulin infusion system is now a well-accepted research tool that is increasingly applied in the clinical setting. This instrument (there are now several commercial variations available) is a small pumping device that delivers insulin into the subcutaneous tissue by a catheter and needle at a preset base rate. Acute increases in delivery rate occur prior to meals, as selected by the patient and physician. Several investigators have demonstrated that in the highly mature, well-motivated patient, the open-loop insulin infusion system can lead to remarkable improvement in overall metabolic control, although true metabolic normality is rarely achieved. The open-loop system appears to be a stepping-stone to the eventual development of the truly complete implantable mechanical pancreas that could fully replace the patient's destroyed beta cells. A number of research groups have spent years attempting to perfect such a method. The frustrations have been great and failures consistent to date. Undoubtedly, however, success will eventually be achieved, allowing insulin-deficiency diabetes to be completely controlled and probably eliminating the complications of this disorder.

Diet is one of the keystones of diabetes therapy. In overweight middle-aged patients with NIDDM, the primary therapeutic approach is caloric restriction and weight loss. Obesity is rarely a problem in the child, adolescent, or young adult with IDDM. Consequently, caloric restriction is not an integral part of their diet plan. The diet in such patients should help achieve four goals:

1. Minimize postprandial hyperglycemia
2. Prevent hypoglycemia
3. Prevent hyperlipidemia
4. Ensure entirely adequate nutrients for full growth and maturation

These objectives are accomplished by spreading the daily calories over the waking hours, utilizing three meals and three snacks in the younger child, and three meals and two snacks (midafternoon and bedtime) in the older child, adolescent, and adult. We recommend that the diet contain approximately 55 percent of its total calories as carbohydrate, 30 percent as fat, and 15 percent as protein. The great majority of the dietary carbohydrates should be in the complex form as starches with a relatively small amount (20 to 25 percent) present as disaccharides or monosaccharides, including sucrose from table sugar, lactose from dairy products, maltose from starches and vegetables, and fructose from fruits. In order to minimize hyperlipidemia (high blood fats) and, it is hoped, eventual atherosclerosis, diet recommendations are for a low-fat diet with a decrease in saturated fats and an increase in polyunsaturated fats. Cholesterol should be limited to 250 mg/day. In order to achieve these objectives in fat content, it is necessary to alter the protein source somewhat from the usual fatty beef or pork to include increasing amounts of chicken, turkey, and seafood.

There is increasing attention to the place of *exercise* and physical fitness in the management of the individual with IDDM. There is little doubt that the very fit individual utilizes energy in a more efficient fashion and thus has a decreased insulin requirement. One would like to conclude that a lifetime of physical fitness will significantly reduce the long-term complications of diabetes mellitus. Although there is some evidence to suggest that this is true, complete confirmation is lacking. However, most clinical diabetologists agree that patients with IDDM should be encouraged to incorporate into their daily routine a program of fairly vigorous physical activity designed to lead to a high state of physical fitness. It is important that such physical activity be planned and incorporated into the daily program in order to prevent excessive variation in glucose concentration.

Hypoglycemia is a predictable occurrence in the patient who exercises excessively without adequate food intake to cover the exercise requirements. Similarly, unless appropriate adjustments of insulin and diet are made in advance, the patient who usually exercises vigorously on a daily basis can expect to be excessively hyperglycemic on those days when exercise is avoided.

Requirements for Management. The patient with IDDM requires insulin administration daily. Most patients currently use plastic disposable insulin syringes with disposable aluminum needles. While the use of disposable equipment adds appreciably to cost, it greatly increases convenience. Disposable needles are sharper and, consequently, accepted more readily by most patients. It is probable that in future years, many patients with IDDM will be treated by insulin infusion pump systems, which although they add to cost, will, it is hoped, lead to improvement in metabolic control.

The patient with IDDM must carry out regular biochemical observations in order to adjust the various aspects of the therapeutic regimen. Urine testing for glucose concentration has been the traditional technique employed by most patients. Urinary glucose concentration is determined semiquantitatively by use of glucose-oxidase-impregnated strips or a chemical-reducing color reaction such as the widely used Clinitest tablet method. We ask our patients to check a minimum of three urines daily. In addition to glucose content, acetone is estimated at least once daily.

Home blood-glucose monitoring is now a widely recommended technique for improving the accuracy of observations on control. Patients are asked to measure the concentration of glucose in their blood one or several times daily using one of several possible glucose oxidase impregnated strips. The equipment necessary to carry out these observations includes sharp lancets for pricking the finger, commercially available impregnated strips, and in some cases, a mechanical device for reading the blood glucose concentration. The cost of the strips averages about fifty cents per determination; the specialized colorimeter costs in excess of $300.

The diet recommended for the child with diabetes is also the diet we strongly urge the entire family to adopt. It may be somewhat more expensive than the general American diet because of the increase in protein content. Although we do not use or recommend weighed diets in our clinic, many centers continue to use weighing, at least initially. The purchase and regular use of food scales further adds to the cost and activity surrounding diabetic management.

These activities and observations should be the direct responsibility of the patient, who should utilize these observations to make decisions regarding overall therapy with the direct supervision and consent of the physician. For the younger child, the parents must make the observations and decisions until the child can become more involved in the decision-making process.

In addition to the observations carried out by the patient and family, other observations must be performed by the physician and his or her team during regularly scheduled visits of the patient with diabetes mellitus. Patients should be seen a minimum of three times annually, with intervening visits if metabolic control is unsatisfactory. Hospitalization is usually recommended at the time of initial diagnosis. If the patient's management is satisfactory, no additional hospital admissions may be required during childhood or adolescence. However, poor metabolic control, hypoglycemia, or diabetic ketoacidosis may be indications for a hospital stay.

The requirements placed on patients with diabetes mellitus and their families in terms of personal observations and decision-making and in terms of the requirements of office, clinic, or hospital visits and the attending specialized studies are associated with high cost and clear infringement on the life-style of both patient and family.

Special Problems and Complications. The complications of diabetes are classified as acute, intermediate duration, or late vascular. These classifications are primarily based on their timing in relationship to duration of disease or rapidity of onset.

Acute complications of diabetes mellitus are a direct result of rapidly developing metabolic changes. They include diabetic ketoacidosis and hypoglycemia. Diabetic ketoacidosis, which results from inadequate available insulin, may develop over a period of a few hours. This may be the result of either grossly inadequate insulin administration or its actual omission for a period of one or more days. More commonly, diabetic ketoacidosis occurs as a consequence of increasing stress, either emotional or resulting from intercurrent infectious illnesses. Patients with diabetic ketoacidosis require hospitalization and careful but vigorous therapy with intravenous insulin, fluids, and the like.

Hypoglycemia may occur very rapidly as a result of (1) excessive insulin administration, (2) inadequate food intake, (3) increased physical activity, or (4) some combination of these. It is seen more commonly in the spring or early summer when children and adolescents with diabetes begin to increase their level of physical activity without increasing food intake or reducing their insulin dose. Hypoglycemia can be especially dangerous in the younger child and may be a factor in central nervous system (CNS) damage. It is also a very special risk in the teenager who drinks excessively. Hypoglycemia occurring in a young person under the influence of alcohol can lead to severe, irreversible CNS damage.

Intermediate-duration complications of diabetes mellitus relate to growth and maturation and to autoimmune disease. Insulin is an important hormone of growth and maturation. Children and adolescents with diabetes do not grow or develop at an optimal rate unless diabetes control is optimal. It is not uncommon to observe a declining rate of height growth and delayed adolescent maturation in the individual with poorly controlled IDDM. Such alterations in growth and development are an absolute indication for vigorous evaluation and improvement in metabolic control. The most dramatic examples of this problem are children with diabetic dwarfism, or Mauriac syndrome.

A number of associated illnesses may occur with diabetes mellitus. This is particularly true of a number of autoimmune diseases, most commonly Hashimoto's thyroiditis but also including thyrotoxicosis, Addison's disease, hypoparathyroidism, and autoimmune inflammatory bowel disease. These disorders must be suspected and the patient properly evaluated for them periodically.

The characteristic *late vascular* lesion of IDDM is a uniquely diabetic lesion, involving small blood vessels throughout the body but causing specific damage in the retina of the eyes, in the kidneys, and in the peripheral nervous system. The mechanism of small-vessel damage is unclear, but increasing evidence points toward inadequacies of metabolic control as a major factor in causation. It is rare to see clinically apparent and important microvascular disease in the child or adolescent, despite several years of diabetes mellitus. However, increasingly sophisticated methods of study are clearly documenting that the small-vessel lesions do have their origin in childhood, when they may begin a relentless progression that continues until clinical disease is obvious in the young adult. This is especially true in regard to diabetic retinopathy, which eventually leads to serious vision-threatening eye damage in a high percentage of insulin-deficient patients with diabetes. Development of visual loss, however, is rarely seen in adolescents with diabetes, although the early microvascular lesions of diabetes mellitus can be detected in more than 50 percent of children and adolescents after five years of the disease. New techniques allow for a longitudinal history of the evolution of diabetic retinopathy and will also allow for greater understanding of the relationship between metabolic control and these alterations. Laser therapy has dramatically improved the outlook of patients with diabetes who have advanced retinopathy. It is hoped that therapeutic techniques may be developed that can be applied to the earliest developmental stages of diabetic retinopathy to prevent progression.

Diabetic nephropathy is the primary cause of death in IDDM. The disease is rarely clinically apparent in the child or adolescent. Persistent urinary protein is a highly reliable indicator of significant renal disease in the diabetic. Urine testing for protein should be routine in the diabetes clinic, and presence of proteinuria on screening tests should lead to quantitative twenty-four-hour estimation of protein loss. Excessive quantitative proteinuria should lead to consideration of renal biopsy and intensive therapy, possibly using an open-loop insulin infusion pump.

Peripheral or autonomic neuropathy is a common accompanying complication of IDDM but is rarely identified clinically in the child or adolescent. Techniques of measuring nerve-conduction time, however, can identify impaired peripheral nerve function in many children with diabetes. Recent studies have suggested that use of the open-loop insulin pump, with its improved metabolic control, may be effective in normalizing peripheral nerve function.

Costs. A recent survey commissioned by the Ames Division of Miles Laboratory (Marks, 1980) estimated the total annual cost of diabetes in the United States for 1979 to be 15.7 billion dollars. Almost half of this amount was due to "Lost Work Days." The next highest category (10 percent) was "Visits to Physicians," followed by "Other Products and Services" (which includes insulin, needles, oral hypoglyemic agents, and urine testing supplies) and "Laboratory Tests." These figures break down to an annual per-capita cost of $2,421.10 for the "average" patient with diabetes with the cost of the insulin-dependent diabetic being 3 percent higher. With the advent of the new but currently accepted insulin techniques, these costs will continue to increase. Home glucose-monitoring equipment, for example, can initially cost approximately $350 with associated supplies costing about $2 a day.

Almost $2 billion is expended for institutional care in short-stay hospital admissions or nursing homes. People with diabetes are hospitalized 2.5 times more frequently and have longer average hospital stays than nondiabetics (National Diabetes Advisory Board, 1980). A 1978 Medicaid survey in Pennsylvania indicated an average hospitalization period of 7.3 days for the total Medicaid population, with a comparable figure of 12 days among all patients, of all ages, who have diabetes and are on Medicaid (Pennsylvania Department of Welfare, personal communication with the authors, 1981).

The patient with diabetes, although burdened with excessive medical costs, is routinely denied the health insurance necessary to cover these costs. Often denial of insurance is made despite a record of good diabetic control. If coverage is granted, patients with diabetes are usually rated far beyond their ability to pay. Unless included in a larger group plan, many diabetics are without any means of protection. Normal costs of health care services often impede the use of preventive health measures. The excessive burden of cost on the person with diabetes often causes treatment to be neglected, which can result in even more excessive future costs.

It is unrealistic to assume that all health services can be reimbursable by third-party payers. Careful selection of coverage of those services that aim at reducing the incidence of diabetic complications could be the most cost-effective approach to reducing the tremendous national economic burden of diabetes.

Role of the Public Sector

Federal Diabetes Program. In 1974, Congress enacted Public Law (P.L.) 93–354, the National Diabetes Mellitus Research and Education Act. The act created a national commission charged with development of a long-range plan to combat diabetes. The commission's plan, based on a comprehensive study of the magnitude of diabetes, specified recommendations for organization and utilization of national health resources. Its goals were to expand and coordinate national research efforts in diabetes mellitus; improve education of patients, professionals, and the general public; promote the control of diabetes; and disseminate information about the disease. The plan evolved after evaluation of the most current scientific information, consultation with more than three hundred experts in the field, and examination of extensive public testimony. It represented the needs of an interacting social system—the patient, the patient's family, the health care provider, the medical researcher, and the general public.

In 1976, Congress approved the long-range plan to combat diabetes and established the National Diabetes Advisory Board (P.L. 94–562) to oversee its implementation and establish priorities for recommended programs. Annual reports of the board submitted to Congress in 1978, 1979, and 1980 describe the accomplishments of the plan. The major focus during that period was on a broad spectrum of basic and clinical biomedical research designed to obtain the information needed to control, prevent, and eventually cure diabetes. This research has resulted in a significant opportunity to reduce excessive morbidity, mortality, and costs associated with diabetes mellitus through improved application of recently available treatment measures.

Public policy at the federal level continues to evolve under the direction of the National Diabetes Advisory Board, redesignated by Congress in 1981 to function for another three years. The success of the goal-oriented biomedical research program in producing new treatment and interventions would indicate continued application of the same approach. Other components of the national diabetes program include eight Diabetes Research and Training Centers throughout the country (they serve as models for patient care and education as well as basic and clinical research), the Diabetes Control Demonstration Projects of the Centers for Disease Control (which serve as the translation mechanism between research and community level care), and the National Diabetes Information Clearinghouse and National Diabetes Data Group (which are the central sources for dissemination of information). These programs must be maintained in order to ensure progress toward improved quality of care and ultimately a cure (*State and Federal Assistance: Resource Directory for People with Diabetes*, 1981; 1976 Health Interview Survey; U.S. Department of Health, Education, and Welfare, 1979).

Financial Assistance Programs. Because the complications of diabetes cover virtually every system of the body, a wide range of services is required to cover disabilities. Several broad-based programs are available, but these meet the needs of children with diabetes in a very limited manner. Not every program is available in every state, and eligibility requirements vary. The following programs may be applicable to children with chronic diseases.

- Supplemental Security Income (SSI) provides monthly financial assistance to blind or disabled persons who meet eligibility requirements.
- Medicaid provides health care services to persons with low incomes.
- Renal disease programs (both state and federal) offer dialysis and transplantation services. Eligibility is based on financial need and severity of renal damage.
- Crippled Children's Services (CCS) provide medical services to children under age twenty-one who are crippled or suffering from conditions that lead to crippling. In many states, eligibility is based on financial need.
- Vocational Rehabilitation Services assist handicapped persons in achieving and maintaining employment. Eligibility is dependent upon the severity of the handicap and the potential for the gainful employment of the individual. Some programs include educational scholarships for handicapped college students. Types and extent of services vary from state to state.

These programs are designed to provide financial relief or palliative measures in crisis situations. Although some children with diabetes experience accelerated complications, most do not develop serious complications prior to young adulthood. Therefore these programs do not meet the needs of the majority of these children.

Categorical State Diabetes Programs. Because the programs just listed fail to meet the needs of the majority of patients with diabetes, several states have begun to develop categorical programs designed to serve this population better.

Four states have already implemented such programs, two of which are directed specifically toward children.

Florida and Connecticut have initiated programs that are administered through their respective Crippled Children's Services. In Connecticut, two university-related diabetes centers provide complete medical, educational, and counseling services. Children eligible for CCS receive services free of charge; others are charged on a sliding scale. In Florida, three centers provide the same services as in Connecticut, but each center sends regional health care teams into the field to conduct clinics and seminars in outlying areas. In addition, Florida provides twenty-four-hour telephone consultation to all patients and their families and to health care personnel.

The Kentucky Diabetes Program is also a university-based program focused on clinical care, training of health professionals, and community outreach. It serves people of all ages with diabetes and operates through cooperative agreements between the state health department, the university, and the Kentucky Diabetes Association. It sponsors a statewide network of diabetes education activities for both patients and professionals and maintains a model patient-referral, education, and treatment center at the University of Kentucky. It is also developing educational materials for people with different levels of learning ability.

In New Jersey, the diabetes program is part of the Chronic Disease Section of the State Health Department. It does not have a clinical component but is primarily concerned with patient and professional education. It provides patient education materials and sponsors symposia for health care professionals.

Under the auspices of the federal diabetes effort, the Center for Disease Control (CDC) sponsors a National Diabetes Control Program. This program is designed to apply public health concepts of disease control at the community level through state health departments. Currently, twenty states have been funded by CDC and are at various stages of implementing local interventions to change the health status of diabetic populations. Several other states are in the process of developing programs to serve the needs of their diabetic populations (Center for Disease Control, 1981).

Other Support Services. Two voluntary health agencies, the American Diabetes Association and the Juvenile Diabetes Foundation, provide support services to people with diabetes and their families. In addition to raising funds for research, both offer educational programs and literature, counseling, meetings, and rap sessions. These programs are administered by local chapters located throughout the country.

The National Diabetes Information Clearinghouse was established by Congress in 1973 to serve as the central resource for the dissemination of educational and scientific information relevant to diabetes. The three major goals of the clearinghouse are to increase availability of accurate diabetes information to health care professionals and to patients and their families, to increase community awareness of diabetes as a major health problem, and to establish a speedy communications network to provide information on new developments, techniques, and programs among the diabetes community. The clearinghouse publishes a regular newsletter and periodically updated bibliographies relating to all facets of diabetes.

Pennsylvania: A Model for the Approach to Public Policy Issues in Diabetes Mellitus. The need to address public policy issues in Pennsylvania arose from a growing awareness of the potential benefits of increased activities at the federal level. Lay leadership of the Pennsylvania diabetes community was able to demonstrate to the governor that the needs of the community were not being addressed at the state and local levels.

During the past forty years, Pennsylvania has ranked among the highest six states in the country with respect to diabetes mortality and has had much higher mortality rates than the nation as a whole. Yet, as of 1979, no state programs existed to address the problems of diabetes in a categorical manner (Tokuhata, 1976). In 1980, Governor Richard Thornburgh created the Pennsylvania Diabetes Task Force. The overall goal of the task force is to reduce diabetes mortality and its complications and their effects by improving the quality of diabetes treatment, care, and education available at the community level in the state. Specifically, the task force has been charged with both collecting data to demonstrate the magnitude of the problem and the areas of need and recommending a comprehensive program to control the adverse effects of diabetes.

Shortly after the appointment of the task force, Pennsylvania was awarded a contract for a Diabetes Control Demonstration Project by the Center for Disease Control in Atlanta. The purpose of the project was to translate recent research advances into community-level health interventions; the task force was to act as the advisory body to the Pennsylvania project. Two projects were immediately undertaken by the task force and the control project staff: a data collection plan and public hearings. The plan included accessing mortality data from commonwealth death certificate records, morbidity and cost data from hospitals in sample counties throughout the state, and resource and services data from multiple sources. The task force felt that input from the diabetic population of Pennsylvania, its health care providers, and the general public was as important as collection of statistical data in assessing the magnitude of the problem. Seven public hearings allowed every citizen the opportunity to express views and make recommendations that would help the task force carry out its charge. Four topics represented leading areas of concern in all seven hearings: patient education, professional education, high costs and need for third-party reimbursement, and psychosocial aspects (Pennsylvania Diabetes Task Force, 1981b).

Based upon the data collection study and the public hearings, the task force developed a comprehensive diabetes plan involving a two-part effort to improve the quantity and quality of care received at the community level by patients with diabetes. The first part of the plan places specially trained teams of multidisciplinary health care practitioners in designated communities to assess needs and develop interventions that address specific problems identified in the community. The second part formulates a "Diabetes Academy" of specialists to provide the community with professional education programs and professional consultative services (Pennsylvania Diabetes Task Force, 1981a).

Public Policy Needs, Impediments, and Recommendations

The majority of cases of childhood diabetes do not begin to develop complications until approximately ten years after onset. Although a small number of children do develop accelerated complications or associated metabolic conditions, this section addresses the needs of the average child with diabetes.

Briefly stated, the goal of treating children with diabetes is to achieve the therapeutic objectives of control designed to prevent or delay complications while developing a life-style that coordinates near-normal activities with effective self-management.

The Therapeutic Team and the Therapeutic Alliance. No longer can treatment of the patient with IDDM by the physician alone be justified. The complexities of this disorder are such that involvement of several health professionals in the therapeutic team is necessary. Because detailed knowledge about diabetes mellitus and its management is prerequisite to the achievement of good metabolic control, the basic function of the therapeutic team is educational. This is true of the physician as well as all other members. However, in most teams, educational leadership comes from a highly skilled and trained nurse-educator whose responsibility it is to educate the patient and family about all aspects of diabetes mellitus including information on causation, pathophysiology, symptomatology, complications and their possible prevention, recognition of hypoglycemia and its treatment, insulin-injection techniques, and urine-testing methods. Usually this individual also serves as the first-line counselor for the patient and family in the area of emotional stress and family problems. The second member of the therapeutic team is the dietician, whose responsibility it is to introduce the concepts of good nutrition in a way that is meaningful to the patient and family and to make specific dietary recommendations that will lead to improvement in diabetic control. Diet instruction takes time and patience. Multiple sessions may be necessary before the family feels confident about diet preparation and selection. The dietician should be available to the patients and the family as needed for specific consultation and should review dietary recommendations and patient status at least annually. The third member of the team is the social worker, whose function is to assist the family in identifying and utilizing community resources and to counsel the family from the point of view of psychosocial needs. In addition to providing assistance in economic areas, the social worker may also expedite procurement of necessary medication, supplies, and special foods. The physician-diabetologist is the fourth member of the primary therapeutic team. The field of diabetes mellitus is rapidly changing. The physician who would function effectively and teach patients and families optimal management practices must spend considerable time keeping abreast of medical literature and applying new observations and methods to his or her practice.

The most important member of the therapeutic team is clearly the patient. Achievement of satisfactory metabolic control (and it is hoped, decreased complications) is largely a result of the patient's knowledge and understanding of the disorder and the emotional acceptance of it and its requirements into his or her life-style. In a very real sense, a contractual relationship should be drawn up between patient, parents, and key members of the therapeutic team, clearly outlining areas of responsibility for each of the participants. Increasingly, the patient should assume control of observational and decision-making aspects of management. Other team members should ideally become consultants for the patient, assisting only with particular problem solving.

In addition to the immediate therapeutic team, there are other team members who should be available for consultation as needed. First among this group is a skilled behavioral scientist, either a child psychiatrist or a clinical child psychologist well-versed in diabetes mellitus and its requirements (Hamburg and others, 1980). The importance of early identification of evolving emotional risks and their management prior to crisis or emotional deterioration cannot be overemphasized. In addition, an ophthalmologist should see the teenager with diabetes on an annual basis with detailed retinal observations carried out as indicated. During the adolescent years, the girl with diabetes should be placed in contact with a gynecologist/obstetrician who is knowledgeable about diabetes mellitus in order to begin her education as it relates to management of diabetes in pregnancy, use of birth control methods, and the like.

It is particularly important for both young men and young women with diabetes mellitus not to be lost to the health care system as they go into and through adolescence. Frequently, such patients who have been faithfully followed by their pediatrician or pediatric diabetologist drop out of the health care system during mid or late adolescence not to appear again for several years until job requirements make medical supervision necessary or in those tragic situations when complications suddenly appear in young adult life. The physician caring for the young adolescent with diabetes must take responsibility for ensuring that the young patient moving into the hands of an internist continues to receive knowledgeable and sympathetic medical management.

Only a small fraction of children with diabetes are fortunate enough to have access to a therapeutic team headed by a well-trained diabetologist. The vast majority of children are treated by pediatricians, internists, or family or general practitioners. Most of these physicians see few children with diabetes within the framework of their own practices. Few have the time, inclination, resources, or knowledge to provide the ongoing educational and counseling components of a multidisciplinary approach. As a result, the treatment received by many such children is fragmented and incomplete (Digon and Miller, 1977).

Since medical centers with multidisciplinary teams and physicians with expertise in diabetes are not available to all children with diabetes, a substitute mechanism must be found to provide comprehensive services. Most public health departments include nurses, nutritionists, and social workers on their staffs. Under the rubric of comprehensive health programs, these allied health professionals are expected to provide services that address all patients and all problems. Specific training in any categoric area is not usually offered, and because of understaffing, the caseload is usually too large to handle. A program providing community-based allied health professionals specifically trained to administer diabetes support services in conjunction with local physicians might well permit a multidisciplinary therapeutic approach to all diabetic children in a relatively inexpensive manner that might even pay for itself in decreased hospitalizations and fewer complications.

Patient Education. For patients with diabetes, the most important component of treatment is education. Both initial and ongoing education are required to produce knowledgeable patients who can participate in management of their own disease.

Most children who have diabetes are diagnosed in a hospital setting. In many cases, the brief inpatient education provided during the initial hospitalization is the only education the child and family ever receive. The initial information provided to the patient and family should cover only what they need to know to begin management. Ongoing education, provided as the family is ready to absorb it, should be available on an outpatient basis. Once again, a multidisciplinary team should present this education in a coordinated manner.

There are few formal education programs addressed to both children with newly diagnosed diabetes and their families. Most inpatient education is administered, in spare moments, by a floor nurse or by a staff dietician who provides a written diet sheet on the day prior to discharge. Often, the impact of diagnosis and the stress of hospitalization have an adverse effect on learning, and inpatient education is not effective. As a result, many families are sent home unprepared to handle the shattering changes in their life-style, and the children involved ultimately become the excessive statistics on hospital readmissions.

Few programs are available to train health care professionals to administer diabetes education. In contrast, extensive patient education materials are available, but no one has attempted to evaluate them by need or target population. By far the greatest impediment to ongoing education, however, is the lack of third-party reimbursement for outpatient education. Inpatient education costs are considered part of the therapeutic program and are usually covered as hospital overhead. Outpatient education generally is not considered reimbursable by third-party payors.

Both inpatient and outpatient education programs should be formalized to include all elements of diabetes management at the proper stages of progression. These programs should be administered by specific diabetes-trained health care professionals, sometimes in group sessions and sometimes on an individual basis. For example, nutritional education is particularly important to adjust a diet to a child's tastes, needs, and time schedule. Assistance is needed to learn how to substitute fast foods and snacks into the diet so the child can relate positively to peers. In addition, the child must know how to adjust the diet during periods of illness, stress, or travel. Periodic counseling is needed to provide individual dietary changes to correspond to growth. The result of good nutritional education can be maintenance of better control and thus the forestalling of diabetic complications.

Improving patient education will require implementation of comprehensive education programs administered with a multidisciplinary approach. One method of accomplishing expansion of diabetes education efforts is development of proper educational centers with outreach programs and mobile units. Another method is to earmark specially trained support personnel to interact with existing professionals in the community to improve community-level education programs. Existing models for each of these approaches have been discussed earlier.

Minimum standards should be established for all diabetes education programs, and an evaluation process should be included to measure effectiveness. Finally, before any program can be successful, health care providers must be educated in diabetes management and third-party reimbursers must accept the concept of education as treatment.

Professional Education. In order to provide good patient education, professionals must be educated first. The lack of general professional education in the field of diabetes has resulted in either poor or unavailable patient care in many areas. The child with diabetes is entitled to care by professionals who are knowledgeable and qualified to administer a comprehensive regimen including treatment, education, counseling, and self-management techniques.

Confusion and controversy within the health care system over appropriate preventive measures for people with diabetes have been a major impediment to effective treatment. Most such people (children included) are treated by primary health care providers. In the absence of a clear therapeutic regimen, these providers frequently fail to take appropriate or timely action that would prevent or delay complications.

Professional school curricula and continuing-education programs are inadequate with respect to diabetes, both in terms of physicians and allied health professionals. Finally, the manpower base of professionals who care for patients with diabetes is inequitably distributed. Little or no specialized or multidisciplinary care is available in rural and semirural areas. Strategies are needed to develop outreach programs that will improve the quality of care in these locations.

Several approaches are needed to upgrade the standard of professional education. Professional school curricula should be evaluated and expanded. Minimum standards should be established for health care providers who treat patients with diabetes. Professional education centers could be established to educate health care professionals in the treatment of diabetic patients. Courses in interpersonal communications skills, counseling, and self-help concepts could be included in the curriculum.

Continuing-education strategies should be developed to reinforce knowledge levels and provide new information. Use of self-assessment methods should be explored, and evaluation measures should be included in any new programs. A permanent system of updating professionals should be established, and more articles on diabetes should be placed in professional journals. Probably the most effective immediate means for improving the quality of professional education would be to include updated diabetes standards of care in testing for licensure and certification and to increase the number of questions on the subject of diabetes.

Psychosocial Support (Hamburg and others, 1980). The emotional burdens on the child with diabetes mellitus and on the child's family are great. The patient soon becomes aware of having an incurable disease that carries with it such frightening potential complications as blindness, loss of limbs, heart disease, kidney failure, and early death. The therapeutic requirements are complex, demanding, and intrusive in the usual life-style of the child or adolescent and the family. Restriction in access to one of the basic requirements of life—food—is a basic tenet of management. The observational and therapeutic requirements necessary to achieve good metabolic control are in direct opposition to the natural movement away from parental supervision and guidance and toward peer-group activities and pressures that characterize adolescence. Emotional disability commonly occurs in the child with diabetes but is especially frequent during the adolescent years. Predictable reactions include rejection of the disease along with the requirements for its management, depression, withdrawal, isolation, hostility and acting out delinquent behavior, excessive risk-taking, and rarely, active psychosis.

During the past decade, there has been a growing awareness of the importance of psychosocial and behavioral factors in determining diabetic patients' adjustment to their chronic condition. More than merely attention to their physical needs is required if they are to cope with the daily demands and potential crises of their disease, to develop responsibility for self-care, and to adopt life-styles to minimize their risk of complications. Problems in the emotional sphere should be anticipated and prevented or minimized by appropriate counseling of the patient and family members early in the course of the disease. Follow-up counseling should continue to be available as needed, particularly in times of stress, during adolescence, or at the onset of complications.

The new awareness of the importance of the psychosocial aspects of diabetes has not yet been translated into action, and today, counseling services for the child with diabetes are virtually nonexistent. Because of the unavailability of trained personnel, current counseling services are not directed at prevention of major problems but are provided only in crisis situations. In the few situations in which preventive counseling is offered, the traditional association of counseling with acute emotional problems often causes the family to reject this option. Furthermore, because counseling has not been fully accepted as part of the treatment process, there is no third-party reimbursement for such services, which makes them inaccessible to the majority of patients.

The primary step must be to include psychosocial counseling as a part of the routine treatment regimen. Training programs are needed to produce knowledgeable professionals. In areas not accessible to diabetes centers, social workers specifically trained in the problems and management of this aspect of diabetes should be available through the public health system. Such services should be third-party reimbursable.

To be effective, psychosocial support for children with diabetes must focus on the entire family. Both management of the disease and fear of eventual complications affect the entire family. In very young children, management responsibilities often fall upon a parent or other family member. The sharing of those responsibilities and their transfer to the patient is not always an automatic part of the maturing process and must be guided through appropriate counseling.

Peer-support systems should be established as a mechanism complementary to professional counseling. Peer counseling and the sharing of experiences provide the child with the assurance that the problem is not being faced alone. Peer support groups are especially valuable to the adolescent with diabetes, who must face all the general problems of adolescence superimposed on learning to manage a chronic disease.

Professional groups, private mental health practitioners, mental health centers, and child guidance clinics need to become more knowledgeable about and sensitive to diabetes and its impact on individuals and families. Research is needed on various psychological approaches to treatment, such as group therapy and behavior modification. The psychosocial aspect of diabetes management should be addressed by public education programs as well as patient education programs because successful emotional development is dependent on both self-perception and the perception of others.

Financial Support Mechanisms. The area of prime importance for which there is no third-party coverage is that of outpatient services. Outpatient education programs are not covered, nor is nutritional or psychosocial counseling. As a result, many patients must be hospitalized to receive these services. Patients who are not hospitalized for such services often appear as later hospital admissions for treatment of diabetic complications.

Another area needing attention in terms of financial support mechanisms concerns day-to-day care of the patient with diabetes. Even without consideration of the catastrophic costs of complications, the cost of routine management of diabetes exceeds the financial capacity of many families. Consequently, many patients avoid doctor visits and urine testing to reduce costs.

Finally, the family or even the young patient who attempts to purchase health insurance to offset some of the costs of diabetic care faces further frustrations. Most health insurance is available to people with diabetes only through large group plans. Individuals are either refused coverage or rated far beyond their ability to pay, even if they can demonstrate that they are under good control. The same problems apply to life and automobile insurance, which creates major problems for families of working or college-bound teenagers who have diabetes.

At the present time, there are insufficient data to illustrate conclusively to third-party payors the efficacy of outpatient education and counseling in terms of lowering the cost of patient care. Furthermore, acceptable minimum standards for third-party coverage of both educational and counseling programs and the professionals who administer them have not yet been developed. Since outpatient education is a departure from traditional reimbursement approaches, careful documentation is needed to illustrate its benefits. The states of Maine and New York have implemented model demonstration projects under the auspices of the

CDC Diabetes Control Program to test the effectiveness of outpatient education programs.

Coverage for diabetic supplies is a major problem mainly to families with income levels not low enough to qualify for financial assistance programs yet not high enough to sustain the burden of long-term medical costs. These families are victims of a gap in health care reimbursement programs. It is primarily these families who suffer also from the inability to obtain individual health insurance.

Third-party payors should be encouraged to study the implications of outpatient education and counseling and to develop policies and financial incentives to encourge these services. Diabetes is an excellent model for development of both programs and standards for coverage that would ultimately apply to all chronic diseases.

Financial assistance programs should be assessed to consider redefining qualifying income levels for families burdened with the ongoing costs of a chronic disease. Health, automobile, and life insurance guidelines should be examined in view of the improved treatment modalities available in diabetes, and applicants should be rated on individual standards of control rather than blanket standards. This process should be monitored through the offices of state insurance commissioners.

Medical Devices. Two new advances in the field of diabetes are rapidly changing the treatment of patients with diabetes.

The advent of home glucose monitoring has provided a method of testing blood-glucose levels that is far superior to urine testing. This new, relatively simple technique enables the patient to measure the actual level of glucose in the blood. This information can be used to provide better diabetic control than has been possible up to now. Home glucose monitoring has already been seen to reduce emergency room visits and hospitalizations and to facilitate normalization of blood sugar levels in pregnant women with diabetes, reducing the risk of congenital abnormalities and neonatal mortality.

Another rapidly developing improvement in diabetes treatment is the automated insulin-delivery system or insulin pump. Many improvements are still needed at the research level, but several current external models are in the process of clinical trials. Enough clinical trials have occurred to verify improved control of blood-glucose levels. Long-term studies to assess the effect on complications are underway. A thrust to make this equipment available to all patients with IDDM should begin now in order to prevent a time lag and unnecessary morbidity once the device has been approved for general use.

Increased general utilization of the above two devices implies strategy changes at several levels of health care. First, primary care physicians must be apprised of the availability and efficacy of the techniques. Second, third-party payors must cover the cost. And third, systems for teaching proper use of the equipment and resulting changes in insulin dosages must be established.

As a prerequisite to utilizing these devices as part of standard therapy, evidence must be assembled concerning their efficacy, costs, and benefits. Then a formal consensus recommending usage should be developed and submitted to third-party payors. Finally, professional education mechanisms (for example, seminars, journal publications) must be developed to teach use of the equipment to health care providers. Initiatives for this program should come from the national level.

Educational Institutions. The child and adolescent with diabetes mellitus have special requirements that must be understood and met by the educational system. These children need to eat on schedule. Many need additional snacks to prevent hypoglycemia. Schools must be aware of these needs and provide the time and place for the child to take care of them. Children do not like to be different. Frequently, school children will avoid their needed midmorning or midafternoon snack because they do not wish classmates to be aware of their disorder. Urine testing may be needed prior to lunch. The child should have the opportunity to carry out this testing in private without interference from classmates or school personnel. Insulin administration will rarely be necessary during school hours, but if it is, the child should be free to give the injection without fear of ridicule or criticism or implication that street drugs are being used. The least the parent should expect is knowledgeable understanding on the part of the health professionals (school nurses and school physicians) and an active desire to provide an optimal atmosphere in facilities on the part of the school personnel.

Knowledgeable school personnel are unfortunately the exception rather than the rule. Few school nurses, physicians, or teachers are adequately educated about diabetes mellitus or its impact on the school-aged child. Many parents of children with diabetes feel the school system regularly erects obstacles for them and their children rather than attempting to solve legitimate problems that lie in the province of the school system. One problem contributing to this situation is the small number of these children enrolled in any one school. At the diabetes prevalence rate of 1.8 per thousand school children, an individual school of one thousand students may have only two children with diabetes enrolled at any one time. However, if children are accepted within the public school system, the school's responsibility is to the entire student body, not merely the majority. Furthermore, the information needed by school personnel to respond to the needs of the child with diabetes is minimal.

The American Diabetes Association and the Juvenile Diabetes Foundation have both made tremendous efforts to provide diabetes education in schools, but without the support of the school districts themselves, results remain fragmented. A truly successful continuing-education program in schools must be advocated from within the educational system. Regular in-service education should include information regarding emergencies and health needs of chronically ill children. Such educational programs should be extended to school bus drivers, cafeteria personnel, and maintenance staff. Organizations and agencies that conduct outside activities for children (for example, Ys, scouting programs, Little League, church, schools) should provide their staffs with similar information. Continuing-education programs should update personnel on new knowledge as well as new approaches to therapy.

Programs within the schools should teach children about chronic diseases in a manner that will help them relate in a positive way to children who have these diseases.

Career Development and Employment (U.S. Department of Health, Education, and Welfare, 1975). Parents should not restrict their view of their child's career future because of diabetes mellitus. They must be positive and optimistic about the future, encouraging the young person to set goals and anticipate achieving them. There are very few occupations denied individuals specifically because they have diabetes mellitus. Two examples would be the commercial pilot and the commercial truck driver involved in interstate traffic. It is understandable why such jobs, which involve lives of others, might be restricted from people with IDDM who, if they became hypoglycemic in such situations, might injure themselves and others. Few other occupations can be eliminated because the applicant has diabetes mellitus. Indeed, there are government regulations that prohibit such restrictive hiring practices.

In the real world, people with diabetes are frequently not employed or are passed over for advancement because of health concerns on the part of management. Unions, for example, may not wish to accept individuals with diabetes mellitus because health insurance rates would be increased if patients with chronic diseases were accepted. Many employers turn away job seekers with diabetes because of fear that they will miss too many work days. Although data indicate a large loss of work days on the part of employees with diabetes, most of this morbidity results from diabetic complications. Individuals who can document good control of their diabetes are no greater risk to the work schedule than any other employees. Often, diabetics are afraid to acknowledge their diabetes to their employers. Working conditions that discourage employees from acknowledging their diabetes also discourage maintenance of good control.

Industry needs programs of general education to clarify all of the misconceptions concerning diabetes and employment. Emphasis is needed in various aspects of the public domain, in industry, and in local, state, and national government regarding the capabilities of individuals with diabetes mellitus to provide a high level of performance at tasks of all varieties.

Additional Needs and Recommendations. Improvement of public information and education about diabetes mellitus should be a high priority of public policy programs. Television and radio spots on diabetes have helped raise the awareness level of the public but have had little effect in actually transferring meaningful information. With respect to children, public information should be directed at providing a better understanding of the disease, which would enable children with diabetes to interact with their peers and the community without fear of ostracism.

An equally important aspect of public education concerns the importance of alerting public employees to emergency procedures applicable to diabetes. Police, firemen, and ambulance and public transportation personnel are potential target groups for this application.

Community organizations such as churches, Y's, and Rotary Clubs can provide a source of referral to other health or social agencies. Diabetes screening within such agencies is probably not a reasonable expenditure of either private or public funds.

Normally, young people with diabetes mellitus do not need specialized housing or other public facilities. However, there are instances in which older adolescents or young adults with diabetes experience severe family conflicts. Immature social skills and poor diabetic control preclude independent living for these young people, yet many group homes will not accept people with chronic diseases. If available, this kind of group living could allow these young people to separate from their conflicted families and begin to work toward independent living while still in a protected environment.

Summary. In the preceding sections, specific impediments to each segment of diabetes care were identified. However, several major recurring problems are common to all areas of diabetes care. These include:

- lack of patient awareness of the availability of treatment and self-help measures that may prevent or minimize complications
- lack of provider knowledge of effective treatment practices
- lack of coordination among diverse parts of the health care system
- inadequate methods to update provider knowledge, skills, and attitudes
- inadequate third-party reimbursement of cost-effective services
- inadequate data on specific diabetes-related issues including measurement of treatment practice

To remove these impediments, two major departures must be made from the traditional approach to public health programs: (1) diabetes must be treated as a categorical disease and (2) a preventive rather than palliative approach must be utilized.

Current public health philosophies suggest that the patient be treated as a total or comprehensive entity. Children who are brought to a community health clinic are treated for their needs at the time of their clinic visit. If they have diabetes, (theoretically) their diabetes is treated. With respect to diabetes, this approach does not work. Granted, it is less costly than a categorical approach in which professionals with specific expertise administer programs, and because the professional staff have general backgrounds, fewer staff are needed and thus lower costs are maintained. But records are not kept by disease category, so there are no data available to evaluate the system, and furthermore, there is no formal program to update the health care providers administering comprehensive care. Educational and counseling aspects are not included in the comprehensive care package. The diverse needs of the diabetes patient are, in and of themselves, comprehensive enough to require the administration of services under a categorical program. A multidisciplinary approach to the treatment, education, and counseling of diabetic patients, administered by specifically trained experts, might seem more costly than a comprehensive care program at the outset, but ultimately it would be the most cost-effective approach in terms of reducing morbidity, mortality, and excess hospitalization.

Traditionally, public health programs in the United States have been based upon health problems that were prevalent in the first half of the twentieth century—these were primarily infectious diseases and sanitation. Programs were designed to administer crisis-oriented or palliative measures. Today, chronic diseases are the leading cause of death and illness in this country, but patterns of health care have not changed to meet the new needs. Chronic illnesses are not cured or alleviated by short-term treatment measures; long-term management and prevention must be the approach.

In a time of rising health care costs and scarce resources, services are being provided only for the crises associated with diabetes (for example, dialysis, kidney transplantation, laser therapy). A preventive approach begun in childhood might preclude the need for many of these costly crisis measures, reduce excessive hospitalization, and ultimately impact on overall diabetes morbidity and mortality. It must be noted, however, that positive results from categorical-preventive chronic disease programs can be measured only after long-term implementation. An important factor in the successful development of such programs is the reassessment of expectations of quick results on the part of the officials who administer them (National Diabetes Advisory Board, 1982).

References

Cahill, G. F., Jr., and McDevitt, H. O. "Insulin-Dependent Diabetes Mellitus: The Initial Lesion." *New England Journal of Medicine,* 1981, *304,* 1454–1464.

Center for Disease Control. "Third Party Reimbursement in Maine, in New York." Diabetes Control Program Update, 1981, *2* (3), 4–5.

Digon, E., and Miller, W. "The Prevalence of Juvenile-Onset Diabetes in Pennsylvania's Schools, 1976." Division of Epidemiological Research, Bureau of Health Research, Pennsylvania Department of Health, August 1977.

Drash, A. L. "The Etiology of Diabetes Mellitus." *New England Journal of Medicine,* 1979, *300,* 1211–1213.

Drash, A. L. "Management of the Diabetic Child." In Stephen Podolosky (Ed.), *Clinical Diabetes: Modern Management.* New York: Appleton-Century-Crofts, 1980.

Drash, A. L., and Becker, D. "Diabetes Mellitus in the Child: Course, Special Problems, and Related Disorders." In H. M. Katzen and R. J. Mahler (Eds.), *Diabetes, Obesity, and Vascular Disease.* New York: Wiley, 1978.

Drash, A. L., and others. "The Natural History of Diabetes Mellitus in Children: Insulin Requirements During the Initial Two Years." *Acta Paediatrica Belgica,* 1980, *33* (1), 66–67.

Drash, A. L., and others. "Descriptive Epidemiology of Insulin-Dependent Diabetes Mellitus in Allegheny County, Pennsylvania." In J. M. Martin, R. M. Ehrlich, and F. J. Holland (Eds.), *Etiology and Pathogenesis of Insulin Dependent Diabetes Mellitus.* New York: Raven Press, 1981.

Hamburg, B. A., and others. *Behavioral and Psychosocial Issues in Diabetes: Proceedings of the National Conference.* National Institutes of Health publication no. 80-1993. Washington, D.C.: U.S. Government Printing Office, 1980.

LaPorte, R. E., and others. "The Pittsburgh Insulin-Dependent Diabetes Mellitus (IDDM) Registry: The Incidence of Insulin-Dependent Diabetes Mellitus in Allegheny County, Pennsylvania (1965-1976)." *Diabetes*, 1981a, *30* (4), 279-294.

LaPorte, R. E., and others. "The Pittsburgh Insulin-Dependent Diabetes Mellitus Registry: The Relationship of Insulin-Dependent Diabetes Mellitus Incidence to Social Class." *American Journal of Epidemiology*, 1981b, *114*, 379-384.

Marks, R. G. "Diabetes: The Expensive Disease." *Drug Topics*, September 2, 1980.

National Diabetes Advisory Board. *The Treatment and Control of Diabetes: A National Plan to Reduce Mortality and Morbidity*. Bethesda, Md.: National Diabetes Advisory Board, 1980.

National Diabetes Advisory Board. "Diabetes in the 1980's: Challenges for the Future." National Institutes of Health publication no. 82-2143. Washington, D.C.: U.S. Government Printing Office, 1982.

National Diabetes Data Group. "Classification and Diagnosis of Diabetes Mellitus and Other Categories of Glucose Intolerance." *Diabetes*, 1979, *28*, 1039-1057.

1976 Health Interview Survey. "Prevalence of Diabetes by Age and Sex, United States." Atlanta, Ga.: Center for Disease Control, 1976.

Pennsylvania Diabetes Task Force. *Pennsylvania Diabetes Plan*. Harrisburg: Pennsylvania Department of Health, 1981a.

Pennsylvania Diabetes Task Force. *A Report of Public Input Meetings of Diabetes in Pennsylvania*, Vols. 1 and 2. Harrisburg: Pennsylvania Department of Health, 1981b.

State and Federal Assistance: Resource Directory for People with Diabetes. National Institutes of Health publication no. 81-2158. Washington, D.C.: U.S. Government Printing Office, 1981.

Tokuhata, G. K. "Diabetes Mellitus Mortality." Bureau of Health Research. Harrisburg: Pennsylvania Department of Health, 1976.

U.S. Department of Health, Education, and Welfare. *Report of the National Commission on Diabetes*, Vol. 1. Washington, D.C.: U.S. Government Printing Office, 1975.

U.S. Department of Health, Education, and Welfare. *Diabetes Data Compiled 1977*. National Institutes of Health publication no. 79-1468. Washington, D.C.: U.S. Government Printing Office, 1979.

Wagener, D., and others. "Pittsburgh Diabetes Mellitus Study: II. Secondary Attack Rates in Families with Insulin-Dependent Diabetes Mellitus." *American Journal of Epidemiology*, 1982, *115* (6), 868-878.

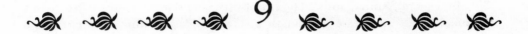

Neuromuscular Diseases

Irene S. Gilgoff, M.D.
Shelby L. Dietrich, M.D.

Children afflicted with neuromuscular impairment, even though they may have different diagnoses, share many common problems regardless of whether the weakness originates within the nerve or within the muscle. These children with muscle disease, who are in need of our care and attention, can be found in wheelchairs in clinic lobbies across the country.

The diversity of neuromuscular diseases gives credibility to the often complex and expensive diagnostic procedures, such as multiple blood studies and x rays, to which these children are often subjected. Specialized tests are also often necessary to differentiate one disease entity from another. In addition, a muscle biopsy, requiring hospitalization and general anesthesia, is sometimes a fundamental part of the diagnostic procedures required. Although diagnostic evaluation may be costly, the gravity of the diagnosis under consideration and the commonly inherited nature of these diseases makes total certainty of diagnosis a strict requirement.

Disorders of the Anterior Horn Cell

Spinal Muscular Atrophy. Spinal muscular atrophy is the name applied to a clinical spectrum of inherited diseases of the anterior horn cell, the site of the connection of the motor (corticospinal) tract within the spinal cord. Involvement at the connection categorizes this disease as a lower-neuron disease.

Accurate statistics on incidence and prevalence of spinal muscular atrophy are not available at this time because children with this disorder are followed by so many subspecialists. Available incidence figures also fail to include children misdiagnosed or undiagnosed. Michael Brooke (1977) reports an incidence of 1 in 15,000 to 1 in 25,000 live births for the severe form of the disease. However, children with the intermediate and mild forms of spinal muscular atrophy are not included in these figures. Brooke estimates the carrier state in the normal population to be about one in eighty.

In general, spinal muscular atrophy is believed to be inherited as an autosomal recessive disease. Although several children within the immediate family may be found to have the disease, no previous family history can be found on either parent's side and both parents are asymptomatic. The parents as a couple, however, face a 25 percent risk of recurrence of the disease in their children. Some rare cases of a mild form of spinal muscular atrophy with an autosomal dominant pattern of inheritance have been reported, but these cases are the exception. No means of detecting the disease carrier is presently available.

Spinal muscular atrophy is divided clinically into at least three different disease entities. In the past, these entities were referred to by such names as Werdnig-Hoffman disease or Kugelberg-Welander disease but are now subdivided into the categories of severe, intermediate, and mild. The severe form of the disorder presents at birth or within the first year of life. Prior to onset, there may be a short time during which the child is noted to be completely normal. The affected infant shows extreme weakness, is floppy, and lacks head control. As is typical in all forms of this disease, the muscles closer to the spinal cord (proximal muscles) are more severely affected than the muscles further away (distal muscles) and the legs are more severely affected than the arms. Children with the severe form may have no movement except in the lower extremities at the ankles and toes and in the upper extremities at the hands, wrists, and possibly elbows. An important aspect of the disease is the severe weakness of the rib muscles, causing these children to be purely diaphragmatic breathers. This fact, combined with severe weakness of the abdominal muscles, renders them unusually susceptible to respiratory infections. The severe form of spinal muscular atrophy was once considered fatal during the first few years of life, but with the availability of effective antibiotics and improved respiratory therapy, including the use of respirators, some of these children are surviving into their second and third decades of life.

The intermediate form of the disease includes children who are able to sit unsupported but unable to walk. They have functioning rib muscles and are therefore less prone to respiratory complications. The weakness seen in these children is generally not progressive, and survival into adulthood is common.

The mild form of the disease is often not diagnosed until adolescence or even later. These children exhibit some muscle weakness (more apparent at the hips than the shoulders) but are able to walk. The prognosis for a normal life expectancy is excellent.

Cases of spinal muscular atrophy that do not fit comfortably into any of the above categories are not uncommonly seen. In general, a mild form of the disease does not progress to a more severe form, and most cases achieve and maintain a plateau for many years. However, rare cases have been described that show clear progression of weakness.

Children with all forms of this disorder have normal intelligence and, as a population group, may be above average. No cardiac problems are found with this disease.

At present, there is no cure. Treatment is directed toward acute and chronic medical care and includes a long-term program of supportive services. Multiple lengthy hospitalizations are often required as are tracheostomies and respirator assistance. Permanent dependence on a respirator is no longer a rare occurrence. With the recent advances in pulmonary medicine, longer life expectancies and more frequent use of expensive medical equipment must be anticipated.

Supportive treatment of the patient includes prevention and treatment of problems that arise secondary to the patient's muscular weakness. Splinting devices and bracing are used in an attempt to prevent contractures of the extremities. If contractures occur, surgical intervention may be necessary. Progressive spinal curvature, often a problem encountered in this disease, is secondary to the weakness of the back muscles and can further compromise the respiratory status of a child already at risk. Curvature can add a significant balance problem to the ambulatory or seated child. Bracing of the back, along with eventual surgical intervention, is often necessary.

For the child who is able to walk, assistance devices may be necessary. Such devices include appropriate bracing. For the nonambulatory child, manual and electric wheelchairs are necessary. However, many other devices exist to improve mobility. Arm supports that are available allow the child increased hand and arm function. Devices that enable the wheelchair-bound patient to retrieve a fallen object or one high on a shelf add an immense measure of independence and security. Special lifts and hospital beds ease the task of the person caring for the child.

The additional stresses placed on the family of a child with severe spinal muscular atrophy are significant. Financial difficulty in meeting the ever-growing medical demands is only one stress area. The autosomal recessive genetic pattern of this disease and the concomitant absence of a family history of the illness means that prospective parents are not aware of the potential for giving birth to a child with a chronic illness or of the problems their offspring may face. Anticipating a normal child, they must quickly restructure their futures to meet the demands of a chronically handicapping disease.

Even families in which there is a child with a mild form of the disease face many stresses. For example, ambulatory children with weakness are clumsy and unable to succeed in physical competition with their peers; prior to diagnosis, such children may have even been labeled lazy and uncooperative. The competitive drives of nearly normal children and their families may be unrealistic, with the children continuously finding themselves set up for failure. Problems such as these make availability of psychological supportive services a necessity in an overall treatment plan for patients with this disease.

Poliomyelitis. One additional disease of the anterior horn cell, poliomyelitis, continues to plague children in spite of immunization that has markedly reduced its incidence during the past twenty years but has not eliminated it.

Because of recent laxity in immunization programs, occasional small epidemics occur within the United States. Furthermore, an unimmunized, susceptible population will continue to exist, both among religious groups with philosophies against immunization and also among immigrants from underdeveloped countries. Rare cases related to immunization are also reported. Other viral infections have occasionally caused a disease clinically identical to poliomyelitis, and no vaccine against these infections is yet available. Although few in number, these children need assistance to improve the quality of their lives. Bracing and surgery offer many of these children their only means of ambulation. Spinal surgery and improved respiratory care are now prolonging the lives of the more severely affected children, and these children with their medical and financial needs should not be forgotten.

Disorders of the Peripheral Nerves

Among the disorders of the peripheral nerves, there are two significant groups seen in childhood: the hereditary peripheral neuropathies (headed by Charcot-Marie-Tooth disease) and Guillain-Barré syndrome (the acute disease of the peripheral nerve).

Charcot-Marie-Tooth is an autosomal dominant disease. In its most common form, it causes weakness of the distal muscles (muscles distant from the spinal cord), but in rare severe forms, significant proximal muscle (muscles close to the spinal cord) involvement may be seen. Generally, the disease exhibits little or no progression for many years, and in some cases, high-arched feet is the only indication that an underlying disease exists. Surgical correction of foot deformities and the use of bracing is helpful when indicated. Although there is no cure, the slow progression of this disease usually permits a normal life expectancy.

Guillain-Barré syndrome is an acute polyneuropathy, the cause of which is unknown, although an autoimmune etiology has been suggested. Beginning with weakness of the distal extremities, it progresses proximally and eventually may involve virtually all the muscle groups, including facial muscles and the muscles of respiration. The normal course of the disease consists of a period of progression, quiescence, and recovery. Recovery progresses in the opposite direction from initial involvement: from the proximal muscles to the distal. Estimates of extent of recovery vary, but approximately 25 percent of children are left with some residual weakness, usually of the feet or the hands. These residual problems may require bracing or surgical correction, or both.

The disease often requires an extended period of hospitalization. The acute and quiescent stages may occur over several weeks, followed by a rehabilitation process that may add many months to the initial hospitalization. To avoid overexertion of impaired muscles and permanent muscle damage, rehabilitation is accomplished through a strictly controlled therapy program. Careful monitoring during both the acute and rehabilitation stages of the disease is the key to a good functional recovery. Although the overall prognosis is good, the disease still carries a 10 percent mortality rate. Improvements in respiratory support systems have decreased the mortality of this disease somewhat. Death from Guillain-Barré syndrome at this time is usually secondary to the involvement of the autonomic nervous system. Shifts in blood pressure and cardiac arrhythmias are often the terminal events. Improvement in management of these complications and the possibility of temporary cardiac pacemakers may further reduce the mortality of this disease.

Disorders of the Muscle

The muscular dystrophies comprise a group of progressive, inherited disorders of the muscle cell varying in severity and pattern of inheritance. Those most commonly seen in childhood include Duchenne's, Becker's, limb-girdle, and facioscapulohumeral muscular dystrophy. In addition, there are several related neuromuscular disorders, such as myotonic dystrophy and myasthenia gravis. Duchenne's muscular dystrophy, a steadily progressive muscle disease, is the most common dystrophy seen in childhood. The actual defect within the muscle cell that causes its eventual destruction is unknown. Current research is focusing on the possibility of a defect in the surface membrane of the cell itself.

Statistics on incidence and prevalence of the disease are extremely variable. Predictions of incidence vary from thirteen to thirty-three per hundred thousand live male births. Within the population as a whole, the prevalence is estimated at about three per hundred thousand.

Duchenne's dystrophy is inherited as a sex-linked disorder, carried by an asymptomatic female, and transmitted to 50 percent of her sons, with 50 percent of her daughters also being carriers with the same potential of continuing the disease for yet another generation. Statistically, the disease is felt to have one of the highest spontaneous mutation rates of any human disease, making complete elimination of the disease through genetic counseling impossible. Accurate prenatal diagnosis is not currently possible, but amniocentesis is available to carrier mothers to determine the sex of the fetus. Carrier detection in female relatives has been attempted through several muscle-enzyme blood tests, but results are crude at best and the possibility still exists of missing females who are carriers.

Duchenne's muscular dystrophy is relentless. The careful observer can see the beginnings of the disease as early as three years of age when the child presents as slower and more awkward than his peers. By age five or six, it is obvious he cannot run or jump, and he never masters the skill of riding a two-wheeled bicycle. Instead of gaining motor control, the boy with Duchenne's dystrophy begins to lose previously mastered skills. Around ten or twelve years of age, ambulation becomes difficult, and eventually, he is confined to a wheelchair. The steady degeneration continues with loss of function in the upper extremities. Death usually occurs around twenty years of age and is secondary to respiratory failure. Because dystrophy is a disease of the muscle itself, cardiac arrhythmias (from damaged heart muscles) may occasionally be the terminal event, although respiratory failure is the much more common cause of death. Recently, respirators have been used in a small percentage of these patients to prevent the natural course of the disease. As a result, some men are still alive in their middle thirties. They remain, however, completely dependent on attendants for all their needs.

Intellectual impairment is seen in a significant number of children with Duchenne's muscular dystrophy. The mean IQ of boys with this disease is found to fall around 85 as opposed to the mean IQ of 100 for the normal population. The intellectual impairment is not progressive. Even though the IQ is lower, the great majority of boys still fall within the educable range. However, the IQ deficit adds school problems to their already obvious physical problems, thereby increasing the young boy's sense of failure and his social isolation.

There is no cure for Duchenne's muscular dystrophy, and there are no medications available that alter the relentlessly progressive nature of the disease. A great deal of research is being done in the area of neuromuscular diseases and multicenter double-blind studies are being carried out on a nationwide basis, but no effective treatment has as yet emerged. Life expectancy for this disease has not changed radically in the past twenty years, although one to five years can sometimes be added to the boy's life by active rehabilitation efforts aimed at maintaining good pulmonary function, by surgical intervention for scoliosis, and by rapid and aggressive treatment of respiratory infections (including vaccination against influenza and pneumococcal disease). But pulmonary failure secondary to muscle weakness is inevitable. Aside from the alternative of full-time respiratory dependency, which can add fifteen to twenty years, there is no effective way of significantly increasing the life expectancy of a boy with Duchenne's muscular dystrophy.

Treatment is aimed, therefore, at amelioration of the secondary problems associated with the disease. Surgical correction of lower extremity contractures, including surgeries involving muscle transfers followed by bracing, have prolonged the years of ambulation for one to four additional years. Spinal curvature, a major complicating event in about 80 percent of these boys, may also necessitate bracing and eventual surgical intervention. Physical therapy and breathing programs are often attempted, but progression of the disease continues.

Much of the treatment program comes to rest on the already overburdened shoulders of the parents because these children eventually can perform no self-care. Families lift the boys, turn them, brush their teeth, dress them, and take care of their toileting needs. Multiple adaptive devices such as lifts to aid in transfer of the boys are essential; they are not luxury items.

The boy with muscular dystrophy must himself contend with multiple psychological issues. Even before a diagnosis is made, the boy is awkward and physically inept and aware of his inability to compete successfully with his peers. Especially painful for a young boy, this can begin a lifelong feeling of failure. School problems, stemming from both physical and mental factors, may add to his feelings of inadequacy. From an awkward ambulator to a wheelchair, the boy's progressive disease may lead him to ever increasing isolation. Even against these odds, however, many of these boys find happy and fulfilling lives. The strength of their families and the involvement of friends, church groups, schools, the Muscular Dystrophy Association, and health professionals, if effectively working together, can become even stronger influences on the child's life than his disease.

Other Muscular Dystrophies. Other forms of muscular dystrophy seen in childhood are Becker's dystrophy, limb-girdle muscular dystrophy, and facioscapulohumeral dystrophy. Less common than Duchenne's, they do occur in the pediatric population. Genetic counseling and other forms of medical assistance, such as physical and occupational therapy, bracing, and surgery may be required to improve the quality of life of these patients. As in Duchenne's muscular dystrophy, there is no cure for any of these diseases. Life expectancy with limb-girdle and facioscapulohumeral dystrophies is generally good because they are less rapidly progressive and usually have significantly later onset than Duchenne's. Becker's muscular dystrophy has a life expectancy of approximately thirty to forty years. No major change in life expectancy has been seen in any of the dystrophies except for some improvement secondary to antibiotic intervention in the event of a pneumonia.

Other Neuromuscular Disorders. Other disorders primary to the muscle (myopathy)—such as congenital myopathies, metabolic myopathies, inflammatory myopathy, and the occasional muscle disease that eludes all diagnostic probing—contribute patients to every children's muscle disease clinic. Myasthenia gravis (a disorder of the neuromuscular junction leading to generalized weakness) and myotonic dystrophy (a disorder in which patients experience difficulty in contracting and loosening their muscles) are also seen in children. Like poliomyelitis, the number of patients each diagnosis contributes to the overall clinic population may be small, but the need for care may be comparatively great. These children should not be forgotten in planning and the organization of services.

Although during the past decade, life expectancy may not have changed radically for many of the neuromuscular diseases, the quality of the patient's life has improved. Bracing and surgery can prolong ambulation. Advances in wheelchairs and other assistive devices have made patients much more independent and thereby greatly expanded their horizons. The advances in scoliosis surgery have saved many of these children from years of pain. Instead of scoliotic curves, which in the past have eventually meant loss of sitting balance and pain in any position, spine surgery has allowed these patients to remain in wheelchairs and be active and comfortable for many additional years.

Issues in Treatment

Because no cure exists for neuromuscular disorders, the goal of treatment is attainment of the most functional state possible, the state at which each individual can accomplish the most in life with whatever physical attributes he or she possesses. Rehabilitation of patients with these diseases requires health professionals from many different fields working together in a coordinated effort.

The necessary physicians include pediatricians, neurologists, geneticists, ortho-pedic surgeons, pulmonary specialists, and occasionally otorhinolaryngologists; to this effort, the skills of physical therapists, occupational therapists, orthotists, respiratory therapists, psychologists, recreation therapists, nurses, and social workers must be added. At first glance, the requirement for so many medical and paramedical specialists may seem unnecessarily costly, but the specialized needs of these patients makes this approach mandatory. A team lacking in only one member is limited from delivering total care. Any public program aimed at helping these children must take into account the unique challenges they present.

Patients and families benefit immeasurably from the comprehensive medical and psychosocial services delivered by these multidisciplinary teams. The convenience of finding all needed services in one location (and even on one visit) lightens the load for families attempting to cope with the burdens of home care, transportation, and the accompanying emotional and physical drain on energies and time. Although fiscal proof of cost-effectiveness of team care is difficult to obtain, the combined expertise and resources of an experienced team discourage unnecessary medical shopping by patients and families, prevent unnecessary medical complications (including unnecessary hospitalizations), and promote rehabilitation.

At the other end of the medical-team spectrum is the solo family practi-tioner, pediatrician, or internist who serves patients living in rural areas of the country, patients who find transportation to established neuromuscular clinics extremely difficult, or patients who reject clinic care. The primary physician may attempt to be a one-person multidisciplinary treatment team, coordinating care for an extremely involved and complicated patient. Identification of such patients and their local medical support systems is, therefore, crucial to good care, as is professional education and assistance for physicians and other allied health personnel involved. It is critical for the quality of life of those patients with progressive neuromuscular disorders that the responsible physician be knowl-edgeable and judicious in applying *specific* techniques of medical care (as well as the orthopedic care that will improve the patient's comfort and decrease or prevent many secondary complications) in order to avoid inappropriate or unnecessary treatment.

It is appropriate to consider family members as sources of clinical treatment because the family is intimately involved in the care of patients with neuromuscular disease—provided the family can sustain the patient in the home. Effective treatment programs must deal with the family stresses that result from a chronically debilitating disease. Personnel specially trained in family counsel-ing and social work and familiar with community and school resources are essential. The psychosocial implications of a disease such as Duchenne's muscu-lar dystrophy are enormous. Family interactions become stressed by the ever-increasing dependency of the child. In addition, a feeling of guilt may often haunt the parents because of the inheritance pattern of the disease and may cause considerable strain on their relationship. Siblings, too, can feel guilt as well as anger.

The Muscular Dystrophy Association (MDA) provides significant assistance for patients of all ages with muscle diseases and offers a wide range of diagnostic and patient services. The MDA sponsors a summer camp program for muscle-disease children, has established a nationwide network of hospital-affiliated outpatient clinics, and supports programs of public education as well as professional education and research. The wide range of neuromuscular disorders covered in the MDA program includes muscular dystrophy, myositis, spinal muscular atrophy, myasthenia gravis, and other myotonias and myopathies resulting from metabolic and endocrine abnormalities. Notable exclusions are Guillain-Barré disease and poliomyelitis. On the national level, the MDA is probably most prominent in the public eye because of its annual telethon and solicitation for funds for research purposes. Recently, conflict has been made public over the approach to fund raising employed in the MDA telethon, which has characterized the typical muscle-disease patient as a child with a severe and crippling form of muscle disease, usually muscular dystrophy. Fund raising and the distribution of funds are areas always open to controversy. To raise funds, the cutest child is selected to appeal to the greatest number of viewers. The older child with more visible disabilities is still too threatening to the average television viewer. Although this "marketing" of the appealing child has its obvious advantages, the public remains uneducated as to the realities of many of these children's lives. Many of the older patients feel rejected by their exclusion. Not only is the older patient, with a respirator and perhaps some deformities, ignored by the fund raisers, that same patient tends also to be less fortunate at the time of fund dispersal. Catch-22 rules often deny such a person any help at all: a person who is not "functional" cannot receive assistance; however, without assistance, that person can never hope to become functional.

The percentage of money heading to research versus direct patient care is another contested area. Items such as electric wheelchairs are many patients' only hope for independence. Competition among manufacturers is not active in the wheelchair market because the demand in numbers is relatively small. Because of this, the cost for an appropriate chair is about $5,800, too expensive for most families. The wait for a chair is about one year. Without the chair, however, these children are prisoners, unable to move their bodies without someone's assistance. Without financial aid for such costly equipment, many families and children are helpless. The explanation that the funds raised each year are going to research to save the next generation often falls on ears of those embittered after many years of struggle.

Depending on individual and family needs, other community volunteer health or social welfare agencies may be called on to provide services. Examples of such agencies include but are certainly not limited to the Easter Seal Association, Visiting Nurse Association, family service agencies, and other agencies offering services or support as needed by an individual patient or family. In metropolitan centers, a variety of such agencies exists, and a skilled and experienced social worker or patient-care coordinator is essential in order to search out the appropriate resource for a given patient. Not to be overlooked is the importance of religious support to many highly stressed families, and it is often a wise move to enlist the cooperation of ministers or clergymen in helping the family cope with care of a chronically disabled or ill child.

A comprehensive program for care of these children aims at making them functional members of society, which requires close collaboration with the educational system. Although special schools are at times the best solution for the orthopedically handicapped child, mainstreaming through Public Law 94-142 has offered other handicapped children many new challenges and opportunities. Sometimes oversheltering in special school environments leaves these children social cripples, creating a more damaging problem than the physical ones. The childhood experience of dealing with an able-bodied peer population is invaluable, easing the adjustment necessary outside the school environment. Public Law 94-142 has made this transition available to large numbers of children for the first time. The achievements of this law are immeasurable. It must be continued.

In order to make P.L. 94-142 a success for the child and the school, education of school personnel about the child's particular needs is essential. Without close contact between medical and school personnel, mainstreaming is often doomed. For example, teachers may have preconceived ideas about a child's ability. Or physical handicaps are often wrongly assumed to imply mental handicaps. And teachers are often fearful that medical problems will occur in the classroom when, in reality, no real danger is present. Even with the most dependent child, proper education of the school staff can allow for effective mainstreaming. Respirator-dependent children, for example, have been successfully mainstreamed. Children with severe neuromuscular weakness are successfully attending college. Many patients from our Orthopedic Hospital clinics, who have weakness of all four extremities, are riding their electric wheelchairs down the halls and competing successfully against able-bodied peers.

It is not just the handicapped child who benefits from mainstreaming. Able-bodied children can become aware of the special needs of their handicapped friends. The reality of difficulties encountered by a wheelchair-dependent person becomes obvious on a personal level when classmates take joint field trips. A peer group of truly socially informed youngsters develops. We have seen classmates learn to suction the tracheostomy of a handicapped classmate. We have also seen handicapped individuals invited to proms and birthday parties. It is in this way, by this interaction, that compassionate youngsters are raised and that our patients can realize their ultimate dream—to be treated normally.

The benefits derived from mainstreaming continue after the educational years. Properly equipped in mind and spirit, handicapped children have learned that they can successfully compete in an able-bodied world. Many of these children have gone on to college. Some are living on their own with attendant care and are successfully employed.

In many cases, locating sources of financial assistance may be more difficult than discovering sources for medical, psychosocial, and recreational services. To estimate medical expenses incurred by patients with hereditary progressive muscular disorders, financial data were obtained from California Children's Services of Los Angeles County, California. By extrapolating medical costs from the first two quarters of 1981, one can expect 220 such patients (or patient episodes of illness) to receive outpatient and inpatient care totaling $433,054 in 1981, or an annual average of $1,968 per patient.

The care of an individual within a family with a chronic and severe neuromuscular disorder may thus place intolerable financial burdens on even a relatively prosperous family. It is important that the family of such a child be assisted in investigating all the possible avenues of financial assistance, beginning with the possibility of finding group medical or health insurance if one of the parents is employed. Many group health insurance plans will cover a disabled or handicapped dependent after an initial exclusion period. The type of medical or health insurance available to a family as well as the fine print provisions of such policies should be investigated very carefully.

Most individuals with chronic neuromuscular disease will both need and qualify for one or more categories of public assistance programs. Medical eligibility and benefits for Crippled Children's Services vary from state to state, as do other health and welfare programs. Availability of these programs and benefits demands careful individual family analysis by a financial counselor (usually a social worker) to assist in appropriate application and in the maximizing of benefits. Helping families and patients cope with the financial realities of life and helping them use the system wisely can do much to alleviate economic hardships.

Through the accomplishments of modern medical technology, an increasing number of children are finding themselves trapped in an especially complex situation. Children who previously would have died of respiratory failure are being placed on respirators that, for many, become permanent attachments. The courts have begun to deal with problems of patients kept on respirators against their will, but no one has begun to address the problems of respiratory patients with normal intelligence who want their lives prolonged by respirators. Often unable to return home from the hospital, they are placed in nursing homes that are frequently ill-equipped to handle them. If not a death sentence, such a nursing home may be a sentence to a life of total isolation and dependency. Acute care hospitals are not appropriate facilities for these chronically ill patients. In this setting, as in a nursing home, the patient's needs are inadequately met. Where are these patients to go?

This dilemma, one of enormous magnitude, is not to be brushed off; the problem will only grow with time. Laws are becoming increasingly strict in placing constraints on physicians. Decisions about whether to prolong life on a respirator or to allow certain death are becoming less the choice of the physician and more the decision of the patient. Many patients will choose life on a respirator. We can offer no simple solution—one does not exist. We can only stress the importance and urgency of initiating recognition of this problem and of beginning the search for solutions.

194

Because a scientifically accurate and precise diagnosis is absolutely essential for both genetic counseling and medical treatment, it is mandatory that the patient and family have such services available to them. Initial counseling may often be provided by a neurologist or pediatrician, with consultation from a geneticist if indicated. Funds for travel and housing for visits to genetic or clinical centers may be a necessary requirement of the medical diagnostic evaluation. The challenge for adequate support of research into prenatal diagnosis as well as identification of the carrier state is quite clear because prevention of subsequent family cases is feasible, at least in theory.

Assuming the correct diagnosis has been reached, proper treatment must be directed not only to the child but also to the family unit. "Total care" includes psychosocial, educational, recreational, and vocational services as well as medical treatment. Many patients with chronic diseases, especially those of the neuromuscular type, seem to slip between the cracks. A case coordinator can avoid this problem by playing an important part in overall treatment and care. Agencies dealing with handicapped children (such as Crippled Children's Services), as well as schools and physicians, must be aware of the need for precise diagnosis in order to prevent the undetected or lost-to-follow-up case from occurring. The hopeless attitude associated with Duchenne's dystrophy has unfortunately stigmatized the entire group of muscle diseases.

Recommendations for Public Policy

Because many Duchenne's dystrophy patients as well as the majority of spinal muscular atrophy patients survive to adulthood, consideration should be given to the extension of Crippled Children's Services to cover these disabled adults. This extension would facilitate rehabilitative efforts including vocational training, counseling, and job placement. Although many adults with neuromuscular diseases have only marginal or limited capacity to work, a positive approach toward the possibility of future gainful work should be displayed, particularly in the adolescent years. Without a positive approach, the young adult capable of employment will be missed. We have a young man with Duchenne's muscular dystrophy who is a college graduate, living independently, and successfully employed with an insurance company. Vocational counseling services must reflect a positive attitude toward muscle disease patients.

Home care is both more economical and more humane for many severely disabled patients, even including those needing respirator support; yet, such care is not feasible unless adequate home support services are available. Such services must include respite resources, daycare for individuals over twenty-one with severely crippling disabilities, and the provision for transportation of patients to out-of-home daycare facilities or sheltered workshops.

In summary, the ability to reach a more precise diagnosis in neuromuscular disease has been generally extended and advanced during the last decade. Formerly, the term *neuromuscular disease* was equated with Duchenne's dystrophy, with the associated concepts of an inexorable downhill course and early demise. Now other, more benign forms of muscle disease are recognizable, and treatment is often available for prevention of secondary complications and for physical rehabilitation of the individual.

Crippled Children's Services (CCS) can do much to stimulate comprehensive multidisciplinary care by funding needed medical and support services on an institutional level. In California, such team care has been supported and encouraged through CCS funding to institutions.

What happens to handicapped children when they become handicapped adults? Many find themselves deserted by support systems. Years of preparing them for life on their own may go to waste because of the untimely withdrawal of medical and emotional support. Chronic handicaps do not disappear with age. Public policy, as embodied in regulations affecting Social Security, Crippled Children's Services, school programs, and public facilities, should be modified to meet the needs of disabled adults. Special attention must be focused on the unique and often agonizing situation of the adult patient requiring total care as well as respiratory support. It is short-sighted public policy to force disabled adults into welfare programs in order to secure medical care. The cost of treatment as well as long-term support for individuals with severe neuromuscular disease is significant, but society, as well as the individual and family, will benefit in both humanitarian and economical ways if coordinated programs between the voluntary and public sector are developed to deal with the needs of this particular group.

References

Blumberg, M. L. "Emotional and Personality Development in Neuromuscular Disorders." *American Journal of Diseases of Children,* 1959, *98,* 303–310.

Brooke, M. H. *A Clinician's View of Neuromuscular Diseases.* Baltimore, Md.: Williams & Wilkins, 1977.

Buchanan, D. C., and others. "Reactions of Families to Children with Duchenne's Muscular Dystrophy." *General Hospital Psychiatry,* 1979, *1* (3), 262–269.

Dubowitz, V. *Muscle Disorders in Childhood,* Vol. 16. Philadelphia: Saunders, 1978.

Pope-Grattan, M. M., Burnett, C. N., and Wolfe, C. V. "Human Figure Drawings by Children with Duchenne's Muscular Dystrophy." *Physical Therapy,* 1976, *56* (2), 168–176.

Prugh, D. G. "Why Did It Happen to Us? A Psychiatrist Explores Chronic Childhood Disability in the Family." In I. Zwerling (Ed.), *The American Family.* Philadelphia, Pa.: Smith, Kline, and French Laboratories, 1979.

Siegel, I. M., and Kornfeld, M. S. "Kinetic Family Drawing Test for Evaluating Families Having Children with Muscular Dystrophy." *Physical Therapy,* 1980, *60* (3), 293–298.

Travis, G. *Chronic Illness in Children: Its Impact on Child and Family.* Stanford, Calif.: Stanford University Press, 1976.

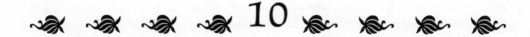

10

Cystic Fibrosis

Norman J. Lewiston, M.D.

We never see this disease in adults. What happens to these kids? Do they outgrow it?

—Professor of Medicine, 1967

All that talent! All that intelligence! Lying there gasping for breath. What a god-damned waste!

-Bereaved parent, 1980

Cystic fibrosis kills kids. Kids have to help kill cystic fibrosis.
—Kristi McNichol, TV spot announcement, 1981

The child will soon die, Whose brow tastes salty when kissed.
—Swiss children's song, Eighteenth century

Although known to folklore for centuries, cystic fibrosis (CF) was not recognized as a disease entity until the late 1930s. Perhaps for this reason, it remains one of the most serious, most common, and least understood genetic diseases affecting children. Although the biochemistry is obscure, it appears that an autosomal recessive gene-linked disorder produces two problems. The first of these is a dehydration of mucous secretions in the ducts of exocrine glands (sweat glands, salivary glands, and pancreas) so that the secreted material is much more viscous than normal. The second is the production of factors that prevent normal immunological mechanisms from clearing bacterial and fungal pathogens from

Note: I wish to thank the Cystic Fibrosis Foundation for permission to quote extensively from many of their publications. Special thanks go to Richard Vodra and Carol Schultz without whose help this chapter would not have been possible. I thank also the hundreds of persons with CF who have taken the time to write or call and share their feelings about their disease.

respiratory secretions. The symptoms of CF are a direct result of one or both of these. Retained purulent respiratory secretions produce progressive lung disease. Retention of exocrine secretions in the ducts of the pancreas and liver results in fibrosis (scarring) of these organs. Viscous mucus in the cervix and fallopian tubes reduces fertility in women with CF. Such secretions probably also are responsible for the nearly universal failure of channelization of the vas deferens in males with CF, with resulting infertility.

CF fits into a number of disease categories. It is congenital, it is lethal, and like epilepsy, it is largely invisible until late in its course. It also can be extremely variable in presentation and severity, ranging from infants born with intestinal obstruction and respiratory distress to adults who for years have carried an erroneous respiratory diagnosis. Most patients survive into their teens or early twenties only to succumb to severe obstructive pulmonary disease. The earlier years are marked with growth failure, respiratory insufficiency, and nagging cough productive of large volumes of green sputum. These occur in a person who otherwise is physically and intellectually normal. The inexorable course of CF and the delayed onset of crippling disease have given CF the label "the most cruel genetic disease known."

CF may present in a number of ways. Twenty percent of individuals with CF are diagnosed as such because they develop meconium ileus (small intestine obstruction) during the immediate postnatal period. Failure of the fetal pancreas to digest the albumin in meconium permits the development of a putty-like substance in the small intestine, resulting in the obstruction. This is a neonatal emergency and usually requires surgical intervention.

Infants who have pancreatic insufficiency but not meconium ileus will fail to thrive. In spite of a vigorous appetite they will appear emaciated and have frequent, voluminous, greasy stools. At this point they are not properly absorbing much of the food they eat. This may progress to hypoalbuminemia and the development of ascites (fluid retention). Older children in whom malabsorption is mild usually will present with recurrent respiratory problems. CF should be included in the differential diagnosis of a small child with recurrent pneumonia. Teenage children with recurrent bronchitis and nasal polyps may have CF as the underlying cause. Physicians should not discard the possibility of CF as a diagnosis because a patient appears too healthy. It is not rare to establish a diagnosis of CF in an adult who has sought medical attention for years because of "bronchitis," "asthma," or another respiratory disorder, even to the point of confinement in a tuberculosis sanitarium because of the appearance of the chest roentgenogram.

Cystic fibrosis is defined as a disease marked by an elevated sweat chloride or sweat sodium concentration and evidence of pulmonary, pancreatic, or liver disease. The diagnosis of CF is confirmed by detecting an increased concentration of sodium and chloride in sweat; thus the salty taste. This is detected by a fairly simple laboratory test with a specificity of at least 99 percent. A brisk rate of perspiration is induced on a small area of the forearm. Sweat is then collected and analyzed for sodium and chloride content by a variety of means. Unfortunately, many clinical laboratories utilize a direct-reading sodium electrode for this purpose, a method with an unacceptably low sensitivity (Shwachman, 1977).

Carriers of the CF gene have no obvious clinical or physiological abnormalities. Sweat-chloride values for this group do not differ significantly from most of the general population. Although several areas of research appear promising, there currently is no dependable means of detecting the carrier state or of antenatal detection of the CF fetus (Littlefield, 1981).

Epidemiology

The CF gene has a prevalence of 0.025 in Caucasians and is present but less common in other races. This means that approximately one out of twenty Caucasians is a carrier for this disease. The projected occurrence of CF in approximately one out of sixteen hundred births (Thompson, 1980) produces about fifteen hundred to two thousand new cases of CF in the United States each year. Exact figures on the prevalence of CF are not available. The patient registry of the Cystic Fibrosis Foundation includes about twelve thousand individuals, but may represent only 25 to 50 percent of all cases in the United States (Jones, 1980). Since the life span of individuals with CF is shortened, these data suggest that approximately one in five thousand Americans has CF but that only one in ten thousand has been diagnosed as having this disorder. Prevalence of CF is similar in countries where the major ethnic background is of European origin. Although CF largely has been unrecognized in Mexico, the incidence in the United States of CF in children of Mexican origin is similar to that of other Caucasian groups.

The serious nature of the disease and the frequency of the carrier state plus the absence of carrier and antenatal detection makes the CF carrier state highly undesirable. Environmental and social factors do not seem to be important in the incidence of CF but, once the disease has presented, may be very important in the likelihood of adherence to the medical regimen and thus to longevity.

Treatment

Therapy for cystic fibrosis is aimed at two general areas—pulmonary disease resulting from chronic bronchitis and malnutrition due to deficiency in pancreatic enzymes. The pulmonary disease usually is more serious and less amenable to treatment, although attention has been focused recently on morbidity related to inadequate nutrition. The treatment described below has increased the life expectancy of the child with CF from less than 6 months in 1953 to 11.2 years in 1966 and 22 years in 1981.

Pulmonary. The pulmonary secretions of virtually every patient with CF become colonized with characteristic bacteria. The resulting low-grade infection adds to the viscosity of the sputum by contributing bacterial debris and white cells. This resultant sputum assumes a glue-like consistency that can be removed only by vigorous cough. Accumulation of secretions can result in segmental lung collapse or distortion of the supporting tissues of the lungs. Several modes of therapy are directed toward these problems: antimicrobials, chest physiotherapy, aerosol mist, oxygen, and hospitalization.

Although colonization of CF sputum by bacteria usually is permanent, several studies have shown that the number of bacteria per unit volume of sputum can be lowered several orders of magnitude by the use of oral antimicrobials. Two specialized uses of antimicrobials in CF deserve mention. Several medical centers have used long-term intravenous catheters to deliver daily dosages of bacteriocidal agents such as gentamicin or tobramycin over periods of weeks to months. Although early results show promise, this is considered to be an experimental mode of therapy. Another means of delivering bacteriocidal drugs is by aerosol. Gentamicin, neomycin, polymixin B, and oxacillin all have been used in aerosol form. This is used in many CF centers although there is little scientific evidence supporting the efficacy of this means of drug delivery.

The viscous nature of CF sputum makes removal by the normal lung mechanisms impossible. Because patients may produce several ounces of sputum daily, efforts to aid lung clearings are important. Sputum can be moved only with a vigorous cough. Posturing to aid in gravity drainage and loosening of sputum plugs with clap percussion (catsup-bottle therapy) is considered to be helpful in assisting the patient to clear the sputum. Positioning and percussion usually are preceded by an aerosolized bronchodilating agent to provide maximal airway diameter. The process, including aerosol, may require as much as forty-five minutes and is frequently prescribed twice daily. Clap percussion requires the assistance of another person; often this can be a family member. Some older patients use a variety of mechanical percussors to perform therapy on themselves. In special circumstances, single adults or very sick children may need the regular services of a home health aide to perform clap percussion. Chest physiotherapy is time consuming, physically tiring, and boring and is therefore the aspect of therapy most likely to be ignored. Unfortunately, it probably is the most efficacious mode of therapy for individuals with widespread disease. Considerable interest in autopercussion, a forced cough starting from the end of a very deep breath, has come from Europe and is being taught in a number of centers.

For many years, it was felt that delivery of moisture to the respiratory tract would aid in loosening secretions. CF patients therefore were instructed to sleep in a plastic tent filled with cooled mist. Clinical experiments in the early 1970s cast doubt on the efficacy of these mist tents, and this means of therapy has been largely abandoned, although physicians still prescribe *intermittent* aerosol therapy in an attempt to loosen airway secretions.

Lung disease inevitably progresses to respiratory insufficiency. Ventilation to perfusion abnormalities may cause low blood oxygen and a considerable loss of tolerance for exercise. The majority of CF patients are unable to respond to low blood oxygen by increasing their red cells (which could carry more oxygen) because of the anemia of chronic infection and other factors. These patients require therapeutic oxygen during sleep and activity. A number of ingenious devices have been developed to deliver oxygen yet permit mobility. These devices carry a small reservoir of liquid oxygen that boils off at a rate matching the need of the patient. The need for an oxygen appliance may be the first obvious physical evidence to the public that the patient is ill.

A viral respiratory illness or failure to perform regular chest physiotherapy can result in pneumonia or in a phenomenon known as gradual deterioration of pulmonary status. This is marked by weight loss, decrease in vital capacity of the lungs, increased haziness of the lung fields on roentgenogram, and low-grade fever. If oral antimicrobials and ambulatory chest physiotherapy are unsuccessful in reversing this process, the patient is hospitalized. In-hospital treatment involves a combination of parenteral antimicrobials directed against the sputum flora and intense chest physiotherapy four times daily. Ten to fourteen days of hospitalization are often needed to reverse the process, restore the vital capacity and chest roentgenogram to baseline levels, and permit weight gain.

Nutritional. Approximately 80 percent of individuals with CF have insufficiency of exocrine pancreatic function. Although the acinar cells appear to be normal, the pancreatic ducts are filled with viscid mucoid material. This prevents the delivery of pancreatic secretions into the duodenum resulting in poor digestion of fat and protein. Treatment of this takes several forms: pancreatic enzyme replacement, vitamins, insulin, and adequate caloric intake.

For many years, CF patients ingested dessicated beef or pork pancreatic material with their meals. Replacement was far from perfect, and many patients selected a low-fat diet to prevent embarrassing fatty bowel movements. Recently, the availability of acid-stable microspheres of pancrelipase has markedly improved the ability of CF patients to absorb fat and thus select a more normal American diet. The capsules of pancrelipase must be taken with every meal including school lunches, which can be a source of contention for most younger children.

Poor fat absorption interferes with absorption of fat-soluble vitamins. These must be provided daily, preferably in a water-soluble form. Infants and older individuals on long-term oral antimicrobials may be deficient in vitamin K and will need biweekly supplementation.

Inflammation and fibrotic changes in the pancreas may result in virtual destruction of this organ and impairment of endocrine as well as exocrine function. The endocrine loss results in diabetes mellitus and a requirement for exogenous insulin for approximately 10 percent of CF patients. The diabetes of CF differs from usual juvenile diabetes mellitus in that insulin requirements are low and ketoacidosis is rarely present. Vascular complications of diabetes in CF are rarely reported.

Two decades ago, the child with CF was characterized as having a voracious appetite. This was true, but it was mostly for carbohydrates. Incomplete ability to digest dietary fat prescribed a diet that was low in this important source of calories. Consequently plasma levels of certain essential fatty acids were low in a number of patients. Additionally, because fat supplies approximately 40 percent of the calories of the normal American diet, total caloric intake for these patients was actually lower than that necessary for normal growth. Two new therapeutic modalities have been useful in improving the fat and caloric content of the CF diet—the availability of pancrelipase (discussed earlier), which permits improved fat digestion, and the availability of palatable nutritional supplements that provide high-fat, high-protein snacks with little bulk. The addition of these supplements to the CF diet has produced satisfactory weight gain and normalization of plasma fatty acids.

Cost of Treatment

The pharmacological and therapeutic needs of cystic fibrosis make this an expensive disease. The Cystic Fibrosis Foundation (1981) surveyed a number of adults with CF to attempt to quantify the actual cost of the disease. Questionnaires were supplied to 2,300 individuals with CF over the age of eighteen. Thirty percent of these (640) responded by mail. Although the survey is thus biased in two ways—age and willingness to respond to a mail questionnaire—it gives a good approximation of the actual cost of the disease in 1980 dollars for the total spectrum of patients. Only the monetary outlay for direct care is discussed here. The total financial impact of the disease on the health care system and on the families of individuals with CF is obviously higher.

Hospitalization. Hospitalization, usually for respiratory complaints, is the most expensive aspect of care. Forty-five percent of respondents to the survey said they had been hospitalized at least once in 1980. The Western Consortium of Cystic Fibrosis Physicians, reviewing clinical records of 981 patients of all ages seen in CF clinics in 1980, reported that 29.7 percent of these patients were hospitalized for CF in 1979. Total hospital days were similar for each group: twenty-one days for the adult survey and twenty-four days for the western group. Since the latter group includes younger children, the figures of 29.7 percent and twenty-four days will be used. Costs for the adult group are representative, however, because the cost of treatment is not age-dependent. The survey used an average-hospital-day cost of $350, certainly very conservative by West Coast standards but probably applicable to a national study. The survey found that the cost of hospitalization ranged from $42 to $75,000; the median cost was $7,285, and the mean was $11,745.

Prescription Medications. The second most expensive aspect of care is cost of prescription medications. This includes antimicrobials, pancreatic enzyme replacements, and aerosolized medicines. The figure derived from the survey is felt to be representative of all ages. The cost of prescription medications ranged from $10 to $18,000; the median was $800, the mean $1,509.

Outpatient Physician Visits. Regular physician visits are encouraged as part of the overall care plan for CF. The frequency of visits varies with each clinic and with the state of health of the individual but ranges from six weeks to six months with a probable average of three months. Chest roentgenograms and pulmonary-function testing are obtained at least annually. The survey found that the cost of outpatient physician visits ranged from $10 to $5,460; the median was $231, the mean $428.

Equipment. Equipment for the care of CF involves mainly items relating to lung care (nebulizers, mist tents, mechanical chest percussors), and virtually every patient requires some equipment for this purpose. Individuals who have severe pulmonary disease may, in addition, require therapeutic oxygen or wheelchairs. The cost of equipment ranged from $6 to $5,000; the median was $180, the mean $409.

Nonprescription Medications. Not all medications suggested for the care of CF are reimbursable by third-party payors. Nonprescription medications include certain vitamins, mild analgesics, decongestants, and other similar items. The cost of nonprescription medications ranged from $4 to $1,400; the median was $520, the mean $127.

Physical Therapy. Although most chest physiotherapy is delivered by members of the patient's immediate family, special circumstances may require the services of health professionals or home health aides. This applies especially to adolescents or to adults who have no immediate family available during times of acute illness. Physical therapy also is important for families with more than one individual with CF when needs for physiotherapy are excessive. Cost of this therapy can vary considerably. It is applicable, however, to no more than about 10 percent of the total CF population, and this figure is used in estimating total cost. The cost of physical therapy ranged from $10 to $30,000; the median was $520, the mean $1,610.

Other Direct CF Health Related Expenses. Respondents to the survey were asked to estimate out-of-pocket expenses relating directly to health care. This included a variety of items, such as transportation to clinic visits and nail polish (to hide cyanotic fingernails), but mostly was for extra food and nutritional supplements not covered by health care plans. These expenses apply to the entire CF population and ranged from $20 to $1,920; the median was $325, the mean $730.

Two other categories of expense should be included in the discussion of total expense for cystic fibrosis. The first is the direct cost of educational and/or vocational counseling for at least one half of the population. This can range from a trivial annual conference with the individual to intensive in-home instruction for the patient unable to attend school. Although no data are available for the population as a whole, the figure of $800 per year for one half of the population is probably close.

The second category is the money spent by the Cystic Fibrosis Foundation for the maintenance of CF Care Centers throughout the country. Although this money is not allocated for direct patient expense, it offsets the cost of patient education, nutritional counseling, exercise programs, and other programs designed to supplement direct physician-patient interaction. In 1980, $2.1 million was spent for this purpose.

The estimate of the total cost of CF care in 1980 (Table 1) is based on the figures just given, with an estimated patient population of twenty thousand. The population is adjusted for hospitalization, physical therapy, and educational expenses. Mean cost figures are used. The annual mean cost is $6,369 per patient, a figure lower than the CF Foundation's estimate of $10,000–$12,000 per year that covers a broad spectrum of disease activity. Individuals with several hospitalizations will have an annual health care cost far in excess of this mean figure.

Table 1. Direct Cost of Cystic Fibrosis—1980.

Hospitalization	20,000 × 29.7% × 24 days × $350	=	$ 49,896,000
Prescription medication	20,000 × $1509	=	30,180,000
Outpatient visits	20,000 × $428	=	8,560,000
Equipment	20,000 × $409	=	8,180,000
Nonprescription medication	20,000 × $127	=	2,540,000
Physical therapy	20,000 × 10% × $1610	=	3,220,000
Other expenses	20,000 × $730	=	14,600,000
Educational/Vocational counseling	20,000 × 50% × $800	=	8,000,000
Cystic Fibrosis Foundation Centers		=	2,100,000
	Total		$127,276,000

The Adult with CF

Adults with CF were a medical curiosity only a decade ago, but now they account for 30 percent of the population known to the CF Foundation patient registry. The expected transition of care from pediatrician to internist has not gone smoothly. There is no internal medicine model for the CF patient whose bronchitis never gets better and whose immune system seems determined to protect the microorganisms in the respiratory tract. Internal medicine is not a nurturing discipline. Patients are expected either to take care of themselves or go to nursing homes. Many adult CF patients cannot accept this philosophy. They require external assistance for chest physiotherapy, sometimes even for house-keeping tasks. Although uniformly given the option of seeking comprehensive care from internists, the majority of adult CF patients voluntarily remain in the care of pediatricians, even into their forties.

A survey of adults with CF (Cystic Fibrosis Foundation, 1979) found that most of the 128 CF care centers in the United States care for adults as well as children. Ninety-five percent of the adults surveyed had received care in a CF care center at some time. Nonetheless, most CF centers do not provide specialized services for adult patients. Less than one third of the care centers provide an adult-oriented service, such as psychological, genetic, and vocational counseling and obstetrical and gynecological care. Although almost four fifths of the adult patients who attended CF care centers expressed satisfaction with them, many patients recommended that the centers place greater emphasis on the particular services needed by adults with CF.

Stress on Child and Family

A fatal illness such as CF is bound to produce stress on individuals and families. Parents may eventually accept cancer, arthritis, or other serious illness because the cause of disease is unknown and thus beyond their control. They accept less well the fact that they have transmitted an awful disease to their child. ("There has never been anything like this in MY family.") Acceptance of the disease and of the child may require considerable assistance from the health care system. Peer support is particularly important in this regard, and parents' groups are an important part of CF care.

The labor-intensive chest physiotherapy that is applied daily reinforces an ambivalent relationship between parent and child—anger for the loss of the hour or so per day required to perform the treatments and relief that there is something physical they can do to retard the course of the illness. This relationship is strained to the utmost by adolescence when the teenager often refuses treatments as a means of achieving control, even at the expense of health. This, of course, is not unique to CF (Korsch, 1973).

Early studies characterized the child with CF as depressed and angry. Frydman (1979) has criticized many of these studies as lacking in proper controls and drawing conclusions from small numbers of patients seen in therapeutic situations. More recent work using sibling or age-matched controls shows the individual with CF in a better light. The major stressors on the individuals are growth failure, poor health, need for repeated hospitalization, and virtual certainty of a shortened life span (Boyle and others, 1973). The medical profession has done only a fair job of counseling individuals for these problems. It is not unusual to receive a written consultation from a mental health professional not familiar with CF stating "this patient is appropriately depressed by his devastating illness"! Fortunately, provision for the mental health of the individual with a chronic illness is becoming a reality. Denning has suggested that denial may be important as a mechanism for coping with fatal illness (Denning, Gluckson, and Mueller, 1976). The subject of mental health services for children with chronic illness has been discussed by Gliedman and Roth (1980) and elsewhere in this volume.

The first external manifestation of CF often is the failure of adolescents to undergo the growth and pubertal changes of their peers. This is probably due to a combination of inadequate nutrition and chronic infection. The individual emerges as the smallest person in the class and is excluded from many of the athletic and social activities that form such an important part of the formative years. Girls may try to compensate for lack of breast development by using padding and wearing long hair styles. Boys may adopt the "little guy" personality and use misbehavior or wit as a means to draw attention. Landon suggests that some of the emotional problems of the adolescent with CF may relate as much to growth failure as to any other manifestations of the disease. He suggests consideration of oral hyperalimentation and/or androgen therapy in selected cases (Landon and others, 1980). Kellerman and others (1980), in a study controlled by adolescents with other chronic illnesses, found that adolescents with CF generally were well adjusted but tended more than the other groups to think about their illness even when they were well. Drotar and others (1980) and Straka and Kuttner (1980) confirmed that as a group, adolescents with CF adjusted adequately and suggested that further studies focus on specific patients rather than the population group.

Education is one area in which children with CF have compensated for lack of physical prowess. Many become scholarly, articulate, model students although the vaunted increased mean intelligence has not been confirmed by IQ testing. Goldberg found CF adolescents to be well-motivated toward vocational goals and realistic in their expectations of what they could hope to accomplish in a job (Basham and others, 1980). A recent CF consumer survey found that 74 percent of adults with CF had academic training beyond high school.

Individuals who finish their educations and are functioning in society may well think of marriage. A consumer survey found that of adults with CF over eighteen years of age about 35 percent were or had been married. Boyle and others (1973) comment on a number of serious emotional problems in this group. Basham, herself an adult with CF, surveyed a number of couples in whom one of the partners had CF. She concluded that these couples had as good a chance as any to have a successful marriage but that regular counseling may be desirable to deal with problems of physical illness, finance, and impending loss.

The successful married couple may wish for children. The vast majority of males with CF are sterile because of failure of development of the vas deferens. Females with CF are fertile. Cohen, diSant'Agnese, and Frielander (1980) reviewed the outcome of 128 pregnancies in women with CF. They concluded that it was possible for women with mild disease to complete pregnancy successfully. Most couples, however, decide to remain childless because of the limited life span of the parent and, in the case of women, of absolute assurance of passing along the genetic trait.

Although CF may be mild at onset, it is progressive and will appreciably shorten the life span of all its victims. The spectre of this overshadows all discussion of the emotional cost of CF. The thanatologic issues of CF are covered superbly by Patterson, Denning, and Kutscher (1973). Kerner, Harvey, and Lewiston (1979) found a high incidence of incomplete mourning in parents who had lost a child with CF and concluded that, although the families had lived with this for, in some instances, many years, they were unable to let the child go. The issue of CF as a fatal disease has been a major one for the CF Foundation. Fund raisers stress CF as a "killer of children" in order to raise money for research. Parents, on the other hand, often conceal the serious nature of the illness, even the diagnosis, from their children. There has been real ambivalence about using the word *fatal* in advertisements for fund-raising events although such usage has become more common during the last few years. Many CF physicians, after frank explanation of the serious nature of the illness, arrange for the parents of a newly diagnosed child to meet with an adult with CF who is doing well.

Sources of Support

Persons with CF may be eligible for a number of public programs. Families who meet financial criteria are eligible for Medicaid as a means of meeting medical expenses. Individuals who are certified as disabled may qualify for Medicare and SSI. Older patients may qualify for a variety of services for the handicapped including vocational rehabilitation and homemaker services. Eligibility for these programs is based on degree of disability and/or rehabilitation potential on an individual basis rather than on disease category. The Cost of CF Survey (Cystic Fibrosis Foundation, 1981)) found that 43.6 percent of adults with CF had applied for some form of disability benefit, usually either SSI or Social Security-Disability Insurance. Eighty-four percent of those who had applied for SSI and 74 percent of those who had applied for Social Security-Disability were successful in obtaining these benefits. Services were applied for from a vocational rehabilitation program by 50.5 percent of all respondents, and 76 percent of these stated they had received benefits. Although there are no data to support this figure, approximately one half of school-age children with CF received some form of educational assistance.

In some states, there are two categorical programs applicable to cystic fibrosis. The first is Crippled Children's Services, which provides care for people under twenty-one years of age. The second program is for care of people with genetic disease after their twenty-first birthday. These programs are administered at the state level and may vary considerably in the quality and quantity of services delivered.

Crippled Children's Services (CCS). The Cystic Fibrosis Foundation (CFF) conducted a survey of state CCS services as applied to children with cystic fibrosis (Cystic Fibrosis Foundation, 1980). All states (but not the District of Columbia) include CF in their CCS programs. There is no correlation between the quality of a state's CCS benefits for people with CF and the size of the state or its general income level. Some relatively poor states have very good programs. Twelve states report that less than half of the known cases of CF are enrolled in the CCS program, and at least four of those states also have below-average expenditures per enrollee. Two states—Mississippi and Missouri—have enacted separate programs for people with CF. CF benefits represent about 2.2 percent of total CCS program spending, but this amount varies widely from state to state, from a low of 0.1 percent to a high of 33 percent. Six states devote less than 1 percent of their CCS budget to children with CF. States report an average expenditure of $800 to $1,000 per child with CF enrolled in the program, ranging from a low of $111 to a high of $3,698. Because the average cost of care for children with CF has been estimated at $6,000 to $12,000 per year, it is clear that CCS provides only partial help to most families.

At least 6,168 young people with CF are enrolled with state CCS programs. If the five states that did not report enrollment figures are assumed to be average, the national total of CCS enrollees who have CF rises to about 6,800 or 69 percent of the 9,906 people under age twenty-one recorded in the CFF Patient Registry. States report caseloads that average 76 percent of the patients under age twenty-one reported in the CFF Patient Registry. This would indicate that most identified cases of CF—those seen in CF care centers—are at least known to CCS programs.

Most states say they provide a full range of services through the CCS program; this includes physician's services, hospitalization, medication, inhalation equipment, lab work, x rays, social work services, and physical therapy services. Less than half of the states provide any help for home health care services. During the three-year period from 1978 through 1981, at least one state in four has had to restrict benefits to people with CF because of financial problems with the CCS program. About half of all states will reimburse their residents for services they receive out-of-state. Less than one in five pays for services to nonresidents.

Most states rely on CF care centers or other physicians to inform patients about CCS benefits; few have outreach programs directed to the general public. Most states provide care through CCS-approved facilities or physicians, including but not limited to CFF-designated centers. Seven states work only through CF care centers, while in two states care is available only through CCS-employed providers. There was found only one instance in which CCS benefits are not available to people attending a CFF-accredited center. Financial eligibility in most states is based on a sliding scale determined by the family's income, outstanding medical expenses, and number of dependents.

The CFF survey recommended that CF programs include these features: physician visits, lab tests and x rays, medication, social work services, inhalation equipment, physical therapy, hospitalization, and home health services. The last item is important as a means for keeping a child close to the family while reducing costs at the same time. In larger states, the cost of transportation to the CF care center should also be included.

Services should be available from all CFF-designated centers, whether or not located in the state of the child's residence. (When services are obtained out-of-state, it may be reasonable to require an in-state doctor to approve the referral.) The provision of out-of-state benefits is especially important for those states without CF care centers or where the CF care center is not conveniently located. The program should pay for prescription drugs purchased from any licensed pharmacy not simply those operated by the hospital in which the CF care center is located.

The program should aim to enroll at least 75 to 80 percent of the known cases of CF among people under the age of twenty-one. Any significant shortfall from this would indicate excessively narrow eligibility standards. Financial eligibility should be evaluated on a sliding scale based on the family's income after medical expenses have been deducted. The survey suggests three ways to determine cost-sharing: having the state pay a declining share of medical costs as family income rises, having family participation be determined on the basis of state income tax liability (for example, the family would be required to pay up to twice its state income tax, with the state absorbing costs above that amount), or assuring that no family is required to pay more than 10 percent (or some other portion) of its income for medical care, with expenses beyond that point being paid by CCS.

A standard CCS program should have a budget equal to at least $1,000 (in 1980 dollars) per child enrolled in the program. CCS need not pay all medical bills for most families with CF, but there will be some families that require much more than the average amount of support. The suggested overall figure should furnish enough money to provide for the most serious cases. Note, however, that some states currently provide more than twice the suggested amount; $1,000 per enrollee should be regarded as a minimum.

Particularly in small states, attention should be given to whether the total amount of money available for CF could be depleted by a long hospital stay by one or two children. A separate budget for CF would not be a good idea in such states, because the amount used from year to year could vary widely. A CCS program should attempt to inform both parents and physicians about the availability of CCS help for children with certain conditions. Especially in states where CCS aid is available only in designated facilities, some physicians may be reluctant to refer their patients elsewhere for care and thus may not inform parents of the CCS benefits.

Care for the Adult with CF. The CF patient who has reached adulthood presents an interesting problem to the health care system. CCS assistance automatically stops at the individual's twenty-first birthday. Many states now provide similar state-supported programs for individuals with certain genetic diseases who have reached age twenty-one. California, for example, provides such assistance for individuals with cystic fibrosis, sickle cell anemia, hemophilia, and certain nervous system disorders such as Friedreich's ataxia. Because these programs are entirely autonomous at the state level, coverage is even more variable than CCS. However, all provide case management and certain services not covered by Medicaid.

Support from the Private Sector. The medical care of most children with cystic fibrosis is financed from the health insurance policies of their parents. The cost of the care of a very sick child can be a real burden to the insurance plan of an individual or a small firm. Parents have lost their jobs after the health needs of their children exceeded the resources of the insurance plan of the company for which they worked. Change of job can be a fiscal nightmare for an involved family if the health care of the new firm excludes coverage of preexisting conditions. Numerous examples of this have inspired legislation for national health insurance that includes coverage of catastrophic illness.

A number of voluntary health organizations are interested in cystic fibrosis. These include the American Lung Association, the March of Dimes, the American Heart Association, and the American Diabetes Association. These groups provide money for professional training, research, and public education. The major support for cystic fibrosis, however, comes from the Cystic Fibrosis Foundation.

CFF is a private, nonprofit foundation devoted to the control and eventual eradication of CF. Founded in 1955 by a group of dedicated parents and physicians, it has developed an extremely vigorous program to support research, education, and patient care. Although it has no major fund-raising event comparable to the American Lung Association's Christmas Seals or muscular dystrophy's Jerry Lewis Telethon, it raises between $16 and $17 million per year in a very well-conducted series of regional events. Approximately $6 million annually is budgeted in support of the national medical program. The remainder is spent at the regional and local levels for program support, education, and legislative action. The medical budget consists of several programs that might serve as models of involvement of a private foundation and the health care delivery system.

Approximately $2 million per year is designated for the support of the 128 CF care centers in the United States. These centers, located primarily in teaching hospitals, meet rigid standards of quality and regionalization. Application for center designation and financial support is made annually to CFF. Peer-conducted site visitation is made approximately every three years. Approved centers then receive financial support according to a complex formula that considers teaching and research activity as well as patient load. This represents approximately $150 per patient served so that a medical center seeing a hundred CF patients would receive an annual grant of about $15,000. This money is not expected to be applied to direct patient care. Instead, it is to be used to establish and conduct CF care center activities that otherwise might not be possible; activities might include parents' groups, peer groups, educational materials, and professional involvement in CFF chapter activities. Efforts of the members of the center committee (all of whom are physician volunteers) to provide regionalization of centers and thus avoid duplication of services in certain geographical areas have attracted the attention of many other agencies interested in this concept. The quality control provided by peer review is of such high quality that center accreditation by CFF is accepted as a hallmark for designation of CCS-accredited pulmonary centers in many states.

Approximately $1.5 million per year is targeted for direct support of research relating to CF. Approximately $200,000 per year is allocated for the Professional Education Committee, which consists of physicians and other professional volunteers who produce and edit a large number of written and audiovisual materials aimed at professional audiences. This committee also helps plan two or three annual professional conferences on subjects of interest to scientists concerned with CF.

The foundation allocates about one hundred thousand dollars per year to the national Consumer Focus Committee, which approaches the medical care of the patient with cystic fibrosis from the point of view of the patient. Activities include the Consumer Representative Program, a data-gathering and educational network of all interested adults who have CF. The committee provides regional workshops for members of the center care teams and provides workshops in mental health issues for a number of caregivers who work with chronic illness.

Since 1965, the foundation has maintained a national patient registry that annually collects demographic data from each known patient with CF. Highly accurate survival tables for individuals with CF have been constructed from these data (Figure 1). In cooperation with the national patient registry, the Western Consortium of Cystic Fibrosis Physicians has begun a multicenter collection of clinical data. The goal is to develop a time-oriented data base that will aid in assessing various means of care delivery. The public policy section collects data on consumer needs and collaborates with other voluntary health organizations in presenting the interests of individuals with chronic disease.

Figure 1. Cumulative Survival Curve for CF.

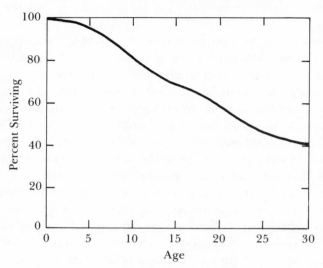

Source: Cystic Fibrosis Foundation, *CF Patient Registry.*

Pressures of CF on Public and Private Institutions

CF may affect the relationship of the individual with public and private institutions. The first such institution may well be the public school system. Younger children with severe disease may be absent from school for prolonged periods yet have a fanatical desire to keep up with their classes and peers. The student may be a social pariah because of the persistent cough and horribly malodorous stools. Teachers also sometimes have extreme difficulty dealing with the child who has a fatal illness, which may cause the child to be either shunned or protectively smothered. Severe illness may curtail school attendance to part-day or even home-based instruction.

The older CF patient offers a challenge to the business world. A great deal of effort is directed at preparing the chronically ill person for a job, yet the adage "hire the handicapped" is honored more in the breach than in the observance. Only exceptional employers will tolerate the need for the person with CF to rest, to stay home during respiratory illnesses, and to go into hospitals several times a year. An equitable means of allowing the individual to work part-time without becoming ineligible for health care benefits is a priority for individuals with CF.

Pressures on the insurance industry have already been mentioned. Although the average annual cost of health care is less than $7,000, a very sick child can accrue hospital bills in excess of $100,000. This can be devastating to the health plan of a small firm with a limited number of employees. The Cystic Fibrosis Foundation has expressed concern about this problem and has favored national health insurance for the chronically ill. The foundation does not endorse any of the bills currently before Congress because none of them solve the problems of chronic illness. Rather, CFF recommends that national health insurance legislation begin with the premise that no family or individual, faced with either catastrophic or chronic illness, should face financial ruin. There are several principles essential to putting this premise into practice:

1. All medical expenses must be counted toward the deductible and the reimbursement formulas.
2. Separate deductibles for hospital and nonhospital expenses should be replaced by a single, integrated deductible, and prescription drug costs should be included in catastrophic coverage.
3. All persons should be eligible for coverage in the program, regardless of health or employment status. Because pre-existing illness clauses usually prevent adults with CF from obtaining private coverage, health insurance legislation should make insurance available to all without regard to pre-existing illness.
4. The needs of people with long-term, expensive diseases should be recognized, perhaps through deductibility periods that extend more than one year.
5. Finally, the reimbursement formula must take appropriate account of the near poor and the chronically ill. Although increasing numbers of CF patients are living into their twenties, their incomes are often low. Health insurance legislation should include an income base deductible for out-of-pocket expenses available to lower income individuals.

Conclusion

People with CF serve as models of a new challenge to the health care system—children with a fatal illness who have survived to adulthood. They are usually not well enough to work full time yet are intellectually and emotionally geared to participate actively in society. They want to be independent, yet require a certain amount of nurturing from public and private sources. A very expensive regimen of outpatient care will add years to their lives. This can be provided but needs to be worked into the total health care system. Meeting the needs of individuals with chronic illness may well be the major task of the health care system in the 1980s.

Chronic illness takes a toll on many segments of the population, including caregivers. There are times in the course of the day when the only progress is lack of deterioration. It seems that the chronically ill get the very last crumbs of the health care dollar and are the first to have their carefully constructed programs cut during a budgetary pinch. What motivates caregivers to work with this patient population? It is, of course, the patients themselves. One of the best descriptions of chronic illness was given by a twenty-nine-year-old man who responded to the Cost of CF survey as follows:

> Having CF and attempting to function in anyway near normal is nearly impossible. The medical expenses which are crippling, the loss of personal esteem, the social repugnance, and psychological burdens aside, this disease is one of the most heart-rending conditions today. It is a physical (not to mention mental and social) handicap without the badges of a handicap: i.e., wheelchair, crutches, braces, etc. It robs the young of

childhood and those who survive longer of the fulfillment of adult life. As a medical professional with the disease, I know the full ramifications, the course it must follow, and the eventual outcome. There is little room for hope.

My only sustaining force is the small fact that something I might do or say as I lecture for the CF Foundation or the personal experiments with which I am involved might in some small way help others that come after me. As I sit here writing this I am cognizant of the fact that a man learns the true meaning of service when he plants shade trees under which he knows full well he never will sit.

References

Basham, C., and others. "Cystic Fibrosis Adults and Marriage." Cystic Fibrosis Club Abstracts, 1980, p. 20.

Boyle, I., and others. "Emotional Adjustments in Adolescents and Young Adults with Cystic Fibrosis." In J. Mangos and R. Talamo (Eds.), *Fundamental Problems of Cystic Fibrosis and Related Diseases*. Miami: Symposia Specialists, 1973.

Cohen, L. F., diSant'Agnese, P. A., and Frielander, J. "Cystic Fibrosis and Pregnancy." *Lancet*, 1980, *ii*, 842–844.

Cystic Fibrosis Foundation. *CF Patient Registry*. Rockville, Md.: Cystic Fibrosis Foundation, updated annually.

Cystic Fibrosis Foundation. "Over-21 Survey." Rockville, Md.: Cystic Fibrosis Foundation, August 1979.

Cystic Fibrosis Foundation. "1980 Survey of State Crippled Children's Services Programs for Children with Cystic Fibrosis." Rockville, Md.: Cystic Fibrosis Foundation, 1980.

Cystic Fibrosis Foundation. "Cost of Cystic Fibrosis Survey Report." Cystic Fibrosis Foundation, March 1981.

Denning, C., Gluckson, M., and Mueller, D. "Psychological and Social Aspects of Cystic Fibrosis." In J. Mangos and R. Talamo (Eds.), *Cystic Fibrosis, Projections into the Future*. Miami: Symposia Specialists, 1976.

Drotar, D., and others. "Psychosocial Functioning of Children with Cystic Fibrosis." *Pediatrics*, 1980, *67*, 338–343.

Frydman, M. "Implications of Cystic Fibrosis for Health Services and the Afflicted." *Social Science and Medicine*, 1979, *13*, 147–150.

Gliedman, J., and Roth, W. *The Unexpected Minority*. New York: Harcourt Brace Jovanovich, 1980.

Jones, M. B. "Years of Life Lost to Cystic Fibrosis." *Journal of Chronic Disease*, 1980, *33*, 697–701.

Kellerman, J., and others. "Psychological Effects of Illness in Adolescents." *Journal of Pediatrics*, 1980, *97*, 126–131, 132–138.

Kerner, J., Harvey, B., and Lewiston, N. "The Impact of Grief." *Journal of Chronic Disease*, 1979, *32*, 221–225.

Korsch, B. "Effects of Chronic Illness on Adolescents and Young Adults," In J.

Mangos and R. Talamo (Eds.), *Fundamental Problems of Cystic Fibrosis and Related Diseases*. Miami: Symposia Specialists, 1973.

Landon, C., and others. "Self-Image of Adolescents with Cystic Fibrosis." *Journal of Youth and Adolescence*, 1980, *9*, 521–528.

Littlefield, J. "Research on Cystic Fibrosis." *New England Journal of Medicine*, 1981, *304*, 44–45.

Patterson, P., Denning, C., and Kutscher, A. (Eds.) *Psychosocial Aspects of Cystic Fibrosis*. New York: Columbia University Press, 1973.

Shwachman, H. "Cystic Fibrosis." In E. Kendig (Ed.), *Disorders of the Respiratory Tract in Children*. (3d ed.) Philadelphia: Saunders, 1977.

Straka, G., and Kuttner, M. "Psychological Compensation in the Individual with a Life-Threatening Illness." *South Africa Medical Journal*, 1980, *57*, 61–62.

Thompson, M. W. "Genetics of Cystic Fibrosis." In J. Sturgess (Ed.), *Perspectives in Cystic Fibrosis*. Toronto: Canadian Cystic Fibrosis Foundation, 1980.

11

Spina Bifida

Gary J. Myers, M.D.
Margaret Millsap, R.N., Ed.D.

Spina bifida is the second most common birth defect after Down's syndrome and affects between one and two of every thousand newborn infants (Stark, 1977). The term *spina bifida* literally means spine split in two (Allum, 1975) and applies to a wide spectrum of similar disorders that have in common a failure of the bony spine (usually the posterior vertebral arch) to develop properly. The bony abnormality, which is only one part of the condition, is often associated with damage to cerebral nerve tissues or failure of these tissues to develop properly, which in turn can lead to a host of serious complications.

The spectrum of spina bifida can vary from minor failures of the bony spine to form properly, which can be seen in up to 25 percent of normal individuals (Sutow and Pryde, 1956), to extensive malformations that affect the majority of the bony spine and its associated neural tissue, the spinal cord. The type of spina bifida midway between these extremes concerns us here because, with treatment, the prognosis for survival and even independence can be surprisingly good, even though it is associated with lifelong disability. This type of spina bifida is termed *myelomeningocele* or *meningomyelocele*. The terms are synonymous and mean a protrusion of the spinal cord and its covering membranes through the bony spine. This accounts for approximately 95 percent of those children recognized at birth as having spina bifida (Lorber, 1977). Even though myelomeningocele is technically a subset of spina bifida, *myelomeningocele* and *spina bifida* are generally used interchangeably by both the public and health care workers. In this chapter, too, the terms are considered the same, and the discussion centers on those forms of spina bifida compatible with survival and associated with neurological and other types of disability. Although spina bifida has been recognized for centuries, it is only with the advent of modern neuro-surgery (especially shunt procedures for hydrocephalus) and antibiotics to control infections that survival of more than an occasional individual with this defect has occurred.

Presentation

Spina bifida is easily recognized at birth, even by the layman. In the midline of the back, over the defective bony spine, there is an area of tissue that appears strikingly different. This tissue is usually thin and delicate, often has raw nerve tissue in its center, and may be filled with watery fluid and protrude like a sac. Occasionally, there is a covering of skin over the sac. The defect may occur any place in the midline of the back, but about 98 percent involve the vertebrae in the lower back below the ribs. Nearly 70 percent involve only the lumbar spine, that is, the spine below the ribs and above the pelvis (Myers, Cerone, and Olson, 1981). The size of the defect is variable and is generally directly proportional to the severity of the associated problems.

If the sac is not well covered with skin, there is an increased risk of infection in the fluid surrounding the brain and spinal cord (cerebrospinal fluid or CSF). This occurs because the normal barriers to invasion by bacteria are not present. If the sac is covered by a membrane, it may tear during delivery. This leads to leakage of the CSF and collapse of the sac. It also increases the risk of CSF infection and the urgency of surgical repair. Closure of the spinal defect drastically reduces the chance of CSF infection, which is the most common cause of death in infants with spina bifida. Consequently, surgical closure of the back should be done as soon as the family has been counseled, understands the situation, and provides truly informed consent.

The birth of a child with spina bifida usually has a profound effect on the family. It is generally an unexpected event that shatters their dreams of the normal baby they anticipated. Parents may react with shock, confusion, anger, frustration, disbelief, or guilt. The infant's very survival is often in question, and both parents and professionals may feel ambivalence about what, if anything, should be done to help the infant. These emotions are not easily or rapidly resolved. In addition, most parents are totally unfamiliar with spina bifida. Educating them about the defect and what the future will hold for the infant and their family is a difficult task. However, they need to be active participants in any decision about treatment because they will bear the major responsibility for the child's long-term care.

In addition, other abnormalities may be present at birth, either as a result of or related to the spina bifida. Hydrocephalus is found in nearly all infants with spina bifida involving the lumbar or higher levels (Lorber, 1961). This usually manifests itself in the first few days or weeks of life by a rapidly expanding head circumference but can be present without head enlargement. Bony malformations of the vertebrae and ribs are also frequent and may be associated with curvature of the spine (scoliosis or kyphosis) or distortions of the chest. The degree and type of neurological impairment related to the bony spinal defect is variable. Total paralysis of the lower extremities (paraplegia) may be present, or there may be movement in some of these muscles. The paralysis is generally associated with poor control of the urinary bladder and may be accompanied by or may lead to dislocation of one or both hip joints, lack of or poor sensation in the lower extremities, and enlargement of one or both kidneys (hydronephrosis). Joint deformities, such as clubfoot, and frozen joints (arthrogryposis) are also common.

Consequently, the infant with spina bifida can present a broad array of physical abnormalities. Each of these needs early delineation, as do the family's strengths and weaknesses, so the health care team can provide an informed opinion and help the family plan for an appropriate treatment. At times, this plan may be a recommendation for only symptomatic support of the infant.

Epidemiology

Spina bifida is one of several defects that affect the developing nervous system. The incidence of spina bifida alone varies widely in different geographical areas of the world. In the United Kingdom (UK), the incidence is 2.5 per thousand births (Record and McKeown, 1949). In the United States, it varies from 0.67 (Janerich, 1973) to 1.64 per thousand (Bigger, Mortimer, and Haughie, 1976). Most authors consider the incidence or occurrence of spina bifida to be between 1 and 2 births per thousand in the United States. The precise figure is difficult to establish because the sources for published data on incidence vary.

The prevalence or number of individuals with spina bifida at one time is difficult to ascertain. Currently, there are no valid estimates of this number either in the United States or elsewhere (Elwood and Elwood, 1980). Much of the incidence data is in reality prevalence at birth, because our knowledge of how frequently spina bifida occurs in the fetus who does not survive to term is limited. In the United States, at least three thousand and perhaps as many as twelve thousand infants with spina bifida are born each year. How many of these infants survive and how long they live is unknown. Their survival is partly related to the vigor with which treatment is pursued. Prevalence rates for spina bifida would be very helpful in overall health care planning but are unavailable.

Risk Factors

Spina bifida is thought to occur during early development of the nerve tissue, around the fourth week following conception. Genetic factors appear to be involved because the recurrence rate in siblings of affected infants is much higher than occurrence in the general population. Simple modes of inheritance do not appear to be present, and a multifactorial or polygenic inheritance has been proposed. In this, the defect (or spina bifida) results from the cumulative effect of several minor gene abnormalities plus environmental factors. The exact mode of inheritance remains to be determined, but etiological heterogeneity is recognized in spina bifida and other neural tube defects (Holmes, Driscoll, and Atkins, 1976). The fact that monozygotic (identical) twins are rarely both affected with spina bifida is strong evidence that genetic factors are not entirely responsible (Laurence, Carter, and David, 1968).

Epidemiologists have favored environmental factors as causative, and a multitude of properly timed insults to pregnant animals have resulted in some newborns having spina bifida (Warkany, 1971). In many, hypotheses such as the presence of unidentified substances in potato tubers (Renwick, Possamai, and Munday, 1974) and hyperthermia (elevated body temperature) during pregnancy (Smith, Sterling, and Harvey, 1978) have been proposed but remain unproven. Spina bifida is known to be more common among lower socioeconomic classes.

There is an increased risk of recurrence in families who have had one child with spina bifida, but other specific risk factors are yet unknown. Unrelated parents with a child who has spina bifida have a 4 to 5 percent risk of recurrence in a subsequent pregnancy, while those with two affected children have a 10 percent risk. If one parent has spina bifida and no affected children, the risk is again between 4 and 5 percent, but it rises to between 10 and 15 percent if the affected parent already has an affected child. Consequently, genetic counseling can be very useful for couples who already have an affected child. Unfortunately, nearly 95 percent of infants born with spina bifida are the first individuals so affected in their family.

Prenatal Diagnosis

In recent years, remarkable progress has been made in diagnosing spina bifida in utero. In 1972, it was noted that in the presence of spina bifida there was an increase in alpha-fetoprotein (AFP) in the amniotic fluid (Brock and Sutcliffe, 1972). This special protein is produced in large amounts by the fetus but only rarely produced by the body after birth. Consequently, any AFP found in the amniotic fluid is almost always of fetal origin, and elevations above normal may indicate a significant fetal problem. Contamination of amniotic fluid with fetal blood is the most common cause of elevated AFP, but a variety of other disorders will also increase it (Crandall, 1981). Ninety-eight percent of open spina bifidas in the United Kingdom collaborative study (Wald and others, 1977) were diagnosed by the AFP level. These studies indicate that amniocentesis is of value in pregnancies where the risk of spina bifida is higher than average. If the amniotic fluid AFP level is normal, the mother can be reassured that an open spina bifida is probably not present; if the AFP level is elevated and other studies confirm a spina bifida, she can choose whether or not to continue the pregnancy.

Because amniocentesis does carry a small risk to both mother and fetus, it does not seem ethically justified in all pregnancies, even if the resources were available to do it. In addition, only 5 percent of infants with spina bifida are born to families who would be counseled to have an amniocentesis. However, sampling of maternal serum might be feasible on a large scale, and AFP can be detected in it. The U.K. collaborative study investigated this by screening pregnancies at sixteen to eighteen weeks gestation. They found that after examination of two separate maternal serum samples and an ultrasound study of the fetus, there were still 2 percent of normal pregnancies subjected to amniocentesis (Wald and Cuckle, 1979). At the present time, widespread screening of pregnancies by this method does not seem feasible.

Ultrasonography has been improved in recent years and can often demonstrate spina bifida in utero (Hobbins and others, 1979). It is especially valuable in determining the exact cause of an elevated AFP because it can confirm gestational age and identify twins and other defects that also elevate AFP levels.

The availability of these prenatal diagnostic techniques for detecting spina bifida has made some prenatal selection possible. Finding the fetus to be normal can be reassuring to the family, but should the fetus have spina bifida, the family can have the option of abortion. Such selection does involve killing the fetus, and the ethical issues are complex and open to personal interpretation (Swinyard, 1978; Smith, 1981). Unfortunately, current use of technology does not help us identify the majority of infants affected with spina bifida before birth. Consequently, the option of feticide is commonly not available.

Description and Course

The infant with spina bifida presents a complex array of defects that vary in occurrence and severity from individual to individual. When describing the defects and what can be expected with each, they have been grouped into general categories.

Spinal Defect. The myelomeningocele sac or opening over the bony spinal defect is generally covered with delicate membranes (meninges). The meninges join with skin near the periphery of the lesion, and in the center, there is raw nerve tissue (neural plaque). The surface is often moist and provides an ideal site for bacterial growth. The closer the lesion is to the anus, the more likely contamination becomes. When the surface of the sac is colonized by organisms, these can pass into the CSF and cause meningitis. They may also move into the fluid spaces inside the brain and cause ventriculitis. If the sac is ruptured, either during delivery or in handling the infant, the risk of subsequent infection increases dramatically. Infection in or around the central nervous system (CNS) is the most common cause of death in the first few weeks or months of life. Risk of infection is greatly reduced by surgical closure of the opening. If the sac is not surgically removed, skin cells from the margins will grow over the surface. Within a few weeks, the sac may have a thin, fragile skin covering. This covering decreases the risk of infection and may account for the long-term survival of some untreated individuals.

Hydrocephalus. Dilatation of fluid spaces of the brain (ventricles) is probably present in most individuals with spina bifida except for some with small sacral defects. It is unusual for hydrocephalus to manifest itself in utero as head enlargement, but ventricular dilatation in utero by ultrasound may be present and can help confirm the presence of spina bifida. Usually, head growth begins shortly after birth and progresses at a variable rate. If progressive hydrocephalus is not halted, then vomiting, irritability, and lethargy will eventually occur, just as they would in the older child with increased intracranial pressure.

Hydrocephalus in spina bifida is generally associated with Arnold-Chiari malformation, a protrusion of the cerebellum out of the skull along with a posterior displacement of the entire brainstem. This results in obstruction of the flow of spinal fluid. About two thirds of such obstructions prevent communication between the inside and outside of the brain. This is termed *noncommunicating hydrocephalus.*

Diagnosis of hydrocephalus can be made on the basis of clinical findings and an abnormally rapid increase in head circumference. The diagnosis can be confirmed by ultrasound, computerized axial tomography (CAT), or contrast studies such as pneumoencephalograms (PEGs) or ventriculograms. Many infants with spina bifida have only moderate degrees of hydrocephalus that may never require neurosurgical intervention (shunting). These infants often survive with normal intelligence and head sizes (Lorber, 1977). Shunting consists of diverting spinal fluid from the brain to other parts of the body, typically by a plastic tube that runs from the brain to other parts of the body (typically from the ventricles to the abdominal cavity). If the shunt is not required during the first few months or year of life, it is seldom necessary later. Because shunt malfunction is an important cause of later mortality in individuals with spina bifida, avoidance of a shunt is desirable.

Spinal Cord Dysfunction. The spinal defect is associated with a variable degree of neurological dysfunction secondary to maldevelopment of the spinal cord and nerves. To this may be added other insults such as postnatal drying and infection of the neural plate, meningitis, and trauma during delivery. The resulting neurological picture can vary remarkably and will depend on the level and pattern of the individuals involved. Two general patterns are commonly recognized. In the first, there is a complete loss of neural function below a given spinal cord level. This results in a flaccid paralysis with loss of reflexes and sensations in muscles receiving nervous input from below that level. This pattern occurs in about one third of patients. The second pattern consists of interruption of the long spinal tracts that carry impulses from the brain although reflex activity is preserved in isolated lower segments of the spinal cord. If any of the long tracts are partially spared, the child may have some voluntary movement or sensation in the lower extremities. About two thirds of patients manifest the latter type.

Neurological dysfunction accounts for many of the deformities seen in the lower extremities, the pressure sores on the feet and buttocks, and the genitourinary problems that are almost uniformly present. The nerve supply to the muscles of the hip is such that different muscles for a given joint are controlled by nerves at different spinal cord levels. Because a neurological lesion may involve only one level, this can lead to a muscle imbalance around the joint (that is, one muscle group would be flaccid and the other normal or spastic). The eventual result of such imbalance will be a deformed joint. This is a particular problem at the hip. The result of muscle imbalance at the hip is dislocation, and the high proportion of defects (98 percent) affecting the lumbar area make this a common occurrence. If hip dislocation is present at birth and not treated, it can adversely affect the formation of the hip joint itself. If it is not present at birth, it may develop as the child grows. Both standing and moving necessitate stability in the lower extremities, and proper hip joint function is essential in achieving this. Stability of the spine and knees, and feet positioned for weight-bearing are also necessary for standing and walking. Motor paralysis at higher spinal levels affects back muscles and contributes to spinal instability and deformity.

The neurological dysfunction also affects sensation, usually all modalities. The pattern of sensory involvement generally coincides with that of the motor deficit. The sensory loss deprives the individual of information from muscles, tendons, and joints. Lack of such proprioceptive and kinesthetic information makes ambulation difficult. In addition, loss of pain, temperature, and other superficial sensations permits trauma, burns, and pressure sores to occur easily and go unnoticed. Casts and orthopedic appliances, which are commonly needed, must be fitted properly and watched carefully to avoid damaging insensitive skin. Loss of sensation also contributes to the disuse atrophy that weakens lower-limb bones and can result in fractures following minimal stress.

In addition, neurological dysfunction affects bladder and bowel control. Except for an occasional defect that involves only half the spinal cord (hemimyelocele), nearly all spina bifida patients have some bladder dysfunction. The neurogenic bladder, like other motor functions, can be either spastic or flaccid. Either type of dysfunction interferes with the two major functions of the bladder, which are storage and evacuation. Inopportune or poorly controlled evacuation leads to incontinence, and incomplete emptying or residual urine predisposes to urinary tract infection. If bladder contraction is not coordinated with relaxation of the external sphincter, pressure within the bladder rises and urine may be pushed back up into the kidneys, and if bacteria are present, kidney infection may occur. This can lead to dilation of urinary tubes and back pressure on kidneys (hydroureter and hydronephrosis). Because the fetus produces urine by the end of the first trimester, damage to the bladder, ureters, and kidneys secondary to the neurological dysfunction may be present at birth. Both hydronephrosis and ascending infection can damage the kidneys and eventually result in hypertension. By age ten, 50 percent of spina bifida patients in one study had hypertension (Lorber and Lyons, 1970). Renal failure is a frequent cause of death in adults with spina bifida.

Genital sensation is also impaired or absent and may interfere with sexual activity, especially in the male where penile erection and ejaculation may be absent. Despite this, sexual interest of adolescents with spina bifida and their concerns about sexual matters are equal to those of the nondisabled (Dorner, 1976).

Effects on rectal control depend on whether there is a total loss of neurological function in the sacrum or whether some reflex activity remains. With complete loss of function, there is total lack of bowel control and a tendency to rectal prolapse (protrusion). Retention of some reflex activity, even in the absence of sensation, usually permits some degree of bowel control.

Associated Malformations and Problems. Children with spina bifida have a high incidence of associated anomalies at birth. Those of the external genitalia or urinary tract are common. Such findings as imperforate anus and congenital heart disease are occasionally seen. However, spinal skeletal defects in addition to the spina bifida itself are particularly common and can result in disabling deformities. The presence of one or more congenital vertebral abnormalities is seen in up to 50 percent of spina bifida infants. The result of these skeletal abnormalities, either alone or in combination with neurological dysfunction of back muscles, can be a severe spinal curvature such as kyphosis, scoliosis, lordosis, or some combination of these curvatures. Some deformity may be present at birth. However, growth of bones and body, gravity, and the changing postures of children as they sit, stand, and move make these deformities a dynamic problem that can change with time, generally for the worse. Spinal stability will eventually be needed in order to maintain an upright posture, whether it be for ambulation or wheelchair sitting.

Psychological, Social, and Behavioral Developments. Despite malformations of the brain such as the Arnold-Chiari and hydrocephalus, there is generally normal intellectual function in about two thirds of children with spina bifida who survive (Hunt and Holmes, 1975; Shurtleff and Foltz, 1972). The intellectual level does correlate with the occurrence of infection in or around the brain, the thickness of the brain at the time the shunt is inserted, and the sensory level of the spina bifida (Hunt and Holmes, 1975). The intellectual level does not seem to correlate with the number of shunt malfunctions or revisions required. When children with spina bifida are compared with siblings or normal peers, their intellectual levels are significantly lower but still fall within the normal range. Visual perceptual problems occur frequently (Tew and Laurence, 1975). These factors, along with lower teacher expectations and others, may account for why the child with spina bifida often functions below age level and intellectual potential.

The child with spina bifida may become dependent and display immature behavior. Language development may result in repetitive, inappropriate chatter that is well constructed but meaningless. This "cocktail party chatter" usually indicates inability to use language appropriately (Swisher and Pinsker, 1971).

The social impact of the child with spina bifida on both family and community is profound. Full understanding of the problem is difficult, even for professionals. For parents, this difficulty is compounded by a host of factors that include the birth itself, the surprise of a defect, their lack of medical background, and the responsibility they face—a responsibility that includes large expenditures of time, physical effort, and money. There are, then, secondary effects on emotional stability and reserves, marital adjustment, and siblings as well.

Treatment and Its Efficacy

Should Treatment Be Undertaken? The first question to answer at birth is whether to treat the infant actively. Even before amniocentesis and selective termination of pregnancy became so acceptable, there was debate on this issue (Lorber, 1971). In England, the following criteria have been proposed as warranting only palliative treatment (Lorber, 1977):

> large mid- or upper-back lesion
> spinal defect clinically apparent at birth
> gross hydrocephalus (head circumference over 90th percentile by at least 2 cm)
> other gross congenital defects
> severe cerebral birth injury or intracranial hemorrhage
> meningitis before or after back closure in the presence of hydrocephalus
> social circumstances of an abandoned or unwanted child, even if condition not so severe

In the United States, similar criteria were also proposed (Shurtleff and others, 1974). However, this approach has been vigorously debated, and a recent review of the issue raises three major concerns (Black, 1979). First, the specific selection criteria for limited or palliative treatment seem inconsistent because other conditions (for example, hydrocephalus or cerebral palsy) producing similar disabilities are generally treated. Thus, such selection criteria seem useful only in the context of a specific disorder affecting many parts of the body, namely spina bifida. Second, the likelihood that infants with spina bifida who are not treated will die early is not as definite as formerly suggested (Feetham, Tweed, and Perrin, 1979). Some may survive many years. This leads to the third concern, which is that those who survive untreated may be more impaired than they would have been had they received treatment.

It is currently a moot point whether the paternalistic attitude of those selecting who will be treated or the empathetic attitude of those who would treat all spina bifida children is best. Even those who exercise selection often disagree on the specific criteria that are used. In addition, both the physician and the parents may be technically guilty of homicide by omission because their legal duty is to provide needed medical assistance to a helpless minor (Robertson, 1978). The issues of whether early selective treatment should be used, what criteria should be used for selection, and the legal status of selection are presently not resolved.

Repair of Myelomeningocele. Emergency closure of the open defect on the back has been proposed, but there is little evidence that urgent surgery improves the outcome. Adequate time to help the family understand the problem and participate in any decision on treatment should be allowed. Following the decision to treat, early surgical repair of the back is usually the initial step. If large back defects are repaired in the presence of progressive hydrocephalus, it may be necessary to place a shunt first. This prevents CSF leakage from interfering with healing of the back. Wound breakdown and infection are not common. Apart from pressure ulcerations over a kyphosis, later problems with the back are unusual.

Hydrocephalus. Progressive ventricular enlargement with clinical symptoms occurs in about two thirds of spina bifida infants and requires surgical treatment. In about one third, the hydrocephalus arrests spontaneously and the complications of surgery and shunts can be avoided (Stark, 1977). Surgery for hydrocephalus consists of diverting spinal fluid from a ventricle in the brain to a site where it can be absorbed. Multiple sites have been proposed, but the abdominal cavity is currently preferred. Shunt malfunction at a later date can result in acute increases of intracranial pressure. This can lead to serious clinical symptoms (vomiting, lethargy, coma) or even death. Apart from mechanical malfunction or separation of the shunt components, problems associated with infection of the spinal fluid or blood and pressure necrosis of the bowel or heart occasionally occur. Once in place, shunts are rarely totally removed.

Urological Problems. Urological problems are present in most children with spina bifida and require regular monitoring to preserve renal function. Urinary tract infection and ureteral reflux to the kidneys are common, often minimally symptomatic, and if untreated, can result in progressive renal deterioration. Routine periodic evaluations of the urine and of the upper urinary tract by contrast radiography are indicated for life.

Urinary diversion to an ileal loop (surgically created pouch of intestine acting as a bladder), thus bypassing the bladder, urethra, and perineum, was used for many years. However, long-term evaluations have decreased enthusiasm for this surgery (Shapiro, Lebowitz, and Colodny, 1975). Reflux from the ileal pouch is characteristic, and a change to the use of the sigmoid colon instead of ileum has been proposed because an antireflux surgical connection can be made. Diversion is primarily used to prevent renal deterioration, but it also provides continence. Incontinence seriously impairs the individual's social acceptability. Attempts to provide continence have also included pharmacological agents, bladder training, urine collecting devices, and surgical procedures ranging from urinary diversion to placement of artificial sphincters and electrical stimulators. Recently, intermittent clean catheterization (ICC) of the bladder has been in use. It can provide dry periods of two to three hours, depending on the individual, and also reduces incidence of infection by reducing the amount of residual urine. The technique of ICC is promising and inexpensive and can be used even with young children. Despite major advances, urological problems remain a lifelong concern that can lead to death from renal failure unless monitored and vigorously treated when necessary.

Gastrointestinal Problems. Fecal incontinence also results from lack of sacral innervation and interferes even more with social acceptance. Regular bowel evacuation, however, can be achieved in most patients by following a consistent routine that recognizes natural reflexes, eating foods with high fiber content and laxative tendencies, and judiciously using oral medications, suppositories, and enemas. Achieving this control may require months or years, and maintaining it is a lifetime effort. With effort and diligence, however, nearly all spina bifida patients can gain bowel control adequate for social acceptability.

Orthopedic Problems. Deformities of the spine and joints in the lower extremities are common, may deteriorate with time, and usually need attention if the child is to be functional and avoid complications from sensory loss. Deformities can result from congenital skeletal defects, imbalance of muscles around joints, or from in-utero positioning. After birth, unbalanced muscle action around joints, growth, fractures, and gravitational effects on the upright spine contribute to increase the orthopedic problems previously present.

At birth and in the early months, any deformity of the feet and dislocation of the hips should receive attention. Casting of feet deformities may correct them or at least lessen the extent of later surgery. In order for one to stand upright, the feet need to be properly positioned and the hips must be stable. If hip dislocation is present early and not corrected, then the acetabulum (hip joint) may form improperly. Even if the hip joint is well developed, muscle imbalance may dislocate the head of the femur at a later time. Regular evaluations are needed to monitor muscle imbalance when there is any motor function, voluntary or not, in the lower extremities. Because the patterns of deformities, defects, and innervation are unlimited, each child is unique and requires an individually tailored treatment plan. Early efforts often utilize casting and corrective appliances. Surgical procedures (frequently multiple—on soft tissues early and bony structures later) are needed by most children. Reduction of the hips, proper joint mobility or fixation, and feet positioned to support weight can generally be achieved with aggressive treatment.

Paralysis from spina bifida impairs mobility to varying degrees. Children with spina bifida needs special devices to aid them in moving about. At the appropriate age, the upright posture can usually be achieved either with conventional braces or by means of a special brace called a parapodium. The parapodium frees the upper extremities while the child is standing, allowing free use of the hands and arms for other activities. Recent advances in bracing have reduced the weight of such appliances and improved their utility. As growth occurs and the child weighs more, bracing becomes more difficult. A wheelchair often becomes an easier means of moving about.

With growth, spinal curvatures become increasingly important. This is especially true when the spina bifida is extensive and located at higher spinal levels. Spinal curvature can affect sitting and standing posture, mobility, and when severe, even heart and lung function. Treatment of spinal curves is complex and lengthy, often involves major surgery, and is not always successful. Following surgery, immobilization of the spine in a total body cast may be required for from six to twelve months. As more infants with large lesions survive, this type of surgery is being performed more frequently.

Outcome

One measure of outcome is simply survival. Modern medical techniques have steadily improved our ability to control or eradicate infections, treat renal failure, and manage hydrocephalus, which are the major causes of death associated with spina bifida. Consequently, the number of individuals with spina bifida who can be kept alive has increased. Even so, one recent series showed that only 60 percent of seventy-six infants operated on soon after birth were still alive at one year of age (Boston and Wilkinson, 1979). In other reported series, which combine infants who were treated with those untreated, from 18 to 43 percent were still alive at one year. Among those infants who are not operated on but only receive supportive treatment, survival averages 20 percent at one year.

A more important question, however, relates to morbidity and the quality of life that survivors and their families can anticipate. Most survivors face a lifetime of medical care and repeated operations. Many are socially isolated as they mature because of limited experiences, incontinence, and physical disabilities. Some families have the strength to provide support, but many do not. Individuals with spina bifida face many obstacles before they are able to learn independence and separate from the family, learn to provide self-care, gain a skill and find a job to support themselves, find accessible accommodation, and master the multiple problems of mobility. These are not only difficult to accomplish but expensive as well. The outlook for such children is improving, but there is a very long way to go.

Stress on Child and Family

The emotional crisis created by birth of a child with spina bifida constitutes one of the greatest challenges any family will ever face. The shock, disbelief, anger, and/or frustration that follows such an event can severely threaten the fabric of any marriage as well as the integrity of the entire family.

Due to the seriousness of the problems and the need for early surgery, the mother and father are usually informed of the infant's condition immediately after birth. Psychologically, emotionally, and physiologically, this is a bad time for both parents. They may hear what the physician tells them but often they fail to comprehend the full implication of the child's condition. Experienced professionals have learned to soften the shock by giving the news to parents in a very general way at first. More explicit information can be provided later (Hare and others, 1966).

The grief seems to be more damaging to the mother because she is denied the pleasure of nurturing her child in the manner she had anticipated. She also finds that most of the time she is the person who must bear the responsibility of caring for the child. Due to the intractable nature of the condition, the mother often feels trapped (Miller, 1968). Her "chronic sorrow" can create a great deal of stress (Olshansky, 1962).

Kolin and others (1971) reported a study of families who had school-age children with meningomyelocele. The sample was small but did yield evidence that the majority of the parents studied had a difficult time adapting to a life that included a child with spina bifida. Eight out of thirteen parents were rated as having a poor adaptation, and six of the couples were divorced or separated. They concluded that "only those parents who had had the opportunity to develop a stable relationship with a minimum of five years of marriage were able to cope successfully with the crisis" (p. 1017). They further concluded that the degree of physical impairment was not the most important factor in the level of adjustment of the family. However, a later study seemed to contradict these findings (Nevin and others, 1979). This study indicated that group supports, activities, and interpersonal relationships are more important for both family regenerative power and family vulnerability to stress. Cohesiveness has also been identified as a significant indicator of family adequacy as well as of its recuperative capacity (Miller, 1968).

Walker, Thomas, and Russell (1971), studied the impact on nine different aspects of family life. This study indicated that genetic counseling and contraceptive techniques were not consistently provided for such families, although there was a definite drop in the birth rate for these women after the birth of one child with spina bifida. The majority of parents included in this study expressed the view that their marital relationship had not been damaged by the birth of the baby. However, most mothers and fathers admitted to increased tension in the family. The study revealed that 73 out of 106 mothers felt fit and well.

The effect on siblings and other members of the family may be marked. Other children may be neglected so the mother can provide care for the disabled child. Many siblings may resent remarks made by their playmates concerning their brother or sister. Some older children worry about the emotional effect on their parents. Care of the child with spina bifida affects the domestic routine of the home, but the Walker study did not confirm a negative effect on the majority of families.

Due to the severity of the condition and the large amount of direct care that must be given to the child with spina bifida, many become emotionally dependent children. Mothers and fathers may become overprotective of the child and find it difficult to allow the child the opportunities needed to learn self-help skills. Such children are often influenced by the way parents and siblings relate to them as well as by the degree of their handicap. They need to participate in peer relationships and to develop self-control and social skills. In order to achieve this goal, opportunities for interaction with other children are necessary, but many times these are not sought by the family because they fear further injury. All children, and especially those with spina bifida, need to achieve success in relationships with others and need the chance to make choices, experience independence, and be allowed to take some prudent risks (Rankin, 1979).

Lack of programs that provide early stimulation and training in self-help skills adds to the stress of both child and family. Many of these children are from one-parent families (usually the mother), many of which have a difficult time providing total care for the child. Transportation to treatment programs is costly and time-consuming. The problem of supervision of other children in the family while the mother attends to the needs of the child with spina bifida also adds to the stress.

Most of these children have average intelligence and will need the same educational opportunities as normal children (Myers, Cerone, and Olson, 1981).

Yet, lack of physical accessibility of school buildings, classrooms, and other facilities has forced many of these children to be placed in isolated classrooms with children who are mentally as well as physically handicapped. In situations such as these, intellectual stimulation is reduced and the children are apt to function at a level below that of their ability.

As the child grows, educational, vocational training, and social opportunities are increasingly difficult to obtain. Needing peer recognition and participation in social and recreational activities of other children, these children will frequently demonstrate noncompliant and socially unacceptable behavior. Many suffer from low self-esteem, and adolescence is a difficult time for them. Lack of attention to their psychosocial needs from infancy onward may account for some of the difficulties they face as they mature.

Preparation for a suitable career or vocation constitutes another barrier for this population. Due to the complexity of the problems they face throughout their lifetime, they are apt to be lacking in academic skills as well as the ability to handle the careers they might aspire to follow. Interruptions in the school curriculum necessitated by their physical problems may force them, even if their intellect is normal, to lag behind others their age. Modifications required to accommodate their physical handicaps cause some employers to ignore the ability of these young adults. The difficulty and disappointment they face is depressing and most discouraging.

Children with spina bifida face an uphill battle. If they survive to adulthood, they will need encouragement and support from their families and their communities. Likewise, the families will need support from friends and their communities if they are to remain intact.

Cost of Treatment

Added to the family's psychological, physical, and emotional stress is worry about the expense of providing care for a child with spina bifida. Very few families have the resources to pay for the medical and support services such a youngster will require.

The cost begins at birth. The child will need care by an intensive care nursery as well as the immediate services of several specialists. A check with three general hospitals in Alabama indicated that the typical bill for a newborn with spina bifida for an average stay of twenty-one days was $6,500 in 1980. This was hospital cost only and did not include the fees charged by the physicians. Those averaged $1,000 for the neurosurgeon's work alone. When there were complications (and this was frequent), the bills for just the first year of life were over $30,000.

Nearly every child with spina bifida will require several surgical procedures. It has been estimated that each child will have at least one operation per year for the first five years of life (Lightowler, 1971). The neurosurgical procedures that are critical to survival of the infant are among the most expensive. Fees for placing a shunt average slightly over $1,000, and revision is often necessary. The child will need to be followed closely by the neurosurgeon for many years.

Most of these children have orthopedic problems that will require surgical intervention, casting, and/or the use of orthopedic appliances. These procedures will necessitate hospitalization, physical therapy, and follow-up care that will add expense. The costs in 1980 of a few of the appliances frequently used are vitrathene jacket, $498; parapodium, $712; spina bifida braces, $680; long leg braces, $278 per leg; and transportation chair, $1,000. Due to kidney and bladder problems, these children will also require the services of a urologist. Fees, x rays, further surgery, and hospitalization add to the expense. Even the cost of transportation to obtain medical care and therapy is no small expense. In addition, many families will need childcare for the siblings while the parents are away from home.

Fortunately, many families have some type of insurance that pays a portion of the expense. Blue Cross/Blue Shield pays 80 percent if the family has major medical. State Crippled Children's Services assume much of the responsibility for uninsured families or pay the 20 percent of the bill not paid by insurance. Many of the children are recipients of Medicaid and are thus provided medical care, social services, and casts.

In 1975, state Crippled Children's Services expended $11,458,000 to treat 9,156 children with spina bifida and/or hydrocephalus (Ma and Piazza, 1979). This represented treatment for only 15.8 percent of the estimated 58,000 children under twenty-one years of age who have these conditions. Based on these figures, more than $80 million was spent caring for these children in 1975. This figure does not include private funds, federal monies supporting their care in other ways, or hospitalization. Considering all of these, the total expenditure is staggering.

Throughout their lifetime, these children will require close medical supervision and special care. If the parents are to have any relief from this responsibility, they will need a great deal of community support. Homemaker services can assist with some of the burden of keeping the family intact. This service is available in some metropolitan areas but is lacking in smaller towns and rural areas. This service requires the family to pay a part or all of the fee charged by the homemaker.

Respite care for the family becomes important if the child lives at home. The constant care and supervision required of the family can create enormous stress. The parents need to be periodically relieved of this responsibility in order to address their personal needs, as well as those of other family members. Again, cost of respite care is a deterrent to many communities and families.

The option of a daycare facility, a residential placement, or home care with help would be ideal but is lacking in most communities. If acceptable facilities can be found to assist families who have children with handicaps, financing may still be a problem. Although most parents would welcome some help with the management of their child on a day-to-day basis, priority is usually given to providing the essential medical care for the child and funds are rarely left for daycare, sitters, or residential care. This burden can become depressing to the family as the child grows and the stresses mount.

It is difficult to estimate the total cost of care for a child who has spina bifida, but the medical expense is staggering. This condition easily qualifies as a catastrophic chronic illness. However, cost in dollars and cents is only one part of the price that families must face. Broken marriages, mental and physical illnesses in families, and the difficult adjustments that must be made also extract a heavy toll from the family.

Challenges to Public Institutions and Agencies

Information pertinent to the care of children with handicapping conditions indicates that there are many problems associated with delivery of service. Services are often fragmented, poorly coordinated, and inadequately planned (National Academy of Science, 1979). Families may face hardships in even entering a system that will help them. Many programs are inaccessible because of location; others provide impersonal treatment or humiliating routines that families find objectionable (Report to the President, 1980).

Medical and social services for families of handicapped children are not as well planned or accessible as services to patients suffering from acute illness. It has been suggested that the existing models of health care for the acutely ill would be adequate for those with long-term chronic conditions such as spina bifida, if only information among health providers were more readily shared. However, it is not easy to believe that a physician working alone can meet all the needs of handicapped children or their families. Even specialty clinics have great difficulty in meeting some of the needs that fall outside their special competence (Gliedman and Roth, 1980).

Due to the diversity of medical, social, educational, and emotional needs, children with spina bifida offer a tremendous challenge to our society. Within the health field alone, responding to their needs is an enormous task. According to Gliedman, "Professional jealousies, distrust, and territorialities separate physicians, nurses, social workers, physical therapists, and education specialists. Thus, multiservice centers and total coordinated plans of care, with one professional assuming responsibility for putting the family in touch with all the pieces and seeing that others fulfill their commitments, are out of the question for most families" (Gliedman and Roth, 1980, p. 403).

This situation needs to be corrected, and it seems increasingly apparent that the remedy will be expensive and will require a sincere commitment on the part of both health providers and families. Currently, services are offered by private practitioners, clinics (both public and private), and official and nonofficial agencies.

Crippled Children's Services (CCS) has provided comprehensive medical care to children with handicapping conditions for many years. Through a network of federal and state grants, this agency has provided care for a large number of children with spina bifida. The service offered varies in the different states, and there is a financial eligibility requirement for patients in most states. Some states maintain a Spina Bifida Clinic that addresses and coordinates the many services the child may need. Other states refer the child to a clinic for each specific problem.

Many states are establishing Spina Bifida Associations as local units of the national organization. This voluntary organization utilizes the knowledge and skills of families and professionals to promote quality care for children with spina bifida and to educate and support their families. The services of this group and others like it, such as the Association for Retarded Citizens (ARC), are being expanded, and their services are not limited to children.

As more children with handicapping conditions are kept at home with their families, the need for more comprehensive services for these citizens becomes more apparent. Families have long been aware of the need for coordinated services within the local community, but society has been slow in responding to this need. These children are more visible today because skilled medical care has kept them alive beyond the neonatal period, techniques and appliances have been developed to assist them with the activities of daily living, and federal law has mandated that they be provided an education. These changes have created an urgent need to look at the total picture and develop a plan that will provide help for the children and their families.

More appears to have been accomplished in the medical field than in other areas. Surgical intervention, multidisciplinary health screening, and comprehensive evaluations have made significant contributions to helping these children and their families, yet much remains to be done, even in the medical world.

Communities must be made aware of the psychological, social, and emotional problems that children with spina bifida face each and every day. Social and developmental support for the child with spina bifida should begin shortly after birth. Infant and parents should be referred to a community agency that offers a program for early stimulation; the parents should be given emotional support and educational information and should be taught techniques that will help the child and the family.

The concept of developing the child's assets through a complete assessment and development of a plan by an interdisciplinary team is basic to the success of any program. Inclusion of both infant and parents in a group whose children have similar problems encourages the parents and provides a social milieu for the children that will enhance their social and emotional development and possibly their physical growth. As plans to encourage development are formulated and families share, these children usually begin to interact with the environment also. This association provides a forceful stimulus for the children to learn as they participate in activities that are designed to help with their development.

Field trips to shopping centers, grocery stores, and recreational facilities within the community are readily available resources that are often overlooked when working with the disabled. As these children and their families become more visible in the community, they should be included more in community plans; in this way, one of the goals of mainstreaming will be addressed early.

Modification of streets, buildings, and recreational facilities to make them barrier-free helps in providing access to facilities within the local community. These changes will also have a positive effect on care of children with spina bifida and their families. Social groups and churches also have an obligation to include children with spina bifida or any handicapping condition in the activities planned for the community. Likewise, their families should not be excluded from participation, either consciously or inadvertently. Coordinated community service councils might be one solution, or the task might be assumed by a group such as a church affiliation.

Recommendations for Public Policy

The complexity of problems children with spina bifida and their families must face requires the concerted effort of many people and agencies if such children are to attain their optimal functioning ability. Recommendations to achieve this goal are proposed in four areas: organization of services, accessiblity of services, attention to total needs of the child, and financial support.

Organization of Services. Due to the fragmentation and lack of coordination of services currently offered to the child with spina bifida, a more effective system of delivery of care needs to be designed. Centers should be established to offer comprehensive care to these children and their families. These should be located so they serve a large area but are not unduly difficult for families to reach. A pediatrician, nurse, social worker, and physical therapist would make an ideal core team who could evaluate the needs of each child and plan and implement a program of care. This team would utilize the services of several medical consultants, such as a neurosurgeon, neurologist, orthopedist, ophthalmologist, and urologist. As the child matures, the services of professionals from other areas such as psychology, speech and hearing, and nutrition would need to be made available. A clinician who is committed to helping these children and their families should coordinate the evaluations, therapy, and services.

Physicians who deliver a child with spina bifida should make immediate referral to the center. A second check on referrals could be made by the Bureau of Vital Statistics when the birth certificate indicates the child was born with spina bifida.

A linkage among the various centers to share information and to track families as they move into different locales would add to the effectiveness of such a network. Such centers would also provide an opportunity for research, education of professionals and lay people, and dissemination of information on prevention. Participation by center staff members in local voluntary organizations, such as the Spina Bifida Association, would add visibility to the needs of these children and their families in the community. Services offered by professionals and lay groups should be coordinated through the centers.

Accessibility of Services. Accessibility of services could be improved by developing spina bifida centers in the most accessible geographic areas of each state. Selection of sites should be based on availability of professionals, transportation accessibility, and interest of the community.

Construction of barrier-free buildings is basic to such centers. However, the human staff is even more critical. A concerned, caring team must be assembled to meet the needs of these children and their families. Clients and their families must be treated with dignity, concern, and empathy, regardless of their background, race, or economic status. The problems these children have are serious and long lasting, and the constant care they require creates a great deal of pressure on the family. Every effort must be made to offer understanding and concern as the child's needs are being addressed.

Attention to Total Needs. Coordinated, concerned care for the child must include attention to both psychosocial and physical needs. Spina bifida is a condition that cannot be cured, but life can be enhanced and made more meaningful for these children if consideration is given to all their needs. Attention to their developmental needs through early intervention programs, concern for a healthy nutritional state, psychological and emotional support, and academic stimulation are a few of the areas that must be considered when planning their care. Parent groups, wherein common problems are recognized and discussed, need to be available. They can be a therapeutic experience and can lend support to meeting the total needs of the child.

Concentration on the talents and abilities of the children, rather than attention to their deficiencies, can help foster development of healthy personalities in these children. They need encouragement and stimulation in order to compete. They, like normal children, need successful experiences, and parents need the encouragement of seeing their children achieve.

Financial Support. The tremendous medical and supportive costs of caring for the child with spina bifida put the condition in the catastrophic category for families. For this reason, provisions need to be made to relieve them of this heavy responsibility. Third-party payments have been one answer that has and can still be a most desirable approach. Federal and state help through special programs such as Medicaid and Crippled Children's Services or national catastrophic insurance may be another answer.

Needs in addition to medical care place a financial drain on these families. Costs of transportation, sitter services, respite care, and countless other expenses add to the burden. Special consideration on income tax, such as is given the blind, might be one way to lighten the load on the parents at a nominal expense to the government. Giving the family a double exemption for the child with spina bifida would be a tangible way of indicating concern for the stress the family is enduring. It might also encourage the family to continue to care for the child at home rather than seek institutional care as the child gets older.

The above recommendations may be idealistic, but they emerge from suggestions in current literature and from experiences with children with spina bifida and their families. They are goals that can be reached if we care enough.

References

Allum, N. *Spina Bifida: The Treatment and Care of Spina Bifida Children.* London: Allen & Unwin, 1975.

Bigger, R. J., Mortimer, E. A., Jr., and Haughie, G. E. "Descriptive Epidemiology of Neural Tube Defects, Rochester, New York, 1918-1938." *American Journal of Epidemiology,* 1976, *104,* 22-27.

Black, P. M. "Selective Treatment of Infants with Myelomeningocele." *Neurosurgery,* 1979, *5,* 334-338.

Boston, V. E., and Wilkinson, A. J. "A Retrospective Analysis of Conservative Versus Active Management in Severe Open Myelomeningocele." *Zeitschrift für Kinderchirurgie,* 1979, *28,* 340-347.

Brock, D. J. H., and Sutcliffe, R. G. "Alpha-Fetoprotein in the Antenatal Diagnosis of Anencephaly and Spina Bifida." *Lancet,* 1972, *2,* 197-199.

Crandall, B. F. "Alpha-Fetoprotein: The Diagnosis of Neural-Tube Defects." *Pediatric Annals,* 1981, *10,* 38-48.

Dorner, S. "Sexual Interest and Activity in Adolescents with Spina Bifida." *Journal of Child Psychology and Child Psychiatry,* 1977, *18,* 229-237.

Elwood, J. M., and Elwood, J. H. *Epidemiology of Anencephalus and Spina Bifida.* Oxford, England: Oxford University Press, 1980.

Feetham, S. L., Tweed, H., and Perrin, J. S. "Practical Problems in Selection of Spina Bifida Infants for Treatment in the U.S.A." *Zeitschrift für Kinderchirurgie,* 1979, *28,* 301-306.

Gliedman, J., and Roth, W. *The Unexpected Minority—Handicapped Children in America.* New York: Harcourt Brace Jovanovich, 1980.

Hare, E. H., and others. "Spina Bifida Cystica and Family Stress." *British Medical Journal,* 1966, *2,* 757-760.

Hobbins, J. C., and others. "Ultrasound in the Diagnosis of Congenital Anomalies." *American Journal of Obstetrics and Gynecology,* 1979, *134,* 331-345.

Holmes, L. B., Driscoll, S. G., and Atkins, L. "Etiologic Heterogeneity of Neural-Tube Defects." *New England Journal of Medicine,* 1976, *294,* 365-369.

Hunt, G. M., and Holmes, A. E. "Some Factors Relating to Intelligence in Treated Children with Spina Bifida Cystica." *Developmental Medicine and Child Neurology,* 1975, *17* (35), 65-70.

Janerich, D. T. "Epidemic Waves in the Prevalence of Anencephaly and Spina Bifida in N.Y. State." *Teratology,* 1973, *8,* 253-256.

Kolin, I. S., and others. "Studies of the School-age Child with Meningomyelocele: Social and Emotional Adaptation." *Journal of Pediatrics,* 1971, *78,* 1013-1019.

Laurence, K. M., Carter, C. O., and David, P. A. "Major Central Nervous System Malformations in South Wales." *British Journal of Preventive and Social Medicine,* 1968, *22,* 146-160.

Lightowler, C. D. R. "Meningomyelocele: The Price of Treatment." *British Medical Journal,* 1971, *2,* 385-387.

Lorber, J. "Systematic Ventriculographic Studies in Infants Born with Meningomyelocele and Encephalocele." *Archives of Diseases in Childhood,* 1961, *36,* 381-389.

Lorber, J. "Results of Treatment of Myelomeningocele: An Analysis of 524 Unselected Cases, with Special Reference to Possible Selection for Treatment." *Developmental Medicine and Child Neurology,* 1971, *13,* 279-303.

Lorber, J. "Spina Bifida Cystica." In C. M. Drillen and M. B. Drummond (Eds.), *Neurodevelopmental Problems in Early Childhood.* Oxford, England: Blackwell Scientific, 1977.

Lorber, J., and Lyons, V. H. "Arterial Hypertension in Children with Spina Bifida Cystica and Urinary Incontinence." *Developmental Medicine and Child Neurology,* 1970, *12* (22), 101-104.

Ma, P., and Piazza, F. "Cost of Treating Birth Defects in State Crippled Children's Service, 1975." *Public Health Reports,* 1979, *94,* 420-424.

Miller, L. "Toward a Greater Understanding of the Parents of the Mentally Retarded Child." *Journal of Pediatrics,* 1968, *73,* 699-705.

Myers, G. J., Cerone, S. B., and Olson, A. L. (Eds.). *A Guide for Helping the Child with Spina Bifida.* Springfield, Ill.: Thomas, 1981.

National Academy of Science. "Toward a National Policy for Children and Families." Report of the Advisory Committee on Child Development, Assembly of Behavioral and Social Sciences, National Research Council. Washington, D.C.: National Academy of Science, 1979.

Nevin, R. S., and others. "Parental Coping in Raising Children Who Have Spina Bifida Cystica." *Zeitschrift für Kinderchirurgie,* 1979, *28,* 417-425.

Olshansky, S. "Chronic Sorrow: A Response to Having a Mentally Defective Child." *Social Casework,* 1962, *43,* 190-193.

Rankin, H. "Handicap: A Parent's Perspective." *Canadian Nurse,* 1979, *75,* 38-39.

Record, R. G., and McKeown, T. "Congenital Malformations of Central Nervous Systems: A Survey of 930 Cases." *British Journal of Social Medicine,* 1949, *3,* 183-219.

Renwick, J. H., Possamai, A. M., and Munday, M. R. "Potatoes and Spina Bifida." *Proceedings of the Royal Society of Medicine,* 1974, *67,* 360-364.

Report to the President—U.S. National Commission on the International Year of the Child. Washington, D.C.: U.S. Government Printing Office, 1980.

Robertson, J. A. "Legal Issues in Nontreatment of Defective Newborns." In C. A. Swinyard (Ed.), *Decision-Making and the Defective Newborn.* Springfield, Ill.: Thomas, 1978.

Shapiro, S. R., Lebowitz, R., and Colodny, A. H. "Fate of 90 Children with Ileal Conduit Urinary Diversion a Decade Later: Analysis of Complications, Pyelography, Renal Function, and Bacteriology." *Journal of Urology,* 1975, *114,* 289-295.

Shurtleff, D. B., and Foltz, E. L. "Ten-Year Follow-Up of 267 Patients with Myelomeningocele." In American Academy of Orthopedic Surgeons, *Symposium on Myelomeningocele.* St. Louis, Mo.: Mosby, 1972.

Shurtleff, D. B., and others. "Myelodysplasia: Decision for Death or Disability." *New England Journal of Medicine,* 1974, *291,* 1005-1011.

Smith, D. W., Sterling, K. C., and Harvey, M. A. S. "Hyperthermia as a Possible Teratogenic Agent." *Journal of Pediatrics*, 1978, *92*, 878-883.

Smith, J. D. "Down's Syndrome, Amniocentesis and Abortion: Prevention or Elimination?" *Mental Retardation*, 1981, *19*, 8-11.

Stark, G. D. *Spina Bifida: Problems and Management*. Oxford, England: Blackwell Scientific, 1977.

Sutow, W. W., and Pryde, A. W. "Incidence of Spina Bifida Occulta in Relation to Age." *Journal of Disabled Children*, 1956, *91*, 211-217.

Swinyard, C. A. (Ed.). *Decision-Making and the Defective Newborn*. Springfield, Ill.: Thomas, 1978.

Swisher, L. P., and Pinsker, E. J. "The Language Characteristics of Hyperverbal Hydrocephalic Children." *Developmental Medicine and Child Neurology*, 1971, *13*, 746-755.

Tew, B., and Laurence, K. M. "The Effects of Hydrocephalus on Intelligence, Visual Perception, and School Attainment." *Developmental Medicine and Child Neurology*, 1975, *17* (35), 129-134.

Wald, N. J., and Cuckle, H. S. "Amniotic Fluid Alpha-Fetoprotein Measurement in Antenatal Diagnosis of Anencephaly and Open Spina Bifida in Early Pregnancy: Second Report of the U.K. Collaborative Study of the Alpha-Fetoprotein in Relation to Neural-Tube Defects." *Lancet*, 1979, *2*, 651-662.

Wald, N. J., and others. "Maternal Serum-Alpha-Fetoprotein Measurement in Antenatal Screening for Anencephaly and Spina Bifida in Early Pregnancy: Report of the U.K. Collaborative Study on Alpha-Fetoprotein in Relation to Neural-Tube Defects." *Lancet*, 1977, *1*, 1323-1332.

Walker, J. H., Thomas, M., and Russell, I. T. "Spina Bifida and the Parents." *Developmental Medicine and Child Neurology*, 1971, *13*, 462-476.

Warkany, J. *Congenital Malformations*. Chicago, Ill.: Year Book Medical, 1971.

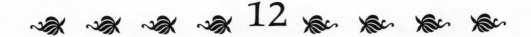

12

Sickle Cell Anemia

Charles F. Whitten, M.D.
Eleanor N. Nishiura, Ph.D.

The recommendations for sickle cell public policies proposed here are based on the premise that public polices for personal health problems are appropriate and justifiable when their absence would result in severely adverse physical, psychological, social, or economic consequences because of either a lack of services or inappropriate practices or procedures related to those health problems.

An understanding of the recommended policies presumes an understanding of the sickle cell problem. Therefore, a brief overview of the sickling phenomenon is presented, followed by policy recommendations, the rationale for each recommendation, and comments on related issues. Since few published studies provide systematically collected data about sickle cell issues amenable to public policies, the recommendations are derived largely from personal experiences and perceptions supported when possible by published data. The recommendations would assure appropriate services and practices in the best interest of the sickle cell population. The policy recommendations have relevance to three groups: potential parents of children with sickle cell anemia, children with sickle cell anemia and their families, and adults with sickle cell anemia.

Sickle Cell Conditions

Since 1948, more than three hundred mutants of normal hemoglobin have been identified. Of these, sickle hemoglobin was the first to be described, is the most prevalent worldwide, and creates the most complex set of health problems.

Note: Research for this chapter was supported in part by Grant HL-16009 from the Sickle Cell Branch of the National Heart, Lung and Blood Institute.

Despite the complexity of its manifestations, this mutation is of the simplest type. There is a single amino acid substitution: valine for glutamic acid in the sixth position of the beta chain of amino acids. The beta chain is one of the two major chains of amino acids (alpha and beta) that are the principal components of the hemoglobin molecule subject to genetic variability.

Inheritance of sickle hemoglobin gives rise to two types of conditions. Sickle cell trait, a benign carrier state, occurs when individuals have inherited the gene for sickle hemoglobin from one parent and the gene for normal hemoglobin from the other. The sickle cell diseases result from the inheritance of the gene for sickle hemoglobin from one parent and the gene for sickle hemoglobin, a gene for another abnormal hemoglobin, or a gene that limits hemoglobin production from the other parent. The most common sickle cell disease is sickle cell anemia, in which the gene for sickle hemoglobin is inherited from both parents.

In the United States, sickle cell conditions occur primarily in black Americans, with a live birth frequency of approximately 8 percent for sickle cell trait and 0.2 percent for sickle cell anemia. A small, programmatically unimportant incidence of sickle cell trait occurs in other U.S. populations, primarily those of Puerto Rican, Cuban, southern Italian, northern Greek, and Sicilian ancestry.

The property of sickle hemoglobin that results in disease is the propensity for its molecules to form microtubules (rods) when sufficiently deprived of oxygen. The rods distort red blood cells from biconcave discs to sickle-shaped forms that have two disease producing properties. First, they are fragile, with a life span of less than 30 days (frequently as low as 6 days) as compared with a normal cell's life span of 120 days. Anemia results from the bone marrow's inability to produce enough blood cells to keep pace with this rate of destruction. Second, the sickle cells are rigid. Rigidity and abnormal shape reduce their ability to be propelled through tiny capillaries and promote the formation of entangled masses of cells (similar to log jams) in larger blood vessels. The obstruction of blood flow produces temporary or permanent organ dysfunction and structural damage.

Sickle cell *trait* rarely produces health problems because sickle cells are rarely present in the circulation. The large quantity of normal hemoglobin (approximately 60 percent) makes it markedly more difficult for sickle hemoglobin molecules to join together to form rods. In effect, the initiation of sickling of sickle cell trait cells requires a greater degree of reduction in red cell oxygen than occurs under normal living conditions. However, sickling of red blood cells in the kidney may occur because of the low oxygen content characteristic of the renal medulla. Sickling in the kidney can have several adverse effects: a decrease in the ability to concentrate urine, a tendency for bleeding, and a higher than normal incidence of infections during pregnancy. However, these symptoms are very slight, sickle cell trait is not considered to be a health hazard, and life expectancy is normal. The virtual absence of health problems under normal physiological circumstances accounts for the fact that physicians do not routinely perform sickle cell tests.

In sickle cell *anemia*, though, the percentage of sickle hemoglobin in the red blood cells is so high (at least 80 percent) that removal of oxygen from hemoglobin results in the presence of sickle cells that are in the circulation at all times. Physical problems result, including anemia, recurrent pain, lowered exercise tolerance, dactylitis (painful swelling of hands and feet in infancy), acute splenic sequestration (sudden pooling of blood in the spleen), increased susceptibility to pneumococcal infections, leg ulcers, breakdown of the head of the femur, growth retardation, delayed onset of puberty, priapism (prolonged and painful erection of the penis), gallstones, and strokes. These manifestations of sickle cell anemia can occur in the other forms of sickle cell disease, such as sickle beta-thalassemia and sickle cell-hemoglobin C disease, but they tend to be less severe than sickle cell anemia.

In the 1940s, elucidation of the genetic difference between sickle cell trait and sickle cell anemia permitted differentiation of these conditions by laboratory tests. The two inexpensive and easily performed tests, the solubility test and hemoglobin electrophoresis, require only a few drops of blood from a finger stick. They positively identify virtually 100 percent of individuals with sickle cell trait. In some instances, more elaborate studies are necessary to differentiate between sickle cell anemia and several of the variants, particularly sickle-beta thalassemia. This distinction is vital for genetic counseling but is rarely necessary for management of health problems.

Because fetal hemoglobin, like normal hemoglobin, reduces the potential for sickling, the first manifestations of sickle cell anemia do not usually occur until the level of fetal hemoglobin decreases to the point that it does not prevent sickling. That usually occurs when the infant is about six months old.

There is a wide spectrum in the clinical expression of sickle cell anemia with respect to the frequency, duration, and severity of pain attacks; incidence of complications; and impact on psychosocial and functional status and life span. Furthermore, there is no basis for predicting the severity of the disease. Even a person's history is unreliable for predicting the future course for life. No reported studies provide a comprehensive picture of the natural history of sickle cell anemia (a cooperative study of the clinical course of sickle cell diseases supported by the National Institutes of Health is under way). However, our experiences in the children's unit of the Wayne State University Comprehensive Sickle Cell Center provide insights concerning clinical expression during childhood.

Since October 1973, we have enrolled approximately 480 children in a comprehensive care program. The average active patient population is about 250. The 33 children who had had a stroke when enrolled receive the same type of care but are not included in the statistical analysis cited here. As of October 1982, 360 of the enrolled children had been followed for a period of three to nine years. We estimate the probability of a child by the age of sixteen sustaining the various major complications of sickle cell amenia, other than pain, as follows:

High probability—more than 50 percent chance
    Growth retardation

Moderate probability—25 to 50 percent chance
  Delay in onset of puberty
  Pneumonia, if the child has not received the polyvalent pneumococcal
    vaccine
  Gallstones—detected by ultrasound technique
  Dactylitis
Low probability—5 to 10 percent chance
  Strokes
  Biliary colic
Slight probability—less than 5 percent chance
  Acute splenic sequestration (infancy)
  Aplastic crises
  Hyperhemolytic crises
  Osteomyelitis
  Aseptic necrosis of the femoral head
  Priapism
  Leg ulcers
  Pneumonia, if the child has received the polyvalent pneumococcal
    vaccine

Pain is the most common symptom experienced by children with sickle cell anemia. Mothers estimate that the number of pain attacks the child had in the year prior to enrollment in the center ranged from none to more than ten pain attacks. Twenty-seven percent reported that their child had not had an attack in the previous year, 60 percent reported from one to five attacks, and 13 percent, more than six attacks. The severity and duration of pain attacks also vary widely. They may last for a week or two, require narcotics for relief, and require hospitalization for the benefit of both child and parents. Or they may last only an hour or two, require no drugs or only aspirin for relief, and be managed satisfactorily at home.

Children may require hospitalization for complications such as pneumonia and strokes. Frequency of hospitalization is highly variable. Of 348 children, 26 percent had never been hospitalized for sickle cell anemia. A majority (55 percent) had from one to five hospitalizations, 12 percent had six to ten hospitalizations, and 7 percent had more than ten. One hundred sixty-five of 355 of the children (46 percent) had been hospitalized at least once during the year prior to enrollment in the clinic. Similar rates of hospitalization were recorded at the Children's Hospital National Medical Center, in Washington, D.C. (Williams, Earles, and Pack, 1983).

Life expectancy is reduced by sickle cell anemia, but data are insufficient to state an average life span. It is not true, as has been commonly believed, that the vast majority of people with sickle cell anemia die in their teens. In fact, a few individuals have lived into their seventies. Of the 360 children enrolled in the Wayne State University (WSU) Sickle Cell Center, 9 have died of sickle cell anemia. Their ages at death were: one year (1), two years (2), four years (3), 11 years (1), twenty years (1), and twenty-one years (1). Seeler (1972) has reported a death rate of 9.1 percent (19 of 207 children) in a five-year period in a Chicago population of 207 children under the age of fourteen with sickle cell disease.

Actuarial calculations from data on a group of patients followed by Powars (1975) in Los Angeles revealed a 10 percent expected death rate during the first decade of life.

Mattson (1972) has cited several causes of emotional stress in children who have long-term illnesses. These conditions apply to children with sickle cell anemia. First, there are the pain, other physical symptoms, and the children's questions about why they are ill; these can contribute to self-blame and blame of other family members. Second are stresses that stem from the treatment procedures. The unfamiliar strange places and procedures can cause anger and anxiety, acting-out behavior, or withdrawal. A third source of stress is the emotional climate. A child's illness often encourages either excessive indulgence and/or resentment of the child due to the illness itself or to burdens the illness has imposed on family members. Emotional stress is also caused by threats of physical impairment, exacerbation of symptoms, and shortened life expectancy. Finally, long-term childhood illness creates stress for the child because of interruptions in normal activities.

Whitten and Fischhoff (1974) have discussed how sickle cell anemia affects children and adolescents. Frequent hospitalizations often make children feel helpless and fearful that they will be abandoned to experience their disease without support. Developing self-esteem and a sense of mastery over the disease and other situations is difficult because of the unpredictability of sickle cell anemia. Frequent interruption of such normal activities as school creates difficulties in competing and in gaining skills necessary for adult functioning.

Adolescents may be passive, dependent, fearful of becoming autonomous, withdrawn from normal relations because of a limited view of their own potential, depressed, and/or preoccupied with death. They may be anxious about slight changes in their condition and experience more pain than can be accounted for by their physical condition. They often lack the universal dreams and aspirations of most young people. Intellectual capacity as measured by standard intelligence tests is not affected by sickle cell anemia (Chodorkoff and Whitten, 1963; Kosacoff, Seligman, and Dosik, 1974), but academic problems are common in children with this disease (Conyard, Krishnamurthy, and Dosik, 1980).

Sickle cell anemia in the child imposes burdens on other family members. Psychosocial inventories of parents (usually mothers) of 174 children at the WSU Sickle Cell Center in 1982 reveal some of these burdens. First, transportation and other arrangements must be made when the child requires medical care. Twenty-three percent of the parents reported problems finding or paying for transportation. Thirty-two of the parents (18 percent) lost days from work when their child was ill, with an average loss of ten days. In addition to the recommended four routine visits a year, many children need additional medical care. During the year before their annual clinic visit, 105 (60 percent) of the children made at least one visit to the emergency room. Those 105 children averaged three emergency room visits, and 8 of them had made ten or more visits in the previous year.

In addition to inconveniences and financial burdens, parents face emotional burdens. Fifty-five percent of the parents reported being frightened by their child's illness at some time; 7 percent felt afraid frequently. Eleven percent and 12 percent, respectively, felt worried and overworked. Less than one third reported no worry at all about the child during the previous year. Ten percent reported a time when they felt their child might die from the disease. Although most children probably did not face a life-threatening situation, parents nevertheless were very fearful when their child had pain attacks or other complications.

One hundred forty-three of the children in the survey had siblings who were two or more years old. Parents of 16 percent of these children thought that siblings were jealous of the attention the child with sickle cell anemia received when ill, and 25 percent thought siblings seemed afraid when their brother or sister was ill.

There is no routine treatment to prevent or reverse the physical problems of sickle cell anemia. We cannot prevent cells from sickling, reverse cells after they have sickled, restore the life span of sickle cells to normalcy, prevent sickle cells from plugging blood vessels, or unplug blood vessels occluded with sickle cells. Current therapy mainly addresses management of manifestations of the disease. Pain is treated with drugs that relieve pain; severe anemia, with transfusions; and infections, with antibiotics. A few preventive measures are effective—for example, regular exchange transfusions reduce recurrences of strokes, and a polyvalent pneumococcal vaccine reduces incidence of pneumococcal infections.

Appropriate health care extends beyond relief of symptoms to efforts to prevent or ameliorate the debilitating psychosocial effects of the disease. Efforts include disease education, anticipatory guidance, adjustment counseling, social casework, academic and career guidance, and assistance in resolving school- and employment-related problems.

To that end, we propose here a set of policies to improve the lives of families with children with sickle cell anemia.

Identification and Counseling

Individuals with sickle cell trait who are of childbearing age should have an opportunity to be identified and counseled.

Rationale. Approximately 1 of 12 members of the black population has sickle cell trait, and approximately 1 of 144 black couples has the potential for having a child with sickle cell anemia with each pregnancy. If they are not aware prior to childbearing that they both carry the sickle cell gene, the first child of 1 out of 576 black couples will have sickle cell anemia. These parents will be faced with the psychological, emotional, social, and economic burden of caring for a child with an incurable illness and reduced life expectancy without having had an opportunity to exercise options with respect to mate selection or whether or not to risk having a child born with the disease.

Since the risk of a sickle cell trait couple having a child with sickle cell anemia (25 percent in each pregnancy) is well established and there are reliable and relatively inexpensive tests to identify carriers, individuals with sickle cell trait have a right to know their sickle cell status and its implications for the health of their children. This is consistent with the current thrust in American medicine for patients to assume greater responsibility for their overall health status. Based on legal judgments against physicians relative to PKU (Wright and Shaw, 1981), we can anticipate that primary care physicians will be vulnerable to malpractice suits for failure to test their patients for the carrier state of severe genetic diseases including sickle cell anemia and to provide or refer them for counseling if the tests are positive.

Comments. Identification and counseling programs should have three components. The first is public education. Because sickle cell trait rarely causes health problems, most people are not aware of the possibility of having it unless they have relatives who have sickle cell disease. Educational programs should provide information to motivate black people in their reproductive years to be tested.

The second component consists of laboratory tests. The solubility test and hemoglobin electrophoresis are relatively inexpensive, easily performed, and positively identify virtually 100 percent of individuals with sickle cell trait.

The third component, appropriate counseling, is crucial. Simply performing laboratory tests and informing a person that he or she has sickle cell trait will not prepare that person for decision making. In fact, testing without counseling is potentially worse than not identifying the condition at all because the public does not understand that there are two sickle cell conditions and that one is harmless. Individuals who are told they have sickle cell trait but are not counseled may interpret the information to mean that they are ill or somehow less than whole. Misconceptions can generate unnecessary anxiety, impair self-esteem, and cause unwarranted alterations in life style and injudicious decisions about marriage and reproduction.

Although there are effective education, screening, and counseling programs in some cities, by and large members of the black population in their reproductive years have not had an opportunity to be identified and counseled. Because of the numbers, we believe that mass screening (defined for our purposes as screening for the individual's personal use and in settings not usually associated with the provision of health care) is essential to meet the needs of the target population in a timely fashion. This recommendation is made with full recognition that mass screening has not been viewed positively by all.

The concerns regarding mass screening relate primarily to the early history of sickle cell screening, which began in the early 1970s as part of the emergence and articulation of black consciousness. It was recognized then that sickle cell disease was a major health problem that had been virtually ignored by the health care system. The outpouring of activity at that time resulted in some misguided efforts.

Some screening programs were developed and implemented by community groups that had little knowledge of the requirements for an effective and acceptable program. Literature contained errors and created unnecessary fear (*A Critical Review of Informational Materials Relating to Sickle Cell Anemia and Sickle Cell Trait,* 1972). For example, the distinction between sickle cell anemia and sickle cell trait was not always clear. Also, the limitations of the solubility test were not appreciated. Although the solubility test only detects the sickle cell gene and does not differentiate between sickle cell trait and sickle cell anemia, it was frequently the only test done. Those tested could gain the impression that they had a disease rather than a harmless carrier state. Further, counseling was frequently either unavailable or lacking in specific objectives, appropriate content, and effective techniques.

There was also the feeling that employers had begun to use sickle cell trait to exclude people from jobs, although few cases were documented. And individuals applying for insurance might volunteer that they had the trait without being aware that some insurance companies (seven of seventy surveyed in 1975) either denied life insurance or had higher premiums for individuals with the trait (National Association for Sickle Cell Disease, 1975). Finally, well-intentioned black legislators introduced bills, which were enacted in some states, that required sickle cell testing either on entering school or as part of a premarital examination. The negativity all this generated naturally created an unfavorable attitude about sickle cell testing.

These factors led some to believe that screening programs should not exist. Another approach was to correct the problems through clarification of the goals; establishment of proper standards and guidelines for education, testing, and counseling programs; and development of counseling protocols and training programs for sickle cell educators, laboratory personnel, and counselors. Using this approach, corrective measures have been implemented under the guidance and leadership of the Sickle Cell Branch of the National Heart, Lung and Blood Institute, the Genetic Diseases Service Branch of the Health Services Administration (U.S. Public Health Service), and the National Association for Sickle Cell Disease, Inc.

Goals of Counseling

The goal of sickle cell trait counseling of individuals in their reproductive years should be to enable them to make informed marital and reproductive decisions that they believe are in their best interest.

Rationale. Two goals have been proposed for the identification and counseling of individuals with sickle cell trait. One goal is to enable individuals to make informed marital and reproduction decisions and the other is to prevent the birth of children with sickle cell anemia.

There are valid reasons that couples with sickle cell trait may elect either to take the chance of having a child with sickle cell anemia or to avoid this possibility. Some will elect to take the chance for various reasons: They wish to have their own biologic children with their current mate; they believe the characteristics of their children are to be accepted as a matter of fate; contraception or abortion are unacceptable practices to them; they believe the course of the disease in their child will be mild; they are willing to cope with the problems the child might have; they are optimistic about the prospects for improved therapy or cure. Other couples with sickle cell trait will reject taking the chance: They have little need or desire to have their own biological children; they believe they should exercise whatever control they can over the characteristics of their children; contraception and abortion are acceptable practices to them; they believe the course of disease in their child could be severe; they are unwilling to cope with the problems the child might have; they are pessimistic about prospects for improved therapy or cure.

Because the determining factors are personal, the decision ought to be made by those who will live with the results of the decision. In addition, there are other reasons for rejecting the preventive goal. First, the intellectual capacity, physical function, and life span of individuals with sickle cell anemia do not warrant a policy to prevent birth of individuals with the disease. Sickle cell anemia only affects the intelligence of a few of the small percentage (about 5 percent) who sustain a stroke. There are no grotesque or dysfunctional physical features. Despite periodic bouts of disability due to pain and other complications, individuals can function normally in the interim. The life span is sufficiently long for the vast majority to be able to live productive, fulfilling lives. Finally, the overall burden of the disease is not uniform and some people with sickle cell anemia are relatively unaffected.

Second, a preventive goal could be easily interpreted by some elements of the black community as an effort to control its growth (genocide). Irrespective of the validity of this claim, the net effect of a preventive thrust would be potentially destructive, for it could create divisiveness within the black community over the desirability of conducting sickle cell testing.

Third, a preventive goal would reactivate a eugenic thrust in reproductive decision making. Discouraging or preventing birth of individuals considered to be genetically inferior has been rejected as an American societal goal.

Comments. So that individuals with sickle cell trait can make informed personal choices, counseling can be conceptualized as having two major components. The first is educationally oriented: The counselor transmits information about the nature of the carrier state, the manifestations of sickle cell anemia, the burden on parents and affected persons, management and prognosis of the disease, how the disease is transmitted, the reproductive odds, and the options with respect to mate selection and reproduction. The objective is to provide adequate, accurate data concerning the trait and the disease to enable informed decisions. The second component is behaviorally oriented: The counselor assists counselees to examine their personality traits, coping abilities, feelings, attitudes, and beliefs about reproduction, contraception, and need and desire to have children. The objective is for counselees to have a clear perception of the personal factors involved in their decisions and to enable personalized decisions.

Nondirective Counseling

Sickle cell trait counseling should be nondirective.

Rationale. Genetic counselors (lay or professional) rarely know enough about all the factors important to their counselees to offer advice on such uniquely personal issues as whether the potential for having a child with sickle cell anemia should influence whom they marry and whether they should take a chance on having children with sickle cell anemia. Further, if counselors provide advice, they are highly vulnerable to being held responsible and criticized if the individual believes the best possible decision was not made.

Advice against having a child can also set the stage for development of deep-seated guilt reactions in those who later, by accident or design, have a child with sickle cell anemia. If serious complications develop, they could be burdened with undue guilt for not having followed advice even though at the time they considered their decision to have a child to be in their best interest. This reaction could inappropriately influence their relationship with the child.

Comments. Counselors must be sensitive to all the covert and subtle ways preference might be communicated or reflected. These ways include the phrasing of statements, the order in which material is presented, the tone of voice and facial expressions when stating key facts, and the timing of eye contact. Furthermore, because perceptions of the severity and burden of the disease can influence the counselee's decision, care must be exercised that both severity and burden are clearly stated; the counselor must recognize the uncertainty that can result from the lack of systematically collected natural history data in a randomly selected population. A completely neutral presentation is extremely difficult to accomplish but every effort must be made to achieve it.

Goal of Mass Screening

The goal of mass sickle cell screening should be to detect sickle trait in people in their reproductive years.

Rationale. Knowledge of sickle cell trait is basically of no value to one's health care or health status. However, knowledge of the potential for having a child with sickle cell anemia can be extremely important for marriage and reproduction decisions. In other words, if individuals plan never to have children, knowledge of the presence of sickle cell trait is valueless. Because most individuals with sickle cell trait are unaware of their status, mass screening of those of reproductive age will be necessary until the identification of sickle cell trait becomes part of routine health care for black persons.

Given the rather limited resources available for outreach testing and the large number to be reached, it is sound to focus efforts on people in the reproductive years. By and large, for those under fifteen years old, it is too early; for those over forty-five, it is too late. Although early teenage pregnancies might argue for testing and informing as early as eleven, it is highly unlikely that choice of sexual partners by eleven- to fourteen-year-olds would be influenced by the partner's sickle cell status.

There is no need to conduct mass screening to detect sickle cell *anemia* beyond infancy. During the first two years of life, lack of awareness could place infants in jeopardy from two complications—death from pneumococcal sepsis or acute splenic sequestration—both of which can occur before there are sufficient manifestations of the disease to lead to its recognition. After infancy, the child with unidentified sickle cell anemia is rarely in jeopardy of preventable lethal or disabling complications. Furthermore, children with sickle cell anemia usually have sufficient sickle cell related health problems to lead their parents to seek medical care for them by the fifth year, when the diagnosis of sickle cell anemia is invariably made.

Mass screening could also detect sickle cell–hemoglobin C disease, which often goes undetected in children and adults (the precise number is not known). These persons have not experienced sufficient manifestations of the disease to lead to a diagnosis. The mild course of the disease does not place them at a substantial disadvantage and would not warrant a mass screening program.

Reproductive Options

Pregnant women who have sickle cell trait should have an opportunity to know whether the fetus has sickle cell anemia and if so to terminate pregnancy if they elect that option.

Rationale. Until recently, couples with sickle cell trait could have children of their own only if they took the one in four chance of having a child with sickle cell anemia. Otherwise, they had to deny themselves the opportunity of having their own biological children.

For many, these two options are highly undesirable. To remain childless forfeits a major source of human fulfillment and gratification. To give birth to a child with a lifetime illness frequently causes psychological reactions such as guilt and resentment as well as financial and social stresses. A third option, now technically available, enables sickle cell trait couples to have their own biological children without giving birth to children with sickle cell anemia. Sickle cell anemia can be diagnosed in utero early enough in the second trimester to permit a legal abortion if the fetus is affected.

Providing an opportunity to ascertain whether the fetus has sickle cell anemia and to terminate the pregnancy if it does is consistent with the principle of self-determination we espouse for all sickle cell related marital and reproductive decisions.

Comments. Two methods are used to make a diagnosis of sickle cell anemia in utero: the determination of the types of hemoglobin produced by fetal red blood cells obtained from the placenta (Baubes, Mears, and Ramirez, 1980) or by a DNA analysis of fetal cells in amniotic fluid obtained by amniocentesis (Chang and Kan, 1982). The first method yields a highly accurate diagnosis but has major drawbacks. Obtaining the specimen through placental aspiration requires a physician specifically trained for this procedure and a forty-eight-hour hospital stay and carries a much higher than acceptable risk of hemorrhage or termination of the pregnancy (up to 5 percent). Amniocentesis appears to yield an equally accurate diagnosis and can be performed on an outpatient basis with a very low risk of termination of the pregnancy, hemorrhage, or infection (0.5

percent). In either case, the laboratory procedures are currently available in only a few research centers. Of the two methods, amniocentesis is the method of choice. To make this option available, amniocentesis and the laboratory analysis must become eligible for reimbursement by third-party payers.

A variety of factors can make it difficult for couples to decide whether to continue or terminate a pregnancy: They may have inadequate or inaccurate information about the disease, amniocentesis, and abortion; they may not have adequately examined their feelings about having children, coping with a child with a chronic illness, and having an abortion; they may feel a high level of anxiety, pressure from family members and friends, and concern about the effect of their decision on others. An appropriately designed and implemented counseling program helps them address these issues and make a decision they can believe is in their best interest. For mothers who elect to terminate pregnancy, counseling is essential to cope with adverse postabortion feelings.

The self-determination goal for prenatal testing implies that testing should be available to couples independent of their decision regarding abortion. Some couples request a prenatal test even though they are undecided about whether to terminate an affected pregnancy. Others want to know their child's sickle cell status even though they have already decided against abortion. In effect, couples may want either to be free of anxiety from wondering if the child will have sickle cell anemia, or in case the fetus has sickle anemia, to have a chance to prepare psychologically for the child. Some change their minds when they learn the results.

Because amniocentesis is relatively free of medical complications for both mother and fetus, provider judgments concerning whether couples have valid reasons for requesting amniocentesis are inconsistent with the goal of self-determination. The Hastings Center Genetic Research Group recommends that prenatal diagnosis should not be denied to a woman at risk who has decided against abortion at the outset (Powledge and Fletcher, 1979).

Voluntary Screening

Sickle cell screening should not be mandated by law.

Rationale. Mandated health procedures or behavior are adopted when two conditions are met. First, is when the adverse consequences to the affected individuals or to those to whom they are exposed are severe, highly likely to occur, and preventable. Second, is when it is unlikely or too risky to take the chance that the health behavior will be implemented voluntarily. Thus, laws require testing for PKU at birth and syphilis prior to marriage and immunizations against smallpox and diphtheria prior to enrollment in school. Can we make a case for mandated sickle cell screening consistent with these conditions?

We have identified three appropriate circumstances for screening for sickle cell conditions: prenatally, at birth, and during the reproductive years. Only at birth is the first condition met. The objective of screening newborns is to enable implementation of a follow-up plan to prevent deaths prior to recognition of the disease that may result from regular health care. In the other two, screening is conducted to provide reproductive options.

The second condition relative to screening at birth has not been adequately explored. Although there are voluntary programs to screen blood taken from the umbilical cord at birth, analyses of their effectiveness have not been published. (Incidentally, the second condition has recently been affirmed by the President's Commission for the Study of Ethical Problems in Medicine and Biomedical and Behavioral Research [1983]: "Mandatory genetic screening programs are only justified when voluntary testing proves inadequate to prevent serious harm to the defenseless, such as children, that could be avoided were screening performed" [p. 6].)

Comments. In a few states, misguided efforts to compensate for the years of neglect of the sickle cell problem led to ill-conceived laws requiring sickle cell tests for newborns, school children, marriage license applicants, and inmates of penal institutions (Rutkow and Lipton, 1973). Fortunately, with the exception of newborn screening the laws have been repealed.

Confidentiality and Insurance

The results of sickle cell tests should not be reported or released to any third party without written consent.

Rationale. Because there are many misconceptions about the health status and functional capabilities of persons with sickle cell trait and sickle cell disease, test results can lead to stigmatization in schools, unjustified job denial, insurance rejection, or higher insurance premiums. Even inclusion of this information in school health records without consent of the parents violates the right to privacy. Therefore, the results of an individual's sickle cell test must always be confidential.

Comments. Funding agencies need to know whether there has been efficient and effective utilization of resources; thus it is appropriate for those who do sickle cell testing to submit data that fulfill this purpose. Information could include the number tested and characteristics of the tested population (for example, age, sex, marital status, race, and residential district); it would be unnecessary and inappropriate to report information, such as names or social security numbers, that would identify individuals.

An extensive review of the relationship between health problems and sickle cell trait reveals no evidence concerning health status or life span that warrants rejecting coverage or assessing a higher premium for life or medical insurance for individuals with sickle cell trait (Sears, 1978).

Governmental Support

Support for education, testing, and counseling should be in part a governmental responsibility.

Rationale. Traditionally, the provision of personal health services has been considered a governmental responsibility when two basic sets of conditions are met: (1) when the lack of service has dire physical, psychological, social, or economic consequences and (2) when a large number of people are not receiving the service because it is unavailable, inaccessible, or prohibitively costly for the individual or requires a population approach. Government meets its responsibility by either requiring, permitting, providing, or underwriting the cost of the service.

The undesirable consequences facing couples having children with sickle cell anemia without awareness of their risks meets the first condition. As for the second, the medical care system in the United States cannot be relied upon to provide sickle cell testing and counseling to all blacks of reproductive age, partly because healthy young adults in this country do not routinely seek health care. Even if all blacks sought medical care before they had children, most probably would not be tested for and counseled about sickle cell disease as a matter of routine. Physicians seldom administer sickle cell tests in the absence of health problems and are even less likely to provide counseling, due to lack of training, the time required, and the nonreimbursable cost.

Thus, without government support of community-based testing and counseling programs, large numbers of persons in the reproductive age group simply will not receive these services.

Citizen Involvement

Black people should participate in the design and implementation of sickle cell education, testing, and counseling programs.

Rationale. Because participation in sickle cell trait testing and counseling programs is voluntary, such programs must be perceived by the target population to be in their best interest. Screening for carriers of a genetic disease that occurs almost exclusively in the black population must be devoid of actual or perceived civil rights, ethical, or cultural factors that could limit participation. The goals must not be viewed as eugenically inspired or as an effort to limit the growth of the black population. This is best achieved by having black professional and lay persons respected by the black community involved in the planning, implementation, and administration of these programs. Black individuals can contribute to the participation in and effectiveness of services through their understanding of the black community and their judgment about how program goals are articulated, when and where to conduct programs, the content of educational materials, and the characteristics of the providers.

Detection at Birth and Appropriate Follow-Up

Parents should have an opportunity to have sickle cell anemia detected in their children at birth and to receive appropriate follow-up care.

Rationale. The infant with unidentified sickle cell anemia may die from either pneumococcal infection or sudden massive pooling of blood in the spleen prior to having sufficient difficulty from sickle cell anemia to lead to detection of the disease. When sickle cell anemia is identified, these complications usually can be detected early enough for successful treatment (Powars, Overturf, and Weiss, 1982; O'Brien, McIntosh, and Aspnes, 1976; McIntosh, Rooks, and Richey, 1980). Until it is commonplace for members of the black population of childbearing age to be tested and thus aware of their sickle cell status before the birth of a child, the most effective way to identify sickle cell anemia early is through routine cord blood screening at the time of delivery of black newborns.

Comments. The screening program must be combined with a management plan in which physicians and parents assume responsibilities. Parents must report immediately to the physician any symptoms such as fever, drowsiness, loss of appetite, and pallor that are evidence of pneumococcal infection or sudden pooling of blood in the spleen. Because these complications are true emergencies, parents cannot sit in a hospital reception area waiting their turn. The physician must instruct the parents concerning warning signs, procedures, and the importance of taking the child to a designated health care facility. The physician must have an effective diagnostic and management plan that is understood by the health care staff and ready for immediate implementation whenever parents bring in the child.

The effectiveness of this approach has been demonstrated. Grover and others (1983), in a report of their experience with newborn screening in New York City, report no deaths among 131 infants with sickle cell anemia followed over the period of ages 8 months to 20 months despite serious life-threatening complications diagnosed in 8 infants. Absence of mortality could be attributed to the comprehensive care the patients and families received.

Services to parents cannot be limited to prevention of death from complications. Parents need to be fully informed about the basis for manifestations of the disease, the risk of sickle cell anemia in future pregnancies, the value of prenatal testing, and the need for comprehensive care (Rowley and Huntzinger, 1983).

The tests used in screening for sickle cell anemia also detect sickle cell trait if present. Thus, parents whose newborns have sickle cell *trait* need to be tested and counseled with respect to the child's as well as their own possession of the gene. The primary focus of the parent counseling will be dictated by whether they are trait-trait or trait-normal couples.

An issue is whether cord blood screening should be limited to populations with a more than incidental prevalence of sickle cell trait. A limit is justified because of the potential for detecting the gene in members of ethnic groups in which it is not recognized and accepted that the sickle cell gene occurs. Although the presence of the gene in a non-Mediterranean Caucasian could be from a mutation, the more likely possibility (and the one likely to be assumed by affected parents) is that the gene is present from unrecognized or undisclosed racial admixture in previous generations. The revelation to white couples that one of them probably has black ancestry could create severe psychological stress and impair the marriage. Incidence of sickle cell anemia in that population is too small for the potential benefit to outweigh the risks.

Another potentially undesirable consequence of routine cord blood screening is the exposure of nonpaternity. Both the racial and nonpaternity issues practically mandate that, if cord blood screening is performed routinely, mothers should be made aware of these two potential by-products and given an opportunity to refuse the test.

Comprehensive Health Care

Children with sickle cell anemia and their parents should receive comprehensive health care.

Rationale. The goal for such children is to have fulfilling and satisfying lives compromised only by unalterable aspects of their disease. A number of factors may undermine this goal: recurrent incapacitating pain, small stature, hospitalizations, teasing by peers, interruption or postponement of pleasurable activities, inability to compete with peers in physical activities, and irregular school attendance and the resultant increased risk of poor academic performance. If these are not addressed satisfactorily, children are at risk to become dependent, to have low self-esteem, and to have a pessimistic outlook. As adults, they are prone to be single, childless, unemployed, and supported by their families or public assistance.

Children with sickle cell anemia need other services in addition to appropriate medical management. These supportive services include disease education appropriate for their age, personal and career adjustment counseling, and assistance in coping with the physical manifestations of the disease, feelings about the disease and its complications, reactions of peers, and school problems.

Parents are pivotal in the child's handling of the disease. In general, parents of these children have imposed upon them care of a child with the potential for developing complications, the most distressing and demanding of which, on a day-to-day basis, are the severe and unpredictable pain attacks. These attacks cause inconvenience, frustration, and hardship by interrupting or preventing many necessary functions, including sleep, essential household chores, job attendance, and recreational activities. Parents are faced with a child who has a shortened life expectancy and a poor outlook for eventual economic self-sufficiency. All of these factors can evoke adverse psychological reactions in parents, including guilt, anger, resentment, shame, denial, helplessness, and frustration. When these are not addressed satisfactorily, parents often overprotect, reject, or have unrealistic expectations with adverse effects upon the child.

Some parents intuitively handle these problems effectively, but in general, parents need help in gaining the knowledge and developing the skills required for satisfactory adjustment and functioning. Care must therefore assist parents in understanding the disease, in helping the child learn to cope with specific problems as well as with the disease in general, in understanding what can happen on a day-to-day basis and how to handle it (anticipatory guidance), in developing goals for the child, in learning to relate to the child from day to day, and in developing the ability to deal with their own emotions in a manner that fosters the child's adjustment. Parents may need help dealing with the costs, arrangements for medical care, household help, transportation, handling the reactions for the child's siblings, and coordination of services. In effect, children and parents need comprehensive care that consists of coordinated medical, psychological, and social services available on a twenty-four-hour basis.

Comments. The extent to which children with sickle cell anemia and their parents receive comprehensive care depends largely on where they receive their health care. There are four principal sources of care. The first is the Comprehensive Sickle Cell Centers funded primarily by the Sickle Cell Branch of the National Institutes of Health. There are ten such centers associated with medical schools and (with one exception) located in urban areas with large black populations. These centers provide a wide range of health services for both children and adults. An example is the Wayne State University Sickle Cell Center (WSU Center).

At the WSU Center, three nurse practitioners are responsible for medical care when the child is ill, visiting and following the progress of the child when hospitalized, monitoring the child's clinical status when well, disease education, and counseling relative to disease, personal relationships, and adjustment. Each nurse has a defined population of patients. The director of the clinic, a pediatric hematologist, supervises and oversees the care of children and provides medical care when the problem exceeds the capabilities of the nurse practitioners. A full-time social worker provides services directly and serves as a consultant to the nurse practitioners. Care is coordinated through the nurse practitioners.

Patient visits, scheduled every three months regardless of whether a child is having medical problems, are used to monitor the clinical aspects of the child's disease and to provide education and psychosocial counseling. Health education combines an age-related planned format for children and family members with a personalized approach. Topics include the pathology of sickle cell anemia, genetics, home management, medical treatment, methods of coping with common psychosocial problems, and clearing up common misconceptions. Clinic personnel meet periodically with hospital staff to educate them about sickle cell anemia and the special needs of hospitalized children.

Hospital outpatient clinics, especially hematology clinics, are a second source of care. These clinics emphasize medical services, although psychological and social services are also available. Clinics are unlikely to screen for psychosocial problems and do not routinely include formal counseling. Continuity with one provider is sometimes lacking, especially when the care is provided primarily by house staff.

Health Maintenance Organizations are a third source of care. Although these organizations have the potential for providing a broad range of services, providers sometimes lack experience with sickle cell anemia because of the small number of cases in their patient population.

Finally, the overwhelming majority of children in the United States with sickle cell anemia, especially in areas without sickle cell clinics or large medical centers, receive their care from private physicians. Recently we surveyed the care provided to children with sickle cell anemia by physicians in seven Michigan cities outside of metropolitan Detroit. Eighty-one children with sickle cell anemia and under eighteen years of age were surveyed. Eighty percent received medical care from a private physician. Their health care was often limited to the treatment of medical problems. A substantial number (35 percent) did not have regular checkups, and went to a doctor only when sick. Nearly half (46 percent) saw no reason to see a doctor when they were feeling well, and 54 percent thought checkups were too costly. Health education and disease adjustment counseling were inadequate. Physicians were more likely to transmit factual information to patients and family members than to counsel them about disease adjustment or general quality-of-life issues.

The survey suggests that many children and parents do not know where to find psychosocial services and that they are more likely to seek help from families and friends than from health professionals. Health professionals and social agencies performed a minor role in coordination of services. Of ninety-nine contacts families made with agencies, 61 percent were self-referrals or referrals by family and friends. Health professionals made only 8 percent of the referrals, and 27 percent of the contacts were initiated by social agencies. Most communities had agencies that dealt with psychosocial problems, but personnel were not trained to serve people with sickle cell anemia and there were no outreach programs aimed at this population.

The comprehensive care provided at the WSU Center is expensive. For example, the laboratory tests cost $148 for tests at the first visit, $24 for those at the quarterly visit, and $97 for those at the annual visit (in 1982). There are additional costs for the initial medical history, detailed psychosocial inventory, physical examination, immunizations, hearing and vision test, health education and psychosocial counseling at the initial visit; the medical history, physical examination, education, and counseling during routine quarterly checkups; and the medical history, physical examination, disease education, psychosocial counseling, and detailed psychosocial inventory at the annual visit.

Of the 278 children with sickle cell anemia who were active at the Wayne State University Comprehensive Sickle Cell Center in 1982, nearly half had their hospital care paid by Medicaid and one fourth had Blue Cross/Blue Shield insurance. Fifteen percent had other insurance or a combination of Blue Cross and other insurance. Four percent used Crippled Children's, 1 percent used Medicare, and 8 percent were not covered or the type of coverage was unknown. These sources are not sufficient to support our staff and provide services. We fund the critical coordination, educational, and psychosocial services primarily through a federal government grant, a United Way grant, and the Medical School. Without specific payment mechanisms, the private medical care system is not likely to provide comprehensive care for children with sickle cell anemia, especially educational and counseling services that take a great deal of practitioners' time. Reimbursement for these services or for nonphysician practitioners is not generally available.

Even if mechanisms for support of personnel in centers and hospital clinics were established, these would not suffice for small communities where the number of children with sickle cell anemia does not warrant the organizational structure and personnel required in centers and clinics. A possible approach is to use personnel in established social service and public health agencies for outreach, health education, disease-adjustment counseling, psychosocial services, and coordination. For example, a social worker in a community social service agency could become the sickle cell coordinator for the community. The part-time salary for this activity could come from a variety of sources including local sickle cell organizations. The coordinator would be trained by personnel in established centers, become knowledgeable about the resources in the community, and provide services or referrals to assure comprehensive care.

School-Related Problems

Children with sickle cell anemia should receive assistance with school-related problems.

Rationale. Children with sickle cell anemia need assistance with school problems both because of the implications of academic achievement for overall adjustment and because of the special school problems sickle cell anemia imposes.

Although intellectual capacity as measured by standard intelligence tests is not affected by sickle cell anemia, many children with this disease have academic problems. Conyard showed poor school adjustment by many children with sickle cell anemia, especially boys (Conyard, Krishnamurthy, and Dosik, 1980). Nishiura and Whitten (1980) reported that one third of the children with sickle cell anemia whom they studied were described by their parents as behind in school and over one half had only fair or poor grades in school. More recently we have collected the standardized test scores of nearly two hundred children with sickle cell anemia and their siblings. Preliminary examination of these data suggests that children with the disease do not do nearly as well as their siblings.

High absenteeism explains many academic problems. A study of 175 children with sickle cell anemia and 171 siblings showed that the children with the disease had an average of thirty absences from school per year compared with eighteen absences per school year for the siblings. Forty-two percent of the children with sickle cell anemia compared to 10 percent of the siblings were absent from school thirty or more days during an average school year (Nishiura, Whitten, and Thomas, 1982).

Doing well in school can be especially useful for children with sickle cell anemia. Many of these children have low self-esteem because of small stature and inability to compete in sports and other strenuous activities. Academic success provides an opportunity for increasing self-esteem and career advantages.

Comments. A program that provides assistance with school-related problems requires cooperation by parents, teachers, and health providers. One of the first tasks is teacher education. Education is best done individually when teachers have a student with the disease in the classroom. Parents should be instructed to take a primary role in educating their child's teacher about sickle cell anemia and the academic and social implications of the disease. Health providers can assist parents with information teachers need. Teachers need to know that the disease is not contagious or fatal, that there are no situations that require immediate action, that a pain attack in the classroom is not an emergency, and that the child will drink more water and use the bathroom more frequently than other children. The only physical characteristics of the disease are yellow eyes and small stature. Children with sickle cell anemia are sometimes teased, and it is helpful to discuss ways of dealing with this. Many of these children become tired easily, and the teacher needs to be aware that the child is not malingering. Some parents or children decide against gym because of the low tolerance of physical exercise. Teachers should accept this wish, although these children should be encouraged to take gym whenever possible. The gym teacher should be informed that such children tire easily and should be allowed to decide when they need to rest.

Some children do not want others to know that they have sickle cell anemia, and the teacher should respect the child's wishes. Teachers should not discuss the child's disease in the classroom unless it is known that the child will feel comfortable with the discussion.

Because intelligence is not affected by sickle cell anemia, teachers should have the same high academic expectations for students with this disease that they have for other students. Children who have frequent absences will need help with the work they miss. A preventive program aimed at helping these children maintain the appropriate skill level for their age despite absenteeism would be useful in their early school years. Careful monitoring of children's skills and attendance, with tutorial assistance when needed, could assure that they attain the basic skills needed for future academic success. Children with sickle cell anemia generally are not eligible for homebound teaching because their excessive absenteeism tends to consist of multiple short absences rather than a single prolonged one.

The source of many academic and attendance problems lies in the family itself. Parents may be overprotective, overly responsive to a child's manipulations, or have low aspirations for their children. They may require reassurance when they are fearful about their child's illness, awareness of how children can use their disease as a way of being allowed to stay home from school, and encouragement to aim at high academic and career success for their child. Sometimes it is necessary to help families deal with severe personal and family problems such as maternal depression or interpersonal conflicts before much can be done about the child's academic problems.

Most children with sickle cell anemia should not be in special education classes. They have no physical or mental handicaps that require a special curriculum, and the psychosocial and educational effects of such placement can be detrimental to their overall development. The health provider has a central role in articulating these facts to parents and school personnel.

Comprehensive Health Care Needs of Adults

Adults with sickle cell anemia should receive comprehensive health care.

Rationale. By and large the psychosocial stresses associated with sickle cell anemia in childhood continue into adulthood, but with additional factors. For many, whether to marry is a difficult decision because of insecurity about their desirability as mates, uncertainty about the long-term attitude of spouses to their chronic illness, and the question of whether the disease will permit them to carry out the role of homemaker or provider. Shortened life expectancy impacts upon their will to plan for the future and for having a family. For some, there is a problem associated with the attitudes and behavior of health care providers with respect to the management of pain. Thus, for a variety of reasons adults as well as children need comprehensive care.

Comments. When pain attacks occur after clinic or physician office hours, patients are usually forced to seek relief at hospital emergency rooms. When adults go frequently to an emergency room and request Demerol (a narcotic commonly used to relieve severe pain), the question arises whether the reported pain is real or whether it is feigned to obtain narcotics. Demerol has been withheld when the latter was considered to be the case. Although drug addiction occurs in individuals with sickle cell anemia, we believe that all sickle cell patients complaining of pain should receive adequate doses of the drug(s) to relieve it. Suspected drug abuse or addiction should be reported to the primary care provider who should initiate and coordinate an investigative and management process. Others who provide care, including the emergency room staff, must be made aware of the investigation and should be instructed to prescribe Demerol for the patient until notified to the contrary.

In general, individuals with sickle cell anemia are encouraged to adjust to pain by carrying on their normal activities as much as possible; thus the severity of pain cannot always be judged by facial expressions or behavior. Some adolescents and young adults have reported to us a paradoxical position with respect to nurses and housestaff when they are in a hospital for treatment of pain. If they cry, they are acting like babies. If they smile or grin and bear it, they are obviously not having severe pain. The primary care provider has a responsibility to assure that all providers know the concepts that underlie the management of pain in sickle cell anemia.

Employment

Adults with sickle cell anemia should receive assistance in becoming economically self-sufficient.

Rationale. Although most young adults with sickle cell anemia have the physical and mental capacity for full-time employment, unemployment is exceptionally high. A 1979 survey of ninety-two nondisabled persons with sickle cell anemia aged eighteen to twenty-five and known to the Wayne State

University Comprehensive Sickle Cell Center revealed that 43 percent of the group were unemployed. At that time, the unemployment rate for black youths in this age category was approximately 25 percent. Twenty-five percent of those surveyed had never worked and 50 percent had never had a full-time job. A survey of persons with sickle cell anemia in outstate Michigan in 1981 showed 68 percent of the respondents over eighteen years of age unemployed. Because the reasons for the high level of unemployment are disease related, a program specifically to help persons with sickle cell anemia find employment is required.

Comments. This program should have two major thrusts. One is for the patient and should focus on disease-adjustment counseling, counseling with respect to academic preparation for jobs, career counseling and guidance specific to sickle cell anemia, vocational education, vocational rehabilitation, and employment maintenance counseling. The other focus should include employer education, job recruitment, and job placement.

Although data are limited, many adolescents and adults with sickle cell anemia appear to lack self-confidence and motivation to succeed in employment. A study of ninety-seven individuals by the Pennsylvania Bureau of Vocational Rehabilitation (*Assessment of Vocational Potential,* 1977) suggests that persons with sickle cell disease lack a sense of control over their own lives. Kumar and his colleagues (1976) observed lower self-esteem in adolescents with sickle cell anemia than in a control group of healthy children. Danlouji (1982) found high rates of social and psychological disability among persons with sickle cell anemia compared with a matched group of diabetics. In our experience, many are reluctant to exchange secure, though marginal, financial support from their families or public assistance for a job. They are afraid pain attacks will prevent regular attendance and they will be discharged.

Many individuals' poor reading and math skills, as well as lack of work experience, make it difficult to achieve their career goals. It is important to help clients evaluate job requirements and personal characteristics needed for the jobs, and to help correct deficits that may interfere with achievement of career goals.

Individuals with sickle cell anemia frequently face a dilemma when filling out a preemployment medical questionnaire. If they disclose the sickle cell anemia, they are afraid they will not be hired; if they fail to disclose it, they fear they will be dismissed for falsification of the medical history. Participants in a conference on "Employment and the Sickle Cell Conditions" (1981) concluded that individuals with sickle cell should disclose not only for legal reasons but also because they otherwise might not get the benefit of employer understanding when employers become better educated about the disease.

The participants made three recommendations: (1) rather than specify that they have sickle cell anemia, persons with sickle cell anemia should write on the medical history form that they have a condition they would prefer to discuss with the interviewer; (2) they should give to the interviewer a letter from their physician stating that in spite of their disease they can perform the job for which they are applying; and (3) they should provide the interviewer or employer with adequate information about the disease.

Are there jobs for which individuals with sickle cell anemia could establish a time bank, working extra hours when they are well so when they are ill they can take compensatory time? This plan would assure the employee of a full income and the employer of a full level of man-hours. Also, the employee's voluntary willingness to work extra hours could foster an accommodating employer attitude concerning that employee.

Employers need to know that there are only two types of tasks employees with sickle cell anemia cannot handle: those that require above-average physical strength and endurance and those that require exposure to cold. Otherwise, from the standpoint of their disease, job performance is entirely related to the frequency of pain and other complications, which is highly variable and may or may not result in excessive absenteeism.

Screening to identify sickle cell trait is unjustified in preemployment physical examinations. The only purpose of preemployment physical assessment should be to identify conditions that would prevent the applicant from performing satisfactorily on the job. The purpose should not be to screen out individuals because they have a handicap. This right-to-employment position is required by federal law for employers receiving federal support and by laws in thirty-three states.

For jobs an anemic individual could not handle adequately, screening to detect anemia is warranted. But anemia should not be an employment issue unless the type of anemia has job performance implications. Individuals who are found to be anemic should be referred to their medical care provider to investigate the cause of the anemia so appropriate treatment can be instituted. In the case of black Americans, it would be appropriate to include a test for sickling in this secondary workup.

Some employees with sickle cell anemia have periods when their rate of absenteeism exceeds that of the average employee without sickle cell anemia. If satisfactory job performance requires a certain level of attendance, some individuals with sickle cell anemia would eventually be unqualified. Valid judgments can be made only through experience with the individual employee. Thus, screening for sickle cell anemia and rejection for employment on these grounds is unacceptable.

The Future

The policies enunciated here are primarily related to the goal of reducing the negative impact of individuals having a single or double gene for sickle hemoglobin. The ultimate goal for any disease is to discover an acceptable cure. In this regard, the outlook for the future is encouraging. There is a substantial level of support from the National Institutes of Health for sickle cell research, an attractive field because the defect is molecular and new information is likely to be of value in unraveling the mysteries of other molecular diseases.

Promising lines of sickle cell research include efforts to gain a better understanding of the properties of sickle hemoglobin, the sickling process, and the types of drugs that may be effective in preventing or reversing the process. In addition, progress is being made in bone marrow transplantation and genetic engineering. These techniques could provide answers to the sickle cell problem.

References

Assessment of Vocational Potential. Harrisburg, Pa.: Pennsylvania Bureau of Vocational Rehabilitation, July 1977.

Baubes, A., Mears, J. G., and Ramirez, P. "Disorders of Human Hemoglobin." *Science,* 1980, *207,* 486–493.

Chang, J. C., and Kan, Y. W. "A Sensitive New Prenatal Test For Sickle Cell Anemia." *New England Journal of Medicine,* 1982, *307,* 30–32.

Chodorkoff, J., and Whitten, C. F. "Intellectual Status of Children with Sickle Cell Anemia." *Journal of Pediatrics,* 1963, *63,* 29–35.

Conyard, S., Krishnamurthy, M., and Dosik, H. "Psychosocial Aspects of Sickle Cell Anemia in Adolescents." *Health and Social Work,* 1980, *5,* 20–26.

A Critical Review of Informational Materials Relating to Sickle Cell Anemia and Sickle Cell Trait. Los Angeles: National Association for Sickle Cell Disease, 1972.

Danlouji, N. F. "Social Disability and Psychiatric Morbidity in Sickle Cell Anemia and Diabetes Patients." *Psychosomatics,* 1982, *9,* 925–931.

"Employment and the Sickle Cell Conditions: Problems/Solutions." Conference sponsored by the National Association for Sickle Cell Disease. Los Angeles: 1981.

Grover, R., and others. "Current Sickle Cell Screening Program for Newborns in New York City, 1979–1980." *American Journal of Public Health,* 1983, *73,* 249–252.

Kosacoff, M. I., Seligman, B. R., and Dosik, H. *Psychological Aspects of Sickle Cell Anemia and Variants.* Proceedings of the First National Symposium on Sickle Cell Disease. National Institutes of Health publication no. 75-723. Washington, D.C.: Department of Health, Education, and Welfare, 1974.

Kumar, S., and others. "Anxiety, Self-Concept, and Personal and Social Adjustments in Children with Sickle Cell Anemia." *Journal of Pediatrics,* 1976, *88,* 859.

McIntosh, S., Rooks, Y., and Richey, A. K. "Fever in Young Children with Sickle Cell Disease." *Journal of Pediatrics,* 1980, *96,* 199–204.

Mattson, A. "Long Term Physical Illness in Childhood: A Challenge To Psychosocial Adaptation." *Pediatrics,* 1972, *50,* 801–811.

National Association for Sickle Cell Disease. "Policies Related to Insuring Individuals with Sickle Cell Conditions." Unpublished report. Los Angeles: National Association for Sickle Cell Disease, 1975.

Nishiura, E., and Whitten C. F. "Psychosocial Problems in Families of Children with Sickle Cell Anemia." *Urban Health,* 1980, *9,* 32–35.

Nishiura, E., Whitten, C. F., and Thomas, J. F. "School Absences and Sickle Cell

Anemia." Paper presented at the American Public Health Association Annual Meeting, Montreal, 1982.

O'Brien, R. T., McIntosh, S., and Aspnes, G. T. "Prospective Study of Sickle Cell Anemia in Infancy." *Journal of Pediatrics*, 1976, *89*, 205–210.

Powars, D. R. "Natural History of Sickle Cell Disease—The First Ten Years." *Seminars on Hematology*, 1975, *12*, 267–279.

Powars, D., Overturf, G., and Weiss, J. "Pneumococcal Septicemia in Children with Sickle Cell Anemia." *Journal of the American Medical Association*, 1982, *245*, 1839–1842.

Powledge, T. M., and Fletcher, J. C. "Guidelines for the Ethical and Legal Issues in Prenatal Diagnosis." *New England Journal of Medicine*, 1979, *300*, 168–172.

President's Commission for the Study of Ethical Problems in Medicine and Biomedical and Behavioral Research. *Screening and Counseling for Genetic Conditions: The Ethical, Social, and Legal Implications of Genetic Screening, Counseling, and Education Programs*. Washington, D.C.: U.S. Government Printing Office, 1983.

Rowley, P. T., and Huntzinger, D. J. "Newborn Sickle Cell Screening—Benefits and Burdens Realized." *American Journal of Diseases of Children*, 1983, *137*, 341–345.

Rutkow, I. M., and Lipton, J. M. "Mandatory Screening for Sickle Cell Anemia." *New England Journal of Medicine*, 1973, *289*, 865–866.

Sears, D. A. "The Morbidity of Sickle Cell Trait: A Review of the Literature." *American Journal of Medicine*, 1978, *64*, 1021–1036.

Seeler, R. A. "Deaths in Children with Sickle Cell Anemia." *Clinical Pediatrics*, 1972, *11*, 634–637.

Whitten, C. F., and Fischhoff, J. "Psychosocial Effects of Sickle Cell Disease." *Archives of Internal Medicine*, 1974, *133*, 681–689.

Williams, I., Earles, A. N., and Pack, B. "Psychological Considerations in Sickle Cell Disease." *Nursing Clinics of North America*, 1983, *18*, 215–229.

Wright, E. E., and Shaw, M. W. "Legal Liability in Genetic Screening, Genetic Counseling and Prenatal Diagnosis." *Clinical Obstetrics and Gynecology*, 1981, *24*, 1133–1149.

13

Congenital Heart Disease

Donald C. Fyler, M.D.

Description of Congenital Heart Disease

Congenital heart disease accounts for the bulk of cardiac illness in children. *Congenital* means present at birth and for that reason the term *congenital heart disease* refers to an abnormally formed heart. Any part of the heart may be malformed. Any of the four valves may leak, obstruct, or be entirely absent. The walls between the chambers may be variably incomplete, allowing intermixture of oxygenated and unoxygenated blood in the newborn. By thirty-five days after conception, the chambers and valves of the heart have formed, and by birth, these structures will have increased thirtyfold, the increase in size being determined by the amount of blood pumped. Any deviation from normal circulation caused by an abnormally formed structure will result secondarily in downstream abnormalities of size. Thus, a chamber with an abnormally formed and obstructing inlet valve at the sixth week of pregnancy receives a reduced flow of blood for the remainder of pregnancy, and so at birth, that chamber may be much smaller than the expected size.

It is important to emphasize that congenital heart defects are uncommon abnormalities of intrauterine development and have no similarity to the acquired coronary artery disease so rampant among adults. Babies do not have heart attacks. Their disorders are fundamentally quite different from those of adults, and many of the surgical procedures used to help children are more complex, often being accomplished inside the heart and rarely concerned with coronary arteries. Among symptomatic infants, death is common. If surgery is successful in the child, it is often possible to anticipate a normal life span, whereas in the adult, surgery is considered successful if the inevitable is delayed.

Between 1950 and 1970, the diagnostic features of many varieties of congenital heart disease were defined. Treatment schedules, including newly invented surgical procedures, were refined and applied to surviving adults and older children. Gradually, fewer children with blue lips, stunted growth, limited physical ability, warped psychological outlook, and constricted social horizons were seen in cardiac clinics. The scrawny infants, short of breath with congestive heart failure, who spent many months in oxygen tents in pediatric hospitals, were seen less often as newer surgical procedures were introduced. By the end of the 1960s, the stage was set for a concerted effort to apply the new knowledge and techniques to children's most lethal cardiac problems—those that cause symptoms in early infancy.

In the 1970s, most infants ill with congenital heart disease survived because of miniaturization of the diagnostic and surgical techniques developed during the preceding two decades. The diagnosis of complex cardiac defects was made with increasing precision, and established surgical procedures were applied with increasing success in very small infants. With improved salvage, it became obvious that systematic casefinding would be desirable. Professional education programs were organized and resulted in hospitalization of larger numbers of new patients. Networks of communication were established among physicians, and systems for patient transport were designed. The desirability of monitoring the success or failure of medical management of children with these uncommon problems was recognized, and some attempts to do this were made (Fyler, 1980; Subcommittee on Standards, American Academy of Pediatrics, 1978). During the 1970s, the costs of providing medical care increased out of proportion to inflation, while at the same time, government funds for patient care and for research became more limited. So, in the mid 1980s, it is appropriate to review the surgical and medical management of children with congenital heart disease and to reconsider the special problems of providing the best medical care.

Etiology. The cause of congenital heart disease is usually described as multifactorial, a term that not only conveniently conceals our ignorance but also recognizes that there are several known etiologic associations. In the majority of patients, there are no etiologic clues; in a minority, useful information is available. For example, maternal German measles (rubella) very early in pregnancy is associated with peripheral pulmonary stenosis and persistent patency of the ductus arteriosus in the child. Rubella immunization, as a public health measure, will decrease the number of infants of this type. Premature birth is also associated with persistent patency of the ductus arteriosus. When the ductus is large, congestive heart failure develops, and intervention with drugs or surgery may be required. A large patent ductus arteriosus in a premature infant accounts for 9 percent of critical heart disease in infants. Here, the prevention of prematurity can be expected to result in fewer infants with congenital heart disease. Children of mothers with diabetes have a greater incidence of congenital anomalies of all types. Which treatment programs for the mother's disease will result in fewer congenital anomalies in the infant is an obvious avenue for investigation. The relation between the use of lithium compounds by the mother and Ebstein's anomaly of the heart in the child is an example of apparent causation of congenital heart disease by maternal use of a drug (Weinstein, 1979). Other drugs are being investigated by epidemiologic techniques at the present time (Rothman and others, 1979). The common thread among these considerations is that when a possible causative mechanism is identified, ways to affect the incidence of congenital heart disease may become available.

Unfortunately, these examples account for only a small portion of the total number of children born with congenital heart disease. More impressive are the number of parents (10 to 25 percent) who report congenital heart disease among relatives (Rowe and others, 1981). A genetic background for congenital heart disease is further supported by the experience of seeing more than one child with the same cardiac anomaly in the same family. The theory that many children have a genetic background that predisposes to congenital heart disease evolved naturally and is generally accepted. The minimal variation in incidence of the different types of congenital heart disease (Fyler, 1980, Table 8) suggests unchanging factors that predispose to the development of congenital heart disease. For example, a constant level of a particular gene predisposing to transposition of the great arteries in the New England states could account for the remarkable constancy of this lesion in this population. Still, the majority of patients and parents provide no indication of an etiologic factor for the child's congenital heart disease. The variations in incidence between children of parents of urban and rural residence (Rothman and Fyler, 1976) suggest the need for further investigation.

Thus, in the 1980s, the etiology of congenital heart disease appears multifactorial, with several factors (of which we are largely uncertain) simultaneously or consecutively involved. Because recognition of an etiologic association can lead to prevention, a continued search for clues using epidemiologic methods is warranted. More fundamental would be a long-range commitment to research into normal and abnormal developmental processes to discover what embryologic mechanisms are involved in the abnormal development of the heart and whether these mechanisms can be safely altered. As these questions are answered, progress in the prevention of congenital heart disease may be possible.

Prevalence. The number of infants hospitalized each year in the New England states because of congenital heart disease has varied little. The greatest variation in new cases over the years was less than twofold during a period of time when casefinding was systematically intensified. Mitchell, Korones, and Berendes (1971) reported that 8 per thousand newborn infants have congenital heart disease. This figure was derived from a count of consecutive births in a widely scattered group of large hospitals in the United States. If the number of stillborn infants is subtracted, the figure is 7.5 per thousand live births, a number identical to that found by Carlgren (1969) in Sweden in a detailed study that spanned thirty years.

Not all children with congenital heart disease require expensive diagnostic and surgical treatment. Some have inconsequential abnormalities, while others require a full range of medical services. The New England Regional Infant

Cardiac Program (NERICP) found that about 3 infants per thousand live births become symptomatic because of heart disease and are hospitalized in the first year of life (Fyler, 1980). Unfortunately, there are no data regarding the other 4.5 per thousand live births. For the 1980s, however, the prevalence of new cases of congenital heart disease is expected to continue to be a near constant function of the number of births.

The more severe anomalies cause both symptoms and mortality early, and there are fewer new patients who require extensive medical services in older age groups. With improving salvage over the years, the number of surviving individuals who have had corrective cardiac surgery for congenital heart disease is presumed to be increasing in the general population.

Diagnosis. Because of the high mortality at a young age associated with some cardiac defects, the relative frequency of the many diagnoses varies with age. The numbers of anatomical and functional variations of congenital heart disease are large, compounding the difficulty inherent in establishing the diagnosis of these uncommon problems because every diagnostic subcategory is rare. Even physicians who have concentrated their efforts on children with congenital heart disease regularly encounter new anatomic and physiologic situations. The well trained cardiologist or cardiac surgeon with limited exposure to children with heart disease will have trouble recognizing some of the possible combinations of congenital cardiac defects known to occur. Thus, the large numbers of anatomical and functional variations result in obvious problems in training and quality control of medical care.

Age at Onset of Symptoms. There are good reasons to believe that most forms of congenital heart disease are compatible with survival of the unborn baby. Because the two ventricles function in parallel during fetal life (rather than in series as is normal after birth), either ventricle may assume some of the workload of the other, abnormal ventricle. Surprising degrees of anatomic abnormality are tolerated before birth.

At birth, the circulation goes through regular changes that provide for separation of the pulmonary circulation from the systemic circulation. Normally, each is pumped in equal volume by separate ventricles. An abnormally small ventricle may not be able to manage, and depending on the degree of anatomic abnormality, the infant may have great difficulty in the first hours, days, or weeks of life. The major life-threatening congenital cardiac defects cause deaths very early, often with only a few hours of obvious symptoms. In 1977, for example, 34 percent of admissions in NERICP were within the first two days of life. Improved salvage is therefore dependent on early recognition and prompt transfer of suspect babies to a medical unit equipped and staffed to handle these problems. As attention has been directed to newborn cardiac problems, the age of new patients with heart disease has been changing. Now 35 percent of all inpatients are less than one year old at first encounter. Whether the present level of early referral in the New England states would continue if all professional educational efforts to promote early referral ceased seems unlikely.

Associated Anomalies. Twenty-seven percent of infants ill with congenital heart disease have other congenital anomalies. Many come to the attention of a cardiologist because the presence of a noncardiac anomaly raised the question of heart disease. Extracardiac anomalies influence the lives and well-being of children with congenital heart disease. The overall increase in mortality because of extracardiac anomalies is small (3 percent) although the increased mortality varies with the type of anomaly. The influence of extracardiac anomalies on the life-style of surviving children is great, whether viewed in terms of growth, motor development, intelligence quotients, or even psychiatric problems. Table 1 shows that children with extracardiac anomalies are more likely to have poor development on these dimensions than are children with heart disease alone. In organizing medical care for children with heart disease, arrangement for management of any other congenital anomalies is an important factor in determining outcome.

Complications. Because congenital heart disease sometimes results in reduced amounts of blood being pumped by the heart and in low arterial blood oxygen, complicating problems resulting from inadequate amounts of blood or blood oxygen may be encountered in any organ system. Perhaps the most prominent complication is poor growth; 26 percent of five-year-old children who have survived symptomatic heart disease in infancy were below the fifth percentile for height (Table 1). How this growth pattern is affected by the timing of surgical intervention and by the particular surgical procedure chosen is unknown. It is reasonable to expect that ideally timed surgery will result in more nearly normal growth. Increased attention to this area of investigation is anticipated.

Cardiac lesions resulting in increased pulmonary blood flow and pulmonary arterial pressure may, over the course of time, produce a permanent pulmonary vascular change that by itself will limit life. In the past, this was increasingly more common with advancing age. Nowadays, with early surgical intervention, development of permanent pulmonary vascular change is much less common. Still, measurements of the factors that advance or delay this process are valuable information for clinicians managing patients who are at risk of this ominous development.

Abnormalities of heartbeat or heart rhythm are rare in children, except among those who have congenital heart disease or among those who have undergone cardiac surgery. Because the new techniques for study of rhythm disturbances offer the possibility of pharmacologic control or even surgical cure, development of specialized study groups for this purpose should be encouraged.

It is not expected that surgical correction will always eliminate the possibility of bacterial infection on the abnormal inner surface of the heart (bacterial endocarditis), yet corrective surgery can be expected to reduce the incidence of endocarditis. The incidence of brain abscess is reduced when low blood oxygen (cyanosis) is corrected or reduced. Similarly, the brain damage produced by unconscious spells caused by low blood oxygen (hypoxic spells) is avoided through early surgical correction.

Table 1. Influence of Infant Heart Disease and of Extracardiac Anomalies (Percentage).

	Height *Equal to or less than 5th percentile*	Wechsler *Intelligence Quotient* *Equal to or less than 69*	Vineland Social *Maturity Scale* *Equal to or less than 53*	Psychiatric *Score**
Heart disease	21	4	6	3
Heart disease plus extracardiac anomalies	26	12	14	9
Without heart disease	5	2.5	5	Unknown

Source: Fyler and others, 1982.
* Children with a score of 5 on a scale of 1 to 5. 1 = no psychiatric problem, 5 = major psychiatric problem.

The delays in motor development demonstrable in five-year survivors of congenital heart disease perhaps do not seriously affect the future well-being of these patients. A clumsy, awkward, skinny five-year-old child with funny speech and a chest scar will not necessarily find those handicaps to be a permanent or major impediment in adult life. Even earlier reparative surgery may avoid the problems of motor limitation and poor growth. Fortunately, the intelligence quotients of these children are normally distributed unless there are overriding extracardiac anomalies such as Down's syndrome.

Survival. The natural history of many congenital heart defects has been incompletely described. The natural course of events is documented for a few defects that do not require surgery and for a few where the natural history was recorded before a corrective surgical procedure was invented. Serious efforts to document natural history have been made, but most studies of natural history were prompted by the introduction of a new surgical procedure and are consequently flawed. It is not possible to know what would have happened if the operation had not been done. So, in the 1970s, the pre- and post-surgical course of each cardiac lesion, rather than its natural history, was the focus of interest.

For critically ill infants with congenital heart disease, the major loss of life is in the first days or weeks of life and is mainly determined by the specific cardiac anomaly (Nadas, Fyler, and Buckley, 1980). The loss of life in infants with ventricular septal defect (VSD) is minimal, while few infants with hypoplastic left heart syndrome survive the second month of life. Those with tetralogy of Fallot (TF) and those with d-transposition of the great arteries (TGA) lie between the two extremes.

Attempts to further reduce mortality require early recognition of the infant at risk and efficient transfer to an appropriately staffed and equipped central hospital. Improvement in survival through better diagnostic and surgical techniques is probable, but for the immediate future, simple dissemination of knowledge already available should produce significant benefit.

Management

Relief from symptoms, even if temporary, is a desirable goal of medical treatment. Prolongation of a limited life-style may be similarly desirable. But correction of a potentially life-limiting cardiac defect in a child is a truly gratifying outcome of medical treatment. As a matter of policy, any child who is likely to develop symptoms by thirty years of age because of congenital heart disease should undergo reparative cardiac surgery if it is available at reasonable risk. This policy is quite different from the usual management of adults who undergo cardiac surgery to relieve symptoms.

Because all cardiac surgery carries some risk, surgical misadventure in an otherwise asymptomatic child may occur. In a sense, some of this surgery is a preventive medical manipulation designed to provide the longest life for the greatest number. It would be easier for the parents if cardiac defects were visible. Defects that can be looked at, even touched, and in which function is visibly deranged are more readily understood. Invisible defects that produce no symptoms are much more difficult to comprehend, and when the outcome is unexpectedly bad, malpractice litigation is a natural consequence. The cardiologist must ensure factual understanding by the parents of what is at stake.

The emotional relationship between a parent and an infant with congenital heart disease is affected by the heart disease. An overly protective attitude or parental denial may emerge. Reluctance to develop a deep emotional tie to an infant who may die is common. Guilt because of these thoughts, as well as the responsibility for having brought a crippled child into the world, may sour the parents' attitude. Although in the past, surgical correction of congenital heart disease was withheld from children who were severely mentally retarded, today children whose life expectancy would be shortened without cardiac surgery are systematically referred for operation regardless of other problems. These considerations lead to the following philosophy of management. In general, all children who will ever need cardiac surgery should have the surgery performed as early in life as is compatible with the best mortality and morbidity attainable. The child and parents should be given the earliest opportunity to get about the business of developing a new person without the fears of a major surgical procedure hanging like a sword of Damocles over their heads. Whenever possible, the time spent awaiting a major cardiac surgical procedure should be as short as possible.

Although all pediatric cardiologists know of families that disintegrated because of children with congenital heart disease, NERICP data show no greater number of divorces in the five years after the births of infants seriously ill with cardiac problems than the numbers expected in the community at large. The child and adolescent with cardiac disease, however, suffer from problems of adjustment. The problem of a negative body image, the dangers of pregnancy, the limited availability of life or health insurance, and the difficulty of obtaining gainful employment are formidable obstacles for these children when they reach adolescence and young adulthood. Who would marry, insure, or hire a person whose heart is abnormal? Such thoughts plague these young people.

If the desirability for cardiac surgery in early infancy is accepted and if, as the author believes, the state of the art for cardiac diagnosis and surgery are far enough advanced to handle most infants with heart defects, it follows that the earlier the infant is referred to a central hospital, the better. Although this conclusion may seem obvious, it has emerged only in the past ten to fifteen years with the demonstration that intracardiac surgery can be performed in infancy. With some exceptions, the size of the child is no longer an obstacle to successful reparative cardiac surgery.

The waiting lists for cardiac surgery common in the United Kingdom are not compatible with this point of view; nonetheless, it is the author's view, and that of the parents he encounters, that the earlier the reparative surgery is carried out the better, provided that surgery is unavoidable and the risk does not improve with growth. Simply to survive is not enough.

Case Discovery. The high mortality associated with congenital heart disease in early infancy is the main reason to arrange the earliest possible referral to a cardiac center. The amount of time available for diagnostic evaluation is often limited by the rapid deterioration of the patient.

In the NERICP, the thoroughness of casefinding and the tendency to earlier referral are largely determined by the nursery nurses. It is presumed that the continuing NERICP education program has some bearing on the improvement in mortality over time (Fyler and others, 1980). Because it is the nursery nurses who have the most frequent contact with the infant and who first recognize that a baby has blue lips or is short of breath, the NERICP professional education effort is directed to the nursery nurse. It is easier to organize and carry out systematic teaching for nurses than for physicians. Because the number of infants sick with heart disease is small and because there is a rapid turnover of nursery nurses, it is necessary to reinforce this kind of educational experience regularly. Older patients are discovered through encounters with practicing physicians, school physicians, and organized programs for examination of athletes.

Communications. Because congenital heart disease is uncommon, appropriate medical facilities and personnel are often some distance from the patient's home or from the local hospital. Day and night access to a cardiac consultant can be provided by using radiobeepers and by scheduling a back-up physician for the cardiologist (Fyler, 1980). Furthermore, it often happens that a child is transferred from one major medical center to another to take advantage of special expertise in managing a particular cardiac defect (15 percent of NERICP patients are transferred from one cardiac hospital to another). The scheduling, transportation, and follow-up of those children must be coordinated at all levels. Interhospital and interprofessional communication is important. All major hospitals, and perhaps all hospitals, should be formed into communication networks that allow ready transfer of data for patient care, for comparison of statistics, and for coordination of patients moving from one hospital to another. Computer networks already designed could handle most of this need without great cost. Networks would be particularly helpful in pediatrics, where most major medical problems are rare and maintaining a full staff of specialists in rare disease is impractical for most institutions.

Transportation. In recent years, much thought and effort has gone into transportation systems for sick infants. These systems have been developed largely for transfer of infants with respiratory distress syndrome (RDS), but they serve also for transfer of infants with cardiac disease. Stabilizing the infant before transfer may be appropriate for RDS babies but is usually a waste of time for infants with cardiac disease. The reason for rapid transfer of an infant with cardiac disease is to learn the diagnosis and carry out cardiac surgery before the infant deteriorates irreparably. Oxygen and suction and support of body temperature may help the infant survive until reaching the central hospital. Sending out a special ambulance to pick up a patient is inefficient at long distances because much time is lost in traveling. At long distance, it is more appropriate for the local ambulance or aircraft to transport the patient to the central unit. In New England, using this philosophy of transporting infants with heart disease, loss of life en route has decreased to zero (Fyler, 1980).

The most frustrating feature of patient transportation systems is lack of regional coordination. Some plan of systematic interdependence among private, state, town, city, police and fire department, and hospital patient transport is desirable. Questions of jurisdiction and the appropriate commitment of ambulances are best decided in advance.

Local Hospital. Congenital heart disease is sufficiently uncommon that any recommendations for special equipment and personnel to help care for these babies at the local level are unwarranted. The local social worker, nurse, pediatrician, electrocardiographic laboratory, and x-ray department can be very helpful, but their help is best arranged on an ad hoc basis as the need arises. In some communities there will be a regular cardiac clinic with a visiting pediatric cardiologist. Often in these clinics, a local physician, adult cardiologist, or pediatrician develops an interest in these children, becomes informed through attending clinics, and provides invaluable service. The requirement for frequent communication with tertiary hospitals is obvious. Indeed, it is the author's experience at a tertiary hospital that a significant part of each day is spent on the phone discussing patients in outlying areas.

Cardiac Hospital. The location of a pediatric cardiac unit depends on the size of the surrounding population, the distance to the nearest comparable unit, the location of the nearest medical school, and regional political factors. Because the equipment and trained personnel are expensive, they are shared with adult cardiologists. Cardiac surgery for both children and adults is performed by the same cardiac surgery team. This arrangement can be a resounding success or a dismal failure. The outcome is partly related to how recently the pediatric cardiologist and cardiac surgeon were trained. With limited patient experience, it is only a matter of years before abilities fade or techniques become out of date. However, deficiencies rarely persist for long because a cardiologist, a cardiac surgeon, and a primary physician are involved with most patients, and it is unlikely that all three would have a persistently unrealistic view of their capabilities. No difficulties ensue unless state, medical school, or hospital authorities insist that, having paid for a cardiac unit, that unit should provide full service. When it is clearly understood that some patients will appropriately be referred elsewhere and some patients will be handled locally, all goes well. Physicians make more accurate assessments of their own capabilities when there is no element of embarrassment in moving a patient elsewhere for further care. When making judgments about where surgery should be performed, it is helpful to have data comparing local and regional experience such as those provided by NERICP. Because these decisions concern sensitive issues, the information used must be demonstrably precise and reliable.

In New England, there have been a variety of evolutionary changes in pediatric cardiology. Of eleven hospitals offering services to infants with heart disease in 1970, one has discontinued all inpatient pediatric cardiology. One has been absorbed by a nearby cardiac unit, and two have discontinued infant cardiac catheterization and cardiac surgery although continuing to do limited childhood surgery. Two provide all services except for limited reparative surgery in infancy.

Five provide full service, although one of these receives virtually all referrals between cardiac hospitals. These modifications in delivery of care in New England were decided by each hospital independently and were coincident with the availability of detailed experience data for the region.

In terms of staff, it is advantageous, on the average, to have board certified individuals in all physician positions. Still, it is apparent that anyone with experience with children with heart disease is superior to another who is board certified and has no experience in the pediatric age group. This is a recurrent problem for those interested in children. Although the child is a small adult, the child's medical problems bear little relation to those of the adult. There is almost nothing about the adult with coronary artery disease that relates to the infant with transposition of the great arteries or most other congenital heart defects. Similarly, with the requirement for large numbers of cardiac surgeons to handle coronary artery surgery and the limited numbers of pediatric patients, it is obvious that all cardiac surgeons will not have the same exposure to infants during their training. The rarity of congenital heart disease, the many cardiac lesions, the variety of surgical operations, and the broad age range of the patients result in continuing new challenges for these surgeons. Consequently, it is difficult to maintain competence among pediatric cardiologists and cardiac surgeons handling minimal numbers of patients with congenital cardiac anomalies.

Thus, although the marriage of adult cardiology and cardiac surgery with infant cardiology and cardiac surgery can be successful, there are problems. Practical solutions vary from sending all pediatric patients away, to trying to care for some or all of them at the local cardiac unit. One solution is to define pediatric patients in terms of age. Thus, some hospitals provide full service to pediatric patients over the age of two years and provide none for infants, while others take only patients over the age of twelve or fourteen. This concept provides a sliding scale where the degree of pediatric expertise or lack of it is balanced by the age of the patient—an unusual yet rational solution.

Another solution is the pediatric hospital in which virtually all personnel and equipment are geared to pediatric use. Usually, only the surgeon is shared with nearby adult hospitals, although there are pediatric hospitals where everyone including the surgeon limits activities to pediatric patients. When the surgeon's experience with infants and children is great, the success rate is likely to be outstanding. Without doubt, the pediatric hospital provides the most satisfying solution for the child, the parents, pediatrician, and pediatric cardiologist, but is only practical where there are large numbers of patients.

Finally, in terms of personnel a variety of skills are highly desirable. It is useful to have on the scene a person whose responsibility is maintenance, largely preventive maintenance, of the ever more sophisticated machines that are being used. The possible value of a specialist, whether originating from pediatrics, anesthesia, or cardiology, is worth considering. Physician's assistants can be used in intensive care units, much as they are used to operate pump oxygenators in operating rooms. Again, it comes down to experience with the special problems of infants more than prescribed training.

Where does the computer fit into all of this? Computer systems can save time and money and perhaps improve efficiency in interpretation of EKGs, catheterization laboratories, interpretation of twenty-four-hour tape-recorded electrocardiograms, word processing, scheduling, and reporting. But a more compelling feature of computers is the ability to sort a morass of patient information. Considering the numbers of possible diagnoses, the potential surgical options, the effects of age on diagnosis and surgical success, it is not surprising that in deciding whether a patient should have an operation, the common experience is to refer back to the outcome of a prior case. Unfortunately, the medical literature reports mainly successes. Plainly, it would be more rational to have all the prior local experience readily available. Maintaining a usable computerized data base should be an acceptable burden, particularly in a large cardiac unit. Indeed, a few such units in the United States could provide adequate services to all others in the country, either through telephone line connections or by making the programming available to all.

Ancillary Resources. Ancillary services commonly utilized by a pediatric cardiology service include social service, nutrition, genetics, physical therapy, play specialists, psychiatry, respiratory therapy, infectious disease specialists, neurology, and dentistry. Most pediatric units have such personnel available. Among these, the dentist is often overlooked, and it is important to remember that systematic dental hygiene can prevent as many episodes of bacterial endocarditis as the use of prophylactic antibiotics during dental extraction. Although a child with a repaired congenital heart lesion may be less likely to get bacterial endocarditis, many congenital cardiac lesions, even when repaired, are suscept-ible to bacterial endocarditis. Whether the total number of susceptible children will increase or decrease as more children survive is not clear. The problem is sufficiently important that it will be necessary to accumulate documentation in the decades to come.

It is important to provide for the child's parents, particularly parents of children at a great distance from the central hospital. Parents of small children are rarely at their peak income, and indeed, many are indigent. Yet they need to be near their child at the time of surgery. Financial aid to provide transportation and a place to stay for those who cannot afford them are needed. The desirability of having the parents participate in the hospital care of the child is widely recognized. A simple room near the hospital or a reclining chair by the child's bed are remarkably valuable assets; even more important is an open and encouraging attitude among the hospital staff. Someone whose job is simply to report on progress in the operating room can help parents bear the hours of waiting. Literature, introductory visits to facilities such as intensive care units, and scheduled information sessions with parents are remarkably helpful. The availability of personnel to counsel bereaved parents some months after the death of the child is important. Although these suggestions are not central to the technical medical care of children with heart disease, they are desirable and cost comparatively little.

Follow-up. Systematic follow-up, which requires slight expense, both benefits the patient and adds to medical knowledge. At long distance, it is clearly better to have the cardiologist visit the local clinic than to have the patients return to the central hospital. Follow-up is more complete, and the educational contact between the primary physician and consultant is productive.

Successful follow-up clinics may have a variety of organizations. The central requirements of a follow-up visit, wherever it is held, are weighing and measuring the child, listening to the heart in a quiet room, and having electrocardiograms and chest x rays. It is also desirable to have a nurse, a social worker, and a nutritionist available and to have other specialty clinics in the same place. A participating local physician, often a pediatrician with an interest in cardiology, adds greatly to a follow-up clinic. Although the primary goal is the welfare of the patient, a secondary goal is feedback of information to all concerned, not the least of whom is the cardiac surgeon.

In follow-up clinics, age related problems are often encountered. Among small babies, poor growth, poor nutrition, and other anomalies may be major problems. In the older child, difficulty with teachers who are afraid the child will have a heart attack in class is common, as are troubles with a compulsive gym teacher. The difficulties for the teenager with a diminished self-image because of heart disease can be overpowering. Pregnancy and contraceptive pills are prohibited at risk of death for women with pulmonary hypertensive vascular disease. The possibility that pregnancy could result in a child with a similar cardiac defect must be considered by all women who have a congenital heart defect themselves.

Whereas in former times, it was a reasonable goal for the cardiac patient to reach the age of twenty-one, today most of these children survive into adulthood. Much data that would be useful in helping young adults with heart disease are therefore unavailable. How many are gainfully employed? Is employment status related to the prior cardiac condition? Are young adults able to get health and life insurance? How many of these cardiac patients have children with congenital heart disease? What is the incidence of late development of arrhythmias? What is the possibility of late, unexpected death? Does a history of surgically cured congenital heart disease influence the chance of developing and surviving acquired heart disease? Systematic follow-up of surviving adults with congenital heart disease is an appropriate study for the coming decade.

Results. Some factors determining survival for children with congenital heart disease have been defined (Fyler and others, 1980). As might be expected, the anatomic problem and the surgical procedure used are major determinants of success. Even among infants with the same anatomic diagnosis, there is greater loss of life among those who become symptomatic in early infancy. Most mortality is early, with a gradually declining mortality after the first few months continuing through the first years of life. Other lesser contributions to mortality are the presence of extracardiac anomalies and low birthweight. Viewed overall, mortality seems to have improved slightly for infants born in recent years.

Quality of life is good. Indeed, when those children with extracardiac anomalies were excluded from consideration, the specific problems attributable to heart defects are poor growth (25 percent of five-year survivors are below the fifth percentile) as illustrated earlier in Table 1 and delayed motor development, which is at least in part associated with poor growth (Fyler and others, 1982). Thus, measures of intelligence, psychologic tests, neuropsychologic measures, and estimations of psychiatric outcome are within expected range, provided the children with extracardiac anomalies are excluded. Those with extracardiac anomalies have a variety of problems that often bode ill for the future and are mainly a function of the extracardiac problem.

Thus, the main impact of congenital heart disease is in terms of survival or not. Among survivors, poor growth may be noticed but the child is otherwise normal provided there are no extracardiac anomalies. Of necessity, the presently available data about survivors involves individuals treated with methods in use ten years ago. Systematic follow-up will be required before the outcome of present-day treatment becomes known.

Organization. The organization of medical care delivery for children with heart disease varies considerably from place to place. In the New England states in 1982, there were nine hospitals serving a population of 12,000,000 with 150,000 births annually and providing services to children with congenital heart disease. Five hospitals provided a full range of services to children with heart disease. There were nine medical schools, two without pediatric cardiology units. Eight of the nine hospitals were affiliated with a nearby medical school. All states have at least one pediatric cardiac hospital. Only a rare baby receives initial care outside the region. In a few instances, children receive care elsewhere in order to take advantage of special expertise.

Each of the states has a Crippled Children's or Handicapped Children's program with wide variation in funding and in definition of who is eligible for care. Naturally, when funds are supplied by a state, there is a tendency to require expenditures within the state. In New England, this results in a series of compromises because the states are small, distances are short, and movement of patients across state borders is common.

There are a number of helpful private organizations. Perhaps most interesting is Parents and Children Together (PACT), an organization formed to learn about and to influence the care of children with congenital heart disease. Summer camps for children with heart defects and special recreational groups for children who are handicapped are found where the population is large and are perhaps a good substitute for simply knowing another family whose child has a similar problem.

Maintaining Competence. The NERICP, because it recorded consecutive symptomatic infants born with congenital heart disease, became a de facto surveillance system for monitoring the care provided in New England. Perhaps the most important finding is that there is a natural tendency for some physicians to remember that results were better than they were. Sometimes there is a tendency to question the validity of monitored data. It is easier to believe that the data are incorrect or that the computer did it than to take seriously the suggestion that treatment may have been suboptimal. If data are to be heeded, they must be unquestionably accurate. Finally, there must be follow-up. Re-evaluation of patients' records is a reliable method of guaranteeing accuracy.

Through trial and error, methods have been developed for acceptable and useful presentation of data. Annual NERICP meetings are held to discuss methods, progress, and controversies about management. On these occasions, the data are extracted for specific topics for the region as a whole, and then, using the same output programs, identical analysis is performed for each hospital. It is useful for each hospital to learn its own results and to have them in a format that can be readily compared with the results of other hospitals in the region.

Who should collect such data? It is the author's opinion that state agencies should not. If figures show a particular hospital is having trouble, a state agency would be required to react even though this might be the first time the hospital had any idea that it was in trouble. On several occasions in recent years, hospitals were noted to be functioning at a statistically poorer level than the region as a whole. In each case, it was apparently not known locally until the data were provided. It does not seem rational to have the difficulties experienced by a hospital known to the government before the hospital learns the news. At the same time, if the state is to subsidize care of the children, it should be mandatory that all experience be submitted to a recognized monitoring system.

Ideally, physicians should monitor themselves. This has worked for NERICP, but whether it might work for comparable groups of physicians elsewhere is unknown. NERICP was formed voluntarily. It is not known what would happen if such an organization were compulsory.

Beyond identification of hospitals having difficulty, data collected are useful for planning where a new clinic should be located, for deciding what facilities a hospital should provide, and for epidemiologic studies. Federal funds substantially in excess of those required to collect NERICP data have been spent on studying the data file or studying retrospectively the patients identified.

There is a need for continuing professional education at all levels. Although surgical teams can learn to do most pediatric cardiac operations well, teams learning new operations must expect to have poor results initially. The problem is that there is not enough patient material for everyone to learn—there may be only enough patients for each team to do one or two operations. Unless limits are set on the number of teams learning these operations, the initial poor results associated with many surgical teams learning new techniques may be a prohibitive burden. To minimize this problem, a possible solution is for surgical societies to set minimum standards for cardiac surgeons who operate on children.

Costs. Medical costs for a child with congenital heart disease are a function of the number of days spent in hospital. Considerable expense is associated with spending several days in specially staffed and equipped hospital areas such as nurseries, intermediate care units, and intensive care units. The data in Table 2 suggest that physicians' fees, the costs of cardiac catheterization, and the ancillary tests are small by comparison with inpatient hospital costs. The costs of follow-up clinics, monitoring the results of care, and transporting patients are negligible. The average per patient units of medical care for NERICP patients and average per patient costs are shown in Table 3.

Table 2. Estimated Charges for Pediatric Cardiac Care (Dollars).

	Hospital	Physician
Outpatient		
Clinic visit	75	50
Electrocardiogram	35	Included in hospital fee
Echocardiogram	100	Included in hospital fee
Sector scan	200	Included in hospital fee
Ambulance	250	
Inpatient		
Intensive care nursery/day	750	—
Hospital bed/day	250	—
Cardiac catheterization	1,370	500
Cardiac operating room	1,500	2,000
Cardiac intensive care/day	890	100/day

Note: Data taken from the Boston area in 1980.

Table 3. Average Units of Medical Care and Costs of Infant Heart Disease, 1968–1973.

Medical Care	Birth–1 Year	1–6 Years	Total
Hospital days per patient	23	17	
Catheterizations per patient	1.06	0.75	
Operations per patient	0.55	0.50	
*Costs**			
Per patient	$ 9,000	$ 3,000	$12,000
Per survivor	18,000	12,000	30,000

Source: Nadas, Fyler, and Buckley, 1980.
* These amounts are in 1979 dollars.

NERICP (Fyler, 1980) surveyed the cost of infant cardiac care in New England for 1975. Reported charges varied widely; within the same city, the charge for use of an operating room varied fivefold. Still, total charges per patient varied only twofold among all the New England hospitals. In general, the highest charges were found in hospitals providing the most services and handling the largest number of patients. The lowest charges were found in the most rural states; the highest estimated charges were approximately twice the lowest estimated (rural) charges per patient. When the average days of hospitalization, the average number of cardiac catheterizations, and the average number of operations were multiplied by the charges reported, figures varying from $3,800 to $7,090 for cardiac care in the first year of life were obtained. The costs per survivor were higher, $7,200 to $16,700. It is the author's impression that costs in 1980 were approximately double those estimated in 1975 and would likely double again by the end of 1985.

Even though there have been some changes in the usual medical management, estimations for hospital days, number of cardiac catheterizations, and cardiac operations in the first year of life are comparable for 1970 and 1980. At the present time, cardiac surgeons tend to use reparative surgical operations in infancy so the need for later secondary operation is less than it was in earlier years. Presumably the total costs will be less, and since several of the common defects are now repaired with single operations, it is likely that this consideration is not trivial.

NERICP infants comprise 3 per thousand live-born babies. Because there are 7.5 cardiac patients per thousand live births, costs of managing the additional 4.5 per thousand patients should be considered. Clearly, these patients are less ill, and most are not expected to contribute greatly to overall costs. For these infants' first year, we estimate an average of one day of hospitalization and three clinic visits at a cost of $1,200.

Twenty-eight percent of the patients have other anomalies, 11 percent of which are of major consequence and so may be considered for other funding arrangements. For example, 4 percent of NERICP patients have Down's syndrome, and their expenses could be attributable to either Down's syndrome or congenital heart disease.

Research

The discoveries of basic research in adult heart disease are often useful to children. For example, research in bacterial endocarditis, electrophysiology, myocardial function, effects of drugs, pacemakers, artificial materials used in surgery, artificial valves, and studies of degenerative disease and hypertension produce information useful in caring for children. Although there are categories of cardiovascular research that have no bearing on pediatric problems, such as studies of coronary artery disease, there are also categories of research important to children that have no bearing on the adult, such as embryologic development of the heart. Because research funding for heart disease is largely controlled by individuals with an interest in adults (and correctly so because adult cardiac problems are so numerous), the possibility exists that studies pertinent only to children will be overlooked. Pediatricians have a stake in all cardiovascular research, but for this discussion, emphasis is placed on research of primary or exclusive interest to pediatrics.

Perinatal Patients. The study of the normal and abnormal features of the developing circulation in the fetus and infant may be termed developmental cardiology. Clinial studies of congenital cardiac abnormalities before and after birth and animal studies of the physiology and pharmacology of pre- and postnatal circulation are fundamental to pediatric cardiology. The techniques of cellular and molecular biology should provide a fruitful approach to the study of the developing circulation. For unclear reasons, the use of molecular and cellular techniques of investigation into cardiologic problems has been delayed while progress in cellular biology in other areas of medicine has been rapid.

These methods of study can be used to learn the mechanisms of normal function in the developing heart and, even more important, the mechanisms resulting in malformation of the heart.

A number of important areas of inquiry should be pursued. They include: (1) the cellular and molecular mechanisms concerned with the circulatory changes from intrauterine to extrauterine life, (2) the mechanisms affecting differences in response to drugs in the fetus, newborn, and infant, (3) appropriate treatment of the newborn with congenital heart failure, (4) epidemiologic factors associated with congenital malformations, (5) the syndrome of persistent fetal circulation, and (6) improved methods, both before and after birth, of cardiac diagnosis such as the techniques of ultrasound, nuclear magnetic resonance, dynamic spatial reconstruction, and Doppler echograms.

Older Children. The response of the growing child to a replacement valve is quite different from that of the adult. The basic processes behind this problem should be studied. Disturbances of heart rhythm following cardiac surgery are not common; nor are spontaneous rhythm disturbances in children common. Still, these problems are frequent enough to suggest the use of newly available electrophysiologic techniques in managing these patients.

Recommendations for Public Policy

Who Should Pay? It is unimaginable that the average family can pay the usual charges for workup and surgery for a child with heart disease. Short of some universal insurance plan, it will be necessary to rely on Medicaid, the Crippled Children's Services, and private insurance plans.

Organization. Regional organization of facilities for children with heart disease should be encouraged. Such an organization involves several hospitals managing a minimum of 1,000 new patients in the region per year. Its basic purpose is to pool resources for the care of the many diverse forms of congenital heart disease. Such an organization should be formally tied to state, federal, and voluntary programs that have overlapping interests. Control should be vested in the physicians.

Systematic monitoring of patient experience can provide evidence for comparative success or failure of treatment. The identified patients could form the basis for clinical research projects.

Shared computing facilities are needed to accomplish monitoring and epidemiologic and systematic follow-up studies. A network of computers that can serve pediatric cardiology needs could also serve for all regional needs in management of rare and uncommon pediatric diseases.

A regional organization can assist in interstate transfer of patients, and in resolution of jurisdictional problems among medical schools, among hospitals, and among states. It can put on educational programs, organize outlying clinics, and assist and encourage the parents of children with congenital heart disease.

It is unlikely that all regions of the United States can overcome animosities built up over years of competition among hospitals or that a single hospital monopoly built up through cooperation with its state and medical school will readily pool its resources with adjoining hospitals in other states. Still, the advantages for the patients, the hospitals, and medical science are sufficiently great that, despite contrary forces, funding patterns that promote this form of organization should be undertaken.

Basic Research. Pediatric cardiologists of the 1980s should concern themselves with developmental cardiology, with the normal and abnormal mechanisms in formation of the heart, as well as the normal and abnormal pharmacophysiology of the developing circulation of the fetus and newborn. The expanding knowledge of molecular and cellular biology can be applied to the following types of problems with reasonable expectation of progress: What is the cellular or molecular basis for the observed physiology of the fetus and newborn? Why is there a difference between newborn and older infants? What are the basic mechanisms behind abnormal development of the heart in congenital heart disease? Can these mechanisms be safely altered?

This focus is not suggested to the exclusion of more conventional basic studies, such as the effects of pharmacologic agents in various age groups, of calcium deposition in blood vessels, studies of lipoproteins and atherosclerosis in children, and studies of rhythm disturbances. Rather, it is proposed that Project Program Grants or Specialized Centers of Research for children with heart disease should have this theme.

Clinical Research. A number of clinical research projects are of prime interest to pediatric cardiologists. The first pertains to diagnostic methods, such as pulsed Doppler echocardiograms, digital subtraction angiography, and imaging by nuclear magnetic resonance. Prenatal diagnostic examination of the fetus should be encouraged. It is imaginable that in the future all babies with prenatally recognized abnormalities will be born in specially equipped and staffed centers. The methods of nuclear magnetic resonance may allow indirect measurement of specific biochemical processes within the living child. If this possibility becomes a reality, the research possibilities are unlimited.

Second, the effect of drugs used during the pre- and post-natal periods should be systematically studied because the effects, the excretion, and the uptake may be different from those in the adult.

Follow-up, for ten to thirty years, is important for surviving children. This is needed if future surgical planning is to be done on a rational basis. Otherwise, prophylactic cardiac surgery to prevent late difficulty in the otherwise well child may be no more scientific than circumcision.

Implementation of Recommendations. It is the author's opinion that programs combining research and patient service are not readily managed by present federal funding organizations. A program including research support and patient care support has the interesting difficulty that one or the other funding agency may disagree. Service programs with associated research tend naturally to favor service, while research programs with associated service tend to favor research. The author favors joint consideration of mixed programs of service and research by a committee of the two types of funding agencies.

The success of the Crippled Children's Services in developing and maintaining high quality medical care for children requires recognition and continued support.

The present NIH system for handling research projects, whether basic or clinical research, has been quite successful. No change is suggested. It is expected that individual grants will continue to be judged on their merits. To promote developmental cardiology, it is proposed that several Specialized Centers of Research grants in developmental cardiology be awarded to pediatric cardiac centers. These programs should be awarded to centers with a demonstrated critical mass of patients and physicians, with creditable clinical and basic research, and with an associated regional organization so a broad impact can be predicted.

How much money should be spent on these programs? Clearly this is a political budgetary decision. Without research, there will be little progress, while unbridled research has no limit in cost. In assessing expenditures for children, it should be remembered that successful management of the small infant may result in a near-normal life span. Therefore, on the basis of years of productive life that result from treatment of congenital heart disease, a greater expenditure for research in pediatric heart disease is appropriate. Successful prevention of congenital heart disease would eliminate the need for pediatric cardiology and surgery.

References

Carlgren, L. E. "The Incidence of Congenital Heart Disease in Gothenburg." *Proceedings of the Association for European Pediatric Cardiology*, 1969, *5*, 2–8.

Fyler, D. C. "Report of the New England Regional Infant Cardiac Program." *Pediatrics*, 1980, *65* (Supplement), 375–461.

Fyler, D. C., and others. "The Determinants of Five Year Survival of Infants with Critical Congenital Heart Disease." In A. N. Brest and M. A. Engle (Eds.), *Pediatric Cardiovascular Disease: Cardiovascular Clinics*. Philadelphia: F.A. Davis, 1981.

Fyler, D. C., and others. "Assessment of Survivors of Critical Congenital Heart Disease." Unpublished data. 1982.

Mitchell, S. C., Korones, S. B., and Berendes, H. W. "Congenital Heart Disease in 56,109 Births: Incidence and Natural History." *Circulation*, 1971, *43*, 323–332.

Nadas, A. S., Fyler, D. C., and Buckley, L. P. "Outcome of Early Management of Infants with Critical Heart Disease." Paper presented at World Congress of Pediatric Cardiology, London, June 1980.

Rothman, K. J., and Fyler, D. C. "Association of Congenital Heart Defects with Season and Population Density." *Teratology*, 1976, *13*, 29–34.

Rothman, K. J., and others. "Exogenous Hormones and Other Drug Exposures of Children with Congenital Heart Disease." *American Journal of Epidemiology*, 1979, *109*, 433–439.

Rowe, R. D., and others. *The Neonate with Congenital Heart Disease.* Philadelphia: Saunders, 1981.

Subcommittee on Standards, American Academy of Pediatrics. "Guidelines for Pediatric Cardiology Diagnostic and Treatment Centers." *Pediatrics,* 1978, *62,* 258–261.

Weinstein, M. R. "Lithium Teratogenesis: The Register of Lithium Babies." In T. B. Cooper and others (Eds.), *Lithium: Controversies and Unresolved Issues.* Lawrenceville, N.J.: Exerpta Medica-Princeton, 1979.

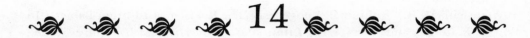

14

Chronic Kidney Diseases

Barbara Korsch, M.D.
Richard Fine, M.D.

Chronic kidney disease in children is relatively rare and usually survivable thanks to recent advances in dialysis and organ transplantation. However, current treatment cannot always avoid the potentially devastating side effects of long-term renal disease in children, notably bone disease and growth retardation. Complications of the disease, coupled with the massive financial demands of treatment, can put tremendous stresses on the young victims and their families. Federal law, passed in 1972, entitled every U.S. citizen, regardless of age, to reimbursement of the cost of chronic kidney disease under Medicare. Yet, despite support by the federal government and by many public and private agencies, there remain important gaps in services for children with kidney disease.

Description of the Disorder

Chronic kidney disease can be defined as an irreversible abnormality of kidney function. Normally, the kidney performs numerous functions: it maintains a fluid balance by controlling salt and water; it plays a pivotal role in the metabolism of various hormones, such as those involved in calcium absorption and red-blood-cell production; and it excretes the waste products of protein metabolism. Although a disease process may affect certain functions of the kidney, most kidney disorders produce damage to all of them. Compromise of the excretory function, however, is potentially the most dangerous because the retained products of protein metabolism cause harm to various organs and can lead to death.

Children with a disease process affecting the kidney may manifest either a consistent impairment of or a progressively declining kidney function. It is important to detect the presence of impaired kidney function in children in order to initiate measures to forestall subsequent decline in kidney function and to minimize the potentially devastating clinical consequences of bone disease and growth retardation. In addition, identification of the child with chronic renal failure is necessary for optimal planning of future treatment.

During the past two decades, the outlook for treatment of children with irreversible renal insufficiency or end-stage renal disease (ESRD) has changed dramatically from one of frank pessimism to cautious optimism. This change has resulted from the development of two therapeutic modalities: dialysis and transplantation. Following our discussion of the disease itself—its epidemiology, etiology, and course—we focus on these treatment strategies. Subsequent sections of the chapter deal with costs of care, psychosocial factors, and the role of social institutions in the care of these children and their families. The final section presents our recommendations for an appropriate public response to the dilemmas posed by ESRD in children.

Epidemiology. The incidence of ESRD in children is relatively low compared with that of the adult population. Depending upon the criteria utilized for accumulating the incidence data, the number of children presenting yearly with ESRD varies from less than 1 to 3.5 per million persons (Scharer, 1971; Meadow, Cameron, and Ogg, 1970). In contrast, the number of adult patients presenting yearly with ESRD varies from less than 45 to more than 100 per million children.

The discrepant incidence data reported in children are attributable to the age of patients included in the data and to the demographic data utilized. If children less than one year of age and those more than fifteen years of age are included, the incidence is higher. Similarly, if only those children who present to a pediatric facility for ESRD care within a specific catchment area are included, the incidence will be lower because those children who died without the opportunity to initiate ESRD care would not be included in the data.

With the passage in May 1972 of H.R. 1, which entitled all individuals in this country, regardless of age, to reimbursement for ESRD care under Medicare, the availability of ESRD care for children has increased markedly. Together with widespread dissemination of information concerning the availability of ESRD care for children to the lay public as well as to the medical community, the lack of financial constraints has facilitated treatment being offered to almost every child with ESRD. Such circumstances do not exist in those parts of the world where financial constraints limit the availability of care. Incidence data from such countries would obviously be an underestimate.

Etiology. The etiology of ESRD in children is somewhat different from that of adult patients and can be broadly categorized into (1) congenital or hereditary disorders and (2) acquired disorders. The congenital or hereditary diseases occur in slightly less than one half of the children with ESRD; however, the single most common problem is a congenital problem, obstructive uropathy (blockage of urine flow from the kidneys) (Habib, Broyer, and Benmaiz, 1973). Acquired lesions primarily involve glomerulonephritis, an inflammatory process of the glomerulus (a basic working element of the kidney where blood is initially filtered to remove wastes) that results in scarring and either a slow or rapid decline in kidney function.

Although the lesions producing obstructive uropathy may occur with increased frequency in some families, the factors that could lead to the development of such lesions are poorly understood, and specific genetic or environmental factors have not been implicated. Of the three most frequent hereditary diseases that ultimately lead to ESRD in children (Alport's syndrome, polycystic kidney disease, and cystinosis) the exact mode of transmission is known only for cystinosis.

A specific etiology for the acquired glomerular diseases leading to ESRD is unknown, with the exception of lupus nephritis. In many instances, an immunologic etiology is inferred from in vitro tests and histologic examination of kidney tissue; however, the specific course of these glomerular diseases remains unknown, and the risk factors have not been delineated.

Course. The course of chronic renal disease in children varies according to etiology. Children affected with congenital lesions are usually born with nephrons (the functioning unit of the kidney) that are either inadequate in number or that function abnormally. These children manifest a slowly progressive downhill course with ultimate development of ESRD at the time when the metabolic needs of the individual are not adequately met by the number of functioning nephrons. In contrast, children with acquired glomerular disease either (1) present with ESRD without prior evidence of renal disease and have a rapid decline in kidney function once clinical symptoms lead to diagnosis or (2) have a prolonged course of kidney disease with stable function followed by a rapid decline once function begins to deteriorate.

Certain factors may influence the rate of functional deterioration. The child with an anatomic obstruction to the flow of urine and dysplastic kidneys may benefit from early correction of the defect. Similarly, children with anatomic abnormalities that predispose to recurrent infection may benefit from careful monitoring for the presence of infection and assiduous attempts to maintain urine sterility. Secondary hypertension will lead to further deterioration of kidney function. Prompt treatment of the hypertension may forestall the rapidity of functional deterioration. Recently, some experimental evidence has shown that hyperphosphatemia and elevated calcium phosphorus product leads to the deposition of calcium phosphate in the kidney that contributes to a decline in kidney function (Ibels and others, 1978). Dietary counseling resulting in lower serum phosphorus level may also lessen the decline in kidney function.

The two most devastating consequences of chronic renal disease in children are the development of bone disease with associated deformities that may prevent adequate ambulation and impaired growth and sexual development with its profound effects on psychosocial adaptation. Assiduous monitoring of various biochemical and radiological parameters of bone disease and prompt therapeutic intervention with Vitamin D and calcium supplementation and antacids to control the serum phosphorus level are helpful in preventing and reversing the development of bone disease (Norman, 1982). This treatment can be administered by a primary physician in consultation with a pediatric nephrologist at a tertiary unit. However, supportive personnel must be available to give adequate psychosocial support in assuring adherence to the therapeutic regimen.

Numerous factors have been implicated in the etiology of growth retardation in children with chronic renal disease (Fine, 1984). The one prominent factor that is potentially correctable is energy intake. Children with chronic renal disease are anorectic and in general consume inadequate calories. Dietary counseling by a sympathetic and knowledgeable dietician is helpful in improving the caloric intake. Additional factors of acidosis and renal osteodystrophy (bone disease) are potentially correctable with careful monitoring of various biochemical parameters. Unfortunately, despite optimal medical and dietary management, it is likely that the child with chronic renal disease will suffer from growth retardation and delayed development of secondary sex characteristics. Psychosocial support for the child and family is important in order to enhance adaptation and prevent maladjustive behavior.

Treatment

The treatment of chronic renal disease can be categorized into (1) treatment directed toward either reversing the primary disease process or preventing deterioration of kidney function, (2) treatment directed toward the secondary medical consequences of chronic renal disease, and (3) treatment directed toward supporting or replacing the kidney once ESRD has developed. In this section we discuss requirements for treatment.

Reversing Disease Process or Preventing Deterioration. Various therapeutic regimens utilizing immunosuppressive drugs have been proposed to forestall the progression to renal failure of various glomerular diseases. With few exceptions, notably membranous nephropathy in adult patients, these regimens have yet to be proven efficacious in controlled therapeutic trials (Coggins and others, 1979). Therefore, once significant glomerular disease occurs, it is unlikely that the course of the disease can be changed.

Surgical correction of congenital obstructive lesions is helpful in maintaining stability of renal function; however, the ultimate fate of children with such lesions is dependent on the degree of dysplasia—that is, on the number of residual intact functioning nephrons (Glassberg and Filmer, 1984). Similarly, prevention of recurrent bacterial infection of the kidney, either by chemoprophylaxis or by correction of ureterovesical reflux, is helpful in minimizing the development of chronic renal disease. In addition, as previously indicated, normalization of calcium and phosphorus metabolism and control of hypertension may have a salutory effect on the rate of progression of renal failure.

Treating Secondary Medical Problems. Many organ systems are adversely effected by the uremic milieu. Treatment is nonspecific and usually ineffectual. The major facet of therapy is directed toward dietary manipulation to attempt to minimize the intake to a level that can be handled by the reduction in kidney function. Adequate dietary and psychosocial support are advantageous in formulating the diet and assuring compliance.

Treatment Following ESRD Onset. Once ESRD has occurred, the child and family members have two primary options: conservative treatment or active ESRD care. Conservative treatment is essentially treatment of secondary problems and the reduction of pain and suffering. Active ESRD care involves dialysis or kidney transplantation.

The rigors of coping with an active ESRD care program may be difficult for some patients and families. This is especially true of children with moderate and severe degrees of mental retardation and those with significant psychoemotional disturbances. Such children adapt less well to the demands of the ESRD care regimen. Parents may elect conservative management in such circumstances. Since conservative treatment will ultimately lead to death, it is important that the family be given maximum psychosocial support in implementing their decision. A similar situation exists with parents of infants or very young children affected by ESRD. Although ESRD care is technically feasible in such children, the long-term outcome is rather bleak. Therefore, parents may choose conservative therapy. Again, significant psychosocial support is necessary in assisting the parents in carrying out their decision.

Active ESRD care is potentially life-saving and consists of dialysis and transplantation. There are two types of dialysis currently available: hemodialysis and peritoneal dialysis. Hemodialysis is the extracorporeal perfusion of an "artificial kidney" with blood to remove certain metabolic substances that are retained by the body because of reduced kidney function. The artificial kidney also permits removal of retained fluid that cannot be excreted because of decreased kidney function. In order to perform the procedure, a vascular access must be available to facilitate repeated access to the patient's blood.

The dialysis procedure is typically carried out thrice weekly for periods of four to six hours. Depending upon the age of the patient and the competence of the parents, the hemodialysis procedure can be carried out in a specialized center or the parents can be trained to undertake the procedure at home. For small children, specially trained personnel are mandatory.

Peritoneal dialysis utilizes the patient's peritoneal membrane for dialysis. Fluid is inserted into the peritoneal cavity and substances that are retained in the blood because of reduced kidney function diffuse into the peritoneal cavity. By varying the osmotic concentration of the peritoneal dialysate, fluid can be removed during the procedure. Repeated access to the peritoneal cavity is obtained by a permanent indwelling peritoneal catheter.

Peritoneal dialysis is especially suited for home dialysis. Intermittent peritoneal dialysis utilizes a machine to generate sterile dialysate and cycles the fluid into the peritoneal cavity. The procedure is performed thrice weekly for periods of ten to twelve hours. Since access to blood is not necessary, it is technically rather simple and can be used for small children at home with minimal risk.

A new adaptation of peritoneal dialysis is continuous ambulatory peritoneal dialysis (CAPD) (Popovich and others, 1976). This adaptation approaches a wearable artificial kidney. Dialysate is instilled into the peritoneum four to five times daily, seven days a week, and dialysis proceeds continuously. No machines are required and the use of plastic bags, which can be easily attached to the body when empty, minimizes the number of connections. With this procedure, the patient is totally mobile and requires minimal professional assistance. The only obstacle to increased utilization of this procedure is the incidence of peritonitis.

Successful renal transplantation restores normal renal function and has the potential of permitting the child to have a normal life (Ettenger and others, 1979). The kidney for transplantation may come from a live, related donor or a cadaver donor. Live, related donors are still used because the success rate remains superior (Gradus and Ettenger, 1982). The major impediment to successful transplantation is immunologic rejection. The body recognizes the foreign antigens of the kidney transplant and attempts to eliminate them (rejection). Various therapeutic regimens can minimize the rejection phenomenon. Currently, however, no regimen is totally successful. Because all the regimens are nonspecific and therefore decrease the body's immune reaction to any foreign substance, the patient has an increased susceptibility to infection. With our current methods of immunosuppression, the five-year graft survival for a kidney from a live, related donor is approximately 75 percent and from a cadaver donor, 40 percent. If the initial transplant is unsuccessful, it is possible for the patient to obtain a subsequent graft. Success rates with second and third cadaver-donor transplants approach that of first cadaver-donor transplants (Fine and others, 1977). Technically, kidney transplantation is possible for most children afflicted with ESRD; however, success remains limited because of the inability to totally suppress the rejection phenomenon.

Requirements for Treatment. Drugs used in the treatment of chronic kidney disease can be categorized as follows: (1) immunosuppressive drugs (prednisone, cyclophosphamide), which are used to prevent progressive deterioration of glomerular disease; (2) antibiotics (ampicillin, trimethoprim-sulfa, Furadantin), which are used to both treat and prevent urinary tract bacterial infections; (3) Vitamin D analogues (Dihydrotachysterol, Rocaltrol), calcium supplementation (calcium gluconate, Os-cal), and antacids (Amphogel, Basaljel, Dialume) to both treat and prevent renal bone disease; (4) antihypertensive drugs (Apresoline, Minipress, Aldomet, Minoxidil, Captoril) and diuretics (Diuril, furosemide) to control hypertension; (5) folic acid and vitamin supplements to supplement dietary restrictions; (6) immunosuppressive drugs to both treat and prevent rejection (prednisone, azathioprine, antilymphocyte serum, cyclosporin).

Dietary restrictions are mandatory to prevent various complications of uremia. These include sodium and fluid restriction to prevent hypertension and congestive heart failure, potassium restriction to prevent hyperkalemia and heart arrhythmias, phosphorus restriction and calcium supplementation to treat and prevent bone disease, caloric supplementation to enhance growth, and protein restriction to limit uremic symptomatology. A highly competent, sympathetic dietician is required to formulate a palatable diet that takes into consideration the individual's preferences and ethnic and social situation.

For the most part, the dialysis equipment in general use for adult patients is utilized for children. However, specially designed devices for vascular and peritoneal access, which are available, are necessary for small children (Nevins and Mauer, 1984). Similarly, special adaptation of existing dialyzer equipment is required for treatment of small children. Whereas only one dialysate bag size is adequate for all adult patients undergoing CAPD, it was necessary to develop at least two or three bag sizes in order to offer this treatment modality to all children (Salusky and others, 1982).

In order to provide comprehensive treatment for children afflicted with chronic kidney disease and their families, it is necessary to have a multidisciplinary group of individuals available to deal with the numerous complex problems that may arise. The coordinator of such a multidisciplinary team is usually a pediatric nephrologist with specialized training in pediatrics and subspecialty training in pediatric nephrology. Evidence of competence is certification by the American Board of Pediatrics and the Subspecialty Board of Pediatric Nephrology. Additional physicians with specialized training in pediatric surgery and urology are required.

Needed allied health professionals with specialized skills and training in dealing with chronically ill children include nursing personnel with special skills in utilization of dialysis equipment, a medical social worker with specific knowledge of ESRD regulations as well as access to community resources, and a dietician with specialized skills in treatment of patients with chronic renal disease. In addition, the availability of medical and associated medical personnel to support patients and families and to assist in the many psychosocial problems that are present in children and families with chronic renal disease is highly desirable.

A tertiary clinical facility is necessary to provide a coordinative role in the management of a child with chronic renal disease. Such a facility must have the personnel and equipment previously described in order to plan and implement an optimal treatment plan for such children. In all probability, a tertiary center that meets the described requirements could serve a population of approximately five million. However, depending on the demography, it is necessary for the tertiary facility to coordinate care with the primary physician and allied health professionals who are in close proximity to the patient's home. Liaison with primary physicians will optimize patient care and minimize traveling to the tertiary facility.

Costs. It is difficult to estimate the annual cost of caring for a child with chronic renal disease. Factors that influence the cost are (1) degree of renal insufficiency, (2) necessity of one or many surgical procedures, and (3) development of potential complications. In a child with stable or slowly progressive chronic renal disease who does not require any surgical procedure during the specific year in question, it is probable that the cost of medical care is between $5,000 and $10,000. As the child approaches ESRD, the annual cost will escalate because the need for medical attention will increase.

Hemodialysis thrice weekly in a center costs approximately $25,000 yearly. However, the actual cost is significantly higher because the cost of medication, physician's fees, and hospitalization is not included in this figure. The cost of thrice weekly peritoneal dialysis in a center is considerably higher because involvement of nursing personnel is required for a longer period of time. Home hemodialysis, home peritoneal dialysis, and CAPD costs approximately $12,000 to $15,000 annually per patient. These figures are also an underestimate because medications, physician's fees, and hospitalization are not included.

The cost of the transplant procedure and the initial year of follow-up care is approximately $25,000. However, the cost may exceed $100,000 if significant complications arise. If the transplant is successful, the cost of treatment during successive years is $5,000 to $10,000 and decreases with time as long as kidney function does not deteriorate.

Stress on Child and Family

There is increasing evidence that any chronic illness in childhood is stressful for both child and family. Yet, chronic renal disease also has its specific effects. From either vantage point, however, it is clear that actual disabilities are sometimes less significant in determining overall adaptation than are the period in the child's growth and development, the child's own personality, the interpersonal relationship and communication pattern in the family, and the attitude of significant persons in the child's life toward the illness and treatment (Korsch, 1958). In this section, we cover briefly some of the general stress of childhood chronic illness and discuss in some detail the stresses peculiar to ESRD.

Nonspecific Stress from Chronic Illness in Childhood. The most helpful approach to evaluating the effects of illness on a young child is first to consider the crucial developmental task and the basic needs for each developmental stage and second to determine how they are influenced by the experiences with the illness and its treatment (Prugh, 1963). Thus, for infants and very young children, the single greatest stress results from the medical need for many separations from the family. This stress is exaggerated by repeated hospitalizations and the exposure to a multiplicity of caretakers. In addition to maternal deprivation or its equivalent, there may be periods of environmental deprivation, as in the intensive care unit or isolation ward of a hospital, which can be very traumatic. Finally, the gratification of being fed when hungry and of having a normal sucking experience is often interfered with by the need for restricted intake or even omission of oral feedings for periods of time. This disruption of the feeding pattern that constitutes such an essential feature of mother-child interaction in the first year of life can lead to deviant development.

Toddlers and young preschool children have their own set of vulnerabilities. Separation is still highly traumatic; in addition, restraint of movement is especially hard on these young children, because locomotion is only developing and these children must test their own power against the world. Toddlers and preschoolers cherish their autonomy above all and are often offended and embarrassed by the degree to which illness and treatment forces them into passivity. Toilet training is often in progress at this stage and may be disturbed by changes in care-taking routines or in sphincter function itself.

The child between three and six years of age suffers from the above stresses and, in addition, is preoccupied with even minor physical injury, blemish, or loss. These children are prone to blame themselves and feel guilty over real or fancied bad deeds or bad thoughts. In this age group, the limited fantasy life and imagination all tend to exaggerate the impact of illness and treatment. These children also have no assurance that painful experiences will ever stop, that assaults by caretakers have any predictable limits, or that the dreary, lonely life in the hospital will ever definitely come to an end.

By the time these children reach school age they tend to become better patients for the caretaking establishment, as well as for themselves. They have more resources; they know what "tomorrow" means and that their parents most probably will not abandon them completely. They can express themselves verbally and can understand what they are told. Although insulted by what is done to them, they also know what they are capable of doing on their own. Increased reliance on peers, siblings, and friends can serve as a source of strength and support during illness in and out of the hospital. On the other hand, children with chronic illness suffer from isolation from peers, school absences, and inability to play and compete physically.

During adolescence, physical illness presents another complex set of psychologic crises (Hamburg, 1983). Adolescents are self-conscious about their bodies and constantly worry lest they do not measure up to their peers. Chronic illness of any kind will inevitably cause a number of frustrations in this respect. Adolescents are shy and especially protective of their privacy. Medical and surgical treatment, with frequent exposure, constant inspection and palpation of body surface, and exploration of various body orifices, contribute to destroying the sense of privacy in these patients. Sexual development, crucial at this developmental stage, often does not proceed normally. When denied the opportunity for normal emancipation, adolescents may have an exaggerated need to rebel. In sick adolescents, this rebellion may be channeled toward the medical treatment. Finally, in adolescence, more than in other age groups, a peer group is the source of reference, support, and meaning in life. The adolescent with a severe illness is often deprived of normal social life, and this may constitute the single most devastating aspect of the illness experience. Normal adolescents achieve a measure of independence from their parents, and this is often impossible for the sick adolescent, at least at the appropriate age.

Temperament and other pre-existing personality attributes of individual children influence in large measure their experience with chronic illness (Korsch and others, 1973). There are certain children who on the basis of a sense of basic trust, security, self-confidence, and competence, cope well with illness. Others, especially those who come from deprived backgrounds and less supportive family situations, may be overwhelmed by fears and depression when they develop chronic physical illness. The better endowed the child is with previous experience, intelligence, good self-esteem, ability to communicate, and competence, the more likely that child can cope and adapt well, no matter how stressful the experience that must be undergone.

Chronic illness in a child is stressful to all members of the family (Korsch and others, 1973). There are no manifestations specific to this kind of stress, but illness usually presents a number of practical and financial burdens that tend to make family life less pleasurable. The parents tend to be less available to each other and to the siblings of the sick child. Siblings, often given less parental attention, are prone to use deviant behavior to attract parental concern. The relationships, communication patterns, and feelings observed in families when a child is ill are usually not essentially different from those existing prior to the child's illness; however, pre-existing problems may become more severe when there is severe stress, and potential conflicts may manifest themselves for the first time.

Specific Stresses of Kidney Disease. In addition to nonspecific features of chronic illness in childhood, there are a number of problems inherent in renal disease and its treatment that have specific implications for child development and family functioning (Korsch and others, 1971). One troublesome aspect of any renal disease, with impairment of renal function, is the *uncertainty* concerning course and prognosis. This uncertainty is difficult even for the physician to deal with, and it certainly creates confusion and added anxiety in patient and family. As a result, a sick child is often handled inconsistently.

In instances in which kidney disease appears abruptly and leads to sudden renal failure, a predictable set of psychological problems arises. With no forewarning of anything being wrong, it is extremely difficult for patient and family to accept the diagnosis and reality of ESRD. Under these circumstances, the patient's reaction to the diagnosis is similar to those described with any catastrophic illness, such as childhood leukemia. Unfortunately, if renal failure develops rapidly, it may be necessary to institute drastic treatment without preparation of patient and family. Bilateral nephrectomy and kidney transplantation may be required before the family or the patient have reached the point of accepting the devastating diagnosis. Serious problems in management develop unless the medical team is attuned to the adaptation problems manifested by patient and family.

A specific feature of renal disease is the anatomic *location* of the abnormality. All considerations of the genotourinary tract are burdened with emotional overlay and irrational fears. The combination of sexual and excretory functions associated with the genitourinary system lead to embarrassment and exaggerated guilt feelings for patient and family. Procedures such as instrumentation, specimen collection, and surgical intervention assume undue importance for patients and family. Loss of control of urination, which causes anxieties in persons of all ages, is more acute in age groups where sphincter control is a more recent accomplishment.

Fear of sexual impotence is ubiquitous among adolescents and young adults. It is often exaggerated in the presence of a malfunctioning genitourinary system. Living in close contact with, and awareness of, one's own waste products is an embarrassment and may be the source of extreme distress, shame, and anxiety in some families. Some children and young people are excluded from school activities and all socialization because of disturbing smells or cosmetic problems related to their genitourinary tract. All these complications of genitourinary disease are magnified in those unfortunate patients who have to live with indwelling catheters, neophrostomy tubes, urine collecting bags, or worse yet, some sort of abnormal collecting system, such as an ileal loop, colostomy, or other unusual anatomical contrivance.

A major complication of long-term renal disease is growth failure and bone disease. The short stature, abnormal gait, and at times, grotesque deformities resulting from abnormal calcium and phosphorus metabolism in the patient with renal disease, are a source of anguish to patient and family. High school students have to face classmates and younger siblings who tower above them. Physically awkward or even grossly handicapped youngsters with normal ambitions in terms of competitive sports and physical prowess can be devastated by their progressive deformities and disabilities, as well as by their persistent failure to grow in stature and stamina. Since medical and surgical treatment for these problems is limited, it is essential that children and families be given maximal support in dealing with these physical disabilities. Patients with renal disease, even more than in some other chronic illness, have additional assaults on body image and self-esteem (Korsch and Barnett, 1961). First, the waxing and waning of edema contributes to the children's perceptions of their bodies as troublesome and unreliable objects. The alternation between grotesque swelling, especially around the abdomen and the eyes, and the wasted, puny appearance that results from diuresis undermines such children's confidence in themselves as physical persons. In addition, side effects of corticosteroids exaggerate the distorted body image of such patients.

A perplexing problem for the health care team treating a child with renal disease that leads to psychosocial complications is the variable course and difficulty in assessing the degree of disability or malaise at a particular moment (Korsch and others, 1971). It is extremely important for the treatment team and family to be aware that there are many reactive behavior disturbances that are related to physiologic changes. Such physiological symptoms may alter the child's behavior unfavorably.

The specific treatment measures required for renal disease have their own set of psychological implications for the growing child. The instrumentation and manipulation involved in the diagnosis and treatment of genitourinary conditions, especially in cases of obstructive uropathy, are painful, embarrassing, and intrusive. Young boys, especially, forced to grow up with catheters and tubes inserted in various natural orifices or iatrogenic surgical openings, have special problems with their body image in general and with their masculinity in particular (Korsch and others, 1973). These difficulties are exaggerated by the tactless approaches of caretakers walking to the bedside and removing bedcovers and dressings, and exposing the vulnerable area to a group of bystanders. The care of stomata or catheters often involves mother and child in close physical manipulation that may place inappropriate encumbrances on the parent-child relationship, especially when the patient is a boy.

Diet restriction and limited fluid intake during certain stages of treatment can be very difficult for the child. Some older children undergoing dialysis become intensively concerned with their intake; others endanger their comfort, and even their lives, by overindulgence in fluids and foods containing excessive sodium and potassium. In the younger child, the restricted diet may become the focus of parent-child conflict, disciplinary problems, and general discord. The child's increased well-being, coupled with corticosteroid medications, tends to make for greatly increased appetite, excessive weight gain, and often severe obesity. There have been individual patients who are so discouraged by their grotesque appearance, their failure to lose weight in spite of repeated valiant efforts to do so, and the social and interpersonal difficulties resulting from their appearance that they welcome the loss of the transplanted kidney and return to dialysis and their former, more attractive physical proportions.

The specific treatment modalities that have powerful social and emotional implications are dialysis and transplantation. The enforced confinement and passivity of patients on hemodialysis and intermittent peritoneal dialysis, the interruption of their daily routines, the awareness of complete dependency on dialysis for life, all produce a wide spectrum of psychological reactions in children and their families. The emotional implications of transplantation are myriad. Even without dealing with the unconscious fantasies associated with the presence of another's organ in the patient's body or with donor-recipient relationships, a number of serious emotional problems are frequently observed. Anxieties concerning rejection of the kidney are never-ending and paramount. Problems caused by attempts at re-entry into a normal social life at home and at school after a prolonged sick-role behavior need to be faced. Family equilibrium can be upset if there has been a live, related family donor. Siblings may show severe emotional reactions. Disfiguring side effects of corticosteroids may be so severe that individual patients, especially female adolescents, may interrupt their corticosteroid therapy against medical advice and risk graft failure (Korsch, Fine, and Negrete, 1978).

Follow-up studies have been undertaken at one dialysis and transplant program at Childrens Hospital of Los Angeles on 135 patients following transplantation. The methods used were systematic interviews with the child and family, personality testing, and clinical assessment. In spite of severe and serious problems encountered by these patients, these studies showed that after one year or more following transplantation, most children and their families had returned to pre-illness adaptation and family equilibrium. These observations were made under conditions where continued attention and support was provided for the patients and family by a comprehensive health care team. Under other conditions, long-term outcome might be less favorable.

Demands and Challenges to Public Institutions

The current treatment modalities for children with ESRD and their families pose dramatic challenges to institutions and agencies. These challenges and demands change as new treatment modalities are devised, as financing is altered, and as the survival and quality of life for patients and families change as a result of innovative treatment approaches.

The challenges to the community vary according to the population served. For example, isolated minority populations, lower socioeconomic groups, and multiproblem families require special programs and additional assistance in coping with problems resulting from ESRD. Over a thirteen-year period of treating children at Childrens Hospital of Los Angeles, there was a marked increase in children from the most deprived segments of the community in our sample, and this was reflected in the increasingly heavy burden on the treatment team as well as on the community. The intact middle-class families and their children usually were able to mount a credible independent effort in relation to financing, support systems, and transportation; they were also able to coordinate the complex surgical and medical care. This was not the case for the single-parent family or the impoverished, unemployed, disorganized families who were heavily dependent on the various community support services. The presence of chronic illness adds to the stresses of their daily life, and they become increasingly dependent financially on governmental agencies.

The financial requirements of patients and families are tremendous. With few exceptions, individual families cannot cover the cost of treatment of ESRD. Improved technology can produce some economy, as is proposed for CAPD, but no matter which kind of combination of therapies is chosen, the cost and expense will overwhelm the patient and family. These costs have to be met by either governmental or community agencies. Categorical programs either on the national or regional level have traditionally covered the largest amount of patient care expenses. But when the cost of research and program development is added, federal and local government agencies must again play a significant role. Voluntary agencies and philanthropic foundations can make a contribution, but this amount will probably never reach sufficient proportions to constitute a major solution to the financial burden imposed by the treatment of ESRD.

ESRD is now the only categorical medical condition for which there is national health insurance in the United States. Those of us who have worked with patients requiring ESRD treatment see the need for this coverage. Yet, we also realize that support for the care of ESRD limits the funds available for other programs focused either on well children or on children with other physical illnesses—illnesses that might require smaller investments producing more tangible long-term results.

In thinking about government and foundation spending related to ESRD care, as in all other aspects of this report, it cannot be overemphasized that anything that could be done to *prevent* the development of renal failure would naturally be the best investment. Treating individual patients can only achieve limited goals.

Furthermore, from a practical standpoint, additional legislative support is required to ensure employment for patients with ESRD who have been rehabilitated and who reach young adulthood where employment is an essential condition for a good quality of life. Legal assurances are necessary to make sure live, related kidney donors will not be discriminated against from the point of view of employment. Additional legislation would be advantageous to assist family planning and childbearing for patients with ESRD.

In addition, legislative and community support should be given to housing that will accommodate home dialysis treatment. Transportation for patients to and from treatment centers needs both financial backing and legislative support. Utilization of home hemodialysis and CAPD, as well as other new treatment modalities, facilitates the ability of patients to lead active lives with assistance from community agencies and institutions.

The responsibility of schools, colleges, and universities in relation to patients with ESRD is twofold: first, these institutions carry the burden of preparing technical and other professional personnel adequately for the actual treatment procedures; second, they must provide access for patients to receive the maximal benefit of education and rehabilitation. Currently, there are many problems related to getting children who are on dialysis into the school system. There are pressures to keep these children on home teaching even though they need to be in a peer group setting. There needs to be education and legislation to make sure that schools and higher educational facilities are open to and will actively seek participation from patients who have been treated for physical illness and who have special needs.

Churches and community organizations need to be mobilized, especially as federal spending for health care becomes less available. A big educational challenge lies in informing relevant groups about the needs and characteristics of the population of patients with ESRD so they can mobilize resources to help patient and family. Typical organizations that need to be involved are the Kidney Foundation as well as other categorical or noncategorical health-related community groups, parent groups, and patient groups.

The media needs to be included in any planning for so needy a group of patients as those with ESRD. A great deal of misinformation is rampant about dialysis and transplant patients. Used well, the media can help correct many of the prevalent misconceptions.

The problem of organ procurement also requires a great deal of attention. In particular, the ethical and moral issues as well as the economic ones involved in transplantation need to be clarified. The laws concerning brain death and organ transplantation need to be revised and disseminated so that opportunities for successful organ transplantation can be optimized.

Recommendations

Children with diseases of the kidney pose unique problems and require specialized facilities and equipment, specifically trained professional personnel, and extra assistance from local community and governmental agencies. When planning health services for children with kidney disease, the aberrations of growth and development, the adverse effects of the family constellation, the age-dependent psychosocial needs, and the technical requirements should all be considered. Any future local, state, or national initiatives directed toward changing the delivery of medical care to patients with kidney disease should include provisions that address the unique problems of pediatric patients.

Although a considerable amount of financial support in the United States is currently provided for all treatment modalities to children afflicted with ESRD, it would be prudent to initiate an additional major research effort directed toward prevention of the diseases that lead to renal failure. Any local, state, or national health care program that includes treatment of children with renal disease should anticipate an increased expenditure of funds in the area of prevention. These funds are required for public and patient education, preventive patient care activities, and basic and clinical research directed toward elucidating an etiology for the various kidney diseases affecting children.

Planning for the delivery of ESRD care must be integrated at the local, state, and national levels. It should be realized that ESRD care has an enormous impact on the local and state agencies from both fiscal and psychosocial standpoints. Programs that are developed without such integration and ignore the factors that affect children and their families will ultimately provide inadequate care and will result in additional financial burdens to the community.

It is imperative that facilities involved in the delivery of health care to children with renal disease be accountable for their services. However, the demands resulting from the current bureaucracy are onerous to patients, their families, and health care providers. The expenditure of some of the funds directed toward assuring financial and patient care accountability could be utilized for other more productive activities. A possible solution for this dilemma is the establishment of regional centers for the delivery of total health care to children with renal disease. Funding would be to the center rather than to the individual patient, and the center would be accountable for its activities only to the regional funding agency.

A major effort is required to educate the public in general and local, state, and public officials regarding the health care services needed to provide comprehensive care to children with diseases of the kidney. Attempts should be made to indicate the differences in the care required by a child in contrast to an adult with kidney disease. In addition, it must be emphasized that provision of only technical components is insufficient to provide comprehensive medical services to children and their families.

The choice of treatment modality made by a child and family is profoundly influenced by the information imparted by the attending physician and allied health professionals. Such members of the health care team are usually biased from the perspective of their limited experience. Therefore, it would be advantageous if a communication system were established to analyze the outcome of the various available treatment modalities on a periodic basis.

Efforts should be made to initiate long-term longitudinal studies that document outcome as well as the quality of life and degree of rehabilitation of a child receiving the various therapeutic modalities. Since the patient population is small, it would be advisable to initiate cooperative studies in order to maximize the quantity of information.

In addition to the general research support advocated above, it would be beneficial if specific research support were directed toward two areas. The major impediment to successful renal transplantation of a child with ESRD relates to immunologic factors. Since the potential for a normal life is greatest in a child with a successful transplant, it would be helpful if specific research efforts were directed toward making a successful transplantation more successful. Secondly, the aberrations of growth and development in children with renal disease have an enormous impact on the quality of life of such children. Additional efforts are required to delineate the factors operative in producing growth and development retardation in such children so that treatment programs can be initiated to forestall or correct these abnormalities.

References

Coggins, C. H., and others. "A Controlled Study of Short-Term Prednisone Treatment in Adults with Membranous Nephropathy: Collaborative Study of the Adult Idiopathic Nephrotic Syndrome." *New England Journal of Medicine*, 1979, *301*, 1301–1306.

Ettenger, R. B., and others. "Renal Rehabilitation of Children and Adolescents with End-Stage Renal Disease." In S. B. Chigatte (Ed.), *Rehabilitation in Chronic Renal Failure*. Baltimore, Md.: Williams and Wilkins, 1979.

Fine, R. N. "Growth in Children with Renal Insufficiency." In A. R. Nissenson, R. N. Fine, and D. E. Gentile (Eds.), *Clinical Dialysis*. New York: Appleton-Century-Crofts, 1984.

Fine, R. N., and others. "Renal Transplantation in Children." *Urology*, 1977, *9* (6 Supplement), 61–71.

Fine, R. N., and others. "Renal Retransplantation in Children." *Journal of Pediatrics*, 1979, *95*, 244.

Glassberg, K. K., and Filmer, R. B. "Renal Dysplasia, Renal Hypoplasia, and Cystic Disease of the Kidney." In P. P. Kelalis, L. L. King, and A. B. Belman (Eds.), *Clinical Pediatric Urology*. Philadelphia: Saunders, 1984.

Gradus, D., and Ettenger, R. B. "Renal Transplantation in Children." *Pediatric Clinics of North America*, 1982, *29*, 1013–1038.

Habib, R., Broyer, M., and Benmaiz, H. "Chronic Renal Failure in Children: Causes, Rate of Deterioration and Survival Data." *Nephron*, 1973, *11*, 209–220.

Hamburg, B. A. "Chronic Illness." In M. D. Levine, W. B. Carey, A. C. Crocker, and R. T. Gross (Eds.), *Developmental-Behavioral Pediatrics*. Philadelphia: Saunders, 1983.

Ibels, L. S., and others. "Preservation of Function in Experimental Renal Disease by Dietary Restriction of Phosphate." *New England Journal of Medicine*, 1978, *298*, 122–126.

Korsch, B. M. "Psychologic Principles in Pediatric Practice: The Pediatrician and the Sick Child." In S. Z. Levine (Ed.), *Advances in Pediatrics*. Vol. 10. Chicago: Year Book Publisher, 1958.

Korsch, B. M., and Barnett, H. L. "The Physician, the Family, and the Child with Nephrosis." *Journal of Pediatrics*, 1961, *58*, 707–715.

Korsch, B. M., Fine, R. N., and Negrete, V. F. "Noncompliance in Children with Renal Transplants." *Pediatrics*, 1978, *61*, 872–876.

Korsch, B. M., and others. "Experiences with Children and Their Families During Extended Hemodialysis and Kidney Transplantation." *Pediatric Clinics of North America*, 1971, *18*, 625–637.

Korsch, B. M., and others. "Kidney Transplantation in Children: Psychosocial Follow-Up Study on Child and Family." *Journal of Pediatrics*, 1973, *83*, 399–408.

Meadow, R., Cameron, J. S., and Ogg, C. "Regional Service for Acute and Chronic Dialysis of Children." *Lancet*, 1970, *2*, 707–710.

Nevins, T. E., and Mauer, S. M. "Infant Hemodialysis." In R. N. Fine and A. B. Gruskin (Eds.), *End-Stage Renal Disease in Children*. Philadelphia: Saunders, 1984.

Norman, M. E. "Vitamin D in Bone Disease." *Pediatric Clinics of North America*, 1982, *29*, 947–971.

Popovich, R. P., and others. "The Definition of a Novel Portable/Wearable Equilibrium Peritoneal Dialysis Technique" (abstract). *Transactions—American Society for Artificial Internal Organs*, 1976, *5*, 64.

Prugh, D. G. "Toward an Understanding of Psychosomatic Concepts in Relation to Illness in Children." In A. Solnit and S. Provence (Eds.), *Modern Perspectives in Child Development*. New York: International Universities Press, 1963.

Salusky, I. B., and others. "Continuous Ambulatory Peritoneal Dialysis in Children." *Pediatric Clinics of North America*, 1982, *29*, 1005–1012.

Scharer, K. "Incidence and Causes of Chronic Renal Failure in Childhood." *Proceedings of the European Dialysis and Transplantation Association*, 1971, *8*, 211–217.

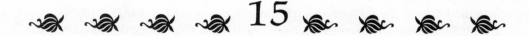

15

Thalassemia and Hemophilia

Margaret W. Hilgartner, M.D.
Louis Aledort, M.D.
Patricia J. V. Giardina, M.D.

Hemophilia and thalassemia are two genetically inherited diseases that require lifelong maintenance with blood products. This chapter considers the health care issues these two diseases have raised and the way public policy related to the delivery of care and research has evolved. We believe consumer advocacy has been the single most important factor in the development of public policy for these diseases. The marked differences in policy that developed for each disorder can be directly related to the effectiveness of individual consumer groups and to the issues these disorders raise in the public arena.

The inherent differences and similarities between the two diseases illustrate the various factors that influence the development of public policy. For example, the incidence and density of the two disorders are quite different. The incidence of thalassemia is one in forty thousand of all live births, with a total population of about one thousand in the United States (U.S. Department of Health, Education, and Welfare, 1979). The geographic distribution of thalassemia is such that the patients are almost all clustered in the northeastern states, Chicago, and San Francisco. Hemophilia has an incidence of one in twenty-five thousand and the total population numbers between fifteen and twenty thousand (U.S. Department of Health, Education, and Welfare, 1972). The geographic distribution of hemophilia is nationwide, although clustered largely on the east and west coasts. The very low density of thalassemia has resulted in a small number of lay and professional people interested in or knowledgeable about the disease and the needs of the patient and family. This small density affects the potency of advocacy groups and, thus, the development of public policy. In contrast, the number of lay and professional people knowledgeable about hemophilia and able to speak for the needs of those with the disease is far greater.

For each disease, patient advocacy was aroused following a scientific advancement that dramatically affected the life span of the patient. For example, public concern for the health and welfare of the patient with hemophilia increased greatly after the development of cryoprecipitate in the late 1960s by Dr. Judith Pool (Pool and Shannon, 1965). Patients with hemophilia bleed because they are missing a blood component necessary for clotting. Pool discovered that a concentrate of the missing clotting factor (Factor VIII) was present in the precipitate found in the bottom of a bag of fresh frozen plasma when it thawed at four degrees centigrade. This simple observation led to the development of an industry capable of producing lyophilized or dried products for the treatment of the two common forms of hemophilia. Similarly, the development of iron chelators (which remove toxic levels of iron) in the early 1970s and the prospect of an extended life span for patients with thalassemia gave hope for longer survival (Barry and others, 1974). This discovery, too, has led to a greater consumer awareness of the issues related to health and welfare of the patient and to development of public policy for the management of the disease.

Thalassemia

Epidemiology. Thalassemia is not one but a group of inherited disorders in which there is an absence or decreased production of one of the normal chains of hemoglobin in red blood cells. Hemoglobin is the protein of the red blood cells that carries oxygen to the tissues. It is made up of heme (which contains iron) and four globin chains, of which there are at least four kinds: alpha, beta, gamma, and delta. Different types of hemoglobin are determined by the combinations of these four globin chains.

The most common form of thalassemia is beta thalassemia, also referred to as Mediterranean anemia and Cooley's anemia. Dr. Thomas Benton Cooley, an American pediatrician, first described this severe anemia in 1925 (Cooley and Lee, 1925; Cooley, 1927).

Although the term *thalassemia* is usually used to refer to beta thalassemia major, several other forms of thalassemia occur, including beta thalassemia minor, alpha thalassemia, delta-beta thalassemia, and so on. In beta thalassemia, there is an insufficient number of beta globin chains, and in alpha thalassemia, there is an insufficient number of alpha globin chains of hemoglobin. In the United States, alpha thalassemia is not as common as beta thalassemia major and minor; it is more frequently found in the Far East and Southeast Asia. The incidence of alpha thalassemia in the United States will no doubt increase with the recent rise in immigration from these areas.

Although beta thalassemia is found predominantly in peoples of the Mediterranean, it may also be found in people with Southeast Asian and African origins. The word *thalassemia* is based on the Greek word meaning sea. It is thought that the defective gene carrying thalassemia was derived over 50,000 years ago in the Mediterranean Basin and may have evolved as a protective mechanism against malaria.

Although approximately two million people now living in Greece and Italy are affected by beta thalassemia, it is a rare disorder in the United States, where approximately one in twenty thousand Americans of Mediterranean extraction are found to have either the disease or the trait.

Incidence and Prevalence of Thalassemia. In 1979, the National Institutes of Health (NIH) Task Force for Cooley's anemia estimated the incidence and prevalence of this rare disorder in the United States (1) by attempting direct enumeration of cases through surveys of medical care professionals and organizations and (2) through projection from the frequency of heterozygotes (carriers) in the population known to be at high risk (U.S. Department of Health, Education, and Welfare, 1979). Attempts to enumerate directly the number of persons homozygous for beta thalassemia gene yielded estimates of between 350 and 700. Although the margin of error in these estimates is large, it seems unlikely that the number of cases afflicted with thalassemia in the United States today exceeds 1,000. Theoretical projections based principally on known frequencies of the carrier state in the at-risk ethnic population ranged from a low of 700 to a high of 3,000. But accurate calculation of the maximum number of afflicted from the frequency of carriers is impossible because it is impossible to determine how many persons of each ethnic group reside in the United States. Development of safe, reliable prenatal diagnostic methods to detect an affected fetus will encourage a greater decline in the number of new cases in this country. However, the current influx of Southeast Asians with a higher incidence of alpha thalassemia along with the beta thalassemia was not anticipated in 1979, and its impact on incidence rates can be assessed only through anecdotal evidence.

The genetics of thalassemia are autosomal recessive, meaning that each parent of an affected child must be a carrier to produce an affected child. With each pregnancy, such a couple has a 25 percent chance of producing an affected child (homozygous state, the severe form), a 25 percent chance of a normal child, and a 50 percent chance of a child with the carrier state (heterozygous) (Valentine and Neel, 1944). The carrier of the defective gene is little affected but may have a greater than normal change of having gallbladder and renal stones, mild anemia, and splenomegaly.

Course of the Disease. The infant with thalassemia appears normal at birth. Signs of the disease first develop a few months after birth and become progressively more severe. By the end of the first year of life, paleness, irritability, poor appetite, and failure to thrive appear. Fever, feeding problems, and diarrhea may occur. These signs and symptoms are caused by the developing anemia, which occurs because the red blood cells are defective, do not contain the appropriate amount of hemoglobin, and break down within a few weeks instead of lasting the normal four months. As the anemia progresses, the body attempts to correct for lack of hemoglobin by increasing production of red blood cells in the bone marrow and in other organs such as the liver, spleen, and lymph nodes.

These organs enlarge as the production of red blood cells increases, resulting in widening of the bone marrow cavities and thinning of the bones, especially of the skull and face. The characteristic facial appearance develops with prominent cheek bones, slanting eyes, prominence of the upper jaw, and malocclusion of the teeth. The long bones of the body become thinner and fracture easily. The abdomen becomes swollen as a result of the liver and spleen enlargement and because of the interruption of normal function caused by iron deposition and tissue scarring. Enlargement of the spleen (hypersplenism) causes the spleen to destroy prematurely all blood cell components, red blood cells, white blood cells, and platelets.

In spite of red-cell overproduction, the body fails to produce or maintain an adequate hemoglobin level; the anemia worsens; tissues receive insufficient oxygen; recurrent infections and failure to thrive occur; and cardiac failure and death eventually ensue.

Nature and Efficacy of Treatment. Periodic blood transfusions are necessary to correct the anemia of thalassemia. They prevent death from the consequences of anemia in the first few years of life, but they do not cure. The accelerated destruction of the transfused red blood cells continues and regular blood transfusions are required every two to four weeks. Children receiving such transfusions to maintain normal hemoglobin levels are relatively active and live fairly normal lives for many years (Pearson and O'Brien, 1975). Most of the changes in facial appearance (resulting from changes in bones of the face and skull) can be prevented by maintaining this physiologic hemoglobin level. However, regular blood transfusions over long periods of time result in complications that lead to death in the second, third, or fourth decades.

The effect of chronic transfusion therapy results in a buildup of the waste products of the destroyed red blood cells; the most toxic of these is iron, which is released from red blood cells and deposited in all tissues. Excess iron is toxic to tissues and destroys normal functioning of all organs. Skin tissue becomes discolored, turning a brownish grey hue. Excess iron in endocrine glands causes diabetes mellitus, calcium deficiency, poor thyroid function, and impairment of sexual development and function. Excess iron in liver causes scarring and cirrhosis as early as five years or as late as thirty years of age. Excess iron in the heart causes rhythm abnormalities, inflammation of the cardiac sac (pericarditis), and heart failure in the second decade of life or earlier (Ellis, Schulman, and Smith, 1954).

Life may be prolonged by the combination of blood transfusions and the removal of excess iron by the early use of a drug known as an iron chelator. Although researchers are investigating the possibility of an oral chelator, the only currently available iron chelator is deferoxamine mesylate (Desferal), which is self-administered by the patient as an infusion under the skin over an eight- to twelve-hour period with the use of a battery operated portable infusion pump (Graziano and others, 1978; Graziano and Cerami, 1977; Poncz, Cohen, and Schwartz, 1984).

When the spleen becomes overactive or hypersplenic, usually between five and ten years of age, splenectomy becomes necessary. Following surgery, these patients are highly susceptible to certain bacterial infections, particularly the pneumococcus. A recently developed vaccine against fourteen strains of bacterial pneumococcus is administered to prevent these infections. In addition, the prophylactic use of small amounts of penicillin daily is also recommended.

Other drugs are also given: daily vitamin E, folic acid, and multivitamin supplemental preparation without iron and with a maximum amount of 100 mg of vitamin C to maintain normal vitamin C levels. Excessive vitamin C has been shown to produce heart failure in patients on iron removal therapy. In addition, all patients are advised to follow diets low in iron content because dietary iron is absorbed ten to twenty times more effectively in patients with thalassemia than normally. They are also advised to drink tea with their meals because tea has been demonstrated to have a mild chelating effect on orally consumed iron.

Thus, the combination of transfusions and iron chelation treatments represents the major scientific advance in the treatment of Cooley's anemia today. There is still no cure for thalassemia, and the life expectancy of patients who are treated with modern therapy from early infancy is currently unknown because successful removal of excess iron by iron chelating drugs is such a recent medical advancement. The average age of death in 1981 was twenty years, recorded in the Children's Blood Foundation Clinic at the New York Hospital.

Discoveries in the last few years have also led to a greater understanding of the molecular defect in the abnormal hemoglobin production and of the genetic defect in the thalassemic gene controlling the hemoglobin production (Weatherall, Clegg, and Naughton, 1965). This information has been applied to improve diagnostic technical skills and to categorize better the heterogenous nature of the thalassemia syndromes. It has also made possible prenatal diagnosis by amniocentesis.

Prenatal diagnosis of thalassemia is currently available at some medical centers in New York, Baltimore, Boston, New Haven, and San Francisco. It can be accomplished by amniocentesis in 75 percent of pregnancies at risk (Kazazian and others, 1980). However, amniocentesis has a 0.5 percent risk of fetal loss. Prenatal diagnosis by studies of fetal red blood cells obtained by fetoscopy is also available, but although quite accurate (error rate of 1.5 percent), the procedure is limited by a 7 percent risk of fetal mortality and by difficulty in obtaining an adequate fetal blood sample in about 8 percent of cases (Mahoney, 1981). Amniocentesis can be carried out at approximately sixteen weeks gestation, and if diagnosis cannot be excluded, fetoscopy can be safely carried out between eighteen and twenty weeks gestation.

If pregnancy develops in a family known to be carriers of the thalassemia gene, health care workers trained in genetic counseling must be available to help the family to decide whether they wish to take the one-in-four chance of having a severely affected infant. Prenatal testing allows parents the option of a therapeutic abortion if the fetus is found to be severely affected.

Requirements for Therapy. Currently, the most advanced blood product available to people with thalassemia is blood that has been frozen, thawed, washed, and repacked. This type of processing removes white blood cells and plasma proteins that may cause transfusion reactions. Careful typing and cross matching for major and minor blood groups by a team consisting of blood banker, nurse, and physician are essential. Use of a unit of blood that can be frozen and stored for months or years is a benefit to those patients who have developed minor blood group incompatibilities and require rare blood types for transfusions.

Researchers are working to improve frozen stored blood. Current trends are to improve the quality of the transfused red blood cells enabling them to survive longer in the circulation of patients with thalassemia and resulting in fewer units of blood necessary to maintain a normal hemoglobin level and a consequent decrease in the rate of iron accumulation. Some researchers are studying the process of making young red blood cells (or neocytes) by flow cytometry, a costly procedure with some risks to the donor; others use a simple but more costly centrifugation technique, using two units of blood for every one processed (Propper, Button, and Nathan, 1980); still others are studying biochemical modification to "rejuvenate" older red blood cells (Valeri and Zaroulis, 1972). All these methods are currently research procedures awaiting the recognition and adoption of their use.

The second major advance in therapy has been the use of iron chelation. Currently, the only efficacious iron chelator available is deferoxamine mesylate (Desferal), a drug that combines with iron in the body, which then excretes it through the urinary system. This drug has been available for more than twenty years, but it was originally limited to intravenous and intramuscular administration. Intravenous Desferal requires patient hospitalization over prolonged periods of time (months) each year to be effective. This mode obviously compromises the social productivity of an individual. When in the late 1970s, the administration of this drug under the skin was found to have remarkably few side effects and little discomfort, a new era of therapy began. Patients and parents are now instructed in appropriate preparation and administration of subcutaneous Desferal. This method is cost-effective and places the transfusion-dependent patient in "negative iron balance," that is, it removes more iron than is administered with transfusion (Graziano and Cerami, 1977).

Research workers are currently investigating the development of a cost-effective iron chelator that can be given by mouth. To date, one oral agent has been shown to be nontoxic, but it is not as effective as Desferal. Costs for evaluating new agents are exorbitant and require a minimum of two years of laboratory preparation and animal work before clinical investigations can be approached. Therefore, progress is slow.

It is obvious from our description of this disease, with its special needs, advanced treatment programs, and medical complications, that a team of highly specialized personnel is required to administer such care; this includes blood processors, blood bankers, specialized physicians, nurses, genetic counselors, psychologists, and social workers. Although some of these services are available in local community hospitals, the availability of and access to specialized blood products; instruction in the use of subcutaneous Desferal; pediatric specialists in hematology, endocrinology, cardiology, surgery, psychiatry, and genetics are generally only found in major medical centers.

Stress on the Child and Family. The single largest study designed to answer the question concerning the impact of thalassemia on the patient and family was developed by the Cooley's Anemia Task Force questionnaire conducted by the Institute for Survey Research of Temple University (U.S. Department of Health, Education, and Welfare, 1979). Seventy-two patients and their families were interviewed to ascertain the impact of the disease on the patient's quality of life and family life. The study was not intended to yield statistically valid information; it merely attempted to obtain a representative view of the family conditions and problems.

Families seemed to see the financial burden as the greatest problem. Seventy-three percent reported a concern "all of the time" about their ability to make ends meet. This response did not necessarily reflect a deficiency in insurance coverage since 64 percent of those interviewed had at least some form of insurance coverage for the patient. Out-of-pocket expenses varied from $50 to $5,650, while families without insurance coverage reported $265 to $10,494 in expenses for medical care and nonmedical associated costs for patient care.

The next biggest problem for the families was the emotional stress associated with the chronic illness, including living with the day-to-day knowledge of a shortened life expectancy for the patient and the logistics of obtaining medical care in the centers. The emotional stress ranged from worry about the wife/mother's depression to the generalized concern about maintaining a "normal" family life. Over half the parents felt a better relationship with their sick children, a fact that was interpreted as meaning a greatly enhanced family cooperative effort for treatment plans. Ninety percent indicated a plan to have no more children, and eighty percent requested a safe prenatal test for thalassemia.

There seemed to be a very high level of frustration associated with finding medical care for the patient with the disease, and more than half of the parents reported difficulty in obtaining routine treatment with which they were satisfied. There appeared to be, however, a great determination on the part of the parents to seek hospital and community supports to which they could turn.

The stress on the patient or child with the disease has not been fully explored. One preliminary study of the coping ability of twenty-five adolescents and young adults has revealed a great concern among these patients about the uncertainty of the outcome of the disease, about the genetic transmission and their own fertility, and particularly about their own body image. Family relationships appear to be the principal support system, but communications are not always open among the family members. The self-esteem and fears about the uncertain prognosis play a major role in patients' coping and the locus of control for autonomy and independence they desire. Much more work needs to be done in this area to help patients cope with these stresses. Private funds are being sought for this effort (R. Woo, personal communication with the authors, 1982).

The demand on public institutions and agencies is not very great because of the small number of patients in any one community. Children with thalassemia may attend regular schools, and with current therapy, those who maintain a normal hemoglobin should be able to enter any physical education program designed for a normal child. They must, however, be given more medical absences than the normal child (every two to four weeks for a regular transfusion program) and must be monitored more closely for intercurrent infections. Housing and public facilities require no special attention.

Career development and future employment are areas as yet untapped. With potential for improved longevity, effort must be put into career development and vocational planning. In early adolescence, both child and family must begin to plan for a career, employment, and self-sufficiency. Although the average age of death in the largest clinic in the United States is twenty years, one quarter of that group is above the age of eighteen years and several are in the fourth decade. Much more effort has to be made by state and local agencies to train and hire these young adults. Little has been done by consumer groups to develop and disseminate information concerning the employability of these patients.

Information and education of the lay public concerning thalassemia is inadequate. A very fine educational film, entitled "Sea of Blood," was made in 1976 by the British Broadcasting Company with the assistance of British physicians. This remains the one piece of material publicizing the problems, inheritance, treatment, and potential improvement in the life of these patients. The Cooley's Anemia Foundation, the Children's Blood Foundation, and other volunteer groups have begun to use this film for the general public and for populations at risk. An important piece of work was done with the Greek Orthodox churches in the New Haven area to screen the congregation for potential carriers and to give genetic counseling to those found to be heterozygotes. However, a fair amount of resistance has been directed at similar proposals elsewhere, despite the assistance of the Greek and Italian lay organizations Ahepa and Unico.

The Cooley's Anemia Foundation has also written several small brochures that describe inheritance, blood needs, and the need for chelation (U.S. Department of Health, Education, and Welfare, 1980a, 1980b). These pieces are the only publications available for public education. Occasional use of the work in research and patient management at the Children's Blood Foundation Thalassemia Clinic at the New York Hospital–Cornell Medical Center has been made by the Greater New York Blood Program. This work is sketchy, but it does introduce the disease and its characteristics to the lay public and to the blood donor in particular. More emphasis needs to be put into development of this work so the lay public can be more aware of the special problems.

Sources of Clinical Treatment. A survey of the facilities available for the treatment of patients with thalassemia was made for the National Heart, Lung, and Blood Institute (NHLBI) by the Institute for Survey Research of Temple University and reported in the Assessment of Cooley's Anemia Research and Treatment (U.S. Department of Health, Education, and Welfare, 1979). The study found that university medical centers or hospitals with university affiliation treated two thirds of the estimated patient population. The remaining one third of patients were treated in community or non-university-affiliated treatment facilities. University centers tend to have at least one physician specifically responsible for and knowledgeable about patients with thalassemia. Specialized (nonhematologic) medical personnel, including cardiologists and endocrinologists, also appeared to be utilized at these facilities. These additional nonhematologic medical personnel did not seem to be utilized or available in the non-university-affiliated facilities. It appears, then, that for at least two thirds of the patient population, multidisciplinary care is available and utilized. For those patients seen at the nonaffiliated facilities, however, care is inadequate—to the extent that the patient has only the facilities of the hematologic equivalent of a "gas station."

The largest clinic (caring for 110 patients, of which 94 are transfusion dependent) is at the Children's Blood Foundation facility at the New York Hospital–Cornell Medical Center in New York City. Smaller clinics with facilities for 10 to 20 patients with multidisciplinary care are available in four other centers in New York and in centers in Boston, New Haven, Philadelphia, Cleveland, Chicago, San Francisco, and Los Angeles. All the larger, well-recognized centers are known to and catalogued by the Cooley's Anemia National Foundation whose headquarters are in New York City.

Sources of Support Services. The same survey points out the lack of specialized personnel and the limited use of social service personnel. Lack of such workers markedly decreases both available third-party coverage for financial relief and the availability of emotional support for family and patient. A need for an in-depth analysis of the magnitude of the need and the numbers of people required for support of the patient's family has long been recognized at Cornell. Individual support and group therapy sessions for adolescents and young adults led by trained personnel need to be established.

Diagnostic services with appropriate laboratory backup are available in all of the university affiliated centers. Screening programs for the at-risk populations, however, appear to be organized by volunteer groups rather than by the treatment centers themselves.

Genetic counselors are used in the larger university centers to help the patient understand the inheritance pattern of the disease and to explain alternate reproductive choices to the families, many of whom expressed a desire for more children but not more children with thalassemia. Counselors are particularly helpful if prenatal diagnosis is desired in subsequent pregnancies.

Educational and diagnostic services, support for genetics counselors, safe prenatal diagnostic services, and help with the financial burden of total patient care were recommendations of the Cooley's Anemia Task Force. These recommendations are now being supported in New York and the New England areas by funds granted through the Genetics Services of the Health Services Administration in response to consumer advocacy. The funds support such personnel as a social worker, a genetic counselor, and a cardiologist.

Vocational rehabilitation services have been found useful to a limited degree. Because of prevailing outdated information concerning the life expectancy of the client, few opportunities are made available to the patient with thalassemia. Unfortunately, discriminatory procedures have been utilized often enough that, in order to avail themselves of what may be open in the employment field, many patients seeking employment will not divulge the true nature of their disease. Although the true efficacy of the chelation therapy currently under study will not be known for a number of years, it seems clear that this form of treatment is becoming widespread and would justify the patient's practice of not fully informing an employer of the problem.

Sources of Financial Assistance. Financial assistance for patients and families is varied and often quite poor. As with hemophilia, private-sector medical insurance is often difficult to obtain for patients with a pre-existing chronic illness. Therefore, a family with a newly diagnosed child with thalasse-mia usually cannot obtain Blue Cross/Blue Shield unless there is a period of open enrollment during which the "pre-existing disorders" clause is waived. There-fore, when the task force report indicated that 64 percent of families reported at least some insurance coverage, it probably referred to inpatient coverage that may or may not include blood transfusions. Many centers and smaller non-university-affiliated centers have often admitted patients for transfusions to take advantage of inpatient blood coverage when such exists. Few patients have outpatient coverage for blood transfusions.

In the New York area, however, through the efforts of a consortium of physicians in the four major treatment centers and the Cooley's Anemia Foun-dation, Blue Cross has initiated an Outpatient Demonstration Program to evaluate the efficacy of the chelator Desferal. At the same time, a period of open enrollment was begun, allowing a broader base of patients to avail themselves of a program that pays for a comprehensive evaluation of disease status four times yearly and for drugs (including use of the chelator, Desferal, in a home setting). It is a model start in financial assistance from the private sector for patients with this disorder.

Public-sector financial support, represented by Crippled Children's Servi-ces (CCS) programs, is varied throughout the country. Some of these programs pay for outpatient comprehensive medical care and some pay for the chelator drug, but many CCS programs do not pay for the battery-operated pumps required for delivery of the drug, and many do not pay for blood. The middle-income patient must seek medical insurance to pay for blood or pay blood cost as an out-of-pocket expense. Furthermore, because of the high cost of care for these patients, the hospitals assuming their care often must accept an unsubsi-dized loss for those patients whose income level excludes them from Medicaid and CCS benefits. For many of the providers involved with these patients, therefore, CCS programs are very unsatisfactory.

For older adolescents and young adults who live beyond the CCS age limit, Supplemental Security Income (SSI) and Medicaid programs provide a living subsidy and payment of total medical care cost. However, these programs, as they are currently structured, do not permit part-time or full-time employment. Instead, they remove all incentive to work or to achieve a sense of self-sufficiency.

Hemophilia

Epidemiology. Hemophilia, a lifelong, inherited disease, first recognized by the Egyptians and then clearly documented in the Talmud, produces significant morbidity, crippling bony deformities with arthritis, and not infrequently, early death. Hemophilia A (classical hemophilia) is characterized by a deficiency of the clotting activity in the presence of a nonfunctioning Factor VIII protein. Hemophilia B is a similar disorder in which a different protein important for clotting (Factor IX) does not function or is absent. Von Willebrand's disease is a deficiency of both clotting activity and Factor VIII protein, with an associated platelet functional abnormality. The first two disorders can be grouped together because of the similarity in clinical symptomatology and outcome. Differentiation is possible only through laboratory testing. Von Willebrand's disease is probably more common than originally thought, although only the patients with severe disease have symptoms similar to hemophilia and require plasma replacement. The mild forms are symptomatic only with severe trauma or oral surgery. The earliest treatment of hemophilia was hypnotherapy (when Rasputin was in favor with the Russian court), a therapy that continues as an adjunctive measure in today's therapeutic armamentarium. Hemophilia is a sex-linked recessive disorder; that is, it occurs only in males but is passed on by asymptomatic mothers.

The incidence of hemophilia in the United States is one in twenty-five thousand males for Factor VIII deficiency and one in forty thousand males for Factor IX deficiency, and this incidence appears to be nationwide and universal. The 1980 projections for the United States were 11,572 patients with Factor VIII deficiency, 2,895 patients with factor IX deficiency, and 3,500 patients with severe von Willebrand's disease (U.S. Department of Health, Education, and Welfare, 1980c). A large proportion of new cases is due to a high mutation rate: Twenty-five percent of new cases occur without a family history of hemophilia. The new mutation has therefore occurred de novo in mother or son. Prevalence, however, appears to be increasing and may be expected to continue to do so because the gene is no longer lethal and more patients with hemophilia are reproducing. Carrier detection of the female can now be accomplished with approximately 90 percent accuracy for hemophilia A and somewhat less for hemophilia B, a more heterogenous disorder. The probability of the carrier state can be determined from the amount of inactive clotting protein present in the female's plasma coupled with the pattern of the disease in the family.

The clinical severity of hemophilia is defined as follows: *severe,* if the patient has frequent bleeding episodes and a history of spontaneous bleeding in more than one joint; *mild,* if the patient has no spontaneous joint bleeding and only experiences bleeding secondary to major trauma or surgery; and *moderate,* if the patient has bleeding manifestations that are intermediate in severity to the above two categories (Hilgartner, 1980). A major national study found that patients with hemophilia in the United States were distributed in the following way by factor-level criteria—Factor VIII deficiency: 55 percent severe, 25 percent moderate, and 20 percent mild; Factor IX deficiency: 25 percent severe, 28 percent moderate, and 47 percent mild (National Heart, Lung, and Blood Institute, 1972).

Course of the Disease. Severe hemophilia is characterized by frequent spontaneous painful bleeding episodes. Bleeding may occur at circumcision but usually does not begin until the toddler begins to walk. Bleeding occurs most often into joints, such as ankles, knees, hips, and elbows; if unabated, it leads to progressive arthropathy, joint destruction, and crippling similar to that seen in rheumatoid arthritis. Bleeding can occur anywhere in the body—into body cavities, into or around any organ, as well as in the joints. If minor or superficial, it can be controlled with pressure; usually it requires factor replacement for control. Before the advent of replacement therapy, all patients with severe disease had significant crippling by twelve years of age and most were wheelchairbound as adults. Death occurred at an early age, frequently due to intracranial hemorrhage.

Patients with moderate disease may bleed with trauma and then continue to bleed spontaneously in a target joint. However, the episodes are usually less frequent than for the patient with severe disease. Patients with mild disease bleed only with severe trauma such as surgery, including dental surgery. Frequency of bleeding or bleeding patterns vary with each patient and throughout the year for any given patient. It is this variability that contributes to the difficulties in coping with the disease (Hilgartner, 1980).

The median age of death in the patient with hemophilia in 1972 as surveyed by the NHLBI study (U.S. Department of Health, Education, and Welfare, 1972) was 11.5 years, or less than half the median age of 26.8 years for the general U.S. male population. With the availability of replacement products and earlier and better treatment, an improved life-style is possible, joint disease is minimal, and life expectancy markedly prolonged. The study done by Dietrich at the Los Angeles Orthopedic Hospital (S. Dietrich, personal communication with the authors, 1979) shows an increase in mean age at death with improved care from 19.6 years in 1968 to 30.7 years in 1974, the period in which concentrates have been used. These data compare favorably with those obtained by Aledort from six centers in this country and in Europe.

Orthopedic disease still occurs because bleeding occurs primarily in joints and most patients develop a target joint—that is, one joint that seems to have problems more frequently than others (Aronstam, Rainsford, and Painter, 1979). Medical care in the form of replacement therapy is used in conjunction with conservative orthopedic care for these target joints where a chronic synovitis has progressed to severe arthritis. Such cases are now benefiting from orthopedic rehabilitation and joint reconstruction. Hip and knee reconstruction is now commonplace. Other joints cannot be reconstructed as successfully at this time.

Approximately 14 percent of patients with hemophilia develop an antibody or inhibitor to the transfused factor (Factor VIII 14.5 percent, Factor IX 2.5 percent), with a peak incidence in the childhood years (Gill and others, 1980). The appearance of the inhibitor is related to infusion of factor, but its presence does not necessarily preclude use of factor for clotting. Inhibitors may be transient and disappear within six weeks, or they may appear with a repeat exposure to factor. Patients with a persistent inhibitor do not bleed more frequently, but their bleeding episodes are often very difficult to control. Products containing activated clotting factors are currently being investigated for treatment of bleeding episodes in these patients. These products, however, are extremely costly.

This lifelong disease makes constant financial and psychological demands on the patient as well as on siblings and all other family members. Most patients, although active and attending school or college or entering the job market, have chronic problems in one or more joints (Guenthner and others, 1980) and have had sufficient exposure through blood product usage to have at least biochemical evidence of liver disease. They are functional at a cost to themselves, their families, and the nation's blood resources.

Nature and Efficacy of Treatment. The unique feature of hemophilia versus other chronic diseases is the continued dependence of these patients on blood products. Bleeding episodes can only be controlled with replacement of the deficient clotting factor, which is obtained from normal human plasma. Plasma can be removed from whole blood and separated into its various components. Because it is prepared from fresh frozen plasma, this Factor VIII component is called cryo(cold)precipitate. The patient deficient in functioning Factor VIII or IX can have the plasma level replaced with an intravenous infusion of one of these components or fresh frozen plasma itself as long as necessary for adequate healing to occur. Type and length of therapy are dependent on the magnitude and site of bleeding. For example, a simple bleed into the muscle requires one small infusion, a bleed into a joint requires a larger dose, and abdominal or central nervous system bleeding episodes may require seven to ten days of daily high-dose therapy (Hilgartner, 1980).

The majority of patients are treated on demand basis, that is, they are treated for each bleeding episode as it occurs. A very small percent of the population are treated routinely every two or three days on a prophylactic program to maintain a low baseline level of more than 10 percent clotting factor and to prevent bleeding (Abildgaard, 1984). A larger number of patients may have short-term prophylaxis for six to eight weeks to allow healing of a damaged joint or persistent synovitis and then return to episodic care. Patients are not put on routine prophylaxis in this country unless they have bleeding episodes on two or more occasions per week.

In a recent study, the average demand for blood products for a large number of patients with hemophilia throughout the United States was about 40,000 units of Factor VIII per patient per year. Patients with severe disease on home care may use almost 60,000 Factor VIII units per year. These figures were corroborated by prior sampling of nonstudy centers (Levine, 1981). It is clear from this evaluation that more factor is used by the more severely involved patient, and that home care patients infuse more often and use more products (Guenthner and others, 1980).

In this country, only approximately 15 percent of the patients with hemophilia use cryoprecipitate for treatment of bleeds. It is used in mild and moderate cases of hemophilia and in patients with von Willebrand's disease. Patients with infrequent bleeding episodes will have a lower risk of developing hepatitis and abnormal liver function using cryoprecipitate because each unit is derived from a single donor blood unit (Levine and others, 1977). In some parts of the country, it is used for almost all patients because of its availability, lower cost, and the concern for conservation of plasma resources. Self-infusion programs with cryoprecipitate are complicated because they require special freezers at home or at work.

Fresh-frozen plasma remains an excellent therapeutic product for mild and moderate cases of Factor IX deficiency where small increments of factor are needed. This product is also useful for patients with von Willebrand's disease. Because of ease of storage, administration, and mobility, concentrates are the favored product for treatment of bleeding episodes for patients on home care programs throughout the world and for hemostatic control of serious bleeding episodes even though they are derived from as many as a thousand donor units and may be contaminated with many viruses. They are preferred for bleeding control during surgery as well because of ease of administration and greater predictability of potency.

Current treatment of hemophilia has moved the patient from being dependent on hospital care to being a more independent, ambulatory person capable of receiving diagnostic and therapeutic programs in an outpatient facility or at home or work. Self-therapy, frequently called home care, has substantially altered the life-style and productivity of these patients. Patient or family members are taught the philosophy of early treatment, the rationale of replacement therapy, and the mechanics of intravenous therapy (Hilgartner and Sergis, 1977). This shift of responsibility for early treatment to the patient or family is made only with those willing and able to accept it. Those entered in a home care program must have periodic examinations with total medical, orthopedic, and dental evaluations, including laboratory tests of liver function and kidney function and for product response and the development of an inhibitor to the replacement product.

Comprehensive Care. Care is best given today by a comprehensive-care team approach (Hilgartner and Sergis, 1977) because the current care of the patient with hemophilia extends beyond crisis intervention during bleeding episodes and management of orthopedic complications. A multidisciplinary approach requires centralization of treatment with regular clinic visits for evaluation and formulation of an individualized treatment plan that incorporates medical, dental, psychosocial, and financial aspects of patient care. The center must have an acute care facility or emergency room facilities as well as concerned medical, pediatric, orthopedic, surgical, dental, and physical therapy personnel familiar with the problems of patients with hemophilia and the special care that may be required. Adequate blood bank facilities with replacement products available on a twenty-four-hour basis are essential, as are special coagulation staff and facilities. Minimum supportive services must include nursing, social service, psychosocial support, vocational and financial counseling, and genetic counseling. One individual must serve as a coordinator of the program, and one individual should identify with an individual patient and family.

Regional hemophilia centers have been organized for two purposes: (1) to provide to the patient and family services and resources that will allow the patient to mature into an independent, self-supporting individual and (2) to collect and analyze data in an attempt to understand the nature of the disease and to improve care. Centers may provide the primary physician, or they may provide secondary or tertiary care as consultants to the primary physician.

This comprehensive-care team approach requires a large number of personnel gathered together in one place. These teams can effectively care for a large number of patients over a wide region. They can also be itinerant, relate to distant primary care physicians, and develop satellite programs. These teams are costly to maintain but are the core for a regionalized network of treatment programs that can assure superior care for patients with hemophilia. It is rare that such a team can be put together and maintained by an institution without outside financial support. In some instances, chapters of the National Hemophila Foundation are helpful in either partial or full support of a single member of the team. In some state hemophilia programs, financial support is given for either personnel or a core state laboratory.

At present, the most important form of support for comprehensive centers in the United States is from the federal government. In 1975, three million dollars was appropriated through Section 1131 of Title XI of the Public Health Science Act for development of a national network of comprehensive hemophilia diagnostic and treatment centers. These grants are competed for, centrally reviewed, and awarded via the Health Services Administration. Twenty-three centers are currently funded; in addition, other nonfunded comprehensive centers exist (*Directory of Hemophilia Treatment Centers,* 1979). Title XI funds are used primarily for personnel that programs could not support on their own. The centers have demonstrated in a short time that more patients are served and more services delivered than previously, and a large number of community agencies have been enlisted to interact with these patients. Almost 30 percent of the nation's patients with hemophilia are served by these centers. Data collected by Levine from the twenty-three regional hemophilia centers in 1980 show the improvement in number of patients cared for, the improvement in health status as measured by days lost from work or school, average cost of care per patient per year with third-party coverage, and the percent of unemployed adults (Gill and others, 1980) (Tables 1 and 2). They emphasize what a regional health care system can do for a relatively low-density population of patients.

Requirements for Therapy. The major requirement for patients with hemophilia is blood and blood products, which translates for them into plasma and its fractionated components: fresh frozen plasma, cryoprecipitate, and the concentrates of Factors VIII and IX. Orthotic devices are for the most part a thing of the past. Braces may be used for temporary support or splints for healing, but multiple extremity braces or long-leg caliphers do not seem to be necessary now that bleeding can be controlled and joints are less diseased. Occasionally,

Table 1. Regional Hemophilia Centers Statistics.

	Historical Control	Fiscal 1980
Average inpatient days per year	14–60	2.4
Average number of hospital admissions per year	6.36	0.71
Average days lost from work or school per year	20–60	8.3
Average cost of health care per year	$8–22,000	$5,252
Average out-of-pocket expense per year	$1–5,000	$388
Percent patients with third-party coverage	74	91
Percent unemployed adults	36	13.6

Note: By way of comparison, the NHLBI Blood Resources Studies of 1972 found that 41 percent of adults with hemophilia were unemployed and receiving public assistance payments.
Source: Levine, 1981.

Table 2. Regional Hemophilia Centers Statistics.

	Year Before HSA Funding	Fiscal 1980
Number of patients receiving regular comprehensive care	1,477	4,768
Number of patients on home therapy	662	2,009

Source: Levine, 1981.

wheelchairs are necessary, as are the orthotic devices for older patients with severe degenerative joint disease; hopefully, these devices will not be necessary for the future generation treated only with replacement material.

Stress on Child and Family. Hemophilia adversely affects the lives of patients in a variety of ways. Most children have had a bleeding episode requiring transfusion by the age of four, and as they grow, they live with the knowledge that they can have a serious bleeding episode that may be lethal at any time. The stress of bleeding, pain, and immobilization, in addition to family separations beginning early in life, tends to affect the psychosocial development of the child (Agle and Mattsson, 1970). These fears, coupled with the overprotectiveness of the family, particularly the mother, can mold the child with hemophilia into a passive, isolated individual whose self-image is poor. Adaptation was found to be poor in 10 percent of a group of hemophiliacs as compared to a physically healthy group, 6 to 7 percent of whom had psychiatric disorders (1976). Five of eight poorly adjusted in a group of thirty-five children with hemophilia were daredevils who had rebelled against oversolicitous mothers and become defiant, overactive boys. Those boys who can adapt and use the experiences gained through normal activities of growth and development to understand their disease and the limitations it may impose usually develop into individuals with good masculine identification and a strong sense of self-worth (1970).

Several authors have described stress, anxiety, and fear as the cause of bleeding episodes. There has been anecdotal evidence for a number of years that stress of any type can be associated with bleeding. For example, the stress associated with school examinations or even holidays may cause bleeding. The connection between the pysche and vascular bed is unknown. However, LaBaw (1975) has documented a decrease in infusion product usage with a relief of anxiety through self-hypnosis. Other mechanisms such as biofeedback to relieve anxiety and pain have been used, without the benefit of supporting studies.

Stress and family adjustment to the disease may influence the place and type of employment of both mother and father. The NHLBI Study reported 11 percent of fathers selected their present jobs because of the child's illness, 20 percent of fathers moonlight to meet costs, and more than one third of mothers who are employed work to help meet expenses. The life-style of many of these families is affected, with financial problems, a need to limit luxuries, a restriction in family size, and a need to live near a good treatment facility paramount in decision making. Even greater is the marital stress that occurs with the birth of a son with hemophilia, which sometimes can cause breakup of the marriage or severe psychological withdrawal of the father (Salk, Hilgartner, and Granich, 1972). Those families that remain intact adapt with different methods to cope with the multiple stresses (Mattsson and Gross, 1966). Agle has catalogued mechanisms of denial and rationalization that parents use to lessen anxiety, despair, and the continual strain of having a chronically ill child with hemophilia (Agle and Mattsson, 1970).

Cost of Treatment. Cost of treatment includes visits to the hospital, physicians' fees, physical therapy fees, and product and infusion materials if the patient is on a home care program. Data collected by Levine and Britten for the period 1960–1970 detailed the cost of care and showed that the primary cost was related to hospital admissions and emergency room fees for transfusions with an average cost ranging from $8,000 to $22,000 per year including surgical procedures (Levine, 1977). The 1972 NHLBI study estimated yearly cost of hemophilia care between $2,400 and $41,000 for product alone including surgical procedures and between $1,000 and $24,000 for medical care (U.S. Department of Health, Education, and Welfare, 1972). The variability is dependent on the severity of the disease, type of treatment, where the treatment is given (whether home care or in an outpatient setting), and material used.

During the last ten years, efforts have been made to extend home care programs to more patients in an effort to decrease the total cost of medical care of these patients at the same time that earlier and better care is given. Levine's review in 1977 showed an overall decrease in cost to $3,500 (Levine, 1977). These costs and the cost of product have risen since 1977 but with a much smaller increment than other medical costs.

The choice of product is frequently a matter of cost. In many centers where a blood bank has a major vested interest in hemophilia, cryoprecipitate is produced cheaply (as little as five cents per Factor VIII unit) and used extensively. In general, however, cryoprecipitate is expensive, and its quality is variable. Concentrates vary in price, at present, from seven to fourteen cents per Factor VIII unit and ten to twelve cents per Factor IX unit. Price varies little from product to product, but a given product may be priced very differently at the place of treatment in various parts of the country at the same time. This is frequently due to long-term contracts by hospital or state programs, volume purchased, or changing manufacturer bids. The total cost of care in 1981 as estimated through a survey of the regional hemophilia centers is on an average $5,252, with $388 an average out-of-pocket expense.

Sources of Clinical Treatment. The NHLBI study showed that in 1970 and 1971 58 percent of patients with hemophilia were treated by physicians who had only one patient with hemophilia under their care, while only 42 percent were seen by specialists in blood diseases (U.S. Department of Health, Education, and Welfare, 1972). One of the mandates of the federally funded regional hemophilia treatment centers was to develop comprehensive programs that might act as consultants to these physicians to help improve patient care. Although only 30 percent of the projected number of persons with hemophilia in the nation are given comprehensive care by these centers (see Table 2), the number of patients seen through outreach programs appears to be increasing each year. However, a large proportion of patients are still receiving only episodic treatment given by local physicians (primarily internists and pediatricians), hospitals, or blood banks that need to be reached by the centers' programs for total evaluation of their patients.

Sources of Financial Assistance. Our nation does not have a uniform system for insuring health care delivery. The poor can avail themselves of Medicaid, SSI, and Crippled Children's Services programs. These programs differ regionally in terms of what they cover, and the latter usually only covers patients under twenty-one years of age. Because factor replacement is most often the major part of the cost of care, its reimbursement is the key part of underwriting care. In almost all of the aforementioned reimbursement programs, factor is reimbursed for inpatient emergency room use only. Underwriting of factor for out-of-hospital care (home care) remains variable and is usually not covered by these programs. Medicaid and Crippled Children's programs reimburse for home care in very selected cases when not covered by Blue Cross, third-party payers, or other private insurance programs. Through the efforts of interested local physicians, the local chapter of the National Hemophilia Foundation, and the local treatment centers, Blue Cross programs authorized payment for home care treatment in the New York City area and for comprehensive care visits in the Rochester area. These, however, are pioneers in providing payment for such services.

The variability of insurance has made treatment centers very aware of the need for evaluating the financial resources of each patient and his family. A treatment program cannot be realistically prescribed without such an evaluation.

Improved care can be provided a patient who is not afraid of incurring medical bills and will follow the prescribed treatment program. When adequate third-party payments can be found for each patient, centers may become financially solvent and programs improved through fee-for-service reimbursement to personnel. Recent publications (Linney, 1979) outline the key elements for financial assessment and counseling. This kind of financial evaluation was the major impetus for the providers through local chapters of the National Hemophilia Foundation and the National Hemophilia office, to begin campaigns to alter policies of third-party payers. These appeals have met with success in many parts of this country. At present, a large number of insurance carriers have altered their policies, and home treatment programs have begun to be underwritten and to flourish. In addition, many union contracts now follow the lead of AT&T to cover home care treatment for patients with hemophilia. This, coupled with state programs that augment reimbursement, has made home therapy a major modality of treatment.

State hemophilia programs have been funded by local grants in twenty-one states (*Directory of Hemophilia Treatment Centers,* 1979). These funds support a variety of needs for people with hemophilia, from product alone (as found in Georgia) to product with some support for a treatment center (as found in New Jersey) to a large statewide program supporting product and multiple centers found in Pennsylvania. Other states, such as New York, have no state program support.

Additional financial support for diagnostic services and counseling is now available through the Genetic Diseases Act. Funds have been made available to support laboratories for carrier detection and the services of a genetic counselor. Carrier studies require a special coagulation laboratory, and the geneticist needs to know the special problems associated with calculating the probability of the carrier state. Counselors must be skilled in explaining the inheritance of the disorders, the probability of carriers in sisters of boys with hemophilia, the obligate carrier state of all daughters whose fathers have hemophilia. Prenatal diagnostic procedures are also explained and discussed, as are all of the reproductive choices for carrier women. To date, portions of the genetics funds have been allocated to the regional centers on a regional basis to support these important services.

Recommendations for Public Policy

The differences between hemophilia and thalassemia in epidemiology and blood demands have been the paramount factors influencing public policy. The incidence and distribution of thalassemia curtails the effectiveness and proliferation of advocacy efforts. For example, thalassemia is currently represented by five organizations: the Cooley's Anemia Foundation with its network of twenty-seven chapters; the Cooley's Anemia Volunteers; Unico, the Italian fraternal organization; Ahepa, the Greek fraternal organization; and the Cooley's Anemia Chapter of the Children's Blood Foundation. Each is relatively isolated with a small constituency and little interaction for the common cause. Hemophilia, on the other hand, is represented by the National Hemophilia Foundation, a nationally coordinated thirty-year-old health agency with more than fifty local chapters that have both lay and medical leadership working for and interacting with the hemophiliac on a local, national, and international level to promote education and improved health care of patients with hemophilia and their families.

The impact on blood resources is substantially different. The demand for packed red cells for transfusions every two to four weeks by patients with thalassemia, if we estimate fifty to a hundred transfusions per year, would amount to something between 50,000 and 100,000 units per year. Because approximately ten million units are drawn per year in this country, the demand by these patients would be 0.5 to 1.0 percent per year; this could reach 2 percent of the national blood resource if neocytes are to be used. This demand could certainly be met without difficulty and with little impact on the blood resource as a whole. Patients with hemophilia, however, can use all the plasma drawn from that ten million units of whole blood. The average figure for consumption of Factor VIII units per year is 40,000 units, and with approximately 15,000 patients with hemophilia in this country, they would need 600 million Factor VIII units or more than 100 percent of the plasma of all blood drawn in the United States if all the Factor VIII units were in cryoprecipitate alone. This figure, of course, does not consider the manufacture of lyophilized (freeze-dried) concentrates or the production of Factor VIII to be used in other countries. However, it is obvious that paid plasmapheresis is necessary to supplement the plasma obtained from the whole blood that is drawn. Hemophilia, thus, has a clear impact on, and need for, the national blood resource.

The manner in which these blood demands will be met and the way in which blood and total medical care costs have been underwritten are also different and important factors. A major difference lies in the interaction between the lay organization and the scientific community and the latter's activity on behalf of the former's needs. For hemophilia, there has been a close liaison between the basic scientist and clinician and a well-demonstrated translation of laboratory advances into the patient care area. The New York Academy symposium in 1975 on State of the Art of Hemophilia Care attests to this fact. Development of those care programs following the discovery of cryoprecipitate and the introduction of lyophilized product is another example of translation of a scientific discovery into improved patient care.

It is certainly true that the scientific community interested in thalassemia has attempted liaison with the lay community for the translation of basic research into improved patient care through multiple symposia (Fink, 1964, 1969; Anderson, Bank, and Zaino, 1980; Zaino, 1974). Through these symposia, patient care has improved in the area of red-cell support, chelation therapy, prenatal diagnosis, and basic understanding of the gene defect in thalassemia. However, the relationship between lay and scientific communities has been a cohesive force in formulating public policy and legislation to ensure adequate supply and to underwrite blood costs, total health care, and continued scientific research only in the field of hemophilia. The scientific community has been able to maintain federal support for research related to thalassemia as shown in the task force report. In fiscal year 1977, seventy-seven projects pertaining to red cell function and metabolism, iron, and iron metabolism as well as patient care projects investigating iron chelators and their efficacy were supported by the NIH. Many of these were funded not because they pertained to thalassemia alone but because the information gained from them might help us understand the basic mechanisms of many red-cell disorders in addition to thalassemia. It has been productive research that has enriched the body of medical knowledge. Nonetheless, the scientific community and lay forces have not developed legislation to underwrite blood products either by federal or local funds for thalassemics, and third-party payment can only be obtained at great cost to the family when open enrollment may waive a pre-existing disease. Funds for comprehensive patient care have been scanty for the thalassemic patient and were only recently allotted to centers in New England and New York through the Genetic Diseases Act. These grants still do not cover the cost of blood and are not nationwide.

The same consortium of physicians and lay people, however, was able to make the Congress aware of the fact that hemophilia could be a model for multidisciplinary care of chronic illness with the subsequent creation of Public Health Science Act, Section 1131, for support of Regional Hemophilia Diagnostic and Treatment Centers. Furthermore, twenty-four state groups have generated sufficient interest through the local Hemophilia Foundation to have state legislators enact laws that underwrite the cost of blood products for patients with hemophilia. Other state groups, as in New York, have negotiated with Blue Cross to cover the cost of transfusion products for home care programs. Attempts to accomplish a similar treatment center plan for thalassemia achieved recognition of the problem of thalassemia with passage of the Cooley's Anemia Bill in the Senate, but the small scientist-lay liaison failed to muster sufficient support to have funds appropriated by the House for enactment of the bill. Instead, interest has been maintained through a single legislator to seek federal research and patient care funds. The former mechanism (active advocacy stemming from a liaison between laymen and professionals) is a broad-based one that has been extraordinarily successful for improving patient care to a moderately large group of chronically ill patients, while the latter mechanism (focusing on a single legislator), although successful for maintaining research support, has lagged behind in obtaining comprehensive care for a low-density chronic illness.

The two groups need to continue efforts begun by the Hemophilia Foundation to formulate discussions that will press for revisions of restrictions in the Medicaid and Medicare laws pertaining to their health care and for catastrophic health plans and national health insurance—plans that may be the ultimate answer for care of these patients and their families. They have already begun to work for the development and implementation of the American Blood Commission, the public sector group whose goal it is to provide safe, effective, affordable blood procured on a voluntary basis for everyone in need.

Both interest groups have pressed for and succeeded in having hemophilia and thalassemia identified in the Genetic Disease Act as diseases with extraordinary unmet needs. Efforts have been made over the past two years to gain support for carrier detection laboratories that provide genetic counseling supported by individual state grants. One third of the hemophilia centers have obtained such support, and centers in New England and New York have such funds for thalassemia. These thalassemia grants also include support for some aspects of comprehensive care. The scope of these grants, however, needs to be expanded and extended to cover a larger portion of the patients at risk and patients with the disease.

Many of the problems associated with these disorders have been faced, and some solutions have been found. However, there are many health care issues and basic mechanisms of disease that still remain as unmet challenges. These include increasing the purity of transfused blood products by removing all causes of hepatitis, developing a mechanism to underwrite the cost of blood and blood products in or out of the hospital, and establishing ambulatory transfusion and care centers. These needs must be coupled with readily accessible and inexpensive carrier detection for the population at risk. The guaranteed diagnosis of the genetic disease needs to coincide with a network of treatment centers that have full comprehensive-care programs. Above all, a better understanding of the impact of chronic illness on the family and the siblings, as well as the ill child, needs to be developed. This last need is critical if we are to formulate support systems that aid the family adjustment to the chronic illness and allow growth and development of the patient into a productive, useful, and contributing member of society.

The still unmet challenges in understanding the basic mechanisms of hemophilia lie in the biochemical description, isolation, purification, and eventual synthesis of the clotting factors and their function in producing hemostatis and in the secondary complications of the disease. For thalassemia, the basic mechanism of hemoglobin evolution must be better understood, and the origin of the gene defect must be known before bioengineering techniques can be utilized to reverse the genetic abnormality. A better understanding of iron metabolism and its role in secondary disease is essential for development of an adequate oral chelator to prevent the secondary disease.

In summary, hemophilia and thalassemia, two chronic blood diseases that create identical patient needs, have had substantially different histories, largely as a result of differences in the public policies that shape the health care system. Care for hemophilia is now far better than that for thalassemia. The key ingredient contributing to this difference has been consumer advocacy. Advocacy efforts themselves have been directly related to differences in the density and distribution of affected individuals. This discrepancy should be recognized in the future development of adequate health care systems for both disorders.

References

Abildgaard, C. F. "Progress and Problems in Hemophilia and von Willebrand's Disease." *Advances in Pediatrics*, 1984, *31*, 137–178.

Agle, D. P., and Mattsson, A. "Psychiatric Factors in Hemophilia: Methods of Parental Adaption." *Haematologia,* 1970, *34,* 89–94.

Agle, D. P., and Mattsson, A. "Psychological Complications of Hemophilia." In M. W. Hilgartner (Ed.), *Hemophilia in Children.* Littleton, Mass.: Publishing Sciences Group, 1976.

Anderson, W. F., Bank, A., and Zaino, E. C. (Eds.). *Fourth Cooley's Anemia Symposium.* New York: New York Academy of Sciences, 1980.

Aronstam, A., Rainsford, J. G., and Painter, M. I. "Patterns of Bleeding in Adolescents with Severe Hemophilia." *British Medical Journal,* 1979, *1,* 469–470.

Barry, M., and others. "Long-Term Chelation Therapy in Thalassemia Major: Effect on Liver Iron Concentration, Liver Histology, and Clinical Progress." *British Medical Journal,* 1974, *2,* 16–20.

Cooley, T. B. "Van Jaksch's Anemia." *American Journal of Diseases of Children,* 1927, *33,* 786–797.

Cooley, T. B., and Lee, P. "Series of Cases of Splenomegaly in Children with Anemia and Peculiar Bone Changes." *Transactions of the American Pediatric Society,* 1925, *37,* 29–30.

Directory of Hemophilia Treatment Centers. New York: The National Hemophilia Foundation, 1979.

Ellis, J. T., Schulman, I., and Smith, C. H. "Generalized Siderosis with Fibrosis of Liver and Pancreas in Cooley's (Mediterranean) Anemia." *American Journal of Pathology,* 1954, *30,* 287.

Fink, H. (Consulting Ed.). "Problems of Cooley's Anemia." *Annals of the New York Academy of Sciences,* 1964, *119,* 369–850.

Fink, H. (Consulting Ed.). "Second Conference on the Problems of Cooley's Anemia." *Annals of the New York Academy of Sciences,* 1969, *165,* 1–508.

Gill, F. M., and others. "The Natural History of Factor VIII Inhibitors in Patients with Hemophilia A: A National Cooperative Study. I. Characteristics of the Population." Unpublished manuscript, 1980.

Graziano, J. H., and Cerami, A. "Chelation Therapy for the Treatment of Thalassemia." *Seminars in Haematology,* 1977, *14,* 127–134.

Graziano, J. H., and others. "Chelation Therapy in β-Thalassemia Major, I: Intravenous and Subcutaneous Deferoxamine." *Journal of Pediatrics,* 1978, *92* (4), 648–652.

Guenthner, E. A., and others. "Hemophilic Arthropathy: Effect of Home Care on Treatment Patterns and Joint Disease." *Journal of Pediatrics,* 1980, *97* (3), 378–382.

Hilgartner, M. W. *Comprehensive Care for Hemophilia.* U.S. Department of Health, Education, and Welfare publication no. 79-5129. Washington, D.C.: U.S. Government Printing Office, 1980.

Hilgartner, M. W., and Sergis, E. "Current Therapy for Hemophiliacs. Home Care and Therapeutic Complications." *Mt. Sinai Journal of Medicine,* 1977, *44,* 316–331.

Kazazian, H. H., and others. "Prenatal Diagnosis of B-Thalassemia by Amniocentesis: Linkage Analysis Using Multiple Polymorphic Restriction Endonuclease Sites." *Blood*, 1980, *56*, 926–930.

LaBaw, W. L. "Autohypnosis in Hemophilia." *Haematologia* (Budapest), 1975, *9* (1–2), 103–110.

Levine, P. H. "The Home Therapy Program at the N.E. Area Hemophilia Center." *Scandinavian Journal of Haematology*, 1977, *31*, 37–51.

Levine, P. H. Hemophilia Diagnostic and Treatment Center Directors' Meeting, San Francisco, March 1981.

Levine, P. H., and others. "Health of the Intensively Treated Hemophiliac with Special References to Abnormal Liver Chemistries and Splenomegaly." *Blood*, 1977, *50*, 1–9.

Linney, D. "Financial Counseling in Hemophilia." The Treatment of Hemophilia Series, National Hemophilia Foundation, New York, 1979.

Mahoney, M. J. "Fetoscopy." *Pediatric Annals*, 1981, *10* (2), 61–68.

Mattsson, A., and Gross, S. "Social and Behavioral Studies on Hemophilic Children and Their Families." *Journal of Pediatrics*, 1966, *68*, 952–964.

Miller, C. H. "Genetics of Hemophilia and von Willebrand's Disease." In M. W. Hilgartner (Ed.), *Hemophilia in the Child and Adult*. New York: Masson, 1982.

Pearson, H. A., and O'Brien, R. T. "The Management of Thalassemia Major." *Seminars in Haematology*, 1975, *12*, 255–265.

Poncz, M., Cohen, A., and Schwartz, E. "Thalassemia." *Advances in Pediatrics*, 1984, *31*, 43–86.

Pool, J. G., and Shannon, A. E. "Production of High-Potency Concentrates of Antihemophilic Globulin in a Closed Bag System: Assay In Vitro and In Vivo." *New England Journal of Medicine*, 1965, *273*, 1443–1447.

Propper, R. D., Button, L. H., and Nathan, D. G. "New Approaches to the Transfusion Management of Thalassemia." *Blood*, 1980, *55*, 55–59.

Salk, L., Hilgartner, M. W., and Granich, B. "The Psychosocial Impact of Hemophilia on the Patient and His Family." *Social Sciences Medicine*, 1972, *6*, 491–505.

Second Conference on Cooley's Anemia. New York: New York Academy of Sciences, 1968.

Third Conference on Cooley's Anemia. New York: New York Academy of Sciences, 1974.

U.S. Department of Health, Education, and Welfare, National Heart, Lung, and Blood Institute. *Blood Resources Studies*. Publication no. 73-416. Washington, D.C.: U.S. Government Printing Office, 1972.

U.S. Department of Health, Education, and Welfare. *Assessment of Cooley's Anemia Research and Treatment*. Publication no. 79-1653. Washington, D.C.: U.S. Government Printing Office, 1979.

U.S. Department of Health, Education, and Welfare. *Cooley's Anemia: Prevention Through Testing*. Publication no. 80-1269. Washington, D.C.: U.S. Government Printing Office, 1980a.

U.S. Department of Health, Education, and Welfare. *Cooley's Anemia: Prevention Through Understanding.* Publication no. 80-1269. Washington, D.C.: U.S. Government Printing Office, 1980b.

U.S. Department of Health, Education, and Welfare. *Study to Evaluate the Supply and Demand Relationships for AHF and PTC Through 1980.* Publication no. 77-1274. Washington, D.C.: U.S. Government Printing Office, 1980c.

Valentine, W. N., and Neel, I. V. "Hematologic and Genetic Study of the Transmission of Thalassemia." *Archives of Internal Medicine,* 1944, *74,* 185–196.

Valeri, C. R., and Zaroulis, C. G. "Rejuvenation and Freezing of Outdated Stored Human Red Cells." *New England Journal of Medicine,* 1972, *287,* 1307–1313.

Weatherall, D. J., Clegg, J. B., and Naughton, M. A. "Globin Synthesis in Thalassemia: In Vitro Study." *Nature,* 1965, *208,* 1061–1065.

Zaino, E. C. (Ed.). "Third Conference on Cooley's Anemia." *Annals of the New York Academy of Sciences,* 1974, *232,* 1–380.

16

Leukemia

Thomas W. Pendergrass, M.D., M.S.P.H.
Ronald L. Chard, Jr., M.D.
John R. Hartmann, M.D.

Cancer can be defined as a group of diseases that originate from a single malignant cell characterized by potentially unlimited growth with local expansion by invasion and systematic extension by a process called metastasis. Simplistically, a normal cell within the body is altered so that control of growth is lost. The relentless growth of these cells results in invasion and injury to normal tissues. Occasionally cells will break away from the original mass and be carried to distant parts of the body. Upon lodging in the new site, a new nest of cancer cells develops. Symptoms of cancer occur because the normal cells are injured or destroyed. Often these symptoms are subtle.

Cancer is an important disease in children. It is exceeded only by accidents as the leading cause of death in children between one and fifteen years of age in the United States. Approximately 130 new cases of cancer occur each year for each million children under the age of fifteen. Of these, approximately 30 percent will be leukemias with an annual incidence of 40 cases per million children under fifteen years of age (Young and Miller, 1975). This means approximately 6,100 new cases of childhood cancer occur each year in the United States, with almost 1,900 of these being childhood leukemia (Young and others, 1978).

Acute leukemia is a cancer of the white blood cells leading to replacement of normal bone marrow elements by undifferentiated or immature cells termed *blasts*. Chronic leukemia is malignant proliferation of differentiated or mature cells. In either acute or chronic leukemia, as the number of these abnormal cells increases, they accumulate in the body. Bone marrow, lymph nodes, liver, spleen,

Table 1. Classification, Distribution, and Incidence of Childhood Leukemia.

Classification	Children's Cancer Study Group (percent of 1,770 cases)	Southwest Cancer Chemotherapy Study Group (percent of 745 cases)	Incidence in Children under 15 Years of Age (rate per million)	
			White	Black
Acute Leukemias				
Lymphocytic	78	86	24.8	10.5
Acute lymphocytic leukemia	44	54		
Undifferentiated and stem cell	34	32		
Nonlymphocytic	19	13	5.5	4.6
Myelocytic	10	9		
Monocytic/histiocytic	8	2		
Myelomonoblastic	--	2		
Erythroleukemia	1	--		
Chronic Leukemias				
Myelocytic (juvenile and adult types)	1	1	0.9	0.8
Lymphocytic	--	--	0.0	0.0
Classification not stated	2	1	4.5	5.9

Note: Table modified from Baehner, 1978; Young and others, 1978. Totals may exceed 100 percent due to rounding.

kidneys, brain, gonads, lungs, and skin become involved over days to weeks if the disease is not treated.

In children, acute leukemias predominate (99 percent acute, 1 percent chronic). The most common acute leukemia is acute lymphoblastic leukemia (ALL) (Baehner, 1978). There are other terms we consider to be the equivalent of lymphoblastic leukemia. These include lymphocytic, stem cell, and undifferentiated leukemia. These varieties of leukemia account for almost 80 percent of childhood leukemia (see Table 1). Acute leukemias of all other cell lines we call acute nonlymphoblastic leukemias (ANLL).

In this chapter, we present an introduction to children with cancer, with special emphasis on those with the most frequent type, leukemia. In addition to describing the disease and its treatment, we consider the impact of having a child with cancer on the family. The cost, both monetary and emotional, for these families and the resources for meeting these costs is described.

Epidemiology of Childhood Leukemia

Incidence and Mortality. Prior to 1916, mortality statistics were essentially equivalent to incidence statistics because most children succumbed to their illness. Therefore, early insights into the etiology of acute leukemia came from analysis of mortality data. In the 1940s and 1950s, mortality appeared to be changing, with the number of deaths attributed to leukemia increasing. Although some of this increase was related to improved laboratory and diagnostic facilities and to better reporting of causes of death, the increase appeared real and was demonstrated in a number of western countries (Hewitt, 1955; Court Brown and Doll, 1961; Cutler, Axtell, and Heise, 1967). By the 1960s, mortality began to plateau and was declining by the end of that decade (Hanson, McKay, and Miller, 1980).

In reviewing the earlier data, age-specific differences in mortality rates were noted. A large peak in mortality rates was present for children between two and three years of age. A smaller, secondary peak occurred during adolescence, mostly due to nonlymphoblastic leukemias. Hewitt (1955) reported that the young-age peak in ALL mortality first appeared in England and Wales about 1940. In 1961, Court Brown and Doll demonstrated that the young-age peak had evolved between 1911 and 1959 and that the greatest increase occurred in the late 1940s and early 1950s.

The British data also revealed racial differences in the age-specific rates. The young-age peak was present only for white children. Further contrast was provided by the lack of any age-specific peak in mortality in Japanese children (Jim, 1968) and Israeli children (Virag and Modan, 1969). These observations suggested that white children had been exposed to an environmental agent that increased leukemia rates in the young-age group. The age-specific mortality peak has been interpreted as evidence for an infecting agent (presumably a virus) and as support for a role for prenatal or perinatal factors, especially host and genetic factors, as causes of childhood leukemia.

When mortality or incidence rates were reviewed by sex, a male excess was shown. Approximately 20 to 30 percent more males than females develop leukemia (Cutler, Axtell, and Heise, 1967). The previously described peaks in age-specific mortality distribution were present for both sexes among whites but completely absent among nonwhites. This suggests that some host factor unrelated to sex is active in white children.

Improvements in the treatment of children with leukemia have resulted in longer survival times (Hanson, McKay, and Miller, 1980). The very high age peak in mortality among young children in the 1950s has declined over time, with the age distribution becoming more flattened.

Since mortality rates no longer reflect leukemia incidence, it has become important to develop new resources for estimating incidence of this disease. These data have been provided by the Third National Cancer Survey (Young and Miller, 1975) and the Surveillance, Epidemiology, and End Results (SEER) Program of the National Cancer Institute (Silverberg, 1981). These data show a continued peak for ALL beginning at approximately two years of age with a maximum in the three- to four-year age group, while the distribution by age of ANLL remains fairly flat.

Hereditary Factors. Familial leukemia has been observed in children and adults. Three or more affected members in a single generation have been reported, as have families with over four generations affected (Gunz and others, 1966; Kaur and others, 1972; Pendergrass and others, 1975; Anderson, 1951). If one member of an identical twin pair develops leukemia, the twin has approximately a 25 percent chance of developing the disease before the age of ten (MacMahon and Levy, 1964; Miller, 1971). When both members develop leukemia, they have generally acquired the disease within months of each other.

There are a number of heritable conditions that can predispose to leukemia. Children with Down's syndrome, Fanconi's anemia, Bloom's syndrome, ataxia telangiectasia, and immunodeficiency diseases have been found to have excessive rates of childhood leukemia. All of these groups are similar in that they have unique genetic constitutions. Identical twins have identical genes. Bloom's and Fanconi's syndromes are genetically induced disorders characterized by frequent breaks in the chromosomes, and patients with Down's syndrome have an extra chromosome. Thus, a potential link between chromosomal abnormalities and the production of leukemia is strongly suggested.

Patients who have abnormal responses to infection may have what is termed immunodeficiency. These immunodeficient states may be characterized by difficulties in making antibodies, in mounting a cellular response to an infecting agent, or some combination of these. Diseases such as infantile X-linked agammaglobulinemia, severe combined immunodeficiency (SCID), Wiskott-Aldrich disease, isolated IgM deficiency, and common variable immunodeficiency have been associated with excessive cancer occurrences. The hereditary patterns of these conditions are quite variable. Although lymphoreticular malignancies predominate, leukemias are common in these patients (Kersey and Spector, 1975).

Other Characteristics of the Patient. Studies on birth weight, birth order, maternal age, and social class have shown that none of these features are consistently predictive of an excess risk of developing leukemia (Wertelecki and Mantel, 1973; MacMahon and Newill, 1962; Fasal, Jackson, and Klauber, 1971; Spiers, 1971; Pendergrass, Hoover, and Godwin, 1975; Szklo and others, 1978).

Geographic Distribution. Blair, Fraumeni, and Mason (1980) examined the patterns of leukemia mortality in the United States between 1950 and 1969, correlating age-specific mortality rates with demographic, industrial, and agricultural data. Although mortality rates were broadly uniform across the country, mortality among whites was 30 to 40 percent higher than among nonwhites, with a tendency to cluster in the north and in south central regions, particularly for cases of acute myeloid leukemia. Regional variations persisted after adjustments for demographic and ethnic differences but appeared limited to males over the age of fifty-five. Among nonwhites, rates were higher in the Northeast and Midwest than elsewhere.

There have been numerous examples of time and space clustering of childhood leukemia cases (Heath and Hasterlik, 1963; McCafferty and others, 1978; Ertel, Newton, and Halpin, 1976). These instances where multiple cases occur in a specific area over a relatively short period of time have provoked considerable interest. Even though many of these have been evaluated for common exposures, both infectious and environmental, little evidence for associations has appeared. Evaluating such clusters is fraught with difficulties;

among them is the problem of defining the population at risk. Often the clusters occur in areas where families are highly mobile. One explanation of the clustering could then be that the children involved were exposed elsewhere, and disease occurrence at that time was strictly a chance event. Equally difficult is defining the geographic area to be included in each cluster. When studies have defined a population or area initially and then looked for temporal associations, no clustering has been found (Ertel, Newton, and Halpin, 1976; Stark and Mantel, 1967; Browning and Gross, 1968). Because of these difficulties, some have suggested that the clusters are statistical and methodological artifacts (Miller and Fraumeni, 1967; Glass, Hill, and Miller, 1968; Lewis, 1980).

Specific Etiologic Agents. The cause of acute leukemia remains unknown, but interactions of genetic, chromosomal, immunologic, and environmental factors appear important. Since few data are available on childhood leukemia alone, the following discussion includes information about both childhood and adult leukemia. Hereditary conditions associated with acute leukemia have already been discussed, so this section focuses on viral agents and environmental factors.

No human cancer-causing virus is known (Temin, 1974; Rapp and Duff, 1974; Henle and Henle, 1974; Deinhardt, 1974). Often, the virus genetic material is incorporated into the cellular material and therefore is not directly measurable. A number of markers or probes have been identified to allow searching for a virus in the cell. These so-called viral footprints have been found in human leukemia, sarcoma, and lymphoma cells. The question remains whether the viral particles were merely passengers or whether they played a causative role in the development of the leukemia process.

One of the best described etiologic agents for acute leukemia in man is exposure to ionizing radiation, high levels of which are clearly associated with an increased risk of leukemia. Survivors of the atomic bomb blasts in Japan who were within 1,000 meters of the hypocenter had a probability of approximately one in sixty of developing leukemia within twelve years of that exposure. Those who were within 1,500 meters of the hypocenter and who were less than thirty years of age at the time of the bombing had significantly shorter time to appearance of their leukemia than persons in the same age groups who were exposed at 1,501 to 10,000 meters from the hypocenter (Bizzozero and others, 1966). Interestingly, these differences were not seen in people over thirty years of age at the time of the bombing.

Radiation was formerly used as therapy in adult patients with polycythemia vera and ankylosing spondylitis (Modan and Lilienfeld, 1965; Court Brown and Abbott, 1955). These patients subsequently had a high probability of developing acute leukemia following their treatment. They were also shown to have persistent changes in their chromosomes, with excessive numbers of chromosomal breaks. These breaks may have a role in producing the leukemia.

The importance of low-level exposures to ionizing radiation is less clear. Definition of minimum doses that are acceptable for radiation exposure in children is debated. This debate began when Stewart demonstrated leukemia mortality was higher among children of mothers who received diagnostic x ray during pregnancy than among offspring of mothers not exposed (Stewart, Webb, and Hewitt, 1958). Concern and interest continue regarding both the procedures for setting safe levels of exposure and for estimating the number of leukemia cases induced (Bross and Natarajan, 1972).

Although a number of chemicals are known to induce or promote leukemia in animals, only occupational exposure to benzene is generally accepted as producing an excess risk of leukemia in man. Even then, the incidence of leukemia is low compared to the frequency of bone marrow hyperplasia (overgrowth) that typically occurs from heavy benzene exposure (Forni and Moreo, 1969). Other compounds that appear capable of inducing leukemia in humans are the anticancer drugs nitrogen mustard and cyclophosphamide. These agents are widely used to treat people with malignancies, those receiving organ transplants, and those with collagen vascular disease. The use of alkylating agents has been associated with development of leukemia following treatment of cancers of the ovary, breast, lung, and brain, and Hodgkin's disease and Wilms's tumor, as well as following treatment of noncancer disorders, such as nephritis, rheumatoid arthritis, and Wegener's granulomatosis (Reimer and others, 1977; Schwartz, Lee, and Baum, 1975; Auclerc and others, 1979). These induced leukemias have appeared as soon as two years following treatment with the alkylating agent.

Little is known about the importance of parents' occupations or drug exposures and the subsequent development of acute leukemia in their offspring. Fabia and Thery (1974) studied children who died with malignancies in Quebec. They found that more of the dead children had had fathers who were employed in hydrocarbon-related industries at the birth of their children than did controls whose birth registration immediately preceded or followed the dead child's birth certificate. Data from the Finnish cancer registry found no paternal occupation associated with cancer and specifically found no association with hydrocarbon-related occupations (Hakulinen, Salonen, and Teppo, 1976). Zack and others (1980) found no excess exposure to hydrocarbon-related occupations among parents with children with cancer in a case-control study in Texas. Blair, Fraumeni, and Mason (1980) found geographical correlation between leukemia mortality and certain manufacturing industries in the United States with the strongest evidence in rubber, leather, and the paint industries.

Summary of Epidemiology of Childhood Leukemia. Although the etiology of acute leukemia is largely unknown, some pieces of the puzzle are clear. The patterns in age-specific mortality rates suggest that events early in life, perhaps even prenatally, may have an influence on developing leukemia in childhood. Racial differences suggest either differences in exposure to certain factors or differences in responses to those factors by white children. Although these differences are not sexually mediated, heredity appears to play a role. Even so, the known familial and hereditary conditions with high incidence of acute leukemia account for well less than 10 percent of all cases in the United States. Viral infections may play a role by contributing to alteration in genetic material through incorporation of the viral genetic material into that of the host cell. The presence of immunodeficiency may allow wider dissemination or enhanced replication of such viruses. Perhaps exposures to substances like benzene or alkylating agents or to ionizing radiation interact with host or viral agents increasing the likelihood of leukemia transformation. We have just begun to unravel this complex interaction of genetic makeup, immune response, and the environment on the development of acute leukemia in childhood. Whether items can be identified to allow prevention of childhood leukemia remains to be seen.

Disease Definition, Treatment, and Outcome

Diagnosis. Diagnosis of leukemia is established by observing an increased percentage of blast cells in the bone marrow. In the majority of new cases of acute leukemia, more than 80 percent of the cells found in the bone marrow are blasts. When untreated, or after treatment failure, these alterations produce anemia, increased risk of infection, and spontaneous bleeding.

Once an excess number of blast cells have been found in the bone marrow specimen, the type of leukemia must be determined. Acute leukemia accounts for more than 30 percent of all childhood cancer and more than 99 percent of childhood leukemia. Untreated cases are characterized by rapid progression leading to death a few weeks or months after diagnosis. Chronic leukemias are much less common. Chronic lymphocytic leukemia does not occur in childhood. Chronic myelocytic leukemia accounts for less than 1 percent of all childhood leukemia. The chronic leukemias are not discussed here.

Therapy of Acute Lymphoblastic Leukemia. The field of cancer chemotherapy began after the demonstration of the favorable effects of folate antagonists on the course of acute leukemia by Farber in 1948. Following discovery of the folate antagonists, other anticancer agents were found. Initial clinical trials were designed to determine the efficacy of these drugs in producing a measurable decrease in amount of disease (Frei and others, 1958; Heyn and others, 1960). Although these trials did show responses with the use of single drugs, there were problems in comparing one agent to another, in part because of the relative rarity of childhood leukemia and the need for treating sufficient numbers of patients to evaluate treatment effects properly. In response to this need, clinical cooperative groups—each involving several medical centers—for the treatment of childhood acute leukemia were developed through the National Cancer Institute. Most research in treatment of leukemia has been carried out through these cooperative groups.

One of the initial tasks of the cooperative groups was establishment of uniform criteria by which response to therapy could be judged. Uniform criteria allowed each cooperative group to evaluate its own clinical trials and to compare its results with those obtained by others. The criteria are paraphrased here.

1. *Complete remission* occurs when the bone marrow, blood morphology, and the physical examination are all normal.

2. An *incomplete remission* occurs either when increased numbers (greater than 5 percent) of blast cells persist in the bone marrow or when anemia, decreased platelet count, or abnormalities of the lymph glands, spleen, or liver are present.
3. *Hematologic remission* means the bone marrow examination was normal whether or not leukemia persists in other sites.
4. *Relapse* occurs when excess numbers of blast cells return after a complete remission has been attained. Relapse may occur independently in the bone marrow, in the central nervous system, or in the testicles.

Remission induction rates went from a zero pretreatment level to between 60 and 70 percent by the mid 1960s. By 1968, it had been established that prednisone, a steroid, was the best single drug for initial therapy for childhood ALL (Freireich and others, 1963; Wolff and others, 1967; Leikin and others, 1968). The next step was to add other drugs to prednisone to enhance the effect. By 1978, 90 to 95 percent remission induction rates could be expected in large numbers of children with ALL who used prednisone and vincristine with or without L-asparaginase (Jones and others, 1977; Ortega and others, 1977). Use of more intensive regimens during induction has not improved the remission induction rate further (Berry and others, 1975; Komp and others, 1975).

Although more children were obtaining a complete remission, the time spent in that state (remission duration) remained unchanged. Lengthened remission durations did not occur until therapy was continued after complete remission induction (Hoogstraten, 1962). This therapy was termed *maintenance therapy*. Along with appreciation of the need for maintenance therapy came improvement in supportive care for the patient. More effective antibiotics were made available for treating infection, and platelet concentrates became available for treating overt bleeding.

Lengthening of remission duration then dominated study goals. Early studies showed that 6-mercaptopurine was useful for maintenance therapy. By the mid 1960s, aggressive maintenance programs had increased median survival time to about two years (Krivit and others, 1968; Burgert and others, 1969). However, during the late 1960s, new problems occurred.

In one study, 51 percent of children were found to develop central nervous system (CNS) leukemia at a median remission duration of seventeen months (Evans, Gilbert, and Zandstra, 1970). Slightly more than half of these occurred during complete hematologic remission. Thus, although maintenance of complete hematologic remission was possible for long periods of time, CNS disease prevented longer complete remission in many patients.

The occurrence of CNS disease was found to be due, in part, to a protective mechanism of the brain that decreases the amount of drug allowed into the brain tissue. To circumvent this problem, medication was given directly into the spinal fluid. Patients receiving repeated doses of cerebrospinal fluid methotrexate during induction and maintenance had significantly longer complete remissions and half the incidence of central nervous system leukemia of those not receiving medications in the spinal fluid (Glidewell and Holland, 1973). These data strongly suggested that some form of central nervous system treatment should be included in the initial phase of therapy. A study begun in 1972, using common induction and maintenance regimens, randomized its patients to receive one of four CNS methods: craniospinal radiation with radiation to the liver, spleen, kidney, gonads, and lower abdomen; craniospinal radiation alone; cranial radiation plus intrathecal methotrexate; or intrathecal methotrexate alone. The results of the study showed that the incidence of central nervous system disease dropped to between 2.5 and 6 percent in all except those children who presented with both white blood counts over 20,000 and who were treated only with intrathecal methotrexate. These children had a 42 percent incidence of CNS leukemia (Hittle and others, 1975). A later follow-up of this study has reported a much higher CNS disease rate among those receiving intrathecal methotrexate alone, regardless of initial white blood count (Nesbit and others, 1975).

Another major contribution of the cooperative groups has been the involvement of the biostatistician in designing treatment protocols and evaluating the outcome. As the groups treated larger and larger numbers of patients, it became evident that certain features at the time of diagnosis could be predictive of outcome. Most important of these prognostic features are age at diagnosis, initial white-blood-cell count, and type of leukemia. Other factors such as enlargement of the spleen, liver, or lymph nodes, central nervous system disease at diagnosis, level of hemoglobin or platelet count, morphology of the cells, and immunologic surface markers have been shown to have prognostic importance but of lesser magnitude (Baehner, 1978).

Even with identification of more homogeneous treatment groups and increasing survival durations, new problems have appeared. Male children with acute leukemia have a poorer prognosis than females, in part because of their risk of isolated relapse in the testicle. As with central nervous system leukemia, children who have testicular relapse are at greater risk of having a subsequent bone marrow relapse (Nesbit and others, 1977; Lendon and others, 1978).

Although there have been dramatic improvements in survival of children with ALL during the last twenty years, several problems remain. Drug resistance may develop allowing leukemia cells to survive exposure to drug concentrations that initially would have killed them. This possibility may be enhanced by a fraction of leukemia cells that persist in a resting phase. In this state, they are relatively insensitive to anticancer agents. Leukemic cells may also be protected in sanctuaries such as the central nervous system or the testis where they escape the lethal effects of the chemotherapy. Progress in the future is dependent on creative research into the etiology, diagnosis, and treatment of childhood leukemia and on clinical trials to document the effects of new agents and new regimens. Because of stratification of patients into smaller groups based on prognosis, the need for cooperative programs to evaluate therapy will continue.

Current challenges include the child who fails to achieve a remission after initial therapy and therapy for the child who suffers a bone marrow relapse. Questions of how long one needs to treat a child who remains in complete remission and what the long-term side effects of the disease and its therapy are remain for those treated successfully. As answers appear for these, efforts to find the minimal treatment that is effective will become necessary.

Therapy of Acute Nonlymphocytic Leukemia in Childhood. Acute non-lymphoblastic leukemia (ANLL) constitutes about 10 to 15 percent of acute leukemia in childhood. Treatment of this disease is much more difficult than that of ALL, and improvements have been much slower to develop. Because of the relatively small number of patients, efforts of cooperative groups have contributed to treatment evaluation. Prior to 1968, the median survival for all patients with ANLL was one and a half months (Freedman and others, 1971). In 1968, a pilot study using intravenous cystosine arabinoside and cyclophosphamide showed improvements in remission induction rates with median remission duration increased to nine and a half months. By 1977, reports of remission induction rates of 65 to 80 percent were common (Chard and others, 1978; Wiernick and others, 1978).

Prognostic factors in ANLL include initial white blood count, sex, and age. These factors seem to be most important for determining remission induction rates. Development of CNS disease has not been as large a problem in ANLL as in ALL. This may be, in part, because children with ANLL do not survive long enough for this complication to arise.

Bone Marrow Transplantation. Bone marrow transplantation involves first finding a tissue-identical family member to serve as marrow donor. The patient then receives lethal doses of chemotherapy and radiation prior to infusion of the donor marrow. This marrow, which is infused much like a blood transfusion, then proliferates in the patient's body. When the marrow is established (engrafted), all blood elements in the patient (host) are made by donor cells. Although substantial problems can occur with infection and pneumonia or reaction of the donor (grafted) cells to the patient (graft-versus-host disease), this elaborate treatment holds considerable promise for the patient who has ANLL or who has relapsed with ALL (Leikin and others, 1969). Because of the requirement for a matched donor, only 25 percent of patients potentially could receive a transplant, but it represents a life-saving procedure for some. Because of the special demands of this therapy, few institutions have committed the resources necessary to support it. Currently the largest experience is that of the Seattle group (Thomas and others, 1975; Thomas, Sanders, and Johnson, 1979).

Summary of Treatment of Childhood Acute Leukemia. Dramatic advances have been made in the treatment of children with ALL. These include better understanding of the anticancer agents and more effective use of them as well as improvements in supportive care. Concerns now primarily revolve around improving remission duration in those children with poor initial risk factors. As more children attain a remission and remain in remission for increasing periods of time, greater attention is given to dealing with the psychological demands of this chronic illness. The consequences of the disease and its treatment on the child's future participation in society will require additional surveillance.

Advances have not occurred so rapidly in ANLL, in part because of its relative rarity. The importance of cooperative group efforts to accumulate sufficient numbers of patients to evaluate new therapy rapidly cannot be overemphasized. This inclusion of therapy involving several different modes (radiation, surgery, and drugs) has also enhanced the improvement in treatment. The combination of the efforts of the oncologist and the radiation therapist in the management of these children is exemplary.

Psychological Impact

The Parents. Among the most difficult aspects of management of the child with leukemia are the psychotherapeutic problems created by the diagnosis. Included with the first priorities following diagnosis are counseling and educating the parents. A frank but sympathetic discussion of the diagnosis should be given in a manner that allows the parents time to give each other emotional support and to ask questions. This informational exchange is likely to require repetition over several days to allow the parents both to integrate the impact of their child's having cancer and to understand the treatment plan. Myths such that leukemia is due to some oversight of theirs, is contagious, or is highly hereditary need to be dispelled. Many parents feel guilt regarding tardiness in seeking medical care. A realistic prognosis for the patient should be described, and the details of therapy should be outlined. Cautious optimism is indicated for the patient with good prognostic factors. Parents often need to be cautioned about sensational reports in the news media regarding immediate cures using nonmedical approaches and about the fanfare that sometimes accompanies more conventional approaches. Discussions of when their child can be expected to return to normal activities and the issues of discipline and overprotectiveness should be included.

During the initial hospitalization and through the next several months of the illness, ample time needs to be allowed for the parents to meet with medical personnel to clarify points made in previous discussions and occasionally to meet with other parents to discuss their situation. Varied patterns of adjustment and adaptive behaviors may protect parents, permitting them to function effectively in the short term. However, constant assessment of these coping behaviors is necessary to be assured that growth is occurring in their ability to deal with their child and the illness. Provision of confident and available physicians with continuity and personalization of care enhances this response.

The Child. The problem of what to tell the child about the disease must also be faced. There is considerable variation in what and how much a child is told. The child's age, the family's approach, and different personal and clinical situations all contribute to this variation. There really isn't a single way better than all others. However, we have learned that methods of the past in which sentiments were strongly against telling a child anything about the disease are counterproductive. Although these may have been appropriate at a time when death would come in a matter of months, they certainly do not apply today when treatment produces longer and longer survivals. Moreover, in spite of not being told of the disease, almost all children come to know the name of their disease and its implications within the first few months of treatment. In those instances where their parents are unable to discuss it, children may react to this secretiveness by feeling lonely, estranged from family and friends, and fearful about the disease and its treatment. They can imagine consequences of the disease or treatment that are worse than reality. Rebelliousness, school problems, and home problems occasionally develop. By contrast, parents who develop an open relationship with their child and frankly tell the child about the disease find that child more accepting of the diagnosis and less fearful.

Children need to have a sense of trust and an understanding of what is happening to them. Discussions about the disease and its treatment depend on the age and maturity of the child. The medical terminology should be explained in an age-appropriate fashion. Immediate and long-term problems in therapy should be briefly outlined. Explanations of procedures such as blood tests, bone marrow aspirations, and lumbar punctures should accompany or precede the procedures themselves. A realistic approach to pain and other physical discomforts is necessary.

The Family. Having a child with leukemia affects not only that child and parents but also the entire family structure. Siblings, grandparents, aunts, uncles, and friends experience many of the same emotional upheavals that parents experience following the diagnosis. Often these anxieties can be dealt with by providing explanations of the child's expected course much as is done for the parents.

Treatment Failure. In those instances when a child sustains a relapse, preparing families for that child's death may decrease the sudden or overwhelming sense of loss. Again, the approach has to be individualized. Several important principles of management should be followed in the care of the dying child. The needs of the child and the family should be approached in a confident and conscientious manner, with the physician available as much as possible. Access to telephone numbers for emergency contact is necessary. When the physician is willing to answer questions and is sensitive to the child's emotional needs, feelings of anxiety, fear, anger, and guilt are minimized. The philosophy of providing ongoing care for the child, despite failure of antileukemia therapy, is key to this approach. An environment of steady, constant support in which honest answers prevail should be encouraged.

Financial Stress. Families can receive additional stresses from the costs, in time and money, of caring for their ill child. Travel to and from clinic or hospital may be a major difficulty during the first few months of therapy. Although this provides for greater contact and some reassurance from the physician, such reassurance is often directed toward the mother who, in most cases, is primary caretaker. In this instance, the father has less information available to him. This may slow his emotional development. Separation because of hospitalization may be an extra strain for siblings and spouse.

The Medical Team. Emotional strain is also a problem for the medical team. The potential for burnout is exceedingly high. To minimize the strain, many institutions have group meetings where physicians, nurses, social workers, and other members of the hospital team can share experiences and frustrations in dealing with families. Other times, members of the team individually provide a sounding board for one another. But even accomplishing adequate communication is a challenge in terms of time and energy required.

Cost of Therapy

Advances in the care of children with cancer have come at considerable expense. Research to provide advances is costly, and treatment itself is an expensive undertaking. To better document cost of treatment, we identified all children who were diagnosed with leukemia at Children's Orthopedic Hospital and Medical Center (COHMC) in Seattle in 1979. The sums discussed here represent costs for inpatient and outpatient care at COHMC but do not include physician fees or fees for care outside COHMC.

Thirty children were diagnosed with leukemia in 1979. Billing records for twenty-four of these were available for review. Six received the majority of their care through their private pediatrician because they lived outside Seattle. Their contribution to the cost of care is clearly an underestimate.

Twenty of the children had ALL; four had ANLL. Three of the twenty with ALL died before September 1981 (at 12.6, 15.6, and 22.7 months following diagnosis). Two children underwent bone marrow transplantation; one died, and one is surviving. Of the children with ANLL, three have died, one after bone marrow transplantation.

Total hospital costs for the twenty-four children through September 1981 were $595,314. On the average, the first year of therapy at COHMC for children with ALL cost $12,334 per patient with a range of $2,000 to $40,825. This latter figure was for a child who died fifteen and a half months after diagnosis. Ten children completed twenty-four months of treatment. The average cost of two years of treatment was $21,114 with a range of $2,958 to $52,343. Only four patients were diagnosed with ANLL, so costs should be viewed as rough estimates. Only one child survived beyond twenty-four months, so two-year costs are not presented here. Average cost for the first year of care (three patients) was $29,337 with a range of $18,788 to $41,911.

Costs for care of children with leukemia are substantial. The costs for a child with ALL exceed $12,000 for the first year and are over $10,000 for the second year. The cost for the third year would be about $8,000 to $10,000. Costs should drop in children in continuous complete remission after three years because chemotherapy ceases in most protocols after the third year of treatment with only follow-up continuing. By contrast, costs for care of children with ANLL and those with recurrent ALL remain high—something over twice that of children with ALL in continuous complete remission. These children require more care in attempting to treat their aggressive disease or to provide comfort in their dying.

A word of caution is necessary regarding these data. Some costs of care were not available to us. We did not have data on costs of care outside our institution.

Physician fees were not included because of difficulty abstracting the data. In addition, costs for investigational drugs provided through the National Cancer Institute and research costs such as funding for secretarial, data management, and other support are not included in our cost estimates. Out-of-pocket expenses for the family for travel, lodging, and time lost from work during treatment represent other financial hardships not included in our estimate. Therefore, our cost estimates should be considered conservative estimates of minimum cost. Actual cost may be much higher.

Demands and Challenges of Care

Sources of Therapy. Most children with cancer are treated in academic pediatric oncology centers. These centers include physicians, nurses, and other members of the health care team. Support by subspecialty consultants, including pathologists, surgeons, and medical subspecialists is required. A radiation oncologist is an integral part of the treatment of children with leukemia. Nurses or nurse practitioners with experience in caring for the hospitalized child as well as those versed in outpatient care of chronically ill children are vital. An oncology nurse-specialist may serve as the liaison between these nursing roles. A psychosocial support team including social workers; occupational, physical, and recreational therapists; psychiatrists; psychologists; and chaplain complete the ideal staff. Additional supportive facilities necessary for the care of children with cancer include a comprehensive blood bank to supply blood products and skilled clinical laboratory facilities to assist in patient management.

Research. Both institutional and cooperative group investigational programs are needed to improve the management of childhood cancer. Investigators in a single institution can provide insight through initial trials of a new agent or a new therapeutic modality, but confirmation of the effectiveness of that treatment likely will involve a clinical cooperative group. The importance of basic science research in the understanding of the etiology and natural progression of this disease cannot be overemphasized.

Supply of Trained Professionals. The pediatric hematologist-oncologist in most institutions has a dual role. He or she not only provides ongoing humanitarian care for patients but also is involved in either clinical or basic research into the etiology or treatment of childhood malignancies. Enough pediatric hematologist-oncologists may have been trained to provide the necessary clinical care (Donaldson, 1978). Of more concern is training adequate numbers of academic physicians to maintain high-quality research. In addition, there is an ongoing need for trained nursing personnel at all levels, from the staff nurse to the oncology nurse specialist to the nurse practitioner. Sources of funding for training such individuals remain precarious.

Sources of Financial Support. Most of the costs of caring for children with cancer are borne by the family. Certainly health insurance assumes a major portion of this burden, but substantial sums remain uncovered. Nonreimbursed expenses include not only the hospitalization and outpatient services not met by insurance or other third parties but also the costs of transportation and housing necessary to visit treatment centers and of time lost from work for parents. Some assistance is available from the American Cancer Society, Crippled Children's Services (in some states), and the Leukemia Society of America. Many centers have developed Ronald McDonald Houses with support of the McDonald Corporation to assist in the housing of patients or parents at low cost. Special educational needs of children with cancer are met even more erratically. Some school districts have excellent home tutoring services; others give little support. Funding for psychological support services is also variable. Most hospitals maintain social work services, but they are often overburdened and provide only for those with extreme needs. Usually manpower and financial support for preventive psycho-therapy or social intervention are scant or absent. Moreover, third-party payors have been erratic in setting payment guidelines.

The major support for research has been the National Cancer Institute (NCI). Through grant and contract mechanisms, competitive funding for indi-vidual research projects, program areas, and cooperative groups has evolved at the NCI. The support for both basic and clinical research efforts grew rapidly with the National Cancer Act; many programs were born and have survived their infancy. Recent inflation and funding restrictions appear not only to place a ceiling on growth but also, in many instances, to cause underfunding of ongoing programs.

Substantial funding has come from the American Cancer Society (ACS). In addition to its patient support activities, the ACS has provided substantial sums for both basic and clinical research. Although generalities are always hazardous, ACS tends to provide more in the way of seed money for new areas or projects and has been less committed to ongoing programs. Other sources of research funding include the Leukemia Society of America (LSA), the drug industry, and small philanthropic foundations. Although salary support is available through LSA, most of the funding through this group serves short-term projects. The major source of funding for personnel development has been the NCI through its Clinical Cancer Education Grants and Research Training Grants. As noted, both ACS and LSA provide some research salary support as well as trainee support for physicians and nurses.

Future Needs. Because the cause (or causes) of acute leukemia has not been determined, vigorous pursuit of the basic etiology of this disease is required. Molecular biologists, virologists, epidemiologists, immunologists, and others must continue to investigate the interactions of hereditary factors, host factors, and viral and environmental factors. Immunologic tools for diagnosis and treatment appear promising.

Bone marrow transplantation has been shown to be effective in late-stage leukemia. Preliminary studies suggest that it is even more effective in children without large tumor burdens. As bone marrow transplants are performed earlier in the course of disease, better understanding of the benefits and complications of this procedure should accrue.

Drug development requires biochemists and pharmacologists. Evaluation of therapeutic effectiveness requires careful clinical trials. Clinical research trials will become more difficult because of the length of time required to tell whether one treatment program is significantly different from another. This is especially true when induction rates and survival rates are at the high levels currently attained in ALL. It is important to maintain a large, strong clinical cooperative program for evaluation of treatment.

As the number of long-term survivors increases, late effects of their disease and of its treatment become more important. Even though we have relatively few patients who have survived their cancer into adulthood, there is some suggestion that second malignant neoplasms may occur at higher than expected rates (Hutchinson, 1972; Meadows and others, 1975). We have little experience to allow us to predict whether they will be at increased risk of other illnesses. Although some children with cancer have had children of their own, we cannot predict fertility rates or carefully quantitate the chance of having children with congenital defects. Nor do we know if their children will be at increased risk of malignancy. Important to the individual is the availability of insurance for future health care needs. Insurance companies have little on which to base rate estimates and have been somewhat erratic in establishing guidelines for insurability.

The intellectual performance of children with cancer is also of concern. Initially these children's school performance can be assessed. But more crucial outcomes will be entry into the job market and becoming productive members of society. Performance there will evaluate whether expenditures made were well spent. Having a whole, healthy child at the conclusion of treatment for cancer is our goal. This goal presents problems beyond ridding the child of the malignancy. Long-term health problems may await survivors. The presence or lack of intellectual and psychological well-being may affect job participation, marriage, or family. These are but a few of the challenges facing us in managing the child with cancer.

References

Anderson, R. D. "Familial Leukemia: Report of Leukemia in Five Siblings, with a Brief Review of the Genetic Aspects of This Disease." *American Journal of Diseases of Children*, 1951, *81*, 313–322.

Auclerc, G., and others. "Post-Therapeutic Acute Leukemia." *Cancer*, 1979, *44*, 2017–2025.

Baehner, R. L. "Hematologic Malignancies: Leukemia and Lymphoma." In C. H. Smith (Ed.), *Blood Diseases of Infancy and Childhood*. (4th ed.) St. Louis, Mo.: Mosby, 1978.

Berry, D. H., and others. "Comparison of Prednisolone, Vincristine, Methotrexate and 6-Mercaptopurine Versus Vincristine and Prednisone Induction Therapy in Childhood Acute Leukemia." *Cancer*, 1975, *102*, 98–102.

Bizzozero, O. J., and others. "Radiation-Related Leukemia in Hiroshima and Nagasaki, 1946–1964: I. Distribution, Incidence, and Appearance Time." *New England Journal of Medicine*, 1966, *274*, 1095–1101.

Blair, A., Fraumeni, J. F., Jr., and Mason, T. J. "Geographic Patterns of Leukemia in the United States." *Journal of Chronic Diseases*, 1980, *33*, 251–260.

Bross, I. D. J., and Natarajan, N. "Leukemia from Low-Level Radiation: Identification of Susceptible Children." *New England Journal of Medicine*, 1972, *287*, 107–110.

Browning, D., and Gross, S. "Epidemiological Studies of Acute Childhood Leukemia: A Study of Cuyahoga County, Ohio." *American Journal of Diseases of Children*, 1968, *116*, 576–585.

Burgert, E. O., and others. "Acute Lymphocytic Leukemia in Children: Maintenance Therapy with Methotrexate Administered Intermittently." *Journal of the American Medical Association*, 1969, *207*, 923–928.

Chard, R. L., Jr., and others. "Increased Survival in Childhood Acute Nonlymphocytic Leukemia After Treatment with Prednisone, Cytosine Arabinoside, 6-Thioguanine, Cyclophosphamide and Oncovin (PATCO) Combination Therapy." *Medical and Pediatric Oncology*, 1978, *4*, 263–273.

Court Brown, W. M., and Abbott, J. D. "The Incidence of Leukemia in Ankylosing Spondylitis Treated with X-ray: Preliminary Report." *Lancet*, 1955, *1*, 1283–1285.

Court Brown, W. M., and Doll, R. "Leukaemia in Childhood and Young Adult Life: Trends in Mortality in Relation to Aetiology." *British Medical Journal*, 1961, *1*, 981–988.

Cutler, S. J., Axtell, L., and Heise, H. "Ten Thousand Cases of Leukemia: 1940–1962." *Journal of the National Cancer Institute*, 1967, *39*, 993–1026.

Deinhardt, F. "Introduction to Virus-Caused Cancer: Type C Virus." *Cancer*, 1974, *34*, 1363–1367.

Donaldson, M. H. "Manpower Needs as Reflected in the Geomet Survey." In M. H. Edwards (Ed.), *Graduate Education in Pediatric Hematology-Oncology: Summary of a Workshop, September 26–27, 1978*. Bethesda, Md.: Division of Cancer Research Resources and Centers, National Cancer Institute, 1978.

Ertel, I., Newton, W., and Halpin, T. J. "Acute Childhood Leukemia— Columbus, Ohio." *Morbidity and Mortality Weekly Report*, 1976, *25*, 77–78.

Evans, A. E., Gilbert, E. S., and Zandstra, R. "The Increasing Incidence of Central Nervous System Leukemia in Children." *Cancer*, 1970, *20*, 404–409.

Fabia, J., and Thery, T. D. "Occupation of Fathers at Time of Birth of Children Dying of Malignant Diseases." *British Journal of Preventive and Social Medicine*, 1974, *28*, 90–100.

Farber, S., and others. "Temporary Remissions in Acute Leukemia in Children Produced by Folic Acid Antagonists, 4-aminopeteroyl-glutamic acid (Aminopterin). *New England Journal of Medicine*, 1948, *238*, 787–793.

Fasal, E., Jackson, E. W., and Klauber, M. R. "Birth Characteristics and Leukemia in Childhood." *Journal of the National Cancer Institute*, 1971, *47*, 501–509.

Forni, A., and Moreo, L. "Chromosome Studies in a Case of Benzene-Induced Erythroleukemia. *European Journal of Cancer*, 1969, *5*, 459–463.

Freedman, M. H., and others. "The Effects of Chemotherapy on Acute Myelogenous Leukemia in Children." *Journal of Pediatrics,* 1971, *78,* 526–532.

Frei, E., and others. "A Comparative Study of Two Regimens of Combination Chemotherapy in Acute Leukemia." *Blood,* 1958, *13,* 1126–1148.

Freireich, E. J., and others. "The Effect of 6-Mercaptopurine on the Duration of Steroid Induced Remissions in Acute Leukemia: A Model of Evaluation of Other Potentially Useful Therapy." *Blood,* 1963, *21,* 699–716.

Glass, A. G., Hill, J. A., and Miller, R. W. "Significance of Leukemia Clusters." *Journal of Pediatrics,* 1968, *73,* 101–107.

Glidewell, O. J., and Holland, J. G. "Clinical Trials of the Acute Leukemia Group B in Acute Lymphocytic Leukemia in Childhood." *Bibliotheca Haemetologica,* 1973, *39,* 1053–1067.

Gunz, G. W., and others. "Multiple Cases of Leukemia in a Sibship." *Blood,* 1966, *27,* 482–489.

Hakulinen, T., Salonen, T., and Teppo, L. "Cancer in the Offspring of Fathers in Hydrocarbon-Related Occupations." *British Journal of Preventive and Social Medicine,* 1976, *30,* 138–140.

Hanson, M. R., McKay, F. W., and Miller, R. W. "Three-Dimensional Perspective of United States Cancer Mortality." *Lancet,* 1980, *2,* 246–247.

Heath, C. W., and Hasterlick, R. J. "Leukemia Among Children in a Suburban Community." *American Journal of Medicine,* 1963, *34,* 796–812.

Henle, W., and Henle, G. "Epstein-Barr Virus and Human Malignancies." *Cancer,* 1974, *34,* 1368–1374.

Hewitt, D. "Some Features of Leukemia Mortality." *British Journal of Preventive and Social Medicine,* 1955, *9,* 81–88.

Heyn, R. M., and others. "The Comparison of 6-Mercaptopurine and Azaserine in the Treatment of Acute Leukemia in Children; Results of a Cooperative Study." *Blood,* 1960, *15,* 350–359.

Hittle, R., and others. "Effectiveness of Presymptomatic Treatment on the Occurrence of Central Nervous System (CNS) Disease in Childhood Lymphoblastic Leukemia (ALL), abstracted." *Proceedings of the American Association for Cancer Research,* 1977, *18,* 143.

Hoogstraten, G. "Remission Maintenance in Acute Leukemia: A New Specific Experimental Design." *Journal of Chronic Diseases,* 1962, *15,* 269–272.

Hutchinson, G. B. "Late Neoplastic Changes Following Medical Irradiation." *Radiology,* 1972, *105,* 645–652.

Jim, R. T. S. "Leukemia in Hawaii." *Cancer,* 1968, *22,* 1060–1064.

Jones, B., and others. "Optimal Use of L-Asparaginase (NSC-109229) in Acute Lymphocytic Leukemia." *Medical and Pediatric Oncology,* 1977, *3,* 387–400.

Kaur, J., and others. "Familial Acute Myeloid Leukemia with Acquired Pelger-Huet Anomaly and Aneuploidy of C Group." *British Medical Journal,* 1972, *4,* 327–431.

Kersey, J. H., and Spector, B. D. "Immune Deficiency Diseases." In J. F. Fraumeni, Jr. (Ed.), *Persons at High Risk of Cancer: An Approach to Cancer Etiology and Control.* New York: Academic Press, 1975.

Komp, D. M., and others. "Cyclophosphamide-Asparaginase-Vincristine-Prednisone Induction Therapy in Childhood Acute Lymphocytic and Non-Lymphocytic Leukemia." *Cancer*, 1975, *37*, 1243-1247.

Krivit, W., and others. "Maintenance Therapy in Acute Leukemia of Childhood." *Cancer*, 1968, *21*, 352-356.

Leikin, S. L., and others. "Varying Prednisone Dosage in Remission Induction of Previously Untreated Childhood Leukemia." *Cancer*, 1968, *21*, 346-351.

Leikin, S. L., and others. "The Use of Combination Therapy of Leukemia Remission." *Cancer*, 1969, *24*, 427-432.

Lendon, M., and others. "Testicular Histology After Combination Chemotherapy in Childhood Acute Lymphocytic Leukemia." *Lancet*, 1978, *2*, 439-441.

Lewis, M. S. "Spatial Clustering in Childhood Leukemia." *Journal of Chronic Diseases*, 1980, *33*, 703-712.

McCafferty, H. G., and others. "Childhood Leukemia—Rutherford, New Jersey." *Morbidity and Mortality Weekly Report*, 1978, *27*, 129-130.

MacMahon, B., and Levy, M. A. "Prenatal Original of Childhood Leukemia: Evidence from Twins." *New England Journal of Medicine*, 1964, *270*, 1082-1085.

MacMahon, B., and Newill, V. "Birth Characteristics of Children Dying of Malignant Neoplasms." *Journal of the National Cancer Institute*, 1962, *28*, 231-244.

Meadows, A. T., and others. "Oncogenesis and Other Late Effects of Cancer Treatment in Children: Report of a Single Hospital Study." *Radiology*, 1975, *114*, 175-180.

Miller, R. W. "Deaths from Childhood Leukemia and Solid Tumors Among Twins and Other Sibs in the United States, 1960-1967." *Journal of the National Cancer Institute*, 1971, *46*, 203-209.

Miller, R. W., and Fraumeni, J. F., Jr. "Leukemia Houses." *Annals of Internal Medicine*, 1967, *67*, 674-676.

Modan, B., and Lilienfeld, A. M. "Polycythemia Vera and Leukemia: The Role of Radiation Treatment. A Study of 1,222 Patients." *Medicine*, 1965, *44*, 305-344.

Nesbit, M., and others. "Influence of an Isolated Central Nervous System (CNS) Relapse on Subsequent Marrow Relapse in Childhood Lymphoblastic Leukemia (ALL), abstracted." *Proceedings of the American Association for Cancer Research*, 1975, *16*, 259.

Nesbit, M., and others. "Prevention of Testicular Relapse by Prophylactic Radiation (XRT) in Childhood Acute Lymphoblastic Leukemia (ALL), abstracted." *Proceedings of the American Association for Cancer Research*, 1977, *18*, 317.

Ortega, J. A., and others. "L-Asparaginase, Vincristine and Prednisone for Induction of First Remission in Acute Lymphocytic Leukemia." *Cancer Research*, 1977, *37*, 535-540.

Pendergrass, T. W., Hoover, R., and Godwin, J. D. "Prognosis of Black Children with Acute Lymphocytic Leukemia." *Medical and Pediatric Oncology*, 1975, *1*, 143-148.

Pendergrass, T. W., and others. "Acute Myelocytic Leukemia and Leukemia Associated Antigens in Sisters." *Lancet*, 1975, *2*, 429–431.

Rapp, F., and Duff, R. "Oncogenic Conversion of Normal Cells by Inactivated Herpes Viruses." *Cancer*, 1974, *34*, 1353–1362.

Reimer, R. R., and others. "Acute Leukemia After Alkylating Agent Therapy of Ovarian Cancer." *New England Journal of Medicine*, 1977, *197*, 177–181.

Schwartz, A. D., Lee, H., and Baum, E. S. "Leukemia in Children with Wilms' Tumor." *Journal of Pediatrics*, 1975, *87*, 374–376.

Silverberg, E. "Cancer Statistics, 1981." *CA: A Cancer Journal for Clinicians*, 1981, *31*, 13–28.

Spiers, P. S. "The Role of Mother's Age in the Risk of Childhood Leukemia." *American Journal of Epidemiology*, 1971, *94*, 521–523.

Stark, C. R., and Mantel, N. "Temporal-Spatial Distribution for Michigan Children with Leukemia." *Cancer Research*, 1967, *27*, 1749–1775.

Stewart, A., Webb, J., and Hewitt, D. "A Survey of Childhood Malignancies." *British Medical Journal*, 1958, *1*, 1495–1508.

Szklo, M., and others. "The Changing Survivorship of White and Black Children with Leukemia." *Cancer*, 1978, *42*, 59–66.

Temin, H. M. "Introduction to Virus-Caused Cancer." *Cancer*, 1974, *34*, 1347–1352.

Thomas, E. D., Sanders, J. E., and Johnson, F. L. "Marrow Transplantation in the Therapy of Children with Acute Leukemia." In American Cancer Society, *Care of the Child with Cancer*. New York: American Cancer Society, 1979.

Thomas, E. D., and others. "Bone Marrow Transplantation." *New England Journal of Medicine*, 1975, *292*, 895–902.

Virag, I., and Modan, B. "Epidemiologic Aspects of Neoplastic Disease in Israeli Immigrant Population: II. Malignant Neoplasms in Childhood." *Cancer*, 1969, *23*, 137–141.

Wertelecki, W., and Mantel, N. "Increased Birth Weight in Leukemia." *Pediatric Research*, 1973, *7*, 132–138.

Wiernick, P. H., and others. "Current Results in Young Patients (PTS) with Acute Nonlymphocytic Leukemia (ANLL), abstracted." *Proceedings of the American Association for Cancer Research*, 1978, *19*, 145.

Wolff, J. A., and others. "Prednisone Therapy of Acute Childhood Leukemia: Prognosis and Duration of Response in 330 Treated Patients." *Journal of Pediatrics*, 1967, *70*, 626–631.

Young, J. L., Jr., and Miller, R. W. "Incidence of Malignant Tumors in United States Children." *Journal of Pediatrics*, 1975, *86*, 254–258.

Young, J. L., Jr., and others. *Cancer Incidence, Survival and Mortality for Children Under 15 Years of Age*. New York: American Cancer Society, 1978.

Zack, M., and others. "Cancer in Children of Parents Exposed to Hydrocarbon-Related Industries and Occupations." *American Journal of Epidemiology*, 1980, *111*, 329–336.

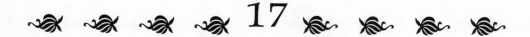

17

Craniofacial Birth Defects

Donald W. Day, M.D.

Craniofacial anomalies (CFAs) represent one of the most frequent types of human birth defects. They are a heterogenous group ranging from the common cleft lip and/or palate to rare and complex syndromes so unique that minimal information exists about their pathogenesis or prognosis. Without regard to its severity or rarity, each CFA takes on additional significance because it affects the human face. No other portion of our body is invested with so much meaning, recognition, and importance. Through the neurosensory functions of our head, we perceive, appreciate, and participate in the world. The face is our window onto life. From our head come our voice, our intellect, and those facial gestures that tell the world so much about the inner person behind the face.

What a marvelous face has man! It is symmetric and beautiful, fluid in movement, expressive in cadence, full of life and intelligence. So much of what we are is written on our faces that rarely do we veil them from view. Therefore, whenever the face is disfigured by a birth defect, the person beneath it must bear additional pain and social stigma (Zapatka, 1982). Fortunately, human courage need not be damaged or diminished by such physical scars. Appropriate psychosocial and physical habilitation can assist the affected individual's inner resolution and cause a reduction of the residual significance of the facial disfigurement.

One can arbitrarily divide craniofacial anomalies into two broad categories based on the presence or absence of isolated facial clefts of the lip and/or palate. This chapter provides information about isolated cleft lip/palate in a section separate from a description of several other common, noncleft craniofacial anomalies. Although their description, etiology, and treatment differ, most craniofacial anomalies (cleft and noncleft) are similar in their effect upon the child and family. Society's response, in the form of clinical support and financial resources for the habilitative process, is also relatively similar. As a result of these

344

similarities, a homogeneous set of policy recommendations can be drawn for all types of craniofacial anomalies.

Cleft Lip and/or Palate

Cleft lip and/or palate represents one of the most frequent human malformations. Its incidence varies between 0.6 to 1.3 per 1,000 births among different racial groups (Battle, 1973). Hence, it is approximately equal to the incidence of Down's syndrome and considerably more common than PKU, muscular dystrophy, and cystic fibrosis. Although clefts are the most frequent single type of craniofacial anomaly, they are not a homogenous entity but rather a spectrum of facial defects.

Since publication of the classic monograph of Fogh-Anderson (1942), most investigators have accepted the concept that isolated cleft of the secondary palate (roof of mouth) is a disorder, cleft palate (CP), separate from that which cleaves the lip. A different genetic disorder, cleft lip and/or palate (CLP), may cleave part or all of the lip, nasal floor, upper dental arch, and roof of mouth (palate). During the past two decades, clinical geneticists have identified more than two hundred different genetic disorders that include facial clefts as part of their manifestations (Cohen, 1978). The etiology, prognosis, and genetic recurrence risk for these syndromes vary greatly from those of isolated clefts. CLP defects can be described as a breech in tissue continuity across the facial midline at the level of the upper lip, anterior nasal floor, maxillary dental arch, and roof of the mouth (bony and soft palate). The nature of CLP defect varies among different children. Some have a unilateral cleft affecting only one side of the face; others have two clefts (bilateral) each of which affects one side of the face. The clefting process may involve the entire lip, dental arch, and palate (complete cleft form) or only a portion of these tissues (incomplete form). Some clefts produce narrow gaps in the tissue continuity, while other clefts cause much wider defects. Therefore, each cleft may be characterized by (1) laterality, (2) completeness, and (3) severity. A particular cleft may be described with any combination of these three characteristics.

Facial structure takes form during the first trimester of pregnancy. Explanations of the development of clefts place different emphasis on the failure of fusion of facial subcomponents or on inappropriate breakdown of previous embryonic tissue fusion planes. However complex the actual cause, the embryonic facial cleft is well established by the end of the fourth gestational month. The etiology of this process involves both environmental and genetic factors. In some cases, one of these factors is clearly the basis for the pathogenesis. For example, CLP is a common birth defect among infants born of mothers exposed to drugs during the gestation (for example, dilantin, alcohol). On the other hand, there are families in which clefting follows a pattern of genetic inheritance with less recognizable environmental influence.

When large samples of human families with cleft-affected individuals are studied, several observations can be made. Most families have only one affected person among close relatives. Offspring of both sexes can be affected by clefting; however, there is slight unbalance of expected sex birth rates with regard to frequency of isolated CLP (more common in males) and cleft palate (more common in females). In families with several affected individuals, the two disorders, CLP and CP, appear to segregate in a manner supporting the concept that these are two separate genetic diseases. There is an increased recurrence risk in families whose affected members demonstrate greater severity of clefting (bilateral versus unilateral and wide, complete versus narrow, incomplete clefts) and those families with females affected by CLP or males with isolated CP.

These observations best support a multifactorial mode of inheritance for human facial clefting. This genetic model proposes that the disease occurs when multiple genes are present that promote clefting and act together with one or more environmental factors (Fraser, 1970), but these genes have not been isolated or identified in a specific manner. Environmental factors may involve the mother's own biochemical milieu in addition to exogenous agents from the environment or the cornucopia of modern pharmacy.

Clefts of the lip and palate cause significant physiologic disturbance in addition to anatomic changes. The "hole" in the palate is part of a very complex developmental and physiologic defect that affects numerous essential human functions: respiration, speech, hearing, chewing-swallowing, and the infantile oral sensory/exploratory behavioral system. In addition, the cleft is centrally placed in the infant's growing face and has significant impact upon the normal pattern of facial skeletal, dental, muscular, and soft tissue growth. The successful habilitation of clefting defects requires surgical and dental efforts to minimize distortions of facial proportion and relationships.

Natural History of Facial Clefting. The natural history of clefting reveals a pattern of complications that affect nutrition; dental, neurosensory, and communication function; educational achievement; and psychosocial adaptation. The last of these concerns is particularly significant because it affects all aspects of human life throughout its entire span. Normal emotional bonding of the parent and infant with a cleft is frequently disturbed (Tisza and Gumpertz, 1962). If the parents have adequate psychologic support and excellent adaptive mechanisms, the disturbance of bonding may be temporary. However, if adaptation is less than appropriate, many aspects of interpersonal relationships may be adversely affected. The consequences are not limited to the infant but frequently spill over to the entire family and produce marital problems, sibling emotional and behavioral disturbances, and conflicts within the extended family. In a family with reasonable psychosocial adaptation, the trauma of the birth defect can be reduced and appropriate parent-infant bonding can occur.

Feeding not only provides nourishment for growth but also is an important part of the human bonding process. Most infants with facial clefts have feeding disturbances. The defect may interfere with production of intraoral suction which, although not essential, is a component of infant sucking. Palatal defects produce abnormal communication between the oral and nasal cavities. Regurgitation and loss of food through the nose may be uncomfortable for the baby, an important loss of caloric intake, and disquieting to the parents. Prior to surgical closure of the palatal defect, the parents can be instructed in specific feeding technics to reduce these problems and their significance.

Disturbances of dental morphology, eruption pattern, and occlusive plane are primary complications of the clefting process. Their significance can be reduced by surgical and orthodontic intervention. Disturbances of dental-facial growth patterns are inherent in these handicaps and may be made better or worse by the selection of intervention strategy.

Only very rare children with unoperated cleft palate develop good speech. The abnormal communication between oral and nasal cavities makes it impossible for the child with CP to develop adequate intraoral pressure for production of certain speech sounds. These children cannot increase intraoral pressure because the air passes through the palatal defect and out the nose. A disturbing hypernasal quality of vowel production and unusual misarticulations of consonant production are created. These unusual consonant substitutions are produced posterior and inferior to the cleft defect. Because the placement is unusual and not utilized in normal speech production, the individual's speech is difficult to understand.

Recent habilitative trends have promoted an earlier age for closure of the palate. The majority of American children with CP have palate surgery between one and three years of age, although many centers repair the palate between eight and eighteen months. A barrier between the oral and nasal cavities can be established at an early age. If this intervention occurs before meaningful speech develops (at six to twelve months), the child has less opportunity to develop defective speech with the characteristic misarticulations. Consequently, minimal or no speech therapy may be required to unlearn the inappropriate speech placements (Dorf, 1982). Recent studies of CP speech development tend to promote early closure of palatal clefts between eight and sixteen months of age.

Children with CP have a substantial risk of moderate, fluctuating, conductive type hearing loss produced by intermittent episodes of serous otitis media. Controversy surrounds the exact etiology of the middle ear fluid and pressure changes. Alterations of eustachian tube function and posterior nasal pharyngeal anatomy are often cited. The problem is particularly severe in young children (three to five years of age) with CP. Placement of plastic ventilation tubes through the tympanic membrane is frequently employed to maintain normal atmospheric pressure in the middle-ear cavity and reduce serous otitis media. These tubes can be placed at the time of cleft lip surgery and replaced if necessary at the time of palatoplasty.

A major secondary complication of clefting is increased risk of faulty self-image and its consequent effect upon ego development, behavior, and educational-vocational achievement. Our face, reflected in the mirror, is usually our first self-identification, which is followed afterward by comparison with other people. The individual with CLP may obtain excellent results from surgery and yet still have facial disfigurement based upon disproportionate skeletal growth of the various facial components. The resultant face may show a surgical scar, flattened asymmetric lower nose, uneven border of the upper lip, or disproportionate forward growth of the upper jaw and mandible. These abnormalities are "up front" for everyone to see and compare with society's normal expectations of beauty. The pleasure with which a person views his or her face (always compared to some other standard) is translated into value points that promote acceptance or rejection of the total body image (Kapp-Simon, 1981). This is extremely important during adolescent years. However, similar issues occur during early school years when peer acceptance is important. Behavioral deviancy, poor social adjustment, and impaired school progress are common secondary complications of this process (Richman, 1976). All of these can be eliminated or at least reduced by appropriate early psychosocial support and counseling for both the child with CLP and the child's parents.

Therapeutic Course for Children with Cleft Palate. Therapy cannot begin without appropriate identification of cases. Approximately one half of infants with cleft palate are not diagnosed during the newborn period (Meskin and Pruzansky, 1967). Individuals with cleft lip are detected almost universally at the time of birth. Equally important for therapy is the nature of the medical referral provided to the family. Naturally, one thinks first about surgical correction of the cleft, but a direct referral to a surgeon may not be the best first decision for the family. Isolated cleft palate may not necessitate active surgical intervention until the child is between eight and eighteen months old. All families in which CLP or CP occur need immediate supportive help, which can best be provided by an interdisciplinary team. There are more than 208 organized cleft palate-craniofacial anomaly teams in the United States (American Cleft Palate Association, 1982). Early referral to such programs provides the opportunity for careful differential diagnosis, treatment planning, contact with third-party funding sources, and parent-infant psychosocial support.

After reaching out to establish support for the family, the cleft palate team's next major task is evaluation of the infant. It might seem that diagnosis is easy. However, facial clefting is complicated by a wide range of cleft manifestations and the possibility of more than one hundred genetic syndromes that must be excluded in the diagnostic process. At this point, the experienced multidisciplinary team can be particularly valuable in clarifying the diagnosis and its prognosis. Members of the team can promote the parent's healthy response to the baby's birth defect, teach them feeding techniques, and start an explanation of the habilitative program for that particular child.

There are numerous surgical techniques (with variable time schedules) employed to repair these facial defects. The plastic surgeon generally plans the surgical closure of the cleft lip at a time between four and eight weeks of age if the baby has gained adequate weight (approximately ten to twelve pounds total weight) and demonstrated a stable health pattern. If the palate is cleft, most surgeons operate when the baby is one to two years old. (Some cleft palate teams now promote earlier closure, in the eight- to eighteen-month range.) Frequently, the team's otolaryngologist joins the plastic surgeon at the operation and performs a microscopic ear examination, with placement of tympanic membrane ventilation tubes if indicated. Surgical revision of the lip and nose may be required in mid to late childhood or adolescence.

Many children with CLP or CP are referred to preschool stimulation programs in their communities. This referral serves many purposes including psychosocial support for the parents, speech stimulation, and promotion of improved and adaptive social skills for the patient. If the child has CLP associated with other birth defects, the stimulation program may provide special habilitative services for the other handicaps. These programs can also assess the child's progress and help prepare a successful entry into regular or special educational programs.

Dental care is an important component of the child's therapy. As the child approaches the adolescent years, active orthodontic care may start. Dental prostheses may be required at various stages of habilitation. Excellent general dental care is necessary to maintain strong and viable teeth without periodontal disease. Frequently, these children do not maintain good oral hygiene, and major dental loss with resultant restorative dental work is often necessary.

Genetic diagnosis and counseling for the parents should be a component of the early visits to the cleft palate team. Over a course of many years of habilitative care, there may be opportunities to reinforce aspects of the genetic counseling. When the patients become sexually active young adults, they frequently have questions about their birth defect and the chance that their offspring might be similarly affected. Perceptive genetic counseling is necessary to provide basic genetic information in their emotionally turbulent teenage years.

Functionally, the cleft palate team needs to be not only *multi*disciplinary in nature but also *inter*disciplinary. Excellent communication among the team professionals allows a homogenous approach to the patient's habilitation, the best utilization of biologic and psychologic data obtained from the patient, and a more holistic appraisal of the patient (Day, 1981). Unfortunately, many patients do not obtain referrals to teams and instead receive piecemeal care from one or more independent health providers. In addition, there are many multidisciplinary teams whose members do not adequately interrelate with each other as they provide patient services. The true interdisciplinary craniofacial anomaly team is uncommon and a real asset when found by the patient and family.

Quality of Life for Individuals with Cleft Palate. Improved quality of life is a central goal for the habilitation of handicapped children. With some chronic diseases, the burden to the patient, family, and society is immense and the long-term prognosis for reasonably normal life is limited. Fortunately, a good prognosis is expected for the vast majority of children with facial clefts and craniofacial anomalies. With early and adequate psychosocial support, they can learn to cope with their residual deformity. Generally, they have normal intelligence and motivation toward achievement (McWilliams and Matthews, 1979). Surgical care may eliminate most of the facial deformity or disproportion. In general, these are children who can be habilitated toward a normal and productive lifestyle (Clifford, Crocker, and Pope, 1972). Their contribution to society far exceeds the help society gives them in their early years of life.

Other Craniofacial Anomalies

There can be an informal division of craniofacial anomalies into cleft and noncleft malformations. Ascertainment bias makes it difficult to determine their relative population frequencies. During the past two decades, there has been a progressively larger volume of patients with other craniofacial anomalies in the caseload of the major centers. These rare syndromes are valuable in craniofacial biology because their evaluation and treatment provides a major impetus toward greater sophistication of basic knowledge.

None of these specific anomalies occur as frequently as simple cleft lip and/or palate. However, in their sum, they represent a patient volume that equals or surpasses the frequency of facial clefts. The following several craniofacial anomalies illustrate characteristics of this category of birth defects and their diagnostic-treatment planning.

Microtia. Microtia is an isolated birth defect consisting of a small and/or abnormally shaped external ear. The middle ear's hearing mechanism is frequently defective, with consequent hearing loss. The more severe variants usually do not have an auditory canal to conduct sound to the middle-ear bones, which may be structurally abnormal. One or both ears may be microtic with asymmetry in the degree of severity. This auricular finding may be part of an oto-facial syndrome (for example, mandibulofacial dysostosis, branchial-oto-renal syndrome) or isolated as the only birth defect. The genetic recurrence risk may vary from 4 percent to 50 percent.

The major habilitative problems are improvement or preservation of hearing and reconstruction of an aesthetically satisfactory external ear. Early identification of hearing loss, determination of its nature, and amplification are essential steps in habilitation. Preschool programs that emphasize auditory training and speech stimulation are helpful. The quality of surgical reconstruction for the most severe microtia still has not reached a level of wide acceptability even though many new techniques have been introduced. Most such reconstructive procedures occur during later childhood or adolescent years.

Facial Asymmetry. Significant craniofacial asymmetry is a frequent component of many CFA syndromes. Plagiocephaly is the generic description for significant asymmetry of the skull and results from an abnormal or premature pattern of maturation and closure of the skull's bony structures. The resultant abnormal shape usually does not have direct or dangerous effects upon the growing brain. However, it may produce a significant facial distortion as it influences facial growth.

There has been substantial progress in surgical therapy for craniofacial asymmetries. Generally these are best accomplished by the massive craniofacial reconstructive techniques that were pioneered in the late 1960s by the French surgeon Dr. Paul Tessier. During previous decades, reconstructive surgery for these children consisted of numerous procedures (frequently between ten and twenty of them) scheduled after most facial growth was completed. Using Dr.

Tessier's techniques, one or two surgical procedures replace the previous multiple procedures.

Hemifacial Microsomia. Hemifacial microsomia is an infrequent but debilitating anomaly that affects any or all of the tissues of the central and lower lateral face (ear, upper jaw, mandible, and dentition). Its expression varies from severe to minimal and may not affect each facial structure with equal severity. This growth disturbance produces a very asymmetric face, severe dental malocclusion, and temporal mandibular joint disease. These last two structural alterations tend to compromise chewing. Ear anomalies usually include variable degree of microtia with hearing loss. The disorder can occur among other family members.

Therapy involves early audiologic assessment and intervention. Orthodontic treatment is linked to surgical reconstruction of the mandible by a maxillofacial (oral) surgeon or plastic surgeon, and final treatment may extend through the young adult period of facial growth. Therefore, these individuals are at particular high risk for development of a faulty self-image and depreciated ego function as the result of their facial defect (Hanus, Bernstein, and Kapp, 1981).

Frontonasal Dysplasia. Individuals with frontonasal dysplasia represent a mixed population whose facial defects are produced by genetic and/or environmental factors. They all demonstrate a wide, flat nasal region between the eyes. The expression of the anomaly ranges from barely perceptible to grotesque appearance in which midfacial structures are not recognizable. Prior to the advent of major craniofacial surgical procedures, the more severely affected children had no chance to lead reasonably normal lives. With current techniques that employ skull and facial surgery, the midfacial sutures are released, excess bone is removed, and the eyes can be repositioned. Partial or complete nasal reconstruction may be necessary.

Craniosynostosis Syndromes. There are almost a dozen recognized genetic syndromes that cause abnormally shaped skull, disturbed pattern of facial growth, and possible limb anomalies. Although rare (incidence is estimated at one in two million adults), Apert's syndrome is typical of this group. In this condition, there is cessation of normal skull growth in a particular geometric axis. With a reduced number of functional bony sutures and a primary disturbance of basal cranial growth, the skull expands into an abnormal shape. These individuals also experience minimal forward growth of the midfacial bones, which causes a reduction of the airway and reduced depth of the bony orbital cavity. These skeletal changes produce orbital proptosis (globe of eye bulges beyond orbital rim) and a chronically exposed cornea. If untreated, many of these children develop eye problems that may lead to corneal scarring, optic atrophy, and blindness.

In addition to these major skull anomalies, individuals with Apert's syndrome have eye muscle imbalance, abnormal palatal structure, dental malocclusion, conductive hearing loss, decreased range of joint motion, soft tissue fusion of digits, and speech problems. Intelligence, which may be normal, is more often mildly reduced. Correction of the eye problems may require reconstruction of the bony orbit, which is accomplished along with reconstruction of the skull and midface bone advancement by the craniofacial surgeon.

Adaptive Stresses for the Handicapped Child and Family

All birth defects create life problems that produce significant stress for both the affected individual and the family. In particular, craniofacial anomalies cause additional intense emotional disturbance for the infant's family because the defect alters facial structure and function. Facial appearance is one of the most influential elements of interpersonal social acceptance. Discrepancy between the individual's actual facial appearance and that individual's perceived self-image is a root cause of many significant personality disorders (Starr and Heiserman, 1977). The family and child must cope with the facial defect prior to treatment, the "changing" facial appearance during prolonged periods of habilation, and physical scars and surgical results that may not produce facial "perfection" (Kapp-Simon, 1981). All of these psychologic stresses are both private, internal concerns and public issues within the larger sphere of the patient's extended family, friends, and peers.

Parents who await the birth of their baby always anticipate a perfect and beautiful infant. For the couple whose pregnancy results in a baby with a craniofacial birth defect, there is usually a flood of emotional anxiety that includes fear, ignorance of factual matters, personal guilt, and grief for the loss of the "perfect baby" who never existed. Human emotional bonding between parent and infant is one of the strongest ties and most significant psychologic events of life. It is the initial step of psychologic and social development. Instead of the recognizable beauty of a baby's face, the parents see a structural alteration they do not understand and that provokes fear and guilt. The rapidity and efficiency with which the parents adapt to the visual and deep emotional stress are major determinants of development of a proper and stable emotional relationship with the child throughout life, self-acceptance as the parents of that special child, and maintenance of a stable marriage with appropriate reproductive potential.

The first step in the habilation of the child must occur at the moment of bonding. At that time of emotional and intellectual confusion, the parents should receive help from an experienced professional. If a proper and effective supportive relationship can be established between the professional and parent, the future habilative process among all these individuals will be stronger and more effective.

The parent and child (in cases of more complex craniofacial anomalies) must adapt to the presence of the altered facial form and function until the appropriate age for surgical intervention. Waiting is very difficult whenever the therapeutic process requires a prolonged period of observable abnormality with its consequent lack of social acceptance. Both child and parent may feel socially defective until the habilative process is more complete and facial appearance more normal.

As the time for habilitation approaches, the parents are informed about surgical details, possible complications, and anticipated results. Then *they* must make a life-shaking and highly stressful decision *for their child*. The parents must decide whether or not they will elect to change their child's facial appearance and all the emotions that they (and the child) have invested in that image. It is an irreversible step, especially momentous for those parents whose children have facial defects more severe than simple facial clefts. That psychological struggle may require a cognitive and emotional evaluation that reopens and unties the fine psychic fabric woven at the time of infant bonding with the handicapped child. For this decision, it is critical that the parents relate to a competent psychologist or psychiatrist who is a member of the craniofacial team. Regardless of the degree of empathy, the surgeon is the child's chief therapist and has an intrinsic conflict if he or she assumes this special therapeutic role with the family.

For individuals with more significant craniofacial anomalies, the child and family continue to undergo extensive psychologic assault during the several years of surgical treatment. During that period, the patient's face is subject to a series of physical changes produced by the sequence of reconstructive surgeries. It is one thing to adapt emotionally to a permanent facial imperfection, accept it, and live with it. However, the contrast is great between that type of reaction and the fluid adaptation necessary to respond to changing facial appearance during several successive surgeries. The changing perception of body image is disconcerting to the patient and frequently occurs during the emotionally unstable adolescent years when a socially respectable facial appearance is of major importance (Kapp-Simon, 1981). Without professional help, the patient's adaptive responses may be overwhelmed with resultant significant psychopathology that may negate the beneficial effects of years of complex and expensive habilitative care.

Beyond the emotional stress produced by birth of a baby with a craniofacial defect, there is the additional crisis of the family's lack of adequate factual knowledge about the handicapping condition and its complications, physiologic consequences, prognosis, and therapy. In optimal circumstances, a knowledgeable professional should be available soon after the child's birth to explain the problem, place it in perspective, and facilitate parental contact with the craniofacial anomaly team. Otherwise the parents must search for a source of information, which may be a traumatic and potentially dangerous situation and can set an emotional barrier between the anxious parents and all future medical professionals. Later professionals may find it difficult to break through the interpersonal barrier erected by the parent who subconsciously always cries out, "Why weren't you present when my baby was born and I needed you?"

Along with the stress caused by psychologic and cognitive factors, there are physical stresses both child and parent must endure and conquer. Many of these babies have significant life-threatening problems that involve feeding, breathing, and communication. Parents must cope with unusual requirements in feeding infants or managing their oropharyngeal secretions. Most laymen and health professionals have very limited experience with such problems. Intense parental anxiety can be provoked until they find a reassuring professional who can teach them the necessary skills. That type of anxiety tends to create a depreciated sense of parental self-worth and interferes with a healthy self-image required for successful adaptation to the child's special needs.

Another tangible source of parental stress is the actual provision of habilitative services for their child. Anxiety, time commitment, and personal and financial sacrifice are the coinage by which parents pay for the child's habilitation. After the immediate reaction to the malformed child, and usually before the numbness of grief has passed, the parent must start the complicated process of searching for competent and empathic professional help. The search is not only for medical assistance but also frequently for adequate and appropriate educational and social experiences for the child. In a few communities, the craniofacial anomaly team is readily available and can help stabilize the child and family while starting contact with educational, governmental, financial, and other necessary social resources. Unfortunately, most children are born into health care systems geographically distant from specialized teams; the child's immediate-care provider may also be unaware of that child's special needs and the presence of competent referral sources. It is all too common that the family itself must seek specialized help.

Family support services that address resolution of deep and complex psychological, social, financial, and educational problems are essential if the total habilitative process is to be successful. Consideration is given here to only a few of these as examples of many possible services. These can be simplified into four groups: (1) educational (preschool stimulation programs, public and private educational systems), (2) psychological services (school counselors, community mental health units, and private clinical psychologists), (3) social-health agencies (state Crippled Children's programs, local boards of health, visiting nurse associations, and so on), and (4) parent support groups (few in number and usually established by successful CFA teams or the American Cleft Palate Educational Foundation).

First, a critically important point should be stressed. Whereas the multi-disciplinary evaluation-treatment team is generally located in a medical center distant from the family's home, child-family support services are best located in or very near the child's local community. The geographic separation of these two related habilitative and support resources mandates that an effective communication system be established. This linkage is often difficult to establish and maintain. Generally, it evolves over a period of years from the experienced needs of several children and their families. On occasion, it may seem easier for the CFA team to develop additional expertise and replace the need for community child-family support services. However, the simple multiplication of such social professionals at the tertiary health care level does not provide the necessary background knowledge of community resources, leverage necessary to extract local help for the child's problems, or immediate availability that may be essential for the family in time of stress. In addition, it is not a cost-effective way to deliver good health care. The highly sophisticated craniofacial anomaly team cannot supplant local support resources and provide the necessary family social services. Success is most probable when both the tertiary care team and community agencies understand their roles and strengths in the child's habilitation and communicate appropriately with each other. Most local health and social professionals are not adequately trained in the complexity of problems children with CFA and their families experience. The large craniofacial anomaly team can support clinical psychologists, speech-language developmentalists, specialized audiologists, and many medical/dental specialists who can teach other individuals in their professional disciplines about craniofacial habilitation.

Habilitative Resources for Clinical Care

There are 258 cleft palate or craniofacial anomaly teams in the United States that are listed in the 1984 directory of the American Cleft Palate Association. By definition, these teams include at least three medical professionals, one from each of the following disciplines: dentistry, plastic-reconstructive surgery, and speech pathology. All states and most territories have such treatment resources available for citizens. Many teams are associated with university medical centers and function as multidisciplinary groups representing five or more medical and allied health fields. Generally the staff meets to evaluate patients only a few times each month. Their clinical experience and the diagnostic characteristics of the patient population tend to support reasonable habilitative services mainly for patients with cleft lip and/or palate and the more simple noncleft craniofacial defects.

Scattered across the nation are several large multidisciplinary craniofacial anomaly treatment centers serving as supercenters for specialized habilitative craniofacial work and the diagnostic evaluations of more bizarre and complex facial defects. These centers, unevenly distributed across the nation, have developed around successful cleft palate treatment programs in combination with a craniofacial surgeon. Both are essential elements. The discipline of craniofacial reconstructive surgery evolved out of plastic surgery as a unique subspeciality during the late 1960s (Jackson and others, 1982), and its disciples are still few in number. They have joined other plastic surgeons and maxillofacial surgeons as the chief specialists for patients with CFA. The merger of craniofacial surgeons and CFA multidisciplinary teams has created approximately twelve major craniofacial anomaly centers in the United States and Canada. About half of them have large clinical volume, but only two or three such centers have a large, diverse, and experienced staff whose full-time function is craniofacial habilitation. One of these programs, the Center for Craniofacial Anomalies at the University of Illinois, is funded by a Maternal and Child Health grant as a regional project of national significance not only for treatment services but also for clinical research into the health delivery system that best provides service at a regional, tertiary care level.

The family of a child with craniofacial deformity has at least three major avenues for clinical habilitative services. They can seek unidisciplinary health care from independent professional providers who do not function as a team. Such care frequently stresses only particular disciplines (commonly, plastic surgery and speech therapy) and rarely anticipates future care needs in an effective, preventive manner. It is a "nonsystem approach" to a highly complex and long habilitative process and is unfortunately the only route found by many parents.

The second major avenue for treatment is through one of the nation's 258 cleft palate/craniofacial anomaly treatment centers. At these programs, the family and child can benefit from a multidisciplinary approach to habilitation. The spectrum of medical/allied health professionals and the team's collective experience vary greatly among different programs. Generally the family's geographical proximity to a particular team is the primary determinant for selection of the center. The nature or complexity of the child's handicap and special service needs may be only secondary determinants.

The third form of health care delivery of habilitative services is represented by the small group of large, experienced, and highly sophisticated craniofacial anomaly supercenters. Their lack of geographical proximity to most Americans and potential referring professionals means that access to their services is difficult for many families. The majority of dentists and physicians who provide primary care for these handicapped children may not know about the existence of the specialized centers or about the unique contribution they can provide for the child with a facial birth defect. Because of problems with health care accessibility, the first two habilitative steps (identification and neonatal support for child and family) may be the most difficult and prohibitive parts of the long treatment process.

Cost of Treatment and Sources of Financial Assistance

Habilitation of craniofacial anomalies is expensive. Many significant factors determine the inevitability of high costs: (1) treatments extend over many years, (2) multidisciplinary care is essential, (3) major components of therapy involve in-hospital surgical procedures, (4) most cases of CFA are complex and require extensive interdisciplinary diagnostic and posttherapy follow-up evaluations, and (5) psychosocial and educational support services are frequently required for the child and/or family.

First, let us consider the expense involved in the diagnostic and evaluation steps of habilitation. A reasonable and average evaluation requires the interdisciplinary efforts of a pediatrician, geneticist, plastic surgeon, otolaryngologist, ophthalmologist, orthodontist, pedodontist, speech pathologist, audiologist, clinical psychologist, nurse, social worker, and numerous clerical and technical helpers. A complete evaluation may require the service of additional specialized physicians (neurosurgeon, neurologist, and so forth) and advanced ancillary laboratory studies (computerized tomograms, chromosomal analysis, special x-ray studies, and so on). Such an evaluation may require two or three visits to the craniofacial anomaly center over a period of several days. The actual cost varies greatly but is generally between $1,000 and $3,000.

The first evaluation is the starting point, at which time certain basic data are collected. Only a few of the largest CFA centers have the experienced professional manpower capable of performing such an evaluation for patients with the more unique or complex craniofacial anomalies. The price for each of these follow-up data collection sessions is somewhat less than that for the original effort ($500–$1,000). It may be necessary to evaluate the child's status every four to six months during the early years of craniofacial growth (birth to six years), during periods of repeated surgical procedures, and during the adolescent period of facial growth.

Dental care is imperative for these children. It includes general preventive dentistry, restorative or pedodontic work, and at appropriate intervals, orthodontic-oral surgical care. Almost all specialties of dentistry may become involved. Dentistry is expensive, and for many patients there is minimal or no insurance coverage. Orthodontic treatment may be staged into two or three periods of months to years in duration and cost from $2,000 to $4,000. In many complex orthognathic surgeries, both the oral surgeon (or plastic surgeon) and the orthodontist are primary participants.

In-hospital surgery is a major expense. There are many different techniques for lip and palate closure that require variable periods of hospitalization (three to seven days). In addition, many patients require surgery of the middle ear, ear reconstruction, additional soft palate surgery (velopharyngeal flap), evaluation for airway problems, and eye-muscle surgery. Some children with CFA have other significant anomalies (limbs, heart, kidneys, and so forth) that require evaluation and therapy. Habilitation of multiple anomalies can lead to numerous hospitalizations at great expense.

It is difficult to give uniform estimates of habilitative surgical expense because of variable surgical practices and fee structures at different CFA centers. The author's experience in a large urban CFA university center provides the following information: cleft lip repair averages four to five hospital days; cleft palate repair averages four hospital days; secondary lip revision averages one to two hospital days; major craniofacial surgery (midface advancement, skull reconstruction, periorbital bone work, and so on) averages two weeks of hospitalization. An average child with CLP might expect: three or four plastic surgical procedures, from one to four otologic surgical procedures (usually tympanostomy ventilation tubes, which may be done in conjunction with the plastic surgical procedure); two periods of orthodontic treatment; and from one to five years of speech therapy in school.

Many cleft lip/palate surgical fees range between $600 and $1,500 for each procedure. Major craniofacial surgery requiring twelve to twenty-four hours of operating time is significantly underpaid. Whenever a public agency is involved in the reimbursement, the fee is rarely more than $2,000 to $4,000 for a full-day craniofacial surgical case.

These children may need speech therapy, special education, clinical psychological services, and hearing aids. Some services may be provided free of charge by public agencies or the school system. However, often the family has to pay for them.

In the case of a major craniofacial anomaly, even a relatively affluent person could not afford to pay all expenses from income. In the midst of their initial reaction to the birth defect, the child's parents would be completely overwhelmed to hear the final price of multiple hospitalizations for surgery, orthodontic treatment, preschool counseling, and years of ambulatory medical evaluations by medical and allied health professionals. Third-party payment for most of these services is essential. Fortunately, many American children have several possible sources of payment for habilitative services.

If the parents are employed, their health insurance may cover part of the child's medical and surgical in-hospital care. The quality of insurance varies greatly, and dependent coverage for the neonatal period may not exist. In addition, there are numerous factors that tend to reduce the percentage of children whose parental insurance represents a helpful resource. Regions of the nation with high unemployment (or underemployment) have less insurance funding for habilitation. The self-employed, partially retired, or those who work for small businesses may have poor insurance coverage. The "working poor" generally do not have adequate insurance and yet are ineligible for public medical assistance programs. And the incidence of divorce and unstable families increases the frequency of one-parent homes with an unemployed (underinsured) parent.

A good health policy may require a sizable cash deposit by the parent as a contribution under copayment plans. Health insurance generally pays for in-hospital/surgical care and less frequently covers ambulatory and diagnostic/evaluation care. Successful surgery requires very careful and extensive outpatient evaluations. Recently, insurance carriers have started to cover more ambulatory care, but these changes are directed most often toward reduction of hospital surgery or emergency care, and less attention is given to diagnostic medical evaluations. In recent years, dental insurance has been provided for many employees, but if available, it usually has substantial modifying conditions that may limit its usefulness for craniofacial patients. Many allied health professionals provide essential diagnostic and therapeutic services for patients with CFA. Most insurance policies severely limit or do not reimburse for nonphysician services. Speech therapy, audiology, genetic diagnosis and counseling, and psychological services are problematic. Therefore, even a good health insurance plan is only a partial financial resource for the parents of these children.

Public aid for medical assistance may pay for ambulatory and in-hospital services. However, aid programs generally reimburse health care providers at a rate below the actual cost incurred for services. Most craniofacial anomaly teams practice within the private (versus public) domain of American medicine. Even government (nonmilitary) and university hospitals rely heavily upon third-party, nonpublic financial resources. Therefore, when public medical assistance programs pay only a portion of the cost of health services provided to their clients, the remainder of the reimbursement must be funded by other governmental (nonwelfare) subsidies, private third-party sources, or directly by nonsubsidized patients.

Each state has a Crippled Children's Services (CCS) program that functions as a financial, social, and medical resource to families of children who have particular chronic handicapping conditions. Each state program varies in the types of service provided, the particular medical conditions considered germane to its mission, administrative relationships to actual medical care providers, and the financial eligibility requirements of clients. Funding for CCS programs is provided by both federal- (maternal and child health) and state-appropriated funds. This money is usually distributed for medical and allied health professional care in a manner that is generous and demonstrates an enlightened understanding of the nature of craniofacial habilitation, its care providers, and its expense. However, the CCS programs resemble public welfare agencies by payment of only part of the actual cost.

A major source of payment for habilitative services comes from indirect, non-patient-related funding. Federal and foundation grant research programs, university professional salary funds, private philanthropy, and simple volunteerism by many people help bridge the sizable difference between all third-party payment sources and actual costs.

In some states, there are funds appropriated by the legislature and administered through vocational rehabilitation or public health departments directed toward payment for habilitative services of adults with CFA defects. Most CCS programs have an upper age limit. Many young adults require extensive facial surgery and orthodontics after their facial growth has matured in the late teen years or early twenties. This is also a period of intensive psychologic and social adjustment. Habilitation may require extensive psychotherapy. Many clients are in vocational schools or college and do not have full-time employment. Those who work may have significant limits placed on their health insurance. Consequently, young adults find themselves in situations that provide minimal third-party payment resources to continue or complete their habilitation. Tens of thousands of dollars, years of habilitative services—and the person's future may hang in jeopardy awaiting some type of administrative decision with regard to the continuation of appropriate habilitative funding for the young adult with craniofacial deformity.

Recommendations for Public Policy

This chapter has described the nature of craniofacial birth defects, the psychological stresses for the patient and the family, the cost to society, and the resources available that allow the existing habilitative system to perform efficiently, be humane, and remain cost-effective. Several assumptions underlie our recommendations:

1. There is a finite limit to the amount of money (public and private) that can be utilized to habilitate individuals with craniofacial birth defects.

2.   There is an insatiable demand upon that finite volume of money, created in part by more sophisticated, expensive medical treatments and a health care delivery system and consumer population motivated by their own self-interest. All parties often behave in a manner that is fiscally irresponsible for the entire system. They too seldom ask the questions, "How much will it actually cost? How will society pay the bill?"

3.   Any administrative system created to promote a program to relieve handicapping conditions will be populated by individuals who by human nature promote their own self-interest in addition to the program's goals for patient habilitation. The usual result is a bureaucracy whose existence may facilitate patient treatment but also costs society a substantial part of the money available for patient habilitation.

4.   Any system developed to provide habilitative services must be flexible, sleek, and willing to accept the challenge of change imposed upon it by the ever-changing nature of governmental funding, general economic conditions, advances in medical technology, and variation in social expectations. In the final analysis, the system must be responsible for a finite amount of society's collective wealth and from that resource improve the caliber of life for those individuals for whom it is responsible.

Given these axioms, it seems difficult to develop a health care delivery system that is practical, humane, and cost-efficient. Most Americans like the competitive nature of our private health care system and reject major attempts by government to organize medical care. Long-term habilitation of infrequent and complex birth defects (such as craniofacial anomalies and myelomeningocele) differs from the common medical and surgical problems treated by competitive community or university hospitals. These patients must be managed through a health care system that has different characteristics. One might propose that the states' Crippled Children's Services collectively develop regional programs for the habilitation of these handicaps. And because of their substantial financial involvement with most of these patients, CCS programs have indirect power to establish an efficient quality health delivery system that is cost-effective. An ideal program would include:

1.   Easy access for all neonates with craniofacial anomalies born in the region, with acceptance of patient transfers from other regions of the nation as families move into the area.

2.   Recognition of existing quality programs, with clustering of them into a regional health care consortium based on their potential contribution to the system and location in the given population's geographical boundaries.

3.   Recognition that different institutions and agencies have varied strengths and weaknesses. In a consortium, they can be woven together into an efficient and fair system.

4.   Development of several craniofacial anomaly treatment programs with linkage to community agencies within each region.

5.   Development of regions in a manner that allows each to have one of the current dozen major craniofacial anomaly centers.

6.   Responsibility on the part of each regional program to the several state

directors of CCS programs for provision of appropriate medical diagnostic and therapeutic care, professional and lay education, and maintenance of a quality, cost-effective program.

If these goals sound ideal but too difficult to accomplish, then we are faced with an inadequate but expanding health system of unequal competing centers. As community hospitals become more sophisticated, many want to possess a craniofacial anomaly team to equalize their status with that of other institutions. Such competitive proliferation may have marginal benefits for the treatment of very common diseases but deleterious effects for rare diseases. The professionals who staff these small volunteer programs have other primary responsibilities and view craniofacial work as an interesting but ancillary activity to their usual work. It is proposed that the collective directors of CCS programs in a region intervene in this developing pattern of proliferation at the community level and establish a better organized referral and treatment system that can accomplish the six goals previously stated.

Organization of Regional Work. At this time, there are approximately one dozen large-volume, highly sophisticated, experienced craniofacial anomaly centers in North America. The directors of CCS programs could establish a regional pattern for the nation, with one of these centers in each region. The center would provide the maximum quality of sophisticated diagnostic and therapeutic services. Major complex craniofacial surgery would be planned at that level. The regional center should not be the prize plum of a particular institution that capitalizes on its success; instead, it should act as the focal point of a consortium composed of many specialists derived from the region's institutions and craniofacial anomaly programs. The regional center's team would be a central tertiary facility for patient care and a major driving force for craniofacial biologic research and education.

Figure 1 demonstrates the stylized relationships within the regional system. The regional center (like any other craniofacial anomaly program) accepts patients for initial diagnosis, treatment, and longitudinal follow-up services. It also has local agencies with which it relates. These community-based groups provide patient and family support services for educational, physical, psychosocial, and financial needs. Public health departments, preschool stimulation programs, and service agencies (for example, Easter Seals rehabilitation units, mental health clinics, and state Crippled Children's clinics) are some of the many valuable community resources with which smaller CFA programs and the regional CFA team can cooperate.

The regional center interrelates with several other craniofacial anomaly programs scattered geographically throughout the region. Although these other smaller programs are not expected to develop a tertiary level of sophistication, they should be competent to diagnose, treat, and follow cases of more common CFA patterns . Both the regional center and the several CFA programs might overlap in some diagnosis and treatment functions. A healthy interchange of these activities would promote optimal treatment near the patient's home. The CFA program level may have cases that would benefit from consultation at the

**Figure 1. Overlap of Relationships Between the Three Basic Elements
of the Regionalized Consortium. Patient Flow Originates in the Community
and May Enter Any or All Elements of the System.**

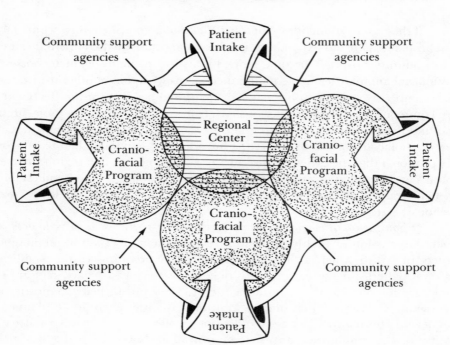

regional center but be better managed by referral back through a local CFA program.

One may ask why regional centers should be designated and supported and the consortium arrangement developed. It seems inevitable that multiple institutions will work in this specialized field of habilitation. It is essential that any child who enters one of these hospital CFA programs receive adequate evaluation and care. With expanding knowledge of these birth defects and the availability of more extensive treatment, each CFA program cannot provide adequate services for the broad spectrum of cases without inordinate overdevelopment of its staff and facilities that is not cost-effective. The equally unacceptable alternative is a system in which professional expertise is limited in order to reduce the cost of service. Patients may not be aware that more appropriate and sophisticated care for their very complex anomalies is available at one of the nation's few supercenters. And a child may receive less than adequate care unless a referral is made to the regional center.

Could an improved referral pattern alone accomplish the same goals? Unfortunately, improved referrals do not address several important elements of a regional system. First, the regional pattern would promote a cooperative approach to the broad problems of craniofacial anomalies. This cooperation would extend from patient services into areas of education, research, improved identification, and financial accountability. A major function of the regional center should be promotion of professional education among all levels of health care providers in the system. Regional center specialists can share their more advanced information and experience to promote more sophisticated services at other CFA programs and local support agencies. This type of cooperation emphasizes the value each component of the system can contribute and tends to reduce the competitive or antagonistic behavior common among several similar institutional agencies that operate within close geographic proximity. A modification of this educational approach can reach local agencies and laymen of the community and result in a heightened level of public awareness about the nature of craniofacial defects and the problems they engender for the child and family. Increased public knowledge augments the more standard methods of patient identification and promotes earlier referral of the handicapped child.

The cooperative nature of this regionalized system tends to provide maximal professional services with a minimum of duplication. This factor keeps the actual cost closer to an irreducible amount of funding required to habilitate these children. The bureaucracy and expense required to operate the system is minimal. Therefore, the regionalized consortium approach promotes the care of the child with CFA and that child's family in an effective, cost-efficient manner.

Funding for Habilitation. I believe that the information presented in this chapter also supports a second set of major recommendations with regard to funding CFA habilitation programs. There should be increased funding coverage of ambulatory services, appropriate funding for allied health professional services, funding based on actual cost experience, and improved state-funded programs for young adults.

The past three decades have witnessed an immense growth in the actual dollar amount required to provide habilitative services to handicapped children. All parties to the treatment of children with CFA (care providers, funding sources, and families) must cooperate and seek reasonable solutions to solve the financial problems related to therapy.

Wisdom encourages the provision of as much service in an ambulatory setting as possible. Yet many public funding agencies and insurance companies pay minimal sums for each service. There has been some improvement in insurance coverage of general ambulatory medical care in recent years, but the response still greatly lags behind reality.

Historically, payment has been directed toward habilitative services provided by physicians and dentists. Frequently a majority of essential services are provided by specialists in audiology, speech pathology, psychology, nursing, social work, genetic counseling, and nutrition. Some of these individuals function along with physicians and dentists and may be supervised by them. Some funding agencies view that relationship as an extension of the physician and pay for these services. However, many of these professionals act independently of the physician and dentist. It is important that their significant contribution be recognized and reimbursed. Even some of the more enlightened public funding agencies reduce their expenses by dodging this issue and refuse to pay appropriate charges for service provided by these allied medical professionals.

The foregoing problem is exaggerated by the most serious action public welfare agencies and state CCS programs perpetrate on individual providers—*underpayment*. There is no legitimate rationale for public health agencies to promote high-level habilitative services and then pay the private health care provider less than actual cost. Yet this is the daily experience of all craniofacial anomaly centers and private health care providers. Someone always pays the bill. Underpayment (a term rarely used by the funding agency) transfers the price for part of the patient's service away from the tax-supported agency's budget and into the nonsubsidized patient's pocketbook. Any resolution of the underpayment problem will require cooperation of both funding agencies and health care providers. The actual costs to maintain the regional program outlined previously should be borne by the agencies (CCS, public welfare, insurance, and so forth) that are supposed to underwrite that habilitative funding. Social agencies, insurance companies, and the health care system need to develop a cooperative system in which all parties can show fiscal responsibility and actual costs can be determined, found in agreement, and properly reimbursed. If the public agency (CCS program) is unwilling to pay full costs, then it should allow a partial payment of the difference between cost and reimbursement formula. Such a copayment by the parent must be evaluated case by case to prevent inordinate hardship to any particular family.

Crippled Children Services programs need to evaluate the potential funding available to their clients after they pass majority age and are no longer eligible for CCS funding support. Informal agreements or legislative action may be necessary in order to facilitate the funding transfer at that time. Although this is only a small percentage of all patients with CFA, the problem is significant and needs to be addressed in each state.

The previously described plan for regionalization of CFA habilitative services would also promote the search for new, non-patient-derived income sources. The regional craniofacial anomaly center, its associated programs, and the region's state CCS programs could cooperate in an effort to raise additional funding from private philanthropic or research sources. Such funds could be directed toward education, research, or special patient services not funded through customary methods.

In conclusion, these two major sets of recommendations would create a more efficient and cost-effective health care system for the habilitation of patients with craniofacial anomalies. Without such alternatives in the delivery system, it is unlikely that major changes in funding patterns will occur. The regionalized system would promote efficiency and improved patient access to the specific level of technical and professional sophistication required by any particular child. The system's actual patient service cost could be determined more clearly and assigned to the appropriate funding source.

References

American Cleft Palate Association. *Membership Team Directory*. Pittsburgh, Pa.: American Cleft Palate Association, 1984.

Battle, C. U. "Special Management of Craniofacial Problems." In R. E. Behrman (Ed.), *Neonatology*. St. Louis, Mo.: Mosby, 1973.

Clifford, E., Crocker, E., and Pope, B. "Psychological Findings in the Adulthood of 98 Cleft Lip–Palate Children." *Plastic and Reconstructive Surgery*, 1972, *50*, 234–237.

Cohen, N. M. "Syndromes with Cleft Lip and Cleft Palate." *Cleft Palate Journal*, 1978, *15* (4), 306–328.

Day, D. "Perspective on Care: The Interdisciplinary Team Approach." *Otolaryngologic Clinics of North America*, 1981, *14* (4), 769–775.

Dorf, D. "Early Cleft Palate Repair and Speech Outcome." *Plastic and Reconstructive Surgery*, 1982, *70* (1), 74–79.

Fogh-Anderson, P. *Inheritance of Harelip and Cleft Palate*. Copenhagen, Denmark: Arnold Busck, 1942.

Fraser, F. C. "The Genetics of Cleft Lip and Cleft Palate." *American Journal of Human Genetics*, 1970, *22*, 336–352.

Hanus, S., Bernstein, N., and Kapp, K. "Immigrants into Society: Children with Craniofacial Anomalies." *Clinical Pediatrics*, 1981, *20*, 37–41.

Jackson, I., and others. *Atlas of Craniomaxillofacial Surgery*. St. Louis, Mo.: Mosby, 1982.

Kapp-Simon, K. "Psychological Adaptation of Patients with Craniofacial Malformations." In G. W. Lucker, J. A. Ribbens, and J. A. MacNamara (Eds.), *Psychological Aspects of Facial Form*. Ann Arbor: University of Michigan, 1981.

McWilliams, B. J., and Matthews, H. P. "A Comparison of Intelligence and Social Maturity in Children with Unilateral Complete Clefts and Those with Isolated Cleft Palates." *Cleft Palate Journal*, 1979, *16*, 363–372.

Meskin, L. H., and Pruzansky, S. "Validity of the Birth Certificate in the Epidemiologic Assessment of Facial Clefts." *Journal of Dental Research*, 1967, *46*, 1456–1459.

Richman, L. C. "Behavior and Achievement of the Cleft Palate Child." *Cleft Palate Journal*, 1976, *13*, 4–10.

Starr, P., and Heiserman, K. "Acceptance of Disability by Teenagers with Oral-Facial Clefts." *Rehabilitation Counseling Bulletin*, 1977, pp. 198–201.

Tisza, V., and Gumpertz, E. "The Parents' Reaction to the Birth and Early Care of Children with Cleft Palate." *Pediatrics*, 1962, *30*, 86–90.

Zapatka, F. "The Elephant Man." *Plastic and Reconstructive Surgery*, 1982, *69* (3), 563–564.

18

Asthma

Fred Leffert, M.D.

Description

Asthma is a chronic obstructive pulmonary disease characterized by an unusual degree of bronchial reactivity to a wide variety of stimuli.

Etiology. The basic cause of the excessive bronchial reactivity that characterizes asthma is unknown. Over the past century, a number of theories have been proposed and discarded (Leffert, 1978). One of the oldest is the concept of asthma as a psychosomatic disorder. Despite much speculation on this point, it has not been demonstrated that there is a personality type or behavior pattern to the child with asthma or that emotional stress alone can produce the alterations in pulmonary reactivity characteristic of asthma (Mattsson, 1975). The personal and intrafamilial stresses observed in many children with asthma appear to be common to children with chronic disease rather than specific for asthma.

A venerable theory only recently discarded is that asthma is an allergic disease. According to this view, the basic defect was a predisposition to become sensitized to inhaled or ingested allergens in the environment. When the sensitized child came into contact with these allergens, the resulting immunologic reaction triggered the release of chemical mediators of inflammation that acted on lung tissue to produce asthma. The more modern view is that, although allergens may be an important stimulus for symptoms in many children with asthma, they are not the basic etiologic agents so that the allergic state per se does not cause asthma. Many children with asthma have no recognizable allergic sensitivities; other children with a high degree of immunologic sensitivity do not have asthma as a manifestation of this condition.

The more recent concept views asthma as resulting from an imbalanace in autonomic nervous system functions. The beta-adrenergic theory of asthma

(Szentivanyi, 1968) locates the defect in adenyl cyclase, a membrane-associated protein that is the receptor for beta-adrenergic stimuli. A quantitative lack or qualitative dysfunction of this enzyme would result in diminished beta-adrenergic responsiveness, thus weakening the normal homeostatic responses (that is, bronchodilatation or widening) to bronchoconstrictive stimuli. A complementary theory postulates cholinergic hyperresponsiveness (leading to excessive bronchoconstriction) as the primary lesion (Kaliner, 1976) so that asthma is produced as a result of exaggerated cholinergic responses to stimuli that do not affect the normal lung. However, although autonomic dysfunction can be demonstrated in asthma, it is not clear whether it is a cause or an effect of the altered pulmonary function.

A disturbance in prostaglandin metabolism has been proposed as an etiology for asthma (Zurier, 1974). Another recent theory suggests that the central defect may reside in the bronchial mast cell, which may have a lower threshold for release of mediators of inflammation by both immunologic and nonimmunologic stimuli (Findlay and Lichtenstein, 1980). At the present time, there is no solidly established or widely agreed upon etiology for asthma. Indeed, there may not be a single etiology. We may be dealing with a number of diseases that have in common the physiologic finding of hyperreactive bronchi with resulting obstructive lung disease.

Pathogenesis. Although the basic etiology of asthma is obscure, a number of stimuli have been identified as frequent immediate triggers for symptoms:

1. *Allergy:* Inhalant antigens such as pollens, animal dander, and mold spores are important triggers for symptoms. Food allergy may contribute to asthma symptoms, but much less frequently than inhalant allergy.
2. *Infection:* Upper respiratory tract infections almost invariably trigger symptoms in children with asthma. Respiratory infections do not appear to be more common in children with asthma than children without asthma, but they often seem more severe in children with asthma because of the associated bronchial symptoms.
3. *Exercise:* This is a very common stimulus for asthma and may cause major problems in school with physical education classes and competitive athletics.
4. *Irritants:* A number of irritant substances may trigger asthma, of which cigarette smoke and aerosol sprays are the most common. Air pollution is a potential aggravating factor, but its contribution to asthma morbidity has not been adequately studied.
5. *Climate:* Fluctuation of asthma symptoms with weather changes is a commonly observed phenomenon, although the mechanism is unknown, and no particular climate has been established as best for asthma.
6. *Emotions:* Although asthma is not primarily a psychosomatic illness, emotional stress may aggravate asthma in two ways: the physiological accompaniments of emotion—crying, laughter, hyperventilation—may trigger symptoms in the sensitive lung. Less frequently, children may "forget" medication or place themselves in situations known to cause asthma for secondary gain.

The preceding are the most frequent immediate triggers of symptoms, although there are many others. Every child with asthma has a unique personal pattern, and this may change as the child grows, even while the basic defect stays the same. Despite the great diversity of inciting factors, a few changes in lung function appear to be the common denominator for all asthma symptoms: increase in tone of bronchial smooth muscle leading to constriction, hypertrophy of bronchial mucus glands with production of large amounts of thick mucus, and inflammation and swelling of the bronchial mucous membrane. All of these changes reduce bronchial caliber and thereby increase resistance to airflow in and out of the lungs. Several major symptoms result from the increased flow resistance:

1. *Dyspnea (difficult breathing):* This may be experienced as shortness of breath, chest tightness, or even chest pain during acute attacks. Or it may take the more subtle form of chronically increased work of breathing, causing fatigue and irritability.
2. *Cough:* Bronchoconstriction and mucus production stimulate the cough reflex, so that intermittent or chronic cough may be a major symptom and, in some children, may be the only manifestation of asthma.
3. *Wheezing:* Turbulent flow through irregularly narrowed airways causes vibration of the column of air and of the bronchi themselves, producing the wheezes and noisy respiration characteristic of symptomatic asthma.
4. *Pseudo-pneumonia:* Rather than acute dyspnea and wheezing, many young children have cough and mucus production as major manifestations. These episodes are frequently associated with fever and upper respiratory tract infection and with mucus plugging of the bronchi, producing densities on chest x rays. These children are often mistakenly thought to have recurrent pneumonia.

There is no typical clinical syndrome for asthma. It may take the form of bronchitis accompanying upper respiratory infections in a child who, otherwise, is entirely well, or it may present as continuous, unremitting wheezing and dyspnea. One child may experience it only as a persistent nocturnal cough, while for another it consists of acute, rapidly evolving episodes of severe dyspnea triggered by exercise, allergen contact, or emotional stress. This great heterogeneity among asthmatic children will have important implications for public policy directed at the disease.

For instance, a very common clinical problem is presented by the child with repeated acute episodes of asthma. Vital to management of this syndrome are education of the family to recognize signs of an impending attack, mastery of relaxation techniques to prevent or minimize panicky behavior during episodes, protocols for home medication, and participation in supportive activities, such as parent discussion groups, to increase confidence and develop proficiency in judging the seriousness of the situation. However, these activities have little relevance for the child whose asthma is manifest as chronic cough or fatigue without acute episodes.

Most of the traditional schemes for classification of asthma approach it from the standpoint of factors that trigger symptoms, so that categories such as allergic asthma, infectious asthma, and the like are commonly used, with only an occasional author viewing the disease in terms of symptom pattern (Turner-Warwick, 1977). My own preference is for the following approach to classification:

1. *Children with good baseline pulmonary function but a high degree of bronchial reactivity.* These are the children described earlier, whose asthma is a series of acute episodes. The overall severity of their disease depends on the degree of obstruction produced by each episode and the frequency of these episodes. Their special needs for management are as previously discussed.
2. *Children with continual obstruction (poor baseline pulmonary function) but less bronchial reactivity.* Their clinical picture may include chronic fatigue, poor growth, and impaired school and athletic performance. The overall severity is determined by the degree of chronic obstruction. The needs of this group include educational techniques that stress to parents and professionals that this syndrome is just as important a form of asthma as the more easily recognized acute attacks and emphasize the need for compliance with a maintenance medication regime over long periods of time.
3. *Children with poor baseline function and marked bronchial reactivity.* This is obviously the most severely affected group. They have acute exacerbations superimposed on chronic obstruction and may be significantly disabled. Although fortunately a small minority of the total asthmatic population, they represent the greatest treatment problems. This group is most likely to benefit from centers for residential care.
4. *Children with normal baseline function and a mild degree of bronchial reactivity.* This is the most mildly affected group. Their needs for medication are intermittent, and they may have symptoms only with unusual stress such as respiratory tract infections or very strenuous exertion. Asthma may not be a major problem for them. Services helpful for more severely affected children may actually be counterproductive for this group because programs such as asthma camps, education and support groups for parents, and special school programs may needlessly stigmatize them.

It must be kept in mind that children often have major changes in their asthmatic syndrome, so that a severely affected infant may be having very little difficulty by school age whereas another baby with mild symptoms over many years may have greatly increased severity in adolescence. We do not yet understand what causes these changes, nor is there any firm evidence that any of our present treatment modalities change the natural history of the disease.

Epidemiology

Asthma is one of the most commonly encountered childhood illnesses, the prevalence having been estimated at 25.8 per thousand (U.S. Department of Health, Education, and Welfare, 1963). It has been estimated that 5 percent of all children under the age of fifteen years have or have had symptomatic asthma (U.S. Public Health Service, 1979). This is probably an underestimate because many asthmatic children are misdiagnosed as chronic bronchitis, recurrent pneumonia, or chronic cough. Death from asthma is uncommon, with ninety-six fatalities in 1972 (U.S. Department of Health, Education, and Welfare, 1972), but the morbidity caused by this disease is enormous. Asthma is the most frequent cause of missed school days, accounting for 23 percent of all days lost in 1963. During that year it caused 7.5 million missed school days, 11.6 million bed days, and 24 million days of restricted activity (U.S. Department of Health, Education, and Welfare, 1963).

The major risk factor determining susceptibility to development of asthma is genetic. The great majority of children with asthma have a family history of the disease and onset of symptoms in infancy. However, assessment of the genetic factors operative in asthma is much more difficult than for conditions such as sickle cell disease or cystic fibrosis. What appears to be inherited is atopy, a constitutional defect predisposing to a group of diseases that includes asthma, hay fever, and eczema. Genetic counseling therefore cannot be as precise as for single-gene diseases and must be based on very crude, empirical risk data (Lubs, 1972).

However, the clinical expression of the disease is not entirely governed by genetic factors because even monozygotic twins may be discordant for asthma. This suggests that environmental factors are also operative and has raised hopes that identification of these factors might allow intervention early in life and prevention or modification of the disease. Two factors that have received extensive study are diet and respiratory infection. Although several studies have suggested that breast-feeding and the avoidance of highly antigenic foods such as cow's milk or eggs during the first year of life reduces the incidence of asthma, other clinical trials have not confirmed this finding, so the efficacy of dietary prophylaxis remains an unproven hypothesis (Halpern and others, 1973). Observation of infants hospitalized for viral bronchiolitis has shown a high incidence of subsequent asthma. Although these patients are a highly selected population, the studies suggest that prevention of viral respiratory infection may modify or prevent subsequent asthma (McIntosh, 1976). However, clinical testing of this hypothesis must await development of effective vaccines against the common respiratory pathogens.

Socioeconomic factors have not been shown to have a major effect on the incidence of asthma, although economic status may strongly influence the quality of care that can be obtained and the ability of the family to implement a treatment plan. Asthma does not appear to favor any racial or ethnic group or to vary with socioeconomic status or region of the country.

Course and Outcome

Asthma has the most variable course of any of the chronic diseases of childhood. It is characterized by remissions and exacerbations occurring at unpredictable intervals. These may occur with changes in life-style or environment or because of intrinsic changes in bronchial reactivity. Although there is a general tendency toward lessening of severity with time, a substantial minority of children do not improve and even worsen as they go into adolescence (Buffum and Settipane, 1966; Martin and others, 1980). Present knowledge does not enable us to predict which children will have a remission of symptoms with age. A number of studies have tried to identify factors early in the course of asthma that might have predictive value (Kuzemko, 1980). For instance, boys appear to be more frequently affected than girls, but they are also more likely to have lessening severity with age, while girls are more likely to have increased difficulty as they go into adolescence. Severity of disease may have some predictive value because the more severely affected children appear to be more likely to retain their asthma as a significant problem as they grow up.

However, such findings represent very broad generalizations based on patterns observed in large groups of children. At present, the physician dealing with an individual patient cannot make firm predictions about a probable future course. The associations so far described are so loose that attempts to group children in terms of predictive factors would not be productive.

As previously mentioned, death is a relatively rare outcome in asthma, given the high prevalence of the disease. There is no evidence that children with asthma, as a group, have a shorter average life span than the general population.

As yet, there is no evidence that any mode of treatment—environmental manipulation, diet, pharmacotherapy, or immunotherapy—alters the natural history of asthma. On the other hand, there is also no evidence that asthma causes irreversible changes in lung function or predisposes to chronic bronchitis or emphysema in adult life so that, even after many years of severe asthma, reversal of bronchial obstruction is still possible (Tooley and others, 1965).

Nature and Efficacy of Treatment

The basic defect in the asthmatic lung remains undiscovered so that therapy directed at this defect is not yet possible, and treatment is directed at modification of its clinical expression. Although all asthma therapy must therefore be considered symptom management, the efficacy of such treatment has been improved so greatly over the past decade that complete control of symptoms is now a feasible goal for most asthmatic children. Even though not yet curable, asthma is one of the most responsive to therapy of the childhood chronic diseases. Asthma therapy takes three general forms: environmental modification, immunotherapy, and pharmacotherapy.

Environmental modification encompasses a variety of maneuvers aimed at preventing contact with allergens and irritants that act as immediate triggers of symptoms. It includes getting rid of pets to which the child may be allergic, avoidance of aerosol sprays, cessation of parental smoking, and reduction of dust and mold concentrations in the home. This may have a dramatic effect in children for whom avoidable stimuli such as animal dander play a major role but is of little use for those for whom unavoidable factors such as weather changes or respiratory infections are important. Many traditional procedures for allergen avoidance have not been proven by clinical trial (Burr and others, 1976), and there is some potential for doing harm with this approach because some environmental control measures, such as major alterations in home heating or air conditioning systems, are quite expensive. Measures requiring major changes in family habits and routines may add to family stresses and may also cause feelings of guilt in parents who cannot fully implement such measures.

Immunotherapy (allergy shots) has been a traditional mode of asthma treatment for many years. It aims at lessening the severity of asthma by reducing sensitivity to allergens that may be involved. There are a number of problems associated with this approach. Because most children with asthma have many stimuli involved in provoking symptoms, it is often very difficult to select those in whom allergy is the major factor. Immunotherapy is an expensive and time-consuming form of therapy that requires at least a year of treatment before any judgment can be made about its benefit. Most importantly, evidence for efficacy is weak despite many decades of clinical use (Lichtenstein, 1978).

At the present time, the most effective approach is pharmacotherapy. The past two decades have seen a sharp increase in research into the pharmacology of asthma, which has resulted in the development of several new agents and more rational and effective use of some of the older medications. This situation has been further improved by recent FDA licensing of several very useful drugs that had been available for the past decade in Europe, Britain, and Canada. The major advantage of pharmacotherapy is that it is effective for all asthma regardless of causative factors, degree of severity, or clinical pattern. The array of medications presently available allows great flexibility so that treatment can be individualized to each child's particular clinical pattern. Problems with pharmacotherapy include drug side effects (although these are rarely a significant problem when they are used with skill and care) and expense. The major problem for the chronically ill child is compliance with a long-term medication regimen (as is true of all chronic disease therapy). Although drug therapy is not curative, the state of the art is now such that complete control of symptoms, normal pulmonary function, and an active life, including participation in athletics, is a reasonable goal for most children with asthma (Leffert, 1980).

Cost of Treatment

The cost of asthma treatment varies greatly. The major variables that determine cost include:

1. *Type of physician:* Secondary level specialists (allergist, pulmonologist) generally receive higher fees than primary physicians (pediatricians, family physicians). Also, the specialist may be more likely to order more elaborate diagnostic studies. However, these high costs may be offset by money saved if better control is achieved by a more knowledgeable physician. Ideally, asthma is most economically managed by a primary physician. Unfortunately, as is discussed later, pediatricians are often not adequately trained in chronic disease management, and the structure of their practice does not permit them to take the time required for optimal management.

2. *Type of therapeutic approach.* Pharmacotherapy is probably the most economic form of therapy. The cost may vary from $25 to $50 a year for a mildly affected child receiving only intermittent therapy to from $400 to $500 a year for more intractable disease requiring daily round-the-clock medication with several drugs. The use of immunotherapy adds to cost for two reasons. The first is the cost of the injections, which may range from $200 to $300 for the first year and from $100 to $200 for subsequent years. The other is the fact that immunotherapy alone is rarely sufficient to control asthma so that pharmacotherapy will also be needed for these children. Most environmental control measures have negligible economic cost, although a few such as major renovation of a heating or air conditioning system may be quite expensive.

3. *Treatment setting:* The greatest single expense in asthma treatment is the cost of inpatient treatment. A few days spent in an intensive care unit for an episode of severe acute asthma costs more than an entire year of intensive outpatient management. Because most hospitalizations for asthma are probably preventable with good outpatient management, the major cost of asthma therapy is the cost of inadequate outpatient management. One children's medical center has estimated that at least 30 percent of their admissions for asthma are preventable and due to failure of physicians, parents, or patients to implement an optimal management plan (Palm and others, 1970). I think this is a great underestimate of the situation.

It is difficult to give an adequate analysis of costs of asthma therapy because there is neither a typical asthmatic nor a standard therapeutic approach. The National Institutes of Health (NIH) estimated a total cost of $806 million in 1975 for all asthma, adult and pediatric (U.S. Public Health Service, 1979). Since children make up about one third of this group, $250 million might be taken as a rough estimate of pediatric asthma expense. It is my personal estimate that at least half of this sum would be saved if every child were receiving optimal care. An important secondary cost of asthma is time missed from work by parents, although I am not aware of any good estimates of this cost.

Stresses on Child and Family

When discussing the stresses on child and family that are part of asthma, the heterogeneity of the disease must be kept in mind. For the child with mild, intermittent symptoms, the impact of the disease may be negligible. The discussion that follows therefore is mainly concerned with the more severely affected child—the patient with daily symptoms, need for continuous treatment, and frequent emergency visits and hospitalizations.

Although asthma is unique among the chronic diseases of childhood in not leading to progressive or irreversible tissue changes, it causes major functional impairment. These range from the very acute—the chest pain, dyspnea, and panic associated with acute attacks—to chronic manifestations of increased work of breathing, such as fatigue, poor appetite, and irritability. A major area of functional involvement is school. Academic achievement may be impaired by asthma-related absences or by fatigue and inattentiveness due to lack of sleep.

Athletics is another problem area, both in school programs and in after-school activities, because exercise is a major stimulus for bronchoconstriction in many children with asthma.

The emotional and behavioral problems associated with chronic asthma are in many ways similar to those of children with other major chronic diseases: feelings of fear, anger, resentment, and inferiority. Also, because flare-ups of asthma can be provoked easily by simple maneuvers such as hyperventilation or coughing or omitting medication, asthma may be used for secondary gain by children in whom emotional problems coexist with their asthma.

Asthma has both physical and emotional impact on other members of the family. Because symptoms commonly flare at night, loss of sleep is a frequent problem for parents. Environmental adjustments such as remodeling heating systems, cessation of smoking, or getting rid of pets are an additional emotional and financial burden. Disciplining the child with asthma can be a problem when parents are fearful of provoking symptoms. The situation may be even more difficult when there are siblings without asthma who resent the extra attention given the affected child. A child with asthma can significantly alter a family's social and recreational activities. It may be difficult to find baby sitters who will stay with the child. The family may avoid activities such as camping trips where medical help is not immediately available. In addition to the normal anxiety of parents with a chronically ill child, parents of children with asthma also bear the burden imposed by the misconceptions and myths that have grown up around this disease. Many parents believe that asthma is a psychosomatic condition and that their child's illness reflects their inadequacy as parents. Some have been led to believe that asthma causes chronic destructive lung disease (emphysema) later in life. The emotional stresses of asthma may do far more damage to the child and family than the reversible physical effects of the disease (Leffert, 1981).

Again, it should be emphasized that these are the problems of asthmatic children whose disease is not well controlled. The situation here is analogous to the economic cost: the major emotional and social cost of asthma is the cost occasioned by inadequate treatment.

Sources of Treatment and Support

Most asthma treatment is conducted on an ambulatory basis by primary physicians (family physicians or pediatricians), although much of it is shared by secondary level specialists (allergists and pulmonary physicians). Other medical specialists, usually involved only during periods of inpatient treatment, include respiratory therapists, nurses, anesthesiologists, and surgeons. Psychologists, social workers, and teachers may be called on to help with the psychosocial problems that may result from asthma or coexist with it and complicate treatment.

Other sources of support include asthma camps (Scherr, 1981) and educational materials supplied by organizations such as the American Lung Association, the National Institutes of Health, and the Allergy Foundation of

America. For children whose problems are so overwhelming as to be beyond the resources of their families and communities, there are residential treatment centers such as the National Jewish Hospital–National Asthma Center in Denver.

There are, to my knowledge, no special sources of financial support for children with asthma. Most medical care is paid directly by parents, by private insurance, or by Medicaid. Children of medically indigent families are usually seen in clinics of municipal or county hospitals. Some asthmatic children are eligible for state Crippled Children's programs, but this varies from state to state. Some institutions, such as residential centers and asthma camps, accept children without regard to ability to pay, the difference being made up by philanthropic contributions.

As is discussed in the next section, it is my strong belief that the major unmet need of many children with asthma is lack of resources that would permit them to receive individual medical care from a personal physican.

Recommendations for Public Policy

There are several areas in which the national government can promote better care for children with asthma. The first is in the area of basic biomedical research. The single most important contribution to the welfare of children with asthma during the past two decades has been the advances in knowledge that have changed the treatment of this disease from a largely empirical enterprise based on tradition to a rational, effective approach based on a clearer understanding of pulmonary physiology, immunology, and pharmacology. Much of this advance has been the fruit of NIH-supported research. There is a great deal yet to be accomplished. Today's asthma therapy, although highly efficacious, is capable only of symptom control and so represents an intermediate stage in the eradication of this disease. More knowledge is needed of the basic mechanics of pulmonary inflammation to allow eventual prevention or cure of asthma. Stronger federal support of research should play a role here.

Another area in which government can have a strong influence is in the training of professionals to care for asthmatic children. The most serious problem faced by these children and their families at present is that many are not receiving state-of-the-art medical care. Asthma therapy has achieved a degree of efficacy sufficient to completely control the disease and allow the majority of these children to function without handicap. With the exception of the problems faced by the small minority in whom the disease is intractable even with optimum management, much of the physical and emotional suffering and economic burden caused by asthma could be prevented if every child were receiving the full benefit of our present knowledge and therapeutic technique. Most hospitalizations for asthma are preventable, as are most emergency room visits, missed school days, sleepless nights, restricted activity, and secondary strains on the family. Millions of dollars are wasted on traditional therapies of unproven efficacy, such as allergen injections. A great deal of morbidity occurs in cases when the diagnosis of asthma is not made and children are treated for chronic bronchitis or recurrent pneumonia.

There appear to be two reasons for the great morbidity exacted by this eminently treatable disease. The first is a result of the recent vintage of much of our knowledge about asthma. There are not yet sufficient numbers of well-trained specialists (allergists and pulmonologists) in this area, either in private practice or on medical school faculties. Many medical schools have no full-time faculty members in these specialties, so that the training of primary care practitioners is inadequate. There has been increasing interest in this area of medicine in the past few years, making it likely that this shortage will eventually be alleviated. Federal policies encouraging more physicians to enter this field might accelerate the process.

A more basic and intractable problem derives from the nature of the medical education system. Asthma is most efficiently and effectively treated on an ambulatory basis by a primary care physician. But medical students and resident physicians receive their training in teaching hospitals where experience with asthma focuses on study of unusual cases, inpatient management of crises, and encounters in the emergency room. This is, of course, not unique to asthma; it represents a common deficiency in the training of physicians in all types of chronic illness. The skills most critical for the successful management of asthma—the ability to establish a therapeutic relationship with a family and maintain it over time, sufficient experience with the natural history of the disease to allow an appreciation of its variability, an understanding of family dynamics as they relate to an illness, and proficiency in communication and education techniques—are not acquired by medical students or resident physicians. The university teaching hospital, with its orientation to the technologically challenging aspects of medical care, does not provide an environment in which these skills are developed. The solution must lie in more innovative approaches to medical education. This is a difficult problem in terms of public policy; it raises the question of whether it is feasible or desirable for government to become involved in shaping medical education at this level. Progress will most likely have to come from within the profession, perhaps from interested groups such as the American Academy of Allergy, the American Academy of Pediatrics, or the American Thoracic Society.

Government might help attack the economic problems that interfere with the care of children with asthma. One of these problems is the reimbursement system that rewards the physician for inpatient care of asthma and for performance of laboratory tests and extensive diagnostic procedures but pays little for extra time taken in the office for education, counseling, and support. The physician derives more economic reward from failures than from successes. This difficult problem is only partly addressed by prepaid health maintenance organizations (HMOs). It will require innovation in the insurance industry to develop payment schedules that recognize the quality of services given and time spent in delivery of service rather than dividing medical care into procedures paid for on a piecework basis.

The other major economic problem is the inability of poor children to obtain quality medical care. It is my strong belief that quality care is provided when each child has a close ongoing relationship with a personal physician. This works well for children whose families can afford the usual fee-for-service arrangement but leaves many poor children unprovided for. Although, theoretically, Medicaid should provide for this group, in practice it is often so poorly administered and reimburses physicians so poorly, that it does not meet this need. There are a number of ways in which government might approach this problem. One might be a "pedicare" system similar to the present Medicare system, which appears to be working well for the elderly.

The school system is a public institution that can make a major contribution to the welfare of children with asthma. Much asthma morbidity occurs in relation to school days missed and academic failure because of illness, inability to participate in athletics, and problems arising around the need to take medication during school hours. Given the high prevalence of this disease, any elementary or secondary school with even a few hundred students will have a significant number of children with asthma. Properly trained school personnel could prevent or minimize much of this morbidity. For instance, many school days are lost when children are sent home because of mild symptoms that could easily be handled by an adequately trained school nurse or even in the classroom by the teacher. Children with asthma can participate in competitive sports if the physical education staff is aware of the mechanisms by which exercise triggers asthma and the techniques that can be used to prevent or attenuate symptoms. Although the school system is the province of local government, incentives could be provided by the federal government to encourage the public schools to meet the needs of these children.

Public policy should also address the needs of the child with intractable and life-threatening asthma. Although such children make up only a small fraction of the total asthmatic population, they are a significant absolute number. These children can benefit from periods of residential care. Institutions such as the National Jewish Hospital in Colorado or the Sunnair home in California are in a precarious position because medical insurance pays for only a fraction of this type of sophisticated, very expensive care forcing these institutions to rely on private philanthropy for support. Also, because they draw patients from the entire country, the distance to be traveled often inhibits families who might benefit. These families could be helped by the establishment of regional centers for residential care of asthma. Such centers would not have to be limited to asthma care and could serve other chronically ill children who might benefit from varying periods of residential treatment. They could serve as regional centers for research, teaching, and patient care in pediatric chronic disease.

Stronger support of basic biomedical research, encouragement of more appropriately trained physicians, more effective use of the public school system, and the establishment of regional chronic disease centers—these are the major areas in which the federal government can help. Both the government and the private insurance industry need to develop more innovative approaches that will give all children access to the private health care system and structure a system of reimbursement that offers more incentive for preventive outpatient management and less for hospital-based crisis management. Other needs of families of children with asthma, such as educational programs and emotional support, can best be addressed on the local level by physicians, parent groups, local medical societies, local chapters of the American Lung Association, and other community-based organizations.

In conclusion, it should be emphasized that efforts directed at improving the care of asthmatic children are particularly productive. Asthma is one of the few diseases whose pathophysiology is entirely reversible, and it is usually possible to return the patient to completely normal function. Few medical problems are so responsive to an aggressive therapeutic approach and so amply repay the efforts made to address them.

References

Buffum, W. P., and Settipane, G. H. "Prognosis of Asthma in Childhood." *American Journal of Diseases of Children,* 1966, *112,* 214–217.

Burr, M. L., and others. "Anti-Mite Measures in Mite-Sensitive Adult Asthma." *Lancet,* 1976, *1,* 333–335.

Findlay, S., and Lichtenstein, L. M. "Measurements of Basophil Releasability in Patients with Asthma." *American Review of Respiratory Diseases,* 1980, *122,* 53–59.

Halpern, S. R., and others. "Development of Childhood Allergy in Infants Fed Breast, Soy, or Cow Milk." *Journal of Allergy and Clinical Immunology,* 1973, *51,* 139–151.

Kaliner, M. "The Cholinergic Nervous System and Immediate Hypersensitivity." *Journal of Allergy and Clinical Immunology,* 1976, *58,* 308–315.

Kuzemko, J. "The Natural History of Childhood Asthma." *Journal of Pediatrics,* 1980, *97,* 886–892.

Leffert, F. "Asthma—A Modern Perspective." *Pediatrics,* 1978, *62,* 1061–1069.

Leffert, F. "The Management of Chronic Asthma." *Journal of Pediatrics,* 1980, *97,* 875–885.

Leffert, F. "Management of the Emotional Consequences of Chronic Childhood Asthma." In B. Berman and K. MacDonnell (Eds.), *Differential Diagnosis and Treatment of Pediatric Allergy.* Boston: Little, Brown, 1981.

Lichtenstein, L. M. "An Evaluation of the Role of Immunotheraphy in Asthma." *American Review of Respiratory Diseases,* 1978, *117,* 191–197.

Lubs, M. L. "Empiric Risks in Genetic Counseling in Families with Allergy." *Journal of Pediatrics,* 1972, *80,* 26–31.

McIntosh, K. "Bronchiolitis and Asthma: Possible Common Pathogenetic Pathways." *Journal of Allergy and Clinical Immunology,* 1976, *57,* 595–604.

Martin, A. J., and others. "The Natural History of Childhood Asthma to Adult Life." *British Medical Journal,* 1980, *2,* 1397–1400.

Mattsson, A. "Psychological Aspects of Childhood Asthma." *Pediatric Clinics of North America,* 1975, *22,* 77–88.

Palm, C. R., and others. "A Review of Asthma Admissions and Deaths at Children's Hospital of Pittsburgh from 1935 to 1968." *Journal of Allergy,* 1970, *46,* 257–269.

Scherr, M. S. "Special Camp Treatment of Asthmatic Children." In B. Berman and K. MacDonnell (Eds.), *Differential Diagnosis and Treatment of Pediatric Allergy.* Boston: Little, Brown, 1981.

Szentivanyi, A. "The Beta-Adrenergic Theory of the Atopic Abnormality in Bronchial Asthma." *Journal of Allergy,* 1968, *42,* 203–232.

Tooley, W. H., and others. "The Reversibility of Obstructive Changes in Severe Childhood Asthma." *Journal of Pediatrics,* 1965, *66,* 517–524.

Turner-Warwick, M. "On Observing Patterns of Airflow Obstruction in Chronic Asthma." *British Journal of Diseases of the Chest,* 1977, *71,* 73–86.

U.S. Department of Health, Education, and Welfare. *Illness Among Children.* Children's Bureau publication no. 405. Washington, D.C: U.S. Government Printing Office, 1963.

U.S. Department of Health, Education, and Welfare. *Vital Statistics of the U.S.* Vol. II-A. Washington, D.C.: U.S. Government Printing Office, 1972.

U.S. Public Health Service. *Asthma and the Other Allergic Diseases.* National Institute of Allergy and Infectious Diseases Task Force Report, National Institutes of Health publication no. 79-387. Washington, D.C.: U.S. Government Printing Office, 1979.

Zurier, R. "Prostaglandins, Inflammation, and Asthma." *Archives of Internal Medicine,* 1974, *133,* 101–110.

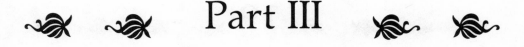

Part III

Populations with Special Needs

Fragmentation of care, lack of access to services, inadequate financial support, and inconsistent provision of primary care are among the problems encountered by chronically ill children in inner-city and rural areas. The particularly harsh effects of these problems on special populations, who also tend to have low incomes, are analyzed in the two chapters in this part.

Ruth E. K. Stein and Dorothy Jones Jessop, in Chapter Nineteen, point out conditions that are general for inner-city residents that exacerbate the situation of people in the inner city who also have to cope with chronic illness: social disorganization, fragmentation of services, lack of financial resources, low social status, and lack of political clout. Stein and Jessop outline health care needs, organizational issues, and professional issues and consider the interaction among them. Policy-relevant implications are then delineated for increasing funds for service provision, improving education, and conducting research on existing service delivery systems.

Chapter Twenty, by James M. Perrin, describes chronic health problems in rural America, highlighting the special health issues of Indians and farm-workers. Perrin documents service needs and problems in rural areas. He notes that the low prevalence rates of certain chronic diseases in rural areas contribute to the difficulties children with chronic illnesses and their families face in trying to obtain needed services. Recognizing the support for rural health services given by government and private foundations, Perrin presents recommendations that focus on the continued need to provide adequate financing to support such services and to improve rural families' access to quality primary care.

19

Delivery of Care to Inner-City Children with Chronic Conditions

Ruth E. K. Stein, M.D.
Dorothy Jones Jessop, Ph.D.

The Select Panel for the Promotion of Child Health has made a landmark contribution in reviewing and documenting issues in child health (1981). A single chapter of this kind cannot substantially expand that background information. It can, however, highlight some of the general findings of that report and other reviews as they apply to the health of children with chronic conditions living in the inner cities of our nation. In seeking to do this, we also have drawn heavily on the clinical and administrative experience of one of the authors in providing care to chronically ill children in two such communities and on the social science background of the other. It is our hope that such applied, hands-on, and interdisciplinary experience may enrich the interpretation of the data and suggest possibilities for future policy.

When we use the term *inner city,* we are speaking of more than a geographic location. Living in an inner city does not mean living on New York's upper East Side or San Francisco's Nob Hill but in the deteriorating and devastated sections of a central city that have been abandoned by all who can leave. What is more, it means belonging to the least favored groups in our society—that is, belonging to a racial or ethnic minority, having little income, and perhaps not speaking English. It often means being black or Hispanic, poor, and culturally different from the mainstream of American society.

It has recently been suggested that, in our society, children with chronic illness and handicapping conditions represent an "unexpected minority" who suffer the results of significant social stigma as well as political disenfranchisement (Gliedman and Roth, 1980). Similarly, the residents of inner cities are sometimes characterized as an "underclass" who are also nonparticipants in the mainstream of our society. Inner-city children with chronic illnesses and handicapping conditions therefore suffer from two types of what Birch and Gussow (1970) call systematic disadvantage.

The thesis of our discussion is that parallels exist between the condition of inner-city residents and people with chronic illness everywhere. We suggest that, when they come together, these similarities reinforce and exacerbate one another and that the superimposition of these factors upon one another—as in the case of an inner-city child with a chronic condition—creates significant needs not adequately addressed by current health policies.

We first examine the characteristics of the inner city and their relationship to health and health care of children and then review briefly the related issues for children with chronic conditions. In each section, we outline the needs, the organizational issues involved in service delivery, and the professional issues that face providers. Subsequently, we consider the ways in which these circumstances interact and, finally, conclude with a discussion of the policy implications for the group of children who live in the inner city and have chronic conditions.

The Inner City and Health

Although generalizations are difficult, compared to the country as a whole, most inner cities have high percentages of blacks and Hispanics; some also have many foreign-born residents and undocumented aliens and hence many non-English speaking residents. Population distributions are often skewed toward large numbers of dependent children and elderly residents who raised families in the area prior to the influx of a new minority group. Unemployment and underemployment are the norm in some inner-city areas, resulting in a disproportionate number of low-income families. Levels of education are lower than the national average. Large numbers of children in the inner city live in single-parent (often female-headed) households. As a consequence of all these factors, inner-city families often depend on public assistance programs for financial support. Many mothers in both single-parent and two-parent households work and may have special problems with childcare arrangements. Inner-city housing often has severe structural deficiencies as well as inadequacies of basic services such as heat, hot water, lighting, or gas. Needless to say, such homes offer little in the way of comfort or aesthetically pleasing amenities. Such neighborhoods have a variety of problems: poor lighting, street noise, heavy traffic, streets needing repair, litter, odors, and rundown, abandoned, and burned out structures (Lash, Sigal, and Dudzinski, 1980; Select Panel for the Promotion of Child Health, Vol. 3, 1981). The quality of water supply and sanitation may be poor. Public transportation and services may be sporadic, nonexistent, or inaccessible. These factors and attendant problems of drug or alcohol use and personal and property crime produce a general and realistic sense of victimization. Information or finances may be lacking for a sound diet, adequate housing, and warm clothing.

At risk of continuing to oversimplify reality, it is also fair to say that, by their very nature, cities tend to be bureaucratic and multileveled. In contrast to rural areas where services are usually organized on a countywide or statewide basis, municipalities (and their subsections) may have several administrative levels that are superimposed on the state and national levels of bureaucracy. Even within a single city, programs may originate from and be managed by different levels within multiple agencies, thus complicating attempts toward integrated functioning. From the viewpoint of the client, this can result in fragmentation, duplication, or gaps in service.

Beyond these generalizations, great variations exist among American cities. There are significant differences in the types of government, political culture, degree of commitment to public services, and manner in which the political leadership approaches problems. There are also differences in age and condition of the available physical resources both in the public and private sectors, as well as variation in the socioeconomic composition of the residents (Millman, 1981). Additionally, there are the state-by-state differences in Medicaid and related programs that affect the delivery of services to inner-city residents. These differences in cities make it difficult to make uniform, detailed policy recommendations that are universally applicable.

Questions regarding the health status of poverty-area residents and the delivery of health services to them are partially addressed by several large-scale national surveys, but the data presented do not completely answer the questions. The Health Interview Survey and Health Examination and Nutrition Survey data are presented in terms of the health of broad categories of people tabulated by race, income, age, or place of residence. Missing, however, are detailed multi-variate analyses providing simultaneous breakdowns by race, income, and poverty-area residence. Thus, inferences must be made from a series of bivariate analyses. Looking at each of these separate variables, it appears that those who are in the less socially advantaged categories are consistently reported to have more health problems and to receive fewer and less desirable types of service than the rest of the population. Moreover, it is generally held that race compounds the effect of income (Dutton, 1981; Select Panel for the Promotion of Child Health, Vol. 3, 1981). The extent to which the separate analyses are redundant or additive is not clear, however. Nor is there a way to tie these data to information collected by administrative units of service delivery agencies.

What we do know from these surveys is that traditional sociodemographic variables such as education, income, inner-city residence, and combination of adults in the home are each individually related to traditional measures of mortality and morbidity (for example, infant death rates, death rates after infancy, premature or low-birth-weight infants, limitation of activity, and self-assessed health status) (Dutton, 1981; Select Panel for the Promotion of Child Health, Vol. 3, 1981). In disadvantaged populations, incidences of birth defects, prematurity, accidents, malnutrition, and infections tend to be above those of the population at large. These populations also have relatively high frequencies of young adolescent mothers and others at high risk for disorders of pregnancy and of parenting.

Unlike the pattern in previous decades, the health problems of the poor are currently similar to those of the rest of the population except that they are more numerous and more severe. Poor children are also more likely to have chronic problems and significant abnormalities (Starfield, 1982; Starfield and Pless, 1980). The Select Panel for the Promotion of Child Health (Vol. 3, 1981) reports a trend since the 1960s toward an increase in the number of children with limited activities within the population and suggests that this increase has occurred more among poor children than among nonpoor children.

Most observers seem to agree that Medicaid, along with other public programs at the federal, state, and local levels, has made medical care possible for many children who otherwise would not receive it, but poor children still receive less medical care than nonpoor children (Starfield, 1981). The programs appear to have succeeded in reducing the differentials in rates of ambulatory care usage; in particular, differences have narrowed in the proportion of children having seen a doctor in two years and in the number of physician visits per year. Poor children now have a greater number of hospitalizations than other children, whereas prior to Medicaid, they were less frequently hospitalized (Select Panel for the Promotion of Child Health, Vol. 3, 1981; Starfield, 1981).

Although there is still some question whether differentials in use of medical care by the poor and by the affluent have been eradicated (Aday, Andersen and Fleming, 1980), all agree that "equity (that is, equal use according to need) has not been achieved" (Select Panel for the Promotion of Child Health, Vol. 3, 1981, p. 61). Minority and poor children (and near-poor children) still receive less medical care than nonpoor children on most measures. Moreover, because of the greater needs of the poor and minority groups, their use in relation to need is even less than the figures show, and they thus have large unmet health needs (Dutton, 1981; Kovar, 1981; Orr and Miller, 1981; Select Panel for the Promotion of Child Health, Vol. 3, 1981). In fact, in 1974, in comparison with the most affluent children, four times as many poor children had unmet health needs (Dutton, 1981).

It is still too early to determine if the narrowing of the gap in access to medical care has reduced the disparities in the health status of poor children as compared to nonpoor children. Davis and Schoen (1978, p. 27) suggest that "better medical care for the poor cannot be expected to show up in reduced prevalence of chronic conditions for decades yet."

When one examines with traditional indicators of quality the types of care being received, there are similarly large differentials between the care of the urban poor and minorities and that of the rest of the population. Poor children are less likely to be cared for by pediatricians and less likely to have a regular source of care. They are more likely to receive care from a variety of sources and are less likely to have telephone contact with the source of their care or to have received certain kinds of preventive care (for example, immunizations or dental care)

(Dutton, 1981; Select Panel for the Promotion of Child Health, Vol. 3, 1981; Starfield, 1981). They are also more likely to receive care in the public sector—in the outpatient facilities of large hospitals—than in private doctors' offices.

The findings of large-scale national surveys just summarized are borne out at the local level as well (Brink and Nader, 1981; Dutton, 1978, 1981; Gilman and Bruhn, 1981; Gortmaker, 1981). Studies based on single communities present more detailed and elaborated relationships between the variables, but because of the specific characteristics of the given inner-city or urban area, the data may not be generalizable to all inner-city populations. What such work particularly suggests is that there are structural barriers that affect the patterns of utilization and that, when such barriers are removed, the utilization behavior of the poor approaches that of other sectors of the community. Gilman and Bruhn (1981) showed with data from Galveston, Texas, that when barriers are minimized, Mexican American and Anglo children, who otherwise have differing care patterns, do not differ in their use of health services in the community. Using data from Washington, D.C., Dutton (1981) found wide differences in access among practice settings. Her analyses suggest that the multiple access barriers typical of outpatient departments reduced the likelihood of visits by 40 percent compared with the barriers typical of individual private practitioners (and by an even higher percentage compared with prepaid group practice). Higher fees are a major barrier to the poor, even when copayment is quite small. Long waiting time, distance traveled, and seeing different doctors on each visit decrease utilization; while scheduled appointments, longer hours, and better off-hours coverage may aid access (Dutton, 1981). Similar factors are reported elsewhere (Harvard Child Health Project, 1977).

These analyses suggest that differences in the place and type of care are important because of what they indicate about other aspects of care that are more difficult to measure. Dutton (1981, p. 388) cites evidence that hospital-based care on which many poor and minority group children depend, "although apparently comparable to that provided in private settings on a technical level, is deficient with respect to the goals of primary care such as accessibility, continuity, communication, and accountability." Although the intent of Medicaid originators was to make the poor competitive in the market for private medical care, it has resulted in the growth of the public sector health services (Orr and Miller, 1981). Rather than mainstreaming the poor, it has had the effect of reifying two separate types of care: private care for the nonpoor and care in the public sector for the poor (Dutton, 1981; Gortmaker, 1981; Starfield, 1981). In fact, use of the private sector by the medically indigent has actually decreased during this period of time (Orr and Miller, 1981).

Medicaid itself does not assure access to care. Not all physicians accept Medicaid reimbursement. Some have limits on the percentage of Medicaid patients they will accept. Others object to the increasing delays in payment, demands for documentation, and limits on fee scales and refuse Medicaid patients altogether. In some settings, practices have been created geared specifically toward Medicaid. These "shared health facilities," or "Medicaid mills," sometimes seem to emphasize fee-generation rather than quality comprehensive care.

Most public facilities accept Medicaid payments. However, they often are understaffed, have high staff turnover, operate in antiquated plants, and have long patient waits for care. Numbers of staff are steadily declining as cutbacks are implemented. In the face of budgets that seem large in absolute dollars, it is easy to forget the implications to the individual patient of losing a single nurse or clerk. However, the net effect of repeated losses in personnel is a serious deterioration and dehumanization of services. In addition, because public facility reimbursement is often paid for on a total service basis (and two services supplied on the same day are reimbursed as a single visit, regardless of the cost of the services), there is a tendency to break elements of service into separate units that take place on two or more different visits at maximal inconvenience to the patient.

With all these deficiencies, there has been some improvement under the social programs of the 1960s and 1970s for those fortunate enough to have obtained them. Gortmaker (1981) has shown, and others have indicated, that sizable proportions of the poor are not covered even though they meet eligibility criteria. Gortmaker suggests that in 1977, 15 percent of the children at poverty levels in the city of Flint, Michigan, were still not enrolled, and Flint was a community that provided better than average health coverage. Davis and Schoen (1978) estimate that nationally about eight to ten million people below the poverty level (or about one third of the poor) are not covered by current federal health care programs, and hence their receipt of basic health care services lags behind that of the rest of the population. They suggest that the number covered at any one time may be even lower, perhaps as low as one half of the poor (1978). These figures do not encompass the additional groups who fall just short of eligibility for Medicaid—the near-poor, who continue to receive the fewest services of any group.

It is difficult for summary statistics to convey graphically the complexity of the real-life situations confronting the individual family in the inner city, including the confusion, the irrationality, and the frustration of the system in which care is given, the intermeshed need-on-need of people's everyday lives, and the coping strategies they develop to come to terms with the situations with which they are faced—situations such as:

- No heat, no hot water, and a baby scalded from water heating on the stove
- Waiting in successive lines at a hospital with one sick child, while another child comes home from school to an empty house
- Telephone calls to Medicaid offices that go unanswered, being put on hold for long periods, and making all those calls from a pay phone because there is no phone at home
- Mail applications lost and requiring a fresh start
- Forms requiring a twelfth-grade reading level when the applicant reads at the eighth-grade level (Peterson, 1981)
- A fifteen-year-old adolescent mother alone with a sick child who requires tracheostomy care at home

Physicians are not trained and medical care facilities are not organized to deal in a total fashion with the range of problems faced by the urban poor. Rather, they tend to address each individual medical problem as if it occurs in isolation and is amenable to a traditional medical remedy.

Children with Special Needs

There are few large-scale epidemiological studies that look systematically at the population of children with chronic conditions, and "no national health survey has included questions which would allow direct estimates of the incidence or prevalence of chronic handicaps" (Ireys, 1981, p. 323). Most work on chronically ill children has been institutional rather than epidemiological in origin and reflects the experiences of specific programs or groups of patients. Pioneering work has been done on selected regions including Monroe County, New York (Haggerty, Roghmann, and Pless, 1975); Erie County, New York (Sultz, Schlesinger, Mosher, and Feldman, 1972); Cleveland, Ohio; Flint, Michigan; and Berkshire County, Massachusetts (Harvard Child Health Project, 1977). However, there is still some uncertainty about generalizing from specific locales to the national population. As with inner-city neighborhoods, there is a lack of detailed multivariate analyses of the relationship of chronic illness and sociodemographic variables by place of residence. The Select Panel for the Promotion of Child Health (Vol. 3, 1981) reports that a special survey in late 1978 of children under eighteen years of age receiving Supplemental Security Income benefits revealed that an unexpectedly high proportion of those living with their families were minority; lived in homes in which the mother was the sole parent, were poor, had received welfare during the previous years; and were multiply handicapped and mentally retarded. This report supports the association between such variables and chronic conditions cited sporadically throughout the literature.

Clinicians who treat the chronically ill note considerable differences between chronic and acute conditions. Chronic conditions require focusing on the individual as a person rather than on a specific symptom or illness (Lefton and Lefton, 1979). The progress and care of the individual with a chronic condition requires the clinician to consider the entire physical and social environment as relevant. Moreover, in successive stages of illness or child development, different components of care become the major focus. Chronic illness creates a need for skill in providing ongoing "care" rather than "cure," whereas acute illness often holds the prospect of cure. Gliedman and Roth (1980, p. 253) suggest that the inability to provide a cure creates "the central ethical dilemma for physicians in chronic medicine."

Additionally, many types of chronic conditions require physicians to have considerable diversity of expertise or to work in complementary fashion as members of a team with other health providers, a role for which they have received no training. The traditional medical model is less applicable not only for these reasons but also because large numbers of nonmedical disciplines and services are needed to maximize the functioning ability of the individual.

Medical personnel customarily think in terms of discrete disease entities. However, as Starfield and Pless (1980, p. 297) suggested, "to describe in detail the specific manifestations of each discrete condition in a single child fails completely to describe the health of the child as a whole. . . . The use of discrete descriptions perpetuates the insidious effect of labeling and the other important social implications of systems of classification of children based on their diagnoses rather than on themselves as individuals."

Pless and Pinkerton (1975) have suggested that it would be preferable to describe children with special needs noncategorically along a series of discrete dimensions, such as the time and nature of onset, the prognosis, the course of the disease, the types of routines required for care, the visibility or stigma, and any special features. Within each diagnostic grouping, there is a great variability along many of these dimensions. Children with many types of chronic conditions may have courses characterized by unpredictable crises that disrupt their lives and require attention or hospitalization. Some conditions are associated with a limited life expectancy or an ever-present threat of death, while others are stable or even improving. Many children with chronic conditions require care beyond that of a normal child on a regular basis and experience associated primary and secondary psychological effects. Although there is undoubtedly great merit in pursuing a disease-oriented approach in seeking biomedical cures for specific conditions, in the areas of health care delivery this traditional approach should be supplemented by one that takes into consideration the commonalities among children across many different diagnoses. All chronic illnesses in childhood are characterized by a potential to disrupt both family life and child growth and development; thus, they share many common features.

Health care delivery for chronically ill children is frequently divided among and between subspecialists and primary care physicians. This often results in duplication or neglect of important areas of care (Kanthor, Pless, Satterwhite, and Myers, 1974; Okamoto and Shurtleff, 1981; Palfrey, Levy, and Gilbert, 1980; Pless, Satterwhite, and Van Vechten, 1978; Stein, Jessop, and Riessman, 1983). In some situations, subspecialists assume total responsibility for the child's medical services, but there is great variation among subspecialists in the degree of attention paid to the provision of primary care pediatric services. Sometimes children, seen regularly in settings where the main focus is on their special needs, fail to receive standard forms of care, such as immunization and assessment of growth and development. This gap may be an even more significant problem for inner-city residents (Palfrey, Levy, and Gilbert, 1980) than for other segments of the population.

Both public and private reimbursement programs pay for high technology interventions for those with chronic conditions; few if any provide reimbursement for coordinative services (Vanderbilt University Primary Care Center and Tennessee Department of Public Health, 1981). When a large number of highly technical services of different types are needed by a family, the parent may be asked to interact with a wide variety of providers and with many agencies, often without any assistance in this task and without sufficient understanding of the relationship of each component of care to the whole.

Moreover, there appears to be a serious shortage of generalists who feel comfortable managing children with chronic conditions. People feel intensely uncomfortable with the thought of chronic illness in childhood, a time when health is the expected norm. Pediatricians seem to share in finding this a difficult task. Recent assessment of house staff training in a pediatric residency program suggests that interns have a fairly negative attitude toward children with chronic conditions and that the area of chronic illness remains a problematic one throughout the year of internship (Adler, Werner, and Korsch, 1980). Two phenomena may result in the generalist pediatrician feeling inexperienced in caring for chronically ill children as a group: (1) the heavy emphasis during training on distinct biomedical needs of children with each specific diagnosis, and (2) the relatively low incidence of each type of chronic illness within the community setting.

The nature of chronic illness poses significant professional problems for those delivering services to children with such conditions. The ongoing nature of the conditions provides little gratification for the health professional trained in the acute medical model who expects that an action will produce improvement. Chronic conditions not amenable to short-term interventions prove frustrating for providers. Many chronic conditions are overwhelming, and health professionals who work with multiproblem situations often experience the phenomenon described as burnout.

This situation is further aggravated by the fact that chronic illnesses also have significant effects on the families in which they occur, and these in turn may make it difficult for the health provider to work with the family. Chronic illness often lowers self-esteem and isolates a family, as parents' guilt and self-blame over producing a child who is not "perfect" interact with the negative reactions of others. There may also be social isolation because of practical difficulties in handling the child's condition (including crises, complicated nursing tasks, or frequent hospital appointments) or because of a family's need to protect itself and the child from the outside world. These experiences may lead to defensiveness, hostility, and anger or, alternately, to great passivity on the part of the family. In either case, the consequences may make it extremely difficult for the health care provider to engage in a meaningful reciprocal relationship with the family.

Finances pose problems for providers and families. The provider is generally reimbursed poorly, if at all, for the time spent talking with a family and evaluating or coordinating information and services for the child with a chronic condition. Because a clinician may view time as money, there is a real disincentive to perform these functions. From the family's perspective, there are significant direct and hidden costs of the child's care. For many conditions, these latter include such items as the inability of a parent to return to work in the absence of the specialized childcare arrangements sometimes needed for these children or in the presence of a demanding schedule of visits to health care facilities. The financial costs of running electrical equipment such as a suction machine or a dialysis unit at home are other examples of hidden costs, ones that will vary with the condition. Few, if any, programs provide financial assistance for hidden costs. The amount of direct costs and the degree to which they are covered by special programs vary by diagnosis. For example, the direct costs of conditions such as end-stage renal failure are fully reimbursed while the costs of others must be borne by the family.

Parallels Between Problems of the Inner-City Resident and Those of the Child with a Chronic Illness

As stated previously, it is the thesis of this chapter that the issues for the inner-city resident and the child with a chronic condition have many similarities and that the problems for the child living in an inner city with a chronic condition are not merely additive. Rather, these effects are compounded, creating a devastating experience both for the child in the inner city who has special health needs and for that child's family.

There are a number of parallels between the problems of each of these groups. The resident of the inner city and the child with a chronic condition are each faced with multiple and complex problems in their day-to-day lives. For each, the organization of services generally ignores the pressing need for services to be interrelated so that problems can be dealt with in their context. Instead, services tend to be arranged in discrete compartments, as if each occurred in a vacuum. Agencies often have individual contradictory and conflicting eligibility requirements and processes. Thus, clients must duplicate similar information for separate agencies. There is little effort to address the group of needs as a totality encompassing the physical, technical, social, economic, and psychological aspects at both the personal and familial levels. The inner-city family of a child with special needs requires, on the one hand, a multitude of specific and diverse services and, on the other hand, an overall plan and coordination that will keep the whole person and family as a focus.

Inner-city residents and those with chronic conditions are faced with a good deal of fragmentation (the division of services into discrete entities, as if the entities had no relationship with one another), an unknown degree of needless duplication of services, and gaps (or omissions) in the availability or delivery of services. Both groups tend to use public sector programs because of a lack of private sector services and a lack of personal resources. Thus, members of each group are enmeshed in a bureaucratic tangle associated with getting assistance within the bureaucratic structures of our municipal governments.

In the area of chronic illness, as in the care of the poor, it may be hard to determine the boundaries of the health care system. Pediatricians generally have moved beyond the one-to-one encounter with a specific illness and have become concerned with issues of environmental health, such as malnutrition and accident prevention. Yet, despite the knowledge that malnutrition contributes to the overall morbidity of children, our society does not accept the principle that provision of food is part of the responsibility of the health care delivery system. Similarly, while we treat the consequences of ingestion of lead paint and consider it our responsibility to ensure that children with lead ingestion are not returned to a lead-laden environment, we have no effective means of ensuring that children do not reside in such environments prior to the identification of lead intoxication. Problems such as these become even more complex in situations in which a child has an identified chronic illness. For example, it is now well accepted that tight control of diabetes mellitus is associated with reduced risk of long-term complications of the disease, and there is little doubt that dietary management is a helpful component in achieving tight control. Yet, the family in an inner city may receive help in paying for insulin and expensive hospitalization when complications occur but is not generally eligible for financial assistance in providing the foods (sometimes beyond the family's budget) helpful in controlling fluctuations of blood sugar. Although we know that families with limited income eat irregularly and often have diets high in carbohydrates, we have no systematic method for helping the family of a child with diabetes provide a more appropriate and consistent diet.

The problems of the urban poor and of the chronically ill transcend traditional professional and disciplinary areas of service delivery, policy, and research. This fact requires multiple disciplines to work together, which in itself is difficult to do productively. Many who provide services obtain some experience in public programs and move quickly on to more "pleasant" environments, where their own professional gains are clearer. The result for public programs is high turnover on the part of the staff and a lack of continuity and personalization of services.

For the inner-city family and for the child with special needs, the most pressing aspects of their problems are not the concrete and technical ones that can be delivered and evaluated in ways comprehensible to policy makers and the public but the more intangible social, psychological, and economic services that are harder for the uninvolved to see as important, harder to deliver, and once delivered, harder to evaluate. These problems have proven to be more intractable than specific technical problems, particularly to simple financial solutions. Moreover, they are not remediable through quick interventions, and they may take a very long time to move toward even partial solutions. The result is frustration, a sense of failure, discouragement for all, and a major obstacle to those trying to establish empirical documentation concerning the effectiveness of remedies.

The problem for residents of the inner city, unlike that for residents of rural areas, is not the lack of tertiary care facilities or highly specialized biomedical equipment. Diverse and highly specialized services, skills, facilities, and providers are often within a fairly small geographical range. But there are still problems of access, such as reliance on public transportation, long trips through multiple fare zones, long waits for services, and impersonal lines blocking the receipt of services from unfamiliar and often changing faces in the revolving-door staffing patterns of many large public agencies.

A further similarity between the chronically ill and the residents of inner cities is that they may fail to participate in services that could help them because of the structural barriers in the organization of care, rather than lack of interest, intrinsic personality differences, or cultural differences (Riessman, 1974; Dutton, 1978, 1981).

There are also a series of parallels between these two groups as concerns their status in the society at large. As the minority and poor residents of inner-city neighborhoods are subject to stigma and avoidance on the part of the more affluent mainstream of our society, those with chronic conditions similarly experience stigma associated with being "ambiguous" people (Preston, 1979). Fear and dislike mingle with concern on the part of the rest of society, resulting in ambivalence. In our culture, the inability to measure up according to many of the traditional yardsticks of success is often perceived as entirely the fault of the individual and hence something for which society blames the victim. In a society where economic and political power go together, the chronically ill and the inner-city resident have both become functionally disenfranchised.

The low prestige of these groups is reflected in the low prestige awarded provision of services to chronically ill and inner-city residents within the respective helping professions. A result is that newer, less experienced members of the profession sometimes provide the bulk of services to the chronically ill and inner-city residents. This is especially so in the health care system, where many public facilities serve as training sites in which trainees provide most of the care, and in municipal agencies whose physical plants are often decrepit and whose pay scales lag significantly behind those of the private sector. An advantage of this situation is that some idealistic young providers identify with and are drawn by the overwhelming nature of the problems some patients face. This sometimes leads them to act as advocates for patients or to join with patients in bending rules or circumventing limitations on services that seem to them not to be in a patient's best interest.

In addition, the chronically ill and the inner-city resident both have at this point in history a low position on the political agenda of our society. For a brief period during the 1960s, the disadvantaged were in the public focus, and multiple programs were developed to try to bring them into full participation in society. Political climates have changed, however, and current politics seem more responsive to the middle and upper classes who are part of the mainstream of society.

In light of the advances in biomedical research, the delivery of medical and social services to larger numbers of people through the programs established in the 1960s, and the advances of economic and social reform of that period, there is a general air of complacency, a sense that things are not as bad as they once were, on the part of mainstream America, both about the inner city and about chronic conditions. This sense that all is well seems always to be accompanied by a disclaimer that states "except for a very small percent" or "except for a small target group." The inner-city family of a child with special needs is often the exception for whom services are poor, fragmented, duplicated, or lacking in important areas. Yet, despite the documentation of persisting problems, compla-

cency exists about the problems of inner-city families with chronically ill
children.

Issues Between the Helping Professions and Inner-City
Families with Children with Special Needs

A wide variety of issues come into play in any discussion about assisting
families of children with special needs. In this chapter, it is assumed that families
have a right to be involved in their child's care and that such involvement is, in
fact, central to the management and best interests of the child. The corollary of
this position is that the role of the professionals and paraprofessionals involved
in care is to serve as facilitators whose responsibility it is to help the family
provide for the needs of the child. In that capacity, health care providers may at
times provide a wide variety of direct services, or they may serve as educators,
supporters, advocates, or advisors.

Moreover, we view the child with chronic health problems as a growing
and evolving individual whose needs vary over time, but one whose most essential
need is to be appreciated as an individual with assets as well as deficits. Thus,
our concept of the health-related needs is rooted in a health model rather than
a strictly medical one. In this light, it is important to note that health
professionals have traditionally been trained in and hence learned to emulate a
model that is authoritative, hierarchical, and institutionally based—a model that
has tended to assume that professionals know best and that the family that rejects
their advice is malevolent or at least very unwise. This paternalistic model tends
to create for the family a situation that fosters progressive loss of control, sense
of failure, incompetence, and dependency. Only recently have some professionals
and families begun to challenge this notion of professional dominance and to
recognize that many families are able to participate as partners in the delivery of
care to their children. The family alone knows the areas in which it has a real
need for assistance. Additionally, involvement of family members as active agents
in the care of the child strengthens the family's ability to cope and their
independence.

As difficult as it may be for a professional to step back into the role of
facilitator, this process is even more monumental in situations such as those
discussed in this chapter. In the case of the inner-city child with a chronic
condition, there are the additional barriers to equal partnership that stem from
cultural differences. For the most part, those in the helping professions are not
drawn from underprivileged, inner-city backgrounds. Hence, there can be serious
gaps in trust and in understanding divergent cultures, life-styles, and priorities.
Often, there are differences in socioeconomic background, social status, and
financial resources. In addition, there is often a difference in dialect or even in
native language.

These differences are vividly perceived when the health provider contem-
plates an active role in the field outside the clinic or office. Most health providers
openly admit a preference for providing care for and talking to families in the

institution rather than in the home territory of the family. Inner-city families are often ill at ease in the intimidating and unfamiliar office that is the professional home of those providing services, and these discomforts become barriers to effective dialogue and to the sharing of responsibility on an equitable basis.

Finally, there is the issue of values: the professional has been trained to make certain judgments about the relative merit of choices. At times, families choose options that are not easily understood or tolerated by the health professional. Treatments or interventions that the professional would choose may be considered undesirable by the family or patient. These implicit and explicit values permeate much of what is undertaken, and as a rule, health professionals have relatively little tolerance for options or values that fail to coincide with their own.

If we accept these premises and the notion that we wish to alter the way in which needs are addressed, what are the possible remedies? It is our view that no single approach will solve these problems. Rather, we would advocate a pluralistic approach to the problems of the inner-city family with a child who has a chronic condition. Although there are many alternative models that may be helpful, there appear to be a number of components that are critical to the success of a model. The specific way in which these components are addressed must be tailored to both the needs of the individuals involved and the needs and structures of the local municipal government.

All models should involve designation of a care coordinator, a responsible person who assumes a central role in coordinating the care and maintaining communications between the range of agencies and individuals involved in providing services for a given child. In some cases, the care coordinator or central person may be a pediatrician or another professional or paraprofessional member of the health care delivery system. In others, it may be a teacher, school counselor, or lay person such as the lay family counselors trained in Rochester (Pless and Satterwhite, 1975). In other situations, there may be a family member who can assume the role. Regardless of who performs the function, the central person or care coordinator must be clearly identified to all and must be acceptable to the family. This person must be familiar with the system and must play a central role in ensuring that the family has access to him or her and to all needed parts of the system. This person should also have a concept of the child as an individual and of the social and physical environment in which the child lives. In addition, the coordinator must have an awareness of the total needs of the family, be able to keep conflicting priorities in perspective, and help to synthesize a coherent plan. Another major role of this person is to serve as an advocate and to help foster independence and coping skills of the family. The care coordinator should be familiar with the range of available community resources and also with the family's own strengths.

Because needs and problems change over time, it may be that no one individual plays the role of the care coordinator permanently, although we strongly prefer continuity when it can be achieved. It seems essential, however, that someone be clearly identified at all times to play this central role and that information be transferred completely when necessary changes do occur. In order to assure that there is no lapse in responsibility in the overall assistive function when a consultation or referral is made from one type of service or specialty to another, it seems advantageous for all contacts between the referrer and the consultant to specify the reason for the referral, a time frame for the completion of the assessment, a mechanism for communication of information to the coordinator and to the family, and an understanding of how the care will be provided and coordinated during the interim. The evaluator in turn should be responsible for completing the assessment expeditiously and comprehensively and for communicating findings to the coordinator. This is true whether the consultation is to establish bureaucratic eligibility for a special program or to obtain a formal medical subspecialty evaluation. Upon completion of the evaluation, the evaluator, coordinator, and family (if the family does not assume the role of coordinator) should agree on a plan. Unless specifically prearranged, it should be assumed that the referrer retains responsibility as care coordinator until a specific alternative is arranged.

In general, it is our bias that a generalist pediatrician, pediatric nurse practitioner, or family physician or practitioner should be involved in the care of the child, especially when a number of specialists provide segments of care. Without such a generalist's involvement, heavy concentration on specific problems, lack of coordination, gaps in the provision of basic services, and at times, conflicting recommendations concerning therapy can become problems.

Some suggest that wherever possible, "a variety of services needed by the poor should be coordinated at one location convenient to the patient" (Aronson, 1981, p. 267). At such a setting, the proper mix of social and health services, laboratory and pharmacy services, economic support, and food and nutrition programs can be organized. Davis and Schoen (1978) indicate that the comprehensive health centers have been remarkably successful when carried out on a demonstration basis. They suggest that the experience of such centers shows that quality health care can be provided within low-income communities, overcoming many barriers that impede access and improving the health status of the community in a cost-effective manner. This has been done using "innovative delivery systems that include the use of health professionals other than physicians, outreach efforts, and community participation in the governance and operation of centers" (p. 206).

The practicality of implementing this for children who need diverse and highly specialized services is still an open question. It may be that, for some children, coordination in a single site is neither feasible nor desirable. To cover these instances, coordinators must have previously developed linkages with highly specialized services that can be called into play in the interests of a given child. An endemic problem for coordinators is maintaining these linkages even though a given service may be activated relatively infrequently. Situations of children with chronic conditions will be unique and will require imaginative and flexible problem solving by coordinators. This requires that the system allow them the discretion to operate in such a fashion.

This chapter has suggested that several types of coordinating services would be desirable in helping children with chronic and handicapping conditions and their families. But this does not mean that there are not many other specific types of assistance families of children with special needs could use. These should be available to be called into play when and by whom they are needed. Aronson (1981), for example, in discussing the special needs of the urban poor, suggests that they need services such as culturally oriented advocacy, outreach translators, escorts, childcare help, and direct or indirect assistance with transportation. In addition to these more general services, children with special needs may require respite services to relieve parents, baby-sitters who are especially trained to perform nursing tasks and who are tolerant of differences, parent groups or children's peer groups for education and support, and/or homemakers. Without the presence of some total plan coordinator, families will not be in a position to know about or utilize services effectively.

It is important to note in this connection that there is some skepticism about wholesale efforts at coordination. It is easy to say that coordination and integration of services are needed, and such efforts are suggested so frequently as to sound facile. At least one recent review (Weiss, 1981, p. 21) suggests that recommending coordination is "in recent years the most popular strategy of reform in the human services arena" and is motivated by its strong symbolic value, rather than by any work suggesting that it is a valuable strategy. Weiss (p. 33) suggests that, in most cases, programs result in little coordination and that "failure to create coordination leads quite naturally to failure of coordination efforts to produce outcomes." In most instances, political and organizational interests, the inertia of the system, and desires to maintain the system and individual autonomy override the rhetoric of coordination. As a result, little, in fact, changes. "On a small scale, in a response to a specific crisis, with an easily bounded target group, or on an informal basis, coordination efforts have been implemented and may even have produced desired results" (pp. 35–36). In spite of these facts, there is some evidence that in the area being discussed, coordination may be desirable and effective (Brewer and Kakalik, 1979; Strawczynski, Stachewitsch, Morgenstern, and Shaw, 1973). The danger to be avoided is that of the coordination service becoming another specialized service and failing to really coordinate.

Another issue is the implication in much of the literature that receipt of services from public facilities is, in and of itself, less desirable than receipt of services from the private sector. And in fact, as we have indicated, receiving care from the public sector is often associated with less desirable kinds of services and fewer of those attributes thought desirable for quality care. Although it may be desirable both in line with the political and economic climate of the country to have care provided when possible within the private sector, it does not follow that all care within the public sector is second-rate. It is not impossible for programs within the public sector to provide good services and to have attributes thought desirable for quality care. For the past ten years, a program of Pediatric Home Care for children with chronic physical illnesses has been in operation at the

Bronx Municipal Hospital through an affiliation with the Albert Einstein College of Medicine. In this program, a team of generalist pediatricians and pediatric nurse practitioners has attempted to provide coordinated comprehensive care to children for whom the severity of the medical conditions and often the seriousness of family and social problems made it impossible or undesirable to function within the traditional ambulatory setting. Team members have provided direct care, coordinated the care of subspecialists, provided health care maintenance, served as advocates on behalf of the patients both within the medical setting and with other service agencies, and provided patient education in self-care and nursing tasks (Stein, 1978). Anecdotally, some private sector patients, when in contact with public sector patients, have indicated a desire to receive such services. A controlled clinical trial of pediatric home care demonstrated increased satisfaction with care, improved psychological adjustment of the child, and decreased psychiatric symptoms in the mother (Stein and Jessop, 1984). This program, which has some elements of the models proposed, has been easier to implement in the public than private sector.

In order to implement a plan of coordinated services for children with chronic conditions, several things are needed. First, it is important to state that although there may be a need for additional resources, money alone does not appear to be the solution. Even within the existing level of funding, there is room for a reordering of priorities. At present, the major portion of money allocated for services to the families of children with special needs is expended in technical interventions such as surgery or hospitalizations, while very little is expended in preventive services, coordination, or support. Considerable money could be saved if unnecessary duplications were avoided and if hospitalizations were reduced. In order to accomplish this, however, it may be necessary to pay for the coordinative efforts of the care coordinator, even when those efforts involve hours of work on the telephone or at a case conference rather than in the operating room or doctor's examining rooms. Financial incentives should be developed to encourage care coordination and to remove the current disincentives to this important set of tasks.

A second priority should be for improved education and reeducation of those in the helping professions so that their aspirations will be those of facilitating and working in a partnership with the families who need their help rather than continuing the dependency-producing patterns that have characterized many programs in the past.

Finally, there is a need for more information and empirical research about the actual delivery of services. In this discussion, we have felt it necessary to rely frequently on inferences from data not specifically targeted to the problem and on the clinical experience of those giving care to chronically ill children; this in itself is evidence of the lack of available hard data on the problems and care of children with chronic conditions in inner cities. There is a need for a child-based information system, and this is especially important in the inner city with the presence of multiple possible sources of care and services. There can be little growth in understanding of needs, service patterns, and their effects without such a system (Zill and Mount, 1981; Silver, 1981).

In conclusion, the problems of the inner-city child with a chronic condition cannot be solved by emphasizing only individual medical needs. Rather, solutions must also include attention to problems of the social and economic realities. In the absence of a major overhaul of priorities with regard to inner-city children with chronic conditions, we must conclude as Birch and Gussow (1970) did so eloquently that "children whose mothers were ill-fed and unready for pregnancy, who are born into poverty and survive an infancy of hunger and illness, are seldom miraculously saved in the third act" (p. 263).

References

Aday, L. A., Andersen, R., and Fleming, G. V. *Health Care in the U.S.: Equitable for Whom?* Beverly Hills, Calif.: Sage, 1980.

Adler, R., Werner, E. R., and Korsch, B. "Systematic Study of Four Years of Internship." *Pediatrics*, 1980, *66*, 1000–1008.

Aronson, S. "The Health Needs of Infants and Children Under 12." In Select Panel for the Promotion of Child Health, *Better Health for Our Children: A National Strategy.* Vol. 4. Department of Health and Human Services publication no. 79-55071. Washington, D.C.: U.S. Government Printing Office, 1981.

Birch, H. G., and Gussow, J. D. *Disadvantaged Children: Health, Nutrition, and School Failure.* New York: Grune & Stratton, 1970.

Brewer, G. D., and Kakalik, J. S. *Handicapped Children: Strategies for Improving Services.* New York: McGraw-Hill, 1979.

Brink, S. G., and Nader, P. R. "Patterns of Primary Care Utilization in a Tri-Ethnic Urban Population of School Children." *Medical Care*, 1981, *19* (6), 591–599.

Davis, K., and Schoen, C. *Health and the War on Poverty: A Ten-Year Appraisal.* Washington, D.C.: The Brookings Institution, 1978.

Dutton, D. B. "Explaining the Low Use of Health Services by the Poor: Costs, Attitudes, or Delivery Systems?" *American Sociological Review*, 1978, *43*, 348–368.

Dutton, D. B. "Children's Health Care: The Myth of Equal Access." In Select Panel for the Promotion of Child Health, *Better Health for Our Children: A National Strategy.* Vol. 4. Department of Health and Human Services publication no. 79-55071. Washington, D.C.: U.S. Government Printing Office, 1981.

Gilman, S. C., and Bruhn, J. G. "A Comparison of Utilization of Community Primary Health Care and School Health Services by Urban Mexican American and Anglo Elementary School Children." *Medical Care*, 1981, *19* (2), 223–232.

Gliedman, J., and Roth, W. *The Unexpected Minority: Handicapped Children in America.* A Report of the Carnegie Council on Children. New York: Harcourt Brace Jovanovich, 1980.

Gortmaker, S. L. "Medicaid and the Health Care of Children in Poverty and Near Poverty." *Medical Care*, 1981, *19* (6), 567–582.

Haggerty, R. J., Roghmann, K. J., and Pless, I. B. *Child Health and the Community.* New York: Wiley Interscience, 1975.

Harvard Child Health Project. *Report of the Child Health Project Task Force.* Vols. 1–3. Cambridge, Mass.: Ballinger, 1977.

Ireys, H. T. "Health Care for Chronically Disabled Children and Their Families." In Select Panel for the Promotion of Child Health, *Better Health for Our Children: A National Strategy.* Vol. 4. Department of Health and Human Services publication no. 79-55071. Washington, D.C.: U.S. Government Printing Office, 1981.

Kanthor, H., Pless, I. B., Satterwhite, B., and Myers, G. "Areas of Responsibility in the Health Care of Multiply Handicapped Children." *Pediatrics,* 1974, *54* (6), 779–785.

Kovar, M. G. "Health Status and Care of Children Living in the Community." Paper presented at the annual meeting of the American Association for the Advancement of Science, Toronto, Canada, January 1981.

Lash, T. W., Sigal, H., and Dudzinski, D. *State of the Child: New York City.* Vol. 2. New York: Foundation for Child Development, 1980.

Lefton, E., and Lefton, M. "Health Care and Treatment for the Chronically Ill: Toward a Conceptual Framework." *Journal of Chronic Diseases,* 1979, *32,* 339–344.

Millman, M. "The Role of City Government in Personal Health Services." *American Journal of Public Health,* 1981, *71* (Supplement), 47–57.

Okamoto, G., and Shurtleff, D. A. "Perceived First Contact Care for Disabled Children." *Pediatrics,* 1981, *67* (4), 530–535.

Orr, S. T., and Miller, C. A. "Utilization of Health Services by Poor Children Since the Advent of Medicaid." *Medical Care,* 1981, *19* (6), 583–590.

Palfrey, J., Levy, J. C., and Gilbert, K. L. "Use of Primary Care Facilities by Patients Attending Specialty Clinics." *Pediatrics,* 1980, *65,* 567–572.

Peterson, I. "Inequity Reported in Welfare Survey." *New York Times,* September 28, 1981, p. A15.

Pless, I. B., and Pinkerton, P. *Chronic Childhood Disorder: Promoting Patterns of Adjustment.* Chicago: Yearbook Medical Publishers, 1975.

Pless, I. B., and Satterwhite, B. "The Family Counselor." In R. Haggerty, K. Roghmann, and I. B. Pless (Eds.), *Child Health and the Community.* New York: Wiley, 1975.

Pless, I. B., Satterwhite, B., and Van Vechten, D. "Division, Duplication and Neglect: Patterns of Care for Children with Chronic Disorders." *Child Care, Health, and Development,* 1978, *4,* 9–19.

Preston, R. P. *The Dilemmas of Care: Social and Nursing Adaptations to the Deformed, the Disabled, and the Aged.* New York: Elsevier, 1979.

Riessman, C. K. "The Use of Health Services by the Poor." *Social Policy,* 1974, *5,* 41–45.

Select Panel for the Promotion of Child Health. *Better Health for Our Children: A National Strategy.* Vols. 1–4. Department of Health and Human Services publication no. 79-55071. Washington, D.C.: U.S. Government Printing Office, 1981.

Silver, G. A. "Reflections on Maternal and Child Health Programs: Reviewing the Literature, 1975–1980." In Select Panel for the Promotion of Child Health, *Better Health for Our Children: A National Strategy.* Vol. 4. Department of Health and Human Services publication no. 79-55071. Washington, D.C.: U.S. Government Printing Office, 1981.

Starfield, B. "Family Income, Ill Health, and Medical Care." *Journal of Public Health Policy,* 1982, *3,* 244–259.

Starfield, B., and Pless, I. B. "Physical Health." In O. G. Brim and J. Kagan (Eds.), *Constancy and Change in Human Development.* Cambridge, Mass.: Harvard University Press, 1980.

Stein, R.E.K. "Pediatric Home Care: An Ambulatory Special Care Unit." *Journal of Pediatrics,* 1978, *92,* 495–499.

Stein, R.E.K., and Jessop, D. J. "Does Pediatric Home Care Make a Difference for Children with Chronic Illness? Findings from the Pediatric Ambulatory Care Treatment Study." *Pediatrics,* 1984, *73,* 845–853.

Stein, R.E.K., Jessop, D. J., and Riessman, C. K. "Health Care Services Received by Chronically Ill Children." *American Journal of Diseases of Children,* 1983, *137* (3), 225–230.

Strawczynski, H., Stachewitsch, A., Morgenstern, G., and Shaw, M. E. "Delivery of Care to Hemophilic Children: Home Care Versus Hospitalization." *Pediatrics,* 1973, *51* (6), 986–991.

Sultz, H., Schlesinger, E. R., Mosher, W. E., and Feldman, J. G. *Long-Term Childhood Illness.* Pittsburgh, Pa.: University of Pittsburgh Press, 1972.

Vanderbilt University Primary Care Center and Tennessee Department of Public Health. "The Role of the Primary Care Provider in the Treatment of Handicapped Children." Conference at Nashville, Tennessee, September 1981.

Weiss, J. A. "Substance vs. Symbol in Administrative Reform: The Case of Human Services Coordination." *Policy Analysis,* 1981, 7 (1), 21–45.

Zill, N., and Mount, R. "National Information Needs in Maternal and Child Health." In Select Panel for the Promotion of Child Health, *Better Health for Our Children: A National Strategy.* Vol. 4. Department of Health and Human Services publication no. 79-55071. Washington, D.C.: U.S. Government Printing Office, 1981.

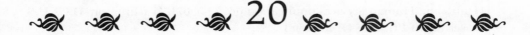

20

Special Problems
of Chronic Childhood Illness
in Rural Areas

James M. Perrin, M.D.

There is little agreement on the definition of *rural*, and especially on the criteria for distinguishing rural from urban areas. The 1970 Census definition of *urban*, for example, included all incorporated communities with more than 2,500 occupants. Others have defined rural people as those living outside Standard Metropolitan Statistical Areas (SMSAs), a definition that increases the number of rural dwellers. By any definition, a sizable portion of the United States population live in rural areas. In 1980, about sixty-three million people (28 percent of the population) were estimated to live in nonmetropolitan areas (Bachrach, 1981).

Certain characteristics of rural life and people affect access to health services and utilization of them. In comparison with urban areas, rural communities usually have a weak economic base with poorer support of public services. There is greater poverty in rural than urban areas, and the population is often skewed toward the old and the very young, with many young adults migrating to cities to enter the work force and leaving behind a rural population with special needs for health and other human services but limited resources with which to purchase them. With greater needs and fewer resources, 40 percent of rural dwellers also live in areas of medical underservice (Lichty and Zuvekas, 1980).

Note: The author would like to thank Drs. Lewis Lefkowitz and Budd Shenkin for their helpful criticism and advice.

Farming remains an important occupation in rural areas, although its character has changed greatly in the past quarter century, with a transition from family farms to corporate farming, increasing mechanization, and greater reliance on migratory workers as the main source of human labor on farms. Farming as an occupation is hazardous, mainly through risk of accident but also through frequent exposure to toxic chemicals, many of whose long-term effects are unknown and may conceivably lead to chronic illness or birth defects in offspring of farmworkers. Another common rural occupation, especially in mountain areas, is mining—also hazardous with a high rate of industrial injuries.

More housing is substandard in rural than in urban areas, and public transportation is almost nonexistent. Although geography often interferes both with access to services and with the development of effective community organizations, many rural areas exhibit important characteristics—especially a sense of community and of the importance of local autonomy and initiative—that can be productive in the development of effective service programs.

Despite these generalizations, rural areas in the United States demonstrate tremendous diversity—from the vast, open, sparsely populated parts of Montana to the many small communities near each other in western New York State to the poor mountainous sections of Appalachia to the relatively affluent midwestern agricultural sections. This diversity creates wide variation in service needs and suggests that policy solutions for rural human services needs are of necessity pluralistic (Sheps and Bachar, 1981).

Epidemiologic Considerations

Rural populations in most of the United States are characterized by great poverty, high rates of chronic illnesses (at least among adults), and poor access to health and related services. Parents in rural areas are more likely to consider their children's health as fair or poor (5.1 percent) than are parents in urban areas (4.2 percent) (Kovar and Meny, 1981). On the other hand, restricted activity and days of school missed per person per year are *lower* in rural areas than in urban ones. Poverty is associated with more illness, and among children with chronic illnesses, greater severity of handicap is associated with more poverty (Davis, 1976; Egbuono and Starfield, 1982). Widespread poverty and limited access to health services suggest more (and more severe) childhood chronic illness in rural than in urban areas. Rural families with childhood chronic illness are faced with a series of special problems that increase even further the burdens of illness. There are, furthermore, certain groups of people living predominantly in rural areas who face increased risks of some chronic handicapping disorders.

The low prevalence of most of the chronic handicapping conditions of childhood means that, in most rural counties, the number of children with any specific disorder is low. As an example, in a county of 10,000 people, one might expect to find three or four children with diabetes, one child with cystic fibrosis, one child with spina bifida, and only rarely children with other handicapping disorders. Indeed, of the conditions described in other sections of this volume, only asthma will be found in a relatively large number of children. Severe asthma in childhood nevertheless would be limited to about ten to twenty children in this county. The problem of low prevalence defines important considerations in the provision of health and related services to rural families.

Farmworkers and Native Americans: Rural Groups with Special Needs

Two population groups that merit special attention are migrant laborers and American Indians in rural areas. Migrant farmworkers in the United States are predominantly blacks traveling along the East Coast and Mexican Americans traveling from home-base areas in Texas and the Southwest to the West Coast and Midwest. Although precise prevalence figures for childhood chronic illness in farmwork populations have been difficult to obtain, it is known that farmworkers are affected by increased rates of acute and chronic infectious diseases (including tuberculosis and parasitic infections), of adult hypertension, and of low-birth-weight infants (often in association with maternal malnutrition). Surveys of farmworkers in South Texas have documented numerous uncorrected congenital deformities, untreated seizure disorders, and similar problems. Because of their occupations, migrant families also face large numbers of work-related accidents for adults and pesticide exposure for both children and adults (Shenkin, 1974). Whether they are at special risk of other chronic handicapping disorders of childhood is unclear, although the problems of family migration create difficulties in provision of adequate educational experiences as well as of needed health and social services.

Almost all farmworker families' earnings are below poverty level. To earn their seasonal wages, they often need to move from area to area, staying for relatively brief periods of time. Indeed, with increased mechanization in many agricultural areas, the need for seasonal workers has diminished, both in the number of workers employed and in the length of time employment is available for harvesting each crop. Housing in work areas is poorly regulated and often offers the barest minimum of privacy, sanitary facilities, refrigeration for food, and safe water supplies. Able-bodied and very young children usually travel with their families, although older children with handicapping disorders often remain in home-base areas with other relatives. Children with chronic handicapping disorders among migrant farmworker families thus often have the additional problem of family separation for a major portion of the year.

Although many farmworkers are Spanish-speaking, most rural health providers are not. Communication, difficult enough with patients not previously known to a practice, is rendered almost impossible by language and cultural barriers. Because of cultural differences, payment problems, and unwillingness to serve transient people, there are many communities in which farmworkers can find no providers willing to see them for either preventive or acute health care.

Access to health care for farmworkers, especially in work areas, is an important problem. First, medical services in rural areas are relatively sparse.

Second, although some studies have shown that the vast majority of farmworker families meet *eligibility* criteria for Medicaid, only about 20 to 30 percent of such families are usually *enrolled* in Medicaid. Enrollment is commonly decided and implemented on a county-by-county basis. To enroll in a specific county, a farmworker often must take half a day or more away from field work, obtain transportation to the local eligibility office, be able to provide adequate evidence of income over the past several months (often very difficult for farmworkers to document), and occasionally indicate an intent to settle in the community. In states with limited eligibility criteria, many families fail to meet one or another of the various eligibility criteria. Relatively few families overcome these major barriers to enrollment. Third, access to medical services, with or without Medicaid coverage, is also difficult. Many farmworkers travel in groups in buses under the control of crew bosses. To obtain needed services, farmworkers are often dependent on the bosses' willingness to provide transportation from the camp to the service provider. Insofar as most providers do not offer services outside of usual daytime hours, farmworkers desiring health services must choose between working and seeing a doctor, especially in an industry in which sick days are not provided as usual benefits and pay is dependent on individual worker productivity.

The federal government has had a limited direct service program for migrant farmworkers and their families since the early 1960s. Called the Migrant Health Program, this program, which was funded in fiscal year 1981 at a level of approximately $35 million dollars (about $35 per migrant family member per year), provides grants for the provision of health services to migrant families throughout the country. Implementation of the program has been varied, from development of comprehensive health centers (usually in home-base areas) to more limited services (often as little as a nurse in a rural health department) in many upstream work areas. Coverage in main work areas is quite variable, and whether the family will have access to health services is often a matter of chance.

In summary, migrant families are characterized by poverty, a higher proportion of chronic handicapping conditions, disruption of family life by traveling, financial barriers, and problems of access to health services.

Native Americans face somewhat similar problems. Although not plagued with the problem of frequent moving, they have a high incidence of acute and chronic health conditions. As an example, their children have an especially high rate of chronic otitis media with associated hearing loss. Certain tribes have especially high rates of congenital deformities, including congenital heart disease, dislocation of the hip, and cleft lip and/or palate. Infant mortality among Native Americans is much above the national average. Trachoma, a chronic or possibly recurring disease, has been an intractable problem for children living on the reservations of the Southwest, even though it is treatable in nonreservation settings. Through the Indian Health Service, Native Americans have access to moderately continuous health care, although it has been characterized by problems in the retention of medical manpower, access in particularly rural areas, bureaucratization, and limited financing. In general, Native Americans have not had freedom to choose among health providers or otherwise to have much direct responsibility in the choice of, say, specialty services for children with chronic handicapping conditions.

Services in Rural Areas

Health Services (Physicians, Nurses, Hospitals, and Health Departments). In general, primary care services are less available in rural areas than they are in urban and especially suburban areas. With increasing specialization during the past twenty to thirty years, including the emphasis on specialization in most American medical schools, increasing percentages of physicians have chosen to remain in urban and suburban settings rather than to enter rural general practice.

In 1975, the ratio of nonfederal physicians to population in urban areas (SMSAs) was 158.7 per thousand compared with 70.4 per thousand in nonurban areas. The smaller number of providers is reflected in larger percentages of children in rural areas not having identifiable sources of care (10.9 percent in rural areas; 7.0 percent in non-inner-city urban areas). In addition, of children with regular sources of care, those in rural areas were much less likely to identify a pediatrician as the source (24 percent) than were families in non-inner-city urban areas (45 percent). Similar trends are found from reviewing utilization data. Urban children average 4.4 physician contacts per year; those in rural areas, 3.4. Immunization rates in rural areas are generally intermediate between those in suburban areas and those in poor urban areas, likely reflecting the relative success of rural health departments in child immunization programs (Perrin and others, 1981). Finally, large portions of the rural population have no form of health insurance (including Medicaid or Medicare), especially among the rural *farm* population (Kovar and Meny, 1981).

To some degree, the problem of less available primary care in rural areas has diminished during the past ten or fifteen years, mainly as a result of three important trends and because of public investment in rural health services described later in this chapter. First, the growing family practice training efforts throughout the country have resulted in increasing numbers of well-trained family physicians, many of whom have made a commitment to practice in relatively small communities. Although family practitioners may settle in urban areas, many training programs have had an emphasis on the preparation of physicians for smaller communities. Second, with the increasing numbers of physicians in all specialties, and probably in association with other secular trends that indicate migration to rural areas, physicians in general are finding rural areas more attractive. Also, it is increasingly difficult for new physicians to enter practice in many urban settings, thus encouraging the exploration of rural opportunities. Third, it has been noted that large numbers of new rural physicians in some parts of the country have been foreign medical graduates (Swearingen and Perrin, 1977), who may have found rural areas more hospitable for practice than urban ones. Although very little is known directly about the quality of medical care provided by rural practitioners compared with urban ones, or by foreign medical graduates in comparison with graduates of U.S. medical schools, one can speculate that someone from an entirely different culture may be less likely than other physicians to attend to the family issues related to childhood chronic illness in the United States. At any rate, despite these positive trends in rural physician migration, it is likely that there will be a deficiency of physicians through the end of the century (Rural Health Committee, 1981).

Rural physicians are more likely to practice by themselves than in groups. Solo practice makes consultation with colleagues less likely and diminishes the probability that a physician will share with colleagues the problems inherent in providing services to children with chronic illness and their families. Although, on the one hand, the increasing numbers of well-trained family practitioners in rural areas indicate a healthy trend, there is an associated tendency for recently trained general surgeons to settle in rural areas, again because of diminishing opportunities in urban settings. To supplement the limited surgical practice available in many rural communities, many of these physicians provide general health services despite very limited training in basic issues of health maintenance, prevention, or especially, the special problems of children with chronic illness. Thus, larger numbers of physicians in rural areas may not lead to better care for chronically ill children.

Simply because of the low prevalence of most of the childhood chronic disorders, physicians in rural areas, whether well-trained or not, are less likely to have had experience with the specific childhood chronic illnesses. Most chronically ill children are, for at least some parts of their health care experience, concentrated in the tertiary care urban health centers. Thus, although urban general physicians and pediatricians may also have limited direct experience with the specific conditions in their practices, they may at least encounter them occasionally by way of their patient care and educational associations with the tertiary care centers. For the rural physician, this lack of experience creates important early identification and referral problems as well as difficulties in keeping abreast of new information concerning unusual diseases.

The problem of early identification is straightforward. Insofar as a physician may not have encountered a case of a specific rare condition within the previous ten years or, indeed, since medical school training (or perhaps ever), his or her index of suspicion of that condition may be low and the ability to differentiate a rare condition from more common disorders may be limited. As an example, one of the problems of rural hospitals with only a couple of hundred newborn deliveries a year is that, even with the very best of nursing staffs, the relatively limited experience with sick babies may mean that nurses fail to identify the rare child with an important disorder and, even when they do, do not know best how to stabilize such an infant and minimize risk.

Problems with referral are very similar. Most rural physicians maintain good consultation links with urban consultants, especially for problems they see frequently in their practice. For rare disorders, though, they may not know the referral sources well, nor are they likely to know what, if any, options they have.

As an example, different tertiary (referral) centers treat children with myelomeningocele differently, some quite aggressively and some much more conservatively. Insofar as a rural hospital delivering some three hundred babies a year will
encounter a case of myelomeningocele only once a decade on the average, it is
unlikely that anyone in that community will be familiar with the approach of
a particular referral institution to the management of the disorder. Thus,
although families and providers should both have the opportunity to participate
in decisions regarding the intent and extent of care, this participation is unlikely
to be possible in the rural circumstance. Similarly, although the rural practitioner is likely to be fairly well acquainted with the cardiologists to whom he or
she refers cardiologic problems because of the frequency of adult cardiovascular
disease, that family practitioner is likely to encounter a child with leukemia only
rarely and will thus have very limited (or no) experience with the consultants
available at the tertiary care center.

The maintenance of knowledge regarding specific chronic illnesses is
another difficult task for the rural practitioner. Although a practitioner may be
motivated to provide ongoing services to children with chronic illnesses in the
community, maintaining adequate knowledge about new developments in such
disorders as cystic fibrosis or diabetes requires extensive continuing education or
excellent communication links with the specialists in the tertiary care center.
From the viewpoint of the family, this is a significant problem. To whom should
the family with a child with diabetes turn when their child has developed
gastroenteritis or has an insulin reaction? To their local physician or to the
tertiary care center sixty miles away? When the four-year-old child with asthma
has a significant attack, should that child go to the local family physician or
emergency room, or would it be better to travel to the allergist or pulmonary
specialist in the urban center? Families, especially with children with exacerbating conditions, need accessible and knowledgeable services. In general, most
studies indicate that families want services relatively close to home, but families
with children with varied chronic conditions report confusion in knowing where
to turn when they need certain kinds of medical services (Okamoto and Shurtleff,
1981).

During the past fifteen years, nurse practitioners have been an increasingly
important group of health providers in rural areas. The need for more rural
health services was one major stimulus to the development of expanded roles for
nurses. Nurse practitioners have worked effectively in many rural settings: in
rural comprehensive health centers, solo nurse practices, county health departments, and private collaborative practices with physicians. Because of special
training in mobilization of community resources and a tradition of a holistic
approach to patient care, nurse practitioners have important skills that may be
limited in physician-only settings. In poorly served rural areas, nurses are often
the only professionals knowledgeable about local community resources that may
enable a chronically ill child to function as well as possible. In some communities, nurse practitioners have met resistance from other primary care providers
(especially physicians) and may not be accepted as real partners in providing

health services. Access to needed referral services at the secondary and tertiary care level has been less of a problem. Studies of quality of primary care provided by nurse practitioners have uniformly found no diminution in quality in comparison with that provided by physicians and often greater quality and breadth of services (Sox, 1979; Perrin and Goodman, 1978). Nurses thus have taken a major role in improving access to primary care in rural areas. They do, however, face many of the same problems as physicians in consulting with chronically ill children and their families; these include isolation and lack of experience with specific conditions and with early identification and referral.

The Rural Health Clinics Act of 1977 recognized the increasing responsibility of nurse practitioners for delivering primary care in rural areas. The act provided a means of reimbursing nurses and physicians' assistants who deliver services in rural primary care settings. Although paperwork burdens have to some extent hampered access to Rural Health Clinic reimbursement, more than three hundred sites were receiving reimbursement by 1981.

As a result of the Hill-Burton program after World War II, which supported much of the construction cost of nonproprietary community hospitals, hospital beds are not lacking in most rural communities (McNerney and Riedel, 1962). Rural hospitals, however, are frequently small (twenty to forty beds) and usually lack any organized pediatric section with skilled pediatric nursing care. Many hospitals do not have a local pediatrician to provide professional supervision for child health services. Indeed, some who favor regulatory approaches to the care of chronically ill children have suggested that they be admitted only to hospitals meeting standards including certain nursing and medical capacities. Doing so, however, means that children facing frequent hospitalization will spend more time further away from their home communities. Other problems of rural hospitals include cost-efficient management of hospitals with relatively few beds and the nationwide shortage of trained hospital nurses—a shortage exacerbated in rural areas. Whether rural hospitals are important for recruitment and retention of medical manpower is equivocal. Large amounts of practice income (encouraging practice stability) are generated via hospital care for patients. Yet, additional hospital responsibilities (such as emergency room coverage and committee responsibilities) can prove onerous to rural providers. It is not clear that small hospitals can maintain efficiency and quality, and in some rural areas, there have been efforts to consolidate or close small hospitals.

In many rural areas, local health departments play an important role in the provision of primary care services, especially to poorer people. With the prevalent chronic illnesses of adults, some health departments have successfully developed programs for long-term management of adults with such conditions as hypertension and diabetes. Such health departments can be an important resource for community-based care for children with chronic illnesses. On the other hand, for those health departments that have ventured into the provision of primary care services, some studies have suggested that health departments provide primary care services less well than they provide traditional well-child services, such as immunizations.

From the viewpoint of children with chronic illnesses, increasing the availability and training of Crippled Children's Services (CCS) nurses in rural health departments, as is occurring in some states, should improve the quality of services available in these agencies, especially if there is effective communication between CCS and primary care staffs. The original Crippled Children's Services legislation recognized the special needs of rural areas and emphasized carrying care to rural populations. The typical CCS service in the early days of the program has been described as two women, one nurse and one social worker, driving in a rickety 1930s Ford down a dusty road to visit a family fifteen miles out of town. Many CCS programs have kept this rural emphasis.

The Select Panel for the Promotion of Child Health also recommended that rural health departments become eligible sites for the placement of National Health Service Corps physicians, a policy change likely to improve services in those agencies. Especially insofar as many extremely poor rural areas lack the economic base to support a physician in traditional private practice, the health department can become an important base for primary health services.

Other Services. Geographic access to health and related services in rural areas is hampered by lack of adequate transportation in many communities. Many communities are isolated, with poor roads, and health services may be distant from the places people live. In mountainous areas, especially, although services may be just over the next mountain range, it may be a fifty-mile drive around the base of the mountains to get there. Even in areas where roads are good, public transportation is almost nonexistent in rural areas, and families needing frequent health services can rarely depend on public sources for their transportation.

Other resources important to children with chronic illnesses and their families are often lacking in rural areas. Importantly, mental health professionals are particularly sparse in rural areas. Social services are often limited to the county welfare agency and only rarely found in hospitals or other community agencies. Similarly, the agencies themselves are relatively few and often poorly staffed and funded. Thus, families find little community support for meeting their therapeutic, transportation, childcare, or other resource needs. Although disease-specific community agencies play an important role in urban areas in family support and obtaining basic resources for children with specific chronic illnesses and their families, few have strong regional or rural components, and they generally have very little impact in rural areas.

The special problems schools face in integrating children with chronic illnesses are exacerbated in rural areas, again mainly because of the issues of low prevalence and lack of experience with chronically ill children. Where urban school systems usually have the opportunity to gain some experience with such children (at least for a few staff members) and to seek consultation from experienced practitioners and community agencies, in rural areas, school personnel will have had very limited experience and will have little knowledge of where to turn for consultation when a child with a chronic illness is in the school.

Public Support for Rural Health Services

The need to improve health services in rural areas has been recognized as a public responsibility for decades. In addition to the Hill-Burton hospital construction program and specific migrant health and Indian health programs, several federal programs have strengthened primary care services in rural areas, mainly through direct support of rural primary care programs. Family Health Centers, an outgrowth of the neighborhood health center developments of the 1960s, include about thirty in rural areas. The Rural Health Initiative Program supports networks incorporating varied federal programs (such as Migrant Health and National Health Service Corps) in rural areas. The Appalachian Regional Commission has supported numerous rural primary care efforts, especially in Kentucky and Tennessee. The Rural Health Clinics Act of 1977 recognized the problems of financial viability of isolated rural practices, especially those dependent in large part on nonphysician providers. The act represented a growing awareness of the importance of financial incentives in maintenance of rural practices.

During the 1970s, the National Health Service Corps has placed many physicians, dentists, and nurses in underserved rural areas. The Corps offers a way for young professionals to try rural practice and has encouraged many to continue in rural settings. Most Corps sites, however, are in very isolated or poverty-stricken areas, for which continuing federal support will likely be necessary. With recent federal cutbacks, the Corps has essentially disbanded. Several states have vigorous rural health office that actively recruit physicians and nurses and at times directly support rural health clinics. Foundations, especially the Robert Wood Johnson and the W. K. Kellogg Foundations, have supported important demonstrations in rural primary care. Johnson has emphasized well-administered small practices with strong physician leadership, while Kellogg has supported satellite primary care activities in association with larger health institutions (Sheps and Bachar, 1981). Although major staffing and financial problems remain in providing access to primary care for rural Americans, these programs have in large measure improved rural health services.

Recommendations

The major health needs of rural Americans remain access to quality primary care services and adequate financing to support such services. Maintaining and strengthening the progress of the past two decades is essential for rural people and should now be coupled with efforts to demonstrate improved health status stemming from publicly supported activities. Continued progress will assure the basic structure of a primary care system for rural areas, without which public programs for chronically ill children in rural areas will make little sense and be impossible to implement. The recommendations that follow are based on the assumption that basic progress in rural health services will continue.

Regionalization. The regionalization of health services has so far been best implemented in the context of perinatal services. Levels of nursery service have been defined, and different nurseries have been accredited to provide certain levels of service. As the intensity of the newborn infant's need increases, the baby is referred to increasingly specialized levels of service. Then, as the baby improves and the need for specialized services diminishes, the infant is referred back to the home community or to a nursery offering less intense services. The benefits of regionalization have included (1) definition of clear referral patterns, (2) improvement of consultation as a result of these referral patterns, and (3) identification of local providers (physicians and hospitals) able to provide ongoing care in rural communities. The nursery physician or nurse in an outlying community knows well whom to call to discuss a problem infant even before the point of transferring a sick child to a more specialized service. A similar model should be developed for the regionalization of care for children with chronic handicapping conditions. Regionalization should include definitions of shared responsibilities and the explicit clarification of what services are provided in a specialized center and what are provided within the home community (Kanthor and others, 1974). Similarly, effective communication between primary and tertiary care providers would be expanded and improved in a regional system, such that primary providers could effectively maintain their interaction with families and support their needs broadly while maintaining adequate knowledge of the specific condition and knowing the means of obtaining consultation with a tertiary specialist when necessary.

As shown in the perinatal experience, regionalization requires changes in usual activities of both primary and tertiary providers. Where primary providers take more responsibility for ongoing patient management (in addition to screening and referral), specialists assume greater responsibility for community physician continuing education and for providing needed information to families and physicians in rural areas. The initial and ongoing evaluation of referred patients in the specialty center should address plans for long-term care and follow-up in the home community. In Iowa, recent experiments in the decentralization of care for children with leukemia have been very promising and may serve as an additional model (Kisker and others, 1980; Strayer and others, 1980). Here community physicians collaborate with specialists and provide most care for children with leukemia (including the administration of most drugs) in the home community. The program has met with patient and family satisfaction and has decreased costs of care for these families.

Community Chronic Illness Support Workers. Nonspecialized support workers aiding families with chronic illnesses should be made available in rural communities. Although there is no purpose for a support person specializing in, say, cystic fibrosis in a small community, a person specializing in *chronic illness* can become proficient in knowing community resources available to families and in gaining access to services and information from urban specialty centers. Support people can come from a variety of backgrounds and do not need particular disciplinary training. They are similar to the family counselor of Pless and Satterwhite (1972). Counselors can be associated with any of a number of stable institutions in the community—schools, the health department, private service agencies. Their tasks are to work with families of children with chronic conditions, to obtain necessary resources for them, to work with schools and other agencies to improve the integration of these families and children, and otherwise to provide support for the families. Given the relative rarity of most chronic disorders in rural areas, support people need to be generalists able to interact effectively with families coping with a variety of different conditions.

Special Groups. Rural populations with special needs, especially farm-workers and Native Americans, continue to need categorical public attention to their health care needs. Although improvement in rural health services in general, and specifically for children with chronic illnesses, will somewhat improve services for farmworkers and Native Americans, the special problems of migrancy, reservation isolation, and language will continue to provide barriers to care for these families. For migratory labor families, expansion of comprehensive health centers in high-migrant-impact home-base areas should continue. In upstream work areas, the emphasis should be on the development of incentives for the integration and easy access of farmworkers into improved health services for all rural people. This can be accomplished through the seasonal addition of staff to year-round community practices and by easing eligibility of farmworker families for Medicaid (potentially by federalizing Medicaid or at least eligibility determination). The development of small, separate units for farmworker care in upstream areas makes little sense and is unlikely to meet the referral and community care needs of farmworker children with chronic illnesses.

The Indian Health Service merits increased funding as a source of care for Native Americans. Present efforts to regionalize the Indian Health Service and to define consultation-referral links with neighboring academic health centers should be encouraged.

Communications and Technology. Application of high technology communication and data systems should be vigorously pursued in rural areas. Despite their isolation, most rural communities are reached by television, and increasing numbers have access to cable networks. Developing technology provides excellent opportunities for community health education, providers' continuing education, and communication among components of an organized regional system.

Training. Some of the preceding recommendations call for special training efforts. Programs to train community workers (counselors) should be developed offering basic education regarding the workings of school, health care, and other relevant community agencies as well as of academic health centers and other referral sites. In general, these workers need skills that will help them coordinate services and recruit resources for involved families.

Education for providers intending to practice in rural areas should take into account the special skills needed for practice there. These include formal training in referral-consultation activities, training in numerous areas in minor surgery and emergency care (often referred to specialists and surgeons in urban areas), and special language skills. Short continuing education courses for rural

providers should be offered to improve skills in early identification of handicapping conditions. Similarly, efforts to train specialists in the consultation process
and in concepts of community health are important.

References

Bachrach, L. L. *Human Services in Rural Areas: An Analytical Review.* Human
    Services Monograph Series, No. 22. U.S. Department of Health, Education,
    and Welfare publication no. 05-76-130. Washington, D.C.: U.S. Government
    Printing Office, 1981.

Davis, K. "Medicaid Payments and Utilization of Medical Services by the Poor."
    Inquiry, 1976, *13,* 127-135.

Egbuonu, L., and Starfield, B. "Child Health and Social Status." *Pediatrics,* 1982,
    69, 550-557.

Kanthor, H., and others. "Areas of Responsibility in the Health Care of Multiply
    Handicapped Children." *Pediatrics,* 1974, *54,* 779-788.

Kisker, C. T., and others. "Health Outcomes of a Community Based Therapy
    Program for Children with Cancer." *Pediatrics,* 1980, *66,* 900-906.

Kovar, M. G., and Meny, D. J. "Volume III: A Statistical Profile." In Select Panel
    for the Promotion of Child Health, *Better Health for Our Children: A National
    Strategy.* U.S. Department of Health and Human Services publication
    no. 79-55071. Washington, D.C.: U.S. Government Printing Office, 1981.

Lichty, S. S., and Zuvekas, A. "Rural Health: Policies, Progress and Challenges."
    Urban Health, 1980, *9,* 26.

McNerney, W. J., and Riedel, D. C. *Regionalization and Rural Health Care.* Ann
    Arbor: University of Michigan Press, 1962.

Okamoto, G. A., and Shurtleff, D. A. "First Contact Care for Disabled Children."
    Pediatrics, 1981, *67,* 530-535.

Perrin, E. C., and Goodman, H. C. "Telephone Management of Acute Pediatric
    Illness." *New England Journal of Medicine,* 1978, *298,* 130-135.

Perrin, J. M., and others. "Kids in the Sticks: Quality of Rural Primary Care."
    In *Annual Program Abstracts.* Philadelphia: Ambulatory Pediatric Asso-
    ciation, 1981.

Pless, I. B., and Satterwhite, B. "Chronic Illness in Childhood: Selection,
    Activities, and Evaluation of Non-Professional Family Counselors." *Clinical
    Pediatrics,* 1972, *11,* 403-410.

Rural Health Committee, American Public Health Association, Medical Care
    Section. "Suggested Policy Statements Presented to Council." *Nation's
    Health,* Sept. 1981, pp. 4-6.

Shenkin, B. *Health Care for Migrant Workers: Policies and Politics.* Cambridge,
    Mass.: Ballinger, 1974.

Sheps, C. G., and Bachar, M. "Rural Areas and Personal Health Strategies."
    American Journal of Public Health, 1981, *71* (Supplement), 71-82.

Sox, H. C. "Quality of Patient Care by Nurse Practitioners and Physician's

Assistants: A Ten-Year Perspective." *Annals of Internal Medicine*, 1979, *91*, 459–468.

Strayer, F., and others. "Cost Effectiveness of a Shared Management Delivery System for the Care of Children with Cancer." *Pediatrics*, 1980, *66*, 907–911.

Swearingen, C. M., and Perrin, J. M. "Foreign Medical Graduates in Rural Primary Care." *Medical Care*, 1977, *15*, 331–337.

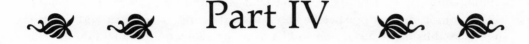

Part IV

Provision of Services
and Professional Training

Children with severe chronic illnesses and their families have complex, special needs that require care by professionals from many disciplines. Part Four begins with an overview of problems inherent in the multidisciplinary care of chronically ill children. Lorraine V. Klerman, author of Chapter Twenty-one, states that interprofessional problems arise in the care of all children but may be exacerbated when a child has a chronic illness. When several professionals are involved in the care of a patient, responsibilities may overlap and some needs may be neglected. Such important needs of chronically ill children as medical management, coordination of care, family support, primary care, and education may be affected. Klerman suggests a variety of approaches that could ameliorate these problems, including structural changes in the delivery system, modification of professional training or utilization of in-service education, and economic incentives to provide services that are needed but not currently available.

In Chapter Twenty-two, Michael Weitzman defines the goals of health services for chronically ill children as the reduction of physical and psychosocial disability and the promotion of optimal functioning. Obstructing the achievement of those goals, however, are the numerous difficulties that chronically ill children and their families frequently experience in trying to obtain health services. Weitzman suggests that the complicated mix of public and private services and the high degree of specialization that typify the health services system may be largely to blame. Weitzman acknowledges that a single approach to the organization of services would be impractical; however, he suggests reorganization of existing community resources as a way of alleviating many delivery problems for children with chronic illnesses. He stresses the need for continuity of access to one medical provider, coordination by one provider, and the availability of comprehensive, quality programs for these children and their families. His recommendations for accompanying policy changes are directed to medical education and child advocacy initiatives.

C. William Daeschner, Jr., and Mary C. Cerreto, authors of Chapter Twenty-three, address the needs of chronically ill children as a prelude to summarizing the current status of medical education. Stating that the major orientation of medical practice has been toward "cure," Daeschner and Cerreto suggest establishing educational and fiscal policy that would reorient the system toward "care" to meet the needs of chronically ill children. The authors describe education models, available and projected, for teaching professionals to care for chronically ill children, including university affiliated centers, chronic disease health maintenance organizations, care-by-parent units, and camps, among others. Recommendations for the education of professionals are presented for five areas: facilities, faculties, financing, curriculum, and research.

Chapter Twenty-four, by Debra P. Hymovich, reviews the several kinds of care that nurses can provide to chronically ill children and their families, including direct care, guidance and support, casefinding, patient education, consultation, coordination, collaboration, client advocacy, and research. In describing the expanding roles of nurses and the specialties that are developing within the profession, Hymovich cites examples such as nurse practitioners, school nurses, clinical specialists, and nurses involved in home care. She points to five policy issues that must be addressed if nurses are to realize their full potential in providing services to chronically ill children and their families. Her recommendations concern nursing education, nurses' roles in comprehensive health assessment and care of children, research, and other areas.

Nursing education is addressed from a historical perspective by Corinne M. Barnes, in Chapter Twenty-five. Barnes describes the main types of educational programs available for those who would enter practice as nurse generalists—baccalaureate degree, associate degree, and diploma. She then discusses the importance of clinical nursing research in the care of chronically ill children, with special attention to the role and function of the clinical nurse specialist. In her summary and recommendations, Barnes addresses specific areas of nursing education that must be examined and acted upon in order to further benefit children with chronic illness.

The mental health of chronically ill children and their families is the topic of Chapter Twenty-six, by Dennis Drotar and Marcy Bush. The authors examine the knowledge base in the areas of illness-related stresses, studies of individual psychological adjustment, adjustment problems in life contexts and pediatric settings, and services and treatment modalities. They then discuss future models for service delivery for chronically ill children that would emphasize integration of hospital-based services with community-centered advocacy and focus on preventive, family-centered mental health services. Finally, Drotar and Bush state that future research should investigate the factors that contribute to children's resilience over time and link family coping strategies to adaptive life outcomes. As future research agendas, objective measures assessing compliance, advanced planning, and documentation of the efficacy of psychosocial interventions can contribute to prevention-focused research concerning the mental health of chronically ill children and their families.

In Chapter Twenty-seven, Susan M. Jay and Logan Wright examine pediatric psychology, a subspecialty within psychology that interfaces with behavioral medicine and that has made contributions to training and research in the area of chronic illness in children. Jay and Wright point out essential content areas that should be incorporated into training programs for psychologists who plan to work with chronically ill children, including normal child development as well as psychopathology and the impact of chronic illness. Psychologists' needs for good grounding in assessment techniques, intervention and consultation skills, and applied clinical research as well as expertise in dealing with terminal illness are also discussed. In conclusion, the authors express support for improvement and expansion of training opportunities for psychologists that can result in the enhancement of the quality of life of children with chronic illnesses.

Claire Rudolph, Virginia Andrews, Kathryn Strother Ratcliff, and Dorothy A. Downes discuss professional training for social work with chronically ill children in Chapter Twenty-eight. After covering the historical development of social work practice, the authors describe current social work education programs, concentrating on training for health care service delivery. An orientation to practice as basic training for social workers dealing with chronically ill children follows. The authors outline psychosocial problems among chronically ill children and their families with which the social worker must be familiar and specify the competencies needed for three types of social work practice—direct, coordinative, and research oriented. In conclusion, the authors state that social work practitioners who serve chronically ill children must have an interdisciplinary theoretical knowledge base and must develop a range of clinical, organizational, analytical, and research skills, as well as the personal skill of recognizing their own limitations.

Chapter Twenty-nine, by Tom Joe and Cheryl Rogers, uses three case studies to illustrate the strengths, limitations, and service needs of chronically disabled children. These case studies demonstrate that chronic impairment or disability denotes an identifiable loss of function, but should not necessarily imply a lack of potential ability to perform. Joe and Rogers assert that impaired children must be viewed as composites of myriad strengths and weaknesses. Applying this new, broader perspective in public and private delivery systems may enable these children to realize their potential and live as productively and fully as possible.

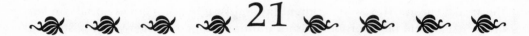

Interprofessional Issues in Delivering Services to Chronically Ill Children and Their Families

Lorraine V. Klerman, Dr.P.H.

Medical care seems to reach its peak of organization, efficiency, and effectiveness in emergency situations. The rescue of an injured president from what seemed certain death is an example with which the general public is familiar. Similar miracles occur daily and often involve children. The most exciting such events can be observed in delivery rooms, neonatal intensive care units, emergency rooms, and operating rooms, but smaller miracles take place in physicians' offices, hospital diagnostic units, and community health centers as pediatricians and others solve the puzzle of what is causing a child's problem and then, in many cases, find a way to lessen, if not totally overcome, it.

But when the issues are more routine, when the problems defy traditional medical or surgical solutions either because no therapy is available or because social and economic issues interfere, when treatment must continue indefinitely or for extremely long periods, or when the condition is one that no one wants to handle, then medical care becomes less effective. As effectiveness diminishes, patients, their families, professionals, and laymen become anxious, concerned, and irritated. This chapter first explores some of the interprofessional issues that

Note: The assistance of Kathryn King, Marty W. Krauss, and Michael Weitzman is gratefully acknowledged.

420

tend to emerge under these conditions, then it examines how these issues affect the care of chronically ill children and their families.

Interprofessional Issues in the Care of All Children

The interprofessional problems that interfere with the optimum care of children with chronic illnesses are not unique to this field of specialized health care. Rather, such problems are generic to the child health area, if not to the entire health field. Interprofessional issues may be exacerbated when the patient is a child suffering from spina bifida, cystic fibrosis, or another chronic illness, but many of the basic problems are evident in dealing with a child who has an acute illness or even with a healthy child.

Lack of agreement about roles and services exists both within and among professional groups. In the medical profession, the general pediatrician and the specialist sometimes vie for patients or, conversely, attempt to unload patients on each other. In some cases, the family physician may want to treat a child who other physicians or the family or friends feel needs the care of a pediatrician. Even when physicians attempt to collaborate, delineation of precise professional roles is often difficult, leading to confusion, poor communication, and dissatisfaction on the part of physicians, patients, and families.

Medicine and nursing are often in disagreement about mutual responsibilities. The pediatric nurse practitioner or child health specialist may believe she or he has the ability to treat independently all but a very few complicated cases whereas the pediatrician may feel that such nursing specialists should only work under close supervision of the physician who makes the original diagnosis, establishes the treatment plan, and checks progress periodically. Even within the more traditional nursing roles in hospitals and clinics, nurses are expected to assume responsibility for supervision of increasingly complex therapies and for detection of subtle changes in patient condition. Because of such responsibilities, and as a result of their longer interaction with children and their families, nurses often want to assume the initiative in roles for which they have been particularly trained—teaching, counseling, and comforting. Even in these tasks, they may find themselves in conflict with physicians who want total control over what their patients and families are told about their condition, prognosis, and treatment.

The public health nurse and the visiting nurse presumably have unique roles in the care of both the sick and the well child. In clinic settings, they sometimes function without a physician's presence, although they work under a set of standing orders. More important, however, is their role in the home. There they provide a variety of therapies, do much health education, help families adjust to children's problems, and observe and listen. The question is to what extent they can or should act upon the information they receive—whether or not they are only an extension of physicians' senses and therefore expected to report to them and wait for their decisions. Parallel problems are experienced by school nurses and by outreach workers employed by many freestanding community clinics.

Other health professionals, especially those concerned with the emotional components of childcare, have roles to play and need to have their responsibilities clarified in relation to physicians and nurses. Social workers can be essential to a family's understanding of their child's problems and their ability to cope effectively with them. But to ensure that the family receives the same information and advice from all concerned and that no aspect of their problems is ignored, the social worker must be kept informed and able to maintain two-way communication with both physician and nurse. Child psychologists may also fulfill this role.

Why are so many individuals involved in the various aspects of patient care? In earlier, simpler days there was only one type of physician (the general practitioner), nurses' tasks were much more limited, and social workers were rare. Interprofessional problems were less frequent, but so were accurate diagnosis and effective treatment. With an increasing ability to detect and cure has come medical specialization and fragmentation of caregiving. Technological advances have increased the cost of medical care and thus led to the development of presumably less expensive nonmedical specialists and paraprofessionals, again fragmenting the delivery of care. Interprofessional conflict and referral of problems to other professionals are the prices children and their families pay for the increased possibility of cure or amelioration of their health problems. Many feel it is worth the price.

Nevertheless, interprofessional issues need not be considered inevitable or insoluble. Roles can be clearly delineated, responsibilities divided in ways satisfying to all, and the needs of children and their families met successfully. But such an outcome requires realization of the dimensions of the problem and sensitivity to the interests of others. It may also require some realignment of financial arrangements.

Special Issues in the Care of Children with Chronic Illnesses

Because of the nature of chronic illnesses, children with these disorders and their families are particularly likely to be affected adversely when interprofessional issues are not resolved. As noted earlier, in times of acute crisis, all members of the health team seem to know their roles and to integrate quickly into a well-functioning team. But when a medical condition continues over an extended period of time, includes multiple interventions by individuals from a variety of helping professions, is complicated by socioeconomic factors, and requires the involvement of family members, there is greater likelihood of more than one person doing the same task and of no one doing others.

The majority of interprofessional problems arise either because more than one individual or profession claims the exclusive right or responsibility to perform a given task or because no individuals or professions are certain a task is theirs: Whose responsibility is it to tell families that a diagnosis is a life-shortening neurological disease—pediatric neurologists, who have all the facts of the particular case and many others at their disposal? or family physicians or pediatricians who have more knowledge of the family's dynamics? Whose task is it to teach the child and the family how to detect early signs of an asthmatic attack, how to deal with it, and under what circumstances to seek medical assistance—the nurse, the primary care physician, or the pulmonary specialist? Who should adjust the medication for juvenile arthritis, epilepsy, or diabetes? And—in the area of neglected responsibilities—it is clear that there are tasks in the care of chronically ill children that no one wants, or feels capable of, or has the time for, or is paid to perform. Examples of such functions are primary care, communication with school personnel, and managing the vegetative or dying patient.

Overlapping Responsibilities

Questions of responsibility can involve tasks of medical management, coordination of care, and family support. They can be found within the medical profession and between physicians and other caregivers. Problems of medical management, coordination of care, and family support are examined here in depth.

Medical Management. Few would disagree that the physician has major responsibility for medical care of the chronically ill child, and apparently, pediatricians feel confident of their ability to manage this aspect of their practices. Only 18 percent of the respondents to an American Academy of Pediatrics survey indicated that their pediatric residency experience in the care of patients with such chronic diseases as diabetes, cystic fibrosis, or rheumatoid arthritis was insufficient. More than 40 percent, however, felt they had had inadequate experience in the care of patients with various manifestations of chronic cerebral dysfunction. Although this may seem high, 40 percent is low when compared with other areas such as care of adolescents (insufficient experience: 66 percent) or care of patients with psychosocial and/or behavioral problems (insufficient experience: 54 percent). This suggests that these pediatricians believed their training in relation to the chronically ill child was adequate. In fact, 74 percent checked that their experience had been sufficient and 7 percent thought it had been excessive. However, only 6.8 percent checked "the handicapped child" as a subspecialty area or special interest. An additional 26.7 percent listed other areas that might involve chronically ill children: cardiology, 7.6 percent; hematology-oncology, 7.7 percent; nephrology, 3.9 percent; endocrinology, 4.0 percent; and pulmonary, 3.5 percent (Task Force on Pediatric Education, 1978).

Other professionals, such as nurse practitioners, psychologists, and social workers believe they should be allowed to share diagnostic and treatment responsibilities with physicians. In a 1976 survey of selected functions of nurse practitioners providing infant and child health care, a question was asked about care for a child with bronchial asthma (mild attack). More than 40 percent of the 307 nurse practitioners responding stated that they would assume health care management for such a case. More than 60 percent would order laboratory tests or other diagnostic procedures, and about 80 percent would perform a physical examination or obtain or update the health history. They were also asked: "For what percent of patients for whom you perform this activity, do you consult with a physician?" More than 40 percent consulted about health care management, over 30 percent about ordering tests and procedures, and over 20 percent about performing a physical examination or obtaining or updating a health history. In cases in which they were participating in the care of a child with common, mild, and usually uncomplicated chronic illness, they were doing it fairly autonomously (Sultz and others, 1978).

Physicians, however, seem reluctant to admit that such delegation is occurring; nor do they generally encourage it. An American Adademy of Pediatrics (1978a) study indicated that among pediatricians who currently employ pediatric nurse associates only 26 percent currently delegate to the associate the physical examination of children with chronic illnesses (interim care), 15 percent the continuing management of such children, and 36 percent home visits to such children. The corresponding percentages among those who do not employ an associate were 4 percent, 5 percent, and 13 percent. When asked what they would do under "ideal" circumstances, the percentages for those employing associates jumped to 34 percent, 26 percent, and 56 percent and for those not employing to 16 percent, 16 percent, and 46 percent.

Educational programs appear to reflect this ambivalence. A recent report noted that although about 80 percent of programs training nurse practitioners prepared them for the care of healthy infants and children and children with mild problems, only about 50 percent taught management of mild chronic illness (Ruby, 1981).

Pediatric psychologists working with pediatricians in hospital or outpatient settings may expect to share with their medical colleagues responsibility for diagnosing psychological malfunctioning in patient and family and for the treatment of depressed or otherwise emotionally disturbed children (Drotar, 1981). Psychological skills are particularly essential in distinguishing between normal, adaptive reactions (such as depression, anxiety, denial, and anger) and maladaptive or long-standing psychopathology (Brantley, Stabler, and Whitt, 1981). Social workers, particularly those working within a team framework, may also wish to participate in these functions (Bergman and Fritz, 1981).

Coordination of Care. A number of other professional groups claim they also coordinate (or should coordinate) the care of the chronically ill child. *The Future of Pediatric Education* stated, "The care of the child with a handicap is usually multidisciplinary and on-going, and the role of the pediatrician is normally that of a coordinator of services. Residents should appreciate the role of other disciplines in the care of the disabled child and develop the ability to work cooperatively with them. They should learn to help parents to understand the need for multiple services and the importance of complying with the multitude of recommendations that may be made. . . . The resident must learn to assist the family in marshalling the community resources for the benefit of children with handicapping conditions" (Task Force on Pediatric Education, 1978, p. 24).

Battle (1972) also stressed this responsibility of the pediatrician in regard to coordination. She first described a pediatrician's role as family advisor and counselor and then stated, "He [the pediatrician] functions among the team members [of specialists] as the coordinator. Once treatment priorities and sequences are set by the team, the pediatrician . . . can distill and transmit this information to the family. This should not prevent their direct contact with the specialist, which they need and have a right to expect. Rather the pediatrician's role is to help the family in a situation which may be overwhelming if they are bombarded with a list of recommendations from a multitude of subspecialists. It is his role to shape the recommendations of the various disciplines into a long-range program" (p. 920).

Battle supported the role of the pediatrician as ombudsman and as being the person in the best position to help the family understand and accept the treatment plan. The absence of mention of other professionals is interesting. It probably reflects the 1972 publication date, which was prior to much of the current interest in team responsibility, as well as the real problems pediatricians experience in developing collaborative arrangements.

Problems in coordination of care between primary care physicians and specialists were made apparent in a mid 1970s study by Pless, Satterwhite, and Van Vechten (1976). They asked seventy-nine pediatricians and general practitioners in New York state whether they usually treated chronic illnesses alone, shared the care with a specialist, or referred to a specialist for continuous care. The six conditions studied were asthma, cerebral palsy, diabetes, epilepsy, heart disease, and rheumatoid arthritis. The percentage sharing with specialists ranged from 89 percent for asthma to 31 percent for diabetes. The percentage of primary care physicians having primary responsibility ranged from 93 percent for asthma patients to 57 percent for those with cerebral palsy. The authors noted extremely limited use of services offering emotional and other family support, such as public health nursing, social work, and psychological or psychiatric services.

The American Academy of Pediatrics suggests that residency learning experiences in areas relevant to coordination of service activities may be inadequate. More than half of the respondents to the academy's survey of pediatricians indicated they felt underprepared for involvement in child advocacy, 64 percent believed they had insufficient training in school health, and 73 percent felt they lacked training in community programs affecting children (Task Force on Pediatric Education, 1978). All three areas are crucial to the comprehensive care of many children with chronic illnesses.

This appraisal is echoed by Budetti and others (1981) who stated, "Presently, physicians have little specific training in working with the handicapped child's environment and coordination of care" (p. 725). They suggest that a system of training and coordination of health care professionals, educators, and psychologists is necessary to meet the needs of children with chronic disability.

Several professions see coordination of services as their responsibility. Nuckolls (1981) noted that nurse practitioners in specialized clinics for chronically ill and handicapped children serve as coordinators of medical care and as providers of primary care. Her definition of the coordination function, however, was markedly different from that of the pediatric establishment. She described nurse practitioners as making home visits, serving as links between hospital and community, and performing special services.

The social worker also has traditionally assumed the coordinator role, with particular attention to community agencies rather than to medical or hospital-based specialists. The physician has usually ordered referrals to or consultations with medical specialists, physical therapists, and similar professionals while the social worker helped the family utilize visiting nurses, home health agencies, school services, and other community-based facilities. Bergman, Lewiston, and West (1979) stressed the coordinating function of the hospital social worker in relation to the chronically ill child. As a clinician noted, however, in reality, it is often difficult to distinguish medical from nonmedical functions and rare to find a clear definition of the roles of the professionals who assume responsibility for coordinating different aspects of the child's and the family's overall care (M. Weitzman, personal communications to the author, 1982).

Family Support. A third area in which several professions claim competence is interaction with the family, particularly support of family members through the trying experiences of coping with a child with a chronic illness. The Select Panel for the Promotion of Child Health (1981) drew special attention to the burdens and challenges borne by parents and siblings of children with chronic illnesses. It recommended that families have "ready access to a wide range of psychosocial support services" (p. 306).

The Future of Pediatric Education assigned the family support function to the pediatrician: "A child's chronic illness has serious impact on the entire family structure imposing emotional and financial burdens. The resident [physician] must be able to recognize these effects and manage them appropriately. . . . Residents should be able to explain to the child and family the nature and prognosis of the particular disease. They should discuss openly and frankly any questions raised by the patient, even if these concern the possibility of death" (Task Force on Pediatric Education, 1978, p. 25). Battle (1972, p. 919) urged the pediatrician to work with the family whose members are experiencing "shock, grief, depression, anger, guilt, and embarrassment" after the birth of a child with a moderate or severe handicap.

Despite these endorsements from the pediatric community, it is questionable that most pediatricians have sufficient training and experience in dealing with psychosocial issues to serve as family counselors under stressful conditions. And Pless, Satterwhite, and Van Vechten (1976) do not suggest that referrals were made to others for counseling. Featherstone (1980) cited numerous examples of insensitivity of physicians to the needs and problems of families, drawing not only on her own experience but also on the publications of other parents of severely handicapped children.

Traditional nursing education, too, does not devote much time to family support issues. Nurses being prepared for community-based practice, such as public health, are more likely to have training in these areas. Nuckolls (1981) specifically cited the use of nurse specialists to counsel parents of chronically ill and handicapped children.

Hospital-based social workers have always worked closely with families, trying to ease their burdens. But usually the brief period of hospitalization and the pressure of coordination functions limit the hospital social worker's functions as a counselor. Many hospitals have both inpatient and outpatient social work services, and communication and coordination of their services can be particularly difficult in the case of children who are hospitalized frequently but who receive ongoing services from social workers located in the outpatient department or community.

When available, pediatric psychologists or child psychiatrists can play an important role in assessment and treatment of the families of children with chronic illnesses, as well as of the children themselves. They can assist families as they react to the child's chronic illness with anger, frustration, anxiety, grief, guilt, and mourning for their child (Brantley, Stabler, and Whitt, 1981). These authors urged the psychologist not only to relate to the child and the family but also to assist the physician who attempts to treat both child and family. The psychologist operates in two roles: "as a generator and provider of clinical information gained through interaction with the child and family and as an interpreter and model to the physician" (p. 232). Brantley and colleagues perceived "the psychologist acting as intermediary between the physician, the patient, and the family. . . . Many families of chronically ill children do not expect their physician to offer suggestions and advice around problems of living with the disease. Hence, they rarely ask a physician for counsel around such issues, although there is often need for psychosocial information and guidance. These needs can often be met by joint patient and family contact with their physician and consulting psychologist, or within parent group meetings run to provide ongoing parent and patient education and support" (pp. 232–233). These activities involve not only family support but also some aspects of coordination of care.

Summary. In at least three areas—medical management, coordination of care, and family support—several professional groups have indicated that they should play a significant role. Physicians, particularly pediatricians; nurses, especially those with specialty training in child health or public health; pediatric psychologists; and social workers believe their training does or should provide them with the skills necessary to assist chronically ill children and their families. This situation should mean that families receive the services they need, but it also has the potential for rivalries, antagonisms, and duplications. Methods for avoiding these pitfalls are discussed later in this chapter.

Neglected Responsibilities

Although competition for patients and patient/family responsibilities may lead to difficult situations, more critical problems can arise when professionals do not want to accept responsibility.

Primary Care. The Select Panel for the Promotion of Child Health (1981) indicated particular concern with the lack of communication among providers and between patients and providers regarding primary care: "Parents often think that when a child sees 'the doctor' he or she is getting comprehensive services. On the other hand, 'the doctor' of the chronically ill child is often a specialist who may assume that the child is receiving primary care services elsewhere. Although this situation is not universal, it occurs frequently and can be ameliorated by clear specification of provider roles. As a system of care is planned, program designers should always consider the coordination of primary care needs of these children with their specialized needs" (pp. 293–294).

A recent study indicates the extent of primary care neglect. Palfrey, Levy, and Gilbert (1980) found that 31 percent of children followed in the specialty clinics of a children's hospital had no source of primary care. Interview data suggested, moreover, that not all the medical needs of these children were being met by the specialty clinic. About 60 percent of the children had perceived medical problems other than those under care, and 38 percent reported that one or more symptoms had not been discussed with any medical provider. Although some problems might have been associated with the patient's chronic condition, many reported with high frequency were unrelated to the specialty problem. Moreover, patients without a source of primary care tended to be older, to live in the inner city, to be self-referred or referred from another hospital source, and to have lost contact with the physician, if any, who referred them to the specialty clinic. Thus children likely to have the most health problems—inner-city adolescents—were least likely to have a source for primary care.

Two other studies of children with special needs have indicated that parents experience difficulties concerning certain nonspecialized aspects of care. In a 1972 study of children with spina bifida, Kanthor and others (1974) found that 68 percent of families felt that neither specialists nor primary care physicians discussed their children's needs for special schooling, adjustment to handicaps, methods of discipline, behavior problems, or the "total child." Eighty percent claimed that neither helped in planning for future schooling, vacations, marriage, and sexual functioning. The authors concluded, "The reported gaps in health care may be related to the false assumption by specialists that the primary physicians would take the responsibility for providing care in many areas and a similar, but reverse assumption by the primary physicians. The greatest deficiencies in patient care occurred in future planning, advice, genetic counseling, and support—aspects of care characterized by the need to listen to the patient and his family, understand, and provide advice on how to deal with actual or potential problems" (p. 783).

Almost ten years later, Okamoto and Shurtleff (1981) conducted a similar study of children with myelodysplasia. Mothers were asked whom they would contact first for each of twenty-four health-related problems. The local physician was chosen in preference to the clinic staff and specialists for only four items: immunization update, suspected ear infection, minor accident, and eating/dietary habits. The authors recognized that problems in determining who is responsible for what may be the result of beliefs and attitudes of all three parties—specialists, community physicians, and parents. Specialists may believe their coordinating role includes primary care, especially for children residing close to the medical center. Community physicians may prefer to have even routine care for children with very special needs handled by the specialty team. Pless, Satterwhite, and Van Vechten (1976) found that for some conditions, such as cerebral palsy and rheumatoid arthritis, about 20 percent of general practitioners would refer to a specialist for continuous care. A smaller percentage of pediatricians would choose not to treat these children by themselves or to share responsibility with a specialist. Finally, parents may feel more confident using the clinic even for primary care because of its knowledge of the many aspects of the child's condition, twenty-four-hour on-call coverage, and subsidized charges.

Clearly, issues of primary care responsibility need to be resolved lest children's needs go unrecognized or expensive and inconvenient sources of care be used unnecessarily.

Educational Issues. Despite the fact that a large percentage of children seen by pediatricians and family practitioners are of school age or eligible for preschool programs, questions about school attendance or performance have not been a routine part of the pediatric workup of either a well or a sick child (Weitzman and others, 1982). The situation has been even more critical in regard to children with chronic illnesses; physicians and other health professionals, in their concern with medical management, have paid little or no attention to educational needs. This neglect has often been coupled with an unwillingness to collaborate with school personnel even when educational issues arise.

The passage in 1975 of Public Law 94–142 (the Education for All Handicapped Children Act) made interprofessional communication around the problems of children with special needs a public issue as well as a private problem. The need for information on which to base decisions about mainstreaming or placement in special classes, about adjustment of school regimens, and about specialized services and the role of schools in delivering them brought health professionals outside the schools in contact with health and education professionals within schools. The interaction has often been difficult. Physicians often resist the efforts of the schools to involve them in this process.

Featherstone (1980) provided a vignette that suggests the multiple origins of physician-school problems. A mother gave her physician a school form to complete so she could obtain special help for her child with a newly discovered hearing loss, and "he rebelled angrily against the demand that he fill out a form which seemed meandering, anonymous, and ultimately useless. His reflections suggest that the paper represented more to him than twenty ill-spent minutes. It reminded him of other assaults on doctors: of legislative regulation and media hostility. He speaks as though the referral form were a weapon in the bureaucratic arsenal, as though the real issue was his autonomy, and his resistance to a mindless, alien machine" (p. 190).

On the other hand, school administrators and others responsible for providing special services complain that physicians do not seem to understand the role of the school or what the school can provide. They cite unrealistic medical treatment plans and the reluctance of physicians to attend meetings at which Individual Education Plans are developed.

Pediatricians are being urged to overcome barriers to school collaboration for the benefit of their patients. "A final challenge that P.L. 94-142 presents to physicians is to communicate and share some of their understanding of children with other professionals. Traditionally, this sharing of information has been difficult. For P.L. 94-142 to succeed, turf issues and professional jealousies need to be displaced in favor of multidisciplinary decision making" (Palfrey, Mervis, and Butler, 1978, p. 824).

Crossland, DeFriese, and Durfee (1981) have suggested a model for the integration of child health and educational services. They note that "health care providers have early and periodic access to children with the potential risk of educationally handicapping conditions while the public school systems nation-wide desperately seek new and more effective ways of finding such children so that early intervention can help prevent serious learning-related disabilities" (p. 211). They proposed that (1) all children have a regular source of primary care, (2) physicians understand the nature and consequences of learning-related handicaps, (3) physicians be taught how to obtain from children and parents information about possible learning-related disorders that might need specialized attention, and (4) appropriate referral sources for diagnostic evaluation and treatment of learning-related problems be available.

Downing (1981) has pinpointed some of the reasons physicians and school personnel have difficulties working together. Physicians employ a medical model that is reactive, individual, and based on organic or trauma causality whereas school counselors are more likely to be proactive, group- and community-oriented, and to have a broader perception of causality. Another area of difference lies in exchange of information. Physicians stress confidentiality and are reluctant to share material with individuals outside their profession, and because school counselors do not often receive information from physicians, they may hesitate about providing them with their data. Economic factors may also operate. School counselors have a public agency point of view while physicians have a private enterprise philosophy. Because physicians may be "giving away valuable time" when they talk to or meet with school personnel, the counselor may have to initiate contacts. Physicians see treatment primarily as an interaction between a patient and medical personnel; counselors are accustomed to involving people of varied backgrounds. Finally, physicians may have to be convinced that school personnel are professionals who can assist in treatment.

The urgent need of chronically ill children for as much education as they can absorb makes it essential that methods be found to bring together the medical and the school community to plan educational programs for these children.

Coordination of Care. Although this chapter has included coordination of care among the areas that many disciplines believe to be their responsibility, it also must be listed among the areas of neglect. Professional pronouncements are clearly in conflict with families' perceptions. The Rand study of handicapped children stated, "Fully two-thirds of the families had difficulty finding appropriate services. Direction is a major problem because in most areas *no one* has all the information needed or the responsibility to coordinate help for families. The result is that there are gaps or delays in the services received, or inappropriate services are delivered" (Kakalik and others, 1974, p. 19).

Families may also contribute to this problem. Featherstone (1980, p. 191) described one pediatrician's frustrations as he tried to coordinate medical care:

> The child has multiple congenital abnormalities. I had endocrine work-ups, neurological work-ups, had a work-up at the L-Hospital, and what I felt to be a very complete work-up. And the family, I guess, just weren't willing to accept that particular conclusion. And came to the point of needing information for something or other and got involved with another developmentalist or endocrinologist . . . one thing I work very hard to do is to avoid fragmenting the child's care. There is nothing wrong with having an endocrinologist involved, an orthopedist involved, but someone has to run the show. Otherwise, it's trite but true, the left hand doesn't know what the right hand is doing. Duplication of services, redundance, etc., and at times even antagonism. . . . And when I got the report I spoke to the family. . . . "Don't do this to your daughter, please. If you want a thousand consults, let me know. I'll send off the information, I'll give them whatever they want." Because as it happened, *very* expensive studies were repeated. Not only repeated, but repeated by the same lab that had done it the first time. . . . "You know, it makes it very difficult." I don't like to run my practice as though, "Do it my way or I'll take my ball and go home," but I think it does tend to undermine the relationship. And if they are going to pay me for my services I think it's certainly a foolishness for them to come, sit down, get my advice, and then go off and do what they want.

Patients Nobody Wants. Perhaps the most tragic cases of neglected responsibilities are the patients no professional wants to manage. The layman reads with horror the medical sagas in novels such as *The House of God* (Shem, 1978) in which much medical time is spent trying to devise ways of getting rid of patients who are time-consuming, troublesome, boring, or otherwise undesirable. "Buff 'em up and turf 'em" becomes the way to manage such situations on an adult medical ward. And the same procedure—an extensive workup (buffing) to indicate that some other service such as surgery or neurology is the appropriate placement (turf)—is known to occur in pediatric services.

Families whose children suffer from severe mental retardation or multiple disabilities that make them unresponsive or difficult to treat often find their physicians losing interest in their care and referring them to other individuals or organizations who supposedly will be of assistance, but who often are not. Families already under extreme stress because of their children's conditions are further exhausted by seeking help no one seems able to give. Clearly, each community needs some individual or agency that can tell such families where assistance is available—or help them adjust to the reality that they must handle their burdens by themselves.

Summary. Although many groups of professionals are interested in the care of children with chronic illnesses, certain types of problems and certain kinds of children are likely to be neglected. Despite the urgent need for such activities, differences in training and outlook make collaboration between medical and educational personnel difficult. Coordination of services is another responsibility that, although claimed by many professionals, is often assumed by the family. And finally, there are the children whose conditions are so hopeless that most professionals try to avoid them. For these children and their families, new, caring individuals and institutions are needed.

Attempts to Solve the Problems

Both types of interprofessional issues—overlapping functions and neglected responsibilities—have negative implications for delivery of high-quality, comprehensive service to children with chronic illnesses and for keeping the costs as low as possible. Program administrators and policy makers, therefore, need to examine a variety of approaches to the amelioration of these problems.

Structural Changes

One set of approaches to inter- and intra-professional problems involves changing the structure of the delivery system. For example, attempts to solve the overlapping or competition problem often involve team concepts or well-developed referral patterns with varying degrees of flexibility or rigidity in task assignment. Approaches to the problem of neglected responsibilities also may take several forms, for example, modifying the responsibilities of existing service providers and developing new types of providers, such as coordinating pediatricians and nonprofessional family counselors.

The Team Approach. Interprofessional teams are relatively common in the hospital or specialty clinic setting. They are also often the structure of choice in health maintenance organizations (HMOs). A priori decisions about delegation of functions, combined with periodic meetings to review individual cases, can lead to rewarding experiences for professionals and comprehensive care for patient and family (C. J. Nicholls, personal communication with the author, 1981). Unfortunately, little effort has been expended in evaluating the team approach in terms of patient satisfaction or possible confusion, of beneficial outcomes, or of costs.

HMOs seem convinced that use of nurse practitioners and other nonphysician professionals reduces use of physicians, and thus the overall cost of care, without negative impact on quality. Maintenance care of chronically ill children is often handled by specially trained nurses in these settings, and social workers and psychologists rather than pediatricians and psychiatrists are assigned counseling and supportive functions.

The rationale and cost/benefit parameters of team practice have not been explored in the hospital setting or community clinic. Referrals, consultations, and team meetings reduce the hours available for direct patient contact. Are they cost-effective? The fact that many team efforts take place in teaching hospitals and that consequently these efforts have both educational and service functions makes analysis difficult. Recent cuts in personnel in community clinics necessitated by reductions in federal funding have disproportionately affected social workers and other nonphysicians, suggesting that administrators and the public are not completely convinced about the utility of these professionals in comparison with physicians.

The team concept is not usually utilized outside of organized settings such as hospitals, clinics, or HMOs. In the world of private, office-based practice, increasing numbers of physicians employ nurse practitioners and delegate certain tasks to them. But relationships with professionals outside the office, including other physicians, may depend on referral systems that often are not fully effective because of failures in communication among the individuals involved: referring physician, professional (physician or other) to whom referred, patient, and family.

Referral Systems. A recent series of articles (Kisker and others, 1980; Strayer, Kisker, and Fethke, 1980; Strayer and others, 1981) describing a shared-management approach to the care of children with cancer, although not directly relevant to interprofessional issues, does suggest that carefully designed referral systems with built-in communication links may promote beneficial, coordinated, and cost-effective care. Families using the shared-management group elected to have their children receive most of their treatment from community practitioners; those in the specialist-management group had all their therapy conducted at the cancer center. Both groups had an initial workup at a medical center's cancer center. In the shared-management system, the community practitioners were contacted by phone and sent copies of therapeutic protocols. Telephone communication between center oncologists and private physicians was available at all times, and the community physicians were urged to seek advice about management. The community physicians completed a one-page report each time the patient came to the office, and the oncologists completed the same report for the community physician each time the child visited the center. Evaluation of the shared-management approach, compared with the usual specialist-management approach, showed no differences in unfavorable outcomes between the two groups, compliance with protocols by community physicians, favorable attitudes by patients and families, reduction in medical and nonmedical costs, and positive reactions from the community physicians who reported that the program provided personal satisfaction, an educational opportunity, and a way to share the emotional load of caring for children with cancer. This model deserves replication in tertiary care centers serving chronically ill children.

Physician Supply. The anticipated oversupply of physicians may have a significant impact on the use of the multidisciplinary teams and referrals as ways of resolving interprofessional issues. Midlevel practitioners, such as pediatric nurse practitioners, were first trained and deployed as a solution to the shortage of physicians. Similarly, widespread use of social workers, pediatric psychologists, and other nonmedical personnel is more usual at times and in places where physicians are in short supply. Such places might include rural areas or inner-city hospitals. Currently, however, the supply of pediatricians and family practitioners is on the increase, while the number of children is declining. Recent studies show that even relatively small communities now have board-certified pediatricians. Furthermore, salaried positions in neighborhood health centers and public hospitals are easier to fill. This physician surplus may worsen the competition for medical management and family counseling responsibilities that might have been handled by nonmedical personnel in times of physician shortage. Or the competition may lessen as pediatricians force other practitioners out of the market, because medical referral is usually required before families accept help from such individuals.

The latter scenario would not seem to be the best approach to the problem, however, because it has been shown that nurse practitioners, social workers, and psychologists perform certain supportive functions as well as, if not better than, most physicians. Because their services usually cost less than the physician's, having pediatricians perform a wide range of nonmedical functions may not be cost-effective. Nevertheless, unless the supply of physicians is checked or some more rational way of distributing tasks is found, nonphysicians may be assigned fewer and fewer tasks in relation to chronically ill children.

Expanding Provider Roles. Battle (1972) has suggested that the pediatrician serve as an ombudsman. She urged pediatricians to assume responsibility for coordination of the team of specialists the child needs as well as for provision of routine and emergency health care and some family counseling.

Alternatively, the specialty clinic or practice might provide comprehensive care rather than only specialized treatment. This would mean assuming the tasks of coordinating care among specialists and of providing primary and emergency care as well. One advantage of this system is that it seems to reflect parental preference. Parents of chronically ill children may feel more comfortable discussing a general problem with a specialist than a special problem with a generalist. The disadvantages include the aura of technological sophistication that often pervades specialty clinics (Palfrey, Levy, and Gilbert, 1980) and specialized practices (which makes parents reluctant to discuss routine matters) and the relative paucity of such facilities (which means that many parents must travel long distances to reach them and makes them impractical as sources of primary care).

New Professionals. Several authors have suggested that new professionals should be trained who would coordinate, manage, or integrate services. Kanthor and others (1974, p. 784) suggested that a "'coordinating pediatrician' could be designated by a number of specialty clinics or community agencies to oversee the provision of health care for handicapped children." The task is described as follows: "This pediatrician would be the counterpart of the proposed community pediatrician in Britain. He would work with supportive staff (for example, social workers and public health nurses), communicate with the specialists and primary physicians, and would himself, if necessary, provide counseling and rehabilitative services. He would have the responsibility to insure that the technical care is provided in full, and to facilitate (through support and effective communication), the greater involvement of the practicing pediatrician."

Pless and Satterwhite (1972) experimented with the use of nonprofessional family counselors for families with chronically ill children. The counselors' functions included listening, educating, counseling, advising, and psychotherapy as well as providing services, coordination, advocacy, and socializing. The program, which involved six counselors and fifty-five children during 1969 and 1970, was judged successful on the basis of acceptability by patients and physicians and greater improvement in psychological test scores among children in counseled families compared with noncounseled controls. The authors list the following advantages of nonprofessionals over professionals: greatly reduced cost, opportunity to select on the basis of personality characteristics, absence of rigid role definitions and of preconceived ideas about worker-client relationships, greater flexibility in hours, and willingness to work with families in their own homes. Despite these plusses, this organizational model has not been widely adopted.

Educational Programs

Among the most frequently offered suggestions for improving interprofessional relations is modification of professional training or utilization of inservice education.

Medical Education. Studies of medical education have revealed how many of the attitudes and behaviors of practicing physicians are developed during the medical school years. If physicians are to be more alert to the possibilities and advantages of sharing their responsibilities with other professionals, as well as more competent in nontechnical areas such as counseling and educational diagnoses, training and experience should begin in the clinical years of medical school. Some schools have instituted such programs, but the problems still remaining suggest that more schools need to develop curricula in these areas and to expose medical students to models of care that involve other professionals. Jennison (1976, p. 6) has summarized some of the problems, as well as suggesting the medical school period as a time for attempting solutions. "Medical educators and academicians have not adequately recognized the need for preparation of physicians to utilize fellow professionals in carrying out comprehensive care. . . . traditionally, the respective roles of physicians, nurses, and social workers have been embroiled in a situation filled with ambiguities and contradictory expectations, particularly as regards chronic disease care. . . . This ambiguous interprofessional situation cannot be resolved until medical educators as well as those responsible for the training programs of other professionals are willing to bring trainees together, during the undergraduate training period, to observe qualified role models and a team in action before the traditional prejudices and blocks to communication have occurred."

Other programs have focused on the residency period as the most appropriate time to inculcate skills. Wolraich and others (1981) developed a program whose objective was to improve the pediatric residents' skills in communicating emotion-ladened information to parents. And in 1982, Wolraich reviewed the literature on the problems physicians sometimes have in communicating with the parents of handicapped children and summarized the problem areas: (1) the physician's knowledge of developmental problems; (2) the physician's attitudes toward handicapped children; and (3) the physician's skills in communicating with parents.

Dworkin and others (1979, p. 712) stressed the role of formal pediatric training in advancing interprofessional skills: "In order to coordinate effectively a variety of services for handicapped patients, pediatricians must have a sophisticated understanding of what each discipline can and cannot provide. If introduced during formal pediatric training, cross-disciplinary education will not only foster more productive communication in later practice, but will also contribute in a major way to the task of teaching pediatricians the principles of child development."

Postresidency Training. Education in these areas, however, cannot be restricted to medical school and residencies. In fact, a survey by Dworkin and others (1979) indicated the importance of clinical experiences for practicing pediatricians. They surveyed pediatricians to determine their perceptions of their training in developmental pediatrics and their preferences for further education. When asked to rate how valuable they found several sources of knowledge in this field, only 8 percent of the respondents stated that medical school was highly valuable, while 30 percent gave residency experience that rating. Postgraduate courses, books and journals, and professional contacts were considered highly valuable by between a third and a half of the respondents. Although clinical experience received the highest rating (86 percent thought it was highly valuable and 13 percent, somewhat valuable), almost two thirds did not regard it as an adequate substitute for formal training. When presented with options for additional education, pediatricians clearly preferred part-time longitudinal clinical experiences (78 percent highly desirable) over a postgraduate course (56 percent) or written material (21 percent). The authors urge medical centers to provide opportunities for such experiences.

The American Academy of Pediatrics, in collaboration with the Office of Special Education, has developed a training curriculum for primary care physicians who serve handicapped children and their families. Although not based on clinical experiences, the project is designed to affect physicians' interpersonal and professional attitudes toward handicapped children and their families, cognitive knowledge about such children, clinical skills related to such children, and interactions with the educational system (Powers and Healy, 1982). This sixteen-hour course has apparently had a significant impact on the participants, and the process of developing the program has served as a model of interdisciplinary collaboration. Project implementation was handled by teams of pediatricians and special educators, and the task forces that focused on issues of related services and the medical information needed by special educators also provided opportunities for interaction between these groups.

Downing (1981) developed a five-step program for improving medical school relationships in one state. Step one was a meeting for school staff led by the counselor and the school nurse. At this meeting the need for improved relationships with physicians was stressed and methods for accomplishing this were discussed. These included observational techniques, teacher limitations concerning medications, and role of counselor and nurse as link between teacher and physician. In step two, a group of physicians were selected who were considered receptive to improving working relations with the schools. Step three was a luncheon meeting attended by these physicians, a school nurse, and the supervisor of pupil services. The services offered by the school district were described briefly, and printed material was provided. A discussion of teacher practices and referrals followed. Step four was immediate follow-through on service requests by physicians, and step five included luncheon conferences at six-month intervals. Downing reported that, as a result of these procedures, school counselors were contacted by physicians more frequently and physicians received useful information from teachers and other school personnel.

Education of Other Professionals. Although the central focus in this section has been on education of physicians, clearly the other professionals involved in treatment of children with chronic illnesses should not be neglected. They also need training in counseling, communication, coordination, and family dynamics. And they, too, need to be made aware of the capabilities and perspectives of other professionals, including physicians.

Economic Incentives

Changes in structural arrangements and even willingness to become involved in postresidency education are more likely if economic incentives are promised. Modification of reimbursement mechanisms is essential if health professionals, and physicians especially, are to spend time working with schools in developing programs for chronically ill children or with families in finding methods of caring for the multiply handicapped child. Most pediatricians find such activities uninteresting, nonproductive, or threatening. Their wish to avoid these activities can be justified on economic grounds. Parents who will pay forty dollars for a fifteen-minute office visit will not pay at the same rate for travel and meeting time while the physician attends the school session at which an education plan based on the physician's assessment of the medical condition is developed for the child. Even filling out forms and making the phone calls necessary to obtain essential modifications of the child's educational program take time from revenue-producing office and hospital visits. Compensating physicians and others for educational and other related services, even though they do not directly involve diagnosis and treatment, would probably be cost-effective in the long run. Because these charges would add to medical care costs, however, they are resisted by insurance companies and other third-party payers.

Effective use of social workers and psychologists by physicians in private practice is also significantly affected by third-party reimbursement policies. State Medicaid policies, Blue Cross/Blue Shield coverage, and provisions of other insurance programs influence physicians' decisions about referring patients and families and families' decisions about whether to seek help from these providers. In 1976, Jennison pointed out the limited or nonexistent reimbursement provided by conventional third-party payment systems to team members in the care of the child with chronic illness and urged the American Academy of Pediatrics to express pediatricians' concerns about this issue at the local, state, and national level. In 1978, the American Academy of Pediatrics (1978b) issued a position paper on "Financial Compensation for Evaluation and Therapy of Children with Developmental Disabilities." Not surprisingly, it stated that physicians should receive third-party compensation for coordination, staffing, and follow-up efforts as well as for counseling and visits to schools on behalf of developmentally disabled children. However, it also stressed the need for third-party compensation for the services of occupational and physical therapists, psychologists, nurses, social workers, speech pathologists, and audiologists, but "only if the diagnostic and therapeutic measures are prescribed by a physician" (p. 602). In 1981, the Select Panel for the Promotion of Child Health also recommended that third-party reimbursement be made available from public and private sources for psychological and other supportive services. Present federal and state retrenchment policies, however, make unlikely the universal implementation of such policies.

Conclusions

Issues of responsibilities and role definitions often interfere with society's ability to obtain comprehensive, high-quality care for children with chronic illnesses. Unfortunately, the consequences of fragmentation, duplication, and neglect of services are seldom addressed directly as matters of public policy. Rather, they are discussed by families and agencies on an anecdotal basis.

This chapter has attempted to document the problems that arise when professionals try, or do not try, to communicate and coordinate their activities. It has also reviewed some of the approaches that have been suggested in order to overcome these problems. The report of the chronically ill child project, of which this is one small segment, may itself provide the impetus for experimentation with and evaluation of the several organizational, educational, and financing alternatives that have been elaborated.

References

American Academy of Pediatrics. "Projecting Pediatric Practice Patterns." *Pediatrics*, 1978a, *62* (supplement), 625–680.
American Academy of Pediatrics, Committee on Children with Handicaps.

"Financial Compensation for Evaluation and Therapy of Children with Developmental Disabilities." *Pediatrics,* 1978b, *62,* 602.

Battle, C. U. "The Role of the Pediatrician as Ombudsman in the Health Care of the Young Handicapped Child." *Pediatrics,* 1972, *50,* 916–922.

Bergman, A. S., and Fritz, G. K. "Psychiatric and Social Work Collaboration in a Pediatric Chronic Illness Hospital." *Social Work in Health Care,* 1981, *7,* 45–55.

Bergman, A. S., Lewiston, N. J., and West, A. M. "Social Work Practice and Chronic Pediatric Illness." *Social Work in Health Care,* 1979, *4,* 265–274.

Brantley, H. T., Stabler, B., and Whitt, J. K. "Program Considerations in Comprehensive Care of Chronically Ill Children." *Journal of Pediatric Psychology,* 1981, *6,* 229–238.

Budetti, P., and others. "Child Health Professionals: Supply, Training, and Practice." In Select Panel for the Promotion of Child Health, *Better Health for Our Children: A National Strategy.* Vol. 4. Department of Health and Human Services publication no. 79-55071. Washington, D.C.: U.S. Government Printing Office, 1981.

Crossland, C. L., DeFriese, G. H., and Durfee, M. F. "Child Health Care and the New Morbidity: Toward a Model for the Linkage of Private Medical Practice and the Public Schools." *Journal of Community Health,* 1981, *6,* 204–214.

Downing, C. J. "Getting the M.D. and the School Counselor Together." *Elementary School Guidance and Counseling,* 1981, *15,* 295–300.

Drotar, D. "Psychological Perspectives in Chronic Childhood Illness." *Journal of Pediatric Psychology,* 1981, *6,* 211–237.

Dworkin, P. H., and others. "Training in Developmental Pediatrics—How Practitioners Perceive the Gap." *American Journal of Diseases of Children,* 1979, *133,* 709–712.

Featherstone, H. *A Difference in the Family.* New York: Basic Books, 1980.

Jennison, M. H. "The Pediatrician and Care of Chronic Illness." *Pediatrics,* 1976, *58,* 5–7.

Kakalik, J. S., and others. *Improving Services to Handicapped Children.* Santa Monica, Calif.: Rand Corporation, 1974.

Kanthor, H., and others. "Areas of Responsibility in the Health Care of Multiply Handicapped Children." *Pediatrics,* 1974, *54,* 779–785.

Kisker, C. T., and others. "Health Outcomes of a Community-Based Therapy Program for Children with Cancer—A Shared-Management Approach." *Pediatrics,* 1980, *66,* 900–906.

Nuckolls, K. B. "Nursing." In Select Panel for the Promotion of Child Health, *Better Health for Our Children: A National Strategy.* Vol. 4. Department of Health and Human Services publication no. 79-55071. Washington, D.C.: U.S. Government Printing Office, 1981.

Okamoto, G. A., and Shurtleff, D. A. "Perceived First Contact Care for Disabled Children." *Pediatrics,* 1981, *67,* 530–535.

Palfrey, J. S., Levy, J. C., and Gilbert, K. L. "Use of Primary Care Facilities by Patients Attending Specialty Clinics." *Pediatrics,* 1980, *65,* 567–572.

Palfrey, J. S., Mervis, R. C., and Butler, J. A. "New Directions in the Evaluation and Education of Handicapped Children." *New England Journal of Medicine,* 1978, *239,* 819–824.

Pless, B., and Satterwhite, B. "Chronic Illness in Childhood: Selection, Activities, and Evaluation of Non-Professional Family Counselors." *Clinical Pediatrics,* 1972, *11,* 403–410.

Pless, B., Satterwhite, B., and Van Vechten, D. "Chronic Illness in Childhood: A Regional Survey of Care." *Pediatrics,* 1976, *58,* 37–45.

Powers, J. T., and Healy, A. "Inservice Training for Physicians Serving Handicapped Children." *Exceptional Children,* 1982, *48,* 332–336.

Ruby, G. "New Health Professionals in Child and Maternal Health." In Select Panel for the Promotion of Child Health, *Better Health for Our Children: A National Strategy.* Vol. 4. Department of Health and Human Services publication no. 79-55071. Washington, D.C.: U.S. Government Printing Office, 1981.

Select Panel for the Promotion of Child Health. *Better Health for Our Children: A National Strategy.* Vol. 1. Department of Health and Human Services publication no. 79-55071. Washington, D.C.: U.S. Government Printing Office, 1981.

Shem, S. *The House of God.* New York: Dell, 1978.

Strayer, F., Kisker, C. T., and Fethke, C. "Cost-Effectiveness of a Shared Management Delivery System for the Care of Children with Cancer." *Pediatrics,* 1980, *66,* 907–911.

Strayer, F. H., and others. "Physician Incentives for Shared Management of Childhood Cancer Patients." *Pediatrics,* 1981, *67,* 833–837.

Sultz, H. A., and others. *Longitudinal Study of Nurse Practitioners, Phase II.* Department of Health, Education, and Welfare publication no. 78-92. Hyattsville, Md.: Bureau of Health Manpower, 1978.

Task Force on Pediatric Education. *The Future of Pediatric Education.* Evanston, Ill.: American Academy of Pediatrics, 1978.

Weitzman, M., and others. "School Absence: A Problem for the Pediatrician." *Pediatrics,* 1982, *69,* 739–745.

Wolraich, M. L., "Communication Between Physicians and Parents of Handicapped Children." *Exceptional Children,* 1982, *48,* 324–329.

Wolraich, M. L., and others. "Teaching Pediatric Residents to Provide Emotion-Ladened Information." *Journal of Medical Education,* 1981, *56,* 438–440.

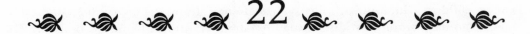

22

Medical Services

Michael Weitzman, M.D.

This century has witnessed profound changes in the health status of American children. At the turn of the century, morbidity and mortality patterns at all ages were dominated by acute infectious diseases such as smallpox, diphtheria, polio, tuberculosis, and similar conditions. Today, each of these conditions causes less than 2 percent of the mortality it caused in 1900 (Fries, 1980). Similarly, the infant mortality rate (defined as the number of children who die in the first year of life per thousand born alive) was 100 in 1900; today it is approximately 13 (Wegman, 1980). The decline in infant mortality and death due to infections has been accompanied by a marked increase in the prevalence of chronic illnesses. In fact, because so many children are now living with chronic illnesses that would have previously killed them, chronic illness has replaced acute illness as the major threat to health in this country and is now the major preoccupation of our health care system. The complex nature of chronic illnesses and their psychosocial consequences have led both to a high demand for health services and to increasing specialization and fragmentation of these services.

Medical research has been quite successful in treating many of these chronic conditions, as demonstrated by the increased survival of children with these problems. Despite this progress, the needs of many children and their families are frequently not being met in systematic and comprehensive ways. Ironically, many of these persistent health care problems are the result of scientific and technical advances and of changes in the health care delivery system that reflect these advances.

Goals of Health Service for Children with Chronic Illnesses

The goals of all therapeutic efforts on behalf of children with chronic illnesses are to minimize the biologic manifestations, complications, and progression of the conditions and to maximize the child's functioning and independence to the extent allowed by the degree of the problem (Pless and Pinkerton, 1975). Often it is possible to intervene at the level of the biologic problem and control virtually all physical manifestations of the abnormal condition. For example, many children with asthma, epilepsy, hematologic disorders, and cardiac conditions can have all or most disease manifestations controlled by medications. In other cases—exemplified by certain types of heart disease, renal disease, or neuromuscular conditions—the major functional manifestations can be successfully curtailed by surgical interventions. And, finally, some children—such as those with spina bifida, muscular dystrophy, or cystic fibrosis—have static or progressively deteriorating conditions that cannot be altered through surgical or medical intervention. The goals for all of these children are basically the same: to reduce physical and psychosocial disability and promote optimal functioning.

In the most basic and general terms, the biologic problem (disease, illness, or condition) may result in both physical disabilities and secondary handicaps. The physical disabilities are the immediate physical manifestations or limitations caused by the problem; secondary handicaps include the negative physical, psychological, and social consequences of the biologic problem. Children with the same primary disability may differ dramatically in secondary handicaps.

Two children with cerebral palsy, for example, may not be able to use their right hands and arms. One child may learn to compensate, using the left arm and hand, and grow up to hold a job and have a family. The other child may develop profound muscular contractures secondary to disuse and lead a life marked by pain, alienation, and daily sorrow. Secondary handicaps can often be prevented and should always be treated.

The child who is functioning and coping well is said to be well adjusted, and the child who is functioning poorly is said to be maladjusted. *Adjustment,* as used in relation to chronic illness, refers (1) to the extent to which the child and family have learned to adapt to the problem and make maximal use of the existing abilities and (2) to a global sense of psychologic balance and freedom from psychiatric and social abnormality (Pless and Pinkerton, 1975). Development and implementation of strategies aimed at promoting adjustment should be viewed as a central concern in the overall therapeutic plan for any child with a chronic condition.

For these strategies to be effective, children, parents, and health care providers must collaborate in their accomplishment. The success of treating chronic illness is limited to a great extent by the degree of compliance with therapeutic regimens. Noncompliance is often a major problem in long-term management of chronic illness (Gordis and Markowitz, 1971; Gordis, Markowitz, and Lilienfeld, 1969). Motivating patients and families toward active participation in therapeutic activities and helping them abandon the "sick role" are often the essential ingredients in managing the medical aspects of care and in preventing severe psychosocial maladjustment (Almy, 1981).

For many chronic problems, compliance involves participation well beyond drug administration or short-term diet restrictions. Children with cystic fibrosis may require dietary supplements and frequent chest physical therapy. Neuromuscular problems such as spina bifida or muscular dystrophy demand parental involvement to stimulate resourcefulness and persistence on the child's part. Children with diabetes mellitus or chronic renal disease may have to adhere to strict diets. Dialysis patients must live near medical centers that have appropriate machines and professionals in order to spend two to three days each week in the hospital. Thus their entire lives must be structured around their treatment plan.

Compliance with medical advice has been shown to be influenced by the nature of the doctor-patient relationship, the degree of patient understanding of the disease, the complexity of the treatment plan, the duration of the illness, and the patient's perception of the severity of the illness (Seligmann, McGrath, and Pratt, 1957; Fink and others, 1969; Becker, Drachman, and Kirscht, 1972; Meyers, Dolan, and Mueller, 1975). Duration of illness and complexity of treatment plan tend to decrease compliance, whereas satisfaction with the doctor-patient relationship and the degree of understanding of the disease tend to increase compliance. It would thus appear that the quality of communication between doctor and patient and the nature of their relationship can greatly affect the motivation and cooperation of children and their parents. Fragmented services, lack of long-term involvement with a particular physician (continuity of care), and present third-party fee schedules (which offer physicians attractive incentives to provide technical services while discouraging efforts to perform as the patient's adviser and counselor) all contribute to making noncompliance a major problem in the management of chronic illness (Almy, 1981; Select Panel for the Promotion of Child Health, 1981).

Health care providers must attend to areas far beyond purely physical concerns if they are to achieve the overall goal of promoting adjustment and maximal functioning in children with chronic problems. In addition to providing and directing these services, families need instructions on age-adequate developmental activities, realistic pictures of their children's prognoses, and help in dealing with their feelings.

Organization of Services for Children with Chronic Illnesses

Children with chronic illnesses receive health services from a wide variety of service arrangements. These arrangements have evolved in the unsupervised and largely unplanned fashion that reflects our health service system in general— one typified by pluralism, local initiative, a high degree of specialization, and a complicated mix of public and private services (Schmidt, 1973). A description of the levels of care and the various service arrangements available is essential to an understanding of the health service difficulties that face these children and families.

Levels of Care

Primary care refers to the range of services that are typically provided by general pediatricians and family practitioners and is the point at which most patients enter the health care system. Primary care services for children in the United States are generally concerned with routine well-child care necessary for prevention of certain diseases. It is also the level of care at which most screening for occult problems is done and referrals are made for more sophisticated diagnostic and therapeutic procedures. In some situations, primary care providers also serve as facilitator, brake, conduit, and coordinator of services provided by other professionals. The accomplishment of this aspect of care requires that one person have long-term responsibility for overseeing and coordinating care (Andreopoulos, 1974; Institute of Medicine, 1978).

Secondary care refers to the range of services provided by medical and other child health specialists (neurologists, hematologists, physical therapists, speech therapists, and special educators to name just a few) available in many urban communities. The focus of the care provided at this level is usually oriented toward a particular problem or set of problems. Providers of secondary care services may provide a one-time evaluation (consultation), share case management with primary care providers, assume responsibility for management of a specific problem or set of problems, or take over all aspects of care.

Tertiary care, the most sophisticated level of care, refers to those services usually available in limited supply and most often associated with medical centers and training hospitals. Tertiary care in particular, and secondary care to a somewhat lesser degree, tend to be segregated from other community resources available to the child and family.

Service Arrangements

The majority of children in the United States receive primary and secondary health care from private physicians in solo or group practices. The range of health-related services these children receive is largely determined by what the physician provides directly and mobilizes from other available resources. Some physicians are quite adept at finding and coordinating services; others devote little energy to needs they themselves cannot meet. Unfortunately, under the private-physician model, there is little incentive for private physicians to form close working relations with other community health services (Andreopoulos, 1974).

As a response to the problems created by the limited range of services any individual can provide, group practices and private clinics have evolved. These arrangements often offer a wider range of services and greater availability (such as at night or on weekends or holidays) than the individual, and in some cases, these arrangements may serve as the foundation for the evolution of more comprehensive and organized health service arrangements. At the present time, however, there is no evidence that such group practices can consistently deliver the range of services required by many children with chronic illnesses.

Much primary care is also delivered in neighborhood health centers, hospital outpatient departments, and prepaid group practices, such as health maintenance organizations. Prepaid group practices aim to provide comprehensive care for enrolled populations and may prove a very useful model for the care of both the general population and individuals with chronic problems. Neighborhood health centers and publicly funded clinics (such as those sponsored by Crippled Children's Services) often offer comprehensive, long-term care but frequently confront significant problems such as serving populations restricted by geographical or categorical regulation, extremely high costs per patient, and difficulty in coordinating different levels of care.

Hospital outpatient departments in urban areas now provide much primary, secondary, and tertiary care. Many have developed comprehensive programs aimed at taking advantage of resources available in the hospital to make needed services readily accessible. Many of these hospital-based clinics, however, are categorical in nature. That is, they only serve individuals with specific biological conditions. In addition, they typically suffer from lack of continuity of care and fragmentation of services. Comprehensive clinics using team approaches would appear to be an ideal model except that relatively few facilities have all the necessary resources or appropriate professionals. In addition, such teams are often assembled using available professionals who have numerous other responsibilities so that the clinic functions only at restricted times. This situation occurs because many children with widely varying conditions require widely different mixes of disciplines and medical specialties, and it is simply not cost-effective to have all team members available at all times.

The Effects of Specialization

Much frustration, dissatisfaction, and possibly even suboptimal medical care result from the usual service arrangements for chronically ill children. Deficiencies exist even in communities with rich medical, social, and other specialized services. As medical understanding and technologies have grown, patients have been directed more frequently to specialists with highly skilled techniques and knowledge. Many chronic problems are so uncommon and medically complicated that the family doctor or pediatrician has tended either to share the child's management with specialists or to turn it over entirely. Children have undoubtedly benefitted from these advances in medical specialization, but the splintering of services that has accompanied them has also had its costs.

It would be foolhardy to blame specialists for many of the difficult and unpleasant aspects of the lives of these children and their families. Indeed, the increased life span of many children with chronic problems and the improvement in the quality of their lives have resulted in large part from scientific and technical advances of an extremely specialized sort. But this specialization has resulted in many problems very difficult to correct. Specific medical needs may be expertly met by specialists, but many other needs central to the child's adaptation are often neglected. Because of this, a medical specialist has been described as a person who knows more and more about less and less (Wechsler, 1976).

Because no one professional can meet all the needs of a particular child or family, the family must depend on a number of professionals. It is recognized that many communities suffer shortages in certain types of professionals while other communities are glutted with them. Urban areas with large medical centers often have many of the necessary services while smaller cities, towns, and rural areas may suffer extreme shortages.

Even in communities with adequate numbers of appropriate professionals, child and family needs may go unmet because of poor coordination and communication between professionals. This may even occur in situations where all the care is rendered under one roof. Excellent care for chronically ill children requires that one person oversee and coordinate all aspects of that care. Yet this rarely occurs, and as a result, certain needs go unattended. One professional attends to one aspect of care and another to another aspect, but many needs do not necessarily fit neatly into the domain of any particular specialty. This is especially true of the child's developmental and psychosocial issues, but it is also often the case for purely medical aspects of the child's care.

As might be expected, many families cannot find services. A large national study conducted by the Rand Corporation found that two thirds of parents of children with hearing and vision impairments report difficulty in finding basic services (Brewer and Kakalik, 1974). Most of these parents also report that no one service provider had all the information necessary or took responsibility for coordinating services. Similar problems are reported by parents of children with cerebral palsy and spina bifida (Kanthor and others, 1974). Even when services are available in a community, parents are often unaware of them, don't know that they are necessary, or don't know how to get them. There is no reason to believe that studies of families of children with other complicated chronic disorders such as congenital heart disease, renal disease, cystic fibrosis, and hematological problems would not reveal the same basic difficulties. A recurring theme in the literature on health services for children with chronic problems is that medical and other health-related technologies are now at a point where they can make real contributions to the lives of many children. Many communities have the services available to use these technologies, but the fragmentation of care resulting from specialization means that many children and families go without services that could benefit them (Brewer and Kakalik, 1974; Kanthor and others, 1974).

Characteristics of Services Desirable for All Children with Chronic Illnesses

Because children with chronic illnesses receive health services from a wide variety of service arrangements, it would be impractical to advocate a single type of approach to the organization of their care. Such an approach could probably not be universally implemented and would not necessarily be in the best interest of all chronically ill children. It would appear that many of the delivery problems faced by these children and families could be alleviated if all service arrangements were designed with certain characteristics in mind. In most situations, these characteristics can be achieved by a reorientation and reorganization of existing community resources rather than by the creation of more services. These characteristics are noted here.

Continuity of Care

Many workers agree that the most important element in management of chronically ill children is establishment of continuity of access to one medical provider (Allen and Lelchuck, 1966; Battle, 1972). Much work has suggested that doctors' inadequate communication with patients and parents contributes to stress, dissatisfaction, and noncompliance with therapeutic regimens (Korsch, Freeman, and Negrete, 1971). Chronic illness necessitates many short-term interactions with numerous professionals. Children who receive their care at university centers have to contend with a staff that turns over yearly (or even more frequently as physicians in training rotate from one service to the next). The lack of long-term involvement with one provider inhibits the development of a warm, trusting, supportive relationship that fosters good communication. The result is parents and children who are frequently left confused, anxious, and angry because their expectations have not been met.

Coordination of Services

Coordination of services provided by multiple medical specialists and other child health professionals is essential to the care of children with chronic problems. Lack of such coordination often results in duplication of services or unmet needs. Coordination can be accomplished by one provider who contacts other agencies, directs patients to appropriate specialists, receives feedback from specialists and interprets it for patients, and in general, takes responsibility for coordinating all aspects of the patient's care. In the case of chronically ill children, it makes more sense to speak to the entire family as the client, so that the number of services is often quite large.

The pediatric literature suggests that the pediatrician, rather than the medical subspecialist or other service provider, is the logical person to conduct and oversee the overall care of children with chronic disorders (Battle, 1972; Mattsson, 1972). Little recognition is given to the fact that many such children receive only specialist care with virtually no primary component. Battle (1972, p. 921) suggests that "the pediatrician is the logical person to serve as ombudsman for the handicapped child. The organization of treatment, and indeed, of daily life, for such a child and his family has such numerous and complex ramifications that it demands the direction of one individual with knowledge and interest in the overall problems of the child as a person and his family. The child's medical care, and ultimately the child himself become fragmented and lost among the various specialties evaluating and treating him unless the pediatrician is diagnosing, organizing, selecting, interpreting, integrating, and implementing the total care." One may disagree about who should fill this role, but it is certainly an essential role and one of the most difficult health service issues to resolve regarding chronically ill children.

Whatever the service arrangement, it is critical that one person oversee all aspects of care and facilitate receipt of needed services. It is important to recognize that, even in communities with adequate numbers of appropriate services and where financial barriers are removed, families do not necessarily seek or obtain needed services. Families need consistent information and coaching regarding necessary services and how and where to obtain them.

The pediatrician, family practitioner, medical specialist, or any other person with long-term involvement can play this role effectively. Some communities have recently begun to employ nonmedical "case managers" to fill this role in geriatric care with reports of some success. Other communities have begun to train "parent professionals," parents of children with chronic illnesses who coordinate care and advocate on behalf of other chronically ill children in the community (E. Boelke of the Effective Parents Program, personal communication with the author, 1981). Some also interpret Public Law 94–142 as a mandate for local school systems to assume this responsibility (Jacobs and Walker, 1978; Palfrey, Mervis, and Butler, 1978). In many cases, however, no one professional assumes this responsibility and the family is forced to organize and oversee their child's package or services without supervision or training. Many families present stories reminiscent of Kafka novels with nightmarelike passages through bureaucratic mazes that leave them stunned and alienated from the very people who are supposed to be helping them.

Comprehensiveness

Chronically ill children and their families have multiple problems and health care needs and require a wide range of services. Obviously, services cannot be used if they are not available. An adequate number of physicians is a very crude index of the adequacy of the overall service system for these children. Although one cannot overlook the importance of the physician in the management of the child's problem, in the majority of cases involving severe medical problems, a single physician is not able to provide the full range of services needed. Therefore, any assessment of the adequacy of available services must include other essential service providers (special educators, respiratory therapists, physical therapists, occupational therapists, and social workers, just to mention a few) as well as detailed descriptions of different categories of physicians required (primary care providers and medical specialists). It is also important to recognize that availability of service is only one factor in determining the quality of services children receive.

Because these children have their conditions through their entire lives, the approach to their care must be to provide an individualized management plan that includes the various aspects of development (physical, emotional, social, and cognitive) and is designed to improve the child's functioning to the maximum allowed by the extent of the disability. Such a task requires a synthesis of medical, educational, and psychosocial approaches and often involves a number of professionals from different disciplines. It is here that we often get into trouble and most frequently fail these children and families. The conceptualization of mental health needs as being separate and distinct from physical health needs is particularly inappropriate for the care of chronically ill children. There is a profound need to shift the focus of health services for chronically ill children away from the present disease orientation to a more comprehensive perspective that promotes interdisciplinary collaboration (Select Panel for the Promotion of Child Health, 1981).

At the present time, most children with severe chronic illnesses receive their care in a fragmented fashion from multiple providers operating out of geographically and organizationally different sites. This situation results in part from the fact that funding and regulation of government supported programs are generally categorical in nature, thereby discouraging evolution of interdisciplinary team approaches. Some medical center programs and programs funded by Crippled Children's Services are comprehensive in scope, but they are the exception rather than the norm, and few have been evaluated or widely publicized.

A general lack of comprehensive programs for children with chronic conditions results in families having to shop around, to use many providers, and even to go without needed services. Comprehensive care, in addition to facilitating receipt of needed services and decreasing the burden on the family as coordinator, may have other very significant benefits. Heagarty and others (1970) found that the cost of comprehensive services was less than the cost for fragmented pediatric care. In one study, they found that children receiving comprehensive care had fewer laboratory tests and x rays than children receiving fragmented services. Another study by the same group showed decreased hospitalization rates, decreased surgery rates, decreased number of visits for acute illness, and higher rates of health maintenance visits among children receiving comprehensive care (Alpert and others, 1968). Other studies, however, have been unable to document clearer benefits for comprehensive services in comparison to fragmented services (Haggerty, 1971; Moore and Frank, 1973; Leopold, 1974).

The specific areas of care desirable in any comprehensive program for children with chronic illnesses are discussed briefly here.

Attention to the Underlying Medical Problem. Many children with complicated medical problems cannot be well cared for by general pediatricians alone. Optimal care for these children requires significant input from medical specialists who have sophisticated diagnostic and therapeutic capabilities. In many cases, a primary care physician may manage the majority of a child's care, with the specialist serving as a consultant and backup for complicated problems. Such a model may work well for such conditions as asthma, diabetes mellitus, certain forms of congenital heart disease, hemophilia, sickle cell anemia, and cystic fibrosis. Other conditions, such as dialysis-dependent chronic renal disease, leukemia, and more complicated forms of congenital heart disease, may require more frequent involvement and increased responsibility on the part of specialists. At this time, there is no consensus on which medical problems require specialist supervision and which conditions allow for management by general primary care physicians. Like many other aspects of the care of chronically ill children, this depends on the individual physician, child, and family. Some primary care physicians see it as their role to remain intimately involved in the most technical aspects of their patients' problems; others relegate virtually all responsibility to medical specialists or drop out entirely.

There are, unfortunately, a number of substantial disincentives for primary care physicians to remain intimately involved in the care of these children. Many chronically ill children have relatively rare problems so that primary care doctors do not see enough of them to feel comfortable handling the medical and technical aspects of their management. It is no easy task to coordinate well-child care, acute care, and specialized care. There is no easy way to obtain reports from all the providers involved to guarantee that all recommendations for further evaluation and treatment are carried out (North, 1979). It is also costly for primary care providers to care for these children. Both general pediatrics and family practice are high-volume practices with low pay per patient visit. The average pediatrician in private practice sees a child for a well-child visit every ten minutes and allots approximately five minutes for each acutely ill child seen (Bergman, Dassel, and Wedgwood, 1966). Medicaid and private insurance plans do not adequately reimburse for primary care visits of chronically ill children. The majority of their physician visits may require a half hour or more, and much of the work, such as coordinating care and communicating with other involved professionals, occurs when the patient is not actually with the physician.

Whatever the arrangement, a common problem is for the chronic illness, itself, to become the focus of care. In most cases, the care directed at the medical aspects of the chronic problem is of excellent quality and commensurate with the standards set by our present knowledge and technology. The condition may be so technically complicated or play such a significant role in the minds of the professionals, however, that it is attended to exclusively, while other aspects of the child's life are ignored and other less dramatic and visible needs go untended.

Attention to Acute Illness. Because most children with chronic problems are managed medically by multiple providers working out of geographically and administratively separate medical settings, parents frequently do not know which provider to choose to manage a crisis, even when they have good access to services. If a child with spina bifida receives medical care in various clinics at a university center, which clinic will be responsible for attending to an acute illness? Should the child have a fever, will the neurosurgery clinic, urology clinic, or orthopedic clinic be responsible for handling this acute problem? The fever may be the result of an illness unrelated to the basic problem (such as an ear infection or pneumonia), or it may be a kidney infection directly related to impaired renal function, or it may be a life-threatening infection of a neurosurgical shunt.

Most specialty clinics at university centers close in the evenings (or meet only for several sessions per week) so these children are often routed to a general pediatric clinic or an emergency room where they must be cared for by providers unfamiliar with their particular problems. Parents are forced to be dependent on the care of physicians they do not know and therefore must advocate for their children in environments they may perceive as being unfamiliar and indifferent. Although adequately trained to make judgments related to normal fluctuations of a condition, the lack of a consistent source of care constrains parents' ability to make judgments about how a given episode fits into the long-term management of their child's problem.

In designing a package of services for an individual child, it is crucial that one physician be identified as responsible for triaging acute illnesses. The family must realize which individual fills this role and know how to reach this physician at all times. The physician assuming this responsibility should be capable of assessing the illness, managing the majority of acute problems, and have easy access to other team members to ensure optimal management of each episode.

Preventive Care and Health Maintenance. The preventive potential of pediatric care is well recognized (American Academy of Pediatrics, 1977). Preventive care and health maintenance activities are essential components of health service for all children, regardless of their health care status. The components of preventive care are

1. *Immunizations.* Immunizations against the common childhood infectious diseases represent one of the most far-reaching advances in medical care in the past century, profoundly altering childhood morbidity and mortality and the nature of pediatric practice. Children with chronic illnesses have the same needs for the standard immunizations as their healthy peers. In addition, vaccines against pneumococcal bacteria and influenza viruses have recently become available for large-scale use in selected segments of the population. Individuals with chronic debilitating diseases and chronic heart or lung disease are especially susceptible to these infectious agents. Pneumococcal and influenza virus vaccines are recommended for these at-risk children, including children with cystic fibrosis and severe asthma and certain children with cerebral palsy. Influenza vaccines must be given annually and pneumococcal vaccines every three years.

   If no one person takes responsibility for monitoring a particular child's immunization status, it is likely that child will be inadequately immunized and remain susceptible to one of these life-threatening infections.
2. *Monitoring Physical Growth and Nutritional Status.* One of the major functions of routine well-child care is to monitor physical growth and nutritional status. All children should be weighed and measured at routine intervals, and the values plotted on growth charts. The American Academy of Pediatrics (1977) recommends that the average child should have this done five times in the first year of life, three times in the second, three times between the ages of two and six, and at least once every three years during the school years. For children at risk for malnutrition (such as those with cystic fibrosis or diabetes mellitus) or for those at risk for obesity due to decreased motor activity (children with neuromuscular problems such as cerebral palsy or spina bifida), attention to this area of health supervision is even more important than for their healthy peers.
3. *Periodic Screening for Acute Diseases.* It is now accepted that various screening tests are essential components of preventive health services for

children as well as adults. Several metabolic diseases such as phenylketonuria (PKU) and hypothyroidism are routinely screened for in the newborn
period. Other problems, such as hypertension, anemia, and vision and
hearing deficits may develop at any time during childhood and must be
screened for periodically. These serious problems are common and frequently amenable to correction or alleviation by health service input.

All children are at risk for hearing and vision problems, and periodic
screening for sensory deficits are accepted as part of the preventive services all
children should receive. Early identification of these problems, with initiation of
effective therapeutic measures, can have considerable influence on cognitive
development, school performance, and social adaptation.

Psychosocial Needs. It is impossible to generalize about how far an
individual pediatrician, family practitioner, or medical specialist can go in
delivering mental health services and when referral to a more specialized mental
health worker is indicated. It depends on the particular physician, the child, and
the family. The medical literature is replete with statements about the desirability
of providing attention to developmental and psychosocial needs of physically
healthy children (Richmond, 1959; McClelland and others, 1973). In addition, it
is recognized that these needs are greatly increased for chronically ill children, yet
there is evidence to indicate that very little time is actually devoted to these areas
either in medical education or in practice (Bergman, Dassel, and Wedgwood,
1966; Bishop, Parrish, and Baker, 1967; Korsch, Freeman, and Negrete, 1971).
This evidence suggests that the social aspects of children's lives and illnesses are
not routinely considered in medical encounters. Yet physicians are in the ideal
position to make substantial contributions to this aspect of the child's and
family's functioning, and there are a number of things in this regard they can
and should do.

First, it is important that the primary care provider or someone else with
long-term involvement do periodic screening and assessment of the child's and
family's psychosocial functioning. These assessments, which form the basis for
counseling or referrals to mental health workers, can be fit into the regular
schedule of routine health care visits (sometimes referred to as well-child visits).
It might appear more efficacious to use objective screening instruments to
monitor this area of the child's and family's functioning, but at present, there are
few such reliable instruments available. Many physicians, however, have long-
term relationships with these families and, over time, get to know them quite
well; under these conditions, they can adequately screen them using informal
interviews.

Second, these children need strategies aimed at promoting psychological
and social adjustment and positive self-image. One of the central goals in the
management of chronic illness is to diminish, as much as possible, the patterns
of self-defeating expectations and behavior that are often complications of
physical disease. Obviously, different children with different medical problems,
disabilities, family situations, and coping capacities will require differing
amounts and types of inputs from social workers, psychiatrists, psychologists,

and educators, as well as from primary care physicians and medical specialists. Often the interventions are quite simple from the perspective of child health professionals, but if the issues are not addressed, the interventions and referrals will not occur.

Third, it is important that someone attend to the psychosocial needs of other family members. It is especially important to provide support and counseling to families when they experience major crises, such as those that occur at the time of diagnosis. It is important because it is humane and because this is the most opportune time to engage the family in a psychotherapeutic alliance. According to crisis theory all crises are time-limited, and the strongest point for the resolution of conflict occurs at the peak of a crisis. Although each crisis is time-limited, crises are cyclical and repetitive in these families. There are acute exacerbations of medical problems, frequent hospitalizations, and profound disruptions and disappointments at many developmental stages.

There is reason to believe that primary care physicians, although not routinely performing these supportive functions, perform them more often than medical specialists; thus, expanding and improving this role fits more neatly into the domain of primary care than specialized care. By the very nature of their work, the orientation of medical specialists is usually focused on disease. Many specialists are unfamiliar and uninvolved with child development theory, the home and school setting of the child, and community factors that impinge on the child's and family's lives. It is this need for a broader view of the child and family as well as the need for coordination of services and continuity of care that makes primary care involvement in the management of chronic illness so attractive.

In any event, physicians must recognize limitations and feel comfortable referring patients to mental health professionals. Routine referrals of all children with chronic illnesses to mental health workers does not appear justified at this time because many seem to do quite well without such professional involvement; yet in many cases, patients do need to be referred to professionals more skilled in these areas than primary care physicians and medical specialists. Thus, physicians must be familiar with mental health workers in the community and feel comfortable collaborating with them.

It would facilitate communication across professional disciplines if pediatricians were to learn more about various psychotherapeutic approaches and have experience collaborating with mental health professionals during their training. Although many pediatric training programs are now beginning to foster such interaction, this is still not universally the case. Too many physicians still leave their training with only a rudimentary appreciation of mental health issues and approaches.

Recommendations

Medical Education

Increasing the number of physicians produced by medical schools should not be thought of as a major solution to the inadequacies of our present system of care for children with chronic problems. More physicians will not solve such problems as geographic maldistribution, lack of comprehensive care, and poor coordination of services.

Medical education has a substantial influence on the attitudes and career goals of medical students and doctors in training. During the past several decades, medical education has been supervised to a large extent by medical specialists, and this has resulted in many significant scientific and technological advances. It has also had a marked influence in generating large numbers of medical specialists and inadvertently fostering fragmentation and disease-oriented approaches to care.

The past two decades have shown significant progress in the area of educating primary care physicians. This progress should be supported and encouraged in the future. If subsequent generations of primary care providers are to be more intimately and effectively involved in the care of these children, there will have to be significant changes in role models for medical students, in their educational experiences, and in the relationship between medical schools and the communities they serve. Increasing involvement and visibility of academic primary care faculty members in the care of these children and the training of pediatricians should be encouraged and supported.

Need for Local Child Advocacy Initiatives

Virtually every community in the United States could benefit from a well-organized child advocacy group. Efforts to foster their creation, perpetuation, and evaluation should be encouraged and supported. Local consumers and providers of health services are most knowledgeable about their community's specialized child health services and needs. The best advocates are enlightened parents, and we should be working toward creation of enlightened parents who are willing to collaborate in the planning of their children's and community's health care services.

Effective organization of services at a local level requires meticulous fact-finding efforts and monitoring of existing programs, together with repeated contacts at all levels of the community. These activities can be both frustrating and draining, and most providers of direct services do not have the time or motivation to be involved in such activities. Therefore, if these activities are to be carried out, they are dependent on government regulation and consumer monitoring in the form of advocacy.

Child advocacy, in this context, refers to efforts that are targeted at institutional barriers, administrative procedures, and budgetary restrictions that interfere with the receipt of services. Public Law 94–142, for example, is a product of child advocacy activities at a national level, supplying the legislative basis for local communities to provide all children with a public education. This legislative act, however, merely begins a process that ultimately must be implemented at a local level. Every community must now implement programs and monitor efforts to meet this new mandate, and this requires continued advocacy work at the community level. Early identification and referral of preschoolers in need of special services, school health services for children with chronic problems, inertia in local health programs and health departments, implementation of existing laws, respite care for families with chronically ill children, the effects of local community practices on children with special problems, poor access to dental services, and serious gaps in the quantity, quality, and coordination of services—these are all areas that could be greatly influenced by an articulate, well-informed, and well-organized advocacy group. Such groups may well be more efficient and cost-effective than creating still another government agency to create and enforce regulations.

In the long run, communities need an impetus, financial support, and organizational leadership to give child advocacy groups a sense of identity at the local level.

References

Allen, J. E., and Lelchuck, L. "A Comprehensive Care Program for Children with Handicaps." *American Journal of Diseases of Children*, 1966, *3*, 229–235.

Almy, T. P. "The Role of the Primary Care Physician in the Health Care Industry." *New England Journal of Medicine*, 1981, *304*, 225–228.

Alpert, J., and others. "Effective Use of Comprehensive Pediatric Care: Utilization of Health Resources." *American Journal of Diseases of Children*, 1968, *116*, 529–533.

American Academy of Pediatrics. Committee on Standards of Child Health Care. *Standards of Child Health Care*. (3d ed.) Evanston, Ill.: American Academy of Pediatrics, 1977.

Andreopoulos, S., and others, *Primary Care: Where Medicine Fails*. New York: Wiley, 1974.

Battle, C. U. "The Role of the Pediatrician as Ombudsman in the Health Care of the Young Handicapped Child." *Pediatrics*, 1972, *50*, 916–922.

Becker, M. H., Drachman, R. H., and Kirscht, J. P. "Predicting Mothers' Compliance with Pediatric Medical Regimens." *Journal of Pediatrics*, 1972, *81*, 843–854.

Bergman, A. B., Dassel, S. W., and Wedgwood, R. J. "Time-Motion Study of Practicing Pediatricians." *Pediatrics*, 1966, *38*, 254–261.

Bishop, F. M., Parrish, H. M., and Baker, A. S. "Functional Role Activities of the Private Practitioner: A Method of Investigating Office Practice and Time Study of the Typical Day of 25 Physicians." *Clinical Pediatrics*, 1967, *6*, 459–463.

Brewer, G. D., and Kakalik, J. S. *Improving Services to Handicapped Children: Summary and Recommendations*. Santa Monica, Calif.: Rand Corporation, 1974.

Fink, D., and others. "Effective Patient Care in the Pediatric Ambulatory Setting: A Study of the Acute Care Clinic." *Pediatrics*, 1969, *43*, 927–935.

Fries, J. F. "Aging, Natural Death, and the Compression of Morbidity." *New England Journal of Medicine,* 1980, *303,* 130–135.

Gordis, L., and Markowitz, M. "Evaluation of the Effectiveness of Comprehensive and Continuous Pediatric Care." *Pediatrics,* 1971, *48,* 766–775.

Gordis, L., Markowitz, M., and Lilienfeld, A. M. "Why Patients Don't Follow Medical Advice: A Study of Children on Long Term Antistreptococcal Prophylaxis." *Journal of Pediatrics,* 1969, *75,* 957–968.

Haggerty, R. J. "Symposium: Does Comprehensive Care Make A Difference?" *American Journal of Diseases of Children,* 1971, *122,* 467–471.

Heagarty, M. D., and others. "Some Comparative Costs in Comprehensive vs. Fragmented Pediatric Care." *Pediatrics,* 1970, *46,* 596–602.

Institute of Medicine. *A Manpower Policy for Primary Health Care.* Washington, D.C.: National Academy of Sciences, 1978.

Jacobs, F. H., and Walker, D. K. "Pediatricians and the Education for All Handicapped Children Act of 1975." *Pediatrics,* 1978, *61,* 135–137.

Kanthor, H., and others. "Areas of Responsibility in the Health Care of Multiply Handicapped Children." *Pediatrics,* 1974, *54,* 779–788.

Korsch, B. M., Freeman, B., and Negrete, V. F. "Practical Implications of Doctor-Patient Interaction Analysis for Pediatric Practice." *American Journal of Diseases of Children,* 1971, *121,* 110–114.

Leopold, E. A. "Whom Do We Reach? A Study of Health Care Utilization." *Pediatrics,* 1974, *53,* 341–348.

McClelland, C. Q., and others. "The Practitioner's Role in Behavioral Pediatrics." *Journal of Pediatrics,* 1973, *82,* 325–331.

Mattsson, A. "Long Term Physical Illness in Childhood: A Challenge to Psycho-Social Adaptation." *Pediatrics,* 1972, *50,* 801–811.

Meyers, A., Dolan, T. F., and Mueller, D. "Compliance and Self-Medication in Cystic Fibrosis." *American Journal of Diseases of Children,* 1975, *129,* 1011–1013.

Moore, J. T., and Frank, K. "Comprehensive Health Services to Children: An Exploratory Study of Benefits." *Pediatrics,* 1973, *51,* 766–775.

North, A. F. "Health Services in Head Start." In E. Zigler and J. Valentine (Eds.), *Project Head Start.* New York: Macmillan, 1979.

Palfrey, J. S., Mervis, R. C., and Butler, J. A. "New Directions in the Evaluation and Education of Handicapped Children." *New England Journal of Medicine,* 1978, *298,* 819–824.

Pless, I. B., and Pinkerton, P. *Chronic Childhood Disorders: Promoting Patterns of Adjustment.* Chicago: Yearbook Medical Publishers, 1975.

Richmond, J. "Some Observations on the Sociology of Pediatric Education and Practice." *Pediatrics,* 1959, *23,* 1175–1178.

Schmidt, W. M. "The Development of Health Services for Mothers and Children in the United States." *American Journal of Public Health,* 1973, *63,* 419–427.

Select Panel for the Promotion of Child Health. *Better Health for Our Children: A National Strategy.* Department of Health and Human Services publication no. 79-55071. Washington, D.C.: U.S. Government Printing Office, 1981.

Seligmann, A., McGrath, N. E., and Pratt, L. "Level of Medical Information Among Clinic Patients." *Journal of Chronic Diseases,* 1957, *6,* 497–509.

Wechsler, H. *Handbook of Medical Specialties.* New York: Human Sciences Press, 1976.

Wegman, M. E. "Annual Summary of Vital Statistics—1979." *Pediatrics,* 1980, *66,* 823–833.

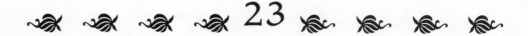

Training Physicians to Care for Chronically Ill Children

C. William Daeschner, Jr., M.D.
Mary C. Cerreto, Ph.D.

Seven to 10 percent of all children live with chronic illness of primary physical origin (Pless, 1968; Rutter, Tizard, and Whitmore, 1968). Although the illnesses vary in severity, visibility, morbidity, and mortality, they share the characteristics of chronicity. These children and their families face physical, emotional, and financial stresses quite different from those faced by acutely ill or healthy children and their families. Their medical needs are sufficiently different to warrant classifying the chronically ill as a distinct minority and to encourage careful consideration of the education of medical professionals to care for them.

Several factors complicate the analysis of medical education. First, the medical disabilities and related care needs involved are extremely diverse. For example, the patient with cleft lip and palate might require multiple plastic surgical procedures in the first years of life, a situation that can drain a family emotionally and financially. Speech therapy and psychological support must follow to prepare the child for school. Throughout the process, the primary care pediatrician must be supportive and anticipate developmental and social problems. Second, because of the pluralism of the American medical care system, sources of care, financing, and other issues are influenced by the patient's age, the nature of the defect, family financial status and geographical location, and the capabilities of the medical institutions to which the patient has access. Third, the chronically ill are a polymorphic rather than clearly defined minority.

Another problem is that the major orientation of medical practice to date has been toward "cure," and fulfilling the needs of the chronically ill demands reorientation toward "care." Meeting this demand requires a major attitude change toward both the physician's role and the goals of medical education. Education for medical practice has traditionally emphasized acute disease of recent origin and limited duration. It has been sufficient, perhaps, that the physician diagnose, treat, and dismiss until contacted about a new problem or for a health maintenance visit. Offices, hospitals, and laboratories have been designed for care of acute illness. The time required for training in acute care of life-threatening diseases leaves little opportunity to pay attention to other aspects of the patient's well-being. Some have not considered the emotional, psychosocial, and financial problems of the chronically ill to be a proper province for physicians and their teachers. This situation is changing: Medical science now permits the physician to prevent, cure, or remedy many acute illnesses, thus permitting increased attention to the needs of the chronically ill. The same advances enable many chronically ill children to live longer and to participate more fully in social and educational activities, thus expanding their need for comprehensive medical care.

This chapter addresses the preparation of physicians to provide health care for chronically ill children and their families, summarizes the current status of such education, and delineates gaps and weaknesses in the present system. It attempts to put into perspective the roles that medical education should play in preparing professionals to serve the chronically ill. Perhaps it also will alert us to the magnitude of the stakes, should we fail.

The Needs of the Chronically Ill

To the subspecialist, children with diabetes, hemophilia, leukemia, and spina bifida have few needs in common; however, the general pediatrician must realize that these children have the same need for anticipatory guidance, learning readiness evaluation, preventive medical care, and care for acute illnesses that other patients do. Therefore, underlying the problems unique to handicapped or chronically ill children are a set of common needs for which medical education should prepare the physician (Kempe and Olmsted, 1978; Kempe, 1978). A brief summary of general medical problems of chronically ill children and their families permits us to examine the appropriateness of the current curriculum and points the way to innovation. Although other aspects of care for the chronically ill impinge on this discussion, those listed here are sources of problems to which educators must be particularly attentive (Pless and Roghmann, 1971):

1. Early and precise problem identification
2. Continuity of care, including identification of a central provider
3. Comprehensive care that includes a multidisciplinary focus
4. Sensitive and flexible care

5.   Skillful anticipatory guidance that includes education of the patient and family and full preventive health care
6.   Economical care

Our goal is to reemphasize to teachers, learners, and planners the subtle but significant shades of difference between the needs of a chronically ill child and those of a child who is neither chronically ill nor handicapped.

Early Identification. The first manifestations of many chronic illnesses are hidden or subtle. Because early and exact identification plus timely intervention can prevent mortality and decrease disability, physicians must maintain a high index of suspicion about the possibility of a developing chronic medical problem and should recognize their responsibilities when genetic transmission is known or suspected. Responsibilities include determining the need for future family planning and providing appropriate counseling for parents, siblings, and relatives.

Continuity. Communication among professionals and with the child and family is enhanced by the continuing presence of a physician skilled in primary pediatric care, particularly when the subspecialists and other health professionals are geographically distant or are not part of a comprehensive care group. The solo practitioner of otolaryngology in a nearby city might, for instance, provide skillful care of otitis media or sinusitis that complicates a case of cystic fibrosis but is not prepared to monitor other aspects of care, and the cardiologist or pulmonologist in a medical center might be sought for advice concerning heart and lung problems secondary to the disease but would probably be unwilling or unable to deal with school problems, nutrition, maturation failure, and the psychosocial stresses on the patient and family. By definition, chronic illness requires prolonged medical care, which is adequate only if a central professional is responsible for overall supervision and assessment.

Comprehensive Care. Most chronic illnesses involve multiple organ systems and require the services of many health care professionals. Almost all chronic illnesses generate secondary problems for the patient and family, who must develop coping skills and may require social, psychological, and educational counseling. These are the areas in which the skills of other health professionals are essential for achieving the best outcome. The primary physician must plan comprehensive, multidisciplinary care and must accept the role of team leader as well as share responsibilities with subspecialists and allied health personnel.

Flexible Care. Some chronic illnesses are progressive; others are highly variable in the degree of disability they create. The physician and members of the medical care team must be able to adjust to changing medical and social needs.

Anticipatory Guidance. Education of chronically ill patients and their families to care for a chronic disability is always important and sometimes critical (Mattsson, 1972). The physician's ability to communicate accurately and effectively is a major factor in successful long-term care. Education of the community is another essential ingredient in a nurturing environment for children with handicaps; the physician-ombudsman has a major opportunity in this area.

Economical Care. Prolonged or extensive medical care is expensive, and the cost usually exceeds the personal or insurance resources of the family. From the beginning, medical care must be provided as economically as is consistent with maintenance of quality.

The Present System for Educating Professionals

Medical education is a lengthy and expensive process. Physicians who provide primary care for children have prepared themselves by investing a minimum of eleven years in education after high school graduation. First, they acquire a bachelor's degree, achieving high marks throughout. Those who obtain admission to medical school face four years of intensive study and evaluation before they receive their doctorate degree, which is only the preface to three or more years of intensive, often exhausting, hospital-based clinical training in preparation for certification as a specialist. Should the trainee aspire to a career in teaching or research, an additional two to three years of fellowship training are required to focus clinical skills and acquire a knowledge of research methodology. The average professional is twenty-eight to thirty-two years of age before beginning to earn a living, pay off debts, and enjoy the fruits of all this labor. But the end is not yet in sight: In order to maintain competence, the physician must invest time and money in continuing education throughout the years of practice. These facts are important to remember as we examine the education of physicians to care for the chronically ill because they play a significant role in determining attitudes, priorities, geographic location of practice, and the type of practice situation selected. They point clearly to the need for economic subsidy of this costly process.

Premedical Education. Premedical studies begin with a broad base of arts and sciences courses but tend to concentrate on science as students move toward their baccalaureates. The student is aware of the intense competition for medical school admission and often selects courses likely to yield high marks and to have content valued by medical school admission committees. These committees tend to require, or at least to treat with great respect, courses that are considered hard science—biology, chemistry, physics, calculus, and so on—and to weigh lightly courses in psychology, education, and the social sciences. Not surprisingly, most medical students begin their study of medicine with a relatively poor foundation in the latter areas and are ill prepared to assimilate teaching directed to the psycholosocial issues in patient care, stress and family dynamics, problems, and school health issues; yet these areas are critical to the health care of chronically ill children and their families.

Medical Education. Throughout medical school the basic biological sciences are emphasized, and little attention is paid to teaching the skills needed to respond to the psychosocial needs of the chronically ill. The integration of social science professionals into the medical student's supervising faculty is late and infrequent, and social science often is viewed by students and other faculty members as a fringe area of knowledge and performance. Only in the later parts of the students' clinical experience do they work with psychologists, social workers, and special therapists. Otherwise, medical school has a dearth of courses and of faculty models that emphasize chronic illness care. Small wonder that few of these teachings rub off on the fledgling physicians (Kutner, 1978).

Students' exposure to chronically ill children in teaching hospitals might be frequent (or even excessive), but the aspects of continuity and comprehensive care are often neglected. Thus a student's ability to diagnose muscular dystrophy or hemophilia or to manage acute diabetic ketoacidosis might not be matched by skills in educating the family and child for long-term care, incorporating other professionals into the patient's management team, or assisting the family to cope with day-to-day life with an incurable illness.

In addition to basic science and clinical instruction, the usual medical school curriculum devotes several weeks to pediatric problems. Because most medical students will not go on to a pediatric residency, the medical school curriculum is designed to provide the background necessary to prepare physicians for a practice that includes infants, children, and adolescents. The experience includes a block for ambulatory care, an equal period assigned to care of a group of hospitalized children, and brief exposure to the care of newborns. In each setting, students are exposed to normal and abnormal children, and they gain, through personal experience and observation of their mentors at work, an appreciation for the effects of chronic illness in young patients. For example, the student observes that the discovery of chronic nephritis in a child can have devastating impact on the patient and family. The student is soon impressed with the needs to be sensitive, thorough, and precise, lest inappropriate communication needlessly increase the burden on the patient and family.

The in-hospital clerkship usually emphasizes the skilled use of diagnostic and counseling facilities and the role of consultants, but the health-care team is modeled with variable success. In the hospital setting, multiple medical disciplines might be involved in a child's care, particularly during diagnostic and treatment periods. Unfortunately, the student is frequently exposed to a patchwork care pattern in which individual teachers seem concerned with only one aspect of the patient's needs and unmindful of the relation of their care to the patient's total well-being. The team leader is often difficult to identify, so that the student might wonder whether anyone is in charge of the whole patient.

This tendency is, in part, related to third-party funding practices, which are largely procedure-oriented. Private foundations, health insurance programs, and federal health services for the economically disadvantaged usually define the exact type of case they will support. Because specific items (diagnostic, radiological, or laboratory studies; anesthesia; surgery; and the like) are more easily defined and given a dollar value, remuneration for them might be designated whereas equally essential but less clearly defined services might not be reimbursed. For example, acute care of the critically ill child with diabetic ketoacidosis is covered by most medical care financing systems, but payment for education of the patient and family for living with diabetes mellitus often is meager or nonexistent. The child with cleft palate might have full coverage from private or public programs for repair of the anatomic defect but might be hard pressed to obtain speech therapy, even though it is essential if the child is to attain acceptable communication skills. The student who observes this situation is likely to conclude, on the basis of the reward system, that procedures are important but that total care is not. This deeply embedded contradiction is a major obstacle to ideal care for the chronically ill as well as to the balanced education of medical students.

In the ambulatory setting, a major barrier to appropriate education of the medical student is the absence of systems for direct financial support of patient services and teachers. As a result, universities find that providing adequate staff for ambulatory services and for supervision of trainees during community-based learning experiences are difficult tasks. Public and private sources often fail to recognize the importance of health professionals other than physicians and so exclude the patient from essential services. The system therefore provides a poor model to the trainee because it cannot demonstrate continuity, balance, and comprehensive service. Medical education is defective because of an unrealistic distribution of financial support in the medical care system as a whole.

Pediatric Residency. The American system of pediatric education is designed to produce physicians who provide high-quality primary and secondary care to all children and who have consultant skills sufficient to identify and sometimes treat life-threatening or uncommon deviations from health (American Board of Pediatrics, 1974). More often, the latter are considered the province of subspecialty (tertiary) practice. Achievement of skills in general pediatrics requires three years' extensive, supervised training after receiving the medical degree, and the training takes place in diverse settings: in hospitals, clinics, nurseries, emergency rooms, and the community. As a natural outgrowth of the scientific and technological revolution of the early 1900s, graduate medical education in the United States has been based principally in acute care hospitals where residents are exposed to acute, serious, and unusual disorders. Residents and members of their supervising faculty have daily opportunities to discuss the origin, course, and management of disease in hospitalized children. Didactic seminars and conferences reinforce and extend knowledge in sessions that often focus on immediate management problems in chronic illness. Subspecialty elective assignments permit in-depth study of specific organ-centered chronic diseases. Overall, the resident becomes highly skilled in diagnosis and acute care of the chronically ill child.

Experiences in clinics and community settings enable the resident to view the chronically ill child in more natural surroundings and to learn from the patients and their families about the problems they experience and the solutions they devise. The indispensability of other members of the health care team—social workers, psychologists, and special therapists—is often more clearly demonstrated here than elsewhere. Comprehensive care, provider continuity, and the importance of counseling and emotional support can be imprinted on the resident during a skillfully supervised ambulatory care experience. But, as in undergraduate medical education, exposure is sometimes woefully brief, superficial, and unbalanced. The resident's role might be that of service provider or passive learner, and the experience might leave a skewed impression of the relative importance and complexity of skills involved in comprehensive, continuous primary care compared with the skills involved in acute subspecialty care of chronically ill children. Many pediatric residency programs address this problem by establishing continuity clinics, in which residents, over two to three years, care for a panel that includes healthy, acutely ill, and chronically ill children. The residents, in essence, maintain a small general pediatric practice under supervision of faculty preceptors. They learn to appreciate the importance of knowing their patients and families and to recognize the confidence a family places in its physician's judgment. The influence of a child's age and developmental level on a chronic illness or handicap is often sharply illustrated, especially when a chronically ill patient encounters school or social problems. Residents learn to be more thoughtful and concise in communications and more sensitive to subtle clues to problems when the patient and family are people they know.

A few residency programs now provide supervised experiences in schools—the child's work environment (Wright and Vanderpool, 1981). Residents discuss the special needs of the chronically ill or handicapped with school personnel, families, and primary medical care providers. Most programs also plan time for observation of adoption agencies, children's homes, juvenile courts, and facilities for long-term schooling or domiciliary care of the chronically ill or handicapped. Unfortunately, these nonhospital experiences are usually brief and might not make a lasting impression on the trainee. Other essential lessons are not ideally modeled in the teaching center, so most trainees are encouraged to spend time in physicians' offices.

Residents' training in care of the chronically ill tends to emphasize initial diagnosis and acute care, with little emphasis on child development and the psychological and biosocial aspects of long-term care. Perhaps one should ask, "Where has medical education failed in preparing professionals to meet the needs of chronically ill children and their families?" The failure certainly is not in the area of science. Research has greatly improved the longevity and life-style of all patients; however, trainees in the teaching hospital environment rarely receive more than glimpses of patients with chronic health problems, and this situation gives them a distorted view of the patient, the problem, and the role of the family. Emphasis is too often placed on major organ dysfunction rather than on needs that must be met for the child to become fully functional. Experiences outside the hospital are often brief and superficial and thus unlikely to influence the fledgling pediatrician's learning priorities or practice habits.

Fellowship Training. Consideration of current pediatric training practices would be incomplete without a look at training beyond general pediatrics for those who will seek careers in teaching and research. Two to three years of additional experience in a specific area is the usual prescription for those aspiring to an academic position. Specific training in the organ-oriented subspecialties is well developed and includes programs in cardiology, hematology, oncology, nephrology, allergy, neonatology, infectious diseases, gastroenterology, neurology, and genetics. But structured training experiences to prepare a faculty member to develop programs that will assure high-quality care for the chronically ill are almost unknown. Although many subspecialties provide skilled long-term care to chronically ill patients, this experience is by no means uniform, especially in situations in which the number of patients is great and technical procedures demand most of the physician's time. Subspecialty chronic care programs might provide strong models of team health care for complex chronic illnesses, but they usually focus so sharply on a disease or on a group of clearly related disorders that they do not prepare trainees for leadership roles in general care of chronic illnesses or handicaps. The few professional leaders in the area of chronic illness were trained in child development, general ambulatory pediatrics, behavioral pediatrics, or child neurology, and they often lack training in such critical areas as physical medicine, social science, or research. Low visibility of training opportunities in this field is another problem, along with the difficulty of obtaining money and staff for fellowships. These problems reflect shortsightedness: The fellowship is the traditional time for the future academician to acquire research skills, and few areas of medical research afford more opportunities than do the etiology, epidemiology, management, and outcome of chronic disease.

Continuing Education of Pediatricians for Care of the Chronically Ill. Practicing general pediatricians are the principal links between the chronically ill child and new medical capabilities. The current situation of pediatric practitioners is well described by Steinhauer (1974, p. 825):

> With improvements in the treatment of the infectious diseases and our ever-increasing ability to sustain life even when we cannot restore health, . . . practicing pediatrician[s] [are] increasingly relied upon to aid in the management of the child who is severely and chronically ill. Here, contrary to parental expectations, [they] cannot cure. But there are a number of things, all of them important, that [they] can do. [They] may be able to control the rate of progression or the frequency and severity of complications of the disease. [They] may do a great deal to help the child compensate for some of the more destructive effects of . . . illness. Finally, and equally important, [they] may be able to help child and family face the limitations, anxieties, and discouragements which accompany the disease, to develop a plan of management which can serve as an antidote to feelings of utter helplessness, and to rise above the feelings of resentment and despair which could otherwise crush and overwhelm them.

As we have already seen, the pediatrician's preparation for this task is weak. Continuing education is a logical remedy and, because medicine's knowledge base is constantly changing, is recognized by pediatricians and their teachers as a lifelong, self-imposed professional obligation. New knowledge must be incorporated into practice, or the pediatrician ceases to be competent. Much of a pediatrician's postgraduate education is gained from one-to-one interaction with patients in an office or clinic practice—listening to patients and families, observing interactions, monitoring progress, and initiating careful trials of new concepts provide valuable insights. Care of the chronically ill initiates this process more frequently than any other area of practice and often presents the general pediatrician with problems for which he or she has little preparation and uncertain skill. The ideal solution is to work as a team member with other health professionals. Such a partnership can produce greater competence and interest in chronic illness for all involved; however, if the physician is ill-prepared to seek help and share responsibility, the team approach can result in hardening of negative attitudes and increased tendency to limit care to acute physical needs.

Formal and informal learning experiences also are common in the pediatrician's activities in hospitals, community-based clinics, schools, and professional societies. Perhaps the most useful is peer interaction in which professionals work together to define or solve a patient's problem.

For didactic learning, most physicians turn to medical texts and journals, which, if carefully selected for quality, permit highly reliable, self-paced learning. This method serves the double purpose of supplying new knowledge and monitoring medical progress so that, as their patients present new challenges, physicians will be able to locate relevant information efficiently. To a limited extent, formal continuing education courses offer practitioners the opportunity to return briefly to the didactic environment of student days. Courses planned to involve the practitioner-student actively in the learning process can add measurably to knowledge and skills.

A Critique of the Present System

The foregoing brief description of the present system shows that all is not well. The system contains weaknesses and gaps that, left untended, will continue to result in less than ideal care for chronically ill children and their families. Issues that must be addressed by those who establish educational and fiscal policy are delineated here.

Premedical Curriculum Revision. Students entering medical training are not well prepared by instruction and attitude to acquire the skills necessary to deal with psychosocial problems, work as part of a health care team, plan comprehensive care, or adjust to the fiscal limitations of the health care system. Faculty of undergraduate and medical education institutions should address these problems jointly. The curriculum at each level should be scrutinized and revised to support the trainee's ability to acquire the skills needed in medical practice. Outmoded and unnecessary curriculum requirements must be eliminated, and where gaps exist, new courses introduced. Each step on the educational ladder should be designed to increase the trainee's motivation and ability to meet the specific needs of chronically ill children and their families.

Attitudinal Issues. The necessity for emphasizing the importance of care over cure is nowhere more evident than in the early stages of medical training. Most young people who select medicine as a career idealistically expect to learn to cure disease. For most chronically ill or handicapped children, cure is not possible; the goal often is maintenance of current levels of functioning or prevention of regression. Professional goal failure erodes the physician's sense of adequacy and can create a sense of hopelessness and an unconscious barrier to full professional commitment to chronically ill patients.

Throughout training and professional life, most pediatricians live with constant pressure to do more than time and resources permit. When the pressure of service to a large panel of patients is so great that every minute must be rationed, the chronically ill child's more complex problems might receive less attention than they deserve. For example, attention to education of an adolescent in relation to sexual activity and the use of alcohol, tobacco, and other drugs might be neglected if the patient has a medical condition—sickle cell anemia, leukemia, diabetes mellitus—that may reduce life expectancy. And, because employment opportunities for the chronically ill or handicapped might be limited, identifying them can be a time-consuming task; career guidance and educational planning therefore might receive lower priority when, in fact, they should be given higher priority.

Most physicians feel special concern and empathy for the child with chronic illness or a handicap. They see these patients more frequently at all ages and know them and their families well; in a sense, they provide a medical home for these special children (Battle, 1972). The exception is the economically disadvantaged child, who often has no medical home. Such patients and their families are a special problem, and the quality of their care is often substandard. The parents frequently are young, only partly educated, and itinerant, a situation that leads to medical services via public and other charitable programs, often of fragmented and uneven quality. Medical records are sketchy to nonexistent, parents' understanding of previous care is incomplete and confused, and much duplication of service occurs. Public funds are available in limited and rigidly defined categories that lead to gaps and unevenness of service—the resources available do not fit the patient's needs. The patient with spina bifida might be well funded for primary and secondary surgical procedures but might have no funds for long-term care, developmental monitoring and school placement evaluation, or counseling regarding adolescent problems. Failure to consider the whole person might result in total failure of the system for that patient. Attitudinal and logistical barriers are difficult to modify, for they are almost invisible and rarely acknowledged. Current public pressure and more open discussion of prejudices and inequality may lead the way to minimizing these problems for the physician and educator as both seek to give optimum care to the chronically ill child.

Logistical Problems. Much of the medical care of the chronically ill is accomplished in teaching hospitals, a situation that creates a heavy logistical burden. A vast excess of patients must be cared for by a disproportionately small trainee and teaching staff. The result is often a shortage of time and energy for students to learn and for teachers to model the more subtle, less urgent aspects of long-term patient care. The combination of excessive responsibility and inadequate staffing is common in ambulatory and community settings and presents a poor instructional model.

Another flaw in the instructional experience is related to the entry of the chronically ill into the medical care system. The family is often not aware of all services available and therefore does not seek appropriate help. For some patients, the combination of fear, financial stress, and lack of knowledge creates a sense of panic and hopelessness that further impedes access to effective medical care. The availability of other members of the health care group may be critical in achieving full utilization of resources and attaining the self-confidence necessary for independent living. Physicians must learn to take the initiative in introducing the patient to the full spectrum of services and to assure access to resources not directly under their control (Battle, 1972). Physicians' education should include experiences to illustrate the ways other professionals can contribute to the needs of the chronically ill or handicapped child.

Medical Records. The chronological medical history of a chronic illness is a complex mixture of recorded medical contacts. For the child with asthma, records might reveal seasonal patterns, environmental influences, and response to medications. For the child with spina bifida, the medical record chronicles operations, acute infectious episodes, growth measurements, and developmental and intellectual milestones reached. The record is the major communication among professionals and the major resource for orienting new professionals. If the patient is fortunate enough to receive all care from a single physician or institution, this critical component is usually available. Yet for many children in our modern, highly mobile society, medical records are not available in a timely manner. Too often, the attending physician must resynthesize the history from the parents' uncertain store of knowledge. The family rarely has exact knowledge of biopsy findings in chronic nephritis, muscular dystrophy, or leukemia. Details of heart catheterization are available in only the most general terms. Additionally, the medical record often documents only observations and procedures related to the physical status of the child. Important educational or psychological data are often not part of the document. This situation does not usually reflect unwillingness among professionals to share information relevant to the patient's care but rather a lag in communication because records must be requested, copied, and moved about the nation. The absence of original data frustrates the student and resident physician and encourages them to guess the details of previous diagnosis and treatment. A simple solution to this problem is modeled by the armed forces, which maintains a personal health file that travels with the service member. A personal health record for each child with a chronic illness could similarly improve medical communication.

The financial status of most teaching hospitals is chronically precarious because of the relatively large proportion of indigent patients and the relative inefficiency of patient care in the teaching environment (Hadley, Mullner, and Feder, 1982). The high cost of comprehensive care of the chronically ill is rarely welcomed by a cost-conscious administration. Operating an educational program in an acute care hospital increases inpatient care costs but is generally acceptable in exchange for improved quality of care, as most of the hospital's operating expenses are generated by these patients. By contrast, education for care of the chronically ill in clinics and community settings provides unacceptable increases in the cost of care delivery and generates little or no compensating income. The broad spectrum of training experiences and supervision is relatively costly yet essential to education of professionals for high-quality care of the chronically ill. Despite efforts by many in the field of curriculum planning to make optimal use of each learning experience, cost of the medical education environment remains a major obstacle for learning experiences outside the hospital. An adequate subsidy is essential if the ambulatory and community environments for medical education are to continue and have increasing utilization.

Economic problems in care for chronically ill children also affect general pediatricians, most of whose contributions to a patient's care are in the areas of diagnosis, management, counseling, and education. These essential professional activities are poorly compensated compared to the more procedure-oriented contributions of other specialities. The frequent response of the pediatrician to this problem is to increase the number of patients seen each day, thus decreasing the time allocated to each and leading to extreme physician fatigue at day's end, a situation conducive to using free time for rest or recreation rather than for professional growth.

Chronic illness is a heavy economic burden to the family as well. The many hidden costs include transportation, home modifications, special equipment, and work time lost by employed members who must give or find care for the handicapped member. Physicians are often reluctant to assess an appropriate charge to these already overburdened families, recognizing that although these patients require more of their time than average, they can afford less. The same problem arises in education and counseling of the patient and family; these ingredients are essential to successful long-term care, yet rarely are they compensated by public programs or health insurance. As a result, physicians experience a relative loss of income and tend to minimize the number of chronically ill children in their practice.

Sharing Professional Responsibility. Pediatricians are generally more comfortable when they are involved in direct care of individual patients. For many chronically ill children, the assistance of coprofessionals is required, and the physician's task becomes as much that of coordinator as of active therapist. Modeling this behavior in the educational setting is important but infrequent because of the absence of budgeted positions for supervising and for nonphysician faculty. For the primary care general pediatrician, supervisory and coordinating functions are rarely renumerated by third-party sources. A careful look at the role of these services in the overall outcome of care would readily demonstrate their importance and provide a sound basis for including their cost in insurance contracts.

The Status Quo. An educational barrier of lesser magnitude is the general reluctance to accept change in direction or emphasis. This attitude is common in medical students, residents, and teachers as well as in the general population.

In part, the desire to preserve the status quo derives from fear that a change in content or process will cause something now in place to be forfeited. Although ineffective curriculum content should certainly be pruned, to believe that the learning approaches suggested would displace traditional curriculum experiences of proven value is unrealistic. Perhaps the real problem for curriculum planners is lack of reward for a more appropriate curriculum. Demonstration grants for projects to achieve improved care of chronically ill children might abolish this problem. Such medical care delivery research might also uncover new economies to be implemented without loss of quality and new ways to minimize the impact of chronic illness on the child and family.

Future of Education for Care of the Chronically Ill

What specific education models are available or projected for teaching professionals to care for the chronically ill child?

University Affiliated Centers. Traditionally, the large medical center teaching hospital has been the central unit for education of both medical students and resident physicians. Although this model provides an excellent environment for acute diagnostic and therapeutic instruction, it rarely models the continuity and comprehensive care necessary for care of chronic health problems. Some years ago, a small group of university affiliated centers for the care of the retarded and handicapped were established by the federal government to bring together all the professionals needed to provide full care for those patients. This "one-stop health service" environment gave high priority to the needs of the individual patient and family. For the student, it created a powerful model of the value of comprehensive and continuous care. The university affiliated facility provided a model for comprehensive, continuous, multidisciplinary care within large university systems. Individual physicians learned a great deal about the diagnosis of certain developmental problems, the family factors involved in living with a child with a chronic condition, and the skills and expertise of various other health professionals. They learned little about such management from an office practice model. Unfortunately, guidelines for funding these programs tended to separate them from the mainstream of medical education, and this potentially rich resource has had minimal impact on the education of general pediatricians. Full integration of these programs into the educational curriculum could heighten attitudes and skills needed for care for chronically ill or handicapped children and their families.

Chronic Disease Health Maintenance Organizations (HMOs). With the current national trend toward health maintenance organizations, it seems logical that, at least in larger cities, there will develop specialized units designed to meet the unique needs of the chronically ill or handicapped in an effective and cost-efficient manner. These, too, would be valuable additions to the education of student and resident physicians. Their presence and integration with centers of medical education could provide a more complete health care system for the chronically ill or handicapped and a balanced educational model.

Care-by-Parent Units. In a few schools care-by-parent units provide a unique opportunity for students to interact with the patient and family in a more homelike environment (Caldwell and Lockhart, 1981). Functionally integrated with the ambulatory care delivery system, the care-by-parent unit at the University of Texas Medical Branch provides needed short-term care at one third less cost and complements efforts to avoid disruption of family life while maintaining quality medical care. For example, this unit has proved to be a convenient place for the child with hemophilia to receive clotting factor supplements, for the child with asthma to recover following an acute episode, for the child with a malignancy to receive chemotherapy, or for education of the child with diabetes after initial acute problems have been controlled in the hospital. The unit can be used for diagnostic procedures such as heart studies, biopsies, or minor surgery. Such units extend the capabilities of ambulatory care units, have proved their value, and are greatly appreciated by patients and their families. Unfortunately, they operate on a tenuous basis because they lack consistent and adequate financial support.

Camps for Chronically Ill Children. A significantly underutilized education opportunity for demonstrating the special medical needs of the chronically ill child is the summer (or weekend) camp. These camps operate near most medical schools and are usually well staffed by recreational and general counselors. Adding staff to meet the chronically ill child's medical needs is a realistic and effective educational opportunity for professionals at all levels. Faculty, fellows, residents, students, and allied health personnel can work together and learn firsthand about the children by being with them around the clock. The intense learning experience usually produces lifelong interest, concern, and deep appreciaton of the chronically ill child as a person. Children's diabetic, renal dialysis, epilepsy, obesity, and hemophilia camps are examples that have clearly demonstrated the educational principle to all learners fortunate enough to participate. For adolescents and young adults, whose needs are different, the long weekend camp or retreat provides a similar opportunity for learning and personal growth.

Chronic Illness as a Curriculum Discipline. Underlying academic problems in planning a curriculum to meet the needs of the chronically ill is unwillingness to recognize chronic illness care as a specific body of knowledge. Chronic illness does not fit the classic concepts of a disease or dysfunction of a discrete organ or system. Traditional organization of teaching along the lines of etiology, pathophysiology, differential diagnosis, and specific management does not attend to all the needs of patients. However, if the chronically ill require a plan of individualized, dynamic, comprehensive, and continuing care, then an entity takes shape. Teamwork and continuity of care are basic objectives necessary to plan a substantive curriculum. The key words are *individual* and *planned.* The student and resident must be led to recognize that these patients are constantly part ill and part well—but never free of a problem that sets them apart. Their families, their social interactions, their educations, and their daily routines are different from those of their peers. Sometimes the secondary and acquired psychosocial problems are more debilitating than the primary disease or handicap. Medical problems take on unusual dimensions and facets. The physician's responsibility is to minimize the differences when possible and to help the patient and family cope when the condition cannot be ameliorated. Viewed in this manner, chronic disease instruction includes sufficient substance to be accorded a substantial place in the medical curriculum.

Visibility. A contributor to low visibility for chronic illness instruction in the medical curriculum is the teaching hospital's tendency to be opportunistic and to use whatever patients and resources it has as models for instruction. Thus, when a chronic illness is encountered, it is usually addressed principally in terms of the acute problem that led to the admission. For example, the child with asthma or congenital heart disease might be extensively studied during symptomatic periods that require sophisticated specialty care but might be relatively forgotten once the acute problem is contained and emphasis shifts to comprehensive and continuing primary care. A significant contributing factor to this care deficiency is the absence of a strong professional advocate on the faculty to teach the student long-term health care planning. The training of primary care professionals for this role must be strengthened. A solution, long used in other areas of medical education, is the educational subsidy via career awards, fellowships, and special planning grants in the field of care delivery to chronically ill children and their families. This approach has worked well in psychiatry, public health, basic research, and several specific clinical areas. It should be given a trial in improving education for care of the chronically ill child at medical school and graduate education levels.

Balancing the Curriculum. A growing number of pediatric residency programs seek to achieve a balanced emphasis on education for acute and tertiary care and for comprehensive care of the chronically ill. This includes planning to eliminate the conflict experienced by the trainee who has concurrent responsibility for the care of acutely and chronically ill patients. The needs of the former often create a sense of urgency that takes precedence in the mind of the trainee over the needs of the chronically ill or handicapped child. To avoid this competition, the University of Texas Medical Branch pediatric residency training program has established a six-month general pediatrics block. During this period, residents have no responsibility other than the study and delivery of general pediatric care. Included in their personal panel of patients are a representative variety of patients with chronic conditions. As in many other programs, residents are relieved of hospital inpatient duties one to two half-days each week throughout the three years of residency to return to the model practice to see panel patients. The learning experience enables trainees to focus full attention on continuous care of chronically ill patients. They also spend time as consultants to public school administrative and health personnel. Faculty and allied health associates with special expertise in child development, behavior problems, adolescent medicine, and community pediatrics are available to assist in day-to-day care of individual patients and families.

Chronic Care Research. Learners generally react favorably to new ideas that are based on research findings. Research training improves patient care and polishes trainees' knowledge and skills. It creates an optimism that things can change and an excitement that new solutions will be found. In general, the cost of well-planned research is small compared to the benefits derived (Pless and Zvagulis, 1981; Nelson and Stein, 1982).

Recommendations: What Can and Should Be Done

Education of professionals to give high-quality care to chronically ill children and their families should be a national health priority. Those who make policy and allocate resources have an obligation to remove these children from "have not" minority status and to give them full opportunity to be productive citizens. As a nation, we have the scientific base and the professional motivation to give better care to this segment of our population, and this goal is worthy and attainable from economic, social, and humanitarian standpoints.

Education of professionals to support these goals can best be addressed in five related parts: facilities, faculties, financing, curriculum, and research.

Facilities for Care of Chronically Ill Children

Needs:

- Teaching and care-delivery centers must be designed to meet the special care needs of the chronically ill child. This task involves planning for convenient access of physicians and other health professionals to each another and to their patients in an ambiance quite different from that of the acute care hospital or clinic, an environment that provides a concentration of the special programs and personnel needed by the chronically ill child. Such facilities would heighten the visibility of chronic care and direct students toward such care as a career.
- Chronic health care programs for children must be consolidated to increase efficiency, convenience, and visibility.

Recommendations:

- Use planning grants to develop innovative methods for consolidation of existing fragmented chronic care and to identify gaps that need to be eliminated.
- Use remodeling grants to upgrade the design of facilities to permit more efficient use of personnel and resources.
- Revise existing chronic illness care guidelines so they no longer arbitrarily separate the care of children with similar basic needs.

Faculties to Teach Chronic Illness Care

Needs:

- Faculty educational programs for care for the chronically ill must be strengthened; this step is essential to overall improvements in the quality of care or of professional education.

- There is a shortage of faculty to plan for chronic care delivery, to communicate chronic care skills to students, and to demonstrate the ideal care of the chronically ill child. The number of such faculty must be increased to a critical level so service and teaching responsibilities can be accomplished without sacrificing research and other essential scholarly activities. Only in this way can chronic illness care programs for children develop the intellectual excitement necessary to attract the best and most motivated trainees.

Recommendation:

- Give priority to the allocation of funds to career development and research grants to support faculty and trainees.

Financing of Chronic Illness Care

Needs:

- The environments for education and patient care are so closely related that medical education cannot be improved without improving these resources. Currently, the teaching hospital's income is tied mainly to in-hospital, acute, procedure-oriented care. This leaves us with a patchwork or hand-me-down system for long-term care of the chronically ill that not only neglects these members of our society but also denigrates the importance of their care in the eyes of students and teachers.
- The current medical education system has little or no fat—it is a lean, sometimes undernourished institution. To redirect funds from established educational activities to chronic care would not be a step forward.

Recommendations:

- Create a separate, broad-based system to assure direct new financing for all aspects of the care of chronically ill children. The system must reward comprehensive and continuous care, at least to the degree that current systems reward procedural aspects of health care.
- Place funding for counseling, coordination of care, and health maintenance on a par with that for other essential aspects of medical care. Present health care financing systems are largely blind to the chronically ill child. New programs must recognize the importance of reaching beyond the hosptial environment into the community (for recreation, education, and social contacts) to permit a full spectrum of care and training opportunities. Shifting educational emphasis in this manner to primary care without new resources would denigrate overall curriculum and quality of care and would serve our children poorly.
- Grant funding only to institutions that show evidence of planning for comprehensive care, attention to psychological needs of children, and community linkages with other childcare agencies.
- Revise guidelines that tend to act as barriers so that chronic care delivery can achieve economy; currently, such guidelines artificially segregate the care of chronically ill children from the care of others with similar needs—such as

social work, psychological counseling, school placement, developmental evaluation, and preventive medical care—simply because their illness or handicap has a different name.

Curriculum

Needs:

- The knowledge that scientist-educators already possess must be integrated with educational goals of curriculum.
- Knowledge and skills required of physicians and others who care for chronically ill children must be carefully examined, and a parallel system for evaluating learning must be established. The next task is to identify the learning environments and experiences that enable the student to progress from objectives to competence.

Recommendation:

- Establish grants or contracts in a limited number of institutions with faculty interested in studying and designing new curriculum elements and new models for care of chronically ill children.

Research

Research is considered last because it is an element of each of the aforementioned needs and of many of the recommendations. Research related to the education of professionals to care for the chronically ill is difficult to find and limited in scope. No field can move forward in the absence of a substantial research and development program.

Needs:

- Research at many levels must be encouraged.
- Current management programs must be examined to see whether they are appropriate and efficient.
- The long-term outcome of medical intervention needs to be critically monitored.
- New approaches to care need to be thoroughly evaluated.

These needs are the traditional responsibilities of faculty, but if investments in research are to be profitable, the professionals involved must be critically prepared through supervised training in research methods.

Recommendation:

- Extend the concept of research awards, fellowships, grants, and contracts into all aspects of the study of the health care of the chronically ill child.

Summary

The pediatrician's goal for treating the chronically ill or handicapped is to help the child and family achieve the best adjustment possible in their particular circumstances. The problems are so important to a significant segment of the population that they are worthy of careful analysis, our best efforts, and a substantial allocation of resources.

Education and the delivery of patient care are intimately linked, dynamic processes. Both the academic community and the public must accept responsibility for implementing and accepting change based on the comprehensive health needs of patients and families. Curriculum revision must be based on careful consideration of goals so that appropriate educational strategies will be selected and bureaucratic and financial barriers to a balanced educational experience will be surmounted. Rigid definitions and categories of support are major barriers both to ideal care and to the education of the physician. Although most educators, students, and practitioners recognize the unique value of ambulatory and community-based care as preparation for pediatric practice, they are frustrated by the absence of a system to finance this training experience.

References

American Board of Pediatrics. *Foundations for Evaluating the Competency of Pediatricians.* Chapel Hill, N.C.: American Board of Pediatrics, 1974.

Battle, C.U. "The Role of the Pediatrician as Ombudsman in the Health Care of the Young Handicapped Child." *Pediatrics,* 1972, *50,* 916–922.

Caldwell, B., and Lockhart, L. "A Care-by-Parent Unit: Its Planning, Implementation and Patient Satisfaction." *Children's Health Care,* 1981, *10,* 4–7.

Hadley, J., Mullner, R., and Feder, J. "Special Report: The Financially Distressed Hospital." *New England Journal of Medicine,* 1982, *307,* 1283–1287.

Kempe, C. "The Future of Pediatric Education." *Pediatric Research,* 1978, *12,* 1149–1151.

Kempe, C. H., and Olmsted, R. W. (Eds.). *The Future of Pediatric Education: A Report by the Task Force on Pediatric Education.* Evanston, Ill.: Task Force on Pediatric Education, 1978.

Kutner, N. G. "Medical Students' Orientation Toward the Chronically Ill." *Journal of Medical Education,* 1978, *53,* 111–118.

Mattsson, A. "Long-Term Physical Illness in Childhood: A Challenge to Psychosocial Adaptation." *Pediatrics,* 1972, *50,* 801–811.

Nelson, R. D., and Stein, R.E.K., "Workshop on Children with Special Needs." In L. V. Klerman (Ed.), *Research Priorities in Maternal and Child Health.* Waltham, Mass.: Brandeis University, 1982.

Pless, I. B. "Epidemiology of Chronic Disease." In M. Green and R. J. Haggerty (Eds.), *Ambulatory Pediatrics.* Philadelphia: Saunders, 1968.

Pless, I. B., and Roghmann, K. J. "Chronic Illness and Its Consequences:

Observations Based on Three Epidemiologic Surveys." *Journal of Pediatrics,* 1971, *79,* 351–359.

Pless, I. B., and Zvagulis, I. "The Health of Children with Special Needs." In L. V. Klerman (Ed.), *Research Priorities in Maternal and Child Health.* Waltham, Mass.: Brandeis University, 1982.

Rutter, M., Tizard, J., and Whitmore, K. *Handicapped Children: A Total Population Prevalence Study of Education, Physical and Behavioral Disorders.* London: Longman, 1968.

Steinhauer, P. D., and others. "Psychological Aspects of Chronic Illness." *Pediatric Clinics of North America,* 1974, *21,* 825–840.

Wright, G. F., and Vanderpool, N. "Schools and the Pediatrician." *Pediatric Clinics of North America,* 1981, *28*(3), 643–662.

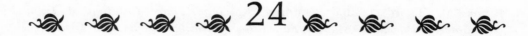

24

Nursing Services

Debra P. Hymovich, Ph.D., R.N., F.A.A.N

Nurses are in a unique position to contribute substantially toward meeting the total needs of families of children with chronic illnesses. They are prepared to understand the medical needs of children as well as the psychosocial needs of children and families. Nursing care strategies are taught that enable nurses to provide direct physical care to children, to assist parents and children regarding management of the child's condition, and to guide and support families. Nurses are taught to use a systematic process of assessing, planning, implementing, and evaluating the care they provide. They function in a wide variety of settings— within institutions as well as in community agencies, in public and private settings, and in interdependent and independent roles. Nurses are prepared to care for children who are healthy and acutely or critically ill as well as those who have chronic illnesses. Graduates of baccalaureate programs are prepared to be consumers of nursing research; nurses with master's and doctoral degrees are prepared to participate in and conduct research.

Although it appears that nurses are in a position to make a significant impact on chronically ill children, their families, and their communities, there is relatively little documentation regarding the effectiveness of this impact. It is evident from various interviews with parents and from my own personal contact with many parents across the country, that nurses are not always providing the care needed by families of chronically ill youngsters. The reasons most often cited for this state of affairs are lack of time, inadequate facilities, other priorities, a fragmented care system, and shortage of nursing personnel. In addition to the limitations existing within the systems in which they practice, it is apparent that

I am grateful for the assistance of Gloria A. Hagopian, R.N., Ed.D., in the preparation of this manuscript.

many nurses have inadequate preparation for managing the multiple stresses associated with childhood chronic illness and its impact on families and on the children themselves.

The purpose of this chapter is to review the literature regarding the role of nurses in providing care to chronically ill youngsters and their families, identify the issues involved in providing this nursing care, and make recommendations for policies related to nursing services for chronically ill children and their families.

A search of the professional literature from 1966 to 1981 yielded 423 articles related to the role of the nurse in the care of children with chronic illnesses. Only 100 articles were listed for the eight years between 1966 and 1974; the remaining 323 articles were written after 1974. The increased number of articles in the last six years in part may reflect the increasing number of nursing journals, but it also reflects a changing focus in nursing to meet the psychosocial as well as physical needs of chronically ill children and their families. The majority of articles are based on experience and include case studies and the opinions of authors regarding the role nurses should play in caring for these children and their families. A small number of articles describe specific programs and their impact on families, and several report needs identified by nurses to improve their nursing care to chronically ill children and their families. Only a few articles published by nurses since 1975 are reports of research findings.

Several recent trends are altering the practice of pediatric nursing within institutions, communities, and society. Changes have come about because of new beliefs concerning nursing and the nurse's role in providing high-quality care and because of technological and scientific advances in medical care. Among the major trends are (1) development of highly specialized areas within pediatric nursing, (2) emphasis on the total needs of the child and the entire family unit, (3) utilization of a systematic and deliberative nursing process in planning and providing care, (4) development of Standards of Care for Maternal and Child Health Nursing Practice (1973), (5) changing patterns of childhood illness and therapy, (6) changes in the roles and relationships of a variety of individuals and groups (including consumers) in planning and providing care, and (7) increasing emphasis on nursing theory and research as a means of improving practice. These trends are reflected in the current and emerging nursing role.

Components of the Nursing Role

Nurses perform certain functions regardless of setting or specialty area. Various components of the nursing role identified in the literature and documented in practice include direct caregiving, providing guidance and support, casefinding, patient education, consultation, coordination, collaboration, and serving as client advocate. The nurse's role as a researcher is also emerging in practice.

In practice, nurses are engaged in many of these components at one time. The complexity of role functions is frequently mentioned. For example, Schnackel (1979) described her role as a pediatric diabetic specialist as one of clinician, consultant, educator, and researcher. Wasteney (1970) provides another example of multiple roles, also in relation to children with diabetes. A school nurse, she provided direct care by treating insulin reactions, taught the child about the condition, supported and guided the mother, and contacted teachers and other school personnel regarding the child's needs.

In an attempt to describe the role components of health professionals working with chronically ill children and their families, Schadt (1980) collected ninety-seven critical incident descriptions from twenty-one registered nurses and five social workers. Analysis of the data revealed five components of the nurse's role: collaboration with others regarding assessment and management of the child's condition, referral of the child or family to others who could provide direct care, and offering support, teaching, and modification of child or parent behavior. Nurses under thirty years of age and those with baccalaureate degrees used support significantly more often than did diploma or master's prepared nurses, while diploma nurses used collaboration more frequently. Nurses tended to use support as an intervention strategy more frequently with younger families and collaboration more often with families of school-aged youngsters. The support category included behaviors such as "lending strength, acting as an advocate, and providing encouragement" (p. 42). Collaboration involved contacting and discussing the family with lay persons and other health care professionals.

Direct Caregiving. The direct caregiving component of the nurse's role spans a wide range of assessment, planning, intervention, and evaluation activities. Direct care includes such activities as obtaining health histories, performing physical examinations, monitoring vital signs, administering medications, performing treatments, preventing infection, and maintaining adequate nutrition and balance. Much nursing literature related to direct caregiving includes discussion of the nature of the chronic condition and its therapeutic management along with descriptions of how to carry out the nursing care. Evidence of the effectiveness of this direct caregiving is presented in the literature primarily through descriptions of personal experience. Actual research documentation of effective outcomes for the child is frequently lacking.

Increasingly, nurses are becoming involved in developing sensory stimulation programs for a variety of infants who are slow to develop (Durand, 1975; Eddington, 1975; Godfrey, 1975). These programs are being developed in home settings as well as in hospitals.

Providing Guidance and Support. Nurses provide guidance and support for the children and their parents and siblings. Activities that reflect the nurse's role in supporting and guiding children include setting limits; preparing children for hospitalizations, procedures, and surgery; and providing sensory stimulation and play therapy. Again, the effectiveness of these activities is documented primarily through case studies and descriptions of personal experiences with children.

For example, Petrillo (1968) concluded that therapeutic play led children to "demonstrate an acceptance of staff members, an ability to participate in their treatments, and a capacity to express their feelings. They are less preoccupied with procedures and illness than was formerly the case, and have a greater capacity for socialization and more interest in play. Tolerance for reasonable periods of separation from parents has also been apparent. Children who are admitted repeatedly for chronic illness adjust more readily since they have already mastered many of their hospitalization fears" (p. 1473). No studies with control groups are cited to validate these conclusions.

Play as an assessment, teaching, and therapeutic tool is frequently used by nurses in outpatient settings (Gnus, 1973; Taylor and Williams, 1980) and inpatient settings (David, 1973; Dittemore, 1973; Knudsen, 1975; Nelson, 1972; Sullivan, 1972). In a case presentation, Conlin (1980) has shown that role-playing activities such as feeding, bathing, and giving injections changed the behavior of one four-year-old from fighting to cooperating with treatments. Studies such as those by Wolfer and Visintainer (1975) and Johnson, Kirchhoff, and Endress (1975, 1976) provide evidence that the guidance and support component of the nursing role can be effective in reducing a child's stress during hospitalization or when procedures have to be performed.

Patient and Professional Education. Nurses in all settings are involved in teaching children and their parents about the child's disease and its treatment, how to perform procedures and provide physical care, observations to be made, normal growth and development, and how to manage psychosocial responses to stress and crisis (Altshuler, Meyer, and Butz, 1977; Bivalec and Berkman, 1976; Leiner and Rahmer, 1968; Leahey, Logan, and McArthur, 1975; Lee, 1978; McFarlane, 1975; Wasteney, 1970).

A number of nurses have documented the effectiveness of their teachings. Altshuler, Meyer, and Butz (1977) describe teaching school-aged children with myelomeningocele and spinal cord injuries to perform clean intermittent self-catheterization. Children were admitted to the hospital for three to seven days to learn the procedure. Parents of preschool children were taught to catheterize their hospitalized youngsters in a twenty-four- to forty-eight-hour period. Close contact with the family following discharge was maintained by the clinic nurse. Of fifty-five children taught the self-catheterization procedure, thirty-seven were dry more than 80 percent of the time and an additional six were dry about 80 percent of the time. Eleven were dry less than 80 percent of the time or the family found the program unacceptable, and one child with hydrocephalus died from an unrelated problem. The authors concluded that "the technique frees [the children] of wet clothing, urine odor, attendant skin problems, and social embarrassment. They are able to participate more fully in peer activities and to feel more like children their own age. The program costs far less than most efforts aimed at maintaining bladder control" (p. 101).

Parfitt and Thompson (1980) described the assessment and instruction necessary before sending a child home on total parenteral nutrition (TPN). The child, a two-year-old girl, was able to be discharged from the hospital, thus saving the family considerable expense and enabling the child to participate in many family activities that are normal at her age. Wheeler (1977) has shown that parents could be taught to carry out home hemodialysis for their eight-year-old son, eliminating the need for the family to travel sixty miles to clinic three days a week and enabling the boy to attend school on a more regular basis.

Pridham (1971), in a case study of a youngster with juvenile diabetes mellitus, stressed the importance of assessing a child's readiness to learn and of applying principles of teaching and learning theories when working with individual children. The nurse's use of age-appropriate tools in teaching children is mentioned by Greene (1975).

Nurses play an active role in providing parents with anticipatory and continuing education. For example, Bindler (1979) described her role in teaching parents of a child with a cardiac defect about feeding practices, symptoms of cardiac distress, medications, and physical, social, and cognitive development. For parents of children with seizure disorders, Slimmer (1979) provided information about the stages of a child's adaptation to a chronic illness and behavior that reflects these stages.

Nurses use a wide range of strategies when teaching parents, including the use of anatomical models, drawings, booklets (Peterson, 1979), audiovisual materials, and demonstrations. Books, such as those of Pohl (1968) and Redman (1980, 1981), have been written to help nurses learn to apply teaching and learning principles.

Nurses teach not only children and their families but also aides and volunteers (Tonyan, 1967), staff nurses (Case, 1969), and community members (Greene, 1975). Stiles, Lierman, and Austin (1982) described a one-year program to prepare community health nurses to work with at-risk, chronically ill and developmentally disabled youngsters. This program, which included a didactic portion followed by a six-month practicum in conjunction with the participants' jobs, resulted in expansion of the participants' direct-care roles in their community as well as their resource, consultation, and in-service education roles.

Casefinding. Nurses play a role in casefinding, both in terms of identifying children with chronic illness and in determining the unmet health needs of handicapped children (Macdonough, 1978) and their families (Hymovich, 1981). In 1968, Healy suggested that much of the public health nurse's casefinding was fortuitous rather than planned. However, Williamson (1978) has described a specific role for the school nurse in screening for early health problems. Little has been written about the nurse's role in discovering secondary psychosocial problems of the child and family. Hymovich (1981, 1983) has developed and is testing a tool to assist nurses in assessing these secondary problems.

Consultation. Nurses describe consultation with colleagues as part of their role in caring for chronically ill children. However, as with other components of the nursing role, the specific nature of this consultation as it pertains to childhood chronic illness is not well documented.

Examples have been described primarily by mental health nurses. Deloughery (1973) described community mental health nurses consulting with teachers of physically handicapped children. The focus of the consultations was on the feelings of teachers, such as isolation, lack of recognition, failure, guilt, and ambivalence. Although there was little documentation of the outcome of this consultation service, at the end of the year the nursing students, teachers, and administrators recommended the program be continued.

Hedlund (1978), a psychiatric nurse, described a demonstration project in which she served as a consultant to nurses working with adult patients in a general hospital. Her primary role was to help these nurses understand the psychosocial aspects of their nursing care. She concluded that following the group discussions the nurses showed improvement in the following areas: data collection, finding explanations for behavior, developing nursing care plans, and communicating. They also demonstrated better understanding of their own feelings and the reactions of their patients, and they were better able to help patients solve problems.

Coordination and Collaboration. Nurses frequently discuss the importance of their role in coordinating the care of chronically ill children and their families and in collaborating with others in order to improve patient care. An example was described by Foley and McCarthy (1976) for children with hematological problems. Collaboration between an inpatient primary nurse and an outpatient clinic nurse promoted continuity of care and facilitated the nurses' understanding of how chronic illness affects children and their families.

In 1972, Hope and Hughes described a collaborative relationship among a public health nurse, a pediatric nurse practitioner (PNP), and two pediatricians in a community, extending the agency's and pediatricians' support and services to children and families. This effort enabled families to receive more comprehensive care than they had before. The pediatricians were able to devote more time to sick children while the nurses concentrated on providing guidance and counseling to adolescents and helping parents with such problems as housing, marital difficulties, and inadequate income.

Client Advocacy. Nurses in a variety of positions and settings function as advocates for chronically ill children and their families. It has been suggested that advocacy is the primary responsibility of clinic nurses working with families of crippled children (Dominquez and Perrin, 1973). Part of the advocacy role involves helping children and families understand and manipulate the systems providing care to them.

An example of how this advocacy component was incorporated into the role of the school nurse was described by Switzer and Kelly (1981). The nurse incorporated parental feeling and opinions into her recommendations to the school's child study team. At the team meeting, the nurse helped parents express their opinions and concerns and encouraged the team to consider the home situation in recommendations. The nurse also helped the family by interpreting the school's programs and positions to the parents.

Research. There is a trend toward increasing emphasis on nursing theory and research as a means of improving practice. Nurses are being prepared at the undergraduate level to critique and use research findings in their practice. At the master's and doctoral levels, nurses are being prepared to conduct independent and collaborative research studies.

Several journals, such as *Nursing Research, Western Journal of Nursing Research, Research in Nursing and Health,* and *Image,* are devoted exclusively to nursing theory and research articles. The clinical application of research findings as well as methodology are also reported frequently in other nursing journals, such as the *American Journal of Nursing, Maternal Child Nursing,* and *Issues in Comprehensive Pediatric Nursing.*

Some recent nursing research has relevance for the care of chronically ill children and their families. Hymovich (1981, 1983) has developed an assessment tool to be used with parents of chronically ill children, and Hart, Fearing, and Graham (1976) suggested nursing interventions based on the relationship of developmental tasks and identity control to adjustment to hemodialysis. Bernard and others (1981) looked at the effects of a physical education program for children with physical disabilities. The impact of childhood chronic illness on well siblings has been studied by Iles (1979) and Taylor (1980). In collaborative studies, nurses have looked at the psychosocial adjustment of latency-aged children with diabetes (Grey, Genel, and Tamborlane, 1980) and evaluated a comprehensive program for handicapped children (Perrin and others, 1972).

Other nursing studies, although not specifically directed toward chronic illness, have implications for nursing intervention. For example, Craft (1981) studied the preferences of adolescents for information providers, Pidgeon (1977) looked at the implications of the characteristics of children's thinking for health teaching, and Hymovich (1980) studied the effects of two types of nursing organization (team and primary nursing) on the perceptions that children, mothers, and nurses had of the nursing role. Nurses have studied the effectiveness of various methods of preparing children for hospitalization (Ferguson, 1979; Wolfer and Visintainer, 1975) and means of altering children's distress behavior during cast removal (Johnson, Kirchhoff, and Endress, 1975).

Expanding Roles of Nurses

Nursing roles and relationships have been changing within the profession of nursing itself, along interdisciplinary lines, and in relation to consumer needs. As noted earlier, specialization in pediatric nursing has been increasing. Nursing specialties are developing along three lines: according to age groups, according to medical problems, and according to practice settings. Changing patterns of childhood illness and therapy are reflected in the emerging nursing specialties. In relation to age groups, for example, the special requirements of premature infants and high-risk newborns and the establishment of neonatal intensive care centers have led to nurses specializing in the care of these vulnerable infants. Other nurses are focusing on the needs of adolescents, while still others concentrate on the needs of preschool or school-aged youngsters. Nursing specialties are proliferating in relation to specific medical problems. Some nurse clinicians or specialists devote their skills to the care of children with problems related to specific systems (such as the nervous or respiratory system), certain organs (such as the heart), or to specific conditions (such as cystic fibrosis, juvenile diabetes, burns, or cancer). Specialty groups are being formed by nurses interested in specific problems, and nurses are becoming more involved in interdisciplinary specialty groups. Other nurses, such as pediatric nurse practitioners, specialize in promoting the health of well children and managing some of their acute illnesses. Nursing specialties have also developed according to the location or setting of the practice, such as intensive care units, schools, or homes and in ambulatory or inpatient hospital settings. Some nurses are transcending traditional settings and are moving between locations (for example, between inpatient and outpatient units or between clinics and homes).

Nurse Practitioners. Perhaps the best known and most widespread change within the profession has been the preparation of the pediatric nurse practitioner (PNP). The PNP role was designed to increase the quality, availability, and accessibility of child health care in the United States. According to the Statement on Scope of Practice, the PNP promotes the psychosocial, physical, and developmental well-being of children by functioning as a practitioner, as a collaborative member of the health team, and as an advocate of child health in the community ("Scope of Practice Statements for PNP's Issued," 1974).

Some evidence supports the effectiveness of adding a PNP to a clinic caring for chronically ill children. For example, Rodgers (1979) reviewed the charts of forty-seven children before, and one year after, a PNP joined the clinic staff. She used seven of Myers's eight criterion measures of good pediatric care: birthweight, gestational age, immunization status, social history, nutritional history, growth chart, and tine test. During the two years prior to employment of the PNP, 95 percent of the records were missing four or more of the criterion measures compared with 21 percent of the records one year after her employment. The PNP was also able to help twenty of twenty-three previously incontinent school-aged children gain improved bowel continence. There was a decrease in the number of long-term hospital admissions (more than ten days) from thirty-five to fifteen and an increase in short-term admissions (less than three days) from seventeen to twenty-six after addition of the PNP to the clinic. It was difficult to document the PNP's effect on psychosocial adjustment of children and their parents because of the lack of precise measurements. Previously unrecognized or untreated psychosocial problems of parents and children were identified by the PNP, but the effectiveness of her intervention was not measured.

Venes and Rodgers (1975) described the functions of the PNP in the Spina Bifida Center at the Yale–New Haven Hospital. The PNP visited the home following the birth of an infant with a myelomeningocele and hydrocephalus to assist the mother in carrying out prescribed therapy. She also evaluated the needs of the infant and family and provided encouragement and reassurance to the parents. Her role in the clinic included obtaining specimens, instructing the mother, working with the school, and administering the clinic.

Wood (1978) described the role of the PNP in an outpatient clinic for children with cancer, and Lee (1978) described a similar role with adolescents with diabetes. Both nurses stressed the teaching role of the practitioner. Wood mentioned the physical assessment and history-taking components of her role whereas Lee stressed her role in assessment, responsibility for total care, collaboration with the physician, and making appropriate referrals. Neither author documented the effectiveness of care in terms of client outcome.

Sedlacek (1978) described the main functions of a school nurse working with children with asthma—assessing the child's health status, planning for a healthful school environment for the child, and managing problems as they arose. Wasteney (1970) described a similar role for a nurse working with a child with diabetes. The nurse treated the child's insulin reactions, taught the child about diabetes and its treatment, supported and guided the mother, and contacted teachers and other school personnel regarding the child's needs. School nurses are also involved in casefinding. One group of school nurses found that students whose handicapping conditions had been monitored and treated still have many unidentified health needs, including vision, hearing, and dental defects as well as subclinical chronic illnesses (Macdonough, 1978).

Continuing education programs are being designed to increase the knowledge base and clinical competence of school nurses, whose role in working with chronically ill and handicapped children has expanded as a result of Public Law 94–142 (the Education for All Handicapped Children Act). One program, described by Procci, Magary, and Tucker (1981), involved 610 school nurses from Los Angeles County who attended a continuing education program developed to assist them in meeting the challenges of the law. The overall program was evaluated by criterion-referenced tests, training session evaluation forms, self-assessment of clinical competence, and observation by supervisors and program staff. Nurses reported increased clinical competence with handicapped children; nursing supervisors observed changes in the nurses' skills and performance levels over the course of the year; and program staff noted greater problem-solving skills and interest in starting new health education programs for handicapped children.

King, Spaulding, and Wright (1974) delineated the functions of the PNP in a clinic for children with diabetes. Direct-care tasks included taking clinical histories, doing physical examinations, and assisting the child in self-care activities. Activities related to the team included functioning as team leader, initiating and coordinating care plans, arranging team conferences, selecting topics and chairing meetings, and deciding which team member clients would see and when they would see them.

Cortez, Mendoza, and Muniz (1975) discussed the expanded roles of nurses in caring for children with cardiac problems. Registered nurses were prepared in an eight-month program as Pediatric Cardiology Associates (PCA) followed by a four-month Pediatric Nurse Practitioner program. The PCAs were responsible for screening and preliminary evaluations of the children, counseling parents, seeing patients in the inpatient areas, and providing home visits following surgery. The PCAs enabled the Children's Heart Program of South Texas to increase its patient population while maintaining a high quality of care. A chart audit indicated that 85 percent of the PCA assessments were accurate as compared with 90 percent of the physician assessments. The authors recommend that "more nurses be trained and work with physicians as P.C.A.s, or their counterparts, to improve the total concept of patient care and health care delivery systems" (p. 29).

School Nurses. A description of the School Nurse Practitioner includes the following functions: screening children for early identification of health problems; performing physical examinations for children in special education classes; and helping handicapped children, their parents, and teachers adjust to the school setting.

The School Nurse Achievement Program, which is the nationwide program designed to prepare nurses to care for handicapped children, is directed by Judith Igoe (1980), a school nurse practitioner in Denver. It consists of programmed learning booklets developed by nurses working with children who have a variety of chronic conditions. The learning modules are designed to provide school nurses with basic knowledge of the diseases, their treatment, and the nurse's role in working with the children. The program has been pilot tested in a number of U.S. cities, and the content has been upgraded to be meaningful for nurses with master's degrees. Documentation of the effectiveness of this large-scale project is not yet available.

Clinical Specialists. Clinical nurse specialists have master's level educational preparation and are able to explore and test the scientific theories on which their practice is based. They are prepared to study and solve complex problems systematically. According to the American Nurses' Association (1980, p. 11), "The nursing specialist is able to synthesize from a broad knowledge base and relate additional theories, knowledge, and skills to the clinical practice role. The nursing specialist participates with others in evaluating availability, accessibility, and acceptability of services to parents and children, and providing leadership in extending and developing needed services in the community."

The Secretary's Committee to Study Expanded Roles of Nurses suggested that, in the future, many nurse practitioners in acute care settings would routinely take health and developmental histories, perform basic physical and psychosocial assessments, translate findings into appropriate nursing actions, and make and carry out decisions about treatment in collaboration with physicians (Lysaught, 1973). There are some clinical nurse specialists who currently carry out these functions in hospital inpatient and outpatient settings.

Schnackel (1979) described her role as a clinical nurse specialist working with children with diabetes. She applied physiological principles and psychosocial and sociological theories in planning and delivering nursing care directly and indirectly to children and their families. As an educator she imparted information to families, nursing staff, and nursing students through formal classes and informal contacts. She also spoke to community groups and was available to nurses, parents, and community members within and outside of the hospital.

The role of a clinical specialist involved in group therapy for parents of children with leukemia was described by Bushman (1976). She and a child psychiatrist served as cotherapists in helping parents explore their feelings about their children, the disease and its treatment, and the personnel with whom they came in contact. Greene (1975) described her role as an oncology clinical nurse specialist. She described herself as skilled in physical assessment; performing procedures such as bone marrow aspirations, lumbar punctures, and venipunctures; providing support to child and family; and serving as a liaison between school and home. She was also actively involved in family and community education.

Home Care: The Impact of Nursing

The trend toward having children cared for in their homes rather than in institutions requires that someone be available to families at the time they need help. Nurses are often the logical people to be called upon because of their role in direct care and patient teaching and because of their availability through visiting nurse associations and public health departments. At times, nurses in outpatient clinics and nurses from hospital inpatient units are available to make home visits.

Schraeder (1979) described preparing the parents of eleven ventilator-dependent children in a pediatric intensive care unit for discharge. Parents were actively involved in developing the plan for their preparation. It was possible to discharge eight of the eleven children, providing them with a more normal home environment without compromising their respiratory status while reducing their cost of care and freeing the hospital beds for others.

The McMaster Diabetic Day Care Centre in Hamilton, Ontario, (King, Spaulding, and Wright, 1974) is an interdisciplinary center established to provide assessment, education, and treatment services to children with juvenile diabetes and their families and to help with the psychosocial problems that interfere with diabetic control. The team is led by a nurse practitioner who initiates and coordinates the plan for each child. The center enabled most newly diagnosed juvenile diabetics to be managed without admission to the hospital, and nearly all the other problems of diabetics could be assessed and treated without hospital admission.

Martinson and others (1977) demonstrated the economic advantage of having home nursing services available to parents of children with cancer. The nurses made recommendations and suggestions regarding care of the child, taught specific aspects of the physical care, provided support to the parents, and helped them maintain a relationship with their dying child. Nurses made home visits and were available to the parents twenty-four hours a day by telephone. The cost of these home nursing services was $25 a day compared with $411 for children who were hospitalized. Lauer and Camitta (1980) have also demonstrated that home care, coordinated and delivered by a nurse, was a "feasible, desired, and effective alternative to hospitalization of many children" (p. 1032). They concluded that "the physical, psychologic, and emotional support required by families [of] children who are dying at home clearly falls into the capability of professional nursing" (p. 1034).

In another study of home care, Klopovich, Suenran, and Cairns (1980) reported that seven children with cancer cared for at home without the assistance of a community health nurse (CHN) had more complications than the seven children whose families were receiving the guidance of a CHN. In addition, the cost of care for children with the CHN was lower than that of the children without such care.

Wheeler (1977) described her role in helping parents of an eight-year-old boy requiring hemodialysis. She was able to allay their initial anxiety about taking their child home, to teach them to carry out the dialysis independently, and to establish appropriate ground rules for behavior of all family members. By being able to care for their child at home, the parents were saved the time and cost of commuting sixty miles to clinic three days a week, and the child was able to attend school more regularly. Similarly, Gross and Algrim (1980) described the beneficial effects of teaching a twelve-year-old boy to participate in home peritoneal dialysis.

Selected Issues of Concern to Nursing

A number of issues need to be addressed if nurses are to realize their full potential in providing services to chronically ill children and their families. Although it is possible to cite examples of how nurses provide a variety of services, it is clear that these practices are isolated and of variable quality. Specific issues to be considered in making policy recommendations are roles and relationships in health care, coordination of services, application of knowledge to practice, stresses in providing care, and the decision-making process.

Roles and Relationships in Health Care. The emerging interdisciplinary roles of nursing and medicine represent a reformulation by both professions in an effort to provide comprehensive care through the best utilization of each profession (Bates, 1970). Medical trends toward family and community medicine attempt to view patients from a broader perspective than just their physical disease. At the same time, nursing is extending its role into primary diagnosis and further into psychosocial care and has established a greater role in physical and assistive treatment areas. The best example of these emerging roles is the collaboration of pediatricians and pediatric nurse practitioners.

The challenges presented by these new role relationships are many, and it is essential to identify the challenges and seek ways to resolve them. Some problems are related to competition that will occur as nurses become increasingly assertive in seeking office space, organizational support, a fair share of the health care dollar, and a fair voice in the decision-making process. Issues related to territoriality and mutual respect need to be addressed, especially if the end result of collaboration and collegial relationships is to occur. "This new relationship will not come easily or naturally because the professions of nursing and medicine have for too long tacitly accepted assumptions and behaviors that are incompatible with the new model. This means simply that change must be planned, consciously accepted, and jointly executed. The fact that some practitioners are already utilizing the collaborative model is proof that it can work; the challenge is to overcome the inevitable inertia accumulated over so many years by dint of our traditional roles and functions" (Lysaught, 1973, p. 42).

Within the profession itself, issues regarding rules and relationships need to be addressed. There are not, as yet, any well-developed models to indicate the most effective and efficient ways to function. The trend toward developing highly specialized areas within pediatric nursing raises many questions for the profession: What types of clinical specialists are needed to care for the chronically ill? Do we need nurses who are generalists in the care of the chronically ill or those who are specialists in selected chronic illness problems, or some combination of these? How will generalists, primary health care providers such as PNPs, and specialists work with one another?

Coordination of Services. The complexity and size of the health care system necessitates good coordination to enable clients to move through the maze and obtain appropriate and necessary care that is of high quality. Children with long-term illness or disabling handicaps usually require a variety of services often widely scattered among different professional groups and public and private agencies and often over considerable distances. To bring diverse services to the aid of an individual child and family requires teamwork and active cooperation based on knowledge, mutual respect, and understanding.

Families of chronically ill children frequently see a variety of professionals, each involved with only a selected aspect of the child's or family's problem. Some families receive most or all of their care from specialists, others from primary care providers, while others have some combination of speciality and primary care plus the support of other services in the community. The result is often fragmented care, with overemphasis on the child's impairment and insufficient attention to all other aspects of family development and functioning. Because a primary focus of nursing is health maintenance, nurses can assume a leadership role in coordination of services to ensure continuity, comprehensiveness, and individualization of care. Nurses have the knowledge and abilities to assume key positions in coordinating such services, especially in view of the trend toward emphasizing the total needs of child and family.

Application of Knowledge to Practice. The theoretical base for nursing practice is derived from many disciplines including the biological, social, and medical sciences. Nursing is now beginning to develop its own theoretical base. The use of knowledge and principles from these various disciplines is synthesized through a systematic process of assessment, planning, diagnosis, intervention, and evaluation. Several trends are clearly evident in nursing as the ability to apply theoretical and factual information in practice continues to increase. All nurses are being taught to use this systematic and deliberative nursing process in providing care to their clients. The scope and depth of its use varies from simple to complex depending on the knowledge base of the nurse and the focus of care. The nursing process is clearly evident in the *Standards of Maternal and Child Health Nursing Practice* (American Nurses' Association, 1973). Equally evident in these standards is the focus on total care for child and family.

Numerous citations in nursing journals describe the underlying basis for intervention strategies identified. For example, knowledge of pathophysiology (including measures to prevent infection; minimize pain, bleeding, and nausea; and maintain hydration) is essential in providing care to children with leukemia (Brown, 1978; Foley and McCarthy, 1976). Other examples of application of knowledge to practice include use of crisis intervention techniques in counseling parents (Everson, 1977) and use of a conceptual framework in providing family-centered nursing care. Sciarillo (1980) described how his use of Hymovich's framework (1979) provided him with a family-centered, rather than child-centered approach to the care of twins failing to thrive. He indicated the outcome of such an approach was improvement in maternal-infant attachment, positive changes in the twins' emotional and cognitive development, and an increased energy level in the parents.

Sharpe (1973) described her work with a blind child and his family over a ten-month period. She was able to encourage attachment and locomotion through her use of research findings on educational techniques in development. As a result of her work the baby, at eighteen months, was able to feed himself, say words, name family members, and walk independently.

As nurses document their use of theory in practice, they also demonstrate the need to update knowledge and skills applicable to the care of chronically ill children and their families. For example, Moore and Triplett (1980) found that nurses wanted more information about students who returned to school after being diagnosed with cancer. The nurses indicated that their knowledge regarding students' physical needs was less thorough than their knowledge of their psychosocial needs.

It remains for nursing to identify and document in much greater detail the manner and extent to which theoretical knowledge is applied in practice. It is also essential to establish the specific knowledge and skill base needed by nurses with different levels of education and practicing in different roles.

Stresses in Providing Care. Caring for chronically ill children and their families can be challenging, rewarding, demanding, and frustrating. The progress made by children is often slow, and the outcome may be further disability, family disruption, and death. The situation often necessitates meeting crises without allowing sufficient time for helping families with long-term needs and goals. The intense care can lead to role stress for the nurse.

Goodell (1980) cites suffering of children, family criticism, and the death of children as sources of stress for the oncology nurse. A recent study (Goodell, 1979) of randomly selected nurses from pediatric oncology units in the United States revealed a staff of young, professionally inexperienced nurses with little background in raising and caring for children. Eighty-three percent of the nurses were under thirty years of age and 66 percent were single. Forty-eight percent had less than two years experience in nursing of children, 43 percent had less than three years experience in nursing, and 69 percent had been in oncology nursing for less than three years. Goodell concluded that there was a high turnover rate of pediatric oncology nurses and a lack of supportive educational programs.

There is a great need to provide supportive services to nurses so they will be able to continue to work with chronically ill children. Support sessions for nurses in neonatal intensive care units have been described by Wooten (1981).

The Decision-Making Process. Decisions regarding the care of chronically ill children and their families depend on society's values and social and political action. Because nursing helps serve society's interest in the area of health, it follows that nurses need to become more actively involved in the policy-making process. Policy decisions have an impact on the practice of nursing. Nurses are learning more about social and political action and the role they can play in the decision-making process. This new role for nurses should be fostered as rapidly as possible.

Policy Recommendations

1. Content pertinent to the care of chronically ill children and their families should be provided at all levels of student education programs in nursing including in-service education and continuing education programs. Necessary content includes
   a. updated information regarding the various chronic conditions and their management; physical and psychosocial impact of childhood chronic illness on children, family members, community, and society; and nursing intervention strategies to minimize the negative impact and enhance family coping abilities to adapt to the stresses
   b. information and skills to apply the principles of teaching and learning, including instruction in the use of print and audiovisual materials
   c. information and skills related to biological, psychological, and social development of families and children
   d. skills to assess and use individual and family strengths to assist families in coping with a child's chronic illness
   e. knowledge and skills related to counseling, crisis intervention, leadership, advocacy, and the consultation process.
2. Utilize nurses more fully in providing comprehensive health assessment and care for children with childhood chronic illnesses. Nurses can
   a. use their knowledge and skills in casefinding, early detection, and prevention of physical and psychosocial problems secondary to chronic illness
   b. obtain complete health histories, perform physical examinations, and help parents and children accomplish their developmental tasks
   c. serve as coordinators of the therapeutic plan and as liaison among the family, health care team, and community
   d. educate parents, children, and community members about child and family development needs and special needs related to the child's condition.
   This recommendation could be implemented through specialized case loads for nurses in health departments and by certification of all nurses working with chronically ill children.
3. Expand opportunities for nurses to provide home care for chronically ill children and their families, including direct physical care, family education and counseling, and coordination of health team members.
4. Include nurses on community decision-making boards that involve child

health concerns. They should become visible by contacting board members and informing them of their interests and skills in working with chronically ill children.

5. Expand nursing research studies to document the needs of chronically ill children and their families and the effectiveness of nursing care provided to them. To accomplish this,
   a. intervention studies are needed, not only to document the current state of the art, but to determine what strategies are effective and under what circumstances they are useful
   b. nursing specialty roles and programs need to be studied to determine cost-effectiveness as well as impact on and value to consumers and the health care system
   c. documentation of the nurse's role through better record keeping is essential in describing the role and its impact on consumers
   d. studies are needed of those children and families who appear to cope well with chronic illness in order to determine the variables that influence their healthy development and functioning; what is learned from these families may suggest more effective nursing intervention strategies for families not coping well.
6. Provide reimbursement of nursing services for chronically ill children by third-party payers. To accomplish this task, nurses need to
   a. provide data to the public to document services provided
   b. organize nursing services so costs for nursing services are separate from institutions' operating budgets
   c. make use of the certification process to establish their credentials.
7. Provide adequate funding to support nursing research efforts, educational programs, and demonstration projects related to the care of chronically ill children and their families.

References

Altshuler, A., Meyer, J., and Butz, M. K. "Even Children Can Learn to Do Clean Self-Catheterization." *American Journal of Nursing,* 1977, *77,* 97–101.

American Nurses' Association. *Standards of Maternal and Child Health Nursing Practice.* Kansas City, Mo.: American Nurses' Association, 1973.

American Nurses' Association. *A Statement on the Scope of Maternal and Child Nursing Practice.* Kansas City, Mo.: American Nurses' Association, 1980.

Bates, B. "Doctor and Nurse: Changing Roles and Relations." *New England Journal of Medicine,* 1970, *283,* 129–134.

Bernard, B., and others. "Exercise for Children with Physical Disabilities." *Issues in Comprehensive Pediatric Nursing,* 1981, *5,* 99–107.

Bindler, R. M. "Home Care for a Child with Physical Disabilities." *Issues in Comprehensive Pediatric Nursing,* 1979, *3* (7), 48–60.

Bivalec, L., and Berkman, J. "Care by Parent." *Nursing Clinics of North America,* 1976, *11* (1), 109–113.

Brown, N. C. "The Child with Acute Lymphocytic Leukemia." *Maternal-Child Nursing Journal,* 1978, *3,* 290–295.

Bushman, P. "Group Support for Parents." *American Journal of Nursing,* 1976, *76,* 1121.

Case, J. "The Team Nurse and the Child with Cancer." *Ohio State Medical Journal,* 1969, *65* (3), 256–258.

Conlin, J. B. "Role-Playing with Paddy." *Nursing '80,* 1980, *10* (5), 136.

Cortez, A., Mendoza, M., and Muniz, G. "The Utilization of Nurses in Expanded Roles to Deliver Pediatric Cardiology Health Care." *Pediatric Nursing,* 1975, *1* (3), 22–29.

Craft, M. "Preferences of Hospitalized Adolescents for Information Providers." *Nursing Research,* 1981, *30,* 205–211.

David, N. "Play: A Nursing Diagnostic Tool." *Maternal-Child Nursing Journal,* 1973, *2* (1), 49–56.

Deloughery, G. L. "Community Mental Health Nurses Work with Problems Related to Teaching of Physically Handicapped Children in a Public School." *Journal of School Health,* 1973, *43* (3), 181–184.

Dittemore, S. "Play Utilized by a Burned Child." *Maternal-Child Nursing Journal,* 1973, *2* (3), 203–214.

Dominquez, B. C., and Perrin, J.C.S. "Advocate for the Crippled Child." *American Journal of Nursing,* 1973, *73* (10), 1750–1751.

Durand, B. "Failure to Thrive in a Child with Down's Syndrome." *Nursing Research,* 1975, *20,* 272–286.

Eddington, C.L.T. "Sensory-Motor Stimulation for Slow-to-Develop Children: A Home-Centered Program for Parents." *American Journal of Nursing,* 1975, *75* (1), 59–62.

Everson, S. "Sibling Counseling." *American Journal of Nursing,* 1977, *77,* 644–646.

Ferguson, B. F. "Preparing Young Children for Hospitalization: A Comparison of Two Methods." *Pediatrics,* 1979, *64* (5), 656–664.

Foley, F. B., and McCarthy, A. M. "The Child with Leukemia In a Special Hematology Clinic." *American Journal of Nursing,* 1976, *76* (7), 1115–1119.

Gnus, M. "A Therapeutic Play Session in a Health Center." *Maternal-Child Nursing Journal,* 1973, *2* (3), 197–201.

Godfrey, A. B. "Sensory-Motor Stimulation for Slow-to-Develop Children: A Specialized Program for Public Health Nurses." *American Journal of Nursing,* 1975, *75* (1), 56–59.

Goodell, A. S. "Perceptions of Nurses Toward Patient Participation on Pediatric Oncology Units." *Cancer Nursing,* 1979, *2* (1), 38–46.

Goodell, A. S. "Responses of Nurses to Stresses of Caring for Pediatric Oncology Patients." *Issues in Comprehensive Pediatric Nursing,* 1980, *4* (1), 2–6.

Greene, P. "Acute Leukemia in Children." *American Journal of Nursing,* 1975, *75* (10), 1709–1714.

Grey, M. J., Genel, M., and Tamborlane, W. V. "Psychosocial Adjustment of Latency-Aged Diabetics: Determinants and Relationship to Control." *Pediatrics,* 1980, *65,* 69–73.

Gross, S., and Algrim, C. "Teaching Young Patients and Their Families About Home Peritoneal Dialysis." *Nursing '80,* 1980, *10* (12), 72–73.

Hart, L. K., Fearing, M. O., and Graham, G. K. "The Relationship of Developmental Tasks and Identity Control to Adjustment of Hemodialysis." *Journal of the American Association of Nephrology Nurses and Technicians,* 1976, *3* (4), 169-172, 177-179.

Healy, H. T. "Variations in Services to Handicapped Children." *American Journal of Nursing,* 1968, *68,* 1725-1727.

Hedlund, N. L. "Mental Health Nursing Consultation in the General Hospital." *Parent Counseling and Health Information,* 1978, *2,* 85-88.

Hope, P. K., and Hughes, A. C. "The Pedi Project." *Nursing Outlook,* 1972, *20* (10), 654-657.

Hymovich, D. P. "Assessment of the Chronically Ill Child and Family." In D. P. Hymovich and M. U. Barnard (Eds.), *Family Health Care.* New York: McGraw-Hill, 1979.

Hymovich, D. P. "How Children, Mothers and Nurses View Primary and Team Nursing." *American Journal of Nursing,* 1980, *80,* 2041-2045.

Hymovich, D. P. "Assessing the Impact of Chronic Childhood Illness on the Family and Parent Coping." *Image,* 1981, *13,* 71-74.

Hymovich, D. P. "The Chronicity Impact and Coping Instrument: Parent Questionnaire (CICI:PQ)." *Nursing Research,* 1983, *32,* 275-281.

Igoe, J. B. "Project Health PACT in Action." *American Journal of Nursing,* 1980, *80,* 2016-2021.

Iles, J. P. "Children with Cancer: Healthy Siblings' Perceptions During the Illness Experience." *Cancer Nursing,* 1979, *2,* 371-377.

Johnson, J. E., Kirchhoff, K. T., and Endress, M. P. "Altering Children's Behavior During Orthopedic Cast Removal." *Nursing Research,* 1975, *24,* 404-410.

Johnson, J. E., Kirchhoff, K. T., and Endress, M. P. "Easing Children's Fright During Health Care Procedures." *MCN: American Journal of Maternal and Child Nursing,* 1976, *76,* 206-210.

King, B., Spaulding, W. B., and Wright, A. D. "Problem-Oriented Diabetic Day Care." *The Canadian Nurse,* 1974, *70* (10), 19-22.

Klopovich, R., Suenran, D., and Cairns, N. "A Common Sense Approach to Caring for Children with Cancer: The Community Health Nurse." *Cancer Nurse,* 1980, *3* (3), 201-208.

Knudsen, K. "Play Therapy: Preparing the Young Child for Surgery." *Nursing Clinics of North America,* 1975, *10* (4), 679-686.

Lauer, M. E., and Camitta, B. M. "Home Care for Dying Children: A Nursing Model." *Journal of Pediatrics,* 1980, *97* (6), 1032-1035.

Leahey, M. D., Logan, S. A., and McArthur, R. C. "Pediatric Diabetes: A New Teaching Approach." *Canadian Nurse,* 1975, *71* (10), 18-20.

Lee, J. "Care and Management of the Adolescent Diabetic." *Pediatric Nursing,* 1978, *28* (5), 42-45.

Leiner, M. S., and Rahmer, A. E. "The Juvenile Diabetic and the Visiting Nurse." *American Journal of Nursing,* 1968, *68,* 106-108.

Lysaught, J. P. *From Abstract into Action.* New York: McGraw-Hill, 1973.

Macdonough, G. P. "Nursing Is the Name of the Game." *Journal of School Health,* 1978, *48* (10), 618.

McFarlane, J. M. "The Child with Diabetes Mellitus." *Pediatric Nursing,* 1975, *1* (15), 6-9.

Martinson, I. M., and others. "When the Patient Is Dying: Home Care for the Child." *American Journal of Nursing,* 1977, *97,* 1815-1817.

Moore, I. M., and Triplett, J. C. "Students with Cancer: A School Nursing Perspective." *Cancer Nursing,* 1980, *3* (4), 265-270.

Nelson, B. S. "Ann's Postoperative Play." *Maternal-Child Nursing Journal,* 1972, *1* (12), 193-196.

Parfitt, D. M., and Thompson, V. D. "Pediatric Home Hyperalimentation: Educating the Family." *Maternal-Child Nursing Journal,* 1980, *5,* 196-202.

Perrin, J.C.S., and others. "Evaluation of a Ten-Year Experience in a Comprehensive Care Program for Handicapped Children." *Pediatrics,* 1972, *50* (5), 793-800.

Peterson, M. C. "Preparation of the Cardiac Child and the Family for Surgery." *Issues in Comprehensive Pediatric Nursing,* 1979, *3* (7), 61-71.

Petrillo, M. "Preventing Hospital Trauma in Pediatric Patients." *American Journal of Nursing,* 1968, *68,* 1469-1473.

Pidgeon, V. A. "Characteristics of Children's Thinking and Implications for Health Teaching." *Maternal-Child Nursing Journal,* 1977, *6* (1), 1-8.

Pohl, M. L. *Teaching Function of the Nursing Practitioner.* Dubuque, Iowa: Brown, 1968.

Pridham, K. F. "Instruction of a School-Age Child with Chronic Illness for Increased Responsibility in Self-Care, Using Diabetes Mellitus as an Example." *International Journal of Nursing Studies,* 1971, *8,* 237-246.

Procci, L., Magary, J. F., and Tucker, A. S. "Meeting the Challenges of P. L. 94-142 Through a Continuing Education Program for the School Nurse." *Journal of School Health,* 1981, *51* (3), 154-156.

Redman, B. K. *The Process of Patient Teaching in Nursing.* New York: Appleton-Century-Crofts, 1980.

Redman, B. K. *Patterns for Distribution of Patient Education.* New York: Appleton-Century-Crofts, 1981.

Rodgers, B. M. "Comprehensive Care of the Child with a Chronic Disability." *American Journal of Nursing,* 1979, *79,* 1106-1108.

Schadt, A. B. "Nursing and Social Work Interventions with Families of Chronically Ill Children." Unpublished master's thesis, School of Nursing, University of Colorado, 1980.

Schnackel, K. "Pediatric Clinical Specialist and Diabetes Nurse Specialist: A Twofold Position." *Nursing Administration Quarterly,* 1979, *4,* 91-95.

Schraeder, B. D. "A Creative Approach to Caring for the Ventilator Dependent Child." *Maternal-Child Nursing Journal,* 1979, *4,* 165-170.

Sciarillo, W. G. "Using Hymovich's Framework in the Family-Oriented Approach to Nursing Care." *Maternal-Child Nursing Journal,* 1980, *5,* 242-248.

"Scope of Practice Statement for PNP's Issued." *The American Nurse*, May 1974, p. 5.

Sedlacek, K. "Helping the Asthmatic Child in School." *Maternal-Child Nursing Journal*, 1978, *3* (4), 207–210.

Sharpe, A. "Helping Parents in the Developmental Rearing of a Blind Child." *Maternal-Child Nursing Journal*, 1973, *2*, 23–28.

Slimmer, L. W. "Helping Parents Cope with Their Child's Seizure Disorder." *Journal of Pediatric Nursing and Mental Health Sciences*, 1979, *17* (2), 30–33.

Stiles, K., Lierman, C., and Austin, J. "Training Community Health Nurses in Care of Handicapped Children." *Journal of Continuing Education*, 1982, *13*, 26–34.

Sullivan, K. "Hospital Play Sessions." *Maternal-Child Nursing Journal*, 1972, *1* (2), 187–192.

Switzer, K. H., and Kelly, J. T. "The Nurse: A Member of the School Team." *Maternal-Child Nursing Journal*, 1980, *9* (2), 109–116.

Taylor, S. C. "The Effect of Chronic Childhood Illnesses upon Well Siblings." *Maternal-Child Nursing Journal*, 1980, *9* (2), 109–116.

Taylor, M. M., and Williams, H. A. "Use of Therapeutic Play in the Ambulatory Pediatric Hematology Clinic." *Cancer Nursing*, 1980, *3* (6), 433–437.

Tonyan, A. B. "Role of the Nurse in a Children's Cancer Clinic." *Pediatrics*, 1967, *40* (30), 532–534.

Venes, J. L., and Rodgers, B. "Yale-New Haven Hospital Spina Bifida Center: Introduction of a Pediatric Nurse Practitioner in a Program of Comprehensive Management." *Connecticut Medicine*, 1975, *39* (12), 801–802.

Wasteney, C. "A Diabetic Child and the School Nurse." *Journal of School Health*, 1970, *40* (5), 239–242.

Wheeler, D. "Teaching Home-Dialysis for an Eight-Year-Old Boy." *American Journal of Nursing*, 1977, *77*, 273–274.

Williamson, M. C. "Staff Development for the School Nurse Practitioner." *Journal of School Health*, 1978, *48* (8), 471–473.

Wolfer, J. A., and Visintainer, M. A. "Pediatric Surgical Patients and Parents' Stress Responses and Adjustment." *Nursing Research*, 1975, *25* (4), 244–255.

Wood, A. "The Pediatric Nurse Practitioner in a Pediatric Cancer Clinic." *Pediatric Nursing*, 1978, *4*, 47–49.

Wooten, B. "Death of an Infant." *Maternal-Child Nursing Journal*, 1981, *6*, 257–260.

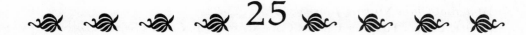

25

Training Nurses to Care for Chronically Ill Children

Corinne M. Barnes, Ph.D., R.N., F.A.A.N

This chapter addresses nursing education and its responsibility for preparation of professional nurses in the care of the chronically ill child. Current levels of educational preparation are presented within a historical framework of key developments in public policy and governmental funding of advanced nursing education programs. Curriculum content specific to nursing care of children, including chronically ill children, is introduced with reference to its relevance to clinical specialization, advanced nursing education, and research. Current trends and recommendations are presented with emphasis on graduate level education.

History

Nursing education plays a critical part in the quality of life and prevention of problems that might occur as a result of an enduring illness. In the history of nursing, focus on children as a special population evolved within the general social movement to improve health care to mothers and children. Early recognition that mothers and children have specialized needs was seen in the establishment of the New England Hospital for Women and Children in Boston in 1862. The economic issue was as prevalent in the 1800s as it is today: "Because there was too often a tendency to degrade the position of a nurse, to bring in untrained people to save hospital expenses, to call upon women of the street in times of stress, to pay nurses very little, nursing as a whole suffered" (Bullough and Bullough, 1964, p. 82).

Educational needs of nursing students were considered secondary to practical hospital experience. Education programs lacked financial support, and less qualified "nursing" personnel were trained in short-term educational courses to care for the chronically ill.

Nurses themselves helped change hospitals by their efforts to improve nursing school standards. By the early 1930s, government programs had heightened public and professional awareness of the important role of nursing in improving the quality of life of children and their mothers.

By 1956, the demand for nursing education at the graduate level led to government support for nurses attending graduate school. Traditionally, graduate education in nursing had been considered preparation for particular functions and positions—primarily teaching and administration. By now, however, although the need for well-qualified nurse administrators with clinical knowledge of nursing of children is still critical to the effective utilization of clinical nurse specialists, the trend has shifted dramatically from the functional preparation of teachers and administrators of the 1950s to the current clinical specializations in nursing.

In a 1980 policy statement, the American Nurses' Association (ANA) noted that, "while demands of the marketplace should be allowed to regulate excess in numbers, the profession must take steps to assure that universities prepare enough specialists in nursing practice to meet the needs for qualified nurse faculty, nurse researchers, and consultants, as well as specialists for direct care practice" (p. 27). With today's financial crisis in higher education, the charge to prepare pediatric clinical nurse specialists in number sufficient for faculty, research, consultant, and practice positions is an awesome task. A balance of quality education as well as a sufficient supply of graduates can be attained only to the extent that criteria of importance to nursing education be adhered to. Criteria proven useful to nursing education in both general academic and professional fields include faculty with intellectual and other qualifications essential to teaching at the graduate level, students with superior intellectual ability as well as the capacity for independent action and thought, an educational climate conducive to intellectual pursuits, and facilities and resources to ensure quality and quantity. Guidelines for criteria for educational programs in nursing are established by the National League for Nursing.

The introduction of specialization in nursing education in general, and in nursing of children in particular, began in the mid 1940s and 1950s. An early program to address the clinical nursing needs of children was developed and introduced in 1946 by Florence Blake (1954). Her study of children at Yale influenced the nature of the program, which she developed at the University of Chicago. The program provided a curriculum of special knowledge and techniques to prepare master's level nurses to understand the behavior of sick children and their parents. Blake's objectives were to teach the nurse to appraise behavior objectively without reacting personally, to learn the needs and conflicts of children at various age levels, to learn about the feelings of children about illness and the disruptive effects of separation from parents, to understand how members of a family interact with each other, and to develop some capacity for introspection. Orientation of the nurse to the child and not to techniques and procedures was the emphasis.

Programs by educators such as Adams, Johnson, and Erickson followed, with different degrees of clinical involvement with children and their families and different degrees of research (Florence Erickson, personal communication with the author, January 1982). Little research was documented before Erickson (1958) published her monograph on the use of play to learn about young children's responses to illness, hospitalization, and treatments. John Bowlby's (1952) report, which focused on the attachment and dependency relationship of infants and young children to their mothers, as well as works by Spitz (1946), Freud (1952), Erikson (1950), Mahler (1965), Piaget (1926), and Robertson (1953), influenced early clinical programs in pediatric nursing.

Additional impetus to the development of nursing curricula grounded in research and theories of child behavior was provided by Bowlby's report (1952, p. 67), which concluded that "to insure optimal physical growth and personality development the infant needs a continuous intimate relationship with a warm, giving mother. . . . Through the infant's attachment to his mother, his personality grows. . . . During the first 3 years of life his mother is his primary object of interest and concern." The report focused on the care of dependent children, emotionally disturbed children, and children ill with physical disease or conditions requiring hospitalizations, and this work influenced pediatric nursing education's direction by examination of the nurse's role.

Nursing Education

The main types of educational programs for entry into practice as a nurse generalist include baccalaureate degree programs, associate degree programs, and diploma programs. Baccalaureate degree programs are generally offered by colleges and university schools of nursing; associate degree programs by community colleges; and diploma programs by hospital schools of nursing. The programs vary in length and curriculum as well as the expected outcomes of the graduate. All three types of programs seek mandatory state approval, and most programs seek accreditation by the National League for Nursing, a voluntary professional organization.

The competencies expected of graduates of the three programs are described in the "Working Paper of the National League for Nursing Task Force on Competencies of Graduates of Nursing Programs" (National League for Nursing, 1979, pp. 11–14). There are differences in the depth and breadth of the knowledge base as well as in the length of the programs, which vary from approximately two years (associate degree) to three years (diploma) to four years (baccalaureate).

Programs vary in the kind of setting utilized: Associate degree and diploma programs utilize the structured setting of acute and extended care facilities; baccalaureate programs use both structured and unstructured settings with equal emphasis on wellness and illness. Nurses graduating from the various programs have varied degrees of knowledge of and practice with pediatric patients. As graduates, their degree of responsibility and liability increases relative to the length of the program. The percentage of requirements in the social sciences, natural sciences, liberal arts, and English is highest in the baccalaureate program. The percentage of nursing courses in the curriculum ranges from 30 percent (baccalaureate) to 67 percent (diploma), with the associate degree program at about 50 percent. The focus of care may include children and new mothers, and the care may range from simple to comlex as the settings change and the expectations become more complex. Importantly, the quality of the specific type of program, not the length, ultimately determines the quality of the graduate and the level of competency, and program quality is strongly related to the quality of the organization and administration, students, faculty, curriculum, resources, facilities, and services within each school.

Chamings and Teevan (1979) recently asked nurse educators in baccalaureate and associate degree programs about perceived differences in expected competencies among graduates. Three areas—conceptual, human, and functional—were noted. Conceptual competencies include activities "requiring the ability to reason, to know and use theoretical content, and to recognize, analyze, synthesize, and evaluate situations in order to plan and implement creative patient care. Human competencies are intellectual competencies merged with technical behaviors in a humanistic fashion and comprise interpersonal and intrapersonal interactions. Functional competencies are primarily psychomotor or technical skills" (p. 18). Results of the study clearly demonstrated differences in the levels of expectation by baccalaureate versus associate degree educators. Baccalaureate degree programs showed higher overall expectations. However, the study did not show a clear pattern of differential response to the question of differences in the *kinds* of competencies expected. Further research is needed to determine whether graduates of different types of programs actually perform differently in practice.

Graduates of these three programs provide much of the nursing care to chronically ill children in acute care settings and in community settings such as public health departments, schools, step-down units, and rehabilitation settings. Therefore, it is important that the programs address the content and skill necessary to prepare graduates for care of chronically ill children. Problems implementing undergraduate education about chronically ill children exist partly because the nursing of children, young and old, has been considered a specialty that is multidimensional in nature and is addressed primarily at the master's level in nursing education programs.

Traditional baccalaureate programs in nursing provide the educational background for master's level study to prepare a nurse to become an expert in one field of practice, such as pediatric nursing. Graduate educational programs prepare the graduate to function as a pediatric nurse specialist in acute care settings and community agencies where children are in need of nursing care: in hospitals, clinics, schools, and public health settings.

An example of one baccalaureate curriculum and its purpose and objectives, one master's curriculum that builds on the baccalaureate, and one doctoral curriculum that builds on the master's curriculum illustrates the progression of programs from basic to specialization in the field of pediatric nursing. Graduates of master's and doctoral programs become faculty in the basic (diploma, associate degree, and baccalaureate) and master's programs. Graduates also take positions in service settings, primarily those providing care for children directly or indirectly. Graduates of all three programs care for children directly or indirectly, and have an impact on the care of chronically ill children.

Baccalaureate Program. The baccalaureate program prepares a professional practitioner of nursing who, through the use of nursing process, can help individuals and groups in varied settings achieve and maintain optimal health. The program provides a foundation for graduate and continuing education in nursing and serves as a stimulus for intellectual and personal development.

Graduates of baccalaurate programs will:

- Apply knowledge from nursing, life sciences, social sciences, and the humanities to the practice of nursing
- Use the nursing process at all levels of prevention at any point on the health continuum with individuals and groups
- Collaborate with others concerned with the delivery of health care
- Use research findings that have value to nursing
- Provide health education for individuals and groups
- Assume an advocacy role in relation to issues of health
- Assume responsibility for their own decisions and actions and for actions delegated to others accountable to the professional nurse in the practice of nursing
- Demonstrate leadership in goal setting and goal achievement in matters relating to health
- Use change process when working with others on matters pertaining to health
- Accept responsibility for continued learning and professional growth

Education for the practice of professional nursing demands a substantial knowledge of the behavioral and biological sciences as a theoretical base. Throughout the program, nursing courses are taken concurrently with courses in the College of Arts and Sciences, which contribute to the educational breadth of the practitioner.

The freshman year establishes the foundation for the study of nursing with an introduction to concepts and theories underlying nursing practice. Clinical study begins in the sophomore year with focus on primary prevention, health promotion, and identification of risk factors. Clinical experiences take place in a variety of settings, such as schools, clinics, neighborhood health centers, and senior citizen centers. The junior year focuses on nursing care of individuals and groups of all ages who are experiencing the stress of illness. Clinical experiences take place in acute care settings and long-term facilities. During the senior year, students' experiences are planned to encourage synthesis of the knowledge of the preceding years. Characteristics of leadership behavior that are introduced in the freshman year and augmented during the years of subsequent study are expanded during the senior year when all students have the opportunity to assume responsibility in a leadership experience.

The program provides a foundation for entry into professional training practice as well as for graduate education. Students who complete the undergraduate program are eligible to take licensing examinations administered by the state boards of nurse examiners. Students who pass the licensure examination are eligible to practice as a Registered Nurse (RN) in the state in which the examination was written.

The baccalaureate program prepares the nurse generalist, although the senior year course allows the student to elect an area of concentration, such as nursing of children. After a year or more of practice in the field of pediatric nursing, the graduate of a baccalaureate program who wishes to specialize in the nursing of children can apply for admission to a master's program with a nursing of children area of specialization. The purpose, objectives, and curriculum of one master's program are described here.

The Master's Program. The master's program provides an organized sequential plan of study leading to specialization in nursing and includes the following components:

- Advanced preparation in medical-surgical nursing, *nursing care of children,* psychiatric-mental health nursing, or adult primary health care nursing
- Preparation in the role of administrator of nursing services, teacher, clinical specialist, or practitioner
- Preparation in research methods
- Foundation for further graduate study at the doctoral level

The graduate of the master's program will:

- Demonstrate mastery of knowledge and skills in an area of clinical specialization
- Critically examine theories and models from nursing and other disciplines for their contribution to the body of knowledge in clinical and functional areas
- Provide evidence of beginning competence as a nurse researcher through empirical investigation of nursing problems
- Contribute to the development of nursing theories by generating researchable questions and testing hypotheses from nursing practice
- Demonstrate competence as a teacher, administrator, consultant, clinical specialist, or practitioner
- Initiate collaborative relationships with other health professionals to bring quality care to the patient/client and to mobilize health and social resources for individuals, families, groups, and communities
- Develop leadership in activities relevant to nursing
- Demonstrate ability to present ideas both verbally and in written form in an articulate, literate, and organized manner
- Take a position on issues relative to nursing practice and health care in the light of scientific knowledge as well as personal and societal values
- Show evidence of accountability for personal nursing practitioners and professional development

The major in nursing care of children is open to nurses who are interested in becoming specialists in the nursing care of children. The program is built on the premise that good nursing care to infants and children is based on understanding of growth and development and of the dynamics of family relationships. Study of well children at various age levels is provided in school or daycare settings in conjunction with courses in child development and childcare. The impact of illness and hospitalization on children and families is studied intensively in hospital and home, and nursing research methods and techniques appropriate to the study of infants and children at various age levels are introduced and developed in a variety of clinical settings.

In response to new technologies, which are commonplace in acute care settings, faculty periodically monitor the need for adequate numbers and kinds of specialists in pediatric nursing. Qualified specialists prepared by universities for direct care practice need curricula that address the challenges posed by the widespread advances in medicine, physiology, and pharmacology. Specialties such as cardiology, oncology, pulmonology, neonatology, and others that involve children constantly force nursing education programs to be current so that graduates can achieve the highest proficiency.

The Ph.D. Program. The Ph.D. program in nursing prepares scholars and researchers who will advance nursing science, thereby influencing the practice of nursing, and who will provide innovative leadership to the profession.

The aim of the doctoral program is to prepare scholars for nursing who will be able to:

- Conceptualize phenomena observed in practice to facilitate further research within specialties in clinical nursing practice
- Evaluate the application of research designs, measures, and statistics to the study of nursing
- Design, conduct, and communicate research relevant to nursing practice
- Translate new knowledge into nursing practice and into formulation of innovative designs to test nursing interventions
- Construct conceptual models and nursing theories that contribute to the science of nursing
- Address the issues and problems related to the delivery of health care and devise solutions collaboratively with clients and health care professionals from related disciplines

The doctoral program is built on the master's program's advanced preparation in nursing care of children. Clinical specializations form the base for the doctoral program. The program of study includes: (1) clinical nursing knowledge and skill unique to the field, (2) research and theory, and (3) supporting courses from related disciplines. The curriculum is approximately three full years.

Graduates of doctoral programs become faculty in university schools of nursing and collegiate schools of nursing that offer baccalaureate, master's, and doctoral programs. Many of them direct graduate programs in the specialty of nursing of children. Others fill positions as directors of maternal-child programs in the community, in health departments, and in government. Still others assume top-level positions as consultants, directors of research in specialty hospitals, and administrators of nursing service departments.

Clinical Nursing Research

Today, nursing education continues its dedication to the development of a professional and scientific approach to the nursing process and nursing care. Preparation in research techniques is a core component of graduate study for nurses. According to the National League for Nursing compilation, *Doctoral Programs in Nursing 1982–83*, twenty-five universities in the United States offer doctoral programs, and more than half include clinical research in their learning environments. Clinical nursing research, particularly in the area of nursing care of children, has far-reaching implications for the care of chronically ill children.

To improve nursing practice in all patient settings, it is essential that knowledge gained through clinical nursing research be organized, validated through scientific inquiry, and eventually applied in the health care delivery systems. Notter (1974, p. 16) defines clinical nursing research as "studies of nursing practice or of the effect of nursing practice on patient care or on individual, family, or community health situations." Clinical nursing research studies began to appear in the literature in the 1960s. In most cases, these clinical investigations were based on doctoral studies and master's theses. From 1961 to 1978, nursing care of children graduate students from the University of Pittsburgh School of Nursing contributed 158 master's theses and 19 doctoral studies to this pool of clinical research findings. Master's theses were in-depth, descriptive case studies of sick children, many chronically ill, who were observed in acute care settings, health care clinics, ambulatory centers, doctor's offices, schools, and homes. Examples of clinical research studies are available in *The Hospitalized Child*, a book of abstracts edited by Diana and Faren Akins and Gillian Mace (Akins, Mace, and Akins, 1981).

Clinical research at the doctoral level in nursing of children addresses researchable problems generated from nursing practice. Doctoral studies are intended to advance nursing science and to add and translate new knowledge into nursing practice. A 1979 ANA survey indicated nearly 2,400 nurses with doctoral degrees, the majority of whom did not produce original research with a clinical focus.

The first Ph.D. program in maternity and pediatric nursing was funded in 1968 by the National Institutes of Health and was directed by R. Rubin and F. Erickson. These pioneers in preparing clinical specialists at the master's and doctoral level described the linkage between nursing care and nursing research as follows: "Nursing care and nursing research are complementary and synergistic. Research is generated from patient need/care problems. Research questions are nursing questions, not medical, social work, or educational questions. Nursing care moves across a broader sphere than the dichotomies of health and illness to include the neither sick-nor-well areas, such as recovery, and the added stress of diagnostic and therapeutic regimes. The target in nursing care is not a virus, a neoplasm, or a fracture, but the person who has any of these and who has to cope with fundamental limitations. The purpose of clinical nursing research is to define precisely the situation of the patient in order to address nursing care effectively and economically in behalf of the patient'' (1977, p. 151).

Rubin and Erickson further describe the setting as anywhere a patient receives or needs health care—home, clinic, or hospital. An illustrative research study was conducted in an intensive care unit (ICU) of a large, urban children's hospital. School-age children's perceptions of ICU phenomena and their levels of consciousness while recovering from heart surgery in the intensive care unit were studied. Seven girls and six boys participated, with data including observations of the children, their drawings of the ICU, interviews, family relationships and dynamics, and pertinent medical histories. Data were analyzed in terms of categories of ICU phenomena (treatment and procedures, persons, events, furnishings, and other general phenomena) and levels of consciousness including alertness, distortion, fantasy, affective memory, and dreams. More than half of the responses were classified as alert and one third as distorted. Children in the ICU remembered deaths of relatives and other highly emotional experiences. The study contributed to the body of nursing science as it was the first nursing study of children's responses to ICU phenomena. Study findings were translated into new and changed attitudes about ICU visiting hours, nurse and physician practices in the ICU, and heightened awareness of parents' needs (Barnes, 1975).

Research continues to be instrumental in the improvement of care for mothers and children. How a small number of mothers responded to their defective newborns was studied by June Kikuchi (1980). She noted that it took mothers longer than one month to become fully acquainted with their congenitally defective infants who were hospitalized at birth. Relevant to nursing practice is the manner in which mothers responded. Mothers sought information about the babies when they could cope with it. They needed to experience some success with feeding them, even though infrequent. Kikuchi noted that in order to be able to begin to mother their newborn infants with congenital defects, mothers also seemed to need the freedom to protest. Nursing has a vital role to play with such ill infants.

Clinical Nurse Specialist: Role and Function

Quality nursing care for chronically ill infants and children requires that providers of care receive a sound educational preparation in the theory and practice of nursing of children, infants, young and school-age children, and adolescents. Clearly, care is provided by nurses with varying degrees of educational preparation, competency, and experience. About 20 percent of the 1.4 million nurses have a baccalaureate degree, some 5 percent hold master's degrees and 0.2 percent the doctoral degree. Thus the vast majority of nurses are prepared by diploma and associate degree programs (Fagin, 1982).

Graduates of baccalaureate programs, referred to as generalists, receive minimal content and clinical learning experience related to the special population of chronically ill children: Curriculum content is integrated into the total curriculum over the four years of the educational program. Opportunities exist for a senior-year synthesizing experience, which may include nursing of children.

To practice nursing in specialty hospitals for children, graduates of all basic programs require long periods of orientation. Basic graduates often receive six full weeks of orientation and may need an additional eight to nine months before they are considered safe and productive practitioners (P. Shafer, personal communication with the author, September 1982). Intensive and extensive orientation of beginning practitioners has become a particular responsibility of staff development units. The long period of time in transition from student to practitioner is due both to the ever-increasing amount of knowledge and complexity of medical and technical advances and to the strain increasing knowledge has placed on content selection for the baccalaureate curriculum.

The recent initiation of the integrated curriculum provides the student a framework within which theory for nursing practice is enveloped and in which the process of nursing bases its existence. The framework provides the faculty a common and specific meaning for the incorporation of content at every level of the curriculum, but it has limited the amount of time spent in specific courses, such as in maternal and child health. The framework permeates every aspect of the curriculum design and every learning experience (Torres and Yura, 1974). Recent graduates appear to have had fewer learning experiences in maternal-child health and nursing care of children than those of five years ago.

In contrast, graduates of master's programs that prepare pediatric clinical nurse specialists have received in-depth knowledge of children and in-depth practice in acute care settings as well as in nurseries, clinics, schools, and the home. Specialized populations of children receive nursing care from knowledgeable, competent specialists—either directly as in a highly complex situation, such as the care of children with organ transplants, or indirectly where clinical nurse specialists have an impact on generalists.

Esther Lucille Brown (1948, p. 73) proposed the future role of the professional nurse as "one who recognizes and understands the fundamental (health) needs of a person, sick or well, and who knows how these needs can best be met. She will possess a body of scientific nursing knowledge which is based upon and keeps pace with general scientific advancement, and she will be able to apply this knowledge in meeting the nursing needs of a person and a community. She must possess that kind of discriminative judgment which will enable her to recognize those activities which have been identified with the fields of other professional or nonprofessional groups." Brown's nurse of the future was to be clinically competent, have leadership qualities, teach and supervise others, and be an agent for change. The idea of the nursing specialist was introduced—with expert clinician her primary role, and teacher, manager, consultant, and researcher her secondary roles.

The American Nurses' Association (1976) defines the clinical nurse specialist as a practitioner holding a master's degree with a concentration in specific areas of clinical nursing. Most educators believe that the function of the nurse clinician should remain closely identified with nursing practice (Reiter, 1966). The education of pediatric nursing specialists must incorporate knowledge of growth and development and dynamics of behavior as well as knowledge of diseases and treatment. Pediatric nurse clinical specialists assume positions in hospitals, schools, and clinics. Their functions span many settings as well as special groups of children, including those with diabetes, cardiac conditions, and leukemia; school-age children in need of ventilator support; and children with renal and liver transplants. Specialists may also work with specific age groups rather than specific groups of conditions. The author of this article, while employed as the first clinical nurse specialist in one children's hospital, gave nursing care directly and indirectly to one child, from age eighteen months to five years, in the hospital, the clinic, the home, and during a transfer from a hospital in one state to a hospital in another state. The continuity of care for the child and the family by one nurse specialist who worked with the health team facilitated the child's admission procedure, treatment in the clinic and emergency room, care in the community, and transfer to an out-of-state hospital. Nurse specialists can be effective as care managers for chronically ill children.

Comprehensive, coordinated, and uninterrupted care are a few of the components of a model that can promote an enhanced health care system for chronically ill children. Two cases involving the care of children and mothers illustrate the complementary nature of pediatric nursing specialization. A four-year-old child, ill since age two from a lye burn, was referred to a nurse specialist (Barnes, 1969a). Lack of recovery and optimal functioning were the main care problems. The clinical nursing research conducted by the pediatric clinical specialist precisely defined the situation of the child and her mother, and after communication with the child and mother, the nursing care needs of the child were effectively addressed. The assessment revealed the child's extreme regression and her mother's lack of involvement in the clinic where she received esophageal dilatations. The inclusion of the mother in the management of her preschool child changed the course of treatment. Initially lost in the complexity of the hospital and hospital care, the child became more compliant with the dilatations after referral to the nurse specialist. The overwhelming stress that caused the child to flee and regress was moderated by permitting her to use her defenses and to use the clinical specialist. It was the clinical specialist who introduced and nurtured this age-appropriate plan for success. The nursing care was effective emotionally, physically, and economically on behalf of the child.

In the case just cited, the demonstration had impact on the service setting because the clinic subsequently hired one clinical specialist to address the nursing needs of lye-burned children and to teach students in the clinical setting. In summary, upon referral, this child with a lye ingestion had been diagnosed as emotionally disturbed and her physician was concerned that her liver would be damaged due to frequent anesthesias for dilatations. The child is now a young adult. She was able to finish high school, marry, and now dilates her esophagus herself. Tabulation of the cost of her care over a two-year period illustrated that, although cost increased with the addition of a clinical nurse specialist, overall costs of care eventually decreased. Not only was the care to this child improved and the quality of her life increased, the cost was ultimately eliminated as she was made independent of the medical system.

Problems in the care of children and mothers continue to merit attention. A second example involves children with congenital heart disease admitted for surgical correction. In the mid 1960s it was observed that some school-age children were not coping well with admission to the hospital for cardiac surgery (Barnes, 1969b, 1972). Parents of these children were unprepared and unknowledgeable, and communication between the parents and their chronically ill children had broken down. Changes and innovative programs were implemented: presurgical and precatheterization parent preparation groups were instituted, and cardiac infant parent groups and pamphlets for educating adolescents with heart diseases were devised. A combined supportive staff of clinical nurse specialists, social workers, physicians, and technicians facilitated care for children and their families in the home, the clinic, the cardiac catheterization laboratory, the operating room, the intensive care unit, and the child's unit. The project provided information that led to improved conditions for children and their families.

In an article on children and illness (on children's thoughts, concepts, and beliefs), Blos (1978) describes children as researchers whose curiosity includes their bodies, how they function, and why things go wrong. For every question there must be an answer, which the child obtains by a mixture of observation, thought, fantasy, previous experience, and prior explanation. Health professionals must learn not only to understand what a child is saying but also to communiate effectively. Blos supports the concept that, with more knowledge of children's responses to illness and its impact on the body, we may be better able to assist children in their mastery of the trauma of long- and short-term hospitalization, chronic illness, and physical handicap. Individual case studies by clinical specialist students demonstrate that the continuous empathic contact with the child and family result in positive outcomes to what seem to be overwhelming situations for the children.

Nursing educational programs that produce clinical nurse specialists for care of infants and children in situations such as those cited need a curriculum that presents a broad theoretical base plus excellent clinical learning experiences (National Commission on Nursing, 1981).

Summary

In summary, the focus of this chapter is nursing education and its involvement in the care of the chronically ill child. Nursing education programs have the responsibility to prepare professional nurses in sufficient quantity and with the necessary knowledge and skill to meet society's needs in this area of specialization. The complex, multidimensional care of the dependent, developing chronically ill child requires a creative, developmentally focused curriculum.

The pediatric nurse clinical specialist, prepared at the master's level, is recommended as the type of professional to deliver comprehensive nursing care to the chronically ill child and the child's family. One illustration of a young child burned with lye suggests the potential of the pediatric clinical specialist for reducing health costs while improving the quality of life for the child. A second illustration of cardiac pediatric clinical specialists demonstrates how clinical nursing research provides the basis for instituting new educational group programs for parents of children with cardiac conditions within one cardiology service. Generalists prepared at the baccalaureate level will continue to care for chronically ill children, and attention to the curriculum to prepare them for this responsibility is needed. Funding for nursing education programs, research programs, and service projects focused on chronically ill children and their families will continue to be critical if adequately prepared nurses are to be produced and knowledge of chronically ill children and better delivery systems are to be documented. Unless funding is forthcoming, it is unlikely that adequate numbers of pediatric clinical nurse specialists will be trained. Today's baccalaureate programs tend to have less and less maternal-child content, and the recent trend toward an integrated curriculum needs to be examined with reference to preparing generalists to care for chronically ill children and their families.

The promotion of continuity of the relationships for infants, children, and parents for optimal development of the chronically ill child is within the scope of the specialist's functions. Continuity of relationship and care for the child in the health care delivery system can be improved. As the infant and/or chronically ill child moves in and out of the many health care settings, continuity for the child/family can be strongly enhanced by the pediatric clinical nurse specialist, who can also assure meeting ongoing preventive health and primary care needs.

Recommendations

1. The recent trend toward integrated baccalaureate and master's programs needs to be examined with reference to maternal-child health curriculum content and clinical experiences. The recent shift to integrate maternal and child nursing content with the rest of the curriculum could result in production of generalists less prepared to respond to the care needs of chronically ill children and their families. Specialization and subspecialization must be reinstated as a high priority in nursing education programs (particularly at the master's and doctoral level), giving attention to the care of the chronically ill child.

2. Notwithstanding substantial attitudinal, financial, and organizational barriers, service settings for chronically ill children must be upgraded to incorporate professional nurses with specialization in the care of children. Such specialists will contribute through direct care, consultation, education, and management positions.

3. New standards should be instituted to reflect new knowledge of this special population of children, and clinical nurse specialists, nurse educators, and

researchers have been at the forefront of developing standards. The challenge is to develop a nursing service/nursing education program to close the gap that presently exists in these critical components of the health care delivery system.

4. Knowledge, skills, and academic credentials of nursing personnel presently providing direct or indirect care to chronically ill children need to be identified through a comprehensive survey. Survey results should be compared against optimal credentials postulated by the American Nurses' Association's Maternal-Child Nursing Division. Responsive public policy should be the final outcome of this survey.

5. The rich body of existing, current, and planned maternal-child nursing research should be examined and further articulated by a panel of maternal-child nursing leaders in order to ferret out qualitative and quantitative findings relevant to professionals responsible for care of chronically ill children and their families. This synthesized body of research must be disseminated to appropriate public and private bodies.

6. Continuity is one of several critical elements in the care of chronically ill children. Recent societal trends indicate that discontinuity of care will be more prevalent in our society due to higher incidence of single-parent families and dual-worker households. A determination must be made about the degree to which continuity of care has penetrated health systems to include the home setting and networks of communications. Public policy and funding strategies that reward systems supportive of continuity would enhance widespread adoption of this philosophy. Existing and planned work of pediatric nurse clinical specialists, supported by nurse practitioners in appropriate settings, will likely have a positive impact on continuity.

7. It is essential that a comprehensive pattern for a unified nursing education curriculum be developed by nursing educators. A position paper will ultimately influence trends underway in the areas of primary, secondary, and tertiary care of chronically ill children. At present, educators have not achieved consensus on didactic and clinical content in maternal-child nursing educational programs. Of interest would be information about programs (baccalaureate) that discontinued the integrated program. Public policy and funding strategies (public and private) are needed to foster and promote development of this consensus for the academic community.

References

Akins, L., Mace, S., and Akins, R. *The Hospitalized Child.* New York: Plenum, 1981.

American Nurses' Association. *The Scope of Nursing Practice.* Kansas City, Mo.: American Nurses' Association, 1976.

American Nurses' Association. *Nursing: A Social Policy Statement.* Kansas City, Mo.: American Nurses' Association, 1980.

Barnes, C. M. "Support of a Mother in the Care of a Child with Esophageal Lye Burns." *Nursing Clinics of North America,* 1969a, *4* (1), 53–57.

Barnes, C. M. "Working with Parents of Children Undergoing Heart Surgery." *Nursing Clinics of North America,* 1969b, *4* (1), 11–18.

Barnes, C. M. "Measurement and Management of Anxiety in Children with Open Heart Surgery." *Pediatrics,* 1972, *49* (2), 250–259.

Barnes, C. M. "Levels of Consciousness Indicated by Response of Children to Phenomena in the Intensive Care Unit." *Maternal-Child Nursing Journal,* 1975, monograph 4.

Blake, F. G. *The Child, His Parents and the Nurse.* Philadelphia: Lippincott, 1954.

Blos, P. "Children Think About Illness: Their Concepts and Belief." In E. Gellert (Ed.), *Psychosocial Aspects of Pediatric Care.* New York: Grune & Stratton, 1978.

Bowlby, J. "Maternal Care and Mental Health." Monograph Series no. 2. Geneva, Switzerland: World Health Organization, 1952.

Brown, L. *Nursing for the Future.* New York: Russell Sage Foundation, 1948.

Bullough, B., and Bullough, V. *The Emergence of Modern Nursing.* London: Macmillan, 1964.

Chamings, A., and Teevan, J. "Comparison of Expected Competencies of Baccalaureate and Associate-Degree Graduates in Nursing." *Image,* 1979, *11* (1), 16–21.

Erickson, F. "Play Interviews for Four-Year-Old Hospitalized Children." *Monographs of the Society for Research in Child Development,* 1958, *23,* 7–77.

Erikson, E. *Childhood and Society.* New York: Norton, 1950.

Fagin, C. M. "The National Shortage of Nurses: A Nursing Perspective." In L. Alken and S. Gorten (Eds.), *Nursing in the 1980's.* Philadelphia: Lippincott, 1982.

Freud, A. "Role of Bodily Illness in the Mental Life of Children." *Psychoanalytic Study of the Child,* 1952, 7, 69–81.

Kikuchi, J. "Assimilative and Accommodative Responses of Mothers to Their Newborn Infants with Congenital Defects." *Maternal-Child Nursing Journal,* 1980, monograph 9.

Mahler, M. "On Early Infantile Psychosis." *Journal of American Academy of Child Psychiatry,* 1965, *4,* 554–568.

National Commission on Nursing. *Initial Report and Preliminary Recommendations.* Chicago: Hospital Research and Education Trust, 1981.

National League for Nursing. *Working Paper of the National League for Nursing Task Force on Competencies of Graduates of Nursing Programs.* New York: National League for Nursing, 1979.

National League for Nursing. *Doctoral Programs in Nursing.* New York: National League for Nursing, 1982.

Notter, L. E. *Essentials of Nursing Research.* New York: Springer, 1974.

Piaget, J. *The Language and Thought of the Child.* New York: International Universities Press, 1926.

Reiter, F. "The Nurse-Clinician." *American Journal of Nursing,* 1966, *66* (2), 274–280.

Robertson, J. "Some Responses of Young Children to Loss of Maternal Care." *Nursing Times,* 1953, *49,* 382–386.

Rubin, R., and Erickson, F. "Research in Clinical Nursing." *Maternal-Child Nursing Journal,* 1977, *6* (3), 151–164.

Spitz, R. "Anaclitic Depression." *Psychoanalytic Study of the Child,* 1946, *2,* 313-342.

Torres, G., and Yura, H. "Today's Conceptual Framework: Its Relationship to the Curriculum Development Process." New York: National League for Nursing, 1974.

26

Mental Health Issues and Services

Dennis Drotar, Ph.D.
Marcy Bush, M.A.

Chronic physical illness is a major life stress that affects the mental health of large numbers of children and their families (Magrab, 1978; Pless and Douglas, 1972; Pless and Roghmann, 1971). Moreover, in concert with recent advances in medical treatment, children with such life-threatening conditions as cystic fibrosis, cancer, myelodysplasia, and renal failure now live longer than ever before and face unforeseen adjustment problems as adolescents and adults (Dorner, 1973; Gogan and others, 1979; Grushkin, Korsch, and Fine, 1973; Rosenlund and Lustig, 1973). For the most part, medical technologies and comprehensive care programs have developed far in advance of a sensitive understanding of their emotional impact. As a consequence, systematic documentation of chronically ill children's adjustment problems and needs for mental health services remains a critical priority in planning humane comprehensive care programs and societal supports for these highly stressed children and their families. Available knowledge concerning the mental health of chronically ill children is a poorly integrated mixture of clinical observations, case reports, and descriptive studies of varying conceptual and methodological sophistication. This report provides a state-of-the-art integration of knowledge concerning the mental health of chronically ill children organized around the following topics: (1) the nature of illness-related stresses and their potential import for mental health, (2) empirical studies of the mental health adjustment of children and young adult survivors, (3) common mental health problems associated with chronic illness, (4) mental health services for chronically ill children, including innovative strategies for preventive intervention in life contexts, and (5) implications for future research.

Illness-Related Stresses

Every chronic illness presents a complex series of interrelated stresses that are potential hazards to psychosocial development, require chronic modes of coping, and vary in psychological significance and cultural meaning (Sontag, 1978). Given the wide variations in adaptation prior to the onset of disease-related stress, in individual coping, and in family and social support (Caplan and Killea, 1976; Cobb, 1976), there is no direct correspondence between a particular stress or set of stresses and a given mental health outcome (Pless and Pinkerton, 1975). However, each of the following stresses has potential implications for chronically ill children's mental health.

Physical Symptoms

Chronically ill children endure various physical symptoms, including pain, shortness of breath, and lethargy, that cannot be completely prevented, become part and parcel of day-to-day existence, and must be managed in ways compatible with normal living. Individual chronic illnesses vary considerably with respect to the organ system affected, the nature and degree of physical symptoms, including physical pain, and the way in which life is disrupted by disease-related symptoms (Mattsson, 1972; Steinhauer, Muskin, and Rae-Grant, 1974).

Each chronic illness has a unique constellation of symptoms that represent a source of anxiety. A chronic illness changes physical appearance in ways that are potentially stigmatizing, restrict mobility, or result in physical isolation, with significant implications for social development (Steinhauer, Muskin, and Rae-Grant, 1974). The symptoms of a chronic illness differ in their responsiveness to variations in family environments. For example, certain subgroups of chronic, psychosomatic illnesses such as asthma (Purcell and others, 1969a, 1969b) or juvenile diabetes (Minuchin, Rosman, and Baker, 1978) are responsive to environmental events and family dysfunction in ways that dramatically affect the course of physical symptomatology.

Treatment Regimens, Hospitalizations, and Physical Procedures

Chronically ill children face treatment regimens that run the gamut from the relatively benign regimen of the asymptomatic child with asthma; to the daily insulin shots needed by the child with diabetes; to the complex, energy draining physical treatments required by cystic fibrosis and end-stage renal failure. The physical demands of treatment regimens also change the balance of interpersonal relationships within the family. For example, chronically ill children and their parents must cooperate in physical treatments that can stimulate dependency or conflict. Moreover, treatment regimens impose special burdens on parents to negotiate their roles and responsibilities, time, energy, and finances and to reconcile career and family demands (Vance and others, 1980; Meyerowitz and Kaplan, 1967; Turk, 1967).

Outside the home, in accord with disease course and the dictates of medical management, a chronic illness may involve periodic or regular visits to physicians as well as hospitalizations. Hospital-based diagnostic and treatment procedures can include injections, surgery, and immobilization that involve actual or imagined assaults to bodily integrity, autonomy, and sexuality, assaults that threaten body image and self-concept (Freud, 1952; Bergmann, 1965; Eissler and others, 1977; Geist, 1979). Physical treatments such as medication can also have serious side effects that disturb physical appearance and physical well-being (Korsch and others, 1971). Finally, hospitalizations remove the child from school and home and require adjustment to an unfamiliar hospital's social and physical environment (Kagen-Goodheart, 1977).

Age of Onset and Etiology

Age of illness onset can have considerable import for child and family adaptation. Chronic illnesses such as cystic fibrosis or congenital malformations are usually diagnosed in early infancy. The diagnosis of a chronically ill or malformed infant ordinarily ushers in a major family crisis characterized by feelings of shock, sadness, anger, and eventual adaptation (Drotar and others, 1975; McCollum and Gibson, 1970). On the other hand, children with a chronic illness diagnosed early in infancy do not have to cope with the implications of the emerging awareness of their disease until their preschool or early elementary school years (Drotar, Mazzarins, and Zelko, 1980). Although physically healthy children's reactions to the sudden onset of a chronic illness have not been systematically documented, diagnosis presents a multifaceted crisis in which the child must adapt to the loss of normal functioning, tolerate and comply with new medical procedures, and struggle with feelings about the meaning of the disease and its treatment (Geist, 1979). Given the difficulty of these stresses, it is no wonder that chronically ill adolescents' retrospective accounts of their reactions to the diagnosis of cystic fibrosis are characterized by strategies that blunt the emotional impact of the disease (Drotar, Mazzarins, and Zelko, 1980).

Etiology of illness may also have psychological meaning for child and family. For example, illnesses such as cystic fibrosis that have an identifiable hereditary component (Wood, Boat, and Doershuk, 1976) entail a sense of parental responsibility for the disease with implications also for the child's interpretation that differs from illnesses of undetermined cause.

Physical Impairment and Deterioration

Illness-related impairments can limit physical activity, capacity to function at work or school, and independence. Although many chronic illnesses afford a very reasonable quality of life, some conditions (such as spina bifida) that involve multiple organ systems and severe physical disability impose a social isolation that cannot be easily overcome (Holroyd and Guthrie, 1979; Dorner, 1973). Similarly, the advanced stages of progressive illnesses such as cystic fibrosis or cancer entail painful losses of physical capacities and cherished activities, and troubling adjustments in life goals (Drotar, 1978). In practice, the determination of expectations for life functioning at a given level of disease severity may be very difficult, especially in instances where both emotional and physical factors disrupt adaptation (Drotar, 1978; Lansky and others, 1975). The levels of life functioning achieved by chronically ill children and adolescents at a given level of disease severity are surprisingly variable. For example, some children with relatively severe disease make rather astonishing progress toward life goals in the midst of extraordinary physical obstacles, while others with relatively mild physical disease become functionally debilitated far beyond the level of their actual physical impairment (Bergman and Stamm, 1967).

Life-Threatening Illness

Life-threatening illnesses pose special psychological threats (Koocher and O'Malley, 1981; Kagen-Goodheart, 1977) different from those usually associated with a chronic disease (Spinetta and Maloney, 1975). For example, the prospect of raising a child with a potentially fatal illness raises extraordinary fears and childrearing dilemmas for parents (McCollum and Gibson, 1970; Friedman and others, 1963; Natterson and Knudson, 1960) who must manage their own anxieties to the extent that they encourage a reasonable level of functioning for their children and do not become unduly preoccupied with the prospect of their death (Koocher and O'Malley, 1981). The death of a chronically ill child is a compelling human tragedy that severely taxes even the most competent families (Drotar, 1977b; Easson, 1970; Koocher and O'Malley, 1981).

Studies of Individual Psychological Adjustment

Given the myriad of illness-related stresses, it is not surprising that mental health clinicians in pediatric settings are frequently called on to work with chronically ill children who present a wide range of childhood behavioral problems including school avoidance and somatic symptoms, overly dependent behavior, depression and suicidal behavior, and learning and behavioral problems (Drotar, 1978; Lansky and others, 1975; Lansky and Genel, 1975; Sterns, 1959; Weinberg, 1970; Drotar, Ganofsky, and Makker, 1979; Spencer, 1968). Unique patterns of psychopathology are not associated with chronic illness. Rather, chronically ill children demonstrate the same general patterns of behavioral disturbance seen in populations of physically healthy children (Achenbach, 1978; Achenbach and Edelbrock, 1978).

One of the most interesting questions concerns the association of mental health disturbance and chronic illness. Although early clinical case descriptions implied that chronic illness was almost always associated with some form of disturbance (Drotar, 1981), more recent controlled empirical studies report a much brighter mental health outlook for chronically ill children. For example, Pless and Douglas (1972) described the medical, educational, and psychosocial status of a large sample of 4,700 children, 518 of whom had chronic diseases, with *chronic disease* defined as a physical, usually nonfatal condition that lasted longer than three months or necessitated a period of continuous hospitalization of more than one month. As a group, children with chronic disorders had an increased number of behavioral symptoms. Twenty-five percent of these children had two or more abnormal behavioral symptoms at age fifteen as compared with 17 percent in the healthy population. Chronically ill children also had more trouble at school and more school absences. Yet (with the exception that children who had experienced early hospitalization had more problems relative to age norms) type of disability or disease characteristics did not relate to maladjustment.

Pless (1979) compared chronically ill children with a matched physically healthy group, controlling for age, race, sex, and socioeconomic status. Children were tested with a comprehensive battery of measures including responses from the child, parents, teachers, and peers and an index of family functioning. The overall rate of excessive maladjustment was much lower than anticipated among chronically ill children as compared with a physically healthy group; but psychological risk increased with age, suggesting that the combined effects of poor health and unfavorable social situations are cumulative over time. The relationship between adjustment and disease severity, however, only approached statistical significance. In general, children with either moderate or severe disorders had an increased risk of severe maladjustment. Children with sensory disorders, such as deafness, were twice as likely to be disturbed as those with general physical or cosmetic problems. The curvilinear relationship between disease severity and adjustment, which has also been found by other investigators (McAnarney, Pless, Satterwhite, and Friedman, 1974), suggests that disease severity based on objective physical criteria may not be as important as personal perceptions of illness in mediating adjustment.

The Isle of Wight study (Rutter, Tizard, and Whitmore, 1970) reported a higher rate of psychiatric disorders (17 percent) among a chronically ill population compared with a physical healthy population (7 percent). The same proportion of chronically ill children had neurotic and antisocial behavioral patterns as the general population. Finally, rates of psychiatric disorder were higher than population norms among children with brain injury, especially children with epilepsy and cerebral palsy.

Recent Studies of Specific Chronic Illness Populations

In addition to these large-scale epidemiological studies, other research has studied the psychosocial adjustment of smaller populations of chronically ill using comparison group designs. For example, Tavormina and others (1976) documented the psychosocial functioning of a group of chronically ill children (with diabetes, asthma, cystic fibrosis, and hearing impairment) on a battery of standardized personality instruments including locus of control, self-esteem, and screening inventories. Chronically ill children performed very much like healthy children in that their functional strengths outweighed psychological weaknesses. Consistent with Pless (1979), the hearing-impaired group stood out as the most psychologically impaired.

Drotar and others (1981b) studied the adjustment of eighty children with cystic fibrosis as rated by parents and teachers compared with that of physically healthy siblings, healthy children, and a group of children with other chronic pulmonary disease. As a group, chronically ill children were rated by parents as having more problems than physically healthy children, but severe adjustment problems were relatively rare. Moreover, children with cystic fibrosis achieved an age-adequate level of adjustment both at home and at school with respect to test norms. Severity of illness did not correlate with either parent or teacher ratings of adaptation.

Klein and Simmons (1979) studied seventy-two children with serious chronic kidney diseases as compared with groups of healthy siblings and a random sample of healthy school children on measures such as physical well-being, ability to perform daily activites, social or interpersonal adjustment, and emotional well-being. The chronically ill group had more learning difficulties and absenteeism and were less physically active but maintained expectable frequency and type of social contacts with peers. Apart from dissatisfaction with looks, chronically ill children's self-images were surprisingly undamaged. No chronic-illness-related differences were found in self-consciousness, self-image stability, sense of distinctiveness, ability to reveal true feelings to others, or perceived level of happiness. Severity of illness as defined by the physician correlated significantly and negatively with some aspects of adjustment. The child's subjective definition of disease severity, however, correlated significantly with almost all of the adjustment measures, underscoring the potential importance of self-perception to successful coping. The most impaired children had lower self-esteem and rated themselves as less popular, more distinctive, more self-conscious, and more anxious.

A series of interesting studies (Spinetta, Rigler, and Karon, 1974; Spinetta and Maloney, 1975) investigated the impact of leukemia on dimensions of personality functioning (anxiety and personal space) thought to be uniquely affected in this disease. Despite the fact that children with leukemia had not been hospitalized more frequently or for greater periods of time than children with arthritis or hemophilia, children with leukemia were more preoccupied with their illness than their chronically ill counterparts and anxious about their bodily integrity and out-of-hospital life. Moreover, the children's sense of isolation, as assessed by a personal space measure, grew stronger as the children neared death.

Finally, recent studies have explored the adjustment of children with chronic non-life-threatening endocrine disorders, which do not have especially arduous treatment regimens. For example, Drotar, Owens, and Gotthold (1980) studied the personality functioning of children with hypopituitarism, a deficiency of growth hormone that causes extremely small stature, compared with a matched group of physically healthy children. Children with hypopituitarism resembled physically healthy children on all measures with the exception of perceived reactions to frustration. Children with hypopituitarism typically perceived less adaptive and less mature solutions to frustrating situations than did peers of average stature. In addition, hypopituitary children emphasized the obstacles rather than the solutions to frustrations. Downey (1979) investigated the adjustment of a group of thirty-two children with adrenogenital syndrome (a relatively rare condition involving a deficiency in enzymes resulting in excessive androgen) as compared with matched groups of children with diabetes and physically healthy children. As a group, the chronically ill children showed adequate self-esteem, sense of sexual identity, and general psychological adjustment but less articulated and mature human figure drawings and less maturity on a standardized test of adjustment.

Mental Health of Survivors

Although not much is known about the mental health of long-term survivors of childhood chronic illnesses, preliminary descriptive studies indicate a reasonable level of overall adjustment, coupled with psychological vulnerabilities in specific areas of adjustment. For example, Fine and others (1978) noted that, although the personality functioning (as assessed by the California Test of Personality) of forty-one children following renal transplantation was not grossly deviant, their social adaptation was deficient relative to a group of normal children of the same age.

Boyle and others (1976) found that a group of twenty-seven adolescent and young adult survivors of cystic fibrosis appeared to function adequately but were emotionally troubled by stresses such as (1) altered physical appearance causing distorted body image and denial of sexuality, (2) strained interpersonal relationships resulting in isolation and marital strain, (3) conflicts over upbringing with their families, and (4) increased awareness of death.

Our own studies (Drotar, Mazzarins, and Zelko, 1980) of eighty young adult survivors (ages sixteen to thirty) of cystic fibrosis documented a wide range of coping styles but a surprisingly high frequency of positive disease-related appraisals (for example, perceptions of disease as challenge) (Pearlin and Schooler, 1978). Many young adults acknowledged the problems, causes, and treatment regimens of their disease yet emphasized their similarity to physically healthy peers. Most coped reasonably well with school and work but reported less frequent dating than might be expected for their ages.

Koocher and O'Malley (1981) reported on 117 childhood cancer survivors who received treatment prior to age eighteen in the most comprehensive study of survivors to date. Although most young adults were in some ways maladjusted, as assessed in a structured psychiatric interview, their psychological functioning generally was not severely affected. Factors related to optimal long-term adjustment included having a type of cancer with relatively short treatment course and a minimum of permanent side effects, a relapse- or recurrence-free recovery period with disease onset during infancy or early childhood, and effective use of denial.

One of the most important but as yet unanswered questions concerns the capacity of social institutions to meet the vocational, academic, and mental health needs of childhood chronic illness survivors, particularly in an era of severe cutbacks in social programs. Because chronically ill adults require special financial help, continued medical care, and vocational planning services to maximize their potential, the quality of their long-term adjustment may depend on the nature and availability of societal supports. For example, in a pilot investigation, the quality of spina bifida survivors' vocational and academic adjustment seemed constrained by the quality of supportive services, including vocational planning and financial subsidy (Glaser and others, 1980). There was a poignant discrepancy between the magnitude and unrelenting nature of the spina bifida population's needs and the unpreparedness of societal agencies to meet these needs. This finding coincides with the anxiety-producing discrimination concerning employment and health insurance experienced by the survivors of childhood cancer (Koocher and O'Malley, 1981).

Adjustment in Life Contexts

Studies thus far reviewed have considered the individual psychological adjustment of chronically ill children independent of their life contexts. However, in that social transactions with key persons in life contexts are potentially important mediators of life stress (Caplan and Killea, 1976), there is merit in considering the adjustment of chronically ill children from a contextual perspective. In this model, the nature and outcome of the child's transactions with persons in relevant life contexts, family, school, peers, and physical treatment (Bronfenbrenner, 1979; Hobbs, 1975) become the critical variables around which research and clinical intervention are organized. In this section, empirical studies pertaining to the mental health of chronically ill children and their families in significant life contexts are reviewed.

Family

The family context is a complex system of transactional influence (Bell and Harper, 1977; Belsky, 1981; Parke, 1979) that provides the chronically ill child's most critical source of emotional support (Caplan and Killea, 1976; Litman, 1974; Litman and Venters, 1979). Moreover, the presence of a chronically ill child exerts a powerful influence on family life, parental self-esteem, and the mental health of each family member (Dorner, 1976; Holroyd and Guthrie, 1979; Meyerowitz and Kaplan, 1967; Pless and Pinkerton, 1975; Turk, 1967; Vance and others, 1980).

Empirical studies have reinforced the importance of family context as a primary influence on children's mental health. Pless, Roghmann, and Haggerty (1972) compared a sample of chronically ill children and a matched group of physically healthy children on a comprehensive battery of measures including responses from the child, parents, teachers, peers, and an index of family functioning. Chronically ill children with the greatest risk for psychological impairment (as judged by a composite adjustment index) were from families with lower family-functioning scores. Hence, family functioning was shown to be an important mediator of adjustment, and one that operated in concert with other variables to affect individual adjustment. Moise (1980) studied the adjustment of thirty-three school-aged children and adolescents with sickle cell anemia as perceived by the patients, their parents, and their teachers. The better adjusted children came from more cohesive families.

Observations by Kucia and others (1979) of family problem-solving indicated that families of well-adjusted children (as judged by physician and parent ratings) demonstrated more creative solutions to a structured problem-solving task than those of maladjusted children. The association of family creativity with positive adjustment is consistent with studies that indicate that families of well-adjusted children are more able to consider alternatives than those of poorly adjusted children (Odom, Seeman, and Newbrough, 1971). In addition, fathers of well-adjusted children displayed more creativity and positive support than those of maladjusted children. This pattern, which occurred only in families of male children, suggests that paternal flexibility and support may have been particularly important to the adjustment of male children. Finally, this study was noteworthy for the *absence* of differences in positive support or communication between families of well-adjusted versus poorly adjusted children and the fact that the families of maladjusted children had higher success scores than had those with adjusted children.

Bush (1981) found a similar relationship between individual adjustment and family measures among juvenile diabetics, emotionally disturbed, and physically healthy children. Moreover, the fact that maternal, paternal, and siblings' ratings of family satisfaction were significantly related to their own individual adjustment indicated that an individual's subjective experience of family may be a salient factor in adjustment. The findings also contrast with clinical descriptions of families of chronically ill children as conflict-ridden or ineffective and indicate that childhood chronic illness does not inevitably disrupt family effectiveness.

Parental Mental Health. Because parents of chronically ill children must cope with extraordinarily difficult life circumstances including compromised finances, restriction of career mobility, and the demands of treatment regimens, it is not surprising that they find the experience stressful (Turk, 1967; Meyerowitz and Kaplan, 1967). Subjective feelings of depression and worry are common (Koocher and O'Malley, 1981; Lauler, Nakielny, and Wright, 1966). Although the subjective stresses of a chronic illness on parents have been well described, the specific effects on parental mental health are less well understood. For example,

Lauler, Nakielny, and Wright (1966) found that most parents experienced considerable emotional upset, with eight of thirty-eight mothers judged clinically depressed. Tropauer, Franz, and Dilgard (1970) also noted maternal depression and guilt but found that most mothers were able to perform effectively despite the stresses with which they were faced. Although such studies suggest an association of childhood chronic illness and parental maladjustment, the implications for children's mental health are not known. For example, among physically healthy children, even severe parental psychopathology does not have a one-to-one relationship with childhood behavior disorders (Anthony, 1969). The way the child is involved in the parental disturbance or stress appears to be more critical than the nature of parental disturbance per se.

Marital Relationship. The demands of a chronic illness stress the parents' relationship and may disrupt their childrearing capacities, ability to support one another, and hence, the mental health of the chronically ill child. For example, Crain, Sussman, and Weil (1966) found that parents of diabetics had less agreement on child management and more marital conflict than parents of healthy children. Parents of children with cancer experience increased marital strain (Lansky and others, 1978), particularly around the time of diagnosis, as do the parents of children who undergo kidney transplant (Korsch and others, 1973). Although clinical lore suggests that chronic illness results in a high rate of family breakdown or divorce (Bruhn, 1977), systematic studies have indicated that the marriages of parents of children with chronic illnesses, including life-threatening conditions, are no more unstable than those of healthy children (Koocher and O'Malley, 1981).

Nevertheless, the consequences of heightened marital strain for the chronically ill child are not well defined. What may be even more damaging than marital strain per se are illness-related changes in family alignments such as parental difficulties in maintaining appropriate boundaries concerning the child's privacy and the development of maladaptive coalitions with one parent to the exclusion of the other (Minuchin, Rosman, and Baker, 1978). One of the most intriguing but ill-understood phenomena is the possibility that the stress of chronic illness may strengthen family unity and adaptation. For example, Pless and Satterwhite (1975) noted that parents felt that chronic illness had been a unifying force in the family, increasing family members' sensitivity to others. In addition, eight of sixteen parent couples of children with hemophilia felt the illness had enhanced family closeness (Markova, MacDonald, and Forbes, 1979), and parents of leukemic children in long-term remission felt the experience had altered their values and priorities in life and generated personal growth (Obetz and others, 1980). A family's capacity to perceive positive meaning in a chronic-illness experience may well be an important mediator of mental health in children (Venters, 1980).

Sibling Mental Health. Physically healthy siblings must cope with the anxieties imposed by their sib's chronic illness, the special parental attention and nurturance given to the ill child, and stresses faced by parents. Clinical observations have suggested that siblings experience adjustment problems (Binger and others, 1969; Mass and Kaplan, 1975), some of which have been documented in controlled studies. For example, Lavigne and Ryan's (1979) study of the adjustment of siblings of cardiology, hematology, and plastic surgery patients indicated that siblings were more withdrawn and irritable than healthy controls. Siblings of children with visible handicaps were more severely affected. Similarly, siblings of spina bifida patients were four times more likely to evidence maladjustment than siblings of controls (Tew and Laurence, 1973), and the physical and emotional health of siblings of children with nephrotic syndrome was more impaired than that of siblings of healthy controls (Vance and others, 1980).

Other recent well-designed studies indicate that the general mental health of siblings of chronically ill children is not necessarily impaired but that their social adaptation may be vulnerable. Cairns and others (1979) found siblings of children with cancer to have "normal" self-concepts but higher perceived social isolation. A well-designed, comprehensive study of families of children with cystic fibrosis, cerebral palsy, myelodysplasia, and multiple handicaps indicated that siblings of disabled children did not manifest higher rates of severe psychological impairment or greater overall symptomatology when compared to control subjects (Breslau, Weitzman, and Messenger, 1981). However, siblings did score significantly higher on two scales measuring interpersonal aggression with peers and within the school. Level of disability or nature of illness did not relate to sibling adjustment. In other recent controlled studies, the adjustment of siblings of cystic fibrosis patients (Gayton and others, 1977; Drotar and others, 1981b) and juvenile diabetics (Bush, 1981) was not found to be impaired relative to comparison groups. Discrepancies in these studies may relate to differences in measures, patient populations, or the nature of comprehensive care afforded to families in various centers. The way a chronic illness affects the long-term relationship among siblings, which is a salient developmental influence (Bank and Kahn, 1976), remains an intriguing but largely unanswered question.

General Family Influences. Because research and clinical observation of family adjustment has generally concentrated on the mental health of individual members, little is known about the generalized effects of chronic illness on the family as a system. However, one area that may be affected by a chronic illness is intrafamilial role patterns. Ritchie (1981) found that, in contrast to families with a physically healthy child, families with an epileptic child had an autocratic matriarchal structure that was more efficient in problem-solving. Crain, Sussman, and Weil (1966) found significantly lower goal consensus and increased role tension of family members of juvenile diabetics in comparison with healthy controls. Moreover, the capacity of family members to perform their usual roles was reduced.

Clinical observations suggest that family members' abilities to discuss the child's disease with one another can be compromised. For example, Turk (1967) found that parents of cystic fibrosis children were able to discuss the child's management with each other but did not discuss the illness with their other children, family, or friends. Sixty percent never discussed the diagnosis with the child. Parents of children in long-term leukemia remission (more than four years) also reported difficulty talking with each other about the illness or discussing it with the child (Obetz and others, 1980). Such patterns of communication may isolate parents from each other, their children, and from social support networks, with negative consequences on children's mental health (Tropauer, Franz, and Dilgard, 1970; Swift and Seidman, 1964). For example, the consistent finding of a positive association between openness of family and parental communication about disease-related issues and childhood adaptation to childhood cancer (Koocher and O'Malley, 1981; Spinetta and Maloney, 1978; Lascari and Stehbens, 1973; Spinetta, Swarner, and Sheposh, 1981) underscores the potential importance of openness of disease-related communication for childhood adjustment.

School

Chronically ill children have intermittent school absences and/or limitations requiring special tutoring or limitations in activity (Pless, 1979). The necessity to take medications or complete treatment regimens in school also singles out the chronically ill child. Although one might expect these stresses to disrupt adjustment, teachers' ratings of the school adjustment of some chronic illness populations (for example, chronic renal disease, cystic fibrosis) are surprisingly positive (Klein and Simmons, 1979; Drotar and others, 1981b). However, school-related psychosocial adjustment may vary with the condition. For example, Spinetta and Spinetta (1980) reported that children with cancer adjusted relatively well but were perceived by teachers as more inhibited, less active, and more cautious than a matched group of physically healthy children. Harper, Richman, and Snider (1980) found that type of physical disability and degree of physical impairment were related to different modes of behavioral adjustment in school in a population of children with cerebral palsy and cleft palate. Children with cleft palate were more impulsive than the cerebral palsy group.

Transitions among hospital, school, and family contexts pose special problems for chronically ill children (Crittenden and Gofman, 1976). For example, parents face a dilemma concerning preparation of teachers for their children's chronic conditions and are often torn between their concerns about wanting to inform school personnel and not wanting to single their child out as special. Moreover, it can be especially difficult for physician, family, and school to determine and coordinate reasonable expectations for academic functioning, particularly in cases where disease severity and emotional factors affect school adjustment.

The impact of teacher attitude and relationship on the adjustment of the chronically ill child has not been studied in depth. Chronically ill children are educated by teachers usually unfamiliar with the disease and its implications for physical activity, socialization, or learning. Faust and Campbell (1979) found that increased personal familiarity with patients did not appear to affect teachers' knowledge and attitudes about childhood cancer. Yet, teachers' concern with children's vulnerability may contribute to unnecessary restrictions or contradictory attitudes toward children with conditions such as spina bifida (Glaser and others, 1980).

Peers and Heterosexual Relationships

Information concerning the special impact of chronic illness on socialization is lacking, with few exceptions (Koocher and O'Malley, 1981). Chronically ill children are called upon to interact with physically healthy children even though hospitalization and physical treatments limit time and opportunities for socialization. The experience of a chronic illness also requires children to make difficult decisions about how much to tell others about their disease, how much to be identified as a well or a sick person, and how to cope with others' reactions to the disease. The manner in which these social dilemmas are reconciled may reveal salient aspects of the child's capacity to understand, accept, and negotiate disease-related stress. Given these difficulties, it is not surprising that socialization may be an area of special vulnerability for the survivors of chronic illness (Korsch and others, 1973; O'Malley and others, 1979; Ganofsky, Drotar, and Makker, 1983). Drotar, Mazzarins, and Zelko (1980) found that young adults with cystic fibrosis perceived others as having a great many misapprehensions about their disease and as equating it with extreme physical vulnerability. Perhaps as a consequence, they preferred not to share information about their disease with others. Limiting disclosure of the disease to intimate acquaintances, which was the preferred strategy of a majority of young adults, appeared to be an adaptive attempt to maintain control of the social impact of the disease, compete in society as a physically healthy person, and cope with realistic social barriers toward obtaining jobs, insurance, and schooling.

Physical Treatment

The interpersonal context associated with physical treatment of chronic childhood illnesses is a potentially salient influence on the mental health of chronically ill children that has not been sufficiently described or studied (Drotar, 1981). The medical care of chronically ill children occurs in many places including ambulatory settings, inpatient hospitals, and specialized treatment settings such as dialysis or intensive care units, each of which has a distinctive subculture (Drotar, 1976). Although physical treatment is optimally given by a continuous team of professionals who attend to psychosocial issues in the child's medical care (Rothenberg, 1976), the *content* and *structure* of comprehensive care programs vary widely. In some settings, physicians and nurses provide the sole ongoing contact with most families while mental health professionals work only with those children judged as having severe adjustment problems. Other programs feature shared professional contact with children and families over the entire course of the illness. Disease-related issues such as the child's physical status or compliance with regimens are the sole focus of some comprehensive care programs. In others, the impact of disease on family, academic, and social adjustment are considered in close conjunction with physical care (Heisler and Friedman, 1981; Drotar and others, 1981a) and with other professional disciplines (Brantley, Stabler, and Whitt, 1981; Drotar, 1976; Koocher, Sourkes, and Keane, 1979; Stabler, 1979). It is important to recognize that pediatricians generally have much more experience with the hospital-based management of chronically ill children's acute physical problems than they do with the continuous care of the chronically ill in home or community settings. Despite cogent pleas for physicians to assume primary responsibility in the care of chronically ill and handicapped children (Battle, 1972), primary care physicians do not generally play a major role in management of children with chronic illnesses with respect to counseling, advising, or coordinating other services (Pless, Satterwhite, and Van Vechten, 1976; Kanthor, Pless, Satterwhite, and Myers, 1974).

Most chronically ill children receive their care in highly specialized centers located in large pediatric training hospitals (Kanthor, Pless, Satterwhite, and Myers, 1974) where structural and organizational problems (Tefft and Simeonsson, 1979; Mechanic, 1972) impede communication among professionals as well as between physician and family members. In the highly subspecialized hospital culture, it is not uncommon for a single professional discipline to have access to only a small part of the total information concerning a chronically ill child and family (Mechanic, 1972). Moreover, the time pressures, emphasis on action, and absence of privacy that are prevalent in pediatric hospitals can severely constrain the quality of caregivers' transactions with children and families (Drotar and others, 1981c). Transactions with chronically ill children and their families may also frustrate physicians (Artiss and Levine, 1973; Ford, Liske, and Ort, 1963) because this work requires communication skills that are not usually emphasized in pediatric training (Haggerty, Roghmann, and Pless, 1975) and an understanding of ethical dilemmas that stimulate great uncertainties for caregivers and families alike (Fox, 1975; Fox and Swazey, 1978; Katz and Capron, 1975).

Although the relationship of the interpersonal context of physical treatment to chronically ill children's mental health has not been studied intensively, available evidence suggests that it is nowhere near optimal. Other potentially dysfunctional features of physician-patient transaction include the emphasis on technical versus emotional issues (Osherson and Amarasingham, 1981) and withholding of information, particularly from patients with serious conditions (McIntosh, 1974).

Adjustment Problems Encountered in Pediatric Settings

Clinicians working with chronically ill children and their families must assimilate a confusing literature concerning the mental health of chronically ill children. Although epidemiological studies consistently indicate that *severe* chronic-illness-related adjustment problems are the exception rather than the rule, mental health professionals in pediatric settings are called on to work with these exceptions. To the extent that clinicians generally see only the most disturbed or stressed of chronically ill children, they cannot obtain a perspective on children who cope adequately with illness. With the exception of clinical reports that concern specific syndromes, the experience of practicing clinicians is not based on empirical studies of presenting problems experienced by chronically ill children at different ages. The complexity of the clinician's task is increased by the fact that certain adjustment problems reflect children's understandable difficulty in coping with the interpersonal context of the hospital environment rather than severe mental health disturbance per se. Nevertheless, the major problems presented by chronically ill children follow certain descriptive patterns (Drotar, 1978; Johnson, 1979), which are the topic of the rest of this section.

Hospital or Illness-Related Reactions

Chronic-illness-related mental health problems often represent acute reactions to stressful experiences. Such reactions are sometimes salient enough to attract the attention of the hospital staff or affect compliance with treatment regimens and necessitate supportive intervention, as in this instance:

> Dan, a 7-year-old child with renal failure, had developed normally and had adequate psychological adjustment prior to the onset of dialysis, which followed a rapidly deteriorating course of renal disease. Despite his positive initial reaction to a discussion about dialysis, Dan displayed an intense, unmitigated panic when dialysis began. His crying was quite upsetting to the staff who requested psychological help for him. However, Dan did not turn out to be an emotionally disturbed child so much as an overly stressed one. His problems quickly abated with extra support and patience and he maintained adequate adjustment subsequently, without additional intervention [Johnson, 1979].

Personality Problems Caused or Intensified by Chronic Illness. In contrast to such adjustment reactions, other chronically ill children experience severe and chronic emotional disturbances that require intensive mental health intervention. For example:

> John, a sixteen-year-old boy with a history of chronic renal failure and a renal transplant, was troubled by excessive anxiety and obsessions centering around sexual and aggressive thoughts. John had long been a constricted and overcontrolled child who had managed to maintain age-adequate adjustment to peers, school and within his family. Although the onset of his renal disease, subsequent hospitalization and transplant were quite upsetting to him, he had managed to bury his feelings and become a model patient. However, John's unresolved anxieties about his condition, sexuality, and body image eventually came to a head resulting in highly disturbing obsessions which he could not contain, even with additional pediatric support. His problems culminated in suicidal threats and necessitated intensive mental health intervention including psychiatric hospitalization and intensive psychotherapy. With individual and group treatment, John's acute problems abated and he was able to resume adequate adjustment [Drotar, 1975b].

Illness-Related Adjustment Problems. The fact that medical regimens can interfere so dramatically with children's autonomy makes compliance inherently difficult. Compliance difficulties can be particularly disruptive in illnesses such as diabetes or renal failure where failure to follow medication regimens can result in physical symptoms necessitating hospitalization. Difficulties with compliance may very much relate to problems in the current family context, particularly stress and disorganization (Minuchin, Rosman, and Baker, 1978). For example, the impact of the family environment on compliance was clearly shown in the case of Al, a thirteen-year-old boy with diabetes who readily admitted that he stopped taking insulin in order to come in the hospital whenever he wanted a rest from the stresses of his quarrelsome parents. Moreover, it is not uncommon for chronically ill children to take out their anger about the constraints imposed by their illness by becoming unmanageable at home and by testing their parents' discipline and authority (Drotar, 1978).

Emotional Problems of Terminal Illness. Although most children and adolescents manage to cope remarkably well with the tragedy of terminal illness, especially when they have the sensitive support of family and professional staff (Koocher and O'Malley, 1981), the emotional upheaval associated with a terminal illness may sometimes stimulate referrals for mental health intervention (Blake and Paulsen, 1981):

> Gail, a 19-year-old young woman, was referred because of her anxiety. She was in the final stages of her disease and faced death within the near future. Her fears about not being able to catch her breath and sadness over life changes that had accompanied her physical deterioration were poignant but understandable expressions of her existential predicament. Gail and her family benefited from some discussion of their mutual worries. To maintain their support and availability throughout the course of her difficult illness, the medical and nursing staff also needed a forum in which to discuss their own feelings about Gail and her family.

Social, Vocational, or Academic Difficulties

The emotional problems of chronically ill children also cause disturbances in academic, social, or vocational functioning. For example, one of the more common adjustment problems associated with a chronic illness is school avoidance, which may be accompanied by somatic symptoms:

> Kate, a twelve-year-old with cystic fibrosis, presented with chronic tiredness and vague pains not explainable by organic factors. Kate had not attended school for more than a year and gradually lost interest in peers and outside activities. Feeling that her peers did not accept her because of her illness, she had given up trying to tell them about it. At home, her parents had gradually given up efforts to involve her in activities. Kate's problems benefited from both individual and family discussions that clarified her isolation and the parents' feeling of grief.

Family Adjustment Problems

A chronic illness affects the life of each family member. Moreover, chronically ill children are often identified by physicians or family members as having individual mental health problems when those problems would be more properly construed as part of family maladjustment. Consider, for example, Jay, a sixteen-year-old with cystic fibrosis, referred for evaluation of poor school achievement:

> Psychological evaluation involving individual, parent, and family interviews indicated that Jay was not really an underachiever, but rather was struggling with excessively high parental standards for achievement predicated on their wish for him to be a supernormal adolescent. His parents harbored a great many underlying illness-related fears concerning his future and his independence, which they undercut in subtle but powerful ways. Outwardly, the parents denied the severity of his illness and not only expected him to behave as if he did not have an illness but also to achieve much more than his physically healthy sister. Since Jay accurately considered himself singled out by his parents, he perceived individually focused intervention as a criticism and an insult. Family-oriented intervention provided a vehicle for Jay and his parents to discuss their differences and achieve a realistic clarification of one another's expectations and feelings.

Summary of Clinical and Empirical Findings

Clinical reports and research indicate that (1) no one personality or adjustment pattern is associated with chronic illness, (2) the personality and adjustment strengths of chronically ill children outweigh their deficits, (3) chronic illness is a life stressor that, in interaction with such variables such as family adjustment, contributes to increased mental health risk but is *not* the sole cause of adjustment problems, (4) for the most part, chronically ill children resemble their physically healthy age mates with respect to mental health, (5) disease severity does not have a simple relation to mental health adjustment, particularly because the subjective meaning of a disease may outweigh objective assessment of disease-related variables as a determinant of adjustment, (6) handicapping conditions involving sensory or motor impairments entail a higher risk for mental health problems than other conditions, (7) specific illnesses appear to have selective effects on various dimensions of psychological functioning, in accord with the special life experiences imposed by symptoms and regimens, (8) young adult survivors of childhood chronic illnesses cope reasonably well with the long-term rigors of the illness but face considerable stress in their social relationships and stumbling blocks in obtaining services such as insurance and vocational training, (9) the family context emerges as a critical influence on children's mental health, (10) school and peer contexts also appear to be important influences on adjustment that deserve priority for future research, (11) although the interpersonal context of medical care experienced by chronically ill children and their families has not been well studied, preliminary evidence suggests that this context does not necessarily facilitate psychosocial adjustment, and (12) chronically ill children present a wide range of problems including hospital or illness-related reactions, such as severe personality problems caused or intensified by illness, reactions to terminal illness, and context-related (social, vocational, school, or family) adjustment problems.

Mental Health Services

Clinical work with chronically ill children requires a perspective that cannot be acquired solely from clinical experience with psychologically maladjusted but physically healthy children (Drotar, 1981). For example, to distinguish between maladaptive and adaptive coping, the mental health clinician must become familiar with the impact of the stresses posed by an individual disease and its treatment regimens. Moreover, the onset of a chonic illness (Geist, 1979) and changes in treatment regimens or physical status present very different stresses; thus, the child's coping should be evaluated against the backdrop of disease severity and physical treatment. Consequently, evaluations of chronically ill children's psychological progress over time may be much more useful than any single evaluation. Many chronically ill children who are severely stressed by crises engendered by the onset of disease, a lengthy hospitalization, or physical deteriorioation show surprising resilience and regain a level of adaptive coping without intensive psychological intervention. However, a protracted retreat from age-appropriate developmental tasks generally signals a more ominous psychological disturbance, which may require more intensive psychological intervention (Drotar, 1975b, 1978). Age-related variations in children's intellectual understanding of disease (Campbell, 1975; Simeonsson, Buckley, and Monsay, 1979), salient emotional concerns (Freud, 1952; Nagera, 1978; Schowalter, 1977), and expectations for management of treatment regimens also require the clinician to acquire knowledge of how developmental processes affect understanding of and adjustment to chronic illness (Whitt, 1982).

The logistics of mental health treatment are complicated by the fact that chronically ill children often live in communities distant from medical centers where their physical care is based. When referrals to community services are indicated, families often require a great deal of support to help them contact professionals who may not be familiar with their child's disease. In fact, community-based mental health professionals may not have had sufficient clinical experience with chronic illness populations to allow them to feel comfortable with service delivery to this population. For this reason, mental health clinicians in comprehensive-care teams in large medical centers have important roles as consultants to community mental health facilities (Brantley, Stabler, and Whitt, 1981).

Finally, the nature of their illness-related experience can also color family acceptance of mental health intervention. Because chronically ill children and their families undergo many procedures over which they have no control, they may need additional preparation and time to consider the meaning of a mental health intervention, lest this experience be seen as yet another violation of personal autonomy (Drotar and Chwast, 1978). Hospital-based professionals' understandable zeal to help a highly stressed child can sometimes lead to premature application of mental health treatment at a time when the child's needs for the continued and reliable presence of family or hospital staff are much more compelling (Drotar and Chwast, 1978). Moreover, the professional staff's work-related stress can lead to counterproductive labeling of a highly stressed but mentally healthy child as emotionally disturbed (Meyer and Mendelson, 1961). In such instances, helping medical and nursing staff recognize how their personal reactions can color their appraisals of children and how they may provide more effective emotional support in the setting can be much more productive than direct psychological treatment of the child's "disturbance" (Drotar, 1975a, 1977a; Drotar and Doershuk, 1979).

Specialized mental health services for chronically ill children are offered by a wide range of professionals (nurses, psychologists, social workers, and psychiatrists) in pediatric hospitals. Such services vary dramatically from setting to setting and are characterized by having developed in response to adjustment problems already experienced by chronically ill children rather than being organized with a preventive focus.

Clinicians employ treatment modalities for mental health problems ranging from treatment specifically geared to chronic illness problems to services that overlap with those offered to physically healthy but emotionally maladjusted children. Unique treatment methods include preventive mental health interventions directed toward mastery of illness-related anxiety, such as helping the child recognize, label, and express feelings through activity and play (Oremland and Oremland, 1973; Petrillo and Sanger, 1972; Kohlberg and Rothenberg, 1970). Potentially helpful methods to prevent adverse emotional sequelae to stressful medical procedures include active strategies, such as information-giving, encouraging expression (Siegel, 1976), correcting fantasies (Schowalter, 1971), and hypnosis (Sarles, 1975). Severe personality problems experienced by chronically ill children may be handled in very much the same way as those of physically healthy children, with the proviso that the child's reactions to the illness, recognition of illness-related stresses, and emphasis on normalization of routine become treatment foci (Drotar, 1975b; Drotar and Chwast, 1978). Family-oriented mental health interventions appear to hold special promise of enhancing day-to-day coping with a chronic illness because they address the main context of the chronically ill child's life (Ablin and others, 1971; Drotar, 1978; Caplan and Killea, 1976; Friedrich, 1977; Litman, 1974; Sourkes, 1977; Stabler and others, 1981). Observations of family problem solving, communication, and coping (Lewis and others, 1976; Liebman, Minuchin, and Baker, 1976; Ablin and others, 1971; Drotar and others, 1981a) can reveal potentially maladaptive family influences (Jaffee, 1978), help structure interventions that minimize the counterproductive labeling of the ill child as the sole focus of disturbance, and support fathers or healthy siblings who may be highly troubled but silent participants in the child's care (Boyle and others, 1976; Cairns and others, 1979).

Preventive Intervention in Life Contexts: Future Models for Service Delivery

Although some clinicians have been highly innovative in developing treatment modalities for chronically ill children, conceptual frameworks that guide treatment approaches have not addressed the special life stresses faced by these children, particularly those that occur in contexts apart from that of physical care. Moreover, since only a minority of chronically ill children develop severe mental health disturbances, services oriented solely to these problems are not sufficient from a public health standpoint. Mental health services should be allocated to address the adjustment strains that are inevitable consequences of an illness for a large number of chronically ill children. In addition, because chronically ill children experience difficulties in the hospital context as well as with peers, in school, and especially in family life, a model service delivery program should integrate hospital-based services with community-centered advocacy.

The present state of the art is characterized by a paucity of empirical demonstrations of the efficacy of service delivery concerning the mental health of chronically ill children. However, long-term clinical experiences with a variety of chronic illnesses attest to the potential efficacy of prevention-focused mental health services in facilitating the quality of professional-family interchange and reducing certain disease-related psychosocial problems such as noncompliance (Drotar, Crawford, and Bush, 1984; Drotar, Crawford, and Ganofsky, 1983; Ganofsky, Drotar, and Makker, 1983). Such services include the following dimensions: (1) design of hospital psychosocial environments to enhance children's emotional expression, sense of efficacy, and understanding (Ack, 1974; Plank, 1971; Adams, 1976; Magrab and Bronheim, 1976), (2) integration of mental health services with the child's medical care (Drotar and Ganofsky, 1976; Drotar and others, 1981a; Koocher, Sourkes, and Keane, 1979; Sourkes, 1977), and (3) organization of physical care to facilitate the child's competencies with life tasks (Hobbs, 1975).

The specific goals of preventive mental health intervention with chronically ill children and their families include (1) mastery of potentially disruptive anxiety related to the disease and its physical management, (2) a reasonable understanding of and adherence to necessary medical regimens, (3) integration of illness into family life, especially the reconciliation of family needs with those of the ill child, and (4) adaptation to hospital, school, and peers. In a preventive model, the clinician functions very much as a guide and advocate for the child and family through the course of the disease, in pursuit of a reasonable level of adaptation. Success depends heavily on the trust between the professional and family. The elusive but powerful concept of trust appears to evolve from the following principles: (1) continuity of relationship, (2) active participation by professional caregivers, (3) mutual participation of child and family, (4) advocacy, (5) a focus on coping and competence, (6) a developmental perspective, and (7) a family-centered focus.

Continuity of Relationship—The Cornerstone of Preventive Intervention

From the families' vantage point, continuity means that they will not be abandoned at any point during the course of the illness, that they will have a familiar person to turn to in times of crisis and with whom to share moments of triumph. From the professional's perspective, continuity provides a critical opportunity for monitoring how a family and child are adjusting to their disease. Continuity of care requires a committed availability in person and by phone, especially at times of crisis. Yet, this commitment does not entail being on call at every moment. Rather, continuity is communicated to children and families in ways that signal commitment of presence: visits during a hospitalization or crisis, remembering a child's birthday, the experience of sharing difficult times. Continuity of relationship allows the caregiver to build on prior transactions, provide feedback to the child and family concerning progress, anticipate future problems, and identify areas that require intervention.

Active Involvement of Professional Caregivers

In preventive work, the caregiver initiates contact with the chronically ill child and family, facilitates information exchange, and defines the nature of the relationship. The professional's initiation and the provision of emotional support and information about the disease help build a sense of security in the midst of an anxiety-laden experience. In addition, the caregiver's understanding of expectable versus deviant psychological reactions can help most families recognize illness-related stress reactions as meaningful and legitimate ways of coping rather than as deviant behaviors. Finally, the anticipation of the emotional impact of developmental and disease-related changes also encourages a sense of mastery. The caregiver must be informative yet not intrusive, must register concern but no alarm, and must respect families' autonomy and capacity to utilize information and resources (Drotar and Chwast, 1978).

Emphasis on Coping and Competence

A coping perspective focuses on the stressful, yet potentially manageable prospect of living with a chronic disease and construes illness as an opportunity for mastery rather than an inevitable disruption. Special advantages in using a competence or coping-based diagnostic perspective to plan preventive mental health interventions include (1) evaluation of the child's coping strategies in terms of whether they enhance or disrupt life adjustment and compliance with treatment regimens, (2) emphasis on strengths in order to communicate a sense of hope and optimism to chronically ill children and their families, who often feel singled out as negative exceptions owing to their illness, and (3) an emphasis on efficacy (what the child and family can do to make positive changes in their situation) as a powerful sustaining force that can contribute to self-esteem (Bandura, 1982).

Family Context as a Unifying Focus of Prevention

Family-centered preventive comprehensive care can be defined as the systematic inclusion of family members in the child's ongoing physical care in ways that encourage family problem solving, decision making, and management of disease-related stress. It appears critical that the child and family negotiate their relationships with caregivers as active partners rather than as passive recipients of treatment. It is important to create an atmosphere in which the child's and family's perceptions are believed and in which families are given clear feedback concerning their responsibilities for treatment regimens and their departures from agreed upon expectations. Inclusion of families in decisions concerning the illness helps promote a sense of control (Nannis and others, 1982) that provides an antidote to the constraint associated with the experience of a chronic illness. Shared decision making and responsibility also allow for more honest transactions in which professional caregivers are not required to have all the answers and family members are encouraged to admit their anxieties.

Advocacy

Advocacy, the use of professional knowledge of a chronic disease to intervene with professionals in other agencies and institutions on behalf of the family, is a critical ingredient of preventive intervention. Advocacy can include explanation of the disease and the health care setting to the family, help with finances, communicating to teachers, or helping create more effective patient-physician interactions. The advocate's direct knowledge of the child's experience facilitates information exchange and ameliorates feelings of helplessness engendered by parents having to separate from their child at a critical juncture.

Preventive Intervention in the School

School is a significant influence on the mental health of chronically ill children, and transitions within hospital, school, and family contexts pose even greater dilemmas for chronically ill children and their families than they do for physically healthy children (Lightfoot, 1978).

Special schooling for chronically ill children may have import for preventive intervention; for example, the decision to obtain home tutoring for a chronically ill child may facilitate short-term physical management, but have negative consequences for long-term socialization. Many chronically ill children are educated by teachers who are unfamiliar with the disease and its implications for physical activity, socialization, and learning. The stigma associated with chronic illness often contributes to systematic discrimination, which may require intervention at a programmatic level. Some of the productive interventions may not involve direct psychological treatment but rather the use of psychological knowledge by the child's advocate in the service of institutional change. School-related preventive intervention on behalf of chronically ill children should thus focus on (1) facilitation of return to school following hospitalization, including normalization of routine, (2) management of the social stresses of illness-related regimens, and (3) preventive educational advocacy with teachers and with the school system (Crittenden and Gofman, 1976).

Enhancement of Peer Socialization

Chronically ill peers can provide an important influence in helping the child master potentially difficult treatment regimens and feelings of deviance. The old-timers can beneficially orient the newcomers. The more experienced patient describes the treatment, dietary restrictions, and medication and shares the inside information, such as how to get along with the staff. The new patient sees that someone else in the same boat has survived the frightening treatments. In addition, the sense of control children and adolescents achieve by being in a more authoritative role with their peers enhances their self-esteem.

Most children who have chronic illnesses know few, if any, other children with the same condition. Attendance at camp for children with the same problem provides an opportunity to meet children like themselves who live each day with similar expectations and restrictions. Seeing other ill children participating in a full range of activities helps many children acquire knowledge about their disease and feel more competent (Harkavy and others, 1982; Primack and Greifer, 1977).

Implications for Future Research

Scientific understanding of efficacy of treatment outcomes and the psychological and physical variables that contribute to mental health outcome within heterogenous populations of chronically ill children is at a rudimentary level. The design of psychosocial research concerning the mental health of chronically ill children requires special methodological perspectives. Because definitive cause and effect experimental research designs are simply not realistic for the study of the mental health of chronically ill children (Shontz, 1970; Gayton and Friedman, 1973), researchers must learn the creative use of comparison group or correlational designs to assess the relationship of disease-related factors (number of hospitalizations, physical pain, treatment regimens, changes in physical appearance) and/or non-disease-related factors (family background, age, prior level of adjustment, stress) to mental health outcome. Moreover, researchers must address the heterogeneity of individual chronic illness populations, which can differ substantially on such variables as disease-related organic problems and anticipated stresses (Wood, Boat, and Doershuk, 1976).

The conceptual frameworks of psychological studies have generally not done justice to the special life experiences of chronically ill children and their families. For example, the interpretation of obtained personality or adjustment differences between chronically ill and a matched sample of physically healthy children (a common research design) poses a very difficult inferential dilemma: are such group differences a psychological deficit or are they an understandable difference in coping that results from exposure to different life conditions (Mohr, 1977)? It is conceivable that test responses that would be ordinarily considered deviant for a physically healthy child may be normative responses for a chronically ill child who faces such very different life circumstances. For example, chronically ill children's discrepant portrayals of human figures may very well reflect accurate appraisals of their compromised physical state rather than a disturbed body image as has been inferred by some (Boyle and others, 1976). Careful interpretation of group differences is especially important because psychological test measures (as well as clinical norms) have been developed on physically healthy populations (Pless, 1979) with variable standardization, reliability, and validity (Pless and Pinkerton, 1975).

The confusing array of potential operational definitions and measures of mental health or personality adjustment also makes it difficult to evaluate findings from different studies. Definitions of adjustment have included (1) freedom from severe psychopathology, (2) normal or age-appropriate personality functioning, (3) acceptance of or adequate coping with disease regimens, and (4) functioning in school, family, and with peers (Pless and Pinkerton, 1975). Each of these definitions has somewhat different implications for study focus and outcome. Integration of differing research perspectives and increased standardization of measures are compelling needs.

Reservations might also be raised about whether the mental health of chronically ill children is best considered from the framework of individual adjustment. Prior research and clinical observation concerning chronically ill children's mental health has often followed a medical model in which psychological problems and the search for psychological causes and treatments are localized *within* the chronically ill child's personality. This paradigm has a number of serious conceptual and methodological flaws including (1) unwarranted assumptions of cross-situational generality (Mischel, 1973), (2) inconsistent reliability and validity of diagnostic categories (Achenbach, 1978; Achenbach and Edelbrock, 1978), (3) negative consequences of labeling (Hobbs, 1975), (4) adherence to a deficit model in which differences from physically healthy peers are generally considered as deficiencies rather than understood as a reflection of special life circumstances and stresses (Mohr, 1977), (5) an emphasis on individual adaptation to crisis, trauma, or stress rather than on coping as a social transaction (Sameroff, 1975; Rutter, 1979, 1981), and (6) failure to consider life-context variables (for example, school, family, health care system) as influences on childhood adjustment and as resources for intervention (Bronfenbrenner, 1979; Hobbs, 1975; Mishler and others, 1981).

Research and clinical intervention concerning the mental health of chronically ill children is sorely in need of a focus that addresses the unique aspects of chronic physical illness. Such clinical research is best construed from a coping and/or competence-based model that focuses on (1) detailed definition of coping strategies (Cohen and Lazarus 1979; Lazarus, Averill, and Opton, 1974; Lazarus, 1980), (2) functional assessments of coping strategies in terms of whether they enhance or disrupt functioning, particularly in social relationships, and (3) similarities and differences in children's and families' objective and subjective definitions of chronic illness and stress. Because coping is a vague, all-inclusive concept that subsumes behaviors across a wide range of adaptive contexts (Lazarus and Launier, 1978; Roskies and Lazarus, 1980), one must differentiate among the *modes* (information seeking or action), *functions* (for example, altering a stressful situation and outcomes), and *effects* (on life adjustment) of coping. Coping strategies can also be functionally categorized as responses that change the situation out of which stress arises, that control the meaning of the experience (for example, positive appraisal), that control stress after it has arisen, or that regulate emotion (Lazarus and Launier, 1978; Pearlin and Schooler, 1978).

Future reseach concerning the mental health of chronically ill children should shift from a preoccupation with identification of deficits to a focus on factors that contribute to children's resilience over time (Rutter, 1979). Such an approach is best exemplified in Werner and Smith's (1982) longitudinal study of physically healthy children who were exposed to severe family stresses yet attained positive mental health. Resilient children were characterized by their responsiveness, ability to engage and retain the attention of adults in a socially acceptable way, and maintain personal autonomy and confidence. As applied to the stress of a chronic illness, these findings suggest the importance of endowing potentially threatening illness-related experience with a positive meaning, as an opportunity for mastery and creation of options (Cousins, 1981) rather than as a negative or limiting experience. For this reason, children's internal appraisal of stressful events—and developmental aspects of how children appraise stress—may be a critical but as yet ill-defined mediating factor in adaptive handling of change, particularly stressful change (Anthony, 1978).

Prospective studies of children at risk for mental health problems (Werner and Smith, 1982; Sameroff, 1975) also strongly emphasize the importance of considering coping as a *transactional process* (Mechanic, 1974) that involves the chronically ill child in competence-enhancing transactions with significant peers and adults over the course of time. Priority areas for future research include identification of those transactional processes that characterize effective coping, the interpersonal contexts in which these processes are likely to occur, and the perceptions of self, others (including family), and the disease that characterize effective coping.

Coping is a process that involves a series of developmental adjustments to life and illness-related changes (Cohen and Lazarus, 1979; Mechanic, 1974), treatment regimens, physical deterioration, and stages of psychological development. Coping is thus best studied from a developmental perspective (Lazarus, 1980) in which children and families are studied over time on measures that link coping strategy to adaptive life outcomes.

The development of objective measures to assess compliance with treatment regimens, management of anxiety, and adaptation to life contexts is another priority for future research. Potentially applicable approaches to the assessment of coping include Koski's (1969) distinction of coping style or mode (external versus internal) from function (constructive versus nonconstructive) among children with diabetes, Johnson's (1979) assessment of the behavior of children with diabetes, Zeitlin's (1980) ratings of behavioral coping strategies in pre-schoolers, Yamamoto's (1979) study of children's perceptions of stressfulness of experience, and Spinetta and Maloney's (1978) classifications of coping strategy in childhood cancer. Finally, the coping strategies of resilient survivors would appear to be a fruitful target area for future research endeavors.

In order to plan services that enhance the mental health of chronically ill children in life contexts, greater attention must be given to identification of factors in school and in medical environments that enhance or disrupt chronically ill children's psychosocial functioning. Moreover, outcome studies of specific psychosocial interventions designed to enhance children's coping skills and management of disease-related stress are very much needed. Such applied intervention research might productively focus on such target areas as the social competencies and problem solving that enhance relations between ill children and important persons in their lives and facilitate stress management (Felner and others, 1981), coping with disease regimens, or self-concept.

The need for advance planning for prevention-focused clinical services that are located in major medical centers but have the capacity to intersect with school, family, and community contexts is especially important given the recent improvements in medical technology (Patenaude, Szymanski, and Rappaport, 1979). With insurance reimbursement tied to mental health services for already identified problems (Iscoe, 1981), it is unlikely that preventive mental health services for chronically ill children will be expanded without concerted efforts toward documenting their efficacy. The lack of documentation of the efficacy of psychosocial interventions with chronically ill children (with certain exceptions—for example, Melamed and Siegel, 1975; Peterson, Hartman, and Gelfand, 1980) may very well go hand in hand with the unfortunate tendency to establish medical care programs without concerted planning for the special intervention, research, and consultation services required to address mental health needs (Brantley, Stabler, and Whitt, 1981). We are convinced that advances in the understanding of the mental health of chronically ill children and their families will not be forthcoming from single studies but will evolve from programmatically applied research in which questions are posed with increasing clarity and measures are slowly refined.

Prevention-focused research with chronically ill children provides a unique vantage point from which to study the factors that enhance or disrupt human resilience under prolonged stress. Moreover, the techniques of intervention that prove effective for management of chronic illness–related stress may suggest principles of intervention that reduce psychologic vulnerability in other stressful life situations (Felner and others, 1981). Certainly, chronically ill children and their families have much to teach us about human resilience, courage, and persistence in the face of prolonged stress and threat (Bluebond-Langner, 1978; Woodson, 1975). Let us hope that we learn to heed their messages.

References

Ablin, A., and others. "A Conference with the Family of a Leukemic Child." *American Journal of Diseases of Children*, 1971, *122*, 362–366.

Achenbach, T. M. "Psychopathology of Childhood: Research Problems and Issues." *Journal of Clinical and Consulting Psychology*, 1978, *46*, 759–776.

Achenbach, T. M., and Edelbrock, C. S. "The Classification of Child Psychopathology: A Review and Analysis of Empirical Efforts." *Psychological Bulletin*, 1978, *85*, 1275–1301.

Ack, M. "The Psychological Environment of a Children's Hospital." *Pediatric Psychology*, 1974, *2*, 3–5.

Adams, M. "A Hospital Play Program: Helping Children with Serious Illness." *American Journal of Orthopsychiatry*, 1976, *127*, 138–145.

Anthony, E. J. "A Clinical Evaluation of Children with Psychotic Parents." *American Journal of Psychiatry*, 1969, *126*, 2–10.

Anthony, E. J. "Theories of Change and Children at High Risk for Change." In E. J. Anthony and C. Chitland (Eds.), *The Child and His Family*, Vol. 6: *Children and Their Parents in a Changing World*. New York: Wiley, 1978.

Artiss, K. L., and Levine, A. S. "Doctor-Patient Relation in Severe Illness." *New England Journal of Medicine*, 1973, *283*, 1210–1214.

Bandura, A. "Self-Efficacy Mechanisms in Human Agency." *American Psychologist*, 1982, *37*, 122–147.

Bank, S., and Kahn, M. "Sisterhood-Brotherhood Is Powerful: Sibling Systems and Family Therapy." In S. Chess and A. Thomas (Eds.), *Annual Progress in Child Psychiatry and Child Development*. New York: Brunner/Mazel, 1976.

Battle, C. U. "The Role of the Pediatrician as an Ombudsman in the Health Care of the Young Handicapped Child." *Pediatrics*, 1972, *50*, 916–924.

Bell, R. Q., and Harper, L. V. *Child Effects on Adults*. Hillsdale, N. J.: Lawrence Erlbaum Associates, 1977.

Belsky, J. "Early Human Experience: A Family Perspective." *Developmental Psychology*, 1981, 17 (1), 3–23.

Bergman, A. R., and Stamm, S. J. "The Morbidity of Cardiac Nondisease in School Children." *New England Journal of Medicine*, 1967, *276*, 1008–1116.

Bergmann, T. *Children in the Hospital*. New York: International Universities Press, 1965.

Binger, C. M., and others. "Childhood Leukemia: Emotional Impact on Patient and Family." *New England Journal of Medicine*, 1969, *280*, 414–421.

Blake, S., and Paulsen, K. "Therapeutic Interventions with Terminally Ill Children: A Review." *Professional Psychology*, 1981, *12*, 655–663.

Bluebond-Langner, M. *The Private Worlds of Dying Children*. Princeton, N.J.: Princeton University Press, 1978.

Boyle, I. R., and others. "Emotional Adjustment of Adolescents and Young Adults with Cystic Fibrosis." *Journal of Pediatrics,* 1976, *88,* 318–326.

Brantley, H. T., Stabler, B., and Whitt, J. K. "Program Considerations in Comprehensive Care of Chronically Ill Children." *Journal of Pediatric Psychology,* 1981, *6,* 229–238.

Breslau, N., Weitzman, M., and Messenger, K. "Psychologic Functioning of Siblings of Disabled Children." *Pediatrics,* 1981, *67,* 344–353.

Bronfenbrenner, U. *The Ecology of Human Development.* Cambridge, Mass.: Harvard University Press, 1979.

Bruhn, J. G. "Effects of Chronic Illness on the Family." *Journal of Family Practice,* 1977, *4,* 1057–1060.

Bush, M. "Family Concept and Adjustment of Siblings and Parents of Children with Chronic Illness and Emotional Disorder." Unpublished Master's thesis. Case Western Reserve University, 1981.

Cairns, N., and others. "Adaptation of Siblings to Childhood Malignancy." *Journal of Pediatrics,* 1979, *95,* 484–487.

Campbell, J. D. "Illness Is a Point of View. The Development of Children's Concept of Illness." *Child Development,* 1975, *46,* 92–100.

Caplan, G., and Killilea, M. *Support Systems and Mutual Help: Multidisciplinary Explorations.* New York: Grune & Stratton, 1976.

Cobb, S. "Social Support as a Moderator of Life Stress." *Psychosomatic Medicine,* 1976, *38,* 300–314.

Cohen, F., and Lazarus, R. "Coping with the Stress of Illness." In G. C. Stone, F. Cohen, and N. E. Adler, and Associates, *Health Psychology—A Handbook: Theories, Applications, and Challenges of a Psychological Approach to the Health Care System.* San Francisco: Jossey-Bass, 1979.

Cousins, N. *Human Options.* New York: Norton, 1981.

Crain, A., Sussman, M. B., and Weil, W. B. "Effects of a Diabetic Child on Marital Integration and Related Measures of Family Functioning." *Journal of Health and Human Behavior,* 1966, pp. 122–127.

Crittenden, M., and Gofman, H. "Follow-Ups and Downs: The Medical Center, the Family, and the School." *Journal of Pediatric Psychology,* 1976, *1,* 66–68.

Dorner, S. "Psychological and Social Problems of Families of Adolescent Spina Bifida Patients: A Preliminary Report." *Developmental Medicine and Child Neurology,* 1973, *15* (supplement 29), 24–26.

Dorner, S. "Adolescents with Spina Bifida. How They See Their Situation." *Archives of Disease in Childhood,* 1976, *51,* 439–444.

Downey, J. "Adaptation of Children with Adrenogenital Syndrome." Unpublished manuscript. School of Medicine, Case Western Reserve University, 1979.

Drotar, D. "Death in the Pediatric Hospital: Psychological Consultation with Medical and Nursing Staff." *Journal of Child Clinical Psychology,* 1975a, *4,* 33–35.

Drotar, D. "The Treatment of a Severe Anxiety Reaction in an Adolescent Boy Following Renal Transplantation." *Journal of the American Academy of Child Psychiatry,* 1975b, *14,* 451–462.

Drotar, D. "Psychological Consultation in the Pediatric Hospital." *Professional Psychology,* 1976, *7,* 76–83.

Drotar, D. "Clinical Psychological Practice in the Pediatric Hospital." *Professional Psychology,* 1977a, *8,* 72–80.

Drotar, D. "Family Oriented Intervention with the Dying Adolescent." *Journal of Pediatric Psychology,* 1977b, *2,* 68–71.

Drotar, D. "Adaptational Problems of Children and Adolescents with Cystic Fibrosis." *Journal of Pediatric Psychology,* 1978, *3,* 45–50.

Drotar, D. "Psychological Perspectives in Chronic Childhood Illness." *Journal of Pediatric Psychology,* 1981, *6,* 211–228.

Drotar, D., and Chwast, R. "Family Oriented Intervention in Chronic Illness." Paper presented at annual meeting of Ohio Psychological Association, Cleveland, Ohio, 1978.

Drotar, D., and Doershuk, C. F. "The Interdisciplinary Case Conference: An Aid to Pediatric Intervention with the Dying Adolescent." *Archives of the Foundation of Thanatology,* 1979, *7,* 79–96.

Drotar, D., and Ganofsky, M. A. "Mental Health Intervention with Children and Adolescents with End-Stage Renal Failure." *International Journal of Psychiatry in Medicine,* 1976, *7,* 181–194.

Drotar, D., Crawford, P., and Bush, M. "The Family Context of Chronic Childhood Illness: Implications for Psychosocial Intervention." In M. Eisenberg (Ed.), *Chronic Illness and Disability Through the Life Span: Effects on Self and Family.* New York: Springer, 1984.

Drotar, D., Crawford, P., and Ganofsky, M. A. "Prevention with Chronically Ill Children." In M. C. Roberts and L. Peterson (Eds.), *Prevention of Problems in Childhood: Psychological Research and Applications.* New York: Wiley, 1984.

Drotar, D., Ganofsky, M. A., and Makker, S. P. "Comprehensive Management of Severe Emotional Reactions of Children with End-Stage Renal Failure." *Dialysis and Transplantation,* 1979, *10,* 983–986.

Drotar, D., Mazzarins, H., and Zelko, F. "Coping Patterns Among Adolescents and Young Adults with Cystic Fibrosis." Unpublished manuscript. School of Medicine, Case Western Reserve University, 1980.

Drotar, D., Owens, R., and Gotthold, J. "Personality Adjustment of Children and Adolescents with Hypopituitarism." *Child Psychiatry and Human Development,* 1980, *11,* 59–66.

Drotar, D., and others. "The Adaptation of Parents to the Birth of an Infant with a Congenital Malformation: A Hypothetical Model." *Pediatrics,* 1975, *56,* 710–717.

Drotar, D., and others. "A Family-Oriented Supportive Approach to Renal Transplantation in Children." In N. Levy (Ed.), *Psychological Factors in Hemodialysis and Transplantation.* New York: Plenum, 1981a.

Drotar, D., and others. "Psychosocial Functioning of Children with Cystic Fibrosis." *Pediatrics,* 1981b, *67,* 338–343.

Drotar, D., and others. "The Role of the Psychologist in Pediatric Outpatient and

Inpatient Settings." In J. Tuma (Ed.), *The Practice of Pediatric Psychology.* New York: Wiley, 1981c.

Easson, W. M. *The Dying Child.* Springfield, Ill.: Thomas, 1970.

Eissler, R. S., and others. *Physical Illness and Handicap in Childhood.* New Haven, Conn.: Yale University Press, 1977.

Faust, D. S., and Campbell, H. S. "Community Attitudes Toward the Child with a Life-Threatening Illness." Paper presented at the annual meeting of the American Psychological Association, New York, September 1979.

Felner, R. D., and others. "A Prevention Program for Children Experiencing Life Crisis." *Professional Psychology,* 1981, *8,* 444–452.

Fine, R. N., and others. "Long-Term Results of Renal Transplantation in Children." *Pediatrics,* 1978, *61,* 641–651.

Ford, A. B., Liske, R E., and Ort, R. S. "Reactions of Physicians and Medical Students to Chronic Illness." *Journal of Chronic Diseases,* 1963, *15,* 785–794.

Fox, R. *Essays in Medical Sociology.* New York: Wiley, 1975.

Fox, R. C., and Swazey, J. P. *The Courage to Fail: A Social View of Organ Transplants and Dialysis.* Chicago: University of Chicago Press, 1978.

Freud, A. "The Role of Bodily Illness in the Mental Life of Children." *Psychoanalytic Study of the Child,* 1952, *7,* 69–81.

Friedman, S., and others. "Behavioral Observations of Parents Anticipating the Death of a Child." *Pediatrics,* 1963, *32,* 610–625.

Friedrich, W. N. "Ameliorating the Psychological Impact of Chronic Physical Disease on the Child and Family." *Journal of Pediatric Psychology,* 1977, *2,* 26–31.

Ganofsky, M. A., Drotar, D., and Makker, S. P. "Growing Up with Renal Failure: Problems and Perspectives." In *Psychonephrology,* Vol. 2. New York: Plenum, 1983.

Gayton, W., and Friedman, S. "Psychosocial Aspects of Cystic Fibrosis: A Review of the Literature." *American Journal of Diseases of Children,* 1973, *126,* 856–859.

Gayton, W. F., and others. "Children with Cystic Fibrosis: Psychological Test Findings of Patients, Siblings, and Parents." *Pediatrics,* 1977, *59,* 888–894.

Geist, R. A. "Onset of Chronic Illness in Children and Adolescents: Psychotherapeutic and Consultative Intervention." *American Journal of Orthopsychiatry,* 1979, *49,* 4–22.

Glaser, N., and others. "Educational and Vocational Attainments of Adolescents and Young Adult Survivors of Spina Bifida." Unpublished manuscript. School of Medicine, Case Western Reserve University, 1980.

Gogan, J., and others. "Pediatric Cancer Survival and Marriage Issues Affecting Adult Adjustment." *American Journal of Orthopsychiatry,* 1979, *49,* 423–430.

Grushkin, G. M., Korsch, B. M., and Fine, R. N. "The Outlook for Adolescents with Chronic Renal Failure." *Pediatric Clinics of North America,* 1973, *20,* 953–963.

Haggerty, R., Roghmann, K. J., and Pless, I. B. *Child Health and the Community.* New York: Wiley, 1975.

Harkavy, J., and others. "Who Learns What at Diabetes Summer Camp?" Paper presented at the meeting of the American Psychological Association, Washington, D.C., 1982.

Harper, D. C., Richman, L. C., and Snider, B. C. "School Adjustment and Degree of Physical Impairment." *Journal of Pediatric Psychology,* 1980, *5,* 377–383.

Heisler, A. B., and Friedman, S. B. "Social and Psychological Considerations in Chronic Disease: With Particular Reference to the Management of Seizure Disorders." *Journal of Pediatric Psychology,* 1981, *6,* 239–250.

Hobbs, N. *The Futures of Children: Recommendations of the Project on Classification of Exceptional Children.* San Francisco: Jossey-Bass, 1975.

Holroyd, J., and Guthrie, D. "Stress in Families with Neuromuscular Disease." *Journal of Clinical Psychology,* 1979, *35,* 735–739.

Iscoe, I. "Conceptual Barriers to Training for the Primary Prevention of Psychopathology." In J. M. Jaffee and G. W. Albee (Eds.), *Prevention Through Political Action and Social Change.* Hanover, N.H.: University Press, 1981.

Jaffee, D. T. "The Role of Family Therapy in Treating Physical Illness." *Hospital and Community Psychiatry,* 1978, *29,* 169–174.

Johnson, M. R. "Mental Health Interventions with Medically Ill Children: A Review of the Literature, 1970–1977." *Journal of Pediatric Psychology,* 1979, *4,* 147–163.

Kagen-Goodheart, L. "Reentry: Living with Childhood Cancer." *American Journal of Orthopsychiatry,* 1977, *47,* 651–658.

Kanthor, H., Pless, I. B., Satterwhite, B., and Myers, G. "Areas of Responsibility in the Health Care of Multiply Handicapped Children." *Pediatrics,* 1974, *54,* 779–786.

Katz, J., and Capron, A. M. *Catastrophic Diseases: Who Decides What?* New York: Russel Sage Foundation, 1975.

Klein, S. D., and Simmons, R. G. "Chronic Disease and Childhood Development: Kidney Disease and Transplantation." In R. Simmons (Ed.), *Research in Community and Mental Health,* Vol. 1. Greenwich, Conn.: JAI Press, 1979.

Kohlberg, I. J., and Rothenberg, M. B. "Comprehensive Care Following Multiple Life-Threatening Injuries." *American Journal of Diseases of Children,* 1970, *119,* 449–451.

Koocher, G. P., and O'Malley, J. E. *The Damocles Syndrome: Psychological Consequences of Surviving Childhood Cancer.* New York: McGraw-Hill, 1981.

Koocher, G. P., Sourkes, B. M., and Keane, W. M. "Pediatric Oncology Consultation: A Generalizable Model for Medical Settings." *Professional Psychology,* 1979, *10,* 467–474.

Korsch, B. M., and others. "Experience with Children and Their Families During Extended Hemodialysis and Kidney Transplantation." *Pediatric Clinics of North America,* 1971, *18,* 625–631.

Korsch, B. M., and others. "Kidney Transplantation in Children: Psychosocial Follow Up Study on Child and Family." *Journal of Pediatrics,* 1973, *83,* 339–408.

Koski, M. L. "The Coping Processes in Childhood Diabetes." *Acta Paediatrica Scandinavia,* 1969, *198* (supplement), 7–56.

Kucia, C., and others. "Home Observation of Family Interaction and Childhood

Adjustment to Cystic Fibrosis." *Journal of Pediatric Psychology,* 1979, *4,* 479–489.

Lansky, S. B., and Genel, M. "Symbiotic Regressive Behavior Patterns in Childhood Malignancy." *Clinical Pediatrics,* 1975, *17,* 133–138.

Lansky, S. B., and others. "School Phobia in Children with Malignant Neoplasms." *American Journal of Diseases of Children,* 1975, *129,* 42–46.

Lansky, S. B., and others. "Childhood Cancer: Parental Discord and Divorce." *Pediatrics,* 1978, *65,* 184–190.

Lascari, A., and Stehbens, J. "The Reactions of Families to Childhood Leukemia: An Evaluation of a Program of Emotional Management." *Clinical Pediatrics,* 1973, *12,* 210–214.

Lauler, R. H., Nakielny, W., and Wright, N. A. "Psychological Implications of Cystic Fibrosis." *Canadian Medical Association Journal,* 1966, *94,* 1043–1048.

Lavigne, J. V., and Ryan, M. "Psychological Adjustment of Siblings of Children with Chronic Illness." *Pediatrics,* 1979, *63* (4), 616–627.

Lazarus, R. "The Stress and Coping Paradigm." In A. Bond and J. C. Rosen (Eds.), *Competence and Coping During Adulthood.* Hanover, N.H.: University Press, 1980.

Lazarus R., and Launier, R. "Stress Related Transactions Between Person and Environment." In L. W. Pervin and M. Lewis (Eds.), *Perspectives in Interactional Psychology.* New York: Plenum, 1978.

Lazarus, R., Averill, T. R., and Opton, E. M. "The Psychology of Coping: Issues of Research and Assessment." In G. V. Coelho, D. A. Hamburg, and T. E. Adams (Eds.), *Coping and Adaptation.* New York: Basic Books, 1974.

Lewis, J. M., and others. *No Single Thread: Psychological Health in Family Systems.* New York: Brunner/Mazel, 1976.

Liebman, R., Minuchin, S., and Baker, L. "The Use of Structured Family Therapy in the Treatment of Intractable Asthma." *American Journal of Psychiatry,* 1967, *131,* 535–540.

Lightfoot, S. *Worlds Apart: Relationships Between Families and Schools.* New York: Basic Books, 1978.

Litman, T. J. "The Family as a Basic Unit in Health and Medical Care: A Social Behavioral Overview." *Social Science and Medicine,* 1974, *8,* 495–519.

Litman, T. J., and Venters, M. "Research on Health Care and the Family: A Methodological Overview." *Social Science and Medicine,* 1979, *14,* 379–385.

McAnarney, E. R., Pless, I. B., Satterwhite, B. B., and Friedman, S. B. "Psychological Problems of Children with Chronic Juvenile Arthritis." *Pediatrics,* 1974, *53,* 523–528.

McCollum, A. T., and Gibson, L. "Family Adaptation to the Child with Cystic Fibrosis." *Journal of Pediatrics,* 1970, *77,* 574–578.

McIntosh, J. "Processes of Communication, Information Seeking, and Control Associated with Cancer." *Social Science and Medicine,* 1974, *8,* 157–187.

Magrab, P. R. (Ed.). *Psychological Management of Pediatric Problems.* Vol. 1, *Early Life Conditions and Chronic Diseases.* Baltimore, Md.: University Park Press, 1978.

Magrab, P. R., and Bronheim, S. "The Child Life Model and Pediatric Hospitalization." *Journal of Pediatric Psychology*, 1976, *1*, 7-8.

Markova, I., MacDonald, K., and Forbes, C. "Impact of Hemophilia on Childrearing Practices and Parental Cooperation." *Journal of Child Psychology/ Psychiatry*, 1979, *21*, 153-161.

Mass, M., and Kaplan, A. "Reactions of Families to Chronic Hemodialysis." *Psychotherapy and Psychosomatics*, 1975, *25*, 20-26.

Mattsson, A. "Long-term Physical Illness in Childhood: A Challenge to Psychosocial Adaptation." *Pediatrics*, 1972, *50*, 801-811.

Mechanic, D. *Public Expectations and Health Care.* New York: Wiley, 1972.

Mechanic, D. "Social Structure and Personal Adaptation: Some Neglected Dimensions." In G. V. Coelho, D. A. Hamburg, and J. T. Adams (Eds.), *Coping and Adaptation.* New York: Basic Books, 1974.

Melamed, B. G., and Siegel, L. J. "Reduction of Anxiety in Children Facing Hospitalization and Surgery." *Journal of Consulting and Clinical Psychology*, 1975, *43*, 511-521.

Meyer, E., and Mendelson, M. "Psychiatric Consultations with Patients on Medical and Surgical Wards: Patterns and Processes." *Psychiatry*, 1961, *24*, 197-205.

Meyerowitz, J. H., and Kaplan, H. B. "Familial Responses to Stress: The Case of Cystic Fibrosis." *Social Science and Medicine*, 1967, *1*, 249-266.

Minuchin, S., Rosman, B., and Baker, L. *Psychosomatic Families.* Cambridge, Mass.: Harvard University Press, 1978.

Mischel, W. "Toward a Cognitive Social Learning Reconceptualization of Personality." *Psychological Review*, 1973, *80*, 252-283.

Mishler, E. G., and others. *Social Contexts of Health, Illness, and Patient Care.* New York: Cambridge University Press, 1981.

Mohr, R. "Paradigms in the Clinical Psychology of Chronic Illness." Paper presented at the annual meeting of the American Psychological Association. Washington, D.C., September 1977.

Moise, J. R. "Psychological Adjustment of Children and Adolescents with Sickle-Cell Anemia." Unpublished Master's thesis, Department of Psychology, Case Western Reserve University, 1980.

Nagera, H. "Children's Reactions to Hospitalization and Illness." *Child Psychiatry and Human Development*, 1978, *9*, 3-19.

Nannis, E. D., and others. "Correlates of Control in Pediatric Cancer Patients and Their Families." *Journal of Pediatric Psychology*, 1982, *7*, 75-84.

Natterson, T. M., and Knudson, A. G. "Observations Concerning Fear of Death in Fatally Ill Children and Their Mothers." *Psychosomatic Medicine*, 1960, *22*, 456-465.

Obetz, W. S., and others. "Children Who Survive Malignant Disease: Emotional Adaptation of the Children and Families." In J. L. Schulman and M. J. Kupst (Eds.), *The Child with Cancer.* Springfield, Ill.: Thomas, 1980.

Odom, L., Seeman, J., and Newbrough, J. R. "A Study of Family Communication Patterns and Personality Integration in Children." *Child Psychiatry and Human Development*, 1971, *1*, 275-285.

O'Malley, J. E., and others. "Psychiatric Sequelae of Surviving Childhood Cancer." *American Journal of Orthopsychiatry*, 1979, *49*, 608–616.

Oremland, E. K., and Oremland, J. D. (Eds.) *The Effects of Hospitalization on Children: Models for Their Care*. Springfield, Ill.: Thomas, 1973.

Osherson, S., and Amarasingham, L. R. "The Machine Metaphor in Medicine." In E. Mishler and others (Eds.), *Social Contexts of Health, Illness, and Patient Care*. New York: Cambridge University Press, 1981.

Parke, R. "Perspectives on Father-Infant Interaction." In J. E. Osofsky (Ed.), *Handbook of Infant Development*. New York: Wiley, 1979.

Patenaude, A. F., Szymanski, L., and Rappaport, J. "Psychological Costs of Bone Marrow Transplantation in Children." *American Journal of Orthopsychiatry*, 1979, *49*, 409–422.

Pearlin, L .J., and Schooler, C. "The Structure of Coping." *Journal of Health and Social Behavior*, 1978, *19*, 2–21.

Peterson, L., Hartman, D. P., and Gelfand, D. M. "Prevention of Child Behavior Disorders: A Lifestyle Change for Child Psychologists." In P.O. Davidson and S. R. Davidson (Eds.), *Behavioral Medicine: Changing Health Lifestyles*. New York: Brunner/Mazel, 1980.

Petrillo, M., and Sanger, S. *Emotional Care of Hospitalized Children*. Philadelphia, Pa.: Lippincott, 1972.

Plank, E. M. *Working with Children in Hospitals*. Cleveland, Ohio: Western Reserve University Press, 1971.

Pless, I. B. "Adjustment of the Young Chronically Ill." In R. Simmons (Ed.), *Research in Community and Mental Health*. Greenwich, Conn.: JAI Press, 1979.

Pless, I. B., and Douglas, I.W.B. "Chronic Illness in Childhood: I. Epidemiological and Clinical Characteristics." *Pediatrics*, 1972, *47*, 405–414.

Pless, I. B., and Pinkerton, P. *Chronic Childhood Disorders: Promoting Patterns of Adjustment*. Chicago, Ill.: Yearbook Medical Publishers, 1975.

Pless, I. B., and Roghmann, K. J. "Chronic Illness and Its Consequences: Observations Based on Three Epidemiologic Surveys." *Journal of Pediatrics*, 1971, *79*, 351–359.

Pless, I. B., and Satterwhite, B. B. "Chronic Illness." In R. J. Haggerty, K. J. Roghmann, and I. B. Pless (Eds.), *Child Health and Community*. New York: Wiley, 1975.

Pless, I. B., Roghmann, K. J., and Haggerty, R. J. "Chronic Illness, Family Functioning, and Psychological Adjustment: A Model for the Allocation of Preventive Mental Health Services." *International Journal of Epidemiology*, 1972, *1*, 271–277.

Pless, I. B., Satterwhite, B. B., and Van Vechten, D. "Chronic Illness in Childhood: A Regional Survey of Care." *Pediatrics*, 1976, *58*, 37–46.

Primack, W. A., and Greifer, I. "Summer Camp Hemodialysis for Children with Chronic Renal Failure." *Pediatrics*, 1977, *60*, 46–50.

Purcell, K., and others. "A Comparison of Psychologic Findings in Variously Defined Asthmatic Subgroups." *Journal of Psychosomatic Research*, 1969a, *13*, 67–75.

Purcell, K., and others. "The Effect on Asthma in Children of Experimental Separation from the Family." *Psychomatic Medicine,* 1969b, *31,* 144–164.

Ritchie, K. "Research Note: Interaction in the Families of Epileptic Children." *Journal of Child Psychology and Psychiatry,* 1981, *22,* 65–71.

Rosenlund, M. L., and Lustig, H. G. "Young Adults with Cystic Fibrosis: Problems of a New Generation." *Annals of Internal Medicine,* 1973, *78,* 959–961.

Roskies, E., and Lazarus, R. S. "Coping Theory and the Teaching of Coping Skills." In P.O. Davidson and S. M. Davidson (Eds.), *Behavioral Medicine— Changing Health Lifestyles.* New York: Brunner/Mazel, 1980.

Rothenberg, M. "Comprehensive Care in Pediatric Practice." *Clinical Practice,* 1976, *15,* 1097–1100.

Rutter, M. "Invulnerability, or Why Some Children Are not Damaged by Stress." In S. J. Shamsie (Ed.), *New Directions in Children's Mental Health.* New York: Spectrum Publications, 1979.

Rutter, M. "Stress, Coping, and Developing: Some Issues and Some Questions." *Journal of Child Psychology and Psychiatry,* 1981, *22,* 323–356.

Rutter, M., Tizard, T., and Whitmore, F. *Education, Health, and Behavior.* London: Longman, 1970.

Sameroff, A. "Transactional Models in Early Social Relations." *Human Development,* 1975, *181,* 65–79.

Sarles, R. M. "The Uses of Hypnosis with Hospitalized Children." *Journal of Clinical Child Psychology,* 1975,*41,* 36–38.

Schowalter, J. E. "The Utilization of Child Psychiatry on a Pediatric Adolescent Ward." *Journal of the American Academy of Child Psychiatry,* 1971, *10,* 684–699.

Schowalter, J. E. "Psychological Reactions to Physical Illness and Hospitalization in Adolescence." *Journal of the American Academy of Child Psychiatry,* 1977, *16,* 500–516.

Shontz, F. C. "Physical Disability and Personality: Theory and Recent Research." *Psychological Aspects of Disability,* 1970, *17,* 51–69.

Siegel, L. "Preparation of Children for Hospitalization: A Selected Review of the Research Literature." *Journal of Pediatric Psychology,* 1976, *1,* 26–30.

Simeonsson, R., Buckley, L., and Monsay, L. "Conceptions of Illness in Hospitalized Children." *Journal of Pediatric Psychology,* 1979, *4,* 77–81.

Sontag, S. *Illness as Metaphor.* New York: Farrar, Straus & Giroux, 1978.

Sourkes, B. "Facilitating Family Coping with Childhood Cancer." *Journal of Pediatric Psychology,* 1977, *2,* 65–68.

Spencer, R. F. "Incidence of Social and Psychiatric Problems in a Group of Hemophiliac Patients." *North Carolina Medical Journal,* 1968, *29,* 332–336.

Spinetta, J. J., and Maloney, L. J. "Death Anxiety in the Outpatient Leukemic Child." *Pediatrics,* 1975, *56,* 1034–1037.

Spinetta, J. J., and Maloney, L. J. "The Child with Cancer: Patterns of Communication and Denial." *Journal of Consulting and Clinical Psychology,* 1978, *46,* 540–541.

Spinetta, J. J., Rigler, D., and Karon, M. "Personal Space as a Measure of a Dying Child's Sense of Isolation." *Journal of Consulting and Clinical Psychology,* 1974, *42,* 751–756.

Spinetta, J. J., Swarner, J. A., and Sheposh, J. P. "Effective Parental Coping Following the Death of a Child from Cancer." *Journal of Pediatric Psychology,* 1981, *6,* 251–264.

Spinetta, P. D., and Spinetta, J. J. "The Child with Cancer in School: Teachers' Appraisal." *American Journal of Hematology/Oncology,* 1980, *2,* 89–94.

Stabler, B. "Emerging Models of Psychologist-Pediatrician Liaison." *Journal of Pediatric Psychology,* 1979, *4,* 307–313.

Stabler, B., and others. "Facilitating Positive Psychosocial Adaptation in Children with Cystic Fibrosis by Increasing Family Communication and Problem-Solving Skills." Research report by the Cystic Fibrosis Foundation, August 1981.

Steinhauer, P. D., Muskin, D. N., and Rae-Grant, Q. "Psychological Aspects of Chronic Illness." *Pediatric Clinics of North America,* 1974, *21,* 825–840.

Sterns, S. "Self-Destructive Behavior in Young Patients with Diabetes Mellitus." *Diabetes,* 1959, *8,* 379–385.

Swift, C. R., and Seidman, F. L. "Adjustment Problems of Juvenile Diabetes." *Journal of the American Academy of Child Psychiatry,* 1964, *3,* 500–515.

Tavormina, J. B., and others. "Chronically Ill Children—A Psychologically and Emotionally Deviant Population?" *Journal of Abnormal Child Psychology,* 1976, *4,* 99–110.

Tefft, B. M, and Simeonsson, R. J. "Psychology and the Creation of Health Care Settings." *Professional Psychology,* 1979, *10,* 558–570.

Tew, B. J., and Laurence, K. M. "Mothers, Brothers, and Sisters of Patients with Spina Bifida." *Developmental Medicine and Child Neurology,* 1973, *15* (29), 69–76.

Tropauer, A., Franz, M. N., and Dilgard, V. W. "Aspects of the Care of Children with Cystic Fibrosis." *American Journal of Diseases of Children,* 1970, *119,* 424–432.

Turk, J. "Impact of Cystic Fibrosis on Family Functioning." *Pediatrics,* 1967, *34,* 67–71.

Vance, J. C., and others. "Effects of Nephrotic Syndrome on the Family: A Controlled Study." *Pediatrics,* 1980, *65,* 948–955.

Venters, M. "Chronic Childhood Illness/Disability and Familial Coping." Unpublished doctoral dissertation, University of Minnesota, 1980.

Weinberg, S. "Suicidal Intent in Adolescence: A Hypothesis About the Role of Physical Illness." *Journal of Pediatrics,* 1970, *77,* 579–586.

Werner, E. E., and Smith, P. S. *Vulnerable but Invincible—A Longitudinal Study of Resilient Youth.* New York: McGraw-Hill, 1982.

Whitt, J. K. "Children's Understanding of Illness: Developmental Considerations and Pediatric Intervention." In M. Wolraich and D. K. Routh (Eds.), *Advances in Developmental and Behavioral Pediatrics.* Vol. 3. New York: JAI Press, 1982.

Wood, R., Boat, T. F., and Doershuk, C. F. "State of the Art: Cystic Fibrosis." *Annual Review of Respiratory Disease,* 1976, *113,* 833–878.

Woodson, M. *If I Die at Thirty.* Grand Rapids, Mich.: Zondervan Corp., 1975.

Yamamoto, K. "Children's Ratings of the Stressfulness of Experiences." *Developmental Psychology,* 1979, *15,* 581-582.

Zeitlin, S. "Assessing Coping Behavior." *American Journal of Orthopsychiatry,* 1980, *50,* 139–144.

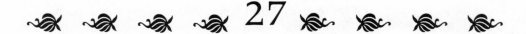

27

Training Psychologists to Work with Chronically Ill Children

Susan M. Jay, Ph.D.
Logan Wright, Ph.D.

The purpose of this chapter is to discuss training needs of pediatric psychologists who work with chronically ill children. Pediatric psychology is a discipline that has made large contributions to training and research in the area of chronic illness in children; it is a subspecialty within psychology that interfaces with behavioral medicine. Although the major emphasis in this chapter is on training needs and issues within pediatric psychology, the content areas and training issues delineated should be applicable to the training experience of any professional concerned with the needs of chronically ill children.

Pediatric Psychology

The recent emergence of behavioral medicine represents a revolution within contemporary medicine as a whole. Developed as a result of the contributions to traditional medicine made by the behavioral sciences, including psychology, behavioral medicine has been defined as the field concerned with development and application of behavioral science knowledge and techniques to diagnosis, prevention, treatment, and rehabilitation of physical health and illness (Schwartz and Weiss, 1977). The development of behavioral medicine resulted, in part, from growing dissatisfaction with the traditional biomedical model (Schneider, 1978).

Along with behavioral medicine and its pediatric counterpart, behavioral pediatrics, there grew—both independently and conjointly—the fields of medical and pediatric psychology. Indeed, pediatric psychology has had a unique identity since the 1960s. When infant and child mortality and morbidity had decreased significantly as a result of medical advances, leaving pediatricians more time to devote to emotional and psychological aspects of development (Routh, 1975), many pediatricians turned to psychology in response to new demands for advice on childrearing and on developmental and behavioral problems. Psychologists became more prevalent in pediatric settings, and training opportunities for pediatric psychologists began to evolve.

Generally, pediatric psychologists function as diagnosticians, consultants, behavior therapists, supportive resource persons, and researchers. Work settings include private pediatric medical practices, hospitals, and developmental clinics. Referrals are often made by pediatricians and include primarily nonpsychiatric patients who exhibit behavioral or developmental problems or physically ill children who have psychological components in their illnesses. Because referrals from pediatricians are generally made early in the development and manifestation of problem behaviors, children seen by the pediatric psychologist tend to exhibit less severe psychopathology than patients seen in traditional mental health settings. Referrals frequently involve assessment of developmental delays, intellectual functioning, and determination of psychological factors in illness. Assessments are problem oriented and aimed toward clinical decision making. Referrals for treatment often include problems such as enuresis, encopresis, compliance problems, food and eating problems, negative behaviors, hyperactivity, psychosomatic problems, family problems, and especially, problems associated with chronic or terminal illness.

Intervention is based on a "primary mental health care" model (Wright, 1979a). Because of high patient volume, emphasis is on prevention, and interventions tend to be economical, pragmatic, and nontraditional (Roberts, Quevillon, and Wright, 1979). Consultation is the primary form of intervention. Direct treatment methods generally include behaviorally oriented or crisis-oriented approaches.

Content Areas

The following section focuses on content areas of knowledge and expertise that should be incorporated into training programs for psychologists who plan to work with chronically ill children.

Impact of Chronic Illness

The effects of chronic illness upon a child and family are pervasive, impinging on almost every aspect of a child's life. Studies have documented findings suggesting that chronically ill children constitute a "high-risk" group in relation to development of psychopathology (Pless and Roghmann, 1971; Sigal, 1974). What are the factors associated with chronic illness that contribute to the development of psychopathology? The psychologist must become aware of these factors so that this knowledge can be used in prevention and early intervention.

Chronically ill children may spend a considerable amount of time in the hospital, which results in school absences, separations from peers and family members, and isolation from normal childhood activities and experiences. The literature on hospitalization in chronically ill as well as acutely ill children documents a significant incidence of adjustment problems related to the experience of hospitalization itself, independent of the reason for hospitalization (Skipper and Leonard, 1968; Belmont, 1970; Nagera, 1978; Wright, Schaefer, and Solomons, 1979). Chronically ill children must also endure frequent medical procedures that may be painful and traumatic. For instance, young children with cancer exhibit extremely high anxiety in relation to bone marrow aspirations and lumbar punctures—diagnostic procedures that are painful, frightening, and often require physical restraint in young children (Katz, Kellerman, and Siegel, 1980). Painful diagnostic procedures, surgeries, and medical treatments (shots, infusions) activate distorted fears of bodily mutilation and disfigurement in young children. Such fears are exacerbated by the young child's misattributions and illogical views concerning painful experiences. For example, young children often perceive painful procedures as punishment for actual or imagined misdeeds (Mattsson, 1972), and such misperception may lead to guilt and/or self-esteem problems. The experience of severe pain early in life and over a long period of time may be the most detrimental factor in the emotional development of chronically ill children. Bergmann and Freud (1966) discussed how painful illnesses and painful medical procedures are to be dreaded in the interest of normal emotional development. Immobilization and restricted activity, over a period of time, may inhibit the chronically ill child's intellectual and emotional development and may result in serious behavioral management problems (Mattsson, 1972) and distorted body image (Korsch, 1961). Enforced dependency and loss of autonomy are common concomitants of chronic illness and may result in regression, rebellion, or depression, particularly in adolescents. Finally, disfigurement and/or impairments in physical appearance resulting from surgeries, medications, or the illness itself may increase self-consciousness, shame, isolation, and depression (Bernstein, 1976).

What factors mediate the impact of such aversive events in a child's development? The psychologist must attempt to assess the factors that distinguish the vulnerable child who copes poorly and exhibits maladjustment from the child who copes well and endures such experiences with no evidence of severe, long-term psychological problems. One important variable in the adjustment of the child and that child's family to chronic illness is the nature of the illness itself (Magrab and Calcagno, 1978). The psychologist must understand the specifics of a given illness in a given child to provide the most effective intervention. Illnesses vary along a number of significant dimensions, each of which holds different implications for the adjustment of the chronically ill child: time of onset, duration, severity (life-threatening or not), need for hospitalization, physical manifestations, and mental manifestations (Magrab and Calcagno, 1978).

Cognitive styles may differentially influence the impact of illness upon a child (Willis, Elliot, and Jay, 1982). Cognitive styles include dimensions such as perceived control over illness (locus of control) and the ways in which one cognitively copes with stress (for example, denial and avoidance versus information-seeking and mastery of stress). Burstein and Meichenbaum (1979) found that children's cognitive styles were related to levels of postsurgery anxiety and distress. Finally, numerous authors have documented the importance of parental attitudes and reactions in influencing the chronically ill child's psychosocial adaptation (Freeman, 1968; Garrard and Richmond, 1963; Maddison and Raphael, 1971). Many authors suggest that parental reactions are a more potent variable in adaptation than the nature of the specific disease (Mattsson, 1972; Prugh, 1963).

Mattsson (1972) described the following coping skills in well-adapted chronically ill children: cognitive understanding and acceptance of illness, compensatory activities and experiences, expressing of illness-related emotions, adaptive denial, and identification with another well-functioning handicapped individual. Mattsson emphasized the influence of familial attitudes and coping skills in determining how well children with chronic illness adjust to their situation.

The psychologist must be cognizant of recent developments and concepts in psychosomatic medicine in order to appreciate the impact of chronic illness on a child's development. The traditional dichotomy of "psychosomatic" versus "real" organic disease is now outdated and has been replaced by the view that *all* disease is multidetermined by interactions among social, psychological, and biological factors (Lipowski, 1977). Psychosomatic medicine emphasizes the concept of the child as a whole and the interdependence of psychosocial and biological factors in illness. Chronic illness may be a function of the interaction of processes at all three levels (biological, social, psychological) or at predominately one level, with reverberations to the other levels (Prugh, 1963). A child's illness may be the sole result of biological vulnerability despite optimal psychosocial experiences, or illness may be precipitated and perpetuated primarily by traumatic and stressful psychological and social experiences that exacerbate biological vulnerability or predisposition.

Regardless of etiology, chronic illness affects all areas of a child's adjustment. Once a child is diagnosed as chronically ill, that child's adaptive and coping capacities also depend on biological, social, and psychological factors. An appreciation of psychosomatic concepts is necessary in effective assessment and intervention by the psychologist. Diagnosis of antecedent-consequential relationships among biological, psychological, and social etiological factors and the weighting of these factors in disease onset and course will determine the appropriate model of intervention (Jay and Wright, 1981). Intervention may comprise primarily psychological modes (therapy), biological modes (drug therapy), social modes (environmental intervention), or a combination of all three, depending on accurate assessment of precipitating and perpetuating etiological factors.

Child Development

Comprehensive knowledge in child development is one of the most important content areas in the training of pediatric psychologists. Children's reactions to illness, pain, and hospitalization differ considerably, depending on the child's emotional and intellectual developmental status.

Illness may interfere seriously with normal development and mastery of developmental tasks (Willis, Elliot, and Jay, 1982). The pediatric psychologist needs an applied understanding of developmental theory to make differential diagnoses between transient adjustment reactions and more severe psychopathology. For instance, the adolescent who reacts to illness with whining, clinging, and tantrums is more likely to be severely delayed in emotional development than the preschool or early school-aged child who exhibits such regressive behavior.

Adequate training in child development would include the study of all major developmental theories, particularly Piagetian, Freudian, and Eriksonian theory. Clinical psychological training too often focuses on psychopathology to the extent that psychologists often begin practicing with a skewed perspective and an inadequate understanding of normal behavior and development. Because pediatric psychologists generally work in nonpsychiatric settings, they are often considered child development specialists, which makes their training in developmental theory even more crucial.

Finally, the integration of developmental theory with clinical practice is important in determining appropriate intervention strategies. The match between the type of intervention strategy and the developmental level of the child can be made with much more precision if a developmental framework is utilized in the decision process (Jay, Brown, and Willis, forthcoming).

Psychopathology

Pediatric psychologists need broad-based knowledge in psychopathology, primarily for the same reasons they need knowledge in normal child development. Pediatric psychologists should be trained in a trichotomous manner incorporating psychodynamic, behavioral, and phenomenological theories of psychopathology. Freudian and neo-Freudian theories concerning psychosexual development and the influence of unconscious processes on behavior can be very useful in understanding and conceptualizing the dynamics operating in a child's behavior. In pediatric settings, behavioral analysis of pathological behavior in terms of behavioral excesses and deficits (Ross, 1974) is a convenient and necessary adjunct to psychodynamic conceptualization because application and intervention can be implemented in a more efficient, less cumbersome manner. Even though pediatric psychologists may not use psychodynamic psychotherapy very often, given the nature of pediatric settings, exposure to and knowledge of psychodynamic theory is important; it gives the psychologist a substantial, well-rounded foundation in psychological theory and practice. Phenomenological or client-centered theories (Rogers, 1961) are perhaps most applicable in psychological work with chronically ill children because nondirective, supportive-guidance approaches are often appropriate for the nonneurotic adjustment reactions and life crises that occur frequently in chronically ill children and their families.

Assessment

Many referrals to pediatric psychologists are requests for psychological evaluation. Referral questions frequently involve assessment of intellectual functioning, behavioral-emotional-social functioning, academic functioning, family functioning, and psychological factors in illness. In order to assess these questions adequately, the pediatric psychologist needs training and expertise in the following assessment techniques: (1) developmental screening tests, (2) intelligence tests, (3) achievement tests, (4) projective tests, (5) diagnostic interviews with children and families, (6) neuropsychological tests, and (7) behavioral analyses. Although the scope of this chapter does not permit discussion of specific tests, other articles describe psychological instruments most relevant to the pediatric setting (Magrab and Lehr, 1982; Walker, 1979; Wright, 1978).

Many referrals involve screening for developmental delays and impairments in intellectual functioning. Some referrals require specialized skills in assessing specific learning disabilities. Although most psychologists are not trained in neuropsychological testing, neuropsychology is a content area highly relevant to work with chronically ill children and should be incorporated into more training programs. Because chronically ill children may have physical or sensory handicaps in conjunction with, or as a result of, their illnesses, the psychologist must also be skilled in the administration of tests designed specifically for handicapped children.

The pediatric psychologist should be able to screen and identify families who are at high risk for development of compliance problems or adjustment problems. Diagnostic interviews are useful in obtaining observations and information concerning reactions to diagnosis, stability of family, sources of emotional support, previous crises and coping methods, and financial and socioeconomic stresses, all of which may be helpful in determining the risk factor in a family (Ablin and others, 1971). Diagnostic interviews using play materials can be useful in obtaining an assessment of a child's emotional and social functioning. Projective tests and more objective measures are available to assess both a child's perceptions of illness and hospitalization and the child's adjustment. Such measures may be particularly useful in evaluating the psychological status of the chronically ill child.

Behavioral analysis is uniquely relevant in assessing the contingencies operating in a child's behavior. For the patient who is exhibiting uncooperative and defiant behavior, one can merely assess the payoffs for negative behavior, which may be subtle but powerful. Once the contingency relationships are discovered, one need only manipulate these contingencies to reinforce more appropriate behavior.

Intervention

The pediatric psychologist must be trained in a wide array of intervention skills because of the diversity of problems and special situations encountered with chronically ill children. Although a psychodynamic orientation can be very useful in understanding and conceptualizing the dynamics operating in a child's behavior, a number of factors related to the nature of pediatric settings (large case load, need for immediate intervention) mandate the need for a training emphasis in behavioral principles, behavioral management skills, supportive therapy skills, group and family therapy skills, and special skills related to the problems encountered with chronically ill children (pain management, preparation for hospitalization and surgery, and anxiety management).

Traditional psychotherapy skills that have proven useful in intervention with chronically ill children include skills in play therapy, group therapy, and family therapy. Play therapy can be helpful in alleviating anxiety and stress-related reactions. Such reactions often occur in conjunction with traumatic medical procedures.

Chronically ill children benefit from structured and unstructured play activities that allow them the opportunity to reenact and master their anxieties and fantasies concerning medical experiences. For instance, the authors have observed children with cancer frequently giving their dolls bone marrow aspirations and lumbar punctures; they gleefully reenact these medical procedures in vivid detail, but in the role of the physician, and they can be observed telling the doll how to cope ("it won't hurt long," "you must lie still," "be a big girl"). Group therapy can be a useful and efficient intervention mode with chronically ill children. Numerous authors have reported the use of group therapy with chronically ill children or adolescents with a variety of illnesses including muscular dystrophy (Bayrakal, 1975), renal disease (Korsch and others, 1971; Magrab, 1975), and cancer (Gardner, 1977; Kagen, 1976).

The pediatric psychologist should receive training in family therapy because the ramifications of chronic illness extend to every member of the family. Entire interaction patterns and adjustment styles can be altered to compensate for chronic illness (Friedrich, 1977). A knowledge of family systems (Minuchin and others, 1975) provides the psychologist with a conceptual understanding of how chronic illness can modify, disrupt, or destroy effective family functioning. Studies have reported a higher incidence of divorce and separation in families with a chronically ill or handicapped child (Kolin and others, 1971; Salk, Hilgartner, and Granich, 1972; Tew and Laurence, 1973). Furthermore, studies have documented a higher incidence of maladjustment among siblings of children with chronic illness (Binger, 1973; Cairns and others, 1979; Lavigne and Ryan, 1979). These findings indicate the need for psychological intervention with families of chronically ill children, particularly at crisis points such as time of diagnosis, relapse or worsening of condition, school entrance, and surgeries. Although use of a family systems viewpoint and implementation of family therapy in pediatric settings has been a relatively recent phenomenon (Bierenbaum and Bergey, 1980), successful results have been reported using structural family therapy with families of children with asthma, diabetes, and anorexia (Minuchin and others, 1975).

Behavior therapy skills are essential in working with chronically ill children. Because some psychological disorders in chronically ill children may be life threatening (for example, refusal of medication), there is no time for relationship building and psychodynamic interpretation. Behavior therapy is the treatment of choice for many disorders such as medical compliance, tracheotomy dependence, encopresis, enuresis, anorexia, psychogenic vomiting, and psychogenic seizures (Wright, 1979b), and behavior therapy skills can be very useful for a number of psychological disorders that may occur in chronically ill children. Simple reinforcement and contingency management programs are useful in eating disorders and other problem behaviors (Palmer, Thompson, and Linsheid, 1975). Behavioral contracting can be effective in compliance issues and family problems (Wright, Schaefer, and Solomons, 1979).

Relaxation training is an effective treatment modality or an adjunct to a more comprehensive intervention program. Relaxation training is particularly effective in reducing asthma attacks in children with asthma (Feldman, 1976; Khan, 1977), in treatment of children's migraine headaches (Diamond and Franklin, 1976), in reduction of epileptic seizures (Seifert and Lubar, 1975), and in asthma (Hock and others, 1978; Knapp and Wells, 1978).

Biofeedback has been a very popular treatment mode in behavioral medicine, particularly with adults. Evidence is accumulating that children can benefit from biofeedback training as well. Biofeedback has been reported as effective in reducing asthma attacks in asthmatic children (Feldman, 1976; Khan, 1977), in treatment of children's migraine headaches (Diamond and Franklin, 1976), in reduction of epileptic seizures (Seifert and Lubar, 1975), and in numerous other childhood disorders (Russell and Carter, 1978). Biofeedback is often used in conjunction with relaxation training for treatment of anxiety and tension.

Pediatric psychologists should be trained in special intervention skills that may have particular relevance for the chronically ill child. These special skills are generally viewed within a behavioral framework and include approaches such as coping-skills training, imagery, hypnosis, and modeling. Many of these approaches are an outgrowth of recent developments in cognitive behavior therapy, which emphasizes the importance of children's perceptions, cognitions, and self-statements in determining behavioral adjustment. Cognitive behavioral techniques have been used in the management of pain and anxiety with adults (Turk, 1978) and offer much promise as intervention approaches with chronically ill children. Cognitive-behavioral techniques as described by Meichenbaum (1977) provide relevant treatment options for children who are forced to cope with stressful and painful procedures. Coping skills training (particularly stress inoculation) can be used with older children. This procedure involves teaching and rehearsing various cognitive methods of coping with pain. Turk (1978) describes a number of coping strategies in pain control applicable to children, including imaginative transformation of content (imagining self as a war hero being tortured by enemy), imaginative transformation of pain (imagining that arm has been filled with Novocain), imaginative inattention (ignoring pain and focusing on a very pleasant image), and distraction (counting ceiling tiles).

For younger children, whose immature level of cognitive development may impede success with primarily cognitive strategies, emotive imagery as described by Lazarus and Abramovitz (1962) may be appropriate in pain and anxiety management. For example, a child undergoing a bone marrow aspiration might be asked to imagine he is Superman's agent and Superman has asked him to undergo the procedure as part of a special secret mission. The meaning of the pain is transformed for the child, and brave, coping behavior is reinforced.

Hypnosis contains elements of relaxation, imagery, and cognition and can be a very potent intervention approach for a variety of problems, particularly anxiety and pain (Gardner, 1974, 1976; LaBaw and others, 1975). Advantages of hypnosis are that most children are easily hypnotized and children can be taught to use self-hypnosis on their own.

Filmed modeling has been reported as an effective treatment approach for fear and anxiety related to medical treatment and procedures. In filmed modeling, the child observes filmed models successfully cope with the medical procedure they are about to encounter. Studies have indicated that modeling is successful in producing significantly lower ratings of stress-related behaviors in children receiving injections (Vernon, 1974), anesthesia before surgery (Vernon and Bailey, 1974), and hospitalization for severe types of elective surgery (Malamed and Siegel, 1975).

The goal of these treatment approaches is to instill within the child a sense of self-control, mastery, and pride in coping with stressful and painful situations. The long-term adjustment of the child with chronic illness may be determined by that child's coping strategies. Cognitive-behavioral techniques offer promise in providing children with effective coping strategies that may mediate the long-term sequelae of frequent stressful, painful, and anxiety-provoking events. Training in such techniques should enhance the effectiveness and flexibility of the psychologist's interventions with chronically ill children.

Pediatric psychologists need expertise in preventive measures as well as in intervention strategies. Hospitalization and surgery present primary opportunities for the psychologist to intervene with the chronically ill child in a prophylactic manner. Vernon and others (1965) delineated three variables that should be included in prehospitalization preparation: (1) information about procedures, (2) encouragement of emotional expression, and (3) establishment of a trusting relationship with the hospital staff. Research suggests that systematic preparation for hospitalization and surgery yields positive results with children and their parents (Visintainer and Wolfer, 1975).

Finally, the pediatric psychologist needs experience and training in crisis intervention because families of chronically ill children generally experience more crises than families of healthy children. Depending upon the adequacy of coping measures, persons may emerge from a crisis with improved mental health (a new healthier equilibrium and new problem-solving methods) or with worsened mental health (Caplan, 1968). Because, as Caplan points out, individuals are more susceptible to influence by others during crisis states, crises permit optimal opportunities for the psychologist to intervene on a preventive basis, helping the family to restore a healthy equilibrium through adaptive coping measures and problem-solving abilities.

Consultation

Consultation skills are perhaps the most valuable skills the pediatric psychologist attains during the training process. Consumers of psychological consultation include medical staff, parents, teachers, and medical students. The consultant most often operates in accordance with one of three consultation models: an independent functions model, an indirect psychological consultation model, or a collaborative team model (Roberts and Wright, 1982). In the independent functions model, the psychologist intervenes directly with the child and takes primary responsibility for assessment and/or intervention. Consultation may include diagnostic assessment, psychological testing, crisis intervention, behavior management, or psychological therapy. In the indirect psychological consultation model, the psychologist assists the consultee (physician, parent, teacher) in dealing with a problem patient and/or teaches or supervises the consultee in intervention techniques; the consultee retains primary responsibility for the patient. This type of consultation involves close collaboration and may include methods such as behavioral management training, parent skills training, and professional advice. This model also includes formal teaching and educational activities through seminars and lectures. In the collaborative team model, the psychologist and consultee engage in mutual problem-solving and decision-making efforts. Cases are handled conjointly, with both parties contributing their skills and expertise. Examples of problems amenable to this approach include medical compliance problems and anorexia nervosa (Roberts and Wright, 1982).

Pediatric psychologists should be trained in each of these consultation models. The type of consultation chosen depends on such factors as the nature of the referral, the relationship between the consultee and the psychologist, the skills and expertise of the consultee, and the intervention setting.

Training in consultation techniques should take place only after the student has received advanced training in child assessment, child development, and intervention techniques, as well as training in chronic illness and its psychological concomitants (Russ, 1978). The psychological consultant needs an applied understanding of systems theory in order to function effectively within pediatric and school settings (Nixon, 1975; Willoughby, 1978). The consultant must have strong interpersonal skills and be able to communicate knowledge in a nonthreatening manner. In medical consultation, psychological consultants need to learn the terminology of their medical colleagues because the medical condition of the child is so intertwined with the child's psychological state. Indeed, Willoughby contends that the pediatric psychological consultant needs to be a "polyglot" who can communicate with team members of various specialties. Effective consultants are highly visible in the consultation setting and make themselves available through participation in hospital rounds, school conferences, and informal discussions concerning individual patients or students (Drotar, 1976).

Medical Consultation. Physicians or nurses often consult with a psychologist when behavioral or psychological problems are manifested by the chronically ill child. The psychologist may intervene directly with the child or collaborate with the medical staff on intervention methods, depending on the referral question. Indirect consultation methods are more cost-effective and include the following: education of medical staff on potential psychological problems in chronically ill children, teaching specific behavioral management skills or other intervention techniques, professional advice, facilitation of intra-staff communication, and exploration of staff reactions to patient care and patient issues.

There are many potential obstacles in training pediatric psychologists to function as consultants in a medical setting (Drotar, 1978). Psychologists and medical personnel are trained very differently, speak different languages, and are taught to function in very different environments. In many medical settings, psychological consultation is sought only as a last resort for the most extreme problem cases. Physician-consultant collaboration may be difficult to establish because of discrepant expectations and negative or narrow-minded attitudes on the physician's part. Many physicians do not believe in or practice according to a holistic psychosomatic approach to medicine (Krakowski, 1979), which makes collaboration more difficult and less effective. Despite these difficulties, pediatricians and psychologists are increasingly recognizing the value and necessity of collaboration in childcare. Problems and resistances should become less pronounced as each discipline experiences the positive benefits that can result from effective collaboration and consultation.

Parent Consultation. Parent consultation is often a primary component of psychological intervention for the chronically ill child. Parent consultation can take many forms, ranging from intensive individual psychotherapeutic work and crisis intervention to indirect group methods focusing on childrearing and behavioral management skills. Parents can work through the mourning process that accompanies the onset of serious illness during childhood or the birth of a child with a serious illness. In order to facilitate parental acceptance of their child's medical condition, the psychological consultant may intervene by providing support, information, and anticipatory guidance. Anticipatory guidance refers to a process whereby the consultant in an ongoing supportive relationship alerts the parent to problems that may occur and helps prepare the parent for potential crisis points, hopefully offsetting serious adjustment difficulties through preventive measures.

Support groups for parents of chronically ill children are an effective form of parent consultation. Parents learn from other parents and often report that it is comforting to realize that other parents endure similar hardships (Knapp and

Hansen, 1973). Parents of chronically ill children may also benefit from structured group consultation concerning behavioral management and childrearing methods (Wright, 1970, 1976).

A problem that is particularly relevant to the care of chronically ill children and that can be addressed effectively through parent consultation is the problem of medical compliance. Research studies have indicated that noncompliance is a problem of major concern to physicians, and estimates of noncompliance range up to 90 percent of patients treated (Bergman and Werner, 1963; Francis, Korsch, and Morris, 1969). The need for intervention is particularly critical in cases in which noncompliance may be life threatening (anorexia nervosa, cancer, diabetes, asthma). Wright (1980) developed a standardized compliance program for parents that can be superimposed on any treatment program and applied to numerous medical disorders. Reviews of parent consultation methods document the efficacy and economy of such consultation approaches (Berkowitz and Graziano, 1972; Johnson and Katz, 1973; O'Dell, 1974). Wright, Schaefer, and Solomons (1979) suggested routine parent consultation as a preventive technique through the use of parent clinics that parents could attend just as they obtain pediatric physical checkups. Schroeder, Goolsby, and Stangler (1975) described a preventive "Call-In Service" in a pediatrician's office through which parents could obtain psychological consultations.

School Consultation. A primary need of the chronically ill child is to live as normal a life as possible within the limitations of the disease. School is a major part of every normal child's life, and many developmental tasks are encountered and mastered through school experience. However, management of the chronically ill child can pose difficult problems for teachers and school administrators. Psychological consultation can provide a useful service for teachers who have a chronically ill child in their classroom.

What needs of teachers of chronically ill children can be addressed through psychological consultation? First, the teacher needs information concerning the child's medical condition, the treatment regimen, side effects of treatment, expected absences from school, and necessary limitations (if any) on the child's activities. The psychologist can serve as a liaison between medical staff and school personnel and facilitate communication concerning the child's illness. Teachers need preparation as well as information in management of chronically ill students. Encountering a student with a colostomy bag or a child who has no hair due to chemotherapy may elicit strong personal reactions as well as management problems. The psychologist can consult with teachers concerning what to do in specific problem situations and can help the teachers become aware of and work through attitudes that may be detrimental to the chronically ill child's adjustment. Kaplan, Smith, and Grobstein (1974) contend that seriously ill children elicit anxiety in school personnel and that, consequently, decisions may be made that compromise the ill child's adjustment needs. But teachers need information, support, and guidance in meeting the chronically ill child's needs because they are generally not prepared in their educational training to cope with such needs. Finally, the psychologist can consult with the teacher concerning children who exhibit behavioral problems. Because children with chronic illness constitute a high-risk group, they are more likely than others to display behavioral and emotional problems. The psychological consultant can educate the teacher on behavioral management techniques that can be used with children who display adjustment difficulties.

Training to Participate in Medical Education. Psychologists need to be trained to impart their skills to physicians, nurses, and other medical personnel in a structured and didactic approach because research has shown that a large percentage of patients who seek medical treatment also have psychological problems. One study indicated that only 12 percent of patients seeking help at a pediatric medical clinic had purely physical problems, 36 percent had purely psychological problems, and 52 percent had combined physical and psychological problems (Duff, Rowe, and Anderson, 1972).

In spite of the need, physicians are not adequately trained in psychological and psychiatric assessment and intervention. Some residents in pediatrics do not have a single lecture on psychological issues during their entire three-year residency (Fink and Strosnider, 1976). Nor are pediatricians adequately trained in child development (Richmond, 1967). Training deficits reported by practicing pediatricians (Toister and Worley, 1976; Weinberger, 1976) included behavioral management skills for frequently encountered problems such as toilet training, food and eating problems, discipline problems, and school difficulties.

Wexler (1976) eloquently contends that the behavioral sciences often fail in their teaching mission because medical students are not taught information that has a functional, applied value. For example, students are often taught psychoanalytic principles in a theoretical manner that has limited applicability to problems within medical practice (Johnson and Snibbe, 1975). Wexler (p. 278) insists that behavioral scientists must choose subject matter that has "a high potential for being translated into usable techniques and information in medical practice." Examples of highly relevant behavioral science content areas would include learning theory and principles of behavioral management, pain management, psychopharmacology, hypnosis, treatment of anxiety and depression, and issues in death and dying.

Community Consultation and Intervention. The chronically ill child's service needs reach beyond what the physician and the psychologist can offer, no matter how comprehensive those services are. A child's total environment must be assessed to determine the needs that exist and to determine services that exist within the community. The fact that chronically ill children and their families constitute a high-risk group has been discussed previously. However, certain demographic factors may increase the risk factor even more. Low-income families, single-parent families, and families without adequate support systems appear to be particularly at risk for psychosocial maladjustment or family dysfunction. Poverty-level families may be crippled by the financial burdens associated with medical care. Single parents, particularly those in lower socioeconomic groups, find it extremely difficult to maintain an independent lifestyle and a steady job when they have an ill child at home or in the hospital. Single parents are often forced to return to their family or to become welfare recipients (Travis, 1976). Chronic illness can also distort family relationships. Travis points out that a common distortion observed in families with a chronically ill child is the father's abdication of responsibility and increased absence from home, in conjunction with an intense alliance between the mother and the ill child. Families without support systems may become overwhelmed with the problems of transportation, childcare, finances, medical crises, and emotional distress.

The numerous stresses and problems associated with chronic illness can be alleviated significantly through utilization of community resources. Families with a disabled child can receive from various sources supplemental income that may decrease or alleviate the financial burdens of medical care. There may be available numerous social services that can alleviate family stress by providing childcare alternatives. Families may qualify for homemaker services, daycare, or foster home care.

The psychologist must be aware of community resources in order to be able to mobilize them for a family. The psychologist often serves as a liaison between medical settings and community agencies. To prevent the disorganization and fragmentation that often occur when families receive services from more than one agency, the psychologist (as a community consultant) can work to establish a coordinated network of services for the chronically ill child. Such an effort requires mobilization and coordination of existing resources as well as development of new services that may be lacking in the community.

Finally, the psychologist can perform a major service to chronically ill children on a community level through public education. Chronically ill children may encounter on a daily basis the ignorance, prejudices, and negative attitudes of persons in the community, and this may cause emotional upset, trauma, withdrawal, and anger in such children. Such attitudes and beliefs arise from ignorance and lack of information—a situation that can be addressed through educational efforts. The media (newspapers, television, radio) can be employed to teach the public relevant facts about chronic illness.

Research

The pediatric psychologist generally receives training in accordance with the scientist-professional model, which proposes that the clinical psychologist be trained as both a professional psychologist and a research scientist. Pediatric psychology represents a frontier for the research scientist in the area of chronic illness and behavioral pediatrics. The majority of psychological studies on chronic illness in children are primitive, consisting primarily of anecdotal reports and clinical observations. There is a dire need for sophisticated scientific studies in the area of chronic illness.

The pediatric psychologist is in a somewhat unique position to generate new research questions and hypotheses. The field is wide open for creative research questions and empirical validation of current psychological methods. A particularly important area of research involves treatment-outcome studies whereby innovative but untested treatment methods of pain, anxiety, and depression (hypnosis, cognitive-behavioral techniques, modeling, preprocedural preparation) are examined in terms of efficacy and cost-benefit ratios. Other topics for research include patient compliance, prevention and early identification of medical psychological problems, and psychological sequelae of chronic illness (Roberts, Quevillon, and Wright, 1979).

Pediatric psychologists should receive training in research design and statistical analysis early in the training sequence. They should be taught to apply the scientific attitude to clinical problems and to translate clinical issues into researchable hypotheses. Training in applied clinical research will serve the pediatric psychologist far better than training in research, which is aimed at studying highly theoretical and abstract hypotheses that have little direct relevance to clinical problems.

Terminal Illness

The psychologist must be prepared to confront what is perhaps the most difficult challenge of all—the process of death and dying in a child. Working with terminally ill children and their families requires not only special professional skills but also (and more important) strong interpersonal skills, emotional stability, and maturity. As Wiener (1970, p. 102) stated, "Meeting the needs of child and parent appropriately, humanely, and yet with equanimity is a task requiring the personnel's repeated re-examination of their own values, attitudes, and convictions about life, dying, and death itself." The professional who does not engage in such self-examination may exhibit inappropriate or detrimental reactions and make a very difficult situation even worse for the child and family. Psychologists should be trained to respond to terminally ill children in an honest, straightforward manner. Research has indicated that children who are allowed to express their fears and concerns about illness and death exhibit less anxiety than those who are not allowed to do so (Waechter, 1971).

Parents with terminally ill children are faced with a number of difficult coping tasks including the following: (1) anticipatory mourning, (2) maintaining a sense of mastery while simultaneously struggling with helplessness, guilt, and anger, (3) helping their child maintain a sense of self-worth, trust, and integrity, and (4) maintaining family stability and integrity (Hoffman and Futterman, 1971). Common reactions include denial, anger, bargaining, depression, and finally, acceptance (Kubler-Ross, 1969). Psychologists must be aware of these difficult coping tasks facing parents and must be able to help them prepare for their child's death in a way that is not detrimental to the child's need for continued support. Specific issues on which parents (and older children) may need consultation involve the decision whether to terminate or continue treatment when death is a certainty (Nitschke and others, 1977) and the decision of whether to die at home or in the hospital.

The psychologist must be trained to consult with medical staff concerning the stress of working with terminally ill children. Physicians and nurses typically receive very little training in death and dying, despite their proximity to circumstances surrounding death (Barton and others, 1972). Reactions of medical personnel commonly include a sense of defeat and failure, guilt, anger, anxiety and withdrawal, and overinvolvement. Such reactions, if not handled with awareness and discipline, may be detrimental to the child's medical and emotional care.

A final point that should be emphasized in training psychologists, (particularly in the area of terminal illness) is the importance of personal empathy and support. As Willis (1975, p. 4) stated, "Professionals working in and out of hospitals need to drop the facade of professionalism and relate to the dying patient as one human being to another. The knowledge and skill we gain through experience in counseling the dying are helpful and should be utilized, but the patients gain comfort not only from our cognitive knowledge solely but from our relating to them on a more personal and intimate level." A survey conducted with parents whose children had died confirms this view. Parents surveyed remembered their caregivers' skill or lack of skill in personal care much more than they remembered the quality of technical care (Geis, 1965).

Training Issues in Pediatric Psychology

We turn now to a discussion of the following questions (Tuma, 1980): What model of training is most appropriate? How is the issue of generic versus specialty training to be resolved, and at what point in the training sequence should specialty training be introduced? How should practicum and internship experiences be integrated into a training program?

Because pediatric psychology is a subspecialty of clinical child psychology, an overview of current training issues in clinical child psychology is appropriate. Tuma provided a comprehensive review of training issues in clinical child and pediatric psychology. A major issue concerns the manpower shortage of specialists trained to work with children and the lack of available services for children. Although 1977 U.S. census data indicated that children under eighteen comprise 30 percent of the total population, less than 1 percent of all psychological service providers work primarily with this segment of the population (Tuma, 1980; VandenBos and others, 1979). In fact, only 10 percent of children and adolescents needing mental health services are served by the present mental health system, according to the Alcohol, Drug Abuse, and Mental Health Administration (1978). One factor contributing to the lack of mental health services for children is the shortage of well-trained clinical child psychologists. The estimated number of additional fully trained clinical child psychologists needed within the next decade is approximately 5,000 (VandenBos and others, 1979), a number *much* higher than the current matriculation of students from training programs in psychology.

If this need is to be addressed, serious consideration must be given to the type of training clinical child psychologists receive. A major problem concerns the lack of uniform recognition of clinical child psychology as a specialty area within psychology. Very few doctoral training programs offer specialized training in clinical child psychology (Roberts, 1982), and psychologists working with children obtain their training in clinical child and pediatric psychology through a variety of programs. The diversity of training programs points to the lack of consensus regarding specific criteria for training programs in clinical child psychology. Furthermore, surveys of programs that claim training in clinical child psychology reveal confusion regarding definitions of clinical child psychology and training needs of clinical child psychologists (Tuma, 1980). One factor contributing to the confusion is the extreme diversity of professional roles performed by clinical psychologists. Cass (1974, p. 470) asks the critical question, "Is there a core of theoretical knowledge and professional skills which can serve as a common denominator for all these roles, for example, is there still a definable clinical child psychology?"

These problematic issues within clinical child psychology also apply to the subspecialty area of pediatric psychology. Although clinical child psychology dates back to the early 1900s, pediatric psychology is hardly fifteen years old, making its identity within psychology even more tenuous. Confusion between the boundaries of pediatric psychology and clinial child psychology still exists, but Tuma pointed out that a major distinguishing factor is the nature of the training setting. Pediatric psychologists receive training in pediatric medical, nonpsychiatric settings whereas clinical child psychologists are more likely to be trained in mental health and psychiatric settings. Currently, there are no doctoral level programs for training pediatric psychologists, who receive their specialty training through a variety of training routes including subspecialization within other psychology programs or postdoctoral training in pediatric psychology.

Although the majority of pediatric psychologists are trained in clinical psychology, 42 percent come from other fields within psychology (Routh, 1977). The high percentage of pediatric psychologists with nonclinical backgrounds raises the issue of postdoctoral training. Routh discussed the problems of American Psychological Association (APA) policies, which require enrollment in a clinical program as well as an APA clinical internship for persons from other programs wishing to respecialize as a clinical psychologist. Routh points out that in pediatric psychology, there is no appropriate graduate training program in which to respecialize. Routh supports the model of postdoctoral training for persons with degrees from programs other than clinical child psychology who wish to specialize in pediatric psychology.

Controversy exists over the issue of predoctoral versus postdoctoral specialization. Although most would agree that clinical child psychology is a specialty area requiring specific skills and training, the issue has not been resolved as to when in the sequence of training specialization should occur. Descriptions and surveys of training opportunities in pediatric psychology can be found in the literature. Ottinger and Roberts (1980) describe one of the few university-based predoctoral practicum programs available in pediatric psychology, which is at Purdue University. More often, training in pediatric psychology is offered within a medical setting. Tuma (1984) edited a directory of training opportunities in pediatric psychology.

An additional issue important to all specialty areas within psychology is the relevance of the scientist-professional training model. This model has been criticized on the grounds that it is antiquated, unrealistic, irrelevant to service delivery, and a hindrance to professional development (Campbell and Hodges, 1975). Professionally oriented training programs have been developed as an alternative model in response to the limitations of the scientist-professional model. Despite the limitations of the scientist-professional model, it would be a foolish and premature move at this point to abolish it. If one takes a historical perspective, clinical psychology grew out of a scientific tradition, and it is this scientific tradition that has made psychology unique among other mental health disciplines. Furthermore, as Korchin (1976, p. 604) stated, "Clinical psychologists have had an uncontested role in mental health research, in large part out of the methodological competence developed in Ph.D. programs."

Leitenberg (1974) reviewed the criticisms of the scientist-professional model and concluded that the problem is not with the model but with the manner in which it has been interpreted and implemented. The model proposes that the psychologist be trained to integrate the roles of scientist and clinical practitioner. Yet, research and clinical practice are taught as separate and unrelated activities in most graduate psychology programs. It is no wonder that most clinicians are not research oriented. Most students are trained in basic rather than applied clinical research and consequently fail to grasp the relevance of a scientific attitude in relation to clinical activities. Leitenberg described a training program that emphasizes applied clinical research and teaches students to integrate research and clinical interests. The adoption of the scientist-professional model as interpreted by Leitenberg would perhaps make the model a more relevant and workable one in psychology training programs.

Currently, most pediatric psychologists receive their specialty training at the internship or postdoctoral level. This model appears to be adequate, given that students reach the internship or postdoctoral level with a solid foundation in core knowledge of psychological theory and methodology. More courses and practicum opportunities at a predoctoral level in behavioral medicine and pediatric psychology are needed to widen students' exposure to the new and expanding interface between psychology and medicine. Strong research training is crucial, given the state of the art in pediatric behavioral research. Although training in pediatric psychology is characterized by confusion, ambiguity, and lack of structure, pediatric psychology is prospering despite the "growing pains" common to any new field.

Problem Areas

The interface between psychology and medicine is expanding, but not without obstacles and difficulties. The pediatric psychologist's major role is a *collaborative*, interdisciplinary one that at times may seem an illusion. Good communication with medical staff is absolutely essential if pediatric psychologists are to be successful in their endeavors. Yet, numerous factors operate to obstruct effective communication. Psychologists and physicians often speak different languages and may have discrepant goals of childcare. Many physicians do not practice according to a holistic, psychosomatic framework, which limits the input and usefulness of psychological services. Physicians may be resistant to working in a collaborative framework, viewing the psychologist as an ancillary rather than integral component in health care of children. Physicians may operate in such a mode because they hold biases and prejudices against psychological services, or more typically, because they are unaware of the skills psychologists have to offer. Psychologists must educate medical staff and prove their usefulness through effective intervention efforts.

Communication problems are not confined to medical-psychological personnel but also occur between mental health specialists. Problems of territoriality and role overlap arise among the disciplines of psychology, psychiatry, and social work, particularly in hospital settings. Flexibility and open communication among these disciplines are essential. As Drotar (1976, p. 81) stated, "A unified approach to mental health teaching, clinical work, and consultation minimizes competitive unilateral efforts that present a confusing and divided picture to our pediatric consultees."

Research in the area of pediatric behavioral medicine is also scant, and many existing studies lack scientific merit. The research in adult behavioral medicine is much more extensive and of much higher quality. For example, Eland and Anderson (1977) conducted a survey of the literature on pain published between 1970 and 1975. Of 1,380 articles on pain, only thirty-three were devoted to pain in children. None of the thirty-three articles related to children's psychological responses to pain or to pain management techniques. The opportunities for research in behavioral pediatrics are unlimited and only await psychologists who are trained to exploit them.

Finally, the demand for psychologists currently outweighs the supply—a situation that compromises the quality of psychologists who work with children. In the area of chronic illness, specialized skills and knowledge are required in addition to traditional psychological skills and knowledge. Such child specialists are too few in number, and many psychologists currently working with children have had little or no formal training in clinical child psychology.

Conclusions

Chronic illness in children is a profound experience that holds the potential for altering or distorting normal development and adjustment. Until recently, the psychological and social needs of chronically ill children have been largely ignored, and attention has been placed primarily on their medical condition. Recent developments in psychology and medicine have resulted in much closer scrutiny of the needs of chronically ill children, and holistic care will, it is hoped, become the rule rather than the exception. The quality of care received by chronically ill children is determined to a large extent by the quality and depth of training of physicians and psychologists who work with them. Increased efforts must be made to ensure quality training. Physicians must receive more training in medical school concerning psychological components of illness and child development. More training programs in pediatric psychology must be established for psychologists who wish to specialize in the care of chronically ill children. Improvement and expansion of training opportunities for physicians and psychologists will serve to improve the medical and psychological care of chronically ill children, consequently enhancing the quality of life for these children.

References

Ablin, A., and others. "A Conference with the Family of a Leukemic Child." *American Journal of Diseases of Children*, 1971, *122*, 362–364.

Alcohol, Drug Abuse, and Mental Health Administration. *Manpower Policy Analysis Task Force Report*. Rockville, Md.: U.S. Department of Health, Education, and Welfare, 1978.

Barton, D., and others. "Death and Dying: A Course for Medical Students." *Journal of Medical Education*, 1972, *47*, 945–951.

Bayrakal, S. "A Group Experience with Chronically Disabled Adolescents." *American Journal of Psychiatry*, 1975, *132*, 1291–1294.

Belmont, H. S. "Hospitalization and Its Effects upon the Total Child." *Clinical Pediatrics*, 1970, *9*, 472–483.

Bergman, A. B., and Werner, R. J. "Failure of Children to Receive Penicillin by Mouth." *New England Journal of Medicine*, 1963, *268*, 1334–1338.

Bergmann, T., and Freud, A. *Children in Hospital*. New York: International Universities Press, 1966.

Berkowitz, B. P., and Graziano, A. M. "Training Parents as Behavior Therapists: A Review." *Behavior Research and Therapy*, 1972, *10*, 297–317.

Bernstein, N. R. "Disfigurement and Personality Development." *Emotional Care of the Facially Burned and Disfigured*. Boston: Little, Brown, 1976.

Bierenbaum, H., and Bergey, S. F. "Family Therapy Training in a Pediatric Setting." *Journal of Pediatric Psychology*, 1980, 5 (3), 263–276.

Binger, C. M. "Childhood Leukemia: Emotional Impact on Siblings." In E. J. Anthony and C. Koupernik (Eds.), *The Child in His Family*. Vol. 2: *The Impact of Disease and Death*. New York: Wiley, 1973.

Burstein, S., and Meichenbaum, D. "Work of Worrying in Children Undergoing Surgery." *Journal of Abnormal Child Psychology*, 1979, 7, 121–132.

Cairns, N., and others. "Adaptation of Siblings to Childhood Malignancy." *Journal of Pediatrics*, 1979, *93* (3), 484–487.

Campbell, L. M., and Hodges, W. B. "Professional Training in Clinical Psychology: A Student's Perspective." *Clinical Psychologist*, 1975, *28* (4), 7–8.

Caplan, G. "Opportunities for School Psychologists in the Primary Prevention of Mental Disorders in Children." In E. Miller (Ed.), *Foundations of Child Psychiatry*. Elmsford, N.Y.: Pergamon Press, 1968.

Cass, L. K. "The Training of Clinical Child Psychologists." In G. J. Williams and S. Gordon (Eds.), *Clinical Child Psychology: Current Practices and Future Perspectives*. New York: Behavioral Publications, 1974.

Diamond, S., and Franklin, M. "Biofeedback—Choice of Treatment in Childhood Migraine." Paper presented at the 7th annual meeting of the Biofeedback Research Society, Colorado Springs, Colo., Feb. 1976.

Drotar, D. "Psychological Consultation in a Pediatric Hospital." *Professional Psychology*, 1976, *7*, 77-82.

Drotar, D. "Training Psychologists to Consult with Pediatricians: Problems and Prospects." *Journal of Clinical Child Psychology*, 1978, *1*, 57-60.

Duff, R. S., Rowe, D. S., and Anderson, F. P. "Patient Care and Student Learning in a Pediatric Clinic." *Pediatrics*, 1972, *50*, 839-852.

Eland, J. M., and Anderson, J. E. "The Experience of Pain in Children." In A. K. Joacox (Ed.), *Pain: A Sourcebook for Nurses and Other Health Professionals*. Boston: Little, Brown, 1977.

Feldman, G. M. "The Effect of Biofeedback Training on Respiratory Resistance of Asthmatic Children." *Psychosomatic Medicine*, 1976, *38*, 27-34.

Fink, P., and Strosnider, J. S. "The Place of Psychiatry and Behavioral Science in the Education of Primary Care Physicians." *Psychiatric Opinion*, 1976, *13* (3), 21-26.

Francis, V., Korsch, B. M., and Morris, M. J. "Gaps in Doctor-Patient Communication." *New England Journal of Medicine*, 1969, *280*, 535-540.

Freeman, R. D. "Emotional Reactions of Handicapped Children." In S. Chess and A. Thomas (Eds.), *Annual Progress in Child Psychiatry and Child Development*. New York: Brunner/Mazel, 1968.

Friedrich, W. N. "Ameliorating the Psychological Impact of Chronic Physical Disease on the Child and Family." *Journal of Pediatric Psychology*, 1977, *2*, 26-31.

Gardner, G. G. "Hypnosis with Children." *International Journal of Clinical and Experimental Hypnosis*, 1974, *22*, 20-38.

Gardner, G. G. "Childhood, Death, and Human Dignity: Hypnotherapy for David." *International Journal of Clinical and Experimental Hypnosis*, 1976, *24*, 122-139.

Gardner, G. G. "Adolescents with Cancer: Current Issues and a Proposal." *Journal of Pediatric Psychology*, 1977, *2* (3), 132-134.

Garrard, S. D., and Richmond, J. B. "Psychological Aspects of the Management of Chronic Disease and Handicapping Conditions in Childhood." In H. E. Lief, V. F. Lief, and N. R. Lief (Eds.), *The Psychological Basis of Medical Practice*. New York: Harper & Row, 1963.

Geis, D. P. "Mothers' Perceptions of Care Given Their Dying Children." *American Journal of Nursing*, 1965, *65*, 105-107.

Hock, R. A., and others. "Medico-Psychological Interventions in Male Asthmatic Children: An Evaluation of Physiologic Change." *Psychosomatic Medicine*, 1978, *40*, 210-215.

Hoffman, I., and Futterman, E. H. "Coping with Waiting: Psychiatric Intervention and Study in the Waiting Room of a Pediatric Oncology Clinic." *Comprehensive Psychiatry*, 1971, *12* (1), 67-81.

Jay, S. M., and Wright, L. "Psychosomatic Disorders in Children." In C. J. Golden, S. S. Alcaparras, F. Strider, and B. Graber, (Eds.), *Applied Techniques in Behavioral Medicine and Psychology*. New York: Grune & Stratton, 1981.

Jay, S. M., Brown, D., and Willis, D. "The Emotionally Exceptional." In R. T. Brown and C. R. Reynolds (Eds.), *Psychological Perspectives on Childhood Exceptionality*. New York: Wiley Interscience, forthcoming.

Johnson, C. A., and Katz, R. C. "Using Parents as Change Agents for Their Children: A Review." *Journal of Child Psychology and Psychiatry*, 1973, *14*, 181-200.

Johnson, W., and Snibbe, J. "The Selection of a Psychiatric Curriculum for Medical Students: Results of a Survey." *American Journal of Psychiatry*, 1975, *132*, 513-516.

Kagen, L. B. "Use of Denial in Adolescents with Bone Cancer." *Health and Social Work*, 1976, *1*, 71-87.

Kaplan, D. M., Smith, A., and Grobstein, R. "School Management of the Seriously Ill Child." *Journal of School Health*, 1974, *54* (5), 250-254.

Katz, E., Kellerman, J., and Siegel, S. "Behavioral Distress in Children with Cancer Undergoing Medical Procedures: Developmental Considerations." *Journal of Consulting and Clinical Psychology*, 1980, *41* (3), 356-365.

Khan, A. U. "Effectiveness of Biofeedback and Counterconditioning in the Treatment of Bronchial Asthma." *Journal of Psychosomatic Research*, 1977, *21*, 97-104.

Knapp, T. J., and Wells, A. L. "Behavior Therapy for Asthma: A Review." *Behavior Research and Therapy*, 1978, *16*, 103-115.

Knapp, U. S., and Hansen, H. "Helping Parents of Children with Leukemia." *Social Work*, 1973, *18*, 70-75.

Kolin, I., and others. "Studies of the School-Aged Child with Meningomyelocele: Social and Emotional Adaptation." *Journal of Pediatrics*, 1971, *78*, 1013-1019.

Korchin, S. *Modern Clinical Psychology*. New York: Basic Books, 1976.

Korsch, B. M. "Psychologic Reactions to Physical Illness in Children." *Journal of the Georgia Medical Association*, 1961, *50*, 519-523.

Korsch, B. M., and others. "Experiences with Children and Their Families During Extended Hemodialysis and Kidney Transplantation." *Pediatric Clinics of North America*, 1971, *18*, 625-637.

Krakowski, A. J. "Liaison Psychiatry in North America in the 1970s." *Bibliotheca Psychiatrica*, 1979, *159*, 4-14.

Kubler-Ross, E. *On Death and Dying*. New York: Macmillan, 1969.

LaBaw, W., and others. "The Use of Self-Hypnosis by Children with Cancer." *American Journal of Clinical Hypnosis*, 1975, *17*, 233-238.

Lavigne, J. V., and Ryan, M. "Psychologic Adjustment of Children with Chronic Illness." *Pediatrics*, 1979, *63* (4), 616-627.

Lazarus, A. A., and Abramovitz, A. "The Use of 'Emotive Imagery' in the Treatment of Children's Phobias." *Journal of Mental Science,* 1962, *108,* 191–195.

Leitenberg, H. "Training Clinical Researchers in Psychology." *Professional Psychology,* 1974, *5,* 59–69.

Lipowski, Z. J. "Psychosomatic Medicine in the Seventies: An Overview." *American Journal of Psychiatry,* 1977, *134* (3), 233–244.

Maddison, B., and Raphael, B. "Social and Psychological Consequences of Chronic Disease in Childhood." *Medical Journal of Australia,* 1971, *2,* 1265–1270.

Magrab, P. R. "Psychological Management and Renal Dialysis." *Journal of Clinical Child Psychology,* 1975, *4,* 38–40.

Magrab, P. R., and Calcagno, P. L. "Psychological Impact of Chronic Pediatric Conditions." In P. R. Magrab (Ed.), *Psychological Management of Pediatric Problems.* Vol. 1. Baltimore, Md.: University Park Press, 1978.

Magrab, P. R., and Lehr, E. "Assessment Techniques in Pediatric Psychology." In J. Tuma (Ed.), *Handbook for the Practice of Pediatric Psychology.* New York: Wiley Interscience, 1982.

Mattsson, A. "Long-Term Physical Illness in Childhood: A Challenge to Psychosocial Adaptation." *Pediatrics,* 1972, *50,* 801–811.

Meichenbaum, D. *Cognitive-Behavior Modification.* New York: Plenum, 1977.

Melamed, B. G., and Siegel, L. J. "Reduction of Anxiety in Children Facing Hospitalization and Surgery by Use of Filmed Modeling." *Journal of Consulting and Clinical Psychology,* 1975, *43,* 511–521.

Miller, P. M. "The Use of Visual Imagery and Muscle Relaxation in the Counter-Conditioning of a Phobic Child: A Case Study." *Journal of Nervous and Mental Diseases,* 1972, *154,* 457–460.

Minuchin, S., and others. "A Conceptual Model of Psychosomatic Illness in Children." *Archives of General Psychiatry,* 1975, *32,* 1031–1038.

Nagera, H. "Children's Reactions to Hospitalization and Illness." *Child Psychiatry and Human Development,* 1978, *9,* 3–19.

Nitschke, R., and others. "The Final Stage Conference: The Patient's Decision on Research Drugs in Pediatric Oncology." *Journal of Pediatric Psychology,* 1977, *2* (2), 58–64.

Nixon, G. "Systems Approach to Pediatric Consultation." *Journal of Clinical Child Psychology,* 1975, *4* (3), 33–35.

O'Dell, S. "Training Parents in Behavior Modification: A Review." *Psychological Bulletin,* 1974, *81,* 418–433.

Ottinger, D. R., and Roberts, M. C. "A University-Based Predoctoral Practicum in Pediatric Psychology." *Professional Psychology,* 1980, *11* (5), 707–713.

Palmer, S., Thompson, R., and Linsheid, T. "Applied Behavioral Analysis in the Treatment of Childhood Feeding Problems." *Developmental Medicine and Childhood Neurology,* 1975, *17,* 333–339.

Pless, I. B., and Roghmann, K. J. "Chronic Illness and Its Consequences: Observations Based on Three Epidemiologic Surveys." *Journal of Pediatrics,* 1971, *79* (3), 351–359.

Prugh, D. G. "Toward an Understanding of Psychosomatic Concepts in Relation to Illness in Children." In A. J. Solnit and S. Provence (Eds.), *Modern Perspectives in Child Development*. New York: International University Press, 1963.

Richmond, J. B. "Child Development: A Basic Science for Pediatrics." *Pediatrics*, 1967, *39* (5), 649-658.

Roberts, M. "Clinical Child Psychology Programs: Where and What Are They?" *Journal of Clinical Child Psychology*, 1982, *11* (1), 13-21.

Roberts, M., and Wright, L. "The Role of the Pediatric Psychologist as Consultant to Pediatricians." In J. Tuma (Ed.), *The Practice of Pediatric Psychology*. New York: Wiley, 1982.

Roberts, M., Quevillon, R. P., and Wright, L. "Pediatric Psychology: A Developmental Report and Survey of the Literature." *Child and Youth Services*, 1979, *2* (1), 1-9.

Rogers, C. R. *On Becoming a Person*. Boston: Houghton Mifflin, 1961.

Ross, A. O. *Psychological Disorders of Children*. New York: McGraw-Hill, 1974.

Routh, D. K. "The Short History of Pediatric Psychology." *Journal of Clinical Child Psychology*, 1975, *4* (3), 6-8.

Routh, D. K. "Postdoctoral Training in Pediatric Psychology." *Professional Psychology*, 1977, *8* (2), 245-250.

Russ, S. W. "Training Child Mental Health Consultants." *Journal of Clinical Child Psychology*, 1978, *7* (1), 65-67.

Russell, H. L., and Carter, J. L. "Biofeedback Training with Children: Consultation, Questions, Applications, and Alternatives." *Journal of Clinical Child Psychology*, 1978, *7* (1), 23-25.

Salk, L., Hilgartner, M., and Granich, B. "The Psychological Impact of Hemophilia on the Patient and His Family." *Social Science and Medicine*, 1972, *6*, 491-505.

Schneider, S. F. "Psychology and General Health: Prospects and Pitfalls." *Journal of Clinical Child Psychology*, 1978, *7* (1), 5-8.

Schroeder, C., Goolsby, E., and Stangler, S. "Preventive Services in a Private Pediatric Practice." *Journal of Clinical Child Psychology*, 1975, *4* (3), 32-33.

Schwartz, G. E., and Weiss, S. M. "What Is Behavioral Medicine?" *Psychosomatic Medicine*, 1977, *39* (6), 377-381.

Seifert, A. R., and Lubar, J. F. "Reduction of Epileptic Seizures Through EEG Biofeedback Training." *Biological Psychology*, 1975, *3*, 157-184.

Sigal, J. J. "Enduring Disturbances in Behavior Following Acute Illness in Early Childhood: Consistencies in Four Independent Follow-Up Studies." In E. J. Anthony and C. Koupernick (Eds.), *The Child in His Family*. Vol. 3: *Children at Psychiatric Risk*. New York: Wiley, 1974.

Skipper, J. K., and Leonard, R. C. "Children, Stress, and Hospitalization: A Field Experiment." *Journal of Health and Social Behavior*, 1968, *9*, 275-287.

Tew, B. J., and Laurence, K. M. "Mothers, Brothers, and Sisters of Patients with Spina Bifida." *Developmental Medicine and Child Neurology*, 1973, *29* (supplement), 69-76.

Toister, R. P., and Worley, L. M. "Behavioral Aspects of Pediatric Practice: A Survey of Practitioners." *Journal of Medical Education,* 1976, *51,* 1019–1020.

Travis, G. *Chronic Illness in Children.* Stanford, Calif.: Stanford University Press, 1976.

Tuma, J. M. "Training in Pediatric Psychology: A Concern of the 1980s." *Journal of Pediatric Psychology,* 1980, *5* (3), 229–243.

Tuma, J. M. (Ed.). *Directory: Internship Programs in Clinical, Child, and Pediatric Psychology.* (4th ed.) Baton Rouge: Louisiana State University, 1984.

Turk, D. "Cognitive Behavioral Techniques in the Management of Pain." In J. P. Foreyt and D. P. Rathjen (Eds.), *Cognitive Behavior Therapy.* New York: Plenum, 1978.

VandenBos, G. R., and others. *APA Input to NIMH Regarding Planning for Mental Health Personnel Development.* Washington, D.C.: American Psychological Association, 1979.

Vernon, D. T. "Modeling and Birth Order in Response to Painful Stimuli." *Journal of Personality and Social Psychology,* 1974, *29,* 794–799.

Vernon, D. T., and Bailey, W. "The Use of Motion Pictures in the Psychological Preparation of Children for Induction of Anesthesia." *Anesthesiology,* 1974, *40,* 68–72.

Vernon, D. T., and others. *The Psychological Responses of Children to Hospitalization and Illness.* Springfield, Ill.: Thomas, 1965.

Visintainer, M. A., and Wolfer, J. A. "Psychological Preparation for Surgical Pediatric Patients: The Effect on Children's and Parents' Stress Responses and Adjustment." *Pediatrics,* 1975, *56* (2), 187–202.

Waechter, E. H. "Children's Awareness of Fatal Illness." *American Journal of Nursing,* 1971, *71,* 1168–1172.

Walker, C. E. "Behavioral Intervention in a Pediatric Setting." In J. R. McNamara (Ed.), *Behavioral Approaches to Medicine.* New York: Plenum, 1979.

Weinberger, H. L. "An Attempt to Identify Frequency of Use of Technical Skills and Procedures by the Primary Care Physician." *Journal of Pediatrics,* 1976, *88,* 671–675.

Wexler, M. "The Behavioral Sciences in Medical Education: A View from Psychology." *American Psychologist,* 1976, *31,* 275–283.

Wiener, J. M. "Response of Medical Personnel to the Fatal Illness of a Child." In B. Schoenberg, A. Carr, D. Peretz, and A. Kutscher (Eds.), *Loss and Grief: Psychological Management in Medical Practice.* New York: Columbia University Press, 1970.

Willis, D. "Silent Presence Is Golden." *Journal of Clinical Child Psychology,* 1975, *4* (3), 3–5.

Willis, D., Elliot, C., and Jay, S. "Psychological Effects of Physical Illness and Its Concomitants." In J. Tuma (Ed.), *The Practice of Pediatric Psychology.* New York: Wiley Interscience, 1982.

Willoughby, R. H. "The Pediatric Psychologist as 'Polyglot'; or Training Students to Communicate Clearly in a Multidisciplinary World." *Journal of Clinical Child Psychology,* 1978, *7* (1), 55–57.

Wright, L. "Counseling with Parents of Chronically Ill Children." *Postgraduate Medicine,* 1970, *47,* 173-177.

Wright, L. "Indirect Treatment of Children Through Principle-Oriented Parent Consultation." *Journal of Consulting and Clinical Psychology,* 1976, *44,* 148.

Wright, L. "Assessing the Psychosomatic Status of Children." *Journal of Clinical Child Psychology,* 1978, *1* (2), 94-112.

Wright, L. "A Comprehensive Program for Mental Health and Behavioral Medicine in a Large Children's Hospital." *Professional Psychology,* 1979a, *34* (10), 458-466.

Wright, L. "Health Care Psychology: Prospects for the Well-Being of Children." *American Psychologist,* 1979b, *34* (10), 1001-1006.

Wright, L. "The Standardization of Compliance Procedures; or The Mass Production of Ugly Ducklings." *American Psychologist,* 1980, *35,* 119-122.

Wright, L., Schaefer, A., and Solomons, G. *Encyclopedia of Pediatric Psychology.* Baltimore, Md.: University Park Press, 1979.

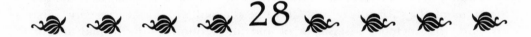

28

Training Social Workers to Aid Chronically Ill Children and Their Families

Claire Rudolph, M.S.W., Ph.D.
Virginia Andrews, M.S.W.
Kathryn Strother Ratcliff, Ph.D.
Dorothy A. Downes, R.N., M.S.W., M.P.A.

Traditionally, a prominent feature of social work practice has been its focus on social problems as phenomena deeply imbedded in environment and society, as well as in personal behavior. The unique function of the social work profession has been to organize and mobilize existing services while working with people on a one-to-one basis. At first, little training was needed to perform these activities. In the early twentieth century, however, when standards for professional education among human services practitioners began to develop, social work joined medicine and nursing in the quest for legitimation: the unique functions and competencies of social work were explicated and its territory defined. Thus, professional education in schools of social work emerged, and curricula were designed to educate and socialize future social workers in the knowledge, skills, and values of social work. Much of the development of social work as a profession can be attributed to the efforts of medical social workers— individuals who originally practiced in hospital settings and who were among the first social workers to advocate professional standards. Their work focused the attention of the profession on the social aspects of health and illness.

Historical Development

Initially, schools of social work were dependent on a practice orientation. When lay personnel in social service agencies sought to legitimate their functions by defining the set of skills that uniquely identified them as social workers, the functions of the "friendly visitor" became the skills of social casework. The casework role included assessment of and intervention for individual and/or family problems. Casework strategies included providing direct services to and coordinating community services for troubled individuals.

Influenced by nineteenth-century scientific methodologies, Mary Richmond (1917) founded the scientific investigation of social problems. She gave credibility to casework as the unique skill of social work. Richmond proposed that casework practice be based on the social worker's assessment of barriers to social functioning that existed within the social context of individuals and families. Intervention, therefore, would be directed toward individual behavioral changes as well as toward changes in social conditions. Such intervention was to become the basis for social work practice. As schools of social work began to develop, they adopted Richmond's conception of casework practice as the generic model for a professional education oriented toward agency practice. As the science of social work continued to evolve, the academic focus broadened, providing a generic education as the basis for training and practice in all fields (for example, subspecialties) of social work.

Although medical social work utilized the basic skills of casework, specialized knowledge of the disease process and of the social causes of illness was also necessary for training. Moreover, the American Association for Medical Social Workers, one of the oldest memberships of social workers representing specialized practice, had included educational criteria beyond generic training (Bartlett, 1961). Social workers in other fields of practice, such as child welfare and mental health, were also beginning to discuss the importance of more specialized education.

By the late 1950s, as Bartlett points out, the gap between the educational curriculum and the need for practice skills became evident. The schools of social work vacillated between offering a generic curriculum focused on skills of social casework, which were presumed to be applicable to all practice settings, and defining specific skills and knowledge areas unique to subspecialty fields. By 1963, a task force of the Council on Social Work Education, the professional organization for social work schools and faculty, introduced the concept of a specialized curriculum to concentrate on subspecialty areas. Recognition of the vast expansion of knowledge in specialized fields, particularly health and mental health, stimulated progress toward acceptance of specialized training.

Medical social work, including mental health, was one of the first areas of specialized practice to move toward a coherent focus of subspecialty training. This movement coincided with the explosion of medical technology and resulted in a need for broadening the subspecialization for social workers in health care. Governmental support for training hastened this development. For example, expanded support for training of social workers in health care settings came about through the Federal Manpower Assistance Act in the late 1960s. The act authorized a program of institutional grants to increase professional enrollment. Scholarship grants were also authorized to finance and improve the quality of professional social work education. These grants prepared students to provide services to the multihandicapped and mentally retarded child (Insley, 1977). By 1976, nineteen schools of social work with health care concentrations had developed.

Finney, Pessin, and Matheis (1976), in their study of health care professionals, found that increasing numbers of social work graduate students had field work in medical and public health settings. Between 1960 and 1970, the number of social workers in health care settings nearly doubled (Bracht, 1974), and social workers were employed at the federal level throughout public health service bureaus, as well as in other social service areas. Social work services were mandated under the Health Maintenance Organization Act of 1973 and the End Stage Renal Disease Program Amendments to Medicare in 1972. Social workers also perform roles in agencies that provide technical assistance to community health area planning organizations or regional health planning agencies. Finney (1976) found that among the staff-level planners, social workers represented the largest employed group. In the late 1970s, federal legislation was designed to broaden access to health care services for various and expanding population groups. Such programs as the Education for All Handicapped Children Act and Supplemental Security Income Program for Disabled Children created additional demands for the services of the social work professional in health settings.

Current Educational Programs

Specialized training for health care service delivery is a recent phenomenon in social work graduate schools. Several approaches to providing specialized education in this field have developed. One approach is a specialization in health within a general school of social work. Such a program stresses clinical skills while incorporating skills in planning and administration (Bracht, 1974).

Several schools of social work have adopted a second approach by designing educational modules that address specific health problems. A module is organized around a practicum and represents a collaborative effort with a specialized health care service system. Hunter College in New York City developed such a module, utilizing both academic faculty and agency personnel as instructors (Tendler and Metzger, 1978). Other examples are found in perinatal social work at Syracuse, New York (Rudolph, 1979), and the primary health care modules at Columbia University in New York City.

A third approach to training is to design a specific course of study on specialized topics. White reports on such a design, which integrates programs of care for child health and child welfare (White, Connely, and Gately, 1978).

Regardless of approach, most training of social work professionals includes an interdisciplinary perspective. The curriculum is taught, for example, by teams of faculty from schools of medicine, nursing, public health, and social work. Such interdisciplinary programs can have a sequentially ordered curriculum that results in a dual master's degree in public health and social work or in public administration and social work (Rudolph, 1979).

The purpose of the health care concentrations in schools of social work is to train social workers to perform a wide range of functions within a variety of health care settings. Such functions include outreach specialists in neighborhood health clinics, providers of home dialysis care, and collaborators on primary health-care teams. Increasingly, social work skills, as part of interdisciplinary team approaches, are employed in highly specialized areas of health care. In perinatal centers, leukemia clinics, and cystic fibrosis programs, social workers link patients and their families with supportive community services.

In July 1975, the Council on Social Work Education proposed the following objectives for curriculum development in health care concentration programs (based on Bracht, 1974):

1. Education for social workers in health care concentrations should be directed toward training social workers to coordinate with other members of health care teams, to provide direct services to patients and their families, and to contribute to planning services.
2. Social work education should incorporate epidemiological approaches and program planning skills.
3. The social work curriculum needs a strong biological and physiological base.
4. Schools of social work need to develop linkages with service systems in medical centers and schools of public health.
5. Schools should be encouraged to develop unique approaches in health care concentrations in order to prepare social workers for specialized practice in health care services; these approaches should include service, planning, and administrative skills.

These objectives have been translated into a core curriculum in which basic understanding of human behavior in the social environment, of public policy analysis, of cultural and ethnic diversity, and of research methods is transmitted during a first year of training. Curriculum specialization builds on this core curriculum through specialized practice tracks either in clinical practice that includes group methods and consultation or in community organization, community planning, and administration and management. Specialized content in health is an integral part of the educational experience in both the clinical track and the community organization and planning track. In recent years, collaboration between schools of social work and schools of public health or public administration has helped expand curriculum components in such areas as psychosocial impact of illness, medical information, health policy, health administration, and research.

As schools of social work become more proficient, they have developed greater expertise in organizing curriculum concentrations for social work practice in health care settings. Attention has been directed toward special health problems among different populations, such as chronically ill children, and toward providing social services to meet their specialized social and medical needs.

Orientation to Education and Training for Practice with Families with Chronically Ill Children

The social, psychological, and biological problems associated with chronic illness in children, and the structure of supportive services for them, have specific implications for the training of future professionals who practice with this population. The educational experience should provide a conceptual framework, knowledge of practical problem-solving skills, and experience with long-term supportive services to such families and their children. The following discussion describes an orientation to practice, recommended as the basis for training social workers who practice with chronically ill children.

There is extensive literature on the concept of the person in the environment as the distinguishing characteristic of the social work perspective (Germain, 1977; Coulton, 1981). This orientation directs attention to the transactions among the members of a family with a chronically ill child and their social environments. These transactions either promote or inhibit the development of individual or family potential (Germain, 1977). Biological, social, and cultural heritage also influences transactions within families and between the family and the environment. Educational content and training experiences should develop the practitioner's awareness of these factors as a tool for understanding the social meaning of physical illness to the child and the family. The demands of care for a chronically ill child have potential for changing the usual manner in which family members relate to each other and to their environment.

The role of the social work practitioner is to promote the maintenance of the family. When working with children and families in stress, the social worker must not only be aware of the specific conditions or events that are perceived by the family as stressful but must also recognize the uniqueness of each family's response, the familial heritage, and the social context (Coulton, 1981). Enhancing the fit between the person and the social world is an important characteristic of the social work perspective in providing service to physically disabled children and their families.

A chronic condition or a significant abnormality need not a priori signify a serious social handicap or emotional disability. The process by which a person or family learns about the condition, the attitudes and behaviors of the family and other social groups toward the facts of physical illness, and the organizational behavior and institutional context in which medical and social health care is provided necessarily influence the extent and form of social disability.

The problems presented by families and children where there is a physical or chronic child health condition need to be approached by the social work practitioner as multicausal. Thus, to meet the needs of chronically ill children, the social work health professional should be well trained in organic illness as well as the psychological and social aspects of health needs.

Problems of Chronic Illness Among Children and Their Families

In the United States, there are nearly seven million children born with severe physical handicaps each year (*Facts,* 1972). Accurate estimates of the proportion of the childhood population now chronically handicapped vary greatly, depending on the definition of "handicapping condition" and the source of information. The sophisticated medical and surgical techniques of our day have dramatically increased the probability of more children surviving with defects and malformations resulting from diseases such as cerebral palsy, cystic fibrosis, and spina bifida. The extent of limitations caused by handicapping conditions cannot be readily assessed because no national health survey has included questions that have been useful in making these determinations (Ireys, 1980); furthermore, there is still little conceptual clarity in defining "disability" among children.

Several surveys have shown that most children with chronic disorders have mild to moderate disability, with 12 to 17 percent facing severe limitations (Pless and Roghmann, 1971). Most of these children now reside in their own homes, and this trend will continue because of limitations on hospital stays and the push toward deinstitutionalization. As a result, it can be anticipated that social workers and other health care professionals in medical as well as nonmedical settings will become increasingly involved in helping maintain the functioning of these families and their children in the community.

A childhood illness represents a personal and familial crisis of varying degree. The impact of a disease, its course, and the response of those affected by it are not easily categorized. Yet, common factors and patterns have been observed, and commonalities can be drawn from the array of diseases of children and the people affected (Travis, 1976).

The impact of a severe illness on the affected child is an equally important factor in the problem of chronic illness. After all, it is the child who first experiences the physical pain and discomfort and, ultimately, much fear and uncertainty. The child's response to the illness may vary with age, ability to conceptualize, physical development, and the degree of daily disruption the illness creates (Travis, 1976).

Adolescence is a particularly vulnerable period in the life of a child. It is both a period of rapid physiological and anatomical change and the time adolescents normally begin to shift allegiance and assess their own values. Peer relationships become more significant models for values and behaviors, so any physical handicap or limitation that separates adolescents from their peers can be stressful. The need for adolescents to experiment with new and different behaviors, and to become psychologically independent of family and other caretakers in their social world can create conflict and tension in adaptations to their illness or physical limitations.

The responses of families to their children's chronic illness can vary with the nature of the illness itself and the implications of the physical condition for future physical and social functioning of the child. The family response is equally affected by (1) the age of the child when the illness first occurs, (2) the cultural meaning of illness, (3) the social and economic resources of the family, and (4) the family patterns of communication and interaction at the time of diagnosis. Each of these factors influences the functioning of the child in the family and the functioning of the family as a unit.

Many families react to the diagnosis of severe illness among children with acute grief, disbelief, mourning, and a sense of loss—not unlike the stages of death and dying. Anger, rejection, or denial as initial responses should be viewed as a means by which the family adapts to and copes with the circumstances and as a time for parents to mobilize their defenses. With time, parents need to begin to define and face the realities of the child's condition (Garrard and Richmond, 1963). A mature adaptation by parents occurs only when parents begin to face their problems with a minimum of stress so their energies can be mobilized to meet the tasks they must face in coping with their problems.

Sometimes, because of their preexisting psychological problems, parents never reach the stage of adaptation and, in fact, incorporate the child's problem into their own psychological problems (Pueschel and Murphy, 1975). If there has been marital discord prior to the diagnosis of the illness in the child, it can be exacerbated. Parents may become distant and create barriers of seeming indifference toward each other; the affected child can become enmeshed in the family transactions and may blame himself or herself for the physical problem and the family responses to it. In effect, the family becomes more disrupted than it was prior to the diagnosis.

Competencies for Social Work Practice with Chronically Ill Children

The concept of the individual or family as part of a broader physical and social world and the knowledge of the impact of a child's illness on family functioning lead to an identification of the competencies that social workers must have to work effectively with these children. These competencies include skills in direct practice, program planning and coordination of services to meet individual and family needs, and research. The development of skills occurs through the acquisition of theoretical knowledge and experience in field settings. Practice situations for social work students are available in hospitals, specialty clinics, public health clinics, and school systems.

With the passage of the Education for All Handicapped Children Act of 1975 (Public Law 94-142), the public schools faced the problem of meeting the needs of physically and mentally handicapped children. The legislation has also resulted in increasing numbers of physically handicapped children in foster care services and group homes. Awareness of the need for this population to be served by many different programs of services should be incorporated into training for professional social work practice.

Direct Practice. Direct practice involves working with the family as a unit. It requires skills in assessing the coping patterns of the family as it responds to the diagnosis of the illness and, later, as it begins to adjust to the demands of the illness. Direct service involves skills in communication, information gathering, and sensitivity to and empathy for the meaning of the problem to the family in the context of its social and cultural milieu. The ecological perspective directs the social work practitioner to assess the interface between the family and its larger context. Discussion of the particular training requirements for the diagnosis phase and the adjustment phase of the coping process follows.

Learning about the diagnosis of a chronic illness and the potential physical limitations of the child is likely to be one of the most stressful times for that child's family. Early intervention during this period reduces the potential that the family will distort the facts concerning the child's condition and helps avoid maladaptive and dysfunctional responses (Parad, 1963). The practitioner learns to intervene at the early stages of diagnosis. The patterns that families use to cope with stress must be understood as the worker tries to build on the positive and functional aspects of family interactions. The practitioner must differentiate the present situation from other crises the family has experienced and must begin engaging the family in a set of problem-solving tasks (Hancock, 1980).

A major task for the practitioner during the diagnosis phase is to be supportive, empathic, and directive at the same time. The practitioner's knowledge about the disease and its impact in relation to the child's age and stage of life is helpful to the family in clarifying their situation. In order to solve problems, families must have the opportunity to vent their anguish, and in order to reconstitute themselves and go on, families may need help in defining their inner strengths and resources. While family members experience their initial grief and anger, perceptions of the illness, their roles, and the roles of others need to be clarified and corrected (Rappaport, 1965).

In general, then, the initial phase of treatment requires that practitioners gather pertinent information about the family, assess the complex relationships and interactions of the family members as they respond to the crisis, and respond sensitively and purposefully in helping the family find appropriate behavioral patterns.

An excellent device for teaching students the meaning and impact of the illness of a child on the family is to have the student accompany the family through the bureaucratic processes involved in gaining access to resources such as Medicaid or the Crippled Children's Services. Students can also learn by listening to explanations of the physical nature of an illness as they are given by physicians to the family. This experience will help students assess the social and physical limitations of a child's illness and provide them with the opportunity to ask the physician pertinent questions in the presence of the family.

Although the diagnosis phase of an illness may represent one of the most traumatic periods for families faced with a child's chronic illness, practitioners of social work should learn that crisis intervention will be an ongoing need as families undergo recurrent tensions during the course of an illness. At times, families must make decisions about whether to treat or not. In the case of multihandicapped neonates, where treatment will permit the child to survive but may leave severe handicaps, the decision may be particularly difficult. Treatment decisions can have a long-term impact on parents and siblings, and practitioners must be sensitive to the family's view of the ethical issues. Furthermore, practitioners must be sensitive to the impact of the health care system on the family during periods when serious decisions about health care must be made.

As the illness progresses, the family makes adaptations to the new situation. The tasks required in helping a family make adjustments to a child's illness are many. Direct services during the adjustment phase should focus on the whole family rather than simply on the sick child. The therapeutic process should activate family members in self-appraisal of their patterns of interrelationships and in finding new ways to relate and communicate when their established patterns are dysfunctional. For example, when a child has a physical problem, dysfunctional alignments may occur between an overprotective parent and child. Overprotecting the child could result in parental overinvolvement with the child, which may lead to further family dysfunction.

In other families, the mother and the affected child may form a coalition that excludes other family members from their interactions. Practitioners should recognize these patterns and begin to intervene by helping families work on their problems as a family. For example, giving a sibling a role in caring for the physically ill child helps that sibling remain an integrated member of the family. The goal of supportive direct services with families of chronically ill children should be to use medical care to normalize the child and family to the greatest extent possible. The social work practitioner should emphasize mainstreaming possibilities that offer opportunities for appropriate achievement rather than emphasizing the illness and its limitations.

Practitioners must learn to select an appropriate intervention to help families develop their own social support and emotional fortitude. One such intervention strategy is group work. Structured group interaction provides the child with a sense of identity, an opportunity to ventilate feelings, and a chance to be educated about the illness. Group work interventions have been reported as a successful treatment mode with some young children with epilepsy (Appalone and Gibson, 1980) and with adolescents who have sickle cell anemia. Parent groups are also useful as vehicles for educating parents about their child's condition and as a means for involving parents in the home care of their child. In some instances, group meetings are meaningful to parents facing the death of a child.

Students gain skill and understanding of group work techniques with physically handicapped children by attending support groups such as Parents of SIDS (Sudden Infant Death Syndrome), Parents of Cystic Fibrosis Children, or groups formed to help arthritic and short-statured children. Observing these groups affords students the opportunity to see the positive effects of providing ventilation and support to these families through group work intervention.

Multidisciplinary teamwork is a significant part of the training of social workers in providing direct services to the family with a chronically ill child. Multidisciplinary teams, which may include both medical personnel and social workers, are part of many health care systems. Students of social work should have the experience of being a part of an interdisciplinary team in order to learn how such teams arrive at decisions. Social work has only recently begun to conceptualize its role on multidisciplinary teams. An important contribution of the social worker is to alert the team to barriers to the child's physical and psychological improvement that result from family functioning and environmental conditions. In turn, it is important that social work practitioners learn that other disciplines can contribute valuable information about the physical processes of childhood illness and realistic expectations for the child's physical functioning. The efficiency of team effort is dependent on communication among team members. Communication skills need to be incorporated in the training of all social work practitioners, but particularly for those involved with interdisciplinary teams.

Coordination of Services. Fragmentation of services is a major problem for chronically ill children and reflects to a large extent the categorical manner in which public supportive services for child health care have developed. A complex, uncoordinated, interconnected maze of services is typical. In many states, the Crippled Children's Services program provides medical and rehabilitation services within the limits of state and local financing. Supplemental Security Income (SSI) gives families with chronically disabled children income support when the family meets the income eligibility criteria. The Education for All Handicapped Children Act provides funds from the federal government to expand state and local educational programs for the handicapped. Much of the federal and state legislation does not define *handicapping condition,* leaving it open to local interpretation. Furthermore, children who have more than one handicapping condition may launch the family into a very long search for sources of needed support because one categorical program definition may not cover all of the child's conditions.

Spina bifida, a condition requiring continuous medical and social health care, provides a good example of the need for social workers to coordinate services. Children with this condition are often unable to function independently and often require a wheelchair. They may be isolated from peers and social contacts if transportation or other community supports to facilitate regular school attendance and normal social interactions are lacking. Frequent hospitalizations associated with this disease are a source of added stress for these children. Services for children with spina bifida can be found under the Crippled Children's Services, SSI, Medicaid, Education for All Handicapped Children, and mental health clinics. Each of these services, however, has separate administrative authority, eligibility criteria, and resources.

In many cases, a family may be eligible for the Crippled Children's Services program, yet not be eligible for Medicaid. Because of the income eligibility of Medicaid and SSI, a family may have to deplete its own resources before they can avail themselves of needed support from these programs. To obtain needed resources, families with chronically ill children often need advocates and ombudsmen. Part of the social worker function is to perform these roles.

Sources of information for practitioners about community resources can be found in the analyses of legislation, annual reports of community agencies, and assessments of communication styles of organizations and bureaucracies. Informal networks among social workers in different agencies can be established through case conferences—an excellent means for learning how to use community resources. Formal and informal interaction among professional groups is another tool for helping families gain access to needed services.

The goal of coordination of services on behalf of families with a chronically ill child should be to bring together those services that can provide both prevention and treatment. These services may include financial, medical, social, and psychological supports. Organizing disparate services requires attention and training, not only in identifying resources and gaining access to them but also in designing mechanisms to maintain the concerted efforts of a variety of services to meet the needs of the family.

Students, through assessing their own field experiences in service systems, should note the responsiveness of settings to children and adults with handicapping physical conditions. Barriers that exist in agency settings, social and legal restrictions, and any differential treatment provided, sensitize students to the institutional constraints that families experience.

The behavioral skills of organizing include negotiating and motivating service systems to develop cooperative relationships on behalf of the client population. The form cooperative arrangements take depends to a large extent on the political climate of a community, the auspices of service provisions, the geographical scope of the effort, and the particular problem addressed. Many of the constraints on the integration of service programs will be imbedded in the authority or jurisdiction that a particular agency has over its goals and resources.

Developing cooperative linkages between child welfare and child health services takes place in an interpersonal arena. It requires leadership skills and the willingness of an agency to take responsibility for starting the process and staying with it until there is a successful outcome. Once these linkages are formed, an agency or a group of workers must take responsibility to maintain coordination. This responsibility should be formalized, if possible. However, the end point of formalization may be a long way down the road. Thus, an alternate mechanism may be put into place while more formal linkages are being discussed.

During the course of their training, students should be taught to evaluate their field experiences from the ecological perspective. They need to be guided through the experience of analyzing agency alignments that they observe, and of recognizing the sources of power and authority that reside within an agency and can be tapped to form cooperative linkages. They should participate in community advisory councils as well as client advocacy groups to ascertain the perceptions that each of these groups has of the other and the possibilities for developing linkages between client needs and agency services.

Case management is a vehicle by which the goals of service provision for an individual family are identified and a primary worker (or agency system) takes responsibility for referring, monitoring, and tracking the family's progress when receiving supportive services from a wide range of community services. The key to effective case management is the ability of practitioners to organize the needed services, set service objectives, and evaluate progress of a family in a timely fashion.

Research. The need for training in research relevant to social work professional activities becomes evident when we observe that no common information system exists across state and federal programs. Services to chronically ill children represent a mixture of public and private auspices that appear oblivious to each other as often as they are complementary (Jackson, 1980). Standard record keeping would be useful in epidemiological studies, as would widely agreed upon definitional criteria for each handicap. Although these issues may be most appropriately identified as management issues, they also constitute a substantial barrier to any intensive research study, including one that would establish basic incidence rates.

Practitioners involved with chronically handicapped children need the skills to establish indicators of social need and to determine target groups in need of services. In the last ten years, these skills have come into focus as local services systems have been required to respond to state and federal regulations for planning care under the Crippled Children's Services and under Title XX of the Social Security Act. Indicators can be used to establish the levels of severity of chronic illness in a child, the progression of conditions, and the degree to which different subgroups in a population are affected. One way to develop more appropriate systems of service is to teach future professional social workers the skills of measuring the usefulness of criteria for identifying disabling conditions and the populations where these conditions are found in order to demonstrate where gaps in service exist.

The time has come to close the gap between practice (which seeks to solve problems of human behavior) and research (which seeks precise routes to knowledge that can be empirically verified). The social work profession must begin to grapple with the persistent dilemmas and issues of social behavior that are too complex for purely subjective analysis. There are many opportunities for practitioners to involve themselves in research, either as participants or as initiators for theory building or evaluation of practice performance.

Unfortunately, social work practitioners have not traditionally relied on the findings of research in their practice, which accounts for some reluctance among professionals to engage in research. Practitioners would rather rely on supervision or consultation than on research findings to guide practice. This phenomenon is partly the result of graduate education that emphasizes apprenticeship learning rather than theory testing. Unless progress is made in knowledge about the art of practice, the social work profession will not contribute significantly to the direction of social care for physically ill children. Only as we systematically define and examine patterns within social phenomena over time do persistent trends and themes emerge that may have significance for directing purposeful social interventions.

Conclusion

To date, the types of manpower needed to meet the health care needs of chronically disabled children have not been determined. Public health estimates generally conclude that there is an adequate supply of medical care personnel. Nevertheless, there is substantial evidence that unmet needs continue to exist, especially among children with handicapping conditions. Solutions to the problem of providing services to the special population of chronically ill children include meeting needs for psychological and social assistance. A continuum of medical, physical, psychological, financial, and educational services is necessary to address the distinctive needs of this population and to enhance their access to health care services. A system for coordinating the training of medical personnel, nurses, and social workers could provide more efficient and effective services to chronically ill children. Social work, by its nature a diffuse profession working across systems of client and health care services, has a unique opportunity to function as an integrating force in linking the needs of the family with the services available from other professional disciplines and from varied institutional resources.

Social work is practiced throughout a system of services that address different aspects of the problems faced by families with chronically ill children. The ecological perspective of the social work profession directs the practitioner to work toward creating a good fit between the needs of the family, the needs of the child, and the expectations of the surrounding environment and toward linking available services in a planned and organized manner. To perform this integrating function, the social work practitioner must have an interdisciplinary theoretical knowledge base and must develop a mix of skills, including skills in clinical services, organizational skills, analytical and research skills, and the personal skill of recognizing one's own limitations.

References

Appalone, C., and Gibson, P. "Group Work with Young Adult Epilepsy Patients." *Social Work in Health Care,* 1980, *6* (2), 23–32.

Bartlett, H. M. *Social Work Practice in the Health Field.* Washington, D.C.: National Association of Social Workers, 1961.

Bracht, N. F. "Health Care: The Largest Human Service System." *Social Work,* 1974, *19* (5), 532–542.

Coulton, C. J. "Person Environment Fit as the Focus of Health Care." *Social Work,* 1981, pp. 5–18.

Facts. New York: March of Dimes, 1972.

Finney, R., Pessin, R., and Matheis, L. "Prospects for Social Workers in Health Planning." *Health and Social Work,* 1976, *1* (3), 7–26.

Garrard, S. D., and Richmond, J. B. "Psychological Aspects of the Management of Chronic Diseases and Handicapping Conditions in Childhood." In H. I. Leif, V. F. Leif, and N. R. Leif (Eds.), *The Psychological Basis of Medical Practice.* New York: Harper & Row, 1963.

Germain, C. "An Ecological Perspective on Social Work Practice in Health Care." *Social Work in Health Care,* 1977, *3,* 67–76.

Hancock, E. "Crisis Intervention in a Newborn Nursery Intensive Care Unit." *Social Work in Health Care,* 1980, *1,* 421–432.

Insley, V. "Health Services: Maternal and Child Health." In J. B. Turner (Ed.), *Encyclopedia of Social Work.* Washington, D.C.: National Association of Social Workers, 1977.

Ireys, H. T. "Health Care for Chronically Disabled Children and Their Families." In Select Panel for the Promotion of Child Health, *Better Health for Our Children: A National Strategy.* Vol. 4. Department of Health and Human Services publication no. 79-55071. Washington, D.C.: U.S. Government Printing Office, 1981.

Jackson, R. C. "Developing Networks in a State-Based System of Health Care for Families." In E. L. Watkins (Ed.), *Proceedings of the 1980 Tri-Regional Workshop for Social Workers in Maternal and Child Health Services.* Rockville, Md.: Office of Maternal and Child Health, U.S. Department of Health and Human Services, 1980.

Parad, H. J. "Brief Ego-Oriented Casework with Families in Crisis." In H. J. Parad and R. R. Miller (Eds.), *Ego-Oriented Casework: Problems and Perspectives.* New York: Family Services Association of America, 1963.

Pless, I. B., and Roghmann, K. "Chronic Illness and Its Consequences: Observations Based on Three Epidemiological Surveys." *Journal of Pediatrics,* 1971, *79* (3), 351–359.

Pueschel, S., and Murphy, A. "Counseling Parents of Infants with Down's Syndrome." *Post-Graduate Medicine,* 1975, *58* (7), 90–95.

Rappaport, L. "Working with Families in Crisis: An Exploration in Preventive Intervention." In H. J. Parad (Ed.), *Selected Readings.* New York: Family Services Association of America, 1965.

Richmond, M. *Social Diagnosis.* New York: Russell Sage Foundation, 1917.

Rudolph, C. "Use of Research as a Basis for Curriculum Development in Maternal and Child Health." Paper presented at the Annual Meeting of the Council on Social Work Education, Boston, March 1979.

Tendler, D., and Metzger, K. "Training in Prevention: An Educational Model for Social Work Students." *Social Work in Health Care,* 1978, *4* (2), 221–232.

Travis, G. *Chronic Illness in Children: Its Impact on Child and Family.* Stanford, Calif.: Stanford University Press, 1976.

White, R., Connely, D. A., and Gately, A. "Interdisciplinary Training for Child Welfare and Health." *Child Welfare,* 1978, *57* (9), 549–563.

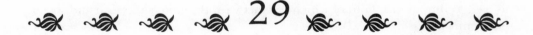

29

Meeting the Service Needs of Chronically Impaired Children: Individual Portraits

Tom Joe, M.A.
Cheryl Rogers, M.Ed.

The subject of this volume—children with persistent disabilities or illnesses—is one that deeply troubles us as a society. The sight of a child in a wheelchair or struggling on metal braces raises a host of emotions. We feel sorry for such children because of the vulnerability created by their afflictions and their status as children; we wonder why such an injustice would befall a young person and view the handicap as a human tragedy. Intermingled with our pity is compassion, an essential ingredient to any effort to help disabled children live full and rich lives.

In itself, however, compassion mixed with pity will not make things better for handicapped children and youth. As a nation, we have failed to develop effective means of helping chronically impaired children maximize their potential. There are many specific areas in which growth is critical. These include the

Note: The authors wish to thank several persons for their help in arranging the case studies used in this paper and for their suggestions on how we might create a more humane world for chronically impaired children: Dr. Frederick J. Kottke, Professor and Head of the Department of Physical Medicine and Rehabilitation, University of Minnesota Hospital; Dr. Dennis D. Dykstra, Instructor, Department of Physical Medicine and Rehabilitation, University of Minnesota; Dr. Arthur F. Kohrman, Director, La Rabida Children's Hospital and Research Center, The University of Chicago; and Dr. James S. Gordon, Chief, Adolescent Services Branch, St. Elizabeth's Hospital, Washington, D.C.

continued development of alternative delivery systems based on the specific needs of individual children, increased understanding of how to maximize individual potential from early life on, and development of strong leadership. Above all, we need to rethink the nature of chronic impairment, replacing a concept that elicits pity and compassion with one that views a handicapped child as having strengths as well as limitations, both of which interact with the child's physical and social environment.

The purpose of this chapter is to make recommendations for structural changes that may result in more effective strategies to help impaired children. We consider the entire repertoire of an impaired child's physical and emotional needs in the belief that the most fundamental needs these children have are ones shared by all children and are not necessarily unique to their particular disability.

Throughout the chapter, we refer to *need* and the *chronically impaired*. Because both of these terms are used to connote a variety of states, it is important to define how we have used them. First, our use of the term *need* is intended to denote the basic elements without which a child cannot live a full and meaningful life. Where *desire* or *want* may be viewed as signifying psychological states over which one has some degree of control, *need* refers to a state that demands some particular fulfillment in order for the child to progress. We do not pretend to be able to distinguish between these two concepts in every case, but the needs to which we refer in this chapter are generally necessary to the vital functioning of the child.

We use the term *chronically impaired* interchangeably with the term *disabled* to indicate the presence of a long-term physical or mental condition that leaves the child unable to perform one or more functions unassisted. Although it denotes an identifiable loss of function, it does not necessarily imply a lack of potential ability to perform. The child may compensate for the impairment with environmental aids, for example, and although blind, may learn to read Braille and walk with a cane. This concept is explored more fully in the text.

To portray the wide range of needs of handicapped children, we have used three case studies, an approach that permits us to capture the richness of these children's lives by describing their particular strengths and weaknesses. These chronically disabled children come from different parts of the country and have different impairments and different needs. Although they are by no means intended to represent all impaired children, from an examination of the lives of these three children, we learned that it is possible to draw some common lessons. The lessons range from how we as a society should view disabled children to how we might develop policies that will meet more adequately the needs of children with chronic impairments and their families.

In order to identify the issues involved in serving these children and their families effectively, we ask several questions. First, who is a chronically impaired child? How do we recognize him or her and how is he or she different from a nondisabled child? This question constitutes the heart of the normalcy-deviancy issue. Second, what do these children need in order to live as fully as possible? Finally, we ask, how can we restructure both our public and private programs and delivery systems so they better serve these children, enabling them to realize their potential and live as productively and fully as possible?

Characterizing the Chronically Disabled Child

An initial response to the question, Who is a chronically disabled child? defines four specific population groups. The first group includes children with chronic physical diseases, such as rheumatic heart disease, renal disease, diabetes, muscular dystrophy, and leukemia. These children often spend long periods of time in the hospital receiving specialized medical services during which they are isolated from usual peer group interaction. The second group consists of children with physical and sensory disabilities, such as blindness, deafness, cerebral palsy, or loss of limb. Third are those with mental retardation and developmental disabilities, conditions that can, in some cases, be traced to organic causes but generally have no known etiology. Many of these children still reside in large-scale institutions built during the nineteenth and early twentieth centuries. Although the U.S. Bureau of the Census (1978) estimates that at least 152,000 children were residents of institutions in 1976, many contend that this number is an underestimate. Fourth are children with serious mental illnesses. These children reside in a variety of settings: correctional facilities, public and private residential treatment centers, hospitals, foster homes, and their own homes.

The number of children in each of the four categories has never been precisely determined, largely because of the great overlap among the categories. One source estimates, however, that approximately ten million children in the United States suffer from some type of chronic impairment (Brewer and Kakalik, 1979). Based on the National Health Interview Survey, the proportion of children limited in activity by a chronic impairment continues to grow, having doubled from approximately 2 percent in the early 1960s to 4 percent in 1976. Although the growth may be explained by several factors including fewer deaths in infancy, greater sophistication in diagnosis, and increased parental awareness, the implications for service resources remain constant.

The increase in the number of children who are classified as chronically impaired may also result, in part, from an increased awareness that health and disability are profoundly affected by environmental and social factors. There is strong evidence that income and family composition affect a child's ability to function. For example, children in low-income families (under $5,000 in 1976) were 1.5 times more likely to be limited in daily activities because of a chronic condition than were children from families with incomes of $15,000 or more (Select Panel for the Promotion of Child Health, 1981, p. 26). The department's National Health Interview Survey found low-income children to be less likely to receive medical care, more likely to have been hospitalized, and if hospitalized, more likely to remain in the hospital longer. Similarly, they found that children without fathers were slightly more likely to be limited in their ability to carry on their major activity than were children with two parents. A high proportion (15 percent) of chronically disabled children receiving Supplemental Security Income

(SSI) were found to be residing in foster care homes and maintained little or no contact with their parents (U.S. Department of Health and Human Services, 1980). All of these findings support the conclusion that we must consider social, economic, and environmental factors in any investigation of a disabled child's life. They also suggest that we should not be surprised to find chronically impaired children in disadvantaged situations (such as in poor families with only one parent).

Beyond these facts, however, the definition of a chronically impaired child becomes less clear. The boundary between a disabled child and a nondisabled child is less a distinct line than a subtle shift on the continuum from normalcy to deviancy. The point at which weaknesses become disabilities is most often a matter of judgment, and even a slight shift in our definitions of deviancy and normalcy can alter radically the number of people considered impaired at any point in time.

To complicate matters further, chronic impairments carry with them a high degree of uncertainty. Physicians, social workers, and others are not always able to make precise diagnoses, nor are they always able to make definitive statements about the prospects for a child's future. For example, if we do not know what the near future may look like for a child with leukemia, but we do know the child is likely to die within ten years, at what point do we consider this child disabled? Or what can we say about how much a child who appears to be mildly retarded will be able to accomplish in a lifetime, given our limited understanding of mental retardation and the infinite variations that exist within the diagnosis?

In addition to our inability to diagnose disability precisely, we have failed to account adequately for the way in which an individual child interacts with the environment and for the fact that different environments will evoke different responses even when the impairment is the same. Two children with the same impairment may function very differently in the world if, for example, one has an assertive personality and strong family support and the other is shy, with little family encouragement for making demands known. It is imperative that we keep in mind children's abilities, strengths, compensatory mechanisms, and immediate environment when we attempt to assess their needs.

Two ideologies have perpetuated the tendency to view chronically impaired children as stereotypes of their disabilities and to treat them without attention to their individual characteristics. One is known as professionalism and the other as the medical model. In the first, certain specialists take responsibility for a child; in the second, impairments are labeled and treated according to medical disease categories. Although professionalism has grown steadily as our scientific knowledge increases, the medical model has remained the predominant framework for viewing and treating disability throughout the past two centuries. Our current system of open-ended public financing for medical care and limited dollar ceilings for social and other nonmedical services is one apparent reason the medical model has predominated. The financial incentives are clearly in the direction of the provision of medical care in the context of the medical model.

The effect of both of these phenomena has been to inhibit a more useful view of the problems posed by chronic impairment, most of which require management from a wide variety of professionals rather than solely by physicians. The distinction between chronic and acute care has been characterized as basically the difference between repeated interaction with an emphasis on continuity of care versus single episodes of care. Purely physical treatment is rarely sufficient. By acknowledging social and environmental factors, the problem extends beyond the child and requires consideration of the child's perceptions of self in relation to others, interaction with others, and modifications of the environment. Although these may be entirely appropriate subjects for intervention, the medical field may not be best equipped to handle them.

In saying this, it is important not to overlook the usefulness of professionals and medical care. We do not underestimate the value of specialists and physicians. Nor do we suggest they be replaced with another unilateral approach. We do, however, advocate a more diverse system.

Unfortunately, we cannot look to the human services system to help us characterize an impaired child. A complex array of programs at federal, state, and local levels of government, as well as in the private sector, presents scores of different and often conflicting definitions of impairment. Federal education legislation defines a handicapped child, for example, as one with a certain impairment who needs special education. Crippled Children's Services defines the child in terms of physical limitation. Title XX uses still another way, and so on. It is not difficult to imagine gaps in services and duplicative efforts that result in some children "falling through the cracks" and others receiving the same services from different agencies.

One way to view chronic impairment among children is to take a developmental approach and ask ourselves what is the best way for all children— disabled and nondisabled—to develop their potential, whatever that might be. The assumption that all children require the same basic resources to support their development is important if we are to avoid the mistake of predetermining deviancy. All children have certain needs, and all children progress through certain stages. It is these fundamental processes that should be the focus of our inquiry for chronically impaired children if we are to avoid stereotyping disabled children as unable to perform certain tasks and thereby immune to traditional theories of child development.

One way to conceptualize the environment of any child is as a set of concentric circles with the child in the middle, surrounded by immediate family and progressive layers of extended family, friends and neighbors, the doctor and other professionals, and eventually the larger community in which the child lives. We then ask how a particular child relates to each of the larger circles. How does a child develop self-image? relate to others in the neighborhood? develop a sexual identity? learn? If we assume a disabled child must pursue the same fundamental objectives as a nondisabled child, we can then focus on the developmental process by which all children come to realize their potential.

In summary, it is not easy to determine who is a chronically impaired child. *Chronic impairment* is a term that varies with the contemporary definitions of normalcy and deviancy. In addition, the label carries a high degree of uncertainty in terms of prognosis, it extends beyond a medical category to include social and environmental factors, and in the end, it is only a partial description of an individual child—a child with many of the same needs as other children and who must undergo many of the same developmental processes as other children, only with a little extra baggage. Beyond these general descriptions, the way to learn well who these children are and what they need is to examine their lives.

The descriptions of the following three children seek to portray the full complexity of their service needs and to illustrate that a detailed understanding of their abilities and disabilities, rather than a particular label, should dictate the services provided. A discussion following the descriptions explores the implications for service prescription in each case.

Ellen

Ellen is a pretty thirteen-year-old girl whom we met, along with her mother, Katy, her stepfather, Larry, and her infant stepbrother, in their suburban Maryland townhouse. With her blue eyes, black shoulder-length hair, pink sweater, and jeans, Ellen looks like any normal teenager. However, Ellen was born with spina bifida—her clothes and hairstyle conceal multiple physical impairments that have been treated with twenty-nine surgical procedures and with many other therapies to provide her with the capability to function as normally as possible.

Mobility and Self-Maintenance. Ellen had clubfeet at birth and no muscles in her lower legs. Operations and follow-up therapy at Children's Hospital in Washington, D.C., and the Georgetown University Hospital spina bifida program were required to correct her feet. Ellen now walks almost normally with the aid of plastic knee-high braces provided through the Crippled Children's Services. The braces have to be replaced periodically as she grows taller. Through Ellen's early years, physical therapy was also provided weekly at Georgetown Hospital to develop her ability to walk, and a muscle transfer from her abdomen to hips was performed to increase her strength and mobility. Ellen's mother and her family were trained by hospital staff to perform daily physical therapy exercises to strengthen Ellen's hips and legs.

In addition to her need for surgery to enhance her mobility, Ellen has required surgery to relieve the pressure of spinal fluid on her brain. A device known as a shunt has been implanted through her skull to regulate the drainage of fluid; the shunt has been replaced periodically during her development. These extraordinary medical/surgical expenses were financed in large part through her parents' Blue Cross/Blue Shield policy, but their own limited resources were also used to pay for her care.

Ellen's neurological damage prior to birth created two major problems for her daily life; first, she did not receive sensations telling her when to void her bladder and risked kidney damage as a result. To correct this problem, an ileostomy was performed during her preschool years. She wears an external ostomy bag, which she has learned to empty at appropriate intervals. Before Ellen could perform this function for herself, her family and her teachers at the local public school assisted her.

Ellen has never developed bowel control, again because of her neurological impairments. She also lacks the coordination necessary to clean herself unaided. At the time we saw Ellen and her family, Ellen was enrolled in a biofeedback program to give her the bowel control she lacks. The program, provided at Washington's Georgetown Hospital with funds from a Kennedy Foundation grant, was apparently succeeding and promised to give Ellen additional independence in the conduct of her daily life.

With respect to the other tasks of self-maintenance, such as bathing, feeding, and dressing, Ellen functions as a normal thirteen-year-old.

Intelligence and Education. Spina bifida is accompanied by severe mental retardation in 30 percent of cases, and most spina bifida children have some learning disability. Ellen's intellectual deficits are relatively minor; she has a learning disability that affects her reading and math performance, but she spells extremely well. The local school system has provided Ellen and other learning disabled students with special classes in reading and math since kindergarten, and she is mainstreamed in classes such as home economics, chorus, shop, and music. Each year, an Individual Education Plan (IEP) with specific goals is developed by Ellen's teachers, reviewed with her mother and stepfather, and carried out to the family's satisfaction. School personnel are hopeful that Ellen will be able to hold a clerical or comparable position as an adult.

Family, Friends, and Self. Ellen's immediate family consists of her mother, Katy, a warm, spirited, blue-eyed blond who works as a dental hygienist; her stepfather, Larry, a tall, rugged thirty-five-year-old who drives a truck for a local firm; and Larry, Jr., an active eight-month-old. Ellen's father and mother have been divorced for three years, and Katy reports that he was never supportive of Ellen's many hospitalizations and special needs. He did not reject Ellen but avoided dealing with her problems from birth onward. Katy managed the physical and emotional strain of Ellen's early years with the support of her own family, particularly her five brothers and sisters. One of Katy's major needs during Ellen's early years was for transportation to and from Children's and Georgetown hospitals—an hour's drive each way from her home. Without such assistance, Katy would have been unable to work full time, which was necessary to pay for Ellen's uninsured medical costs and to help maintain the household. Katy's father was also crucial to her for emotional support and provided loans when needed to pay for disposable medical devices (for example, ostomy bags) and expenses related to Ellen's other conditions.

Throughout our meeting, the importance of Katy's family in meeting Ellen's special needs was emphasized. There were occasions when additional help was provided through federal and state programs as well: Katy received Medicaid to cover hospital costs at one point in Ellen's course of treatment, and the

Crippled Children's Services program has provided orthopedic devices, such as braces, throughout Ellen's development. Katy was informed of opportunities for assistance through Children's Hospital staff and through her priest. Social services funds were not made available for some of Ellen's needs because the family did not meet income eligibility criteria.

Katy and Larry together earn approximately $20,000 a year. Although this permits few luxuries, they do not anticipate any additional surgery or extraordinary expenses for Ellen and are very optimistic about her future.

Ellen's mother was very pleased to report how warm the other children and teachers are toward Ellen. Indeed, Ellen has not had the social and emotional problems that might be expected of a multiply handicapped child who has undergone repeated hospitalization. Rather, she is outgoing and is not self-conscious. We can speculate that the continuity of her life in a stable community, surrounded by an extended and loving family throughout her developmental years, has been significant in producing this positive result.

Summary: Ellen. Ellen will always wear knee-high braces in order to walk, will always require a shunt to relieve the pressure of spinal fluid on her brain, and will always use an ostomy bag or some other device to compensate for her impaired bladder function. Through a combination of sophisticated surgery, physical therapy, appropriate special education, some publicly and privately funded medical assistance, and a warm, accepting, supportive family, Ellen can look forward to a nearly normal and independent life.

Beth

Beth is a nine-year-old who, until recently, lived a very normal life with her family in a suburb in the western part of the country. She has one older sister, age thirteen, and one younger brother, age seven. Her father works for Westinghouse Electric Corporation, and her mother is involved in civic activities and volunteers part-time at the local library. Beth is in the fourth grade, does well in school, and has several good friends. She is a member of a Girl Scout troop and goes to a ranch just outside of town on weekends to ride horses with her best friend. Beth's developmental history has been normal, and her family has no knowledge of any history of chronic illness.

Onset of illness. One night at eleven o'clock, Beth's mother, who was in the family room watching television, noticed that Beth had gotten up to go to the bathroom several times since she had gone to bed at nine. Her mother wondered to herself why Beth should be nervous, if indeed this was causing her frequent trips to the bathroom. She went into Beth's bedroom to ask Beth if she felt all right, and Beth, already back in bed, murmured that, yes, she was fine and quickly fell back asleep. At around midnight, when Beth's mother and father went to bed, they checked Beth again and noticed that she was breathing hard. Beth's father was up again around four o'clock and checked Beth's room. He tried to wake her, but she was completely unresponsive. He and his wife rushed Beth to the emergency room. Intravenous solutions were immediately ordered, several shots were administered, Beth was placed in an intensive care room, and her parents were deluged with questions. After a two-and-a-half-hour vigil, the doctor came into the waiting room to tell them that, although he would have to wait for confirmation from further tests, he felt almost certain that Beth had diabetes.

Beth's parents were shocked. They thought of diabetes as predominantly occurring among adults—not children and certainly not Beth, who was strong and healthy. But gradually, over the next several days, Beth's mother began to piece together evidence to which she had been oblivious. For example, she remembered that Beth had mentioned she had lost four pounds when the school nurse weighed her two weeks ago, yet to Beth's mother she had appeared to be eating and drinking as much as she always did. She also remembered wondering why Beth was going to the bathroom so often at night. When she later talked to Beth's teacher at school, her teacher corroborated the fact that Beth had been asking to go to the bathroom quite a few times each day. Beth also later confessed that she had wet her bed the night before she went to the hospital but had been embarrassed to tell her mother. All of these events convinced Beth's parents that she actually did have diabetes, although this conviction evolved slowly over the days following the doctor's diagnosis.

Beth's Reaction. When Beth first woke up twenty-four hours after being admitted to the hospital, she reflects now that she was a little scared. She knew her parents were worried about her, she felt awful, and most of all, she did not like the IVs set up around her bed. Her doctor came in later that day to try to explain what was happening. He told her that her body was a complicated machine that sometimes needed to be fixed. He assured her that they could fix it. He explained in simple terms what her pancreas does and that she now was not producing enough insulin but that she could get extra insulin from shots. Beth says she froze when she learned she would have to have shots every day for the rest of her life. Her doctor also told her she would have to check her urine daily by collecting it in a jar and comparing the color to a chart after dropping a chemical tablet in it. He also told her what kinds of foods she should eat and not eat. After all this bad news, he assured Beth that she would be able to ride horses and go to school and play with her friends just as before, as long as she took her shots and watched her diet.

Beth cried for a while when the doctor left. Her mother and father took turns staying with her for the next several days. At one point, she said to her mother, "Please don't be mad at me." A nurse who was in the room later tried to tell her that diabetes was not her fault, that it's not something one can bring on by being bad.

Beth stayed in the hospital for six days. During this time, she underwent numerous tests and spent several hours each day learning how to take care of herself. A nurse specially trained in diabetes education spent an hour with her each morning explaining the importance of the pancreas and giving Beth and her mother dietary instructions, which included taking midmorning and midafternoon snacks. She also showed Beth's mother how to give Beth her insulin shots each morning and how to collect a urine specimen four times a day. Beth's mother was instructed to call the doctor each afternoon with the reports on the urine analysis. After four weeks, these calls would decrease to twice a week.

Beth went back to school the Monday after she returned home from the hospital. Her mother had talked to her teacher, who readily understood the dangers of stigma. Her teacher thought it would be most inconspicuous if Beth were to eat her midmorning snack at her desk when the 10:30 recess began, after which she could go out on the playground. This seemed to work fairly well, although Beth could not escape explanations to her friends who wanted to know why she had to eat in the morning.

Beth's Family's Reaction. Following the eventful night of Beth's semicomatose admittance to the hospital, her parents went through several stages of adjusting to the news that Beth had diabetes. Beth's father described his feelings as akin to mourning. Although Beth's life was by no means in jeopardy, her father's image of her as a perfect child was suddenly devastated, causing him considerable sorrow and grief. At the same time, Beth's mother and father experienced feelings of guilt. Beth's father admitted he had been troubled at first by the fact that his great aunt had died of diabetes at the age of eighty-two, thinking it may have been hereditary on his side of the family. Beth's mother similarly wondered whether she had let Beth eat too much sugar. Most severe were the feelings of self-blame on the part of both of Beth's parents that such a traumatic and acute event was required to discover Beth's illness.

Beth's siblings also found themselves having to adjust to her newly discovered condition. Her older sister, Susie, threw a tantrum one night several weeks after Beth had returned from the hospital. Susie resented all the attention Beth was getting and accused her parents of spoiling her "little brat sister" by catering to Beth's every wish. Joseph, Beth's seven-year-old brother, was less aware but complained about having to eat meat and vegetables every night instead of his favorite spaghetti, which his mother no longer made.

Summary: Beth. Once Beth adjusts to her new daily routine of insulin shots, snacks, and prescribed diet, her parents and the medical staff are confident that she will probably lead a normal life with few limitations. Although Beth can be considered fortunate in that she can compensate for her chronic illness through daily injections, this is not to underestimate the impact that chronic diabetes will have on her life. She will have to be more responsible about diet, exercise, and her general health than most children.

Joey

Joey is an engaging twelve-year-old boy with muscular dystrophy, an inherited disease characterized by progressive weakness of the muscles that control body movement. We first met with Joey's mother, Doris, in her spacious apartment in one of the older private apartment complexes in northwest Washington, D.C. Later, we met Joey at school with two of his teachers. At the time of our talks, Joey had been wheelchair-bound for a year. For the most part,

Joey's diagnosis and medical care have been provided through the Children's Hospital in Washington, D.C.

Mobility and Self-Maintenance. Joey began to have noticeable mobility problems—stumbling and falling—at age three. The physicians his mother consulted at that time assured her that nothing was wrong. When he started school, his teachers felt he should be evaluated, which ultimately resulted in a diagnosis of muscular dystrophy at age six by Children's Hospital staff.

The extensive testing required to arrive at this diagnosis was financed partly through Doris's private insurance and partly from her wages. Joey was found to have the Duchenne form of muscular dystrophy, which has its onset between ages two and six, begins in the lower trunk, and typically progresses rapidly. In most cases, the child must use a wheelchair by adolescence and cannot raise the arms above the head. Most children with Duchenne's muscular dystrophy die before age twenty-three.

Joey was able to walk, with increasing difficulty, until his eleventh birthday when he was finally forced to use a wheelchair. He also now wears braces on his lower legs. His ability to move about at present is dependent on the presence or absence of architectural barriers, on the availability of transportation with special lifts, and on others' help. For example, he cannot move the chair up the three steps into his apartment building, so his mother or someone with whom arrangements have been made in advance must be present to assist him. The cab driver who transports Joey from his after-school recreational program performs this role two or three days a week, and the school bus driver does so on the remaining days. Joey is able to let himself into the apartment, where he occupies himself with schoolwork or television until his mother returns from her job one or two hours later. At the time of our meeting, Doris was considering asking the owners of her apartment building for permission to install a ramp, which would be paid for by the local Muscular Dystrophy Association. Doris does not focus on Joey's prognosis; she prefers to deal with his situation one day at a time as a way of preserving her ability to cope with the increasingly demanding and frightening future. At the time of our meeting, Joey was losing muscle strength in his arms and could not rise from a prone position without help.

Joey is still capable of feeding himself and can put on his own socks and shirt. He uses a commode chair at home and can usually transfer himself from his wheelchair to the commode chair alone, although this is becoming increasingly difficult as he loses strength in his arms and upper torso. When he is at school, he requires assistance in toileting from staff at the school's health unit. Joey's mother is able to move him from his wheelchair to the bathtub but does not know how his bathing will be managed when he gets bigger. All that is certain at this point is that Joey's ability to care for himself will erode over time and special supports and training will be required if he is to live outside an institution.

Intelligence, Education, and Speech. Since Joey's condition was diagnosed at age six, he has attended a public special education school. Although Joey appears alert and involved with his schoolbooks, he functions at the second- to third-grade level. Joey's speech is intelligible, and he is fully capable of producing complete, correct sentences when prodded to do so by his teachers. However, his speech is exceptionally slow. His teachers report that extreme slowness characterizes all of his actions: writing, completing workbook tasks, moving himself from the physical therapy room to his classroom, and the like. His mother has been told by Joey's physician that marked slowness is often associated with muscular dystrophy.

With the exception of one year, Joey has been promoted through the grades but has made little progress in developing his reading and math skills. His mother is concerned about Joey's lack of progress, and his teachers are frankly baffled concerning Joey's intellectual status. His speech and writing suggest mental ability within the normal range, but this impression is confounded by his extreme slowness. His school records revealed that Joey's intellectual ability had never been evaluated other than through standardized achievement tests. Both teachers had repeatedly requested that Joey be evaluated but had been told that intellectual/psychological tests for Joey were a low priority in relation to tests for other children at this time. There has been no communication between Joey's physicians and the schools concerning the extent of Joey's abilities and what steps should be taken to provide education appropriate to his abilities or limitations. At the time of our visit, no prevocational plans were being developed for Joey despite the concerns of his teachers. Apparently, neither the school nor the health care system had any plans to develop and pool information with which to chart a path for Joey's future.

Family, Friends, and Self. Joey's mother and father have been separated since Joey was four years old. Doris described Joey's father as an irresponsible person, an alcoholic, who does not provide financial or emotional support. She does have a brother and sister in the area but feels they are too busy with their own lives to offer much support or involvement with Joey except in emergencies. By and large, Doris has confronted the problems of Joey's increasing disability alone.

Since Joey's early years, Doris has had to make the transportation, recreation, supervision, and other arrangements common to all single parents. Above and beyond these normal service needs, Doris has had to make arrangements appropriate for a mobility-impaired child. Joey must also see his primary physician in the Muscular Dystrophy Unit at Children's Hospital every six months, and wheelchair, braces, and other devices must be obtained. Many of these services have been provided through the Muscular Dystrophy Association and the Crippled Children's Services program.

The local Muscular Dystrophy Association sponsors a variety of functions and support groups for parents, but Doris is rarely able to attend because she has no transportation. Doris holds a white-collar job paying approximately $10,000 a year; Joey receives $150 per month in Supplemental Security Income (SSI) benefits and is eligible for Medicaid. Doris first learned of the SSI program through the social service specialist in Joey's school. Obtaining SSI benefits is the most negative experience she has had in connection with Joey's disability.

Local Social Security Administration officials by law requested proof of Joey's disability and found him ineligible for reasons she does not understand. The school social service worker and Joey's physician at Children's Hospital intervened on her behalf to get Joey enrolled and were ultimately successful. However, during the week of our meeting, the local Social Service office had requested a meeting with Doris to review Joey's case, and she feared a reduction in benefits. At another point, Joey's mother became personally involved with other parents in petitioning the government of the District of Columbia to retain a summer camp for handicapped children. This effort was eventually successful.

Joey's teachers and his mother all reported that he gets along well with his peers; for example, there is some good-natured teasing of Joey in the school setting because of his characteristic slowness, to which he responds with exaggerated whining as part of the game. When we met him, he was not shy but rather diffident. In general, Joey is not socially aggressive but interacts well when the occasion arises. His mother has given a great deal of attention to ensuring that Joey has opportunities for activities and socializing; he participates in the after-school activities program even though Doris must pay a cab driver to transport him home; he often attends movies with a teenager in the neighborhood whom she pays to accompany him; and he attends the summer camp sponsored by the District of Columbia school system.

Summary: Joey. As Joey's skeletal muscles continue to deteriorate, his mobility and ability for self-care will diminish. He has been fortunate in having access to Children's Hospital for diagnosis, monitoring, and orthopedic treatment. His social needs have been addressed through the public school after-school system and by his mother's efforts to arrange activities for him. His basic support resources have been augmented by the SSI program, including Medicaid, although getting on the rolls proved to be highly complex, confusing, and unpleasant for his mother. As is the case with many victims of this progressively disabling condition, needs for assistance will increase. Joey's mobility assistance and personal care have become more and more problematic, and his independence may hinge on Doris's ability to locate these services on a regular, affordable basis. In addition, Joey's current or future intellectual abilities and performance have not been adequately assessed by the health or educational systems, so appropriate education plans have not been developed.

Service Needs of Disabled Children and Their Families: A Synthesis

The descriptions of Ellen, Beth, and Joey highlight the various needs of each child. Yet, their medical labels tell us very little about what services they need. Joey's diagnosis of muscular dystrophy does not convey the increasing needs he has for special equipment and architectural modifications. Ellen's medical history does not suggest the extensive, time-consuming travel necessary to get her to a specialized medical center for therapy.

Children have their own strengths and weaknesses—for example, each presents the professional "system" with a unique set of needs that must be addressed in different ways. It is not enough to say, for example, that Ellen needs a biofeedback program, Beth needs diabetes management skills, and Joey needs more muscle support. As we have seen, each needs a wide variety of services.

Beth and Ellen need special instruction in how to take care of their health. Beth needed an intensive period of learning about diabetes and its effects, how to give herself shots, and what diet to follow. In addition to health training, some of the children required training in basic self-care. Ellen had to learn how to use her ostomy device and develop bowel control; Joey had to learn new techniques for self-care as his condition worsened.

Joey will need in-home services in the future. He could also benefit from having someone help him bathe and dress at home each day. Because of his continuing growth, bathing Joey and attending to his personal needs will soon become impossible for his mother alone. Ellen's mother would have required extensive support services in her early years had it not been for her family.

Another area of need appearing in all three cases is parent education. Beth's parents needed immediate instruction in the effects of diabetes and how to manage Beth's condition. Thereafter they could have benefited from ongoing counseling during their period of adjustment. Ellen's mother and her family were taught the importance of physical therapy and home techniques as well as how to manage her bladder problems when she was too young to care for herself. Joey's mother has had some assistance in learning how to manage his disability and has created her own solutions for specific problems. More parent education and support is available to her through the Muscular Dystrophy Association, but as a working single parent with no transportation, she has not been able to take much advantage of it.

Future Directions

Each of these children lives in an imperfect world, as we all do. We do not presume to be able to eliminate their problems altogether, for we cannot ever completely abolish sorrow and pain. But we can alleviate them by modifying the public policies and the programs that serve these children.

Our purpose in presenting these snapshots of chronically impaired children has been to derive some general recommendations for restructuring public policies and practices. Doubtless if we had chosen other children, very different specific interventions would have emerged. Nevertheless, several of the most important directions for public policy that emanate from these stories are offered here, and together, they could form a beginning step toward helping Ellen, Beth, and Joey and other children in similar situations.

Our primary conclusion involves a new way of looking at what these children need. This perspective can be characterized in terms of four dimensions, all of which must be considered simultaneously when we think about what we can do to serve these children well: first, the full range of services that might be required to meet the many needs of a disabled child; second, tailoring a service to the unique needs of a child; third, ensuring access to the service in terms of geographical location and transportation; and fourth, assuring timeliness so the child receives the service when it is needed.

The most typical model used to conceptualize the service needs of impaired children is the continuum of care, a conception that was originally applied to the elderly. A continuum of care most often reflects a range of care options corresponding to a range of severity. For children, however, (and one could probably argue the point for elderly persons as well) the continuum of care should not be considered a linear concept that only progresses from the least to most severe. Children with less severe impairments, such as Beth or a mildly retarded child, may have needs as wide-ranging as those of more severely impaired children. Only when all of these dimensions are considered together is it possible to develop an accurate profile of the needs of the target population with whom we are concerned.

We must try to avoid prescribing single services for disabled children. Too many chronically impaired children are given only special educational services or medical rehabilitation when they additionally need respite care for their parents or financial assistance or technological adaptations. All of our proposed changes must therefore recognize the multiple needs posed by any single impairment.

At the same time, we must consider ways to permit services to be tailored to the unique needs of any one child. There is no substitute for individualizing services; it is not enough to provide a predefined service to all children with a common impairment or degree of severity.

From our case studies, we also saw that geographical access to services is still a major problem and deserves attention from public policy makers and planners. Our suggestions for reform must recognize that services are useless unless they are accessible. Finally, we must recognize the importance of providing timely services—timely in the sense of prevention, early treatment, and assuring availability of service when it is needed.

The importance of including all four of these elements in our efforts to serve chronically impaired children can best be seen in relation to the current pattern of service delivery. We now continue to rely largely on labels that result in single services being provided. Discrete categorical services have been developed that, over the years, have taken on lives of their own; whole industries and professions have grown up around them so that we now have such specialties as medical social workers and in-home attendants. Yet these discrete services will not solve the many problems of disabled children; indeed, they seem to stymie our efforts to find a better approach for helping them. Instead of pursuing a single-service strategy and recommending expansion of one or another, we must elevate the policy debate to a broader level that recognizes the full range of needs these children have in the context of the four dimensions just described. The suggestions that follow are intended to reflect this broader perspective.

Create a Network of Trained Caregivers. In addition to the highly trained medical specialists who have done so much for children like Ellen, Beth, and Joey, we need to expand our efforts to train a network of persons who are really the primary caregivers for disabled children, and others, including family members, who are important to those children. These may be respite care workers or other in-home workers. This idea has been espoused in many forms for several years; we offer no new insights but merely repeat the urgency with which it should be pursued.

Previous research has taught us much about the reactions of families to the handicapping condition of a child. The birth of a handicapped child or the onset of a chronic disability is a period of enormous stress for parents and siblings. Parents experience tragedy, anger, guilt, shock, and denial. We know that the socioeconomic status of parents and other factors affect the family's ability to cope with such stressful situations. However, the need for support systems and for help in managing the child is universal for all families, regardless of their social or economic status.

It is usually the child's parents who assume the primary responsibility of caring for their child—whether chronically impaired or not; and it has been the mother who traditionally spends most of her time with the child. We have already hypothesized that parent education might have had a beneficial effect on Ellen, Beth, and Joey.

Foster families make up another prime group that needs training to handle a chronically impaired child. Under the present foster care system, financial negotiations often counsel many families to accept a foster child. If these families were trained to understand better the nature of the child's impairment and were given management skills to help a child develop to full potential within that particular foster family, many families would be in a better position to decide whether or not to accept such a child. If they did accept one, they would also be able to offer that child a successful experience. Efforts to identify parents willing to participate in educational workshops and efforts to organize groups of these parents according to different types of care needed should be a first step in developing a network of trained caregivers.

The goal in training both natural and foster parents is to transfer skills and knowledge from the professional to the parent. Parents are the primary advocates for the child; they need to learn how to gain access to the system in order to obtain needed services. Joey's mother's difficulty in getting SSI benefits points up the need for parent education and advocacy. Most importantly, parents can provide the consistency to follow the child through years of different service agencies and professionals. It is especially important for these children to have long-term advocates who can ensure appropriate treatment when the child is transferred among agencies. Even when the child must reside in an institution, parents or parent surrogates can become advocates on their behalf.

Although families are the primary caregivers for chronically impaired children, other individuals from either formal or informal institutions could also help fill some of the needs of these children. For example, friends of the family or paraprofessionals could be trained to help provide respite or other in-home services. A network of trained persons in the community should be developed so the child receives services in his or her own home or neighborhood and does not have to go outside the community. Many of the services these children need are not highly technical in nature. Such a person in Joey's neighborhood could create devices for Joey to use to reach distant objects in the kitchen or to move himself into the bathtub. Beth's problem is perhaps most susceptible to assistance from a trained outsider. Because her major difficulty is managing her diabetes, she could greatly benefit from a trained community worker who could see Beth and her family at home periodically to ensure that Beth is taking care of herself and to answer any questions. A highly trained physician or even a registered nurse is probably needed only to monitor Beth's condition not to provide ongoing support directly. A well-informed person—perhaps another diabetic teenager in the community—could be extremely useful. A network of trained persons as a resource upon which families of impaired children can call when necessary is a feasible goal that surely deserves more sustained attention.

Encourage Technological Modification of the Environment. In the first section of this chapter, we defined disability as a highly relative judgment that, depending on numerous factors, falls somewhere on the continuum from normalcy to deviancy. Many impairments—indeed, all impairments if we speak theoretically—cease to impair functioning if we merely modify the environment. If a ramp were installed in the entryway to Joey's apartment, the complex arrangements now required to ensure that he can enter his home would not be necessary.

Our scientific and technological capacity in this country can only be described as amazing. The proliferation of space, electronic, nuclear, and medical technology in our country over the past several decades continues to astound even the most sophisticated of lay persons. With all of this amazing capacity, we should be able to devise new technologies that will allow chronically impaired children to have a greater degree of control over their immediate environments. If there be a more humane goal for all our technological splendor, let it be known.

Several problems impede the development, distribution, and marketing of technologies to modify the environment for impaired children. First, a limited market demand requires considerable up-front market capital. The purchasing power of disabled consumers is less than that of nondisabled persons, and many devices must be financed through third-party payers, often causing payment delays and limiting the kinds of equipment that can be purchased. The specialized nature of many products and the need for individual fitting also create difficulties in distribution. Government regulations and lack of venture capital further inhibit the process. Clearly, new strategies to foster public and private sector cooperation are needed to overcome some of the these barriers.

Another problem, far less practical and more philosophical, involves the dilemma of deciding when to modify the child and when to modify the environment. It is not always that easy to determine precise future prospects. In Ellen's case, the heroic efforts to strengthen her hips and to correct her clubfeet were judged—rightly—to be successful in enabling her to walk with the aid of braces.

The danger of choosing automatically to modify the environment—as in a case of use of an electric wheelchair—becomes evident when one considers the vastly different life of a child who can walk as opposed to one who must use a wheelchair. Although we do not want to eliminate real options by wrongly assuming that a child will never perform some function independently, neither do we want to deny that child compensatory aids that open the world to entirely new horizons. This is an individual judgment practitioners have been making for decades. With our increased technological capacities, we can only hope that professionals will be ever more sensitive to the tradeoffs inherent in their decisions.

The challenge for policy makers in the future is to translate technological knowledge into usable and affordable devices for persons with disabilities. Clearly, the public sector cannot do this alone; nor can we expect the private sector by itself to overcome the marketing, development, and distribution problems mentioned earlier. It is in their mutual interest, however, to work together to apply existing knowledge and to develop new technology that will help impaired persons, especially children, overcome their functional limitations. In the best of all worlds, government would supply the incentives and private corporations would initiate bold new ventures directly applied to the disabled. Our challenge is to devise mechanisms that will bring this scenario to reality.

Help Parents Finance Care for Chronically Impaired Children. The financial burden on families with chronically ill children is often tremendous. The skyrocketing costs of health care are sure to leave impoverished all but the very wealthy and the very poor who qualify for government aid. The lowest of low-income families will be eligible for Medicaid and SSI, and in some states, those with slightly higher incomes will be deemed medically needy and therefore eligible for Medicaid. The majority of poor persons, however, are those who may not quite fit these criteria yet who do not have the ability to meet large medical rehabilitation bills. On the other end of the spectrum are those with private insurance or private resources sufficient to meet the costs associated with disability. Even for these families, however, the ongoing costs of maintaining a chronically impaired child and adapting the environment as necessary could be subsidized partially by public funds.

One strategy would be to provide tax credits to families who care for a disabled child in their own homes. Tax credits may serve as an incentive for such care when parents have a choice. Currently, some parents cannot afford to care for a disabled child at home and have no choice but to send the child to a public institution where Medicaid or special education pays for their care. If these parents were offered a tax credit to help pay for the costs of caring for the child at home, they might then be in a position to do so. This would encourage in-home care of children (which, in gross oversimplification, is generally better than institutional care) at the same time as it reduced the public funds required for institutional and foster care. The number of children who could be adequately cared for in their own homes if afforded financial assistance is a research question that merits attention.

Another area for financial assistance is the technological devices that help many of these children overcome barriers in their daily functioning. A voice-controlled wheelchair is a good example of a device whose cost is prohibitive for most families. Yet it might mean the difference between institutional living and independence for some children. In addition to a tax credit for caring for an impaired child at home, there should be a tax credit for purchase of such equipment.

In another context, a tax credit could also help parents who are already caring for an impaired child and depleting their own resources. Parents should be encouraged to keep working. A tax credit perhaps would enable them to pay for some in-home or occasional respite care. Determining eligibility guidelines for a tax credit scheme is another subject for further research. Rather than relying on strict medical criteria, a scheme should be developed whereby a child is determined eligible when the particular environment is considered as well as the child's needs.

Restructuring Existing Services Programs. The current array of categorial services needs to be reexamined and restructured to improve the distribution of existing resources on behalf of impaired children. No new categorial programs are needed, nor it is necessary to specify further eligibility requirements through the definition of new subgroups of children. Instead, we need people who are knowledgeable about these programs to develop new ways of deploying existing resources across current categorical lines so they better meet the needs of children like Ellen, Beth, and Joey.

Under the current array of programs such as Vocational Rehabilitation, Medicaid, Title XX, foster care, and SSI, chronically impaired children are often only an implicit concern; for example, their benefits originated as an outgrowth of benefits for adults. Only in Public Law 94–142, the Education for All Handicapped Children Act, and amendments to the Elementary and Secondary Education Act have disabled children been an explicit concern for federal policy. In other programs, states may decide what benefits they will provide to which clients, creating a highly variable situation in which some children may be lucky while others go unserved or underserved. The magnitude of the problems caused by impaired children—both in human and economic terms—suggests that they should receive national recognition and explicit attention in each of our existing human services programs.

The task here is to create better distribution patterns and more creative use of existing resources. The lack of physical and occupational therapy in rural areas and the lack of community alternatives in major metropolitan areas point to the need to reexamine how current services are distributed. One program, special education, will serve as an illustration.

Public Law 94–142 was passed in 1975 to ensure that needed services are made available to every handicapped child in the country through the local school district—no matter where the child happens to live. Unfortunately, the intent of Public Law 94–142 still has not been fully realized. Several problems have impeded full implementation, the most notable of which is lack of funds. Federal funding has remained well below the level needed to assure adequate services in all local school districts. Hence, many small towns that have only a handful of handicapped children cannot afford to have a full-time physical and occupational therapist. Yet, one of the reasons school districts find themselves unable to provide sufficient services is that, rather than use other human services funding sources, they continue to assume total financial responsibility themselves. There is evidence that other agencies have taken advantage of special education's mandate to solve their own budget problems and to let special education be held accountable for all cost of care to handicapped children. A more appropriate division of financial responsibilities for special education and other service systems is sorely needed. Some states have begun to do this, although the obstacles are formidable.

Assuring availability of services in rural areas is a difficult endeavor even when other human services programs share in the financing. Much has been written about alternative special education delivery systems in rural areas, and many school districts have successfully formed collectives or consortiums or made other arrangements that pool either resources or children so services can be rendered in a cost-effective manner. As more successful experiences become known, and as parents come to learn of their rights to receive appropriate services for their chronically impaired children, other rural districts may be able to provide similar additional services.

In the current attempts to place human services funds into block grants, the mandate of Public Law 94–142 comes into jeopardy. We must continue to fight for a federal legislative guarantee that all handicapped children will receive a free, appropriate public education in the setting most conducive to their optimal growth. At the same time, we must forge linkages of services, fill gaps in services, eliminate duplications, and establish shared funding arrangements. A single agency must maintain consistent accountability over time for any given child so he or she is not bounced back and forth among agencies.

An example of how to redeploy existing resources on behalf of chronically impaired children involves the financing of in-home attendants and service workers. Under Medicaid personal care services, Title XX in-home services, AFDC special needs allowances, and SSI attendant services, adult and elderly disabled persons are provided this care. These same programs could just as easily be used to finance attendants and in-home supports for children.

Effective delivery of services to impaired children is perhaps the most critical element with which policy makers should be concerned. Yet, effective delivery can only be assured if the basic structure and organization of various service programs allow for it. It is essential that we break the current pattern of categorical labels and discrete services and look to the more comprehensive and individual needs of chronically impaired children.

If we are to alter the futures of the next generation of Ellens, Beths, and Joeys, we must test various means of restructuring programs, training parents and paraprofessionals, and devising financial incentives for expanded application of technology. Model projects could be established in several communities to package mutliple programs in such a way as to facilitate comprehensive care tailored to the unique needs of any one child. Such an endeavor would serve two purposes.

First, it would show the efficacy of combining the current multitude of programs serving these children. Second, it would test the effectiveness of new programs such as those for which ideas were put forth earlier: creation of a network of trained persons in the community and institution of a system of tax credits for parents caring for disabled children. Outpatient services would be linked to inpatient services, and financing mechanisms would accommodate outpatient services, many of which are not now covered. Links with the private sector are another essential component. Longitudinal data on these children would be collected so the outcomes of comprehensive care could be measured.

We do not attempt to spell out the elements of this effort beyond our suggestions in the preceding pages; yet it is clear that steps must be taken to experiment with various program models. Detailed planning necessary for implementation remains to be done.

Conclusion

Portraits of three disabled children have reinforced many of our pre-existing biases and evoked several new concerns. We have seen the full complexity of the wide-ranging needs these children have. The inadequacy of viewing impairment through a medical label became acutely evident in discussions with Ellen, Beth, and Joey. At the same time, the importance of looking at an impaired child as a composite of myriad strengths and weaknesses became ever more clear. In our own minds, Ellen, Beth, and Joey are not disabled; they are children with amazing capacities and tremendous emotional warmth, struggling to adapt to an environment that is not always friendly.

In these times of austere federal and state budget cuts, we cannot afford to use limited funds unwisely. The urgency with which we must maximize public dollars so that disabled children have as fair a start in life as possible cannot be overestimated. It is past time to consider new theories about how better to serve these children; we must act now or resign ourselves to another generation of lost children who have been born with or acquired chronic impairments. We have all seen too many children who cannot get the services they need where they need them. Also, we have seen too many children who have not been given the necessary alternatives to allow them to live in the community. Each of us can no doubt add to this list with our own examples of children who are getting less than they deserve.

References

Brewer, G. D., and Kakalik, J. S. *Handicapped Children: Strategies for Improving Services.* New York: McGraw-Hill, 1979.

Select Panel for the Promotion of Child Health. *Better Health for Our Children: A National Strategy.* Vol. 3: *A Statistical Profile.* Department of Health and Human Services Publication no. 79-55071. Washington, D.C.: U.S. Government Printing Office, 1981.

U.S. Bureau of the Census. "1976 Survey of Institutionalized Persons." *Current Population Reports,* Series P-23. Number 69. Washington, D.C.: U.S. Government Printing Office, 1978.

U.S. Department of Health and Human Services. Unpublished data from the Social Security Administration, 1980.

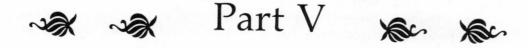

Part V

Educational and Vocational Issues

In recent years, schools have greatly expanded their programs for children with special health and educational needs, yet educational policies and programs require further improvement to deal with the particular problems of children with severe chronic illnesses. The chapters in Part Five present issues and prospects for the education of chronically ill children.

In the first chapter in this part, Deborah Klein Walker and Francine H. Jacobs present a historical perspective of the American education system relating to chronically ill children and summarize advances in this system and legislation currently in effect. Describing a range of available educational options and placement patterns for students with individual chronic conditions, Walker and Jacobs delineate the academic, social, and management difficulties confronted by chronically ill students and by the schools that serve them. School policies and programs of particular importance to children with special health needs are analyzed, including educational placement, provision of medical and related services, school nurse programs, school-based training about chronic illnesses, and physician-school relationships. The authors provide recommendations for educational service delivery, future policy, and research.

Susie M. Baird and Samuel C. Ashcroft, in Chapter Thirty-one, detail sections of the Education for All Handicapped Children's Act of 1975 (Public Law 94–142) as they relate to chronically ill children. The authors raise several major policy questions: Should chronically ill children as a group be considered "handicapped" for educational purposes? Should the guarantees and protections of Public Law 94–142 be extended to children not in need of special education? What should the policy of the school system be with regard to coordinating internal factions? What should the policy of the school system be with respect to collaborating with other community agencies and professionals? The needs of chronically ill children are discussed, and issues, problems, and options for meeting these needs are presented. Baird and Ashcroft also highlight innovative practices across the country and offer recommendations addressing policy issues.

Chapter Thirty-two, by Judith S. Mearig, highlights policy issues in education and assessment of the cognitive abilities of chronically ill children. It then examines the dynamics of particular chronic illnesses—including most of the "marker" illnesses of the Vanderbilt study—and presents an optimistic outlook for improvement in cognitive development for these children when proper education is provided for children, families, and society. Mearig describes psychological dynamics affecting cognitive development that are common to serious chronic illnesses, emphasizing that environmental intervention can make significant differences. In conclusion, Mearig explains how public policy committed to cognitive development and school learning of chronically ill children will benefit the child, the family, and national economic interests.

Phyllis R. Magrab, in Chapter Thirty-three, emphasizes a developmental perspective in documenting needs and providing programs of quality care for chronically ill children and their families. Magrab asserts that age and development should be the basis for linkages among health, education, and social services systems at the community level. She states that during children's school-age years, the changing needs of children and families are especially significant and points out the enormous need for public policy that will enlarge the roles of comprehensive programs designed to provide continuity of care during those years.

The last chapter in Part Five provides a categorical review of existing programs and institutions that offer or have the potential to offer employment-related services to chronically ill children and youth. Paul Hippolitus, the author of Chapter Thirty-four, notes the limitations in these programs and institutions as well as specific problem areas for the chronically ill. He discusses distinct elements in the employment process, including basic preparation, skills training, employment policies, job placement, and financial reward, and he defines their relationship, including barriers, to the pursuit of a work-life for these young people. In conclusion, Hippolitus presents four broad policy initiatives that address the issues and problems outlined in the chapter.

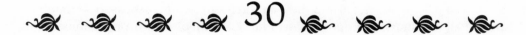

30

Public School Programs for Chronically Ill Children

Deborah Klein Walker, Ed.D.
Francine H. Jacobs, Ed.D.

Attention to the educational needs of chronically ill children is a relatively recent development in American education, beginning in a limited fashion at the turn of the century. Prior to that time, high mortality rates, societal attitudes toward the chronically ill or delicate child, and the view of public schooling as a privilege rather than a right, kept all but the mildly impaired out of the public system. Reversals in these trends—advances in medical sciences that have improved survival rates for some conditions, increasing public acceptance of people who are different and disabled, and legislation establishing education as an entitlement for all children—have allowed for the entrance of many chronically ill children into mainstream education.

School systems currently enroll children with many varieties and degrees of chronic health impairment, and their presence in some cases has forced schools

Note: The research reported in this chapter was supported by funds provided by the Charles Stewart Mott Foundation, the Cleveland Foundation, and the Maternal and Child Health and Crippled Children's Services Research Grants Program, Bureau of Community Health Services, Department of Health and Human Services (#MC-R-250437). The authors would like to thank the parents and staff members of the following local and state voluntary agencies who were interviewed: Muscular Dystrophy Association; Heart Association of Greater Boston; Massachusetts Cystic Fibrosis Foundation; Leukemia Society of America—Greater Boston Chapter; National Kidney Foundation of Massachusetts; American Diabetes Association—Massachusetts Affiliate; Juvenile Diabetes Foundation—Greater Boston Chapter; American Lung Association of Boston; Prescription Parents, Inc.; and Massachusetts Spina Bifida Association.

into previously uncharted territories. Services once thought to be clearly outside the responsibility of the public schools are now legally mandated: administering medications; providing physical, occupational, speech, and language therapy; transporting children to school buildings; revising classroom protocols and curricula to suit an individual child's physical capacity. The assignment during the school day of tasks related to these children can require delicate negotiations among administrative, support, classroom, and school health professionals. In addition, school personnel must now engage in frequent and close communication and collaboration with community medical providers; and issues of differential status and power between educators and physicians that have made this relationship difficult in the past complicate this critical component to educational planning for the chronically ill student.

This chapter traces historical and philosophical determinants to current school programming for chronically ill children. It describes the range of available educational options and placement patterns for students with chronic conditions at several grade levels. The more commonly experienced problems arising from these conditions are detailed; these include difficulties the child faces in academic, social, and management areas, as well as those the school confronts in its attempt to plan and program effectively. Finally, recommendations that focus on the most efficient means of delivering educational services are presented along with suggestions for future policies and research studies.

Historical View

Historical accounts of chronically ill children receiving public education are scant through the early twentieth century, suggesting that previously these children were not identified as requiring special attention. That is not surprising, given that the American educational system of the eighteenth and nineteenth centuries was, in general, fundamentally uninterested in and unresponsive to any needs outside the mainstream. The schools of that time reflected national prejudices toward members of any minority groups (blacks, Chinese, "foreigners," handicapped, and the like) and either excluded them as a matter of routine or included them begrudgingly and without providing special assistance or instruction.

For handicapped children in particular, public authorities moved from total exclusion in the eighteenth century to the development of residential institutions for some few children with certain disabilities in the 1800s. Special schools for the deaf, deaf and dumb, and blind were the first to appear (Fiske, 1976; LaVor, 1976); toward the 1850s, facilities for the "idiotic and feebleminded" were constructed (Ballasalle, 1976). Because neither federal nor state governments required communities to offer education to these children, institutions sprang up in response to locally voiced interest. Concern for these children and their academic progress was a far less salient factor in the great proliferation of institutions during that century than a commonly held belief that these unsightly, abnormal people should be kept from public view (Gearheart and Weishahn, 1976; Gliedman and Roth, 1980).

Such institutions were not established for chronically ill children, probably for several reasons. To begin, few children with the conditions under discussion survived to school age. Children with illnesses such as cystic fibrosis, spina bifida, congenital heart disease, and sickle cell anemia died virtually at onset, which was at birth or soon afterward (see Gortmaker's discussion in Chapter Seven). For children with conditions developed in later childhood (for example, kidney disease, leukemia, diabetes) the primitive state of medical treatments gave them little functional time between onset and death; they would have been unlikely to be able to continue schooling after diagnosis even if school officials had encouraged it. Finally, even conditions with better long-term prognoses were far more disabling day-to-day (Gearheart and Weishahn, 1976). For example, a child with hemophilia who could not be treated with concentrated blood products would be put to bed for weeks after bleeds (Jones, 1974). A child with asthma endured full seasons alternating between suffering and recuperating from attacks. No doubt many children chose not to attend public schools, either remaining illiterate or being privately tutored when possible.

The lack of therapeutic treatments conspired with poverty to keep the numbers of chronically ill children seeking public education relatively small. However, the organization of school life and prevailing pedagogical philosophy also are implicated. Although we have no early firsthand accounts of the experience of chronically ill children enrolled in regular classes, it is known that responsiveness to individual student needs in scheduling, class attendance, and required attentiveness was not a goal of the system during that period. It is likely that these children performed poorly in academic subjects, failed at school, or were encouraged to leave largely because of frequent absences and the inability to participate fully in regular class activities. Architectural barriers and transportation difficulties also contributed and were not mediated by the schools. Communities did not plan for these children or anticipate their needs in any way.

By the turn of the century, forces outside the control of local school boards required them to become more responsive to wider varieties of students. Compulsory school attendance laws, passed primarily to help communities socialize the waves of new immigrants arriving in this country, were applied to children with disabilities as well. Although school authorities still retained the right to exclude from the system those who appeared not to benefit from public instruction (without having to define the basis upon which that determination could be made) (Weintraub and others, 1976), the wholesale exclusion of identifiable groups was no longer supported broadly.

Although there arose some commitment on the part of the school to educate disabled children, there continued to be little interest in having them in regular classes. Special classes and nonresidential special schools developed as a middle ground between institutions (which still enrolled the blind, deaf, and severly retarded) and regular school placements (Gearheart and Weishahn, 1976; Rhodes and Sagor, 1976). The quality of instruction and resources in these classes were often meager by comparison with normal classes; they were the dumping ground for children unsuccessful in the regular track, sufficiently different (foreign language speakers), or disabled (visually impaired but not blind, hearing-impaired but not deaf) to require modification of the regular class routine and curriculum (Aiello, 1976; Dunn, 1968).

Health-impaired children entered the special education sector for the first time during these years and contributed more defensible rationales for use of the special class or school (Gearheart and Weishahn, 1976; Love and Walthall, 1977). Tuberculosis and polio epidemics ravaged the school-age population; the threat of contagion, especially in densely populated urban districts, warranted segregated classroom arrangements (Connor and others, 1976). In contrast to the courses of other catastrophic diseases, these children did survive; their cognitive capacities remained intact, although many were affected motorically or in terms of vitality and endurance. The illnesses were so widespread that the necessity to accommodate sufferers or survivors could not be ignored by school systems. Hospital- and sanatorium-based classes, home tutoring, and specially paced curricula in segregated classrooms all became fairly common educational options.

Arising from similar stimuli, laws instituting school health programs were passed in all states during the period from 1880 to 1940. When education became compulsory, school health emerged as a professional activity and an organized service. At the turn of the century, large public health departments in major cities, such as Boston and New York, responded to outbreaks of disease by appointing medical inspectors to make sanitary inspections of school buildings and school children. Schools handled the large numbers of detected health problems— contagious diseases and physical problems—by introducing school nurses, who demonstrated that they could reduce absenteeism due to contagious disease and play a major role in the control of contagious diseases by "daily medical inspection of all children in the classroom, treatment of minor problems, and referral to the physician for confirmation of the diagnosis of major problems, followed by exclusion and home visits to ensure provision of care" (Lynch, 1977, p. 91).

During the first half of the twentieth century, limited physical examinations by physician medical inspectors and screenings by school nurses successfully identified much of the obvious physical pathology of school children. During the late 1920s, a shared philosophy of school health emerged from meetings between the American Medical Association and the National Education Association: the role of the school was to inform parents of a detected defect and advise the parents to take their child to a physician (it was assumed most children had one). School health programs were not to include treatment but could include screening, referral, and health education (Lynch, 1977).

The epidemics prevalent at the turn of the century created a groundswell of interest and involvement in serving the special educational needs of children with physical disabilities. Attention focused initially on the child debilitated from tuberculosis, polio, and rheumatic heart disease, although gradually the specially designed facilities, equipment, classroom procedures, and curricula were used for children with other health impairments and orthopedic problems. The number of children with other health impairments also was increasing, not because of epidemics, but on the contrary, because of medical advances that heightened their chances for survival. The introduction of antibiotics, the sophistication of surgical procedures, and improved prenatal care all contributed both to the increased visibility of chronically ill children as a distinct class and to the changing patterns of conditions needing special educational arrangements (Mackie, 1969; Segal, 1971).

Some children who twenty years earlier could not have attended school at all were now enrolled in the regular classroom, needing only only periodic special attention from the school nurse or counselor. Children with diabetes, who by the 1920s could inject the insulin their bodies failed to produce, were among that group; and in the place of polio and tuberculosis victims were children with congenital defects or multiple impairments, such as spina bifida, whose life courses had only recently been elongated to include the school years (Griffiths, 1975). The effects that chronic conditions had on academic potential and school success changed rapidly in the 1950s and 1960s, and it was often difficult for schools to synthesize recent medical information and to arrive at appropriate educational programming for physically handicapped or health-impaired children. Special classes, separate schools, and homebound or hospital instruction remained the major options.

The integration of mildly affected children into mainstream regular education no doubt occurred; however, schools continued to exclude, altogether, certain of the more impaired children if there was no arrangement considered to be suitable for them or if the system simply was unwilling to purchase the needed service (Brewer and Kakalik, 1974; Task Force on Children out of School, 1970). In 1953, there remained thirteen states with no classes at all for crippled (physically handicapped) children (Love and Walthall, 1977). A 1964 study of educational opportunities for homebound physically impaired children in North Carolina found only 20 percent receiving any instruction, and the majority of those were being schooled at private expense (Arwood, 1964). Local prerogative continued to dictate the quality, extent, and form of education for the chronically ill child.

Special Education Legislation

The inequities in the educational system experienced by the chronically ill were mirrored in the school experiences of many other handicapped children. Yet, because their rights to an appropriate education had not been established by law, dissatisfied parents had little formal recourse. During the 1960s, existing state codes generally left decision-making responsibilities for most placements to the local educational units. States continued to maintain institutions for the severely handicapped and occasionally chose discrete disabilities to fund in local segregated programs. Thus, a full complement of services might be available for children with one type of disability, while those in other subgroups (for example, the multihandicapped or moderately retarded) were ignored (Blatt and Garfunkel, 1971).

Similarly, the federal government had little apparent interest or involvement with these issues, preferring to rely on state mandates and revenues to serve these children (Cohen, Semmes, and Guralnick, 1979). Prior to the 1960s, federal legislation provided only for vocational rehabilitation for young disabled adults and funded a few specific facilities and programs for blind and deaf children (LaVor, 1976). No comprehensive legislation treating all disabilities equitably and adequately existed at either the federal or state level. Parenthetically, federal involvement in school health activities was also minimal during that period (Lynch, 1977).

In time, the inadequacies of the general and special education system became a rallying point for parents of handicapped children, educators, civil rights activists, and the children themselves. At the national level, the civil rights movement of the 1960s, the War on Poverty, and the rash of accompanying legislation brought attention to the conditions of America's disenfranchised (Blanton, 1976). Educational programs for some handicapped children were provided through Title I of the Elementary and Secondary Education Act (ESEA), passed in 1965 to give aid to school systems with large numbers of disadvantaged students. One part of the law (Public Law 89-313) provided federal funds to state agencies to provide education to handicapped children and youth in state operated and supported schools (LaVor, 1976).

Federal involvement in school health activities was also minimal during that time. Amendments to the ESEA made health funds available to schools with a large educationally disadvantaged population. Much of the money was used to pay for food for children and for the salaries of school nurses and physicians. In 1974, the intent of monies under this act was clarified to be first for educational purposes and only second for health purposes. Thus, resources for health services for poor children had to be found from other funds. In 1971, under Title 8 of the ESEA, demonstration projects including medical, dental, nutrition, and mental health services were funded in selected areas with large numbers of low-income families. Eighty percent of the twenty-three projects funded have been continued under the auspices of local agencies.

During the late 1960s and early 1970s, handicapped persons became identified increasingly as a class of individuals with legitimate demands of the human services systems. For example, one of the strongest statements guaranteeing them the rights of other citizens was enacted into law in 1973 in Section 504 of the Vocational Rehabilitation Act. The law was critical for physically disabled and chronically ill children, in requiring that all public buildings, including schools, be made accessible to handicapped persons. Until passage of Section 504, physically disabled and chronically ill children had been grouped together in a few special schools that were physically accessible because most school buildings where regular classes were held were not architecturally designed to permit access to the physically disabled (Van Osdol and Shane, 1974).

During the first half of the 1970s, many states had developed comprehensive special education codes that were mirrored in the Education for All Handicapped Children Act of 1975 (Public Law 94–142) (Weintraub and others, 1976). Three major factors created the social climate for such a radical overhaul of legislative involvement with handicapped children. Perhaps the most important impetus came through the courts; cases proliferated, alleging denial of equal protection under the law (Fourteenth Amendment) regarding educational opportunities for handicapped children Weintraub and others, 1976) and injury to children by misclassifications, labeling, tracking, misdiagnosis, exclusion, and poor placement. The right to a free, publicly supported education for all handicapped children eventually was established through judicial rulings. [1]

The court cases demonstrated the second (and related) impetus to changing special education practices—the coalescence and increasing militancy of parents and advocates on behalf of handicapped children. The differential treatment of children with handicaps, based on local school priorities, caused some families to move from community to community in search of appropriate programs or to shoulder excessive private tuition costs. Organizing other interested citizens, these parents began to exert political pressures on local and state elected officials. In many states, these groups are credited with getting the issues related to special education into the public forum (Budoff, 1975; Weintraub and others, 1976).

Finally, the mid 1960s and early 1970s saw a growing skepticism among some well-respected special educators as to the effectiveness of traditional special education practices, such as the assignment to special classes of children with a variety of disabilities (Dunn, 1968), the acceptance of single-test evaluations (Mercer, 1974; Senna, 1973) and the "eternal" quality these evaluations and placements tended to acquire. From this internal professional fermentation came redefinitions of special education and the concepts of individuation of instruction, prescriptive teaching, and mainstreaming (Jacobs, 1979).

---

[1]Parents sued for damages resulting from their exclusion from the decision-making processes concerning their children's educations and from the absence of any formal appeals or grievance procedures. The landmark exclusion case was the *Pennsylvania Association for Retarded Children* v. *Commonwealth of Pennsylvania* (1971), in which a class-action suit was brought on behalf of thirteen severely retarded children who were receiving no public education. The court instructed Pennsylvania to provide free, appropriate education to all children, regardless of the severity of the disability (Weintraub and others, 1976).

Other precedent-setting cases were heard during the early 1970s. *Mills* v. *Board of Education of the District of Columbia* (1972) was settled in favor of seven school-aged children (and their mothers), who were expelled from school without parental input or appeal. *Diana* v. *State of California* (1970) tackled the misclassification issue. The plaintiffs, nine Spanish-speaking children, had been placed in classes for the mentally retarded on the basis of IQ tests administered in English. When retested in Spanish, their scores were found to be within the normal range of intelligence. The court ordered the Board of Education to develop placement procedures free from culture bias. Almost every state had similar cases, and pressure grew on state legislatures to rectify inequalities by legally binding state statute. See Weintraub and others (1976) for an overview of these laws and cases.

Unmet educational needs of chronically ill children and the potential impact of new legislation on their schooling were not addressed during this reformulation period as thoroughly as were those of other handicapped children. Even as a composite group, the numbers of chronically ill children were small relative to other populations (for example, the mentally retarded or learning disabled); furthermore, there were separate organizations for each discrete condition so that members became organized around narrowly defined issues rather than identifying elements common to other health impairments and advocating as a larger group. Additionally, parents of chronically ill children whose conditions did not usually produce severe cognitive, orthopedic, or communication difficulties (the traditionally considered "education" problems) were not clear about the extent to which special education legislation should relate to their children. For example, did a child with diabetes or asthma need the protection of special education legislation to receive appropriate schooling? Questions of eligibility and necessity confused both representatives of health-impaired children and educational policy makers.

Central Requirements in Current State Mandates

The new state special education codes support, both implicitly and explicitly, the movement toward deinstitutionalization, mainstreaming, consistent parental involvement, and equal access to education for handicapped children. They commit local school districts to a system of identification, evaluation, and placement for all children within a specified age range, minimally six through seventeen years of age. Typically, schools must conduct yearly census counts and document their efforts to find children with potential educational handicaps. They must perform multifaceted evaluations based on standard test results, teacher observation, parent report, and expert testimony. Most states hold that no single diagnostic tool may be used to determine placement. Children found to need services must have individual plans written for them with corresponding placements. Reevaluations must occur at regular intervals. Every state code requires varying degrees of parental involvement, but at a minimum, parents must be notified of all school actions taken concerning their children and of their rights to appeal any school decisions. The State Educational Agency is named as the titular coordinator of services.

Federal Special Education Legislation: Public Law 94-142

A parallel movement at the federal level to ensure educational opportunites for handicapped children culminated in the passage of the Education for All Handicapped Children Act (Public Law 94-142) of 1975. The findings of Congress that "one million [of the eight million handicapped children] are excluded entirely from the public school system, and more than half do not receive appropriate educational services which would enable them to have full equality of opportunity" (Section 601) provided the ratonale for Public Law 94-142 requiring that states provide a full complement of diagnostic, evaluative, and remedial programming for each identified child. Within ten years, from 1965 to 1975, education for the handicapped had changed from a voluntary, exploratory endeavor to an issue of basic civil rights that Congress could not ignore (Fiske, 1976; LaVor, 1976).

P.L. 94-142 is, to a great extent, a composite of model state special education codes, and it incorporates, at a minimum, the components of state codes mentioned earlier. The act became effective in October 1978 for children ages six through seventeen and for children ages three through twenty-one in 1980 and provided that the existing state codes extend services to children of these ages (for example, where there are mandated kindergartens). States must submit plans detailing how the goal of full educational opportunity is being sought for each child. Public Law 94-142 goes further than many state statutes in due process requirements protecting the rights of handicapped children and their families.

Other salient aspects of the law are:

- *Eligibility*—The law encompasses a wide spectrum of children with handicaps, including those who are "mentally retarded, hard of hearing, deaf, speech impaired, visually handicapped, seriously emotionally disturbed, orthopedically impaired, or other health impaired children, or children with specific learning disabilities, who, by reason thereof, require special education and related services" (Federal Register 42 (163)). States are to limit their requests for reimbursements from federal government special education funds. Up to 12 percent of their population aged six through seventeen can be identified for this purpose as handicapped.
- *Priorities for services*—States are to serve handicapped children currently *not* receiving any education first and the children within each disability category having the most severe handicap and receiving inadequate education second.
- *Rules for placement*—Children with disabilities must be educated in the least restrictive environment possible: that is, with their nonhandicapped peers to the maximum extent possible. Placement into special classes, schools, or residential programs may be made only when the nature and severity of the handicap precludes integration into a regular class or school setting (Jacobs and Walker, 1978).
- *Related services*—Other services defined by the evaluation team as necessary may be included in the individual educational program and must be provided by the responsible educational agency. These services include "transportation and such developmental, corrective and other supportive services as are required to assist a handicapped child to benefit from special education . . . speech pathology and audiology, psychological services, physical and occupational therapy, recreation, early identification and assessment of disabilities in children, counseling services, and medical services, for diagnostic and evaluation purposes . . . school health services, social work services in schools and parent counseling training" (Section 602).

Local and state agencies must engage in vigorous efforts at finding children in their areas who are not receiving the appropriate services. Child identification activities are to be described in detail in state plans.

Chronically Ill Children in Relation to Special Education Laws

In general, parents promptly inform school health and/or administrative staff about their children's chronic illness, either when the child first enters school or at the point when a condition appears (Guyer and Walker, 1980). These are important data for schools to have, even if the condition is mild or well-controlled by medication, for at a minimum, schools need to develop and disseminate to classroom and support teachers emergency procedures to handle the unlikely acute episode or unforeseen illness-related situation. Apart from these precautions, the mildly affected child receives the regular complement of school services.

Chronically ill and physically handicapped children also are eligible for special education: Public Law 94–142 clearly includes them as potential beneficiaries. Federal regulations (45 C.F.R. sec. 121a.5) defining the eligible group of "other health-impaired" offer examples of the range of conditions to be considered in this category: "chronic or acute health problems such as a heart condition, tuberculosis, rheumatic fever, nephritis, asthma, sickle cell anemia, hemophilia, epilepsy, lead poisoning, leukemia or diabetes, *which adversely affects a child's educational performance.*" Children so designated may receive the full range of evaluation and educational services, including [specially designed] classroom instruction, instruction in physical education, home instruction, and instruction in hospitals and institutions," as well as the necessary related services (45 C.F.R. sec. 121a.14).

However, as with other disabilities covered by federal and state laws, there is a functioning (or severity) condition applied to the eligibility; this "adverse effect test" means that the handicap has to be serious enough to impede successful progress in a regular education program (Comptroller General, 1981a, 1981b). A slight limp, a transient behavior problem, or myopia corrected by glasses would not qualify. The application of this measure of functional impairment is appropriate and necessary for chronically ill children. The child who wheezes on rare occasion does not need to involve the schools in the costly, time-consuming special education process; that child should be identified by the school health department but served in the regular education sector. But then what should happen with the child with more severe asthma who at times needs medication and a modified physical education program but otherwise operates well in regularly scheduled classes? Do those difficulties related to asthma constitute a functional impairment that hampers schooling? And do the services that child needs belong within special education?

The legislation gives little guidance to schools on how to determine functional impairment. Because the condition is thought of as a medical problem, many states require physician input, not only to describe the illness to the evaluation team but also to assess the extent to which the condition interferes with learning.

With certain conditions or physical disabilities, the physician can be quite sure that special educational arrangements will be needed. For many others, however, the recommendation needs to be related to that particular school's organization, available support personnel, and physical plant. A physician's assessment of educational concomitants of an illness is probably less valid in this situation than that of a variety of school professionals who are well acquainted with educational programming, scheduling, and curricula. Yet the requirement that an outside authority—the physician—be involved sets up the potential for conflict between the two groups and highlights the medical aspects of a child's condition. [2]

The legislation does not detail which complement of school services is considered regular education with some support and which is considered special education. Most special education students have clear cognitive or learning deficits that cannot be accommodated by the regular curriculum; children with retardation and serious visual or auditory impairments are among them. Cognitive limitations such as retardation should not be presumed for chronically ill children or physically handicapped children. Necessary modifications to curriculum, scheduling, or classroom procedures are often idiosyncratic, episodic, and limited to a few discrete activities.

If a child with diabetes needs to have a gym class at a different time of day from classmates, should scheduling be a concern of special education? or can it be arranged within the general education framework? Is a child whose leukemia has been in remission for more than a year a special education student because it is still necessary to see a school social worker regularly for supportive counseling? When a child with asthma needs daily medication administered in school, is that a school health or a special education function? These questions are not answered in special education legislation; in fact, what might once have been dictated by common sense now must be negotiated within school departments, largely because of the "related services" statutes in Public Law 94-142 and state codes.

[2] There has been increasing attention to the relationship between physicians and educators, especially regarding the education of children with disabilities. For many reasons, medicine historically has enjoyed the highest status among human service professions; this position has allowed physicians to be viewed as experts even in areas where their training, objectively considered, is inadequate. Nonetheless, in the past, physicians played a major role in evaluating disabled children for school placements; school personnel were, at the same time, reverential and resentful. They needed health information but they felt better trained to evaluate and plan educational programs. The special education laws have attempted to correct this situation by assigning primary responsibility for special education to the school district, without legislating physician involvement in most cases; in many state codes, however, physicians are still considered the experts regarding the chronically ill. In general, physicians are disgruntled about their lack of legislative involvement in these laws. On the other hand, because some educators find medical diagnoses largely irrelevant to educational prescriptions (Connor and others, 1976; Crossland, DeFriese, and Durfee, 1981) and physicians' understanding of school programming inadequate, even this requirement to involve physicians appears unsatisfactory (Jacobs, 1979). Neither group is altogether satisfied by the roles the legislation assigns to the other or itself (Low, 1979; Palfrey, Mervis, and Butler, 1978).

These laws have a related services component that allows auxiliary services such as school social work, physical therapy, speech therapy, transportation, and school health services to be required if a special education student needs them to fulfill academic potential. Many special-needs children require these services *in addition* to program modifications. Suppose, however, that a child needs only related services, as is the case with some chronically ill children and with, for example, many speech-impaired children who need only regular speech and language therapy (Comptroller General, 1981a, 1981b). Should these children be counted in the special education population? Rationales to include them under the special education rubric have been that their needs, however transient or focused, will be better served and that the inclusion ensures that serious attention will be paid to their individual progress. Although most schools are prepared to deal with administration of medications and emergency procedures through school health services, they are not mandated to do so by federal statute. Schools can refuse to give the medicines and require parents to come to school or make other arrangements. Special education legislation *does* protect against such a situation, and perhaps, all chronically ill children needing related services should be covered in order to address the lowest common denominator of schools.

Further, the requirement to convene an evaluation team and to develop educational plans provides in-service training opportunities for teachers and staff. Although children with leukemia may need only social services, it is beneficial for their teachers and counselors to think comprehensively about their experiences in school, perhaps integrating discussion into the classes in which they are enrolled. The required engagement of school personnel constitutes consciousness-raising, which may best be accomplished through this legislation.

On the other hand, schools offer many related services regardless of requirements, and these services are, in fact, seen as the special province of departments outside of special education: for example, pupil personnel services (including career and personal counseling) and school health (Foster and others, 1977; Wold, 1981). To require enactment of the whole special education process in order to secure services that would have been forthcoming anyway appears to many a waste of public dollars and precious school time.

The related services component has engendered strong feelings from many quarters; opposition to its inclusion centers around its open-ended provisions, which are at public expense. Few taxpayers would deny that some physically impaired or chronically ill children need the whole range of related services including transportation, supportive therapies, and counseling. However, it can be argued that schoolwork of virtually all chronically ill children could profit from their receiving personal counseling related to their disabilities. Some parents of able-bodied children have reacted angrily to the defunding of intramural sports, elementary school art and music programs, and extracurricular activities in order to support special education programming. Growing constituent backlash appears organized primarily around expenditures for related services, which are viewed as luxuries.

The inability to arrive at consensus on who should be receiving related services has fueled a growing movement to deregulate this component at the federal level (Office of Special Education, 1981). A recent in-depth study of the implementation of Public Law 94-142 in nine states (Education Turnkey Systems, 1981) found extreme variations in the way states defined and delivered related services; the major determinant of the levels of related services in Individual Education Plans (IEPs) was the level of state funds appropriated for special education. Thus, it was concluded that it is unrealistic to expect uniform provision of related services, and that a federally directed attempt to standardize practice in this area could increase opposition, not only to providing related services but also to funding other aspects of special education.

Potential Problems for Chronically Ill Children in Schools

Chronic illnesses and physical disabilities can cause special problems during the school day; they can also heighten the concerns and difficulties that virtually all children experience in the academic and social spheres. This section attempts to generalize about major categories of problems across conditions, levels of severity, and ages; it should not be taken as predictive for an individual child or particular condition.

Scholastic Achievement. Children with chronic illnesses or physical impairments as a group are expected to be of normal intelligence. This rule does not hold for children whose impairments have central nervous system involvement; for them, the likelihood of retardation is higher than for the healthy population. Of the eleven marker conditions under discussion here, only spina bifida is clearly associated with retardation, and 20 to 50 percent of children with spina bifida have limited intellectual abilities (Hunt and Holmes, 1975; Lauder and others, 1979; Pless and Pinkerton, 1975). Children with muscular dystrophy score consistently lower on intelligence tests, although it is undetermined whether these scores represent true organically based retardation or secondary pseudoretardation resulting from maladaption to the illness (Pless and Pinkerton, 1975).

Although retardation is not a prevalent problem among chronically ill children, population-based data from the English study on the Isle of Wight (Rutter, Tizard, and Whitmore, 1970) evidenced significant differences in achievement between chronically ill and healthy groups of children with normal intelligence. Underachievement and poor scholastic performance are thought to be major concomitants of chronic illness and, according to Pless *(Care of Children with Chronic Illnesses,* 1975), are correlated with social class, parents' education, and family size. In a Pennsylvania study, an estimated 33 percent of chronically ill children with low socioeconomic status were underachieving compared with only 12 percent of those in the higher socioeconomic group (Sultz and others, 1972).

Some chronically ill children are more likely than children with other disabilities or nonhandicapped peers to experience academic difficulties resulting from interrupted school attendance. Asthma, hemophilia, cystic fibrosis, nephrosis, leukemia, and sickle cell anemia have all been associated with excessive absences (Parcel and others, 1979; Weitzman and others, 1982). Asthma is among the major causes of school days lost and accounts for one quarter of the absences reported for all chronically ill students (Green and Haggerty, 1975).

Difficulties with school work arise from prolonged, lengthy absences and from frequent but brief and episodic absences. Both are disruptive to learning content material and to sustaining peer relationships that make school attendance appealing. In most states, children absent for more than two weeks receive homebound or hospital instruction under the egis of the special education department. This required waiting time does not help the child with frequent intermittent absences to keep current on academics, and for this child, the potential to develop school phobia appears greater (Drotar, 1978; Pless and Pinkerton, 1975).

Achievement-related effects of absences often extend from the period prior to a planned absence (for treatment, surgery, or diagnostic testing) through some amount of time after the child returns to school. The anticipation of missing schoolwork and therefore falling behind can cause anxieties making it difficult to concentrate while still in school. Painful or exhausting episodes of illness or treatments can leave the child fatigued, unhappy, or distracted. Finally, additional pressures related to making up missed work can have a downward spiraling effect on the child's condition; children with conditions such as asthma or diabetes, for example, can have more difficulty managing their diseases when under stress (Foster and others, 1977; Griffiths, 1975). Children can despair of ever being able to catch up to classmates and compete academically (Green and Haggerty, 1975).

Some children with chronic illnesses exhibit limited endurance or ability to concentrate due to the disease itself or to medications taken for its control. These children should receive an education designed with these effects in mind, and it is likely that children with more permanent, obvious limitations are served under special education codes. Other children, however, experience temporary or gradual reduction in energy or mental alertness, which may not be known to or acknowledged by the children, their families, or their teachers. Their constitutional inability to participate in classroom instruction can be misinterpreted as transient, willful behavior and therefore not treated with the consideration it merits.

For all children, psychological well-being promotes the learning process, and well adjusted children with high self-esteem and expectations of success perform better in school than equally intelligent children with fewer positive psychological indicators. Until the 1960s, some researchers suggested that, because chronically ill children were at greater risk for emotional difficulties than healthy children, they were more likely to experience school failure as a result of psychosocial maladjustment (Pilling, 1973). More recent research challenges this basic hypothesis, indicating that the range of psychopathology in many children with chronic illness approximates that of healthy children (Gayton and others, 1977; Pilling, 1973; Pless and Pinkerton, 1975). Therefore, it should not be assumed that these children are maladjusted or that underachievement is virtually unavoidable as a result.

On the other hand, chronic illnesses do present psychological impediments to academic success for some children. The expression of these difficulties varies by age, knowledge of condition and prognosis, requirements for special modification, and family factors; clear trends are difficult to establish. Yet it is commonly acknowledged that low self-esteem related to being disabled among able-bodied peers, frustration with limitations on activities or levels of energy, and anxiety over career options and future plans can contribute to a lack of motivation—a "Why bother?" attitude.

Other children develop low expectations for their academic careers based, in part, on the well-intentioned overprotectiveness and oversolicitousness of parents and teachers (Schiefelbein, 1979). Parents may convince the teacher to excuse children unnecessarily from examinations and homework; teachers may inappropriately relax grading standards or discipline (Stearns, 1981; Lansky and others, 1975). These behaviors can diminish such children's concepts of themselves as competent, independent persons and can convey the message that they cannot succeed in school without preferential treatment (Foster and others, 1977). In fact, given the limitations in endurance or mobility some of these conditions entail, academics should be cultivated for these children as an area ripe for their expression of excellence and competence (Shock, 1976).

Psychological Difficulties in the School Context. Outside the family, the school is the major context in which children develop their sense of self and their understanding of their place in relation to peers. Virtually all children at some point experience difficulties in negotiating this social environment and in establishing friendships that allow for the expression of their personal differences. In the elementary school years, children often strive to conform to the norms set by their small circles of friends; during adolescence, they are conscious also of the larger community and its expectations for their behavior, appearance, and achievement. Issues related to appearing or being different, restrictions on activities, requirements for special tutoring, poorly developed athletic skills, anxieties over sexual matters, and school learning and career planning are concerns that chronically ill children share with many others. Nonetheless, the courses and treatments of certain conditions obviate these problems for chronically ill children in the school environment, and merit attention in this section.

Daily management requirements or scheduling changes often are implicated in the school adjustment problems that chronically ill children experience. Problems arise not only for children who need substantial architectural and programmatic modifications because of physical impairments or limited stamina but also for children whose conditions demand very little attention during the school day. Simply being different by virtue of needing to take medication (for example, for asthma or diabetes), having even minor or transitory restrictions on physical education and sports (for example, cystic fibrosis or hemophilia), or needing to follow dietary regimes (for example, diabetes) can cause major difficulties.

Adolescence is singled out as a particularly trying time; youths are increasingly sensitive to how peers react to their differences, however subtle those differences appear to adults. Peer pressures at school to be "one of the gang" sometimes result in poor control (as in diabetes and asthma) and in otherwise avoidable medical emergencies requiring school absences and hospitalizations.

Although family members often have difficulty adjusting to the chronically ill child who looks different, concern for the child's emotional well-being and acceptance of the fact of the illness help most close relations overcome this reaction. Classmates in school, on the other hand, are often frightened by visible impairments and disinclined to be supportive or compassionate. Healthy children may ignore visibly ill children—not including them in activities and friendships—or may taunt and ridicule them because of their appearance. Short stature related to cystic fibrosis, loss of hair due to chemotherapy for leukemia, and facial deformities involved with cleft palate can elicit hurtful peer reaction, and without intervention from teachers and friends, these children can experience school as a painful process.

Not only the chronically ill child's academic performance can suffer as a result of overprotectiveness or low scholastic expectations of well-meaning teachers but also the child's emotional status can be affected by teachers' attitudes, making school a particularly lonely or unhappy experience (Stearns, 1981). Teachers often lack information on relatively rare conditions and, in some cases, place unnecessary restrictions on a chronically ill child struggling to normalize the school experience. As Schiefelbein (1979, p. 26) notes regarding children with cancer, "Many teachers isolate children in class because of their mistaken notion that cancer is contagious." Because teachers are in good positions to support chronically ill students and to have a positive effect on peer attitudes, lack of information and of opportunity to work out their own feelings about the child's condition is especially unfortunate.

Provision of Services for Chronically Ill Children in Schools

Schools must provide each chronically ill child with an appropriate set of educational and supportive services based on an evaluation of that child's developmental status and perceived academic potential. Because of the wide variation in functioning, individualized evaluations and placement decisions are critical. Nonetheless, some common patterns of service needs and program choices emerge, corresponding to the more common school-related difficulties.

This section provides an overview of the special programming arrangements and modifications most frequently considered for the chronically ill student, keeping in mind that the most normalized or ordinary school program is preferred. Because there are few systematically collected data on these issues, much information reported here derives from practice-oriented literature (medical and educational) and from interviews with key informants (including professionals and parents) particularly knowledgeable about services to children with chronic conditions.

Prevalence of Chronically Ill Children in Schools. The initial step a local educational authority (LEA) must take in planning for chronically ill children is to determine how many children with various illnesses will be in the schools during a given year. For the most part, with the exception of asthma, the chronic illnesses considered here are extremely rare and occur infrequently within a school-age population. Yet the survival of many of these children has increased over the past twenty years so that school systems can expect children with all of these chronic conditions to matriculate in its elementary and secondary schools.

In general, an LEA could use the conservative prevalence estimates developed by Gortmaker (see Chapter Seven), although these estimates may underestimate asthma and leave out the many other chronic conditions for which similar planning is needed. About 2 percent (based on estimates of 21.58 to 24.97 per 1,000 children from birth to twenty years) of a school population might have one of the eleven chronic conditions; one half of these (or 1 percent of the total population) would be children with asthma and the other half would have one of the other ten conditions under consideration. Thus, a large, urban school system with 40,000 children might expect to have 400 children with asthma and 400 children with the other chronic conditions in their schools in any given year.

Even though in aggregate the LEA may enroll considerable numbers of chronically ill children, at the individual school or class level there are few children, and teachers have limited exposure to specific conditions. An elementary school teacher with a classroom enrollment of thirty children will have had three children with asthma and three with other chronic conditions in the classroom during a ten-year period. The typical senior high school subject teacher with five classes of thirty students each will have seen a slightly greater number of chronically ill children (fifteen with asthma and fifteen with other conditions) during the same ten years.

These estimates assume that children with chronic illnesses are mainstreamed to the fullest extent possible into regular classrooms. If, however, these children are placed routinely into special classes or special schools, the estimated number of chronically ill children in the care of regular classroom teachers is reduced.

Educational Placements for Chronically Ill Children. Depending on the determination of individual learning needs, the chronically ill child will be placed in one of the following class and school placements, listed in order from the least restrictive to the most restrictive (Reynolds, 1962):

- Regular school, regular class, home school district
- Regular school, regular class, out of district
- Regular school, regular class, special education resource teacher
- Regular school, part-time special class
- Regular school, full-time special class
- Regular school, regular class, limited program

- Homebound, tutoring, hospital program
- Special day school
- Residential school

Because the chronic conditions considered here are not highly associated with mental retardation (a reason for automatic placement in some special education classes), the main determinant of whether a child would benefit from something other than normal classes is the extent to which the illness impedes learning or daily functioning. Table 1 gives an overview of the levels of functioning and program modifications associated with various levels of severity of chronic conditions. Only children with moderate and severe levels of impairment need to have some special education classroom placements, and even then, some children can be placed successfully in regular education classrooms appropriate for their academic abilities if the necessary related set of services is provided.

Although placement decisions are made on an individual basis, Table 2 presents the expected type of placement for a majority of children with a particular chronic illness (Gearheart and Weishahn, 1976; Griffiths, 1975). Most children with chronic illnesses will benefit by placement in a regular classroom. Children with physical disabilities, such as muscular dystrophy and spina bifida, will likely need some combination of special and regular classes. Finally, all of these children could at some point need homebound or hospital classes.

The numbers of children (by disability category) served in various special education placements in each state and territory are reported annually to Congress by the Office of Special Education. However, these statistics are virtually impossible to interpret because of the lack of consensus regarding the two relevant categories—orthopedically impaired and other health-impaired. In fact, no available study of special education lists the actual conditions included in a particular category's prevalence rate. In actuality, many states aggregate the estimates for the two categories into a physically impaired category and an otherwise health-impaired category (see the appendix to this chapter).

In the 1979–80 school year, the percent of children aged three through twenty-one served under Public Laws 94–142 and 89–313 was 0.16 for the orthopedically impaired category and 0.25 for the other health-impaired category. Less than one quarter of the children with a physical handicap and with a health impairment who are in need of special education services are being served under federal mandates, according to estimates of the Office of Special Education (1980) and past prevalence estimates of the children in need of special education (Kaskowitz, 1977; Mackie, 1969).

During school year 1977–78, 50 percent of the other health-impaired children, ages three through twenty-one, and 37 percent of the orthopedically impaired children were served in regular classes. More than one quarter of both groups of children were in separate classes. The remainder—23 percent of the other health-impaired and 33 percent of the orthopedically impaired children— were in separate school facilities or other educational environments, including homebound and hospital instruction. These aggregate statistics are difficult to

Table 1. Level of Functioning and Program Modifications Associated with Severity of Impairment.

	Level 1 (Mild)	Level 2 (Mild to Moderate)	Level 3 (Moderate)	Level 4 (Severe)
Is the child handicapped?	No	Possibly	Yes	Yes
How does it affect the child's functioning?	Health impairment does not interefere with day-to-day functioning and learning.	Health impairment does not interfere with learning, but there is a possibility of unusual episodes or crises.	Health impairment either presents frequent crises, or else so limits the child's opportunity to participate in activities that it interferes with learning.	Health impairment is so severe that special medical attention is regularly needed. The child's opportunity for activity is so limited that he or she may not be able to participate in a regular classroom.
Must the program be modified?	No	No change in program planning is necessary. Be aware of the potential for unusual occurrences. Report them to the parents or doctor. Know any first-aid procedures that might be required.	Activities will have to be modified to allow a health-impaired child to participate. Staff must know proper first-aid procedures and be prepred to deal with children's questions about crises.	Extensive staff and program alterations are necessary to accept child into program. Home- or hospital-based programs may be more appropriate. Classroom support from medical services will be necessary if child is in classroom.

Source: Healy, McAreavey, von Hippel, and Jones, 1978.

Table 2. Classroom Placements Needed by Children with Various Chronic Conditions.

	Classroom Placements			
Chronic Condition	Regular only	Special only	Both regular and special	Homebound/ hospital
Asthma	XX			X
Diabetes	XX			X
Cystic fibrosis	XX			X
Hemophilia	XX			X
Leukemia	XX			X
Sickle cell anemia	XX			X
Congenital heart disease	XX			X
Kidney problems	XX			X
Cleft palate	XX	X	X	
Muscular dystrophy		X	XX	X
Spina bifida		X	XX	X

XX Most frequent placement
X Possible placement during school career, depending on course of illness or condition

interpret because no attempt is made to classify the type of children in various placements by diagnosis, severity of condition, or services needed. Furthermore, placement patterns vary dramatically by state. For example, Idaho and Pennsylvania serve less than 1 percent of their school-age children with mental retardation in regular classes with support services, while Alabama, Louisiana, and South Dakota serve more than 75 percent. In Delaware, less than 5 percent of physically impaired children are served in regular classes; in contrast, Rhode Island places 97 percent of the same type of children in regular classes (Office of Special Education, 1980). The wide state variation in numbers of children served is due to several variables, including historical practices, financial incentives, regular school personnel's preferences, availability of other health and support services, and noncompliance with the law.

Information about the educational placements of children with specific chronic conditions is very scant. The largest source of information about placement of these children in the United States comes from the Community Child Health Studies conducted in the late 1970s in three communities (Genesee County, Michigan; Berkshire County, Massachusetts; and Cleveland, Ohio) (Gortmaker and others, 1980; Walker, Gortmaker, and Weitzman, 1981). Educational placements of school-age children with various chronic conditions are presented in Table 3, as reported in interviews with parents in random household samples. If the parents responded that their child had a chronic condition from a list of twenty-two conditions read to them, they were asked if the child's condition affected ability to attend school or do any of the things a child of that age usually does. Children whose parents reported that the condition interfered with activities are likely to be the children for whom special educational services

Table 3. Percentage of Children, Ages Six Through Seventeen, with Chronic Conditions Enrolled in Regular or Special Education.

Condition	Michigan (1977)				Massachusetts (1980)			
	Number of Children	Regular	Special	Both	Number of Children	Regular	Special	Both
Asthma	148	93.2	1.4	5.4	21	76.2	0.0	23.8
with functional impairment	37	86.5	2.7	10.8	6	66.7	0.0	33.3
Diabetes	6	66.7	0.0	33.3	1	100.0	0.0	0.0
with functional impairment	0	--	--	--	0	--	--	--
Kidney trouble	68	86.8	7.4	5.9	45	80.0	0.0	20.0
with functional impairment	15	86.7	6.7	6.7	0	--	--	--
Heart trouble	55	80.0	9.1	10.9	18	61.1	5.6	33.4
with functional impairment	8	75.0	25.0	0.0	1	100.0	0.0	0.0
Trouble speaking	70	68.6	14.3	17.1	24	29.2	29.2	41.6
with functional impairment	10	20.0	70.0	10.0	7	14.3	71.4	14.3
Birth defects	15	86.7	13.3	0.0	8	50.0	0.0	50.0
with functional impairment	7	71.4	28.6	0.0	1	100.0	0.0	0.0
Epilepsy	28	71.4	17.9	10.7	6	16.7	50.0	33.3
with functional impairment	10	60.0	40.0	0.0	2	0.0	100.0	0.0
Cerebral palsy	5	40.0	40.0	20.0	4	25.0	75.0	0.0
with functional impairment	3	33.3	66.7	0.0	1	0.0	100.0	0.0
Mental impairment	28	20.8	62.5	16.7	3	0.0	100.0	0.0
with functional impairment	22	13.6	68.2	18.2	3	0.0	100.0	0.0
All children	2,175	94.4	1.9	3.7	601	84.0	2.5	13.4

Source: Community Child Health Studies, Harvard School of Public Health (Parent reports, Genesee County, Michigan, 1977; Berkshire County, Massachusetts, (1980).

might be necessary. Those children with a functional impairment were more likely to be in special classes than were children with the same condition but without functional impairment. The estimates of class placements for the children with a condition and a functional impairment are close to the national prevalence estimates for health-impaired and orthopedically impaired children.

Class and school placements for clinic-based samples of children with cystic fibrosis, spina bifida, cerebral palsy, and multiple handicaps in the Cleveland metropolitan area in 1977 were studied by Case Western Reserve University School of Medicine and Harvard School of Public Health for the Community Child Health Studies. The trend in placements is as one would expect: the majority of children (64 percent) with a health impairment such as cystic fibrosis were in mostly regular classes, either in a school with only regular classes (64 percent) or in a school with both regular and special classes (32.8 percent). Only a small minority (3 percent) were in special classes in an integrated school and none were in a special school. On the other hand, children with a physical impairment such as spina bifida and cerebral palsy tended more often to be in special classes in a regular school setting (41 percent) or in a special school (16 percent); less than half were in regular classes in the regular school (21 percent) or integrated school (22 percent).

Related School Services Needed by the Chronically Ill Child. Daily management issues surface for many chronically ill children. Therefore, schools need to be in close communication with the medical care system—usually the child's primary care physician—about the child's health status. The questions schools frequently ask physicians so they can best plan the educational program for the chronically ill child are as follows (Levine, Clark, and Maroney, 1979; Van Osdol and Shane, 1974):

1. Does this child's present condition require any specific physical restrictions? Can this child participate in physical education classes without restrictions? Can this child participate on any sports teams without restriction? Are there any specific physical activities that are absolutely contraindicated for this child?
2. Is the child presently taking medication? How will the medication affect the child's behavior? Has the medication been increased or decreased recently?
3. Is the child's physical or health problem improving or worsening? What is the prognosis for the child for future planning of education and jobs? Has the condition been permanently stabilized?
4. Is there a need to shorten or modify the child's school day? To what extent should the school provide rest periods for the child? How often should the child rest, and what type of rest period should be provided?
5. Does the child's condition require modifications of diet?
6. Are there special emergency precautions that school personnel should be prepared to meet?
7. Is there a possibility of self-injury, such that the child might need protective equipment, for example, a helmet? Does the child use a wheelchair or other equipment, such as standing tables? Can the child be removed from the wheelchair or braces? If so, how often?
8. Should this child have preferential seating in the classroom?

9. Does this child need physical, occupational, and/or speech therapy?
10. Does the child need assistance with toileting?
11. Does the child's present condition require specific approaches or cautions on the part of school officials? Should the child receive special counseling or guidance at this time?
12. What is the child's understanding of the problem? How has it been explained to the child? Are further explanations or continuing reinforcements necessary?

Depending on the answers, almost every chronically ill child will need extra consideration in school. The range of special services potentially needed include allied health support (such as toileting, physical therapy, and speech and hearing therapy) and psychologically oriented therapies, specially tailored career and vocational counseling, transportation, and modifications in class scheduling and classroom environment. Most of these services traditionally have been provided through the pupil personnel and school health sectors of the school system; others, such as transportation and the adaptation of physical environments, are relative newcomers and are thought of as clearly being special education's responsibilities. In fact, virtually all these extras are mandated as special education in the controversial "related services" statute of Public Law 94–142; nonetheless, they continue to be considered support services to regular education in many local districts.

Chronically ill children use many of these services, yet there are few systematically collected data available to show their provision through these two sectors. Lauder and others (1979) reported that the percentage of children with spina bifida receiving special services were as follows: transportation (84 percent), toileting assistance (79 percent), bus aid (76 percent), accessibility (63 percent) remedial instruction (58 percent), physical therapy (50 percent), counseling (29 percent), and speech and hearing therapy (13 percent). The availability of transportation and toileting assistance was especially important in placement proceedings.

Pyecha (1979) investigated the types of related services delivered to all handicapped children under Public Law 94–142. About 13 percent of handicapped children served in the public school received related services, which did not include speech therapy (Office of Special Education, 1980). About 10 percent received one related service and 3 percent received two or more services. The type and frequency of the related services specified in the IEPs were transportation (5.5 percent), medical services (4.2 percent), counseling (2.2 percent), psychological services (1.2 percent), occupational therapy (1.0 percent), physical therapy (0.9 percent), social work service (0.7 percent), audiology (0.4 percent), and parent counseling and training (0.2 percent). The medical services included those provided by nurses, along with visual examinations and diagnostic evaluations.

In general, related services were more often specified in the plans for handicapped children in special schools than for those in regular schools, and historically, many related services have been offered only at special-school sites. Although segregated arrangements conflict with the P.L. 94–142 goal of education in the least restrictive environment, some school districts continue to place children needing several or highly specialized services in these schools. The number of children receiving related services is less than the number who need them, in large part because the provision of related services is based on what is available rather than on what is needed (Blaschke, 1979).

The following discussion outlines related services (excluding school health services, discussed in the section that follows this) school districts provide for chronically ill children. Table 4 gives an overview of the related services needed at times by children with several conditions.

In general, chronically ill children do not require the allied health therapies; exceptions include the more physically disabled children who may need physical therapy alone (for example, spina bifida) or in combination with occupational or speech therapy (for example, muscular dystrophy, cerebral palsy). Some children with facial disfigurements, including those with cleft palate, also require speech and language therapy. These therapies usually are provided by itinerant therapists who work in several schools during the week, or by resident therapists attached to special schools for physically or multiply handicapped children.

Many chronically ill children do not require placement in special classes or special schools. They may, however, need modifications in their school schedule or physical environment. Many adaptations can be made easily in the regular school setting, thus allowing for full participation with nonhandicapped peers. Some examples include large-print electric typewriters, classes scheduled on the ground floor to avoid stairs, and adjustments made to water fountains and rest rooms so they are accessible for the handicapped.

As noted earlier, acknowledging the psychological aspects of chronic illness and physical disabilities is as important as attending to the physical and medical components. Negotiating typical developmental milestones (entry to school, puberty, and the like) may be more difficult for chronically ill children, and counseling services sensitive to potential problems are often necessary. Counselors must keep abreast of the child's condition and help the child plan course schedules realistically, given the functional impairments (Foster and others, 1977).

Career counseling must reflect an understanding of present and future functioning. For example, a child with cystic fibrosis or a heart condition should not be counseled to enter a vocation that requires heavy lifting and physical exertion. Children whose conditions require frequent monitoring or treatment in tertiary care settings should be encouraged to apply to colleges near medical centers.

Although it is imperative to be realistic with children in career counseling, counselors must be careful not to curtail prematurely the chronically ill child's dreams or hopes by reifying poor prognoses before they occur. This is especially true for children with illnesses such as leukemia, muscular dystrophy, cystic fibrosis, and sickle cell anemia, which are considered terminal diseases. Inform-

Table 4. School-Related Services Needed by Children with Various Chronic Conditions.

Chronic Conditions	Support Therapies*			Schedule Modifications	Modified Physical Education	Transportation	Building Accessibility	Toileting/ Lifting Assistance	Counseling Services		
	S/L	OT	PT						School	Career	Personal
Asthma				X	X				XX		X
Diabetes				X					XX	XX	XX
Cystic fibrosis				X	XX				XX	XX	XX
Hemophilia				X	XX				XX		X
Leukemia				X	X				XX	XX	XX
Sickle cell anemia				X	X				XX	XX	XX
Heart disease				X	X				XX	X	X
Kidney problems				X	X				XX	X	XX
Cleft palate	X								XX	X	X
Muscular dystrophy	X	X	X	X	XX	XX	XX	XX	XX	XX	XX
Spina bifida	X		X	X	XX	XX	X	XX	XX	X	XX

XX Frequently a needed service

X Sometimes a needed service

* S/L = Speech/Language; OT = Occupational therapy; PT = Physical therapy

ants stressed the need to treat these children as having a future worth serious planning, in spite of the poor survival statistics because any individual child may, indeed, beat the odds for a period of time. The power of positive thinking cannot be trivialized for these children; guidance counselors are uniquely situated to promote it.

Finally, chronically ill children will often need more counseling on personal issues, such as peer acceptance, sibling problems, and family issues, than will the child without a chronic illness (Foster and others, 1977; Pless and Pinkerton, 1975).

School Health Services. Many of the needs of chronically ill children are presently met by the resources of the school's health program. In addition to services provided for the total school population (for example, screening, health education) chronically ill children often need special services from school health personnel. The organization of health services within a school and within a school district can affect the quantity and quality of services delivered to the individual child.

To a large extent, the nature of school health services is determined by who provides the health services at the building level as well as by how these health professionals are related to other health providers at both the building and the overall administrative levels (Guyer and Walker, 1980). There is wide variation within school districts and among states in the way school health services are delivered and in local and state school health policies. No federal statute or set of health codes governs what occurs in schools. In most cases, the school health program is administered by the local board of education and school personnel; in a minority of cases, they are administered by the local health board or by a dual arrangement (Wolf and Pritham, 1965). Often, the administrative staff of school health services at the district level is located in a bureaucratic hierarchy different from that of special education and, in many cases, from that of other pupil personnel services (for example, counseling, social work, psychological services) thus compounding communication and policy problems within the district between ancillary service providers who are especially important to the care of the chronically ill child.

Most of the school health literature assumes that the two individuals responsible for the direction of a good school health program are the school physician and the school nurse. Although the exact details of the school physician's role may vary (Eisner and Callan, 1974; Kappelman and others, 1975; Nader, Emmel, and Charney, 1972; Nyswander, 1942; Wagner, Levin, and Heller, 1967), Murdock (1967) points out that a physician can serve a school health service in one of four capacities: full-time medical director, part-time medical director, school physician, or consultant.

The exact role of the physician is to some extent determined by the role of the school nurse and the type of school health model implemented by the system. The two major models are the health organizer model and the nurse practitioner model (Office of Child Health Affairs, 1976). In the health organizer model, the school is seen as the organizing link between a child in the school and community health resources. In this case, the role of the nurse is to ensure that the child receives comprehensive care through an adequate system of referral, which necessitates record keeping and follow-up by written notices, calls, or home visits. In the nurse practitioner model, the pediatric nurse practitioner provides comprehensive care to children, using an adequate record-keeping and follow-up system and backed up by local physicians. Innovative school health programs based on nurse practitioners delivering primary care in the schools and linking the school program to the community have been developed (Nader, 1978).

The school nurse's responsibilities include health protection and safety; health appraisal, referral, and follow-up; maintenance of health records for each child; counseling and guidance; health education of students, faculty, and parents; faculty-staff conferences; community relationships; and administration, including planning, evaluation, and research (School Nursing Committee, American School Health Association, 1967). Lynch (1977) divides nurse activities into three areas: (1) administrative functions (for example, program planning, program organization and implementation, budget preparation, and program evaluation), (2) problem management functions (including management of family, school, and community resources to resolve health problems of students), and (3) consultation functions—evaluation of course content and the provision of information to school personnel for health teaching. In practice, the nurses' functions are often reduced to scheduling, assisting, first aid, and clerical functions—all of which any trained school person could do. These functions often leave insufficient time for nurses to engage in activities for which they are trained, for example, special counseling on health conditions, health education, and in-service training (Guyer and Walker, 1980).

To facilitate efficient, effective school health services, the inclusion of a health assistant has been recommended by some (Guyer and Walker, 1980; Nader, Emmel, and Charney, 1972; Nutting, Reed, and Shorr, 1975; Randall, Cauffman, and Schultz, 1968; Rosner, Pitkin, and Rosenblath, 1970). A well-trained paraprofessional usually can advise on first aid and injury or illness at the building level, can maintain child health records, and can manage the school triage system to community agencies and individuals.

School health services for chronically ill children have rarely been implemented in school settings according to the comprehensive model presented in the literature. Barriers to development of adequate school health services include lack of community services, poor communication between school personnel and physicians, inadequate funding, and insufficient training of school personnel.

In addition to the specific health services sometimes needed by children with chronic illnesses, Wold (1981) suggests the following examples of the actions school nurses should take in their roles vis-à-vis handicapped children:

1. *As manager of health care within school health program*—Lead and/or participate in interdisciplinary conferences to plan child's IEP and monitor progress in achieving stated educational goals. Apply principles of staffing and delegation to meet handicapped students' health needs while at school.

2. *As deliverer of health services*—Develop and implement appropriate nursing care plans for handicapped students based on careful assessment of their health status and needs. Provide for safe and effective administration of indicated treatments, medications, and other therapies for handicapped students at school.

3. *As advocate for children's health rights*—Serve as advocate for particular handicapped students to ensure school's responsiveness to their educational and health needs. Become politically active and involved to pass legislation providing legal and financial support for equal and adequate educational opportunities for handicapped students.

4. *As counselor for health concerns of children, families, and staff*—Provide supportive counseling to families of handicapped students. Provide one-to-one and/or small group counseling for handicapped students. Provide individual and/or small group counseling for handicapped students' non-handicapped peers, teachers, and other school personnel.

5. *As educator for school/community health concerns*—Provide health information and anticipatory guidance for teachers and other school staff to enable them to plan learning activities consistent with handicapped students' needs and limitations. Provide health education for handicapped students in such areas as nature and extent of their handicap, self-care activities, coping strategies, and sexuality. Provide health education for families of handicapped children regarding such topics as self-care, family dynamics and coping, nature and extent of handicap(s), rationale for prescribed therapies, and availability of community resources.

Although there are limited studies about who delivers which school health services to chronically ill children (Guyer and Walker, 1980; Nyswander, 1942), most schools view the school nurse as the case coordinator for chronically ill children.

In well-organized school health programs, the nurse keeps a confidential listing of children with chronic illnesses that is shared with all school personnel who interact with those children. To ensure that this information is used discreetly, the list of names and conditions is not circulated as such; instead, the nurse contacts each of the individuals involved and personally shares the appropriate medical information. Bryan (1980) describes such a system for sharing medical information for special education students, who are designated with a medical status number from 0 to 9, indicating the functional severity of the child's condition and the likelihood that the child will have a medical emergency.

Most schools keep cards containing telephone numbers of parents or guardians to be contacted in a medical emergency. However, training of school personnel who might be present when a child has a medical emergency (for example, an asthma attack, epileptic seizure, or insulin reaction) is inconsistent across schools. Although the school nurse or school physician usually is responsible for the in-service training of individuals or groups, in truth, other demands on their time greatly reduce their level of involvement in such training. The importance of emergency procedure training for school personnel who interact with chronically ill children cannot be overemphasized, especially because the school nurse or physician is usually absent from the school when the emergency arises. In fact, most emergencies occur on playgrounds and thus immediately involve the teacher on duty and the school secretary.

Another major responsibility of school health services for chronically ill children is the administration of medical treatments or medication. Policies concerning medication are determined at the local school level or by state codes; the majority of states have no legislation or regulations concerning the use of prescribed drugs in schools (Courtnage, 1982; Kinnison and Nimmer, 1979). In some states, such as Massachusetts, the only state laws regarding administration of medications in schools are those for controlled substances; the policies for all other drugs are left to the local school system. Although there are guidelines and models for adequate policies (American Lung Association of Massachusetts, 1980; "Medical Emergencies and Administration of Medication in Schools," 1978), there is wide variation among schools in how they administer medications and whether they have official policies. In some districts, only a qualified nurse is able to dispense medicines; in others, a designated nonmedical person can dispense the medication if a written note from the child's physician is on file. In some states, the requirement to have a nurse dispense the medication holds true only for certain types of drugs; other medications can be dispensed by a variety of adults on the premises. In practice, it seems appropriate for a nurse to have this responsibility if the school has a full-time nurse; however, in those districts where there is none (a situation true in many districts today) or where the nurse's training would be better used in health counseling and health education, a policy designating someone else as the dispenser seems more efficient.

In a descriptive study of school health services in the elementary schools in Flint, Michigan, in 1978, Guyer and Walker (1980) found that school personnel's anxieties about chronically ill children becoming ill and having medical emergencies were usually much greater than the actual risk. Because nurses were not in the school on a full-time basis, the school personnel who knew most about these children in regular classroom placements tended to be the principal, the secretary, and the home school counselor, who performs many of the functions of a health assistant and community worker.

School-Based Training About Chronic Illnesses. All segments of the school community would benefit from general training about chronic illness and from targeted training about particular diseases evidenced in its population. Often local school administrators acknowledge and act upon the need to convey specific information about individual children's conditions to the teachers involved. The data collection and sharing that accompany the special education evaluation process also serve to educate school professionals about the illnesses of those few children covered by those mandates.

Other aspects of school personnel training are neglected by many districts. These aspects include exploration of teachers' feelings about having chronically ill students in their classes (especially those with terminal or catastrophic diseases), provision of brief or episodic supportive counseling for teachers needing or requesting it, opportunity to discuss societal prejudices toward chronically ill children and to describe how school practices inadvertently reinforce negative attitudes or stereotypes, and development of guidelines on dealing with the families of ill children based on an understanding of both family systems and school systems. Although it is understandable that schools attend primarily to issues that ensure the individual child's daily safety and education (strictly speaking), this policy is short-sighted in not providing a nurturant environment for future chronically ill students.

A substantial body of research has accrued on the socioemotional effects of mainstreaming—both to the disabled child and to that child's classmates (Winefield, 1979). Although the results of individual studies are contradictory, it is clear that the *immediate* advantageous effects to all involved anticipated by special education advocates do not occur routinely or exclusively. Children are schooled first in their parents' attitudes, which often reflect the culture's continuing (albeit lessening) aversion to or condescension toward the disabled. School officials admit to social problems within some integrated classes, yet rarely do schools intervene directly in issues of peer rejection, isolation, or scapegoating. Nor do schools attempt to educate children about handicaps or chronic illnesses in a preventive fashion so that, if such children are enrolled in future classes, the school context is welcoming and understanding.

Several curricula have emerged nationally with those purposes in mind. Developed for varying age groups and skill levels, these classroom guides present exercises, discussion topics, suggestions for media aids, and speakers, all of which are meant to sensitize and educate children about handicaps and the experience of being handicapped. In some communities, these curricula are presented by classroom teachers who integrate them into standard subject materials; in others, such as the Understanding Handicaps Program of Newton, Massachusetts, new parent volunteers are trained by veteran parents to implement the program in their local public elementary schools. Preliminary evaluation results from this Massachusetts program suggest that the program has a positive effect on attitudes and an increase of knowledge in the fourth graders involved.

In sum, there remain many areas of training about chronic illness that are not addressed systematically in the majority of American schools. Budget constraints, overworked and demoralized faculty, and the pressing needs to instruct about emergency procedures for specific children overshadow the potential benefits to be derived from enlarging the focus of training efforts.

Physician Involvement with Schools

Both the medical and educational communities feel uniquely invested in chronically ill students. Physicians often develop close relationships with these children and their families based, in part, on the seriousness of their illnesses and the frequent contact they demand. As a rule, physicians are more comfortable and competent in the traditional medical world of physical examinations, diagnostic tests, and medication requirements. Medical advances have dramatically improved the duration and quality of these children's lives, and technical medicine is critically important to them. For these reasons, physicians often expect to coordinate the professional services these children receive, not only from medical colleagues but also from mental health, allied health, and educational specialists.

Some school personnel also lay special claim to this group of children. School health services originated largely to deal with chronically ill students, and presently much of the health provider role at a local school is organized around emergency and daily care, counseling, and schedule modification needs of ill children. By law, the special education department also must serve some segment of this population. Although schools may not be altogether pleased with the comprehensiveness of mandates for the chronically ill student, school personnel at all levels stress the appropriateness of trained school-based (rather than community) professionals making educational programming recommendations. There is little willingness to share with physicians this coordination position.

Although some debate the appropriate role for physicians in educational decisions regarding chronically ill children, their roles as primary referral agents cannot be minimized. This is especially true for doctors of young primary school children because they are often the only professionals with health or psychosocial information on these children.

Physicians do not fill this role to the extent school personnel would like. They are accustomed to dealing with the schools in a hierarchical rather than cooperative manner (Nader, 1974), conveying to schools only information deemed by the individual practitioner as appropriate. Special education mandates of the 1970s have not substantially altered this traditional posture. The intentional withholding of information school personnel would like no doubt reflects doctors' genuine concern for their patients' privacy and confidentiality; the doctor is reluctant to jeopardize a trusting relationship with a family built carefully over time. On the other hand, the protection physicians believe they are according their families when they choose neither to inform the school about a condition nor to urge the parents to do so may not be in the child's best interests. For example, what a teacher interprets as distracting, disruptive behavior on a child's part may be the side effects of medication. The child's schoolwork suffers, and the teacher has no opportunity to share observations of the child's behavior with the prescribing physician who might be able to correct the dosage.

Furthermore, some parents of chronically ill children explicitly request that physicians keep information confidential, partly because difficult situations may arise for children whose illnesses become too public. The issue is complex; parental desire for confidentiality in rare instances conflicts with the school's ability to ensure the child's safety. If, for example, a child whose diabetes is not known to the school experiences an insulin reaction, the child's health may be endangered. Physicians are uniquely situated to allay many parental anxieties about disclosure of such information to school health authorities.

A physician may need to advocate for patients if a school district is delinquent in providing necessary services. Representing the child's interests in this way is encouraged in the legislation and is a role that primary care physicians, of all extraschool professionals, might best fill. However, assuming this position requires familiarity (which many physicians have not developed) with the organization of schools, the availability of special program options, the range of academic subjects, and the legislative requirements. Training in school-related areas is imperative for physicians who wish to be engaged with schools for the benefit of chronically ill students.

Recommendations

The special needs of chronically ill children in schools are served either through special education departments or through general education with supportive school health and pupil personnel services. Great local and state variation in the assignment of children with different conditions and functioning levels to either department results from the varied interpretations of eligibility for special education and from the preference in some communities for using the well-established school health and support services. Our recommendations, therefore, focus primarily on developing uniform jurisdictional policies within schools concerning chronically ill children.

1. The intent of Public Law 94-142 and state special education statutes to apply the condition of adverse educational effect to eligibility for services appears appropriate for chronically ill children. Children with moderate to severe impairments—that is, those whose illnesses eventuate in school failure, chronic absenteeism, complicated scheduling, or architectural adaptation requirements—should be evaluated and placed through the special education process. Some state and local educational authorities have interpreted Public Law 94-142 quite broadly to include as eligible chronically ill children with only mild impairments; we characterize this position as an overinterpretation of these laws. The chronically ill child whose condition only mildly or infrequently affects schooling—children who occasionally require medications or who need modified gym classes—are most appropriately served by the regular education system, utilizing counseling and school health services. A great percentage of children with asthma and diabetes and some children with hemophilia, heart disease, cystic fibrosis, leukemia, sickle cell anemia, and other illnesses could be well served in mainstream education without proceeding through the costly and potentially stigmatizing special education process. The due process protection and wide range of services afforded by Public Law 94-142 should be reserved for moderately to severely disabled children requiring complex, comprehensive, or previously unavailable educational services.

2. To ensure that chronically ill children with mild impairment receive necessary services within each school district, each state should adopt explicit school health codes for this group of children; these do not exist presently. Although a parallel federal statute might assure the maximum protection for these children, there is no precedent or mechanism for implementing such a mandate. State school health codes, which the local school systems would be required to adopt, should minimally include procedures and policies in the following areas:

- Medication Procedures. Each local school system must have an explicit written medication policy on record, allowing for administration of medication in schools by a variety of persons—teachers, aides, and secretaries, as well as school nurses—with orders from a physician on file. In addition, the school must provide an appropriate, safe place for storage of medicines and a private area for medical procedures (such as insulin injections).
- Case Registry. The school system should keep a listing of all students with chronic illness, so that school personnel associated with that child can be notified and trained specifically if necessary. This system should include mechanisms for identification and tracking of children while in school. Discreet use of this information must be assured at all times.
- Emergencies. Policies for handling medical emergencies should be detailed, as should the specific procedures for training school personnel who come in contact with the child.
- In-Service Training. Procedures for training school personnel about chronic illnesses should be incorporated into locally designed policies.
- Case Coordination. Each child with a chronic illness should have a designated school-based coordinator; in most cases, we recommend this be the school nurse. At a minimum, this person should help assure that the appropriate complement of services is delivered and that effective communication between relevant school personnel (especially the classroom teacher) and community persons occur.

3. The physician's role in educating chronically ill children needs to be reexamined and clarified. The physician has health-related information on chronically ill children (general health status, medication needs and potential effects of medication, prognosis, and limitations in activities) that schools must have for proper placement and programming. The transfer of this information to the schools and the fostering of two-way communication between schools and physicians are appropriate functions for the physician. The physician might advise about placements and act as the patient's advocate when the child is not receiving appropriate education. In general, however, the physician's role should be consultative rather than decision-making, with the doctor viewed as a valuable support to schools rather than as case coordinator or central educational program planner.

4. Within the school, there are many training needs regarding care of chronically ill children, and efforts to educate and sensitize should be directed to both school personnel and other students. Training related to children's conditions should be required of all school personnel who come in contact with them; this training should be under the direction of a school nurse or physician. Equally important is the development of specific curricula or techniques designed to explore and modify student and teacher attitudes about chronically ill and physically handicapped children. Finally, supportive personal counseling may be required for school personnel involved with the education of children with terminal or progressive illnesses.

5. More flexible policies regarding the use of homebound and hospitalized instruction should be adopted. The waiting period of two to four weeks before qualifying for homebound services is not in the best interest of chronically ill

students, especially those who are absent frequently for only short periods of time. Homebound instruction might be provided to those chronically ill children whose school-based programs are shortened due to limited endurance.

6. Although it is difficult to advocate for increased research and evaluation monies in an era when services are being defunded, we feel that certain discrete educational intervention studies with chronically ill children, especially the moderately or severely impaired, would produce sound, cost-effective educational models for programming and placement. Of high priority would be studies to document what is currently happening to chronically ill children in schools as well as experimental studies designed to assess the efficacy of selected interventions, such as educational placements and related services.

7. Communication among schools, health practitioners, state and local agencies, and programs for chronically ill children should be facilitated. Improved relationships will avoid duplication of services and help coordinate case management. Cooperative arrangements are especially important in an era of diminishing support for public education. Without this cooperation, we fear that children served best by other agencies or the private medical sector will be dumped on the schools, so that their "free" services can be provided to these children.

Appendix

The following table lists the eligibility categories in individual state special education statutes that apply to chronically ill children and the percentage of children ages 3-21 served under P.L. 89-313 and P.L. 94-142 in Other Health Impaired (OHI) and Orthopedically Impaired (OI) categories for the school year 1979–80.

State	Category That Allows for Special Education Services	Percentage Served	
		OHI	OI
Alabama	Crippled and those having other physical handicaps not otherwise specifically mentioned herein.	0.07	0.05
Alaska	Exceptional children are markedly different from peers. Physically handicapped are those children whose known or diagnosed physical impairment is so severe as to require . . .	0.07	0.18
Arizona	Physical handicap . . . Homebound and hospitalized—certified not to attend school for not less than 3 school months	0.12	0.17
Arkansas	Crippled and otherwise health impaired . . . because of problems, need special education	0.10	0.10
California	Orthopedic or health-impaired physical illness	0.88	0.38
Colorado	Long-term physical impairment or illness	0.00	0.13
Connecticut	Exceptional children means children who deviate either intellectually, physically, socially, or emotionally so markedly from normally expected growth development patterns	0.16	0.09
Delaware	Physically handicapped children means children who suffer from any physical disability making it impractical . . .	0.02	0.24
Florida	Crippled or other health-impaired	0.00	0.18
Georgia	Physically handicapped Hospital or homebound	0.14	0.05
Hawaii	Person by reason of physical defects cannot attend . . .	0.00	0.10
Idaho	Physically handicapped . . . chronically ill . . . homebound student	0.28	0.24
Illinois	Physically handicapped . . . any physical disability	0.12	0.23
Indiana	Physical . . . disability	0.04	0.08
Iowa	Children who are crippled . . . have heart disease or tuberculosis or who, by reason of physical defects cannot attend . . .	0.00	0.12
Kansas	Exceptional children, persons who differ in physical characteristics to the extent that . . .	0.17	0.08
Kentucky	Exceptional children . . . differ in one or more respects . . . physically handicapped children	0.15	0.09
Louisiana	Physically handicapped including . . . cerebral palsy, crippled, and other health-impaired children	0.18	0.09
Maine	Physically handicapped	0.14	0.15
Maryland	Mentally, physically, or emotionally handicapped	0.24	0.14
Massachusetts	Temporary or more permanent adjustment difficulties or attributes arising from . . . physical factor	0.54	0.03
Michigan	Physically or otherwise health-impaired . . . homebound, hospitalized	0.00	0.22

State	Category That Allows for Special Education Services	Percentage Served	
		OHI	OI
Minnesota	Crippled . . . who is otherwise physically impaired in body or limb	0.21	0.16
Mississippi	By reason of defective . . . physical condition	0.00	0.07
Missouri	Physical problems	0.12	0.08
Montana	Physically handicapped children are those children who need . . . to compensate for such physical handicaps as cardiac impairment, cerebral palsy, chronic health problems, or other physical handicaps	0.07	0.08
Nebraska	Physically handicapped	0.00	0.16
Nevada	Handicapped minor . . . one who deviates educationally, academically, physically	0.13	0.18
New Hampshire	Physically handicapped children whose ability is or *may become* restricted by reason of a physical defect or infirmity	0.12	0.12
New Jersey	Orthopedically handicapped, chronically ill	0.17	0.15
New Mexico	Exceptional children means children whose abilities render regular services of the public schools to be inconsistent with their educational needs	0.01	0.07
New York	Physically handicapped	1.20	0.23
North Carolina	Children with special needs . . . any child who because of temporary or permanent disability from intellectual, sensory, physical factors . . . Physically handicapped or other impaired including hospitalized, homebound	0.08	0.10
North Dakota	Crippled or otherwise health-impaired	0.05	0.09
Ohio	So crippled as to be physically unable to properly care for himself without assistance . . .	0.00	0.17
Oklahoma	Children with special health problems	0.06	0.06
Oregon	Crippled or physically handicapped means a disability that has been diagnosed as permanent or that is extended over a two-month period	0.14	0.27
Pennsylvania	Exceptional children deviate from the average in physical . . . to such an extent	0.01	0.11
Rhode Island	Physically . . . handicapped	0.12	0.12
South Carolina	Orthopedically handicapped: impairment that interferes with the normal functions of bones, joints, or muscles to such an extent and degree as to require the school . . . physically handicapped children mean children of sound mind and of legal school age who suffer from any disability making it impracticable or impossible for them to benefit . . .	0.01	0.14
South Dakota	Because of physical or mental condition . . .	0.01	0.12
Tennessee	The physically handicapped and/or other health-impaired including homebound, hospitalized	0.18	0.14
Texas	Physically handicapped child: child of educable mind whose bodily functions or members are so impaired from any cause they cannot be adequately . . .	0.11	0.10
Utah	State Board of Education shall determine	0.03	0.06
Vermont	Handicapped child: educational needs cannot be adequately provided . . .	0.19	0.26
Virginia	Handicapped children includes those who are physically handicapped	0.05	0.05

State	Category That Allows for Special Education Services	Percentage Served	
		OHI	OI
Washington	Handicapped child . . . by reasons of physical handicap	0.16	0.13
West Virginia	Exceptional children differ from the average or normal in physical, mental characteristics	0.20	0.08
Wisconsin	Physical, crippling, or orthopedic disability	0.07	0.11
Wyoming	Having a mental, physical, or psychological handicap	0.10	0.11

Note: Number of children ages 3–21 years served as a percent of estimated Fall 1979 enrollment (ages 5–17).

Sources: Council for Exceptional Children, 1974; Office of Special Education, 1980.

References

Aiello, B. "Up from the Basement: A Teacher's Story." *The New York Times,* April 25, 1976.

American Academy of Pediatrics, Committee on School Health. "Medical Emergencies and Administration of Medication in Schools." *Pediatrics,* 1978, *61,* 115–116.

American Lung Association of Massachusetts. "There are Solutions for the Student with Asthma." Boston: American Lung Association of Massachusetts, 1980.

Arwood, F. "An Inquiry into the Educational Opportunities of Physically Homebound Children in North Carolina with Proposals for a Home Instruction Program." *Dissertation Abstracts,* 1964, *24,* 3159.

Ballasalle, N. "Legislative Provisions for the Education of Handicapped Children in Massachusetts, 1820–1972." Qualifying paper, Graduate School of Education, Harvard University, 1976.

Blanton, R. L. "Historical Perspectives on the Classification of Mental Retardation." In N. Hobbs (Ed.), *Issues in the Classification of Children: A Sourcebook on Categories, Labels, and Their Consequences.* San Francisco: Jossey-Bass, 1975.

Blaschke, C. *Case Study of the Implementation of P.L. 94–142.* Arlington, Va.: Education Turnkey Systems, 1979.

Blatt, B., and Garfunkel, F. *Massachusetts Study of Educational Opportunities for Handicapped and Disadvantaged Children.* Boston: Commonwealth of Massachusetts, 1971.

Brewer, G. D., and Kakalik, J. S. *Improving Services to Handicapped Children.* Santa Monica, Calif.: Rand Corporation, 1974.

Bryan, E. "Use of Medical Information in School Planning." *Journal of School Health,* 1980, *50,* 259–261.

Budoff, M. "Engendering Change in Special Education Practices." *Harvard Educational Review,* 1975, *45,* 507–526.

The Care of Children with Chronic Illnesses. Report of the 67th Ross Conference on Pediatric Research. Columbus, Ohio: Ross Laboratories, 1975.

Cohen, S., Semmes, M., and Guralnick, M. "Public Law 94-142 and the Education of Pre-School Handicapped Children." *Exceptional Children*, 1979, *45*, 279-287.

Comptroller General. *Disparities Still Exist in Who Gets Special Education.* Washington, D.C.: U.S. General Accounting Office, 1981a.

Comptroller General. *Unanswered Questions on Educating Handicapped Children in Local Public Schools.* Washington, D.C.: U.S. General Accounting Office, 1981b.

Connor, F. P., and others. "Physical and Sensory Handicaps." In N. Hobbs (Ed.), *Issues in the Classification of Children: A Sourcebook on Categories, Labels, and Their Consequences.* San Francisco: Jossey-Bass, 1975.

Courtnage, L. "A Survey of State Policies on the Use of Medication in Schools." *Exceptional Children*, 1982, *49* (1), 75-77.

Crossland, C. L., DeFriese, G. H., and Durfee, M. F. "Child Health Care and 'The New Morbidity': Toward a Model for the Linkage of Private Medical Practice and the Public Schools." *Journal of Community Health*, 1981, *6*, 204-215.

Drotar, D. "Adaptational Problems of Children and Adolescents with Cystic Fibrosis." *Journal of Pediatric Psychology*, 1978, *3*, 45-50.

Dunn, L. "Special Education for the Mentally Retarded: Is Much of It Justifiable?" *Exceptional Children*, 1968, *35*, 4-22.

Education Turnkey Systems. *P.L. 94-142: A Study of the Implementation and Impact at the State Level.* Vol. 1. *Executive Summary.* Arlington, Va.: Education Turnkey Systems, 1981.

Eisner, V., and Callan, L. B. *Dimensions of School Health.* Springfield, Ill.: Thomas, 1974.

Fiske, E. "Special Education Is Now a Matter of Civil Rights." *The New York Times*, April 25, 1976, p. 1.

Foster, J. C., and others. *Guidance Counseling, and Support Services for High School Students with Physical Disabilities: Visual, Hearing, Orthopedic, Neuromuscular, Epilepsy, Chronic Health Conditions.* (Rev. ed.) Cambridge, Mass.: Technical Education Research Centers, 1977.

Gayton, W. F., and others. "Children with Cystic Fibrosis: I. Psychological Test Findings of Patients, Siblings, and Parents." *Pediatrics*, 1977, *59* (6), 888-894.

Gearheart, B. R., and Weishahn, M. W. *The Handicapped Child in the Regular Classroom.* St. Louis, Mo.: Mosby, 1976.

Gliedman, J., and Roth, W. *The Unexpected Minority: Handicapped Children in America.* New York: Harcourt Brace Jovanovich, 1980.

Gortmaker, S. L., and others. *Community Services for Children and Youth in Genesee County, Michigan.* Boston: Community Child Health Studies, Harvard School of Public Health, 1980.

Green, M., and Haggerty, R. J. (Eds.). *Ambulatory Pediatrics.* Philadelphia: Saunders, 1975.

Griffiths, M. I. "Medical Approaches in Special Education." In K. Wedell (Ed.), *Orientations in Special Education.* New York: Wiley, 1975.

Guyer, B., and Walker, D. K. *School Health Service in Flint Elementary Schools.* Boston: Community Child Health Studies, Harvard School of Public Health, 1980.

Healy, A., McAreavey, P., von Hippel, C. S., and Jones, S. H. *A Guide for Teachers, Parents, and Others Who Work with Health Impaired Pre-schoolers.* Belmont, Mass.: Contract Research Corp., 1978.

Hunt, G. M., and Holmes, A. E. "Some Factors Relating Intelligence in Treated Children with Spina Bifida Cystica." *Developmental Medicine and Child Neurology,* 1975, *17,* 65-70.

Jacobs, F. H. *Identification of Preschool Handicapped Children: A Community Approach.* Boston: Community Child Health Studies, Harvard School of Public Health, 1979.

Jacobs, F. H., and Walker, D. K. "Pediatricians and the Education of All Handicapped Children Act of 1975." *Pediatrics,* 1978, *61,* 135-137.

Jones, P. *Living with Hemophilia.* Philadelphia: Davis, 1974.

Kappelman, M., and others. "The School Health Team and School Health Physician." *American Journal of Diseases of Children,* 1975, *129,* 191-195.

Kaskowitz, D. H. *Validation of State Counts of Handicapped Children.* Vol. 2: *Estimation of the Number of Handicapped Children in Each State.* Menlo Park, Calif.: Stanford Research Institute, 1977.

Kinnison, L., and Nimmer, D. "An Analysis of Policies Regulating Medication in the Schools." *Journal of School Health,* 1979, *49,* 280-283.

Lansky, S. B., and others. "School Phobia in Children with Malignant Neoplasms." *American Journal of Diseases of Children,* 1975, *129,* 42-46.

Lauder, C. E., and others. "Educational Placement of Children with Spina Bifida." *Exceptional Children,* 1979, *45* (6), 432-437.

LaVor, M. "Federal Legislation for Exceptional Persons: A History." In F. J. Weintraub and others (Eds.), *Public Policy and the Education of Exceptional Children.* Reston, Va.: Council for Exceptional Children, 1976.

Levine, M. D., Clark, T. A., and Maroney, E. F. *Child Health and Education: A Compendium of the Relevant Questions.* Boston: Children's Hospital Medical Center, 1979.

Love, H. D., and Walthall, J. E. *A Handbook of Medical, Educational, and Psychological Information for Teachers of Physically Handicapped Children.* Springfield, Ill.: Thomas, 1977.

Low, M. B. "The Education for All Handicapped Children Act of 1975: A Pediatrician's Viewpoint." *Pediatrics,* 1979, *62,* 271-274.

Lynch, A. "Evaluating School Health Programs." In A. Levin (Ed.), *Health Services: The Local Perspective. Proceedings of the Academy of Political Sciences.* Vol. 32. New York: The Academy of Political Sciences, 1977.

Mackie, R. *Special Education in the United States: Statistics 1948-1966.* New York: Teachers College, Columbia University, 1969.

Mercer, J. R. "A Policy Statement on Assessment Procedures and the Rights of Children." *Harvard Educational Review,* 1974, *44,* 125-141.

Murdock, C. G. "A Report of the Committee on School Physicians of the American School Health Association: A Manual for School Physicians." *Journal of School Health,* 1967, *37,* 395–399.

Nader, P. R. "The School Health Service, Making Primary Care Effective." *Pediatric Clinics of North America,* 1974, *21,* 57–73.

Nader, P. R. (Ed.). *Options for School Health: Meeting Community Needs.* Germantown, Md.: Aspen Systems, 1978.

Nader, P. R., Emmel, A., and Charney, E. "The School Health Service: A New Model." *Pediatrics,* 1972, *49,* 805–813.

Nutting, P. A., Reed, J. C., and Shorr, G. I. "Non-Professionals and the School Age Child." *American Journal of Diseases of Children,* 1975, *129,* 816–819.

Nyswander, D. B. *Solving School Health Problems: The Astoria Demonstration Study.* New York: Commonwealth Fund, 1942.

Office of Child Health Affairs, Department of Health, Education, and Welfare. "School Health." Working paper. Washington, D.C.: Department of Health, Education, and Welfare, 1976.

Office of Special Education, U.S. Department of Education. *Second Annual Report to Congress on the Implementation of Public Law 94-142: The Education for All Handicapped Children Act.* Washington, D.C.: U.S. Government Printing Office, 1980.

Office of Special Education. "Briefing Paper: Initial Review of Regulations under Part B of the Education of the Handicapped Act, as Amended." Washington, D.C.: U.S. Department of Education, 1981.

Palfrey, J. S., Mervis, R. C., and Butler, J. A. "New Directions in the Evaluation and Education of Handicapped Children." *New England Journal of Medicine,* 1978, *298,* 819–824.

Parcel, G. S., and others. "A Comparison of Absentee Rates of Elementary School Children with Asthma and Non-Asthmatic Schoolmates." *Pediatrics,* 1979, *64,* 78–81.

Pilling, D. *The Child with a Chronic Medical Problem—Cardiac Disorders, Diabetes, Hemophilia: Social, Emotional and Educational Adjustment; An Annotated Bibliography.* New York: Humanities Press, 1973.

Pless, I. B., and Pinkerton, P. *Chronic Childhood Disorder: Promoting Patterns of Adjustment.* Chicago: Year Book Medical Publishers, 1975.

Pyecha, J. *A National Survey of Individualized Education Programs (IEPs) for Handicapped Children.* Research Triangle Park, N.C.: Research Triangle Institute, 1979.

Randall, H. B., Cauffman, J. G., and Schultz, C. S. "Effectiveness of Health Office Clerks in Facilitating Health Care for Elementary School Children." *American Journal of Public Health,* 1968, *58,* 897–905.

Reynolds, M. C. "A Framework for Considering Some Issues in Special Education." *Exceptional Children,* 1962, *28,* 367–370.

Rhodes, W., and Sagor, M. "Community Perspectives." In N. Hobbs (Ed.), *Issues in the Classification of Children: A Sourcebook on Categories, Labels, and Their Consequences.* San Francisco: Jossey-Bass, 1975.

Rosner, L., Pitkin, O. E., and Rosenblath, L. "Improved Use of Health Professionals in New York City Schools." *American Journal of Public Health,* 1970, *60,* 328-334.

Rutter, M., Tizard, J., and Whitmore, K. (Eds.). *Education, Health and Behavior.* London: Longman, 1970.

Schiefelbein, S. "Children and Cancer: New Hope for Survival." *Saturday Review,* May 14, 1979, pp. 11-16.

School Nursing Committee, American School Health Association. "The Nurse in the School Health Program: Guidelines for School Nursing." *Journal of School Health,* 1967, *37,* 2A.

Segal, S. S. *From Care to Education.* London: Heinemann Educational Books, 1971.

Senna, C. (Ed.). *The Fallacy of I.Q.* New York: Third Press, 1973.

Shock, N. *The Child with Muscular Dystrophy in the School.* Boston: Muscular Dystrophy Association, 1976.

Stearns, S. E. "Understanding the Psychological Adjustment of Physically Handicapped Children in the Classroom." *Children Today,* Jan.-Feb. 1981, pp. 12-15.

Sultz, H. A., and others. *Long-Term Childhood Illness.* Pittsburgh, Pa.: University of Pittsburgh, 1972.

Task Force on Children out of School. *The Way We Go to School: The Exclusion of Children in Boston.* Boston: Beacon Press, 1970.

Van Osdol, W. R., and Shane, D. G. *An Introduction to Exceptional Children.* Dubuque, Iowa: Brown, 1974.

Wagner, M. G., Levin, L. S., and Heller, M. H. "The School Physician: A Study of Satisfaction with His Role." *Pediatrics,* 1967, *40,* 1009-1013.

Walker, D. K., Gortmaker, S. L., and Weitzman, M. *Chronic Illness and Psychosocial Problems Among Children in Genesee County.* Boston: Community Child Health Studies, Harvard School of Public Health, 1981.

Weintraub, F. J., and others (Eds.). *Public Policy and the Education of Exceptional Children.* Reston, Va.: Council for Exceptional Children, 1976.

Weitzman, M., and others. "School Absence: A Problem for the Pediatrician." *Pediatrics,* 1982, *69,* 739-746.

Winefield, R. "Examining Teachers' Attitudes Toward the Practice of Mainstreaming Handicapped Children." Qualifying paper, Graduate School of Education, Harvard University, 1979.

Wold, S. J. "Tertiary Prevention: Mainstreaming Handicapped Children." In S. Wold, *School Nursing: A Framework for Practice.* St. Louis, Mo.: Mosby, 1981.

Wolf, J. M., and Pritham, H. C. "Administrative Patterns of School Health Services." *Journal of the American Medical Association,* 1965, *193,* 95-99.

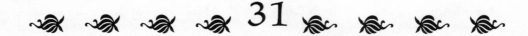

31

Need-Based Educational Policy for Chronically Ill Children

Susie M. Baird, M.Ed.
Samuel C. Ashcroft, Ed.D.

Major Policy Issues and Questions

Children who have chronic illnesses should be able to participate fully in public school programs that address their individual learning needs. Children should have available to them supportive services that facilitate both their physical participation in schools and their intellectual and social development. To meet these challenges, there is a need for renegotiation between special and regular education and between education and other community agencies, specifically, health care agencies.

Precedents Established by Public Law 94–142. Public Law (P.L.) 94–142 redefined the meaning and the mission of public education in the United States and generated precedents that are of importance to children with chronic illnesses. These precedents may be summarized as follows:

1. Access to public education is considered a Constitutional right under the equal protection clause of the Fourteenth Amendment.
2. Education may be broadly defined. In addition to schooling in traditional academic subjects, education is also considered to include development of adaptive behaviors and other skills necessary to equip a child with the tools needed in life (*Fialkowski* v. *Shapp*, 1975).
3. Education programs should be devised according to specific individual needs rather than gross categories of exceptionality.

4. Education should take place in the least restrictive environment, which means "that to the maximum extent appropriate, handicapped children, including children in public or private institutions or other care facilities, are educated with children who are not handicapped" (45 C.F.R. sec. 121a.550(b)).

5. School demissions (exclusions, expulsions, and so forth) should be preceded by due process procedures and accompanied by alternative means of providing services.

6. Parents should be involved in placement and program planning decisions.

7. Supportive services (related services) necessary for an individual child to benefit from an educational program should be provided.

Are Chronically Ill Children Handicapped? Not all handicapped children are eligible for service under P.L. 94–142. *Handicapped children* are those evaluated as "mentally retarded, hard of hearing, deaf, speech impaired, visually handicapped, seriously emotionally disturbed, orthopedically impaired, other health impaired, deaf-blind, multi-handicapped, or as having specific learning disabilities, who because of those impairments need special education and related services" (45 C.F.R. sec. 121a.5(a)). If a child's impairments do not interfere with the ability to learn in a regular classroom environment, that child is not considered to need special education. Because related services are defined as services required to assist a handicapped child to benefit from special education, a child who does not quality for special education is therefore ineligible for related services.

Two categories of the law apply specifically to chronically ill children: *orthopedically impaired* and *other health-impaired,* defined as follows:

"Orthopedically impaired" means a severe orthopedic impairment which adversely affects a child's educational performance. The term includes impairments caused by congenital anomaly (for example, club-foot, absence of some member, etc.), impairments caused by disease (for example, poliomyelitis, bone tuberculosis, etc.), and impairments from other causes (for example, cerebral palsy, amputations, and fractures or burns which cause contractures) (45 C.F.R. sec. 121a.5(6)).

"Other health impaired" means limited strength, vitality or alertness, due to chronic or acute health problems such as a heart condition, tuberculosis, rheumatic fever, nephritis, asthma, sickle cell anemia, hemophilia, epilepsy, lead poisoning, leukemia, or diabetes, which adversely affects a child's educational performance (45 C.F.R. sec. 121a.5(6)).

The regulations are clear that eligibility for special education is based on an impairment that "adversely affects . . . educational performance"; they are not clear on how this phrase should be defined.

Chronically ill children as a group illustrate a major dilemma posed by P.L. 94–142. Those with handicaps such as mental retardation are unquestionably eligible for service under mandatory special education laws. Those who evidence no unusual learning problems may not meet eligibility criteria for P.L.

94-142. However, many students in the latter group require certain physical accommodations, as well as other supports, in order to participate in and benefit from school. They may need related services without needing special education. Yet by definition there can be no related services without special education.

Certain needs of chronically ill children can be addressed by schools. Many of these were detailed by Walker and Jacobs in Chapter Thirty. We here discuss further issues and problems involved in meeting these needs and consider options for meeting each need, together with advantages and disadvantages of various courses of action.

Need for Specialized Instruction

In addition to instruction in traditional academic areas, children who have chronic illnesses may need specialized vocational and career preparation and instruction in such nontraditional areas as disease management, adaptive physical education, nutrition, use of leisure time, and care of appliances. The individualized education program (IEP) has been used to ensure the availability of needed instruction.

Issues and Problems. For children who qualify for special education services, the IEP is an appropriate vehicle for identifying needs and outlining goals and objectives for meeting them. Although the IEP is not a legally binding performance contract demanding educational accountability, it is viewed as an agreement to provide the particular services listed. In theory, the IEP is to include all services needed by the child to achieve maximum potential; these services are not to be limited only to those services available.

Although P.L. 94-142 does not require that schools absorb all costs of providing the services listed in the IEP, the law does specify that the services are to be provided at no cost to parents and that the education agency is ultimately responsible for making these services available. As a result, some education agencies have had to assume costs for services traditionally offered by other agencies, and schools have become reticent about recommending all the assistance a child may need (Craig, 1981). The services ultimately listed in a child's IEP may reflect the knowledge and tenacity of the parent or child advocate more than the needs of the child. Too often, IEPs call only for services that are available already rather than for services the child actually needs.

Options for Meeting the Need. The IEP is limited by the fact that it is required only for students enrolled in special education. In parts of the country, interest has been expressed in extending the IEP concept to all students, not just to those in special education. North Dakota has recently taken just such action (Mirga, 1982), although with an average pupil-teacher ratio of fourteen to one, North Dakota's teachers face considerably fewer obstacles in developing IEPs for all students than do teachers with larger classrooms in more densely populated states.

The health education component of school health programs may be an option for teaching children directly about their illnesses. Although the idea is appealing, most health education programs concentrate on subjects such as drugs, alcohol, and tobacco or venereal disease rather than disease management and related concerns. Only five states—Florida, Illinois, New York, South Carolina, and Virginia—mandate comprehensive school health education and the content to be taught in specific grades (Castile and Jerrick, 1979). These curricula discuss chronic illness, at best, in very limited ways.

Need for Continuity of Programming Despite Frequent or Occasional Absence from School

For chronically ill children, keeping up with course work is difficult when there are prolonged absences because of hospitalization or illness. This task is no less difficult when the student misses a day one week, two days the next week, and perhaps four days at the end of the month.

Issues and Problems. Home and hospital school programs are often the only means of providing educational services to chronically ill students during periods of absence. Such programs are characterized by great diversity in rules, requirements, and quality. In 1981, we mailed questionnaires regarding educational provisions for chronically ill children to chief state school officers in all fifty states, the District of Columbia, seven trust territories, and the Bureau of Indian Affairs (Baird, Ashcroft, and Dy, 1981). We found wide variation among states in the minimum number of days a student must be absent before becoming eligible for home and hospital instruction. Some states (Montana and South Carolina) reported no minimum absence requirement, while others (Indiana, Texas, and Washington) mentioned four weeks as the minimum length of absence necessary. Wisconsin requires that the student's absence from school be anticipated to be over 30 days. These absence requirements generally refer to consecutive days missed and are not flexible enough to include frequent absences of shorter duration.

P.L. 94-142 regulations define *special education* as education needed "to meet the unique needs of a handicapped child, including classroom instruction, instruction in physical education, home instruction, and instruction in hospitals and in institutions" (45 C.F.R. sec. 121a.14(a)(1)). Some states interpret this definition to mean that before home/hospital instruction can be provided to students, they must first be evaluated and classified as handicapped. Presumably, upon return to school, these children go back to their regular classrooms, if appropriate. Unless they had previously qualified for special education, they are no longer considered handicapped. The State of Washington, in its *Rules and Regulations* (1980, p. 23) deals with the problem in this way: "A student who is not otherwise handicapped . . . who qualifies pursuant to this subsection shall be deemed 'handicapped' only for the purpose of home/hospital instructional services and funding and may not otherwise qualify as a handicapped student for the purpose of generating state or federal special education funds."

Some administrators have considered out-of-school students to be temporarily handicapped and have suggested that Section 504 of the Rehabilitation Act of 1973 (P.L. 93–112) may be invoked to guarantee continued educational programming. According to the National Association of State Directors of Special Education and the National Association of State Boards of Education (1979, p. 10), "Section 504 protects students with temporary handicapping conditions, such as a broken leg, and requires development of an individualized program (not necessarily an IEP) for those students. The intent is to assure that temporarily handicapped students continue to receive a free appropriate public education during the time they have an impairment."

Most states require the teacher to spend only three hours per week with home/hospital students. Such brief services—often available only after long waiting periods—seem cruelly inadequate for meeting the chronically ill child's needs for continuity of programming.

Options for Meeting the Need. The Chronic Health Impaired Project (CHIP) of the Baltimore City Schools is an important model for providing home/hospital educational services. Federally funded under the Elementary and Secondary Education Act (ESEA) Title IV-C, the program is open to all students who attend public, private, and parochial schools within the Baltimore City area and who have chronic illnesses that interfere with school attendance and performance. Full-time CHIP teachers visit children participating in the program each day they are absent from school; no minimum number of days missed is required. These teachers attempt to cover the same material that would have been studied in school, thus allowing these children to be marked present on the school roll. In addition to home and hospital instruction, CHIP offers individual, group, and family counseling; vocational, academic, and career guidance; referral services to social and health agencies; a peer tutoring program; monthly parent meetings; and home visits by a parent liaison worker.

CHIP offers the additional advantage of avoiding stigmatization of students. Its composition of 90 percent regular education students and 10 percent special education students reflects roughly the proportions of regular and special education students in most school systems.

Technological models are gaining attention for meeting chronically ill students' needs for home and hospital instruction. The oldest example is teleteaching, which uses the school-to-home telephone. The device requires a costly special hook-up that permits two-way communication (Grandstaff, 1981). Dial access includes taped lectures students can dial at will. Telelecture, teletutoring, and the teleclass consist of teachers lecturing by phone to groups of students. Development of more sophisticated computer technology offers the promise of better teaching models for home/hospital students in the future.

An interesting rule change has been considered in Florida. Individual education programs would be developed for students diagnosed as chronically ill or students who experience repeated intermittent illness. A prime consideration would be that the home or hospital setting becomes the student's school.

For effective teaching, the parent or guardian shall provide a quiet, well-ventilated setting where teacher and student will work; establish a schedule for study between teacher visits; and ensure that a responsible adult be present during the instructional period in the home.

For effective teaching, the hospital teaching setting shall provide appropriate space for the teacher and student to work and allow for the establishment of a schedule for student study between teacher visits [Florida response, Baird, Ashcroft, and Dy, 1981].

This proposed regulation places emphasis on responsibilities of nonschool personnel in contributing to a chronically ill child's educational program.

The extended school year is another option to provide continuity of programming. Some handicapped students have won this service through litigation brought under P.L. 94-142 (for example, *Armstrong* v. *Kline*, 1980). At least two states—Illinois and Rhode Island—offer summer tutoring to students who, for health reasons, are unable to complete the school year.

Need for Supportive Services

Many chronically ill students need supportive services in school, including special diets (for students with asthma, diabetes, or advanced kidney disease), physical therapy and special transportation (for students with juvenile rheumatoid arthritis), special physical handling (for students with spina bifida or muscular dystrophy), social work and liaison services, counseling, and in-school administration of medicines and treatments such as catheterization.

Issues and Problems. The related services provision of P.L. 94-142 has been one of the most controversial parts of the legislation. The definition of *medical services* has been particularly troublesome. Although the law specifically limits these services to those necessary for diagnostic and evaluation purposes, some education officials have argued that many related services listed in the regulations are medical rather than educational because "by common experience and understanding, such services are frequently delivered by 'medical' staff (therapists, nurses, doctors . . .), in medical settings (clinics, hospitals . . .) or with medical equipment or procedures (catheters, sanitary conditions . . .)" ("Related Services, and Medical Services Requirements under Current Legal Standards," 1981, p. 17). The legal meaning of *medical services* under P.L. 94-142, however, includes only services provided by a licensed physician; services that can be provided by nonphysicians are not considered medical services and thus may be an educational responsibility.

Not surprisingly, arguments over provision of related services have reached the courts. The National Center for State Courts calculated that from 1977 to mid 1981, 756 lawsuits citing P.L. 94-142 were filed across the country, and a large percentage of these cases dealt with related services. The case of Amber Tatro, a young Texas child with spina bifida, illustrates these arguments (*Tatro* v. *Texas*, 1980). Because Amber needs clean intermittent catheterization at regular intervals during the day to participate in school and because education officials in the Dallas suburb where she lives have opposed providing this service, her parents have spent over three years in legal battles. The school superintendent has commented that the sticking point in that case is not cost but practicing medicine without a license (Covington, 1982). He contends that, if schools are forced to provide catheterization, they might eventually have to offer dialysis and even more expensive treatments.

Responsibility for payment is a major stumbling block in securing appropriate supportive services for chronically ill children in school. Having no mandate like P.L. 94-142 to ensure provision of services to handicapped children, nonschool agencies have sometimes shifted onto the schools fiscal responsibility for services they provided previously.

Although P.L. 94-142 states that special education and related services are to be "provided at public expense and without charge to parents," the regulations provide also that nothing in the law "relieves an insurer or similar third party from an otherwise valid obligation to provide or to pay for services provided to a handicapped child" (45 C.F.R. sec. 121a.301). Insurance companies have argued that the responsibilities of public schools should not be funded through insurance contract benefits and that such payments violate the no cost to parents provision of P.L. 94-142 because parents pay the premiums. Families have been reluctant to use private insurance benefits, fearing "higher premiums, lack of future coverage, or exhaustion of coverage limits" (Trott, 1980, p. 19). Some parents have questioned schools' practices of labeling various services as therapy in order to bill insurance companies. In 1980, the Secretary of Education issued a policy interpretation stating that education agencies could not require parents of handicapped children to use private insurance proceeds where the parents would incur financial loss and suggesting that, with minor exceptions, use of insurance must be voluntary on the part of parents.

Still another issue in providing supportive services is availability of appropriate personnel. Rural areas may experience particular difficulty in recruiting and retaining skilled physical therapists, occupational therapists, audiologists, and other personnel. Often teachers are required to provide related services, raising concern about liability in matters such as administration of medicines and catheterization; educators are not always "equipped to manage health problems in the classroom" (Select Panel for the Promotion of Child Health, 1981, p. 78).

Transportion is defined as a related service under P.L. 94-142. Special bus transportation for chronically ill students who are also handicapped is generally available throughout the United States, although length of bus rides and availability of special equipment such as lifts may be variable. Some states offer special transportation to nonhandicapped chronically ill students who cannot tolerate long bus rides; the District of Columbia requires medical certification for this service, and New Jersey mandates that the transit time between school and home be no longer than one hour (Baird, Ashcroft, and Dy, 1981).

Options for Meeting the Need. Perhaps the most frequently used recourse for meeting the need of chronically ill children for supportive services is litigation under P.L. 94-142. Few legal recourses are available to the child who is not eligible for service under P.L. 94–142, however. One observer has expressed the view that making the availability of related services "contingent upon the need to profit from special education borders on the ludicrous" (Makuch, 1981, p. 273). The need for such services exists independently of the need for special education.

An innovative school health project offering promise for chronically ill children is the School Health Corporation developed by the Robert Wood Johnson Foundation in the Adams County School District of Commerce City, Colorado. The project is a nonprofit corporation that is separate from the school district and uses a nurse practitioner as the main health care provider. Students and employees in the school district who pay the yearly membership fee of twenty dollars may receive the following services: physical examination, immunization, health counseling/health education, sick-child care, necessary laboratory tests, twenty-four-hour year-round telephone consultation, and referral to necessary specialists. Not included in the membership fee are medications, ambulance services, x rays, sutures, surgery, hospitalization, or specialist treatment. Health services in the eleven schools in the district are provided by three school nurse specialists, ten health aides, three nurse practitioners, one part-time health educator, and one part-time pediatrician (Clark, 1982). Chronically ill children, like other students, can have their routine medical needs met in school for a minimal fee. Such an arrangement seems practical because no special school placements are required and health professionals, rather than teachers, provide the direct medical care.

Need for Coordination of Services and Therapies

There is a need for coordination of services for chronically ill children in schools. Coordination of therapies and services is essential if chronically ill children are to receive maximum benefit from participating in school.

Issues and Problems. One problem in promoting coordination of services is the attitudes, feelings, and stereotypes that inhibit communication among teachers, parents, and health professionals. Part of the problem, as Erickson (1982, p. 1) pointed out, is that "medicine and education constitute two very different 'cultures' with different philosophies, traditions, values, expectations, languages, work-rhythms, and work-views. Professionals working within each of the systems reflect all of these differences and frequently have a poor perception of the complexities of the other system: the organization structure, the decision-making processes, and how the system 'works.'"

Considering the deeply rooted differences in the health and education systems, it is not surprising that a number of respondents to our survey noted "lack of clear definition of school and hospital functions" as a major problem in providing services to chronically ill children.

The question of accountability arises when several systems are involved in the care of children with chronic illnesses. Discussing conflicts generated by P.L. 94–142, Schipper (1980, p. 289) noted that activities such as physical and occupational therapy—usually delivered in accordance with a physician's prescription—are now being written into IEPs and are open to educational due process: "The problem of finding a physician who will agree that the objectives for his prescription be developed by nonmedical personnel and further agree that his prescription be subjected to a non-medical review is an imposing barrier to educational agencies meeting this demand. In some states, this situation is compounded by the difficulty in finding a physical therapist who will willingly violate the state's Medical Practices Act and provide services without a medical prescription." Although "accountability [may be] resolved through due process hearings," school officials complain that other public agencies participating in special agreements may not feel that they also are accountable, since "agreements' legally binding requirements are *ambiguous*" (G. Zittel, personal correspondence with the authors, 1981).

Options for Meeting the Need. Several states have developed team approaches to interagency coordination. In 1978, the U.S. Bureau of Community Health Services funded six collaborative projects for providing health and educational services to handicapped children. The Health/Education Collaborative Project in Connecticut has brought together local education agencies and the public and private health care sectors to develop a coordinated system for serving young handicapped children from birth to age six. The service component of the project includes organization of a Medical/Development Child Find system to promote early identification and appropriate referrals for high-risk children. In addition, regional Community Resource Teams include representatives from various agencies that provide services to handicapped children. Rather than serving a case management function, the teams operate in an advisory capacity to clarify diagnostic and service issues and to determine interagency responsibility. A significant advantage of this model is that it capitalizes on existing resources; the only additional expense is the coordinating role, which can be provided by specifically allocated in-kind services.

All too often the case manager role falls on parents, who may have to "painstakingly piece together a program for themselves and their children. It is not unusual for the mother of a handicapped child to consider advocacy with agencies and schools her full-time job" (Select Panel for the Promotion of Child Health, 1981, p. 77). Although parents may wish to function as their child's case manager, it hardly seems fair to demand that they do so, especially without providing the routine kinds of support that a professional case manager would expect (such as salary, ready access to individuals and information, and collegial status).

Other attempts to coordinate services have included state activities such as the Louisiana effort to mandate agreements between schools and Maternal and Child Health agencies as well as Public Health agencies when such agreements are necessary for provision of free, appropriate public education. The Crippled Children's Services (CCS) program in Alabama is located within the State Department of Education and offers linkages between special education programs and services such as physical therapy and school nursing. Many states have experienced problems in developing effective ties between education agencies and other service providers such as Crippled Children's Services, however. Only about half the states have formal agreements between these agencies, and the agreements vary greatly both in specificity and in their influence on patterns of service delivery (Ireys, 1982). Ireys found that reasons for lack of agreements include New Jersey's first dollar, turf issues, and professional credentials as well as the California CCS limitation of providing physical therapy only to children who are physically handicapped and who will benefit from therapy. The degree to which state education agencies control the activities of local schools is variable; in Idaho, for example, Ireys' report shows that 115 separate school districts operate as 115 fiefdoms—no uniformity. Interagency cooperation on the state level is thus limited by structures and attitudes that inhibit collaboration, although some states have made considerable progress toward resolving these problems.

Need for Physical Access to Safe Schools and Classrooms

Because of their health problems and because of the physical limitations of some chronically ill students, issues surrounding classroom environment and location take on special significance. Students with leukemia or sickle cell anemia may need protection against undue exposure to infection. Students with juvenile rheumatoid arthritis, muscular dystrophy, or spina bifida may experience difficulties climbing stairs or walking long distances.

Issues and Problems. Thirty-two states suggest standards for the environmental quality of schools (Castile and Jerrick, 1979). These standards address subjects such as fire prevention, safety codes, sanitation, and food services. Standards vary from state to state and are generally written to describe minimally acceptable conditions rather than the more carefully planned arrangements that chronically ill children may require. Problems such as "unenforced legislation, lack of funding for legislation, human error, or other factors" (p. 6) complicate efforts to evaluate nationwide school environmental health standards.

Making major building modifications for chronically ill students who need them presents a challenge to many communities. Students are often grouped because of their need for classroom accessibility rather than their need for educational programs. Yet installing ramps and elevators for all children in wheelchairs, widening toilet stalls, and building low water fountains in every school building in a district may represent a significant investment by education agencies that are sometimes scrambling for funds simply to pay teachers' salaries.

Options for Meeting the Need. The Rehabilitation Act of 1973 (P.L. 93-112) offers federal statutory support for modifying school buildings and transportation systems to accommodate students with physical handicaps. Section 504 of this act requires that recipients of federal funds provide persons who are handicapped with the same quality of services and opportunities as they provide persons who are not handicapped. Section 502 mandates barrier-free buildings for handicapped persons. Existing facilities are required to meet standards of accessibility within specified time periods, and new facilities are to incorporate barrier-free design features in their construction. Enforcement authority for these sections is located in the Office of Civil Rights.

It is important to note that the definition of *handicapped* under these sections is more general than that provided by P.L. 94–142. *Handicapped persons* are those with physical or mental impairments that limit one or more major life activities; *major life activities* involve functions such as "caring for one's self, performing manual tasks, walking, seeing, hearing, speaking, breathing, learning, and working" (45 C.F.R. sec. 84.3(j)).

Despite the comprehensiveness of these mandates, progress toward reaching their goals has been slow. Primarily because of the substantial costs to renovate school buildings, districts have not approached such projects with enthusiasm and have frequently applied for waivers and exemptions. In some cases, they have been allowed to provide only one barrier-free building in a community rather than making all schools barrier-free.

Some chronically ill children require only subtle modifications to school buildings, such as access to safe bathrooms, avoidance of temperature extremes, and adaptation of playground routines. These modifications can often be worked out by school personnel without incurring major costs. Travis (1976, p. 313) reported an example of an innovative principal and teacher working together to facilitate the adjustment of three children with hemophilia: "This school adapts itself to their needs. An entire class has been moved from one floor to another to eliminate stairs. Extra sets of books are provided, so the boys can have books at home and not carry them (recommended by authorities for all children with hemophilia). The boys are kept in regular classes, provided with home teachers when they cannot attend, and treated with normal expectations."

Need for Training and Support of School Personnel

Chronically ill children may be served by a number of school personnel in addition to classroom teachers. Depending on the size and sophistication of the school system, children with health problems may spend time with physical therapists, occupational therapists, school psychologists, school nurses, school nurse practitioners, health aides, health educators, and other professionals and paraprofessionals. Many of these persons, particularly those working in education-related rather than health-related disciplines, may have little experience in caring for children with chronic illnesses.

Issues and Problems. Professional preparation programs often lack:

- course work related to legal disability and ethical considerations of health services provided by school personnel
- course work and practica related to the development of procedures for evaluating the effects of medication and medical treatment in the classroom
- course work and practica related to the development of interdisciplinary teamwork [Trahms and others, 1977, p. 348].

In addition, school personnel may lack training in development of appropriate educational goals and objectives for children with chronic illnesses and in dealing with the emotional and social programs that sometimes accompany these children's diseases.

It might be expected that since preservice training programs are inadequate for preparing school personnel to work with chronically ill children, then in-service training programs would address some of these deficiencies. Yet a surprising finding of our survey was that there appears to be relatively low demand across the country for in-service training in medical matters. The rarity of chronic illness and the tendency of many chronically ill students to miss substantial periods of time in school or to drop out altogether may account for the limited interest in in-service training.

Options for Meeting the Need. One option for developing a cadre of qualified personnel to serve chronically ill students is improved training experience. Slonim (1982, p. 2) noted that "interdisciplinary *training* must precede interdisciplinary *services;*" she believed that professionals must be taught during the undergraduate and graduate years to collaborate with other professionals. Interdisciplinary training—involving "mutual respect, sensitivity, and the sharing of knowledge and skills among disciplines"—should include child development theory and clinical experience, family systems theory, communications theory, change theory, issues in public policy, and group/team process skills.

Freund, Casey, and Bradley (1982, p. 348) observed that most training tends to be narrowly focused and categorical in nature: "Physicians are trained by other physicians to deal with medical aspects; teachers are trained by other teachers to deal with educational aspects; and psychologists are trained by other psychologists to deal with psychological aspects. Training in most of the helping professions tends to be focused on exclusive concepts and methods, with little attention given to the thinking and techniques used in other professions to deal with human problems. . . . As a result, problems may not be understood fully or treated in their entirety."

The Department of Rehabilitation and Special Education at the University of Arkansas includes in its master's level teacher training program a required course entitled "Medical Problems in Child Development." The course, taught by a special educator and a pediatrician, covers medical aspects of problems and treatments, referral procedures, and consultation skills. More courses that span professional disciplines would seem important for meeting the need for training and support of school personnel in serving chronically ill children.

No college or university course should be expected to cover all the information a teacher would need to know to teach any child with any chronic illness. Some teachers may encounter their first chronically ill student ten years after receiving the diploma, and what they have learned might have little applicability to one particular student and class. Coursework should focus on general issues of interdisciplinary teamwork, legal liability and ethical considerations, medical perspectives, and so forth. With a solid foundation of this kind, school personnel can proceed to work out programs for individual students with individual illnesses.

All too often, teachers are simply left on their own to organize and carry out a chronically ill child's school program. Most teachers need opportunities for consultation, and some may need emotional support. The special education consultant may be helpful; pediatricians or specialists in chronic illness could function as classroom consultants and child advocates in much the same way that psychologists and applied behavior analysts do now.

Other types of technical assistance could include computer-based information services such as the School Practices Network (SPIN), Exceptional Child Education Resources, Educational Resources Information Center (ERIC), MED-LINE, and PRE-MED. Information on chronic illness could be compiled and made accessible to educators and others working in schools so that exemplary practices and innovative projects could be easily disseminated.

Most state education agencies sponsor regional teacher centers, materials centers, and/or curriculum libraries for use by school personnel. These, too, could be modified to include a section on resources for meeting the needs of chronically ill children in school. Regional centers that offer technical assistance to teachers of handicapped students are another possible repository for such materials.

Conclusion and Recommendations

The presence of a well-designed, smoothly functioning system of services for chronically ill children in school has enormous implications for the quality of life of these children and their families. Efforts to provide a more supportive school environment for chronically ill children may result in a more supportive school environment for all children. Despite the fact that several communities have responded to these children in unusually creative and caring ways, the school system as a whole lacks the flexibility and the need-based policy focus that these children must have to receive maximum benefit from school participation.

We have discussed six major policy-relevant areas in delivering appropriate educational services to chronically ill children. In reviewing certain policy questions, we suggest the following responses. First, as regards determining whether chronically ill children as a group should be considered handicapped for educational purposes, we believe that they should not. Defining a new category of children to be served by schools, developing a new set of rules and regulations for dealing with this particular population, and prescribing uniform practices to be used with all chronically ill children are activities that are not well suited to the realities of the 1980s.

Rather than isolating students with chronic illness into a special educational category, we would prefer efforts directed at making schools more sensitive to and more effective for all students. Chronically ill children, whose needs are so great and yet so diverse, provide a crucial test for schools. Developing community plans and programs to enable children to participate effectively in schools cannot help but influence the school's response to all children who have special needs.

Second, we believe that stretching P.L. 94–142 to include nonhandicapped children in need of related services is a disservice both to these children and to the handicapped children that public law was designed to serve. We would suggest that P.L. 94–142 continue as a protector of educational opportunity for handicapped children. However, we recommend that its related services portion be shaped into a new statute requiring that all students be provided the related services necessary for them to benefit from education. The new law would be separate from P.L. 94–142 and would represent a commitment to meeting children's needs for supportive services whether handicapped or not. The problems and successes in implementing the related services provision of P.L. 94–142 could guide the shaping of the new law. We propose that a task force of parents, educators, administrators, nonschool agency representatives, legislators, and private citizens be appointed to draft the legislation so that consumer as well as official representation will be given proper attention.

Third, schools must adopt new policies for coordinating internal factions (regular education and special education). A more blended system would involve letting go of the notion that special education and regular education are separate service delivery systems with different technologies and different goals. Chronically ill children as a group point out the need for renegotiation between the two systems so that "in the decade ahead, *special education* could become general education and *general education,* special" (Corrigan and Howey, 1980, p. 200).

Fundamental to the renegotiation process is the P.L. 94–142 policy that all children are educable and that school programs should be designed to meet children's needs, rather than that children should be appropriate for school programs. Working from this policy assumption, regular and special educators can develop new relationships. Ideally, students would be able to move into and out of special education as necessary rather than being permanently placed in a special education track. Regular and special educators can serve as consultants to each other in developing plans for individual children.

Finally, we believe that chronically ill students would be well served by school policies that encourage and support collaboration with parents, other community agencies, and professionals, especially health care providers. Improved interdisciplinary training and problem-solving are two important activities in this effort. Perhaps most critical is fostering a sense of community ownership of the problems these children have and the community provision and understanding of the resources for meeting these problems. If chronic illness is viewed as a community concern rather than an individual or family concern, then agencies must respond first to children's and families' needs and second to their own problems and territorial interests. The community resource teams we have described present an intriguing option for bringing agencies together to develop their own solutions to the special problems and needs that exist in their regions.

Our examination of issues involved in delivering educational services to chronically ill children convinces us that public schools can develop workable strategies for meeting these children's school-related needs. Although some solutions are costly, a surprising number are not; they involve simple adjustments in routines or practices. We believe that schools can rise to the challenge of providing more supportive environments for chronically ill children and, in so doing, can provide more supportive environments for all children. We cannot overlook the needs of chronically ill children if we are to continue to espouse goals of equal educational opportunity and free, appropriate public schooling for all our children.

References

Armstrong v. *Kline,* 476 F. Supp. 583 (E. D. Pa. 1979), affirmed 485 F.2d 1298 (3d Cir. 1980).

Baird, S., Ashcroft, S. C., and Dy, E. B. "Survey of Educational Provisions for Chronically Ill Children." Unpublished manuscript, Vanderbilt University, 1981.

Castile, A. S., and Jerrick, S. J. *School Health in America: A Survey of State School Health Programs.* (2d ed.) Atlanta, Ga.: Bureau of Health Education, Center for Disease Control, Public Health Service, U.S. Department of Health, Education, and Welfare, 1979.

Clark, D. "Colorado School Health Program." Paper presented at Symposium on Education and Chronically Ill Children, Vanderbilt University, Nashville, Tenn., 1982.

Corrigan, D. C., and Howey, K. R. "The Future: Creating the Conditions for Professional Practice." In D. C. Corrigan and K. R. Howey (Eds.), *Special Education in Transition: Concepts to Guide the Education of Experienced Teachers.* Reston, Va: Council for Exceptional Children, 1980.

Covington, R. "Handicapped vs. Public Schools." *Suburban Woman,* 1982, pp. 10-11.

Craig, P. A. "Provision of Related Services: A Good Idea Gone Awry." *Exceptional Education Quarterly,* 1981 *2* (2), 11-15.

Erickson, J. "Health and Education as Systems: An Overview of Organizational Issues." Paper prepared for Chronically Ill Child Project, Vanderbilt Institute for Public Policy Studies, Vanderbilt University, Nashville, Tenn., 1982.

Fialkowski v. *Shapp,* 405 F. Supp. 946 (E.D. Pa. 1975).

Freund, J. H., Casey, P. H., and Bradley, R. H. "A Special Education Course with Pediatric Components." *Exceptional Children,* 1982, *48* (4), 348-351.

Grandstaff, C. L. "Creative Approaches to Compliance with P.L. 94-142 and Home/Hospital Programs." *DPH Journal,* 1981, *5* (1), 37-44.

Ireys, H. T. "Report on Responses to CCS Questionnaire." Unpublished manuscript, Vanderbilt University, 1982.

Makuch, G. J. "Year-Round Special Education and Related Services: A State Director's Perspective." *Exceptional Children,* 1981, *47* (4), 272-274.

Mirga, T. N. "Dakota Considers Tailor-Made Instruction for All Pupils." *Education Week,* 1982, *1* (22), 6.

National Association of State Directors of Special Education and National Association of State Boards of Education. *Answering Your Questions About P.L. 94–142 and Section 504*. Washington, D.C.: National Association of State Directors of Special Education and National Association of State Boards of Education, 1979.

"Related Services and Medical Services Requirements Under Current Legal Standards." *Focus on Special Education Legal Practices*, 1981, *1* (2), 13–19.

Schipper, W. "Financial and Administrative Considerations." *Journal of School Health*, 1980, *50* (5), 288–290.

Select Panel for the Promotion of Child Health. *Better Health for Our Children: A National Strategy*. Vol. 2. Department of Health and Human Services publication no. 79-55071. Washington, D.C.: U.S. Government Printing Office, 1981.

Slonim, M. "Policy Issues Involved in Providing Educational Services to Chronically Ill Children." Paper presented at Symposium on Education and Chronically Ill Children, Vanderbilt University, Nashville, Tennessee, 1982.

State of Washington. *Rules and Regulations for Programs Providing Services to Children with Handicapping Conditions*. Olympia: Department of Public Instruction, 1980.

Tatro v. Texas, 625 F.2d 557 (5th Cir. 1980).

Trahms, C. M., and others. "The Special Educator's Role on the Health Service Team." *Exceptional Children*, 1977, *43* (6), 344–349.

Travis, G. *Chronic Illness in Children: Its Impact on Child and Family*. Stanford, Calif.: Stanford University Press, 1976.

Trott, D. C. *Policy Positions on Selected Issues Concerning the Education of Handicapped Children*. Vol. 1. Washington, D.C.: Closer Look, 1980.

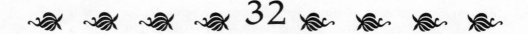

32

Cognitive Development of Chronically Ill Children

Judith S. Mearig, Ph.D.

All aspects of development impinge upon one another, and nowhere is this more evident than in the development of children with a serious chronic illness. In spite of this fact, individuals encountering chronically ill children commonly consider impaired intellectual functioning an inherent aspect of the illness rather than a result of interaction among many developmental factors. The distinction between these two ways of perceiving intellectual functioning is particularly important. The former perspective implies that the level of intellectual functioning is immutable; the latter suggests that environmental intervention, especially education, can alter intellectual functioning and even the course of cognitive development. Because all facets of development interact, the nature of those factors influencing intellectual functioning are never identical, even in the case of two children with the same illness. In facilitating the cognitive development of a child, it is important to assess the child's present intellectual functioning and potential. Furthermore, knowledge of the specific cognitive problems commonly associated with a chronic illness may permit their prevention or reduction.

This chapter first highlights issues in education and assessment of chronically ill children. It then examines the aspects of particular chronic illnesses that make a child vulnerable to difficulties in intellectual functioning or cognitive development. Finally, it explores dynamics that are common to all the illnesses and that can affect significantly the pattern of cognitive development.

Issues in Education and Assessment

Educational Accommodation. Education is an important mechanism whereby chronically ill children may achieve independence. Children's experiences at school influence the development of their self-concepts. In the case of chronically ill children who may experience little control over their health, educational achievement provides an opportunity for the development of feelings of control, mastery, and accomplishment. Isaacs and McElroy (1980, p. 319) stress the importance of the school experience: "The child's definition of his own intellectual development largely depends on the extent of interaction with a sufficiently stimulating environment. This includes meaningful relationships with peers, attainable goals, and optimal academic achievement that does not exclude the child because of illness." Furthermore, educational opportunity may determine whether or not these children are economically self-supporting as adults.

In the past, children have made many of the accommodations to school themselves. Today, under Public Law 94–142, the Education for All Handicapped Children Act, individual programming is required for children whose chronic illness in some way affects their learning or other behavior in school. However, many schools are limited in knowledge, experience, and financial resources, and states vary in how they organize services required to meet individual needs of children designated as handicapped. Moreover, most chronically ill children require much flexibility in their programming because of the changing nature of their illnesses.

Some chronically ill children, whose intellectual functioning is potentially at least average, have been placed in classes for the retarded. Many, whether in special or regular classes, have not had supportive services that they need. There are a multitude of reasons that some of these children score low on intelligence tests and do not function consistently near their potential in the classroom, not the least of which are disruptions in developmental sequences related to their chronic illness. For example, children with severe cleft palate may not speak intelligibly until after the age of six when a series of surgical procedures and speech therapy has been completed. They might be expected to have not only retarded language development for at least a few years but also different communication patterns and extended dependency on their parents.

Parents can face a dilemma if they believe in mainstreaming but the educational program and social acceptance for their child are minimal in the public school. Some teachers and children are not prepared to accept a child with an unusual appearance or physical condition, often because they have had no experience. Negative attitudes likely will pass if young children are not only integrated but also can absorb feelings of communality with chronically ill children or disabled children from adults in their lives to whom they look for direction (Snyder, Apolloni, and Cooke, 1979). But the parents of an older child with chronic illness must make a decision about placement under existing conditions.

Attitudes and values concerning children with disabilities often underlie classification schemes and educational programs that schools arrange (Hobbs, 1975). Varying more than the ultimate learning capacity of children is the amount of investment required on the part of school and society to bring about the learning (R. Feuerstein, personal communication to the author, 1981). Limiting of a child's eventual opportunities in society can occur in integrated as well as segregated settings. Shapiro (1981) points out that mainstreaming children in gym, art, and music, while at the same time giving them a limited academic education, does little to prepare them for independent economic and social status in our society.

Continuity of instruction is extremely important for chronically ill children who attend school but must be absent periodically. Hospital education programs vary greatly, some being very elaborate and others nonexistent. In the latter case, the public school must provide a program. Homebound instruction in many states is inadequate, not only in number of hours provided but also in eligibility requirements. Children who are chronically absent sometimes must wait a certain number of days before they are eligible for instruction at home. Periodic absences can often be anticipated and home teaching built into the child's individual educational plan (IEP) or otherwise authorized on an "as needed" basis. If states have inhibiting rules about eligibility for homebound instruction, under Public Law 94–142 short but chronic absences can be covered by tutoring as a related service. This is written into the IEP and does not have to be reviewed at the time of each absence. Children are entitled to an IEP even if they do not require any other related service or a special instructional program in the classroom.

The decision that a child with a steadily deteriorating condition should leave school for permanent home teaching is a major one. Once this move is made, all aspects of a child's life can change; for example, resistance to infection may decrease and the child may receive less exercise. Certainly the family's role changes. Someone now must be home with the child all the time, and few families can afford to pay an outsider to take this responsibility. Today, schools are often willing to keep disabled children longer if they have some experience and know they can cope. Having had such children over a period of years, they may be able to adapt gradually to their changing needs. Also, peers may help in a chronically ill child's care and come to feel that that child is an integral part of their class.

It is important that capable and innovative teachers be employed for homebound instruction. In addition, closed-circuit television links with the classroom are valuable. These are more effective than telephone connections because they allow the child to see the gestalt of what is occurring as well as to interact verbally. Visual contact between the teacher and children in the classroom and the child at home can vary according to the child's condition.

For children who cannot participate in a group learning situation through closed-circuit television, one-to-one instruction can be supplemented by television observation of classroom proceedings, audiovisual aids, and some form of discussion with peers. Classmates can be encouraged to visit the homebound child for both social and cognitive activities. The child can also supplement instruction interrupted by fatigue, attacks of illness, or treatment procedures by using programmed self-teaching materials.

Assessment of Intelligence and Cognitive Development. Class placement and educational programming for chronically ill children should be based on pertinent criteria. Assessment for this purpose cannot focus on standardized test scores. Knowledge of past history and present functioning of a child in real life, direct observational data, understanding of the dynamics of the chronic illness, and reasoning and integration abilities of the examiner may supplement, supersede, or even contradict information gained through testing. Further, the time dimension can be important in testing children with chronic illness. At what stage developmentally in this child's life and in the progression of the chronic illness does the testing occur?

Basic beliefs about the nature of intelligence can affect interpretation of assessment data. For example, professionals often have viewed intelligence of boys with Duchenne's dystrophy as a component of the genetic defect and accepted scores on intelligence tests as a reflection of this. They have paid relatively little attention to possible effects of the psychodynamics of the disease on cognitive development and academic learning (Marsh and Munsat, 1974; Karagan and Zellweger, 1978).

Standardized test norms and administration format may be just as inappropriate for chronically ill children as they are for those who are culturally and socioeconomically deprived. Chronically ill children may have atypical experiences, delayed developmental milestones, and physical symptoms and treatment interfering with test performance as well as school learning. Educators have been eager to have standardized procedures to assess mental capacities in order to sort children into what are perceived as practical instructional categories. But often overlooked is that the statistical probability of underlying scores refers to a group average. An individual child's performance has to be interpreted in a much more comprehensive context. Low scores are always more suspect than high scores. What can be useful as indicators of potential on standardized tests are peaks of performance. Some traditional tests can be used creatively with chronically ill children if comparison or classification are not primary goals. It is important that selection of tests be individualized to the child and to the purpose of the assessment. The Special Education Assessment Matrix (SEAM) (Lambert, 1980), a regularly updated reference guide to more than seventy recommended tests for assessing needs of exceptional children, can be helpful in this selection.

Feuerstein (1979a, 1979b) and his colleagues have developed special materials to make the transition between testing and teaching of cognitive process (as opposed to context), and they emphasize cognitive modifiability. With regard to assessment for the purpose of developing an instructional plan, Feuerstein's (1979a) analysis of deficient cognitive functions is much more productive than results of intelligence or other standardized test results. These deficient cognitive functions are divided into three phases (input, elaborational, and output) that are examined in great detail through Feuerstein's (1979a) Learning Potential Assessment Device. Whereas many culturally deprived and neurologically impaired children are often most deficient in the input and output phases, the present writer believes that chronically ill children can have significant difficulty in developing the reasoning processes involved in the elaborational phase. The rationale for this belief is presented in the latter part of this chapter.

Feuerstein believes that deficient cognitive functions are modifiable in most children with proper instructional techniques and effective mediated learning experience (MLE). He defines *MLE* as "the interactional processes between the developing human organism and an experienced intentioned adult who, by interposing himself between the child and the external sources of stimulation, 'mediates' the world to the child by framing, selecting, focusing, and feeding back environmental sets and habits. The action of the adult and his activity in restricting the stimulation field and interpreting it to the infant or child constitute the major difference between mediated learning and nonmediated, direct exposure learning" (p. 71). Feuerstein refers to MLE as the critical or proximal determinant of learning. Distal determinants include such factors as genetic background, organicity, socioeconomic status, environmental stimulation, and emotional state. Although important as triggers, these factors, even if positive, will not bring about effective learning unless the quality and quantity of MLE is adequate (R. Feuerstein, personal communication with the author, 1981). A systematic instructional program based on mediated learning may have to be introduced if parents, ordinarily the first and best mediators, have not had the time or motivation to provide these experiences in everyday interactions with their child. Moreover, sometimes parents have been led to believe their child's learning potential is too low to benefit from their teaching.

Dynamics of Particular Chronic Illnesses Related to Difficulties in Cognitive Functioning

In discussing the dynamics that can make a child vulnerable to impaired cognitive functions, the results of selected studies on intelligence and school performance are reviewed. In general, there has been more research about illnesses that pose considerable problems in these areas of functioning than about illnesses that do not. However, the dynamics of some illnesses have not received the attention they deserve.

Asthma. Asthma, the most common chronic illness (affecting two to three million children), can indirectly generate difficulties in cognitive development. Certain medications can affect cognitive functioning: Antihistamines can induce either drowsiness or excitability, and adrenalin and some other drugs can cause tremors, nausea, vomiting, restlessness, headache, and personality changes; possible side effects of steroids include decreasing memory and learning problems.

Dunleavy and Baade (1980) reported very mild to mild brain-damaged behaviors exhibited by some children with severe asthma on the Halstead Neuropsychological Test Battery for Children. These included problems in visualizing and remembering spatial configurations, incidental memory, and planning and executing visual tactile motor tasks. The authors attributed their findings to hypoxic-induced brain abnormalities due to loss of consciousness and prolonged cyanosis possible during a severe asthma attack. They found no relationship between drug usage and neuropsychological test performance. However, Suess and Chai (1981) responded that side effects of corticosteroid and theophylline medications may be responsible for lower performance found on the above tests and indicated that preliminary findings supported their hypothesis. Dunleavy (1981) acknowledged that dosage level of a drug may be a factor. Apparently the question remains to be resolved.

Academic achievement is often affected by the large number of days missed from class by children with asthma. According to the National Institutes of Health (Strunk and Boyd, 1980), asthma leads all chronic illnesses in causing school absenteeism. Freudenberg (1980) estimated that twenty-eight million school days were lost in 1975 due to asthma. The child's motivation to catch up is often lost after successive absences. Although good home instruction is important, many of these children are not absent long enough at a given time to qualify for a home teacher. Bhat and others (1978) found that children who received care in a hospital outpatient clinic missed almost twice as many school days a year as those treated by private physicians, underlining the problems faced by low-income families that use outpatient clinics when coping with a chronic illness such as asthma. However, the study did not find significant differences in school achievement or frequency of school problems in the two groups.

Bakwin and Bakwin (1948) believed that children with asthma may sometimes function above average intellectually. Because of restriction of physical activities, they may be in close interaction with adults and may benefit from this stimulation (and mediated learning?). Mitchell and Dawson (1973), in a study of 288 children with asthma aged seven years and older in Aberdeen, Scotland, found a higher mean IQ (102) in these children than in the general population (95) in all social classes, but particularly in families of semiskilled and unskilled workers.

There are other possible relationships of asthma to children's school success. Parental overprotection can be an adaptational response to a chronic, unpredictable illness. This can arouse much anxiety in the child (Parker and Lipsombe, 1949) and may retard the child's development of independent thinking ability. Creak and Stephen (1958) pointed out that heightened sensitivity to praise and blame makes it difficult for these children to accept their educational problems, some of which develop because of chronic absence from school. Moreover, although stress cannot create an asthmatic condition, it can trigger an attack in a child having asthma. Further, Creer and Yoches (1977, p. 552) observed that both children and teachers often stigmatize a child with asthma, "treating him differently, restricting activities, isolating the child, or limiting social interactions." Also, about 40 percent of the parents in Freudenberg's (1980) study reported school problems for their children wtih asthma. The two most common were long or frequent absences and reading difficulties.

A direct link with learning problems can occur when allergies underlying the asthma cause otitis media and impaired hearing, especially for word sounds. Speech articulation problems can develop if the child cannot hear well enough to distinguish word sounds correctly when initially learning to talk. Even after the otitis media is corrected and the child's physical hearing has improved, incorrect pronunciations for certain words may continue because this was the way the words were originally learned. Difficulty in learning to read the words in the early school years is another common problem, especially if a phonetic approach is stressed. Hearing ability of children with allergies often fluctuates as upper respiratory congestion comes and goes. Their performance in reading activities and in hearing directions in class thus varies.

In summary, the learning difficulties associated with asthma would seem to be able to be controlled or compensated for by ensuring continuity of instruction, by not emphasizing phonetic approaches in teaching reading to children with middle-ear congestion, and by providing emotional support for the child and the child's family.

Cleft Palate. The sequence of language development and communication itself can be disrupted if cleft palate surgery and speech and language therapy are not perfectly timed with the child's developing communication needs. If important restorative surgery cannot be done until the age of five or six and the child is only able to begin to talk clearly after subsequent therapy, there are tremendous implications for all areas of development.

Hearing loss as well as speech problems emanating directly from the atypical mouth formation and subsequent slow language development are common in cleft palate, the degree depending on the severity of the cleft and harelip. Smith and McWilliams (1968) reported that eighty-six boys and fifty girls between the ages of three and eleven with cleft palate were, as a group, below average on the Illinois Test of Psycholinguistic Abilities. In a review of other studies reported in the same paper, Smith and McWilliams found that weaknesses in language tended to become more pronounced with age. Richman (1980) found more language disability in children with only cleft palate (not a cleft lip). These children had poorer verbal mediation requiring categorization and associative reasoning, which lead Richman to believe that the neuropsychological correlates were different for the two groups. She cited the need for more research.

Goodstein (1968) concluded from his own research and a review of other studies that children with cleft palate as a group were mildly to moderately impaired intellectually, with verbal deficits greater than deficits in the performance area. However, the mean IQs ranged from 94 to 99, and Goodstein stressed that a given child could score much higher.

Harper, Richmond, and Snider (1980) compared the degree of physical impairment as it may affect behavior in school in 124 children between the ages of ten and eighteen with cleft palate and cerebral palsy. They were matched for sex, age, IQ, grade level, and socioeconomic status. On the Behavior Problem Checklist, children with cleft palate were described as more impulsive than children with cerebral palsy. This, perhaps, is not surprising if children with cleft palate take longer to develop verbal means of dealing with their world. Mildly impaired children of both groups in the study could inhibit impulses better than those who were severely impaired. This again is not surprising because language impairment is frequent among severely impaired children with cerebral palsy, and both groups could become frustrated if meeting their needs through the usual channels, verbal and physical, was difficult. Feelings of helplessness in carrying out a plan, motorically and verbally, could be another factor in their impulsivity, as could perceived reactions of other people to their physical appearance.

A cleft palate and lip receiving immediate and continuous attention through the formative years can have a very different outcome. Starr (1980) reported no significant differences between attractive and less attractive (based on full face photographs) groups of forty-nine subjects ten years and older on the Children's Behavior Checklist, their ratings of self-esteem, and their attitudes towards clefting. Starr hypothezied that this finding, different from that in many previous studies, may have been due to the good lip repairs the present children had.

Cystic Fibrosis. There are no particular direct cognitive vulnerabilities associated with cystic fibrosis. However, a steady progression in school learning is often difficult because debilitating illness can occur periodically (sometimes requiring hospitalization) and home teaching cannot replicate all that goes on in school, especially in laboratory courses.

Lawler (1966), in a study of eleven children with cystic fibrosis, found that all had average or above average intelligence. Three were in the superior range, six were bright-normal, and two were average. However, most were functioning below these levels in school. Depression (as reflected on the Rorschach) seemed to be a major factor. Another likely contributor, again, is periodic absence from school.

Higher education and specialized vocational training are becoming a reality for children with cystic fibrosis, many of whom are living longer. Adolescents and their families must continue to strive for a balance between respiratory safety and self-actualization. This writer interacted recently with a high school senior who long has been determined to enter the nursing profession and is about to enter college for this purpose. She and her family believe that her desire and commitment outweigh the risks of respiratory infection she will assume if she is in hospitals a large amount of time.

The biggest drawback to success in cognitive pursuits for children with cystic fibrosis would seem to be fatigue, minimal motivation to work toward a future goal, and lack of continuity in educational programming due to periodic and sometimes protracted absences from school.

Congenital Heart Disease. There are some dynamics of congenital heart disease that are important for understanding cognitive functioning. Chazan and others (1951) noted that more intelligent children homebound due to illness might read on their own and improve their performance on a Verbal Scale, whereas slower children who cannot utilize their time this way might fall even further behind. Today, of course, we would assume some kind of educational program is provided for children restricted to their homes, although the quality as well as the number of hours provided may vary. In the study by Chazan and others, there are a disproportionate number of children with IQs below 90, and nine out of forty-three children were below 70. The authors cited loss of schooling, physical fatigue, slower reaction time, poor manipulation of objects, and anxiety as reasons for the lower quotients. If the mother is very anxious about the child's well-being, the above authors noted that she may consciously or unconsciously restrict the child's physical and social mobility, and hence opportunities for experiential learning.

Mothers of twenty-two out of forty-three children in the Chazan study were considered spoiling, overprotective, or neglectful. The mean IQ of their children was 81. The children with the lowest IQs also had the most severe neurotic problems. In twenty-four cases where a grave warning about the child's condition was given to parents, the mean IQ was 85—perhaps, the authors surmised, because of anxiety produced in the parents by these ominous predictions. Again, surgery and medication have reduced some of these situations during the past thirty years. However, when they do occur, it is possible the parents may have reduced their mediated learning experiences for the child because of a pessimistic outlook. Or, they may have lost some of their effectiveness as mediators because the child attributes helplessness to them since they cannot prevent the pain, immobilization, and separation from them.

Chronic heart disease fits Seligman's (1979) concept that situations that produce chronic feelings of helplessness are characterized by lack of predictability and control. Children cannot see a heart defect and can only understand its ramifications by fairly mature cognitive processing.

Too often, we have been quick to blame parents for their anxiety rather than being empathic and helping them deal with it. Their anxieties do go back ultimately to objective fears. Moreover, parents are not always aware of the range of behaviors open to them. Minuchin (1980), Hobbs (1975), and Switzer (1978) have presented constructive strategies for professionals to consider in working with parents of chronically ill children.

The more intelligent children in the study by Chazan and others (1951) often showed a precocious verbosity, possibly due to self-centeredness or to spending much time with adults. They also watched television a great deal.

Linde, Rasof, and Dunn (1967) compared four groups of children: (1) 98 with cardiac malformation, marked cyanosis (blueness from underoxgenation of blood), and physical handicap; (2) 100 with only congenital heart disease; (3) 81 unafflicted siblings closest in age; and (4) 40 unaffected children chosen at random. The mean IQs for the four groups were, respectively, 96.1, 104.4, 119, and 110. The cyanotic children's IQs ranged from 49 to 145. Some were in special schools. During testing, these children showed lower cooperation, less social and self-confidence, a shorter attention span, and less physical activity. These children had experienced a delay in walking but not in talking. They scored lowest of the four groups on tests of early development emphasizing sensory motor tasks. Cyanotic children did better in later years when more verbalization (especially reasoning, concept formation, and recall) was called for. The authors concluded that the intellectual performance of cyanotic children cannot be predicted from early scores. Although cyanotic children remained lower in their scores than noncyanotic children, they did improve. Sociological and sex factors did not account for the differences between groups.

Myers-Vando and others (1979), studying twelve children aged eight to sixteen, found that cardiac illness had a depressive impact on attainment of Piaget's clay and water physical conservation task but not on their conceptualization of illness causality. However, five of twelve children had only mild symptoms and few physical limitations, so real differences between them and the control group can be questioned.

Linde, Rasof, and Dunn (1967) noted higher values of hemotological variables in cyanotic children, suggesting that lower arterial oxygen saturation may be a primary factor in delay in early mental development. But even more plausible, the authors stated, is the possibility of associated physical incapacity of the child leading to curtailment of the types of experience sampled on test items (as suggested by Chazan and others [1951] earlier). Finally, the indirect effects of the child's self-imposed limitations could be as important as parental protectiveness and restriction, especially during the first two years.

Rausch de Traubenberg (1970) also found a deficiency in perceptual and motor functioning in cyanotic children. She, too, hypothesized that, although an organic susceptibility produced by an inadequate blood flow could be responsible, irregular schooling and lack of stimulation had to be considered. Thus, except in extreme cases, physiological factors are probably less important than environmental ones when children with congenital heart disease have cognitive development or school learning problems.

Diabetes. There was a time when it was believed that children with juvenile diabetes might be above average in intelligence (Joslin, 1937; Teagarden, 1939; White, 1932; West, Richey, and Eyre, 1934), in part because they were trying to compensate for their physical illness. McGavin and others (1940) hypothesized that children with diabetes appeared brighter because they were short in stature for their age. Further, they may have seemed mature for their age because people assumed that a certain level of responsibility was required for them to give themselves insulin injections and to weigh food. These writers found an average distribution of intelligence, however. Shirley and Greer (1940) and Boulin and others (1951) reported below average intelligence. Kubany, Danowski, and Moses (1956) found an average distribution of intelligence and no unusual personality abnormalities on the Minnesota Multiphasic Personality Inventory. Bennett and Johannesen (1954) talked about an intellectual constriction and less creativity developing with age in children with diabetes (based on Rorschach responses) but gave no explanation of the dynamics involved.

Selective sampling in particular socioeconomic and educational groups seems to be a major variable responsible for differing results. When these variables are controlled, the distribution of intelligence does not differ significantly from that of children without diabetes, according to Kubany, Danowski, and Moses (1956). Exceptions in the negative direction could be due to deteriorating effects of diabetic coma. In addition, certain dynamics of diabetes can make children vulnerable to poor school performance. For example, general energy level may vary from time to time, and somatic as well as psychological tension may increase as insulin shock or diabetic coma is approached. The uncertainty connected with these latter two possibilities is another factor that could detract from concentration. Further, a general state of dependency, decreasing a child's initiative in academic learning, may develop as a result of being dependent on insulin or of feeling the lack of control over bodily reactions. Today, there is more flexibility in adjusting insulin and diet, but for some children, this is difficult and feelings of helplessness and dependency are strong. In any event, the mother is usually the initial depriving individual as well as the person who may subject a very young child to injections regularly. Her laying the foundations for the child's higher cognitive processes through mediated learning could be difficult because of this negative aspect of her role.

Bruch (1949) noted that diabetes taxes emotional resourcefulness and stability to a high degree. Moreover, children cannot forget for a single day that they have diabetes. Further, it is hard for some children to believe they are not perceived as different by their peers. The peak incidence of onset of juvenile diabetes at age eleven (Travis, 1976) also leads into a vulnerable developmental period for the child in terms of self-concept, identity, and volatile emotions.

Some children with diabetes suffer significant visual loss and must have corrective lenses adjusted regularly. However, it must first be determined whether visual difficulty such as blurring is due to the diabetes going out of control, in which case it should improve when insulin balance is restored (Travis, 1976). An interaction of glandular and developmental upsets can be quite disconcerting to thinking and concentration, especially in adolescence.

In summary, except for possible visual impairment or extreme effects of diabetic coma, any cognitive difficulties experienced by children with diabetes appear to be related to emotional concomitants of the disease. Research indicates that these children's scores on intelligence tests follow a normal distribution when socioeconomic and educational variables are controlled. However, dynamics of the disease can depress school performance at times.

Sickle Cell Anemia. McCormick and others (1975) reported deficits in intelligence in ten- to sixteen-year-old children with sickle cell trait, who are carriers of the anemia but not ill themselves. However, Kramer, Rooks, and Pearson (1978) questioned the research design and, in their own assessment of fifty matched pairs of carrier children three to five years of age on the Peabody Picture Vocabulary Test and the McCarthy Scales of Children's Abilities, found no significant differences in scores. These authors noted that many previous studies did not employ adequate controls for birthweight, age, Apgar scores, and socioeconomic status.

The sudden pain experienced by children who are ill, however, can disrupt cognitive functioning at times. There also can be severe neurological disorders, such as transient or even permanent blindness, convulsion, or coma (Travis, 1976). Although not every pain, respiratory infection, or bout with fatigue requires the child to miss school, teachers must be alert to serious attacks and precipitating causes. Strenuous exercise, body contact sports, exposure to infection, and stress should be avoided. Fatigue sets in easily. Even long school bus rides can contribute to sluggish circulation, especially when children sit with their knees bent, which can result in sickling or an occlusion. Cognitive activities are very important for these children, Travis points out, because they will not be able to work outdoors or in any vocation requiring physical exertion.

Vaughn and Cooke (1979) noted that one of the greatest concerns of parents is absenteeism from school. It is important to begin instruction at home or in hospital immediately, although the primary goal is to avoid the absence in the first place.

Adolescence can be a difficult time for children with sickle cell disease because of delayed sexual development, small size, general fragility, and the uncertainty of survival. Some children do not live beyond the age of twenty. Meeting academic, emotional, and social objectives and setting vocational goals may be difficult, but planning is important.

In summary, the dynamics of sickle cell anemia can generate disruption of various kinds in cognitive learning. Yet success in this area is important because physical activities of these children must be limited.

Hemophilia. Interaction of critical stages of development with episodes of bleeding can be damaging to self-concept and feelings of mastery in boys with hemophilia. The stages of beginning autonomy in preschool years and puberty may be times when the child is particularly vulnerable (Travis, 1976). The teacher of a child with hemophilia must be prepared to act quickly if a bleeding episode occurs. Avoiding strenuous play and contact sports is a necessary precaution. As is true in sickle cell anemia, manual labor for children with a severe type of hemophilia is not possible. The two most common problems for adults with hemophilia are obtaining employment and adequate medical insurance (Demiano, Inman, and Carrigan, 1980). Therefore, a good academic education is vital. Katz (1970) found in a study of adults with hemophilia that 34 percent had not finished school and 6 percent had no public schooling.

Serious bleeding episodes that may lead to long absences from school and even hospitalization should be avoided. Travis (1976) pointed out that in recent years the easier accessibility to cryoprecipitate has helped. But the amount of time a boy will be out of school still varies considerably among individuals. Moreover, repeated bleeding in knee and hip joints can cause orthopedic problems requiring the boy to be on crutches or in a wheelchair for a long period of time. Going up and down stairs can be a problem, as can changing classes when jostling can occur. These children need a reasonable amount of physical exercise because bleeding is less frequent if muscles surrounding the joint are kept strong (Demiano, Inman, and Carrigan, 1980).

Travis (1976) noted that, because of the discontinuity of their educational progress due to frequent absences, boys with hemophilia often have been put in special education classes for which they do not qualify cognitively or emotionally. Children with hemophilia usually have normal to above average intelligence but often are underachievers (Olch, 1971; Katz, 1970). This underachievement could be due not only to absenteeism but also to low expectations and lack of independent cognitive learning skills. A high dependency on the teacher may transfer from the close and dependent relationship with the mother typical in boys with hemophilia.

In summary, it would appear that low academic performance may result from prolonged absences from school due to bleeding crises as well as from a dependent learning style emanating from the usually intense learning relationship the boy has with his mother.

Childhood Leukemia. Sachs (1980) pointed out that major factors in school for children suffering from leukemia are pallor and fatigue, the need for rest periods and snacks, nausea, systemic weakness, and acceptance of the illness by other children and teachers. Also, testing and treatment of leukemia can be frightening or painful. Hair loss frequently affects overall self-image, especially in adolescents. Reactions can include lack of concentration on schoolwork or submersion in academic pursuits to block out and compensate for perceived negative self-image.

Extra help may be needed for the child before and after short absences, although out-of-school instruction should be available if these absences are frequent. Sachs (1980) noted that some researchers have reported school phobia in children with cancer (Futterman and Hoffman, 1970; Lansky and others, 1976). Teachers cannot always accept the symptoms, the poor prognosis, and the kinds of changes that occur in a child with this disease (Kaplan, Smith, and Grobstein, 1974). In these instances, it should not be surprising if the teachers' expectations and manner of instruction were affected.

The psychodynamics and treatment of leukemia periodically involve much pain, both physically and psychologically, as well as great fatigue. Acceptance by peers and success in school are possible with teacher modeling and flexible instructional planning. Teachers themselves need much support to be maximally helpful to children suffering from leukemia.

Spina Bifida. As medical management of spina bifida has improved, so has the opportunity for cognitive development and academic achievement. Surgery and shunts have reduced much negative impact of myeloceles and hydrocephalus on neurological functioning, and some cases of hydrocephalus arrest spontaneously. On the other hand, medical advances have allowed more infants with complicated spina bifidas to survive. Not all past studies controlled for or even acknowledged the importance of education, life experiences, mediated learning, absence from school for illness and surgery, and situational factors affecting performance on intelligence tests as well as cognitive functioning itself.

Tew and Laurence (1975) studied a group of fifty-nine children at the age of five in Great Britain (forty-eight with myelocele, nine with meningocele, and two with encephalocele and congenital hydrocephalus), thirty-one of whom had shunts for hydrocephalus. They found that, although the latter group were the lowest on the Wechsler Preschool and Primary Scale, even those without hydrocephalus had below average scores on this test. Performance IQs were lower than verbal IQs. Scores on tests of visual perception, reading, and spelling followed a similar pattern. Arithmetic scores were the lowest of all.

Anderson and Spain (1977) maintained that most chldren with spina bifida are in the dull-normal or borderline intelligence range, with marked differences depending on the severity of the hydrocephalus. They considered the impression that many children with spina bifida are bright to be due to those children's good verbal fluency, syntax, and memory, although they state that verbal skills generally are less affected by the illness than performance skills. Whether the school curriculum could be responsible for lower performance of these children on many standardized tests is unclear.

Anderson and Spain also reported a high incidence of ocular defects, especially squint, along with poor eye-hand coordination, figure-ground discrimination, detail perception, and fine motor control. Feuerstein's (1979a) deficient cognitive function model may be relevant here because Anderson and Spain noted that poor strategy and impulsivity may have been responsible for poor performance on these tests and that better strategy might be taught. Deprivation of experiences also was cited, with the importance of the preschool years being stressed.

Burns (1967) studied assessment results and school placement in Liverpool, England, of seventy children with varying degrees of severity of spina bifida. Sixty-four were considered educable. Twenty had meningomyelocele and could walk normally; twelve of these were in regular school. Forty-two had lower-limb paralysis of some degree, with forty having meningomyeloceles and two having encephaloceles. All of these children were listed for education in a special school for the physically handicapped. Six of the fourteen children unable to stand in callipers were the ones out of the group of seventy who were considered ineducable. On the Stanford Binet or Merrill Palmer Scales, the range of intelligence quotients was from less than 20 to 148. The average IQ of the sixty-four children for whom school was considered appropriate was 87.2. Twenty-three of these children were able to attend regular school. Thirteen of the fourteen in school at the time were making good progress; the other had a physical problem thought to be emotionally induced. Thirty-eight children with multiple disabilities were recommended for a school for the physically handicapped, one for a school for the educationally subnormal, and one for a school for the blind. Only eight children out of thirty-nine with IQs between fifty and eighty-nine were considered physically fit to attend school at the age of five, as were fifteen of the twenty-five children with IQs from 90 to 120 and above.

Lauder and others (1979) state that one major asset of most children with spina bifida is their intellectual ability, although their average IQs are below those of nonaffected siblings and perceptual and cognitive dysfunction is common. These authors examined educational placement of thirty-eight children with spina bifida in New York State, half of whom had shunts for hydrocephalus, five years after the placement mandate for handicapped children in 1969. Twenty-seven of the children had no learning disabilities. Most of the rural children had been placed in a least restrictive class and had individualized programs, although few specialized services were available. Most city pupils were in regular classes with supplementary service. In suburban areas, the children were less integrated.

For the total group, 60 percent of the thirty-eight children attended regular classes, 34 percent in their own districts; 13 percent were in special education classes full- or part-time; and 21 percent were in regular classes with instruction from a special education resource teacher. The authors stressed the need for more individualized assessment and programming and the importance of the interrelationship between home and family for effective educational programming.

Scherzer and Gardner (1971) of the Cornell University Medical Center evaluated fourteen children with meningomyelocele in the beginning school years. They found eight with intelligence in the low to high average range, three mildly retarded, and three moderately retarded. The median IQ was 88. Social quotients and intelligence quotients were not related to hydrocephalus, which in all but one case had spontaneously arrested, but these quotients correlated well with social class. These authors concluded that, with appropriate interventions, many children with meningomyeloceles can develop the intellectual capacity to master major cognitive and social tasks. Scherzer and Gardner noted that hydrocephalus may have a predictable negative effect only in the more severe cases requiring surgery.

The average intelligence quotient, then, of children with spina bifida is below average. On the whole, status of the hydrocephalus does seem to be a factor in the differing results of various studies, but education and experience also affect these children's performance on standardized tests. Many specific cognitive functions can be affected in spina bifida, and there is great variation in individual children's physical, cognitive, and educational strengths and weaknesses. An intelligence quotient that represents an average of performance in various ability measures may be of dubious value for an individual child. Similarly, the average IQ of a group of children with spina bifida will be depressed by extremely low scores of children who have severe neurological dysfunction. Individual assessment and programming are very important.

Duchenne's Muscular Dystrophy. This writer has challenged the theoretical assumptions and research procedures leading to the long-held position that below-average intellectual potential is an integral part of Duchenne's muscular dystrophy (Mearig, 1979), a disease for which the etiology has yet to be identified. The variation in explanations for below-average intelligence in these children suggests a lack of convincing evidence for any inherent relationship. The assumption that intelligence test scores imply a genetic deficit is also unwarranted. Particularly questionable is the hypothesis that a verbal deficit is to be expected. Marsh and Munsat (1974) and Karagan and Zellweger (1978) are some of the more recent investigators to support this hypothesis, based on Wechsler Intelligence Scale scores and class placement in school.

Marsh and Munsat (1974, p. 121) offered the following generalization: "Partial corroborative evidence of a generalized intellectual deficit may be inferred from the fact that 23 of 34 dystrophics studied were placed in school classes below those of their age-related peers." However, cause and effect are difficult to separate here, especially given the low expectations some school systems have had for these boys and the role that standardized test scores usually play in placement decisions.

Moreover, few studies in earlier years considered the inappropriateness of administering standardized assessment instruments to these boys in light of their frequent shyness and anxiety in new psychological situations. Timing also was poor if intelligence scales were administered in a clinic setting after blood and other tests were done and in the atmosphere of the boys' progress and prognosis being discussed with parents.

Prosser, Murphy, and Thompson (1969), Rossman and Kakulas (1966), and Sherwin and McCully (1961) found no significant differences in verbal and performance scores on the Wechsler. In fact, the latter two authors considered the verbal IQ to be a more valid indicator of intellectual potential. Marsh and Munsat (1974, p. 121) argued that "the verbal deficit in Duchenne's muscular dystrophy appears to be a relatively generalized one that interferes with verbal subtests measuring fund of general information, practical knowledge and judgment, verbal abstract thinking, expressive vocabulary, mentally calculated arithmetic problems, and rote learning." Yet, this statement is merely a listing of what each Wechsler Intelligence Scale for Children verbal subtest is purported to measure. If Marsh and Munsat's (1974) and Karagan's (1979) conclusions that a genetically or central nervous system–induced deficit in verbal function is seriously to be considered, careful studies of children's *earliest* language development are in order.

Champanay, Lieters, and Lachanat (1980) reported lower verbal than performance functioning on intelligence tests and stated that the greater the degree of scholarly or verbal content in the test, the lower the mean intelligence quotient will be. However, these authors went on to say that often there is a fall in interest shown in intellectual or scholarly activities when walking stops. But eventually the child can recover these interests if his parents and the people in his environment also show interest in intellectual and scholarly activities. The child can become stabilized if he is striving toward a goal and has something to do that he will be able to continue to do for a long time.

The present writer, in a study of eighty-five boys with Duchenne's dystrophy in three kinds of educational settings in rural, urban, and suburban areas, did not find the lower intelligence test scores reported by most other researchers on the Wechsler Intelligence Scales (Mearig, 1979). All IQs except the full scale and performance ones for the urban sample were within the average range of intelligence. When tests other than the Wechsler were included, these two IQs also fell at the lower end of the average range. Also, the rural and suburban verbal (98.16 and 97.98) and full scale IQs (96.13 and 94.56) were significantly higher than those reported by Marsh and Munsat (1974). They reported verbal IQs of 85.31 and 87.55 for mild and moderately to markedly impaired boys, respectively, and 90.37 and 87.44 for the full scale IQs.

The nearness to 100 of the rural and suburban mean verbal IQs in the writer's sample does not support the verbal deficit that Marsh and Munsat cite. The lower verbal IQ (90.17) for the urban sample is still higher than theirs and perhaps can be explained by some very low scores of children who exhibited learning disabilities having no known connection to the dystrophy. Otherwise, the educational program in this public school for physically handicapped children might be a factor because the staff had to teach children with a wide range of handicaps. The children in the rural sample went to a variety of public schools in which all but a few of the boys with muscular dystrophy were mainstreamed. Those in the suburban sample attended an independent though partially publicly funded school for physically handicapped children with a strong academic curriculum. Thus, many dimensions must be considered in evaluating intellectual potential and cognitive functioning in boys with Duchenne's dystrophy. In addition to educational programming and expectancy, there may be a developmental or psychodynamic explanation related to the growing helplessness and short life span for any deficits that do exist.

School is important for these boys. Besides maximal development of the one aspect of their functioning this writer believes is not affected by the dystrophy, the structure and concentration required in academic work mean the boys are less likely to become overwhelmed by thinking about the prognosis of the dystrophy. In addition, school is often the only opportunity for these boys to develop social relationships outside their families. Finally, exposure to many other children in school keeps up the boys' resistance to respiratory infections that could otherwise lead to pneumonia and death. With good preventive and crisis care, a number of boys now live well into their twenties, and some go to college or obtain employment. A major chore for involved families every morning is to get these boys ready for school, and having to dress for cold weather complicates matters. Although schools are obligated to transport these children, the exact time of their arrival for classes does not seem to be specified. Sometimes they arrive late because the van cannot start early enough to pick everyone up in time for the opening of school. Stairs are a barrier for boys in wheelchairs, so all classes must be arranged on the first floor or an elevator must be available. Arrangements have to be made for toileting the boys during school, something friends often are willing to help do. However, many boys use a bottle successfully and otherwise wait until they return home in the afternoon.

Needless to say, children who are kept upright and mobile enjoy a different learning environment and have decreased physical complications, such as weight gain, constricted or congested chests, curved backs, and pressure sores. Having observed almost a whole school population of boys with muscular dystrophy walking with braces, after surgery, for three to seven years longer than usual, this writer concludes that the medical outlay and intensive exercises necessary following surgery are well worth the effort in terms of both the physical well-being and cognitive development of these boys.

Common Dynamics of Serious Chronic Illnesses Affecting Cognitive Development

Discussed in turn are eight dynamics of serious chronic illness that can significantly affect the pattern of cognitive development: reactions of other people to the physical appearance of children with certain chronic illnesses, high energy expenditure, disruptions in developmental sequences, mediated learning difficulties, deprivation of a past-present-future perspective, the egocentric nature of verbalization, minimal need of generalization and abstraction, and barriers to acquisition of control over one's own life. The latter three are closely related and are discussed as a group.

Reactions of Other People. Reactions of other people to the physical appearance of children with certain chronic illnesses can retard cognitive development. Self-concept, identity, expectancy, and learning opportunities are important intervening variables in this process. Actual behavior of the child is obviously important in the reactions of others, but so are more static physical characteristics. Examples are Duchenne's dystrophy, spina bifida, and severe cleft palate. Whatever the rationale, some people assume that cognitive impairment automatically accompanies these physical disabilities.

High Energy Expenditure. A straightforward but often overlooked dimension in chronically ill children's cognitive functioning and school performance is energy expenditure. A chronically ill child must cope daily with physiological aspects of the illness, making necessary and time-consuming adaptations, adjusting to new or exacerbated symptoms, and dealing with anxiety in anticipation of the next stage of the illness—possibly even death. There is only a certain amount of energy remaining for cognitive pursuits.

Disruptions in Developmental Sequences. Palmer (1970, p. 23) pointed out, "Although diseases and injuries may be devasting at any time in the child's life, it is important in an assessment to note the ages at which the child suffers such trauma. There may be more psychological injury, for example, just when the child is learning to walk or talk, or the year he enters school, or at puberty." Late adolescence, when one's identity is being stabilized and plans for adulthood made, is another crucial stage. And certainly occurrences such as the birth of a sibling or a divorce could be times of vulnerability. Moreover, Pope-Grattan, Burnett, and Wolfe (1976) suggested from their study of human figure drawings by children with Duchenne's dystrophy that a child in a transitional stage of the disease may feel more insecure than when definitely in one stage or another.

Erikson's (1950) developmental stages demonstrate the interaction of biological, psychological, and sociological components of development and are useful in understanding how cognitive development can be disrupted by chronic illness. Kessler (1966) also has elucidated how all aspects of development are interwoven. For example, disruption in psychological equilibrium can occur in the boy with Duchenne's dystrophy around the age of five if Erikson's locomotor stage (when the boy often begins to feel a deterioration of recently acquired gross motor control), initial exposure to formal school expectations, and separation from family every day all come together in time.

Piaget (1954) stressed the orderly progression of the development of intelligence beginning with direct experiencing of the environment during the sensory-motor stage. This is followed by the preoperational stage, the one often disturbed in the early stages of Duchenne's dystrophy. Schorer (1954) noted that, if physical movement is hindered at any age when the transfer from physical to symbolic manipulation should occur, the transfer may take place awkwardly and result in impaired intelligence.

The transition to a daily existence in a wheelchair can be another time of ego crisis for a physically disabled child. Next, the emotional vulnerability of adolescence with concerns about sexuality, identity, and independence can be intensified for boys and girls with a debilitating or fatal illness. A poor self-concept, loss of control over one's physical functioning as well as over the environment, awareness of early death, and increasing dependency upon parents—especially boys upon mothers when peers are becoming more independent and finding other females with whom to develop a relationship—all these interfere with concentration and consume energy.

Mediated Learning Difficulties. Lemkau (1981, p. 4) stated, "If there is interference with stimulation, unbalanced stimulation, or insufficient stimulation at the internal level which is severe enough during a critical developmental period, failure to develop the function of integration might result, so the child has less meaning to give subsequent experiences though the brain has many functional connections." Feuerstein's concept of mediated learning experience (MLE) may explain how this meaning is acquired. For Feuerstein (1979b), exposure to stimulation is not enough: "Mediated learning experience allows the development of the prerequisite cognitive schemata to enable an individual to derive maximum benefit from direct exposure to sources of stimulation" (p. 19). "An interaction that provides mediated learning must include an intention on the part of the mediator to transcend the immediate needs and concerns of the recipient of the mediation by venturing beyond the here and now, in space and time. Indeed, it is the intentional nature of the interaction that is the defining characteristic of a mediated interaction" (p. 20).

Let us examine why chronically ill children may not receive this kind of MLE. First, if parents are informed in conjunction with a diagnosis in infancy that their children's learning potential or life expectancy is limited, they may not provide the kinds of verbal and nonverbal MLE that can lead to the capacity to utilize maximally all incoming stimulation. On the other hand, some parents identify too closely with their seriously ill children because of guilt, sorrow, or simply having very close interaction with them. If so, effective MLE will be difficult to provide because a certain amount of emotional detachment is required to lead these children gradually into new learning experiences that will result in becoming more independent learners. Moreover, it is not easy to organize increasingly difficult tasks in which children can succeed when the course of the illness takes them in the opposite direction. Teachers in school can be affected by the same dynamics and expectations.

There is a pragmatic reason why a child with a serious chronic illness may receive less MLE, a reason similar to that for a socioeconomically deprived child or one with many siblings. (Needless to say, if all three of these conditions exist, providing MLE is an extraordinary challenge.) The parents are kept busy focusing on the most basic needs, and for a chronically ill child these can be considerable. Just getting through the day can be exhausting, so there is very little time or energy left for MLE. Someone else is needed to help with one or the other of these responsibilities.

Next, children who regularly experience painful or frightening hospitalization from an early age can easily have their mediated learning experience disrupted, not only because of what may be perceived as desertion by parents but also because hospital personnel may do little MLE at all. In fact, events in the hospital (some causing pain) may seem to the child to have no logic or predictability because previous experiences are usually not applicable.

Whether or not in a hospital, young children with serious chronic illness may be late in establishing logical cause-effect relationships. They may not comprehend what caused their illness and what periodically precipitates specific symptoms. Or they may wonder how they have been "bad" enough to bring about this "punishment" (Bergmann and Freud, 1965). The combination of not being able to understand or control what is happening to them physically and also suspecting that they have done something bad to bring it about, can make children feel helpless, guilty, and insecure.

Parents naturally may develop a pattern of reassuring these children that they are "good" in spite of the "bad" things (chronic illness and its treatment) that are happening to them. Such reassurance is desirable for emotional security because essentially these children are asking, "In spite of my physical weaknesses (flaws), am I good enough to be loved?" The children, in turn, may seek extra reassurance from parents every time they dare initiate a new activity, asking, in essence, "Is what I am doing good or bad?"

Thus, when later instructed in reasoning tasks involving generalization and abstraction, some children at first may not even be able to focus on the critical elements of the problem. Rather, they want to approach a solution in terms of its goodness or badness, being most concerned with how the adult, especially a new one, will react. The objective correctness of an answer holds little reinforcement for them.

Deprivation of a Past–Present–Future Perspective. Feuerstein's (1979a) concept of cultural deprivation is also relevant for understanding cognitive development in chronically ill children. His concept is not the same as the one used in the United States, which implies socioeconomic deprivation; rather, he is talking about children being deprived of their cultural heritage. Parents with whom he worked in Israel had experienced a major disruption in their cultural identity and were often unsure of their future, to the extent that they could not adequately transmit their culture to their children. In some cases, they did not think the culture was worth transmitting. But in Feuerstein's cognitive development framework, this link between past, present, and future is very important. If culturally deprived children do not experience this intergenerational continuity, their sense of one event leading to the next and, thus, development of their higher cognitive processes can be inhibited.

In the case of the chronically ill child, the parents may not transmit a cultural or family generational continuity because they have been told the child's future is very limited. They also may not see this child as capable of transmitting their heritage because they have been conditioned by family and the larger world to believe the child cannot fill this role. Moreover, the past–present–future relationship within the child's life may be given a different connotation by the parents.

Three Processes in Cognitive Functioning. The past–present–future perspective leads into three interrelated processes in cognitive functioning: the egocentric nature of verbalization, minimal need for generalization and abstraction, and barriers to acquisition of control over one's own life.

Any skill, cognitive or otherwise, usually shows substantial improvement only when there exist motivation and opportunity to practice it. In the case of some chronically ill children, these conditions are not met. For example, some clearly nonretarded boys with muscular dystrophy have trouble expressing themselves fluently, particularly when sequencing or conveying objective information of any complexity. It seems that, because of physical discomfort and dependency, many of these boys' verbalizations remain basically emotive and egocentric. They may practice little of what Watzlawick, Beavin, and Jackson (1967) designated as the denotive or objective level of communication except when specifically required to do so, as in school. The emotive nature of many communications can also be part of the self-centeredness these boys may retain. This can be due to protracted anxiety about physiological changes of which they are not in control as well as the inability to participate in many group activities that would make them naturally more other-directed. Boys with muscular dystrophy can be slower in developing denotive verbalization particularly because overt symptoms of the disease often appear around the age of four or five, when this level of communication is only rudimentarily established. If the boys must compete for attention with brothers with muscular dystrophy and other siblings, the emotive quality of verbalization could be pronounced.

Children with a debilitating or fatal chronic illness might also be slower in developing generalization and abstraction abilities. Meng (1938) described the effects of a poor body image on these functions. In addition, there may not be any great need to generalize and abstract, so the child will have little practice. Two factors seem to be involved. The first is the reality that in everyday functioning the child with a deteriorating condition can have a difficult time moving from a concrete level, spending considerable time dealing with immediate problems or crises. Contrary to what usually occurs with increasing age, opportunities lessen for making decisions based on generalizations of past experiences and for predicting an outcome, both functions involving abstraction.

These children have diminishing control over what will be done each day, as well as over the future. In fact, they may know they have no long-term future. Moreover, they become increasingly dependent on someone else for execution of the decisions they are able to make in their lives. Thus, there is little motivation to practice the extraction of critical meanings or commonalities from experiences or to predict in the sense of managing present behaviors to reach future goals. As a result, the ability to abstract suffers. This will be especially true if, as indicated earlier, parents and teachers share a pessimistic view of the future that causes their manner of teaching not to be one productive of good mediated learning experiences.

Finally, beyond the initial stages of abstraction, we usually come to rely on verbal handles. If disabled children's verbalization remains egocentric and emotive longer than usual because they utilize it mainly to get immediate needs met by other people, they may be slower in developing abstract verbal concepts. Thus, three components—emotive and egocentric language, nonabstract cognitive functioning, and increased dependency—complement and reinforce one another.

Not all children with serious chronic illness have all these difficulties. Many, in fact, develop both a constructive perspective and effective coping techniques with the help of steadily maturing higher cognitive functions nurtured by a supportive environment. The hope is that sensitivity on the part of professionals, parents, and society to the possibility of problems will bring about conditions that will prevent or at least help children compensate for their vulnerabilities.

Conclusion

Society should have a commitment to provide the best possible care for chronically ill children who cannot develop cognitively to a level enabling them to care for themselves. This commitment is based on a moral value of the intrinsic worth of every human being and cannot be negated by economic considerations.

However, it would appear that the majority of chronically ill children who live into adulthoood can develop cognitively to at least a self-sustaining level, given good mediated learning experience, high enough expectations, a holistic assessment of their individual learning dynamics and an understanding of these dynamics by significant adults in their lives, an individualized education program that has academic integrity and continuity, and a support system for themselves and their families in the many dimensions of their lives that affect cognitive development and school learning. If increased independence of functioning is the result, national economic interests can only be served by investing fully in chronically ill children's cognitive development. The first step is for public policy to make this commitment.

References

Anderson, E., and Spain, B. *The Child with Spina Bifida*. Hampshire, England: Methuen, 1977.

Bakwin, H., and Bakwin, R. "The Child with Asthma." *Journal of Pediatrics,* 1948, *32,* 320-323.

Bennett, E., and Johannesen, C. "Psychodynamics of the Diabetic Child." *Psychological Monographs,* 1954, *68,* 1-23.

Bergmann, T., and Freud, A. *Children in Hospital*. New York: International Universities Press, 1965.

Bhat, B., and others. "Study of Social, Educational, Environmental, and Cultural Aspects of Childhood Asthma in Clinic and Private Patients in the City of New York." *Annals of Allergy,* 1978, *41*, 89–92.

Boulin, R., and others. "The Mental and Affective Development of the Diabetic Child." *Exerpta Medica Pediatrica,* 1951, *5*, 15.

Bruch, H. "Physiologic and Psychologic Interrelationships in Diabetic Children." *Psychosomatic Medicine,* 1949, *11*, 200–210.

Burns, R. "The Assessment of School Placement in Children Suffering from Encephalocele and Meningomyelocele in the City of Liverpool." *Developmental Medicine and Child Neurology* 1967, *13* (Supplement), 23–29.

Champanay, A. M., Lieters, J., and Lachanat, J. "Les Myopathes Duchenne de Boulogne: Intelligence et Scolarité" [Duchenne's Muscular Dystrophy: Intelligence and School Performance]. *Journal de Neuropsychiatrie de l'Enfance et de l'Adolescent* [Journal of Neuropsychiatry of Children and Adolescents], 1980, *28* (2), 539–546.

Chazan, M., and others. "The Intellectual and Emotional Development of Children with Congenital Heart Disease." *Guy's Hospital Reports,* 1951, *100* (4), 331–341.

Creak, M., and Stephen, J. "The Psychological Aspects of Asthma in Children." *Pediatric Clinics of North America,* 1958, *5* (3), 731–747.

Creer, T., and Yoches, C. "The Modification of an Inappropriate Behavior Pattern in Asthmatic Children." *Journal of Chronic Diseases,* 1977, *24*, 507–513.

Demiano, M., Inman, M., and Carrigan, J. "Hemophilia: The Role of the School Nurse." *Journal of School Health,* 1980, *50*, 451–454.

Dunleavy, R. "Neuropsychological Correlates of Asthma: Effect of Hypoxia or Drugs?" *Journal of Clinical and Consulting Psychology,* 1981, *49*, 135–136.

Dunleavy, R., and Baade, L. "Neuropsychological Correlates of Severe Asthma in Children 9–14 Years Old." *Journal of Consulting and Clinical Psychology,* 1980, *48*, 214–219.

Erikson, E. *Childhood and Society.* New York: Norton, 1950.

Feuerstein, R. *The Dynamic Assessment of Retarded Performers: The Learning Potential Assessment Device, Theory, Instruments, and Techniques.* Baltimore: University Park Press, 1979a.

Feuerstein, R. *Instrumental Enrichment: An Intervention Program for Cognitive Modifiability.* Baltimore: University Park Press, 1979b.

Freudenberg, N. "The Impact of Bronchial Asthma on School Attendance and Performance." *Journal of School Health,* 1980, *50*, 522–526.

Futterman, E., and Hoffman, I. "Transient School Phobia in a Leukemic Child." *Journal of American Academy of Child Psychiatry,* 1970, *9*, 477–493.

Goodstein, L. "Psychological Aspects of Cleft Palate." In D. Spriestersbach and D. Sherman (Eds.). *Cleft Palate and Communication.* New York: Academic Press, 1968.

Harper, D., Richman, L., and Snider, B. "School Adjustment and Degrees of Physical Impairment." *Journal of Pediatric Psychology,* 1980, *5* (4), 377–383.

Hobbs, N. *The Futures of Children: Recommendations of the Project on Classification of Exceptional Children.* San Francisco: Jossey-Bass, 1975.

Isaacs, J., and McElroy, M. "Psycho-Social Aspects of Chronic Illness in Children." *Journal of School Health,* 1980, *50,* 318–321.

Joslin, E. *Treatment of Diabetes Mellitus.* (6th ed.) Philadelphia: Lea and Febiger, 1937.

Kaplan, D., Smith, A., and Grobstein, R. "School Management of the Seriously Ill Child." *Journal of School Health,* 1974, *44,* 250–254.

Karagan, N. "Intellectual Functioning in Duchenne Muscular Dystrophy: A Review." *Psychology Review,* 1979, *86* (2), 250–259.

Karagan, N., and Zellweger, H. "Early Verbal Disability in Children with Duchenne Muscular Dystrophy." *Developmental Medicine and Child Neurology,* 1978, *20,* 435–441.

Katz, A. *Hemophilia: A Study in Hope and Reality.* Springfield, Ill.: Thomas, 1970.

Kessler, J. W. *Psychopathology of Childhood.* Englewood Cliffs, N.J.: Prentice-Hall, 1966.

Kramer, M., Rooks, Y., and Pearson, H. "Growth and Development in Children with Sickle-Cell Trait: A Prospective Study of Matched Pairs." *New England Journal of Medicine,* 1978, *299* (13), 686–689.

Kubany, A., Danowski, T., and Moses, C. "The Personality and Intelligence of Diabetics." *Diabetes,* 1956, *5,* 462–467.

Lambert, N. (Consulting ed.). *Special Educational Assessment Matrix.* New York: McGraw-Hill, 1980.

Lansky, S., and others. "A Team Approach to Coping with Cancer: The Behavioral Dimension." In M. Sachs, "Helping the Child with Cancer Go Back to School." *Journal of School Health,* 1980, *50,* 328–331.

Lauder, C., and others. "Educational Placement of Children with Spina Bifida." *Exceptional Children,* 1979, *45,* 432–437.

Lawler, R. "Psychological Implications of Cystic Fibrosis." *Canadian Medical Association Journal,* 1966, *94,* 1044–1048.

Lemkau, P. "Influence of Handicapping Conditions on Child Development." *Children,* 1981, *8,* 43–47.

Linde, L., Rasof, B., and Dunn, D. J. "Mental Development in Congenital Heart Disease." *Journal of Pediatrics,* 1967, *71* (2), 198–203.

McCormick, M. K., and others. "A Comparison of the Physical and Intellectual Development of Black Children with and Without Sickle-Cell Trait." *Pediatrics,* 1975, *56,* 1021–1025.

McGavin, A., and others. "The Physical Growth, Degree of Intelligence, and the Personality Adjustment of a Group of Diabetic Children." *New England Journal of Medicine,* 1940, *223,* 119–127.

Marsh, G., and Munsat, T. "Evidence for Early Impairment of Verbal Intelligence in Duchenne Muscular Dystrophy." *Archives of Diseases in Childhood,* 1974, *49,* 118–122.

Mearig, J. "The Assessment of Intelligence in Boys with Duchenne Muscular Dystrophy." *Rehabilitation Literature,* 1979, *40,* 262–274.

Meng, H. "Zur Socialpsychologie der Körperbeschädigten" [On the Social Psychology of the Handicapped]. *Schweizer Archiv für Neurologie und Psychiatrie* [Swiss Archives of Neurology and Psychiatry], 1938, *40,* 328–344. As cited by F. P. Conner, H. Rusalem, and W. M. Cruickshank, "Psychological Considerations with Crippled Children," in W. M. Cruickshank (Ed.), *Psychology of Exceptional Children and Youth.* (3d ed.) Englewood Cliffs, N.J.: Prentice-Hall, 1971.

Minuchin, S. "Structural Family Therapy: Activating Alternatives Within a Therapeutic System." In N. J. Long, W. C. Morse, and R. G. Newman (Eds.), *Conflict in the Classroom.* (4th ed.) Belmont, Calif.: Wadsworth, 1980.

Mitchell, R., and Dawson, B. "Educational and Social Characteristics of Children with Asthma." *Archives of Diseases in Childhood,* 1973, *48,* 467–471.

Myers-Vando, R., and others. "The Effects of Congenital Heart Disease on Cognitive Development, Illness Causality Concepts, and Vulnerability." *American Journal of Orthopsychiatry,* 1979, *49* (4), 617–625.

Olch, D. "Effects of Hemophilia upon Intellectual Growth and Academic Achievement." *Journal of Genetic Psychology,* 1971, *119,* 63–74.

Palmer, J. *The Psychological Assessment of Children.* New York: Wiley, 1970.

Parker, G., and Lipsombe, P. "Parental Overprotection and Asthma." *Journal of Psychosomatic Research,* 1949, *23* (5), 295–299.

Piaget, J. *The Construction of Reality in the Child.* New York: Basic Books, 1954.

Pope-Grattan, M., Burnett, C., and Wolfe, C. "Human Figure Drawing by Children with Duchenne Muscular Dystrophy." *Physical Therapy,* 1976, *56* (2), 168–176.

Prosser, E., Murphy, E., and Thompson, M. "Intelligence and the Gene for Duchenne Muscular Dystrophy." *Archives of Diseases in Childhood,* 1969, *44* (234), 221–230.

Rausch de Traubenberg, N. "Psychological Aspects of Congenital Heart Disease." In E. J. Anthony and C. Koupernik (Eds.), *The Child in His Family.* Vol. 2. New York: Wiley, 1970.

Richman, L. "Cognitive Patterns and Learning Disabilities in Cleft Palate Children with Verbal Deficits." *Journal of Speech and Hearing Research,* 1980, *23,* 447–456.

Rossman, N., and Kakulas, B. "Mental Deficiency Associated with Muscular Dystrophy: A Neurological Study." *Brain,* 1966, *89,* 769–787.

Sachs, M. "Helping the Child with Cancer Go Back to School." *Journal of School Health,* 1980, *50,* 328–331.

Scherzer, A., and Gardner, G. "Studies of the School Age Child with Meningomyelocele: Physical and Intellectual Development." *Journal of Pediatrics,* 1971, *47,* 424–430.

Schorer, C. "Muscular Dystrophy and the Mind." *Psychomatic Medicine,* 1954, *26* (1), 5–13.

Seligman, M. *Helplessness.* New York: W. H. Freeman, 1975.

Shapiro, H. "Society, Ideology, and the Reform of Special Education: A Study in the Limits of Educational Change." Paper presented at the American Orthopsychiatric Association Annual Meeting, New York, 1981.

Sherwin, C., and McCully, R. "Reactions Observed in Boys of Various Ages (10 to 14) to a Crippling, Progressive, and Fatal Illness (Muscular Dystrophy)." *Journal of Chronic Diseases*, 1961, *13* (1), 59–68.

Shirley, H., and Greer, I. "Environmental and Personality Problems in the Treatment of Diabetic Children." *Journal of Pediatrics*, 1940, *16*, 775–781.

Smith, R., and McWilliams, B. "Psycholinguistic Abilities of Children with Clefts." *Cleft Palate Journal*, 1968, *5*, 238–249.

Snyder, L., Apolloni, T., and Cooke, T. "Integrated Settings at the Early Childhood Level: The Role of Nonretarded Peers." *Exceptional Children*, 1979, *14*, 262–266.

Starr, P. "Facial Attractiveness and Behavior of Patients with Cleft Lip and/or Palate." *Psychological Reports*, 1980, *46* (2), 579–582.

Strunk, R., and Boyd, J. "The Student with Asthma." *Today's Education*, Nov.-Dec., 1980, pp. 64–67.

Suess, W., and Chai, H. "Neuropsychological Correlates of Asthma: Brain Damage or Drug Effects?" *Journal of Consulting and Clinical Psychology*, 1981, *49* (1), 135–136.

Switzer, R. "Perspective of Parents of Disabled Children." In J. S. Mearig and Associates, *Working for Children: Ethical Issues Beyond Professional Guidelines*. San Francisco: Jossey-Bass, 1978.

Teagarden, F. "The Intelligence of Diabetic Children with Some Case Reports." *Journal of Applied Psychology*, 1939, *23*, 337–346.

Tew, B., and Laurence, K. "The Effects of Hydrocephalus on Intelligence, Visual Perception, and School Attainment." *Developmental Medicine and Child Neurology*, 1975, *17*, 129–134.

Travis, G. *Chronic Illness in Children: Its Impact on Child and Family*. Stanford, Calif.: Stanford University Press, 1976.

Vaughn, W., and Cooke, D. "Help for Students with Sickle-Cell Disease." *Journal of School Health*, 1979, *49*, 414.

Watzlawick, P., Beavin, J., and Jackson, D. *Pragmatics of Human Communication*. New York: Norton, 1967.

West, H., Richey, A., and Eyre, W. "The Study of Intelligence Levels of Juvenile Diabetics." *Psychology Bulletin*, 1934, *31*, 598.

White, P. "Diabetes in Childhood." In E. Joslin, *The Treatment of Diabetes Mellitus*. Philadelphia: Lea and Febiger, 1932.

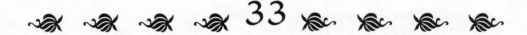

33

Psychosocial Development of Chronically Ill Children

Phyllis R. Magrab, Ph.D.

The care of a child with a chronic or disabling illness represents a challenge to the family, health care professionals, and the entire service delivery system. The posture we as members of a society take regarding the well-being of these children and their families determines the quality of comprehensive care we make available, the public and private resources we allocate for their care, and the nature and availability of service providers.

Individuals who would design public policy to meet the needs of chronically ill children and their families must integrate two major conceptual frameworks—an ecological model and a developmental approach. Such an integration will permit an understanding of the evolving needs of both the child and the family through the various life-cycle stages. Although this chapter focuses on the developmental perspective, the relationship of the chronically ill child to the immediate environment (the ecology) is integrally related to this approach. The socialization of a child consists primarily of a developmental phenomenon involving transactions between the maturing child and the impinging environment. The life of every child is shaped by transactions among the child and parents, extended family, caregivers, and friends and is influenced by the external environment and the interaction of events as they relate to each of these spheres.

Kagan (1971) proposes a model of psychological development in children, suggesting that the process of socialization is accomplished through four basic mechanisms: the desire for affection and positive regard, the fear of punishment or rejection, the desire to identify with respected and admired persons, and a general tendency to imitate the actions of others. This socialization process is interdependent with the responses of the family and others in the environment to the child's socialization needs. The intervention of a chronic illness alters the normal socialization process through its effects on both the child and the family.

The structure of the family, the parameters of the illness, and the developmental needs of the child all interact, determining the effectiveness of the family's ability to cope, and manner of doing so, and the transaction between the child and the family in the ongoing socialization process. The ability of the family to respond to the emotional and the physical needs of a chronically ill child is determined in large part by the level of stress and the family's ability to cope with that stress. The existing relationships within the family, the family's stability, and the family's broad network of support affect its role in the socialization process of the chronically ill child. The nature of different illnesses creates burdens of varying levels of intensity for the family including such financial burdens as the expense of blood plasma to people with hemophilia; such housing adaptations as those needed by people with spina bifida and muscular dystrophy; such physical demands as lifting, dressing, feeding, and extra housecleaning encountered by people with cystic fibrosis, asthma, and spinal cord damage; and such disruptions in family routines as special dietary planning needed by children with renal disease and diabetes. These burdens influence the family's ability to cope with the needs of the affected child.

Talbot and Howell (1971) succinctly summarize the major reactions a family may have to a child with a chronic illness. These include:

Parental disappointment, shame, or guilt

Parental resentment or anger over the burden

Parental anxiety leading to overprotectiveness, overrestrictiveness, overindulgent care

Overconcentration of attention on the sick child resulting in underattention to needs of other family members, fatigue, depression, and family impoverishment

Distortion of family life with respect to where to live and what to do

Sibling resentment of the sick child as the recipient of special and favored attention; also shame caused by having an abnormal sibling

Sibling vulnerability with respect to parental transference of overprotective attitudes and practices to them, and if the sick child is not expected to live, grief and depression in anticipation of the outcome

These family reactions will affect the socialization process of the chronically ill or disabled child in ways that vary with the child's age. Unfortunately, the overall impact of a chronically ill child on a family system is usually more disintegrative than integrative, disrupting the lives of all the family members and exacerbating the developmental risks to the child.

Consideration of the ecological model reveals that the network of extended family and friends comprises a key resource for the reduction of burdens and stresses on the immediate family. Individuals within the network can provide emotional support, assist with daily life activities, and attend to needs of other family members. Identification of such sources of support and assistance should be an integral part of health care planning. Creative health care planners could develop fiscal resources for items as simple as the provision of transportation for significant others who assist in caregiving or the provision of payment to relatives who provide care. Means for effective and systematic incorporation of the participation of extended family and friends in the care of the chronically ill child should be guided by consideration of the developmental needs of the child. As the needs of the child vary from one developmental stage to another, so will the needs of the family.

The quality and availability of comprehensive health, social, and educational services will have a potent impact on the effect of the broad external environment on the socialization of chronically ill children. The fragmentation of services and the lack of coordinated care available to this group of children continue to be significant problems. A system providing continuity of care throughout the life cycle of these individuals has not been developed. Treatment plans rarely incorporate appropriate responses to young children's needs to resolve their feelings of guilt around their illness or adolescents' needs to continue their bids for independence. Children's perceptions of their illness, and the adaptations that they make, evolve out of the characteristics of the illness itself, available environmental supports, and their own intrinsic developmental, psychological, and social capabilities. Thus, to plan for life-cycle care of chronically ill children, health care planners must be sensitive to the interaction between chronic illness and developmental needs.

A Developmental Overview and Chronic Illness

The child is a changing, growing organism moving on a psychological continuum toward increasing independence and cognitive capacity. Development proceeds, by and large, in an orderly, sequential, and cumulative manner leading to increased skill and mastery of the environment. Nonetheless, the child remains vulnerable at each stage of development to the interaction of external stress with the developmental process. Stubblefield (1974) points out that mastery of frustrations and disappointments normally occurring during the various developmental periods is dependent on children's expectations and hopes that they will grow older, stronger, and better able to solve problems. The doubt chronic illness casts on these expectations may significantly disrupt the course of development.

Hughes (1976) suggests that the course of chronic illness challenges eight basic emotional needs of children: (1) love and affection, (2) security, (3) acceptance as an individual, (4) self-respect, (5) achievement, (6) recognition, (7) independence, and (8) authority and discipline. Each of these takes on a special meaning at the various stages of development of the child and with respect to the special features of the existing medical condition. Restrictions in daily activities, interpersonal communication, education, and plans for career and marriage are concrete features of particular illnesses that have major effects on the developmental process (Talbot and Howell, 1971).

A developmental framework, helpful in understanding children's perceptions of and reactions to chronic illness, consists of developmental stages influenced by psychosocial and cognitive determinants. The works of Erikson and Piaget are useful in providing such a framework. Basically, children move along a continuum of psychological growth from trust and complete dependency to growing autonomy, mastery, and a secure sense of self. Cognitively, children develop an understanding of abstract concepts and of normal reasoning through stages of primitive logic and concrete thinking. The particular stage of development of children has an enormous impact on the way they cope with illness or disability. Table 1 summarizes, for each of five age levels from infancy through adolescence, the key psychological characteristics that affect children's responses to and understanding of chronic illness.

There are major parameters of illness that interact with developmental and psychological considerations. These are the age of onset, the severity (that is, potential threat to life and degree of pain), the physical manifestations, the effect on intellectual functioning, the course and type of treatment, and the need for hospitalization. An evaluation of potential impact of a chronic illness within each of the developmental stages must incorporate these features. Consider, for example, the difference between the birth of an infant with spina bifida and the onset of renal failure or osteosarcoma (malignant bone growth) in adolescence. The birth of an infant with a chronic illness or handicapping condition, such as spina bifida, represents a special adjustment for the family and a need for ongoing attention to the child's developmental requirements. The sudden onset of a disease such as renal failure or osteosarcoma in adolescence presents a sharp contrast to the former instance. The family and the child have to readjust their normalized life expectations and cope with the life-threatening nature of the disease.

Planning comprehensive care for chronically ill children requires consideration of the child's concept of illness and death, the child's reaction to hospitalization and treatments, and age-appropriate psychological issues. Table 2 summarizes the key developmental features in each of these areas as a prelude to a more detailed discussion of the several developmental periods.

Infancy. The identification of a chronic illness or handicapping condition in infancy represents a unique situation. For the child, there looms the need of continued intervention and support, and the family must adjust to the disappointment of not having a normal child. Because the infant is totally dependent on the caretaking response of the family, intervention must focus primarily on the parents and siblings. The infant's experience of illness consists of a generalized perception of pain and discomfort when either is present and of an ongoing sense of disruption in the environment.

Parents must cope with their feelings of grief for the loss of the anticipated normal infant, must come to accept the infant as their own, and must face the uncertainty of the future. Drotar and others (1975) describe parents' reactions to

Table 1. Psychosocial and Cognitive Determinants of a Child's Perception of Chronic Illness.

	Psychosocial development	Cognitive skills
Infancy (birth–1 year)	Establishing trust Establishing attachment Emerging affective expression	Movement toward coherent organization of sensorimotor actions Relating actions to specific effects on the environment Simple problem solving
Toddler (1–3 years)	Developing autonomy Differentiation of emotions Emergence of self-concept Parallel play to interactive play	Development of symbolic imagery and genuine representations: words and images distinguished from the thing signified Egocentric thinking Primitive logic based on "centered" thought: attending to only one aspect of the problem at a time, neglecting other important ones; thus, distorting the conclusion
Preschool (3–6 years)	Initiating Increased social interaction with adults and children Sex role imitation Personality definition Cooperative play Conscience development	Intuitive thought Increased verbal skills to permit verbal mediation and more advanced concept formation More complex representations, thought, and images, including ability to group objects into classes according to perception of their similarity
School age (7–11 years)	Industry Mastery Developing peer relationships Developing moral attitudes and values Crystallization of sex role identification	Ability to mentally represent a series of actions Development of rules of logical thinking: ability to think in rational terms, ability to reason separately about part of the whole, ability to serialize
Adolescence (12–18 years)	Establishing social maturity and heterosexual relationships Career choice Emotional choice Emotional control Establishing beliefs and values	Ability to deal with abstractions and probabilities Generalized orientation toward problem solving (systematic generation of hypotheses for testing) Deductive reasoning Ability to evaluate the logic and quality of one's own thinking

Adapted from Johnson and Magrab, 1976.

malformed infants and document a process that appears also to hold true for parents of children born with a chronic illness. They describe five stages of adaptation: shock, denial, sadness and anger, equilibrium, and reorganization. The initial shock or disbelief is often accompanied by immobility or numbness.

Table 2. Developmental Aspects of Chronic Illness.

Age	Psychological Issues	Concepts of Illness	Reaction to Hospitalization	Perception of Death	Intervention Approaches
Infancy	Importance of parent-child bonding; need to be as close physically as is feasible; possibility of anaclitic depression and developmental delays	Generalized perception of discomfort and pain	Need to have parents close by; parents seen as powerful; parents' presence and reactions provide best support in handling fear, pain, and separation; simple explanations useful for maintaining trust	Emotional impact evokes fear of separation and anxiety	Need for information presented in a clear, warm, sympathetic manner to parents by person who will continue to be available; need for substitute caretaker if separation is required
Preschool	Need to bolster sense of mastery and prepare for medical procedures, separation, etc.; possibility of regressions, fears	Illness is a punishment for bad behavior; magical view; adults could magically cure if they wished to	Presence of parents continues to be of primary importance; hospitalization perceived as rejection or punishment; fears of mutilation; treatment may be seen as hostile or punishment; concerns with bodily penetration by surgery or injections	Death may be personified; often seen as violent, comes as retaliation for being bad; may not be permanent; dead people continue to live; may be confused with separation and sleep	Encourage play and fantasy to help young children explore experience and feelings about illness; support and encouragement to sustain developments in areas of eating, toileting, sleeping fears
School-age	Can utilize knowledge and understanding of the body, causation of illness, and the process of treatment; need for honest explanations; need to continue to produce and learn	Self-causation of illness from disobedient or imprudent behavior still occurs but may take longer to express; can begin to understand body processes and functions	Primary concern is lack of body control and mastery; feelings of inadequacy; may become demanding and rebellious to maintain semblance of control; knowledge about illness effective in handling anxiety	Begins to understand irreversibility of death; becomes more real, final, universal, and inevitable; may be able to escape through use of one's wits, skill, or speed (early school-age); differentiation of living and nonliving	Explanations and drawings are useful in gaining cooperation and allaying anxiety; reality can be used more effectively to aid coping

Table 2. Developmental Aspects of Chronic Illness, Cont'd.

Age	Psychological Issues	Concepts of Illness	Reaction to Hospitalization	Perception of Death	Intervention Approaches
Adolescence	Beginning to deal with issues of illness as an individual; relies less on family support; difficulty with compliance with medical regimes proposed by adults (rebellion that may jeopardize health); intense preoccupation with body changes, and sexuality exacerbated; concerns about being "different" heightened; may impair ability to plan for the future	Focus on discrete symptoms rather than overall impact of illness; ability to intellectually question and deal with information about illness; may use denial of illness or overcompensation in areas not affected	May be seen as threat to independence; conflicts over control issues becoming a focal concern; separation from family and peers may interfere with developmental task mastery; concern about status in peer group after hospitalization	More able to acknowledge one's own fragility; may be viewed as philosophical problem of life or challenged and denied by risk-taking; idea that death is not permanent may linger (suicide seen as retaliation but reversible)	Importance of full information about diagnosis and illness; denial useful in coping; emphasis on enhancing control and mastery of illness management; participation in groups to alleviate feelings of isolation

Source: Magrab and Lehr, 1981.

Often parents' fears of what the child will be like are exaggerations of the reality (Klaus and Kennell, 1976). Parents may avoid their infant, and feelings of anger or sadness may be tied to feelings of guilt. In particular, feelings of guilt for having caused the illness may be intense for families when the onset of illness is during infancy.

The withdrawal of parents from their infants that frequently accompanies these first three stages is especially poignant because the child's primary psychological task during this period is development of attachment and trust. Klaus and Kennell (1976) stress that the immediate newborn period is a particularly sensitive time for initiation of patterns of parent-infant responsivity and attachment, although others suggest that patterns established during this period are modified or reversed in later periods (Svejda, Campos, and Ende, 1980). It is important that health planners train hospital staff to recognize this stage of withdrawal of the parents, to encourage parents to express their feelings, to identify these feelings as normal, and as soon as possible, to guide parents in establishing physical and emotional contact with their newborn infant. This type of intervention can be critical in moving parents to the stages of equilibrium and reorganization. Parents eventually should begin to accept their infant's condition, gather and process information, and begin to reframe their expectations and plans.

The severity of the illness may necessitate frequent or long-term hospitalization, which accentuates the threat to the attachment and bonding process. The classic studies of Harlow and Harlow (1966) suggest that the attachment process is crucial to the infant's psychological well-being. Significant alterations in the expected parent-infant relationship may result from disruptions caused by frequent hospitalizations, the parent's response to the infant's condition, and the anxiety generated and may jeopardize the infant's psychological development. To whatever extent possible, health care professionals must help families of frequently hospitalized infants maintain a consistent presence in the infant's life and maximize the opportunities for parents to provide their infant with love and attention.

Early bonding, or lack thereof, may influence the greater incidence of child abuse in low-birth-weight (Klein and Stern, 1971; Martin and Beezley, 1974; Mitchell, 1977) and premature infants (Martin, 1976; Newberger and Hyde, 1975; Stern, 1973). Some hypothesize that subsequent child abuse may be related to the prolonged separation of mother and infant during the initial hospital stay (Klein and Stern, 1971). Williams (1978) summarized preabusive characteristics to include congenital defects, mild neurological dysfunction, developmental deviations, atypical response patterns, and infant irritability, all of which suggest a possible early disruption in the attachment process. The provision of professional assistance to families may serve to prevent other serious secondary emotional and social problems.

Both long-term and transient psychological effects may accompany the onset of an illness. Planning for care must address these possible implications. For example, the long-term neurological implications of a chronic condition such as spina bifida are well known. A continuous health care strategy addressing these implications is essential.

Such chronic illnesses as congenital heart disease require more limited services and may have only a transient effect on psychological development. Although infants with congenital heart disease—particularly those who are cyanotic (having deficient oxygenation of blood or a great reduction in blood passing through the capillaries)—display delayed cognitive development (Feldt and others, 1969), researchers find no difference in cognitive skills between normal and cyanotic children (Linde, Rasof, and Dunn, 1966). Further, surgical correction of congenital heart defects is associated with either a maintenance of prior IQ scores or a postoperative increase in IQ (Landtman and others, 1960; Stevenson and others, 1974; Whitman and others, 1973).

Key resources are needed to plan health programs for infants with chronic conditions and their families. The families must gradually prepare for a lifetime of care for the child. Becoming educated advocates for their child's needs must begin at the outset. Accessing services is not usually easy, and understanding the health and social service systems can be an awesome task. If good case management procedures for transitions that will be needed as the child's developmental needs change are developed at this early stage, very burdensome stresses on families can be diminished.

Continuity of care should begin with good follow-along and follow-up procedures upon the identification of a chronic condition. Often there will be a need for services from multiple specialties. Initiation of both comprehensive and continuous developmental monitoring of the special psychological issues that emerge for chronically ill children should begin in infancy (or as early as the illness is identified). Families need the guidance and support provided by stable and cohesive professional input. Unfortunately, our service delivery system for the care of chronically ill infants is still fragmented, and the ideal of quality interdisciplinary care is far from a reality. An important consideration in establishing public policy is the recognition of the need of families and infants with chronic diseases for lifetime planning and continuity of care. It is critical that interdisciplinary follow-up be established in infancy to meet the needs of these children and their families.

Young Children: Toddlers and Preschoolers. During the early years of development, children who become chronically ill or become aware of a condition existing since infancy are faced with incorporating this new knowledge into their emerging sense of self. Although they have begun to experience themselves as separate and autonomous from their parents, young children tend to view experiences in an egocentric or intuitive way, utilizing only a very primitive concrete logic. They still do not completely differentiate between themselves and the world.

Bibace and Walsh (1979), in examining developmental stages of the child's conception of illness, identify three characteristics of this preoperational stage: incomprehension, phenomenism, and contagion. Incomprehension describes the child's attempt to explain illness by relating irrelevant experiences. Phenomenism describes the child's attempt to define illness in terms of a single external symptom such as a sensory experience that the child had at one time associated with the illness. Contagion describes the ability of the child to explain illness in terms of an external experience that is more immediately in the world of the ill person without drawing a causal link. An example is given of asking the child, "How do people get measles?" and the child responds, "From other people. You walk near them."

Many have pointed out that, on a psychodynamic level, young children view illness as a punishment for bad behavior and hold the magic belief that parents or other adults could cure the illness if they wished to. Aversive treatment procedures (considered hostile attacks) are also thought of as punishment for wrongdoing (Prugh and others, 1953). Because young children are concerned with hunger, warmth, and physical contact (Kagan, 1971) and are motivated primarily by sensory experiences, the impact of painful medical procedures can have substantial effects on personality development, particularly because children interpret sensory discomfort as punishment. They also perceive death as a form of punishment for either real or imagined misbehavior. Children do not consider death permanent and often confuse it with sleep. The sense of guilt that can emerge from young children's view of their illnesses, medical procedures, and thoughts of death may overwhelm and pervade their adjustment to their illness.

Repeated or prolonged hospitalization for a chronic illness during this age period can cause significant anxiety and may arouse fears of abandonment in children. Separation is the most common basis for anxiety in children under four years of age (Prugh and others, 1953; Godfrey, 1955; Robertson, 1970). Robertson characterizes young children's responses to this anxiety as a sequence of protest, despair, and detachment. Children may lose confidence in parents and feel a loss of security (Godfrey, 1955).

The role of the parent is thus a very significant one during this period. Young children need continual reassurance that they are loved, that the illness is not a punishment for misdeeds, and that parents will be available. Simple explanations based on the child's reality are extremely important to alleviate the child's fears. Parents must realize that chronically ill young children are also struggling with the normal developmental tasks of autonomy and separateness by initiating activities and ideas in a meaningful way while still maintaining a strong attachment to parents. Chronic illness can inhibit this process and exacerbate the struggle between parent and child.

Some chronic illnesses typically occur or are diagnosed during the early years. For example, half of the children who will develop asthma do so before five years of age (Gordis, 1973), the peak incidence of rheumatoid arthritis is between two and four years of age and eight to eleven years of age (Calabro and Marchesano, 1967), and hemophilia is usually recognized as the young child begins to explore and to experience falls. The adjustment and reaction of parents and siblings to changes in life patterns accompanying identification of a chronic illness in a young child have long-term implications. Parents initially may become overprotective of the ill child, unresponsive to siblings, and generally overwhelmed by the prospect of a lifetime of caring for a chronically ill child.

The nature of the condition itself will suggest specific threats to the psychological development of the child. For example, asthmatic children usually must have rooms that are free of dust and somewhat barren. Sometimes children will be required to spend extended time in this environment and will consider this experience abandonment and separation. For children with cystic fibrosis, the toilet-training process—a typical arena for the autonomy struggle between parent and child—may become even more difficult because of the odor of the excretions. Korsch and Barnett (1961) describe the effect on social develoment of the lethargy and malaise accompanying kidney diseases in young children and point to children's great need at this age for physical activity and exploration. Allowing children with hemophilia the normal range of exploration and initiating experiences can be difficult for parents. It is important to recall the earlier discussion concerning the young child's fear of abandonment and the interpretation of pain as punishment when planning health care policy concerning chronic conditions that may require surgical correction during the early years; these include congenital heart disease and orthopedic handicaps. Hospital procedures, the size and management of intensive care facilities, and the preparation of the child and family for the ordeal will influence the psychological effects of the surgery. Anticipatory guidance for families and for the children themselves—including hospital visits, written material, and other preparatory techniques—can ameliorate the emotional effects of the experience. Comprehensive care plans for young children with chronic illness must reflect an understanding of the emotional and social needs of this age group as well as the special needs we have been discussing.

Normalization of the life of the chronically ill child is an important goal of service planning. Families continue to need usual services such as daycare and preschool programs along with coordinated health and social services. Although numerous federal programs (such as Head Start; Early and Periodic Screening, Diagnosis, and Treatment; the Social Sciences Block Grant; Title V of the Social Security Act; and community mental health centers) offer services to young chronically ill children, these programs are usually poorly coordinated at the community level. As a result, families have difficulty gaining access to their services. Few models of comprehensive service delivery to families with chronically ill children exist. Information and referral services that assist in locating and facilitating access to the combination of services and resources meeting the needs of handicapped children and their families should be expanded and mandated specifically to target chronically ill children.

School-Age. During the school years, children are faced with developing a sense of mastery over their environment, acquiring new skills and knowledge, establishing moral attitudes and values, and sustaining fulfilling peer relationships. School-age children have the ability to reason rationally and logically, they have achieved a major developmental shift in their ability to differentiate clearly between self and world, and they focus on external real events. During this time, a chronic illness, as a result of related restrictions and increased dependency, may substantially interfere with the acquisition of new skills and the ability to maintain meaningful peer relationships.

Bibace and Walsh (1979) identify two major characteristics of the Piagetian concrete operational stage in the child's conception of illness: contamination and internalization. Contamination describes the child's inability to differentiate between mind and body; hence contact with dirt or germs, or good or bad behavior can be identified as the cause of illness. An example cited by Bibace and Walsh is the response to the questions, "What are the measles and how do you get them?" The child answers, "They are bumps on your body, and you get them by rubbing up against someone else who has the measles." Often children of this age conceptualize the cure for illness as something coming into surface contact with the body, such as rubbing medicine on measle spots. Internalization describes how the child perceives illness as within the body and the source of an illness as an external contaminant.

According to psychodynamic theory, children of the early school years (ages six through eleven) still consider illness punishment or the result of disobedient or imprudent behavior, but they no longer consider parents and other adults omnipotent. School-age children struggle to gain control over their environment and can suffer extensive effects as a result of the loss of control accompanying an illness. Jessner, Blom, and Waldfogel (1952) describe the fear of loss of control of impulses or body mastery exacerbated by fear of loss of a sense of body integrity. Children may become rebellious in an attempt to regain control.

Children of this age understand that death is permanent. Although they accept the finality of death as a separation from this life, they do not consider death as the end of physical existence. Children whose illnesses become life-threatening during this time may come to their own conclusions regarding the possibility of their own death.

School-age children are able to understand simple, honest, and specific information about their illness. Labeling the illness and explaining its symptoms can help the child cope. Children of this age can utilize information about causation, diagnosis, and treatment to reduce anxiety. They need to be encouraged to express their fears and negative feelings; they need reassurance that parents and others will help them deal with their illness.

School-age children should participate as much as possible in their own care and in decisions affecting their treatment; such behavior will help them maintain their sense of control and mastery. The importance of normalized school and life experiences for chronically ill school-age children cannot be overemphasized. Effective and continuing communication among the family, school, and health sector is especially important. Often this communication depends on random factors such as the parent's understanding of the child's needs, the parent's ability to intervene for the child, and the established relationship between school and health provider.

In particular, the health care team must provide ongoing feedback to the family through an identified team member. A school liaison contact person from the health team should have systematic and regular contact with the classroom teacher and with special school resource programs. The schools must establish periodic meetings with the family to monitor the child's progress. Ideally, the school, health care team, and family should meet together several times a year to review the changing needs of the child and family.

At this age of mastery and industry, school is is the child's primary arena for achieving new skills and developing effective peer relationships. Significant disruptions in school attendance will require supplemental educational input at home. The importance of providing the child with every opportunity for a normalized school experience cannot be overemphasized. The direct and sensitive education of the child's peers by the classroom teacher can help school-age children cope with their reactions. The fears of teachers must be addressed by the health community through education and ongoing support.

Biases concerning the academic ability of chronically ill children may subsequently influence their academic performance. Physicians, parents, and others often perceive chronically ill children as less intelligent than their healthy peers and thus expect less learning and achievement (Korsch, Cobb, and Ashe, 1961; Cleveland, Reitman, and Brewer, 1965; Linde, Rasof, and Dunn, 1966; McAnarney and others, 1974). Researchers suggest that underachievement results from factors other than school absences (Dorner and Elton, 1973; Green and Hartlage, 1972; Katz, 1970; Lauler, Nakielny, and Wright, 1966; Olch, 1971; Rutter, Tizard, and Whitmore, 1970. Children with hemophilia, juvenile arthritis, cystic fibrosis, diabetes, ulcerative colitis, sickle cell anemia, and rheumatic heart disease demonstrate at least average intellectual ability (Ack, Miller, and Weil, 1961; Allain, 1975; Cleveland, Reitman, and Brewer, 1965; Chodorkoff and Whitten, 1963; Fisher and Fogel, 1973). Children with most of these conditions, however, display academic achievement significantly lower than that of their peers even though they display adequate intellectual functioning.

Clearly, there must be a stronger interface between health and education professionals to respond adequately to the multiple needs of school-age children. Education must become a part of the interdisciplinary health care team to assess the educational needs of chronically ill children, develop linkages between the health and educational systems, plan educational programming for these children, assist teachers in the education settings to implement appropriate educational strategies, and provide continuity of educational planning through follow-through for these children. The need for training programs for educators who can participate effectively in the interdisciplinary systems serving handicapped children and their parents is evident.

Public Law 94-142 and companion legislation force educational agencies, medical agencies, and social service agencies to interact in new and challenging ways as they strive to serve handicapped children. Bringing into practice the principles mandated by P.L. 94-142 and Section 504 of the Rehabilitation Act of 1973 has created havoc in the various service delivery systems (Elder and Magrab, 1980). The initiation of efforts to improve collaboration by developing understanding between the school system and the Early and Periodic Screening, Diagnosis, and Treatment programs and between the school system and Maternal and Child Health Programs represents a needed step toward more effective coordination. A significant need remains to develop stronger linkages between the health and education sectors to meet the needs of school-age chronically ill children.

Adolescence. The period of adolescence is a time when young people are immersed in defining a coherent sense of self. Adolescents are finalizing concepts and body images, and they can be devastated by the effects of a serious or chronic illness. They have a normal preoccupation with bodily function and bodily changes, a preoccupation that can be heightened for those adolescents whose body image is threatened by the presence of an illness or chronic condition. Adolescents are still in a formative period, but like adults, are coping with issues of career, sexuality, and marriage. The challenge of the future, although stressful for most adolescents, can be especially stressful for chronically ill adolescents who may harbor strong doubts around their ability to obtain a job, their sexual potency, and their relationships with their peers. The important task of the adolescent period, that of developing independence from the family, becomes significantly thwarted by the presence of a serious or chronic illness.

Adolescents live intensely in the present and are attuned to peer pressure; thus, the most disconcerting dimensions of an illness may be those that arouse a feeling of differentness from peers. The physical manifestation of a condition may create the most poignant response. Often for the adolescent cancer patient, fear of death may have less effect than fear of alopecia (loss of hair), and for the renal transplant patient, concern over the effects of steroid treatment will be more worrisome than the threat of rejection of the kidney.

Adolescents may develop a more philosophical view of illness and death. They understand the universality and permanence of death, and they can be very sensitive to the meaning of death. They may be more able to acknowledge their vulnerability. On the other hand, rebelliousness typical of adolescents may be expressed in an exaggerated flirtation with death resulting in extreme risk-taking or failure to comply with medical regimes. It is not uncommon for adolescent hemodialysis patients to violate their dietary program or for diabetics to skip treatments.

Relationships with parents, physicians, and other adults may become increasingly hostile as adolescents attempt to assert their independence. The parent's natural desire to nurture and protect the affected adolescent conflicts with the adolescent's need for decreased dependency. Adolescents may reject support from family members and become angry and bitter about their condition.

Adolescents cope with illness in a variety of ways. Moore, Holton, and Marten (1969) describe denial, intellectualization, compensation, and anger as typical responses. Denial allows the adolescent patient to live as if normal. Research with long-term cancer survivors (Koocher and others, 1980) indicates that denial can facilitate long-term adjustment. Yet, there are implicit dangers in extreme denial, as in the case of the adolescent with cystic fibrosis who begins smoking or the renal patient who indulges in pizza binges. Adolescents may intellectualize, studying obsessively about their disease and possibly becoming emotionally constricted or overcontrolled. They may attempt to compensate for their illness by intense academic striving or unique physical accomplishments. This behavior results in problems if the adolescent selects medically contraindicated activities. Anger is a functional response to illness. Expression of anger can indicate the emotional security of the adolescent to express appropriate feelings, but anger can become maladaptive if it persists and interferes with daily functioning or medical compliance.

Helping adolescents maintain their self-esteem is a critical aspect of care at this time: They have a need for privacy, information about their illness and procedures, truth, and respect. It is especially important that adolescents develop skills for self-care. For example, home care may be a desirable goal for the hemodialysis patient, but the family will need training in the technology as well as psychological support when issues such as noncompliance arise. When adolescents are in hospital-based programs, health care providers should maximize adolescents' participation in their own care (for example, by expecting their assistance in the maintenance of machines) to help develop their sense of independence and control.

The sense of hopelessness about the future may cause adolescents to experience their most severe feelings of depression. The adolescent with cystic fibrosis has a limited adult life to anticipate, and along with a shortened life span comes poor opportunity for employment and remote possibility of marriage. The girl with diabetes, particularly, fears marriage, sex, and pregnancy (Travis, 1976). A major study of hemophila patients reported that 34 percent did not complete high school (Katz, 1970). Because of profound feelings of alienation and isolation, adolescents with chronic illness may find participation in support groups helpful.

The physiological and psychological onset of adolescence may be delayed for some of these teenagers—for example, hemodialysis patients, whose disease has persisted through childhood. These youngsters can benefit from programs, similar to that developed by the National Kidney Foundation (Jacobstein, Lehr, and Magrab, 1981), designed to prepare them for adolescence and to supplement their daily experiences around dating, social interactions, and job seeking. The public and private sectors must cooperate in these efforts. Adolescents whose disease strikes during the adolescent period will also need crisis counseling. Liaison work between the school and the health care team can facilitate appropriate service delivery.

Perhaps one of the key public policy issues for adolescents with chronic diseases is building linkages between services for children and services for adults that will provide for continuity of care for the adolescent. At the community level, there must be both horizontal and vertical coordination of health, social, and vocational planning services. Vocational services, adult mental health capabilities, and adult health services for chronically ill individuals must be available for an orderly transition of care and support. The changing role of the family and the issues of full life-cycle planning must be addressed in the planning of comprehensive services.

Summary

The fragmented nature of the service delivery system, the evolving and changing needs of chronically ill children, and the existence of few comprehensive programs designed to provide continuity of care to these children result in an enormous need for development of public policy to address these problems. Creation of networks among public and private resources must be accomplished to provide for optimal development and growth of chronically ill children and to reduce the short-term and long-term burdens of families. Particularly at the community level, linkages must be established across the health, educational, and social services systems. Different linkages benefit different age groups. Parents of infants need coordination of health and social services programs and the establishment of good information, referral, and follow-along services. Parents of school-age children need concerned liaison between the health and educational systems and specially trained educators serving in new roles. For adolescents, the transition to adulthood places particular demands on linkages between adult and child services programs. Public policies must be established that will prompt needed services and promote access to care at all age levels. Services must be organized to meet developmental needs and must include adequately trained individuals who understand the specific needs of chronically ill children.

To date, chronically ill children have been a neglected group in the establishment of public policy. The hidden handicaps of these children have kept them out of view of mainstream services. Now, as professionals emphasize the provision of quality care to these children and their families, it is essential that we take a developmental perspective in documenting their needs and in establishing programs.

References

Ack, M., Miller, I., and Weil, W. B., Jr. "Intelligence of Children with Diabetes Mellitus." *Pediatrics*, 1961, *28*, 764–770.

Allain, J. P. "A Boarding School for Hemophiliacs. A Model for the Comprehensive Care of Hemophilic Children." *Annals of the New York Academy of Sciences*, 1975, *240*, 226–237.

Bibace, R., and Walsh, M. "Developmental Stages in Children's Conception of Illness." In G. Stone, F. Cohen, and N. Adler (Eds.), *Health Psychology: A Handbook*. San Francisco: Jossey-Bass, 1979.

Calabro, J. J., and Marchesano, J. M. "Current Concepts in Juvenile Rheumatoid Arthritis." *New England Journal of Medicine*, 1967, *277* (13), 696–699.

Chodorkoff, J., and Whitten, C. F. "Intellectual Status of Children with Sickle Cell Anemia." *Journal of Pediatrics*, 1963, *63*, 29–35.

Cleveland, S. E., Reitman, E. E., and Brewer, E. J., Jr. "Psychological Factors in Juvenile Rheumatoid Arthritis." *Arthritis and Rheumatology,* 1965, *8,* 1152-1158.

Dorner, S., and Elton, A. "Short Taught and Vulnerable." *Special Education,* 1973, *62,* 12-16.

Drotar, D., and others. "The Adaptation of Parents to the Birth of an Infant with a Congenital Malformation: A Hypothetical Model." *Pediatrics,* 1975, *56,* 710-721.

Elder, J., and Magrab, P. *Coordinating Services to Handicapped Children: A Handbook for Interagency Collaboration.* Baltimore, Md.: Paul H. Brookes, 1980.

Feldt, R. H., and others. "Children with Congenital Heart Disease." *American Journal of Diseases of Children,* 1969, *117,* 281-287.

Fisher, K., and Fogel, B. "Psychological Correlates in Children with Ulcerative Colitis." Paper presented at the American Psychological Association Convention, Montreal, Canada, 1973.

Godfrey, A. "A Study of Nursing Care Designed to Assist Hospitalized Children and Their Parents in Their Separation." *Nursing Research,* 1955, *4,* 52-70.

Gordis, L. *Epidemiology of Chronic Lung Disease in Children.* Baltimore, Md.: Johns Hopkins University Press, 1973.

Green, J. B., and Hartlage, L. C. "Comparative Performance of Epileptic and Nonepileptic Children and Adolescents." *Diseases of the Nervous System,* 1972, *32,* 418-421.

Harlow, H., and Harlow, M. H. "Learning to Love." *American Science,* 1966, *52,* 244-272.

Hughes, J. "The Emotional Impact of Chronic Disease: The Pediatrician's Responsibility." *American Journal of Diseases of Children,* 1976, *130,* 1200-1203.

Jacobstein, D., Lehr, E., and Magrab, P. *Adaptation Training Manual for Use with Adolescent Renal Dialysis and Transplant Patients.* Washington, D.C.: Kidney Foundation of the National Capital Area, 1981.

Jessner, L., Blom, G. E., and Waldfogel, S. "Emotional Implications of Tonsillectomy and Adenoidectomy on Children." *Psychoanalytic Study of the Child,* 1952, *7,* 126-169.

Johnson, R., and Magrab, P. "Introduction to Developmental Disorders and the Interdisciplinary Process." In R. Johnson and P. Magrab (Eds.), *Developmental Disorders: Assessment, Treatment, and Education.* Baltimore, Md.: University Park Press, 1976.

Kagan, J. "Personality Development." In N. B. Talbot, J. Kagan, and L. Eisenberg (Eds.), *Behavioral Science in Pediatric Medicine.* Philadelphia: Saunders, 1971.

Katz, A. *Hemophilia: A Study in Hope and Reality.* Springfield, Ill.: Thomas, 1970.

Klaus, M. H., and Kennell, J. H. "Maternal-Infant Bonding." In M. H. Klaus and J. H. Kennell (Eds.), *Maternal-Infant Bonding.* St. Louis, Mo.: Mosby, 1976.

Klein, M., and Stern, L. "Low Birthweight and the Battered Child Syndrome." *American Journal of Diseases of Children,* 1971, *122,* 15–18.

Koocher, G., and others. "Psychological Adjustment Among Pediatric Cancer Survivors." *Journal of Child Psychology and Psychiatry,* 1980, *21,* 163–173.

Korsch, B., and Barnett, H. L. "The Physician, the Family, and the Child with Nephrosis." *Journal of Pediatrics,* 1961, *58,* 708–715.

Korsch, B., Cobb, K., and Ashe, B. "Pediatricians' Appraisals of Patient's Intelligence." *Pediatrics,* 1961, *27,* 990–1003.

Landtman, B., and others. "Psychosomatic Behavior of Children with Congenital Heart Disease. Pre- and Postoperative Studies of Eighty-Four Cases." *Annales Paediatriae Fenniae,* 1960, *6,* 1–78.

Lauler, R. H., Nakielny, W., and Wright, N. A. "Psychological Implications of Cystic Fibrosis." *Canadian Medical Association Journal,* 1966, *94,* 1043–1046.

Linde, L. M., Rasof, B., and Dunn, D. J. "Attitudinal Factors in Congenital Heart Disease." *Pediatrics,* 1966, *38,* 92–101.

McAnarney, E. R., and others. "Psychological Problems of Children with Chronic Juvenile Arthritis." *Pediatrics,* 1974, *53,* 523–538.

Magrab, P., and Lehr, E. "Assessment Techniques in Pediatric Psychology." In J. Tuma (Ed.), *Handbook for the Practice of Pediatric Psychology.* New York: Wiley, 1982.

Martin, H. P. *The Abused Child: A Multidisciplinary Approach to Developmental Issues and Treatment.* Cambridge, Mass.: Ballinger, 1976.

Martin, H. P., and Beezley, P. "Prevention and the Consequences of Child Abuse." *Journal of Operational Psychiatry,* 1974, *6,* 68–77.

Mitchell, R. G. *Child Health in the Community: A Handbook of Social and Community Pediatrics.* Edinburgh, Scotland: Churchill Livingston, 1977.

Moore, P., Holton, C., and Marten, G. "Psychological Problems in the Management of Adolescents with Malignancy. *Clinical Pediatrics,* 1969, *8,* 464–473.

Newberger, E. H., and Hyde, J. N. "Child Abuse: Principles and Implications of Current Pediatric Practice." *Pediatric Clinics of North America,* 1975, *22,* 695–715.

Olch, D. "Effects of Hemophilia upon Intellectual Growth and Academic Achievement." *Journal of Genetic Psychology,* 1971, *119,* 63–74.

Prugh, D., and others. "A Study of the Emotional Reactions of Children and Families to Hospitalization and Illness." *American Journal of Orthopsychiatry,* 1953, *23,* 70–196.

Robertson, J. *Young Children in Hospital.* 2d ed. London: Travistock, 1970.

Rutter, M., Tizard, J., and Whitmore, K. *Education, Health and Behavior.* London: Longman, 1970.

Stern, L. "Prematurity as a Factor in Child Abuse." *Hospital Practice,* 1973, *8,* 117–123.

Stevenson, J. G., and others. "Intellectual Development of Children Subjected to Prolonged Circulatory Arrest During Hypothermic Open Heart Surgery in Infancy." *Circulation,* 1974, *50,* 54–59.

Stubblefield, R. "Psychiatric Complications of Chronic Illness in Children." In

J. A. Downey and N. L. Low (Eds.), *The Child with Disabling Illness*. Philadelphia: Saunders, 1974.

Svejda, M. J., Campos, J. J., and Ende, R. N. "Mother-Infant Bonding: Failure to Generalize." *Child Development*, 1980, *51*, 775–779.

Talbot, N. B., and Howell, M. C. "Social and Behavioral Causes and Consequences of Disease Among Children." In N. B. Talbot, J. Kagan, and L. Eisenberg (Eds.), *Behavioral Science in Pediatric Medicine*. Philadelphia: Saunders, 1971.

Travis, G. *Chronic Illness in Children*. Stanford, Calif.: Stanford University Press, 1976.

Whitman, V., and others. "Effects of Cardiac Surgery with Extra Corporeal Circulation on Intellectual Functioning in Children." *Circulation*, 1973, *48*, 160–163.

Williams, G. J. "Child Abuse." In P. R. Magrab (Ed.), *Psychological Management of Pediatric Problems*. Baltimore, Md.: University Park Press, 1978.

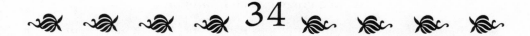

34

Employment Opportunities and Services for Youth with Chronic Illnesses

Paul Hippolitus, M.A.

Work. A career. A job. Employment. Short, clear words in our vocabulary, they mean so much. Most of our lives are spent working. School years and retirement flank work like bookends. Work is an important dimension to life both to the individual and to society as a whole. Yet, ask a disabled youth how often he or she has been asked by relatives or professionals, "What are you going to be when you grow up?" Chances are, they will respond, "Never!" People seem afraid to ask such a question for fear of focusing attention on the child's disability and limitations. The conditioning that results for all concerned is a negative feeling about eventual employment.

This lack of acknowledgment of potential is only the beginning of a series of obstacles, barriers, and negative attitudes that will block the path of a chronically ill youth who can, like everybody else, work. This chapter explores this subject and examines policy issues with respect to how disabled youth fare in the institutions and programs that open the doors to the world of work and fulfilling careers.

The chapter has three sections. The first is a categorical review of nine existing programs and institutions that offer or have the potential to offer employment-related services to chronically ill children and youth. These include special education (elementary and secondary), vocational education, higher education, vocational rehabilitation, sheltered workshop programs, public work programs, job service or employment security, affirmative action programs, and union apprenticeship training programs. The second section views employment as a process consisting of five distinct elements: work preparation, work development, work placement, work security, and work economics. The final section develops more general statements relating to common attitudes and issues and offers a focus for policy makers for future action.

Existing Programs and Institutions

Special Education—Elementary. Tremendous growth has occurred in elementary special education since the full implementation in 1978 of the Education for All Handicapped Children Act, Public Law 94-142. Prior to 1978, it was estimated that only one half of our nation's handicapped children were being served. During the four years that followed, practically every handicapped child received services. During this period of rapid growth, the first priority was full service (that is, special education for the large number of handicapped children not being served prior to 1978). Other issues, such as attention to career-related instructional needs, have not yet been fully addressed, despite the law's mandate that "each public [education] agency shall take steps to insure that its handicapped children have available to them the variety of educational programs and services available to nonhandicapped children . . . including . . . industrial arts, consumer and homemaking education, and vocational education." The law adds, "The above list is not exhaustive."

Few elementary or middle-school special education programs offer industrial arts programs for chronically ill children. Further, in local education agencies, where career education is integrated into the curriculum, special education students are accommodated. Both program dimensions are critical elements to the career development of disabled persons and need to be incorporated, as the law states, just as they may be for nonhandicapped students. This is a crucial policy issue for two reasons. First, the work preparation process is developmental and begins during the elementary years. Second, omission of career education and industrial arts could be argued to deny a handicapped child an appropriate education—the most basic guarantee of P.L. 94-142.

Special Education—Secondary. Secondary special education is the last formal program available to every chronically ill child and youth during the important transition all youngsters must make from school to work. No other program is mandated to serve every handicapped youngster. This uniqueness alone should inspire secondary special education to meet the challenge of work preparation.

At best, approximately 31 percent of senior-high level special education students (ages sixteen to twenty-one) have prevocational or vocational instructional objectives in their individualized education plans (IEPs). Only 2.6 percent of elementary-age special education students receive prevocational instruction. Because of the generally ineffective academic preparation during the elementary years, high school special education teachers feel pressure to make up ground that may have been lost during the elementary years. So, instead of devoting precious class time to industrial arts, for example, time is spent on basic math and measurement skills that should already have been taught.

There is another explanation for the limited attention to career preparation at the secondary special education level. Special education, as a profession, had its genesis in the elementary field. Nearly all university-based special educational training programs offer only early childhood or elementary special education programs. Most secondary level special education teachers come from the elementary ranks; they have not received adequate instruction in the course objectives, techniques, and content of a secondary program. This professional deficit reduces the effectiveness of secondary special education to provide prework instruction to chronically ill children and youth.

Studies by the Office for Special Education on the high school–age handicapped adolescent highlight the result of these shortcomings. The studies found that the dropout rate for handicapped high school special education students was four to five times higher than the dropout rate for all others. Many experts believe this is due, in large measure, to the perceived irrelevance of the special education program on the part of the special education student, who feels that programs focus on academic instruction and neglect vocationally oriented instruction. The studies also found that each year approximately 650,000 special education students are graduated or terminated their eligibility. Of this number, 21 percent will become fully employed, 40 percent will be underemployed and at the poverty level, 8 percent will be in their home and idle, 26 percent will be unemployed and on welfare, and 3 percent will be institutionalized. Only 21 percent will be successful at making the transition from school to work!

Vocational Education. Vocational education is taught in many settings: at the secondary level; postsecondary, at either a vocational school or in a college; and at the work site, such as apprenticeship training programs. Such education is a valuable and necessary resource for the employment preparation of chronically ill youth.

Fortunately, as a consequence of compliance activities precipitated by Section 504 of the Rehabilitation Act of 1973, we have data on the participation of handicapped youths in vocational education. These data document the low level of handicapped participation in vocational education. Approximately 2 percent of the national vocational education student population is handicapped, compared to the 9.5 percent expected prevalency rate reported by the Office for Special Education of the U.S. Department of Education. A breakdown of handicapped students in vocational training, by settings, shows handicapped students comprising:

- 2.7 percent of students in comprehensive high school vocational education programs
- 1.0 percent of those in junior or community college vocational education programs
- 3.8 percent in area vocational centers
- 2.0 percent in adult education vocational education programs
- 0.4 percent in apprenticeship training programs associated with vocational education programs

Participation is low in spite of aggressive and prescriptive legislation designed to help chronically ill youth gain access to these programs.

Consequently, it is important that we look beyond the legislation to understand what is wrong. As in the case of secondary special education, vocational education is not receiving handicapped adolescents adequately prepared for the coursework. The failure to prepare special education students for the vocational education option is especially serious because admission to vocational education is selective and competitive. Vocational education's accountability for funding is based on the number of admitted students who successfully complete the instructional program. This accountability and the oversubscription of students for a limited number of seats motivates admissions personnel to select only the best prepared students. Since secondary special education has, in most instances, not adequately prepared its students for vocational education, many students fail to gain admission. This circumstance adds to the problems created by disability or handicap.

Most vocational instructors have not received training on how to serve chronically ill children. They have not been taught about the employment and training potential of disabled people, nor have they been taught how to modify instructional strategies, facilities, or equipment to meet the special needs of chronically ill youth. Lack of information creates fears and suspicions in vocational educators and administrators as to what to expect of disabled students, making them reluctant to admit chronically ill students.

This defensiveness is intensified when advocacy groups exert pressure on vocational education to serve handicapped youngsters. The principal reason for this intensified defensiveness is the misconception on the part of recent advocacy efforts that all that is needed is pressure to get the special needs students into the program. Too often, the advocates fail to understand the necessity not only to provide the program with qualified and well-prepared students but also to cooperate with vocational education in order to ensure that the special needs of these students are both understood and effectively met.

It is important to recognize the variance in needs among chronically ill youth. Many handicapped youngsters who need and could benefit from vocational education could never be adequately served in the regular program even if elementary and secondary special education were to do their job effectively. The severity of the disability is a critical factor. Therefore, a continuum of program options is needed. For the less severely ill, the regular vocational education program is applicable. For the severely handicapped student, a specialized program may be needed. And there are those in between these extremes who require modified regular or special programs.

Higher Education. Careers in business, government, medicine, law, engineering, social services, and others demand successful completion of college degree programs. Data on participation of handicapped young people in higher education were collected during 1978 by the American Council on Education. Approximately 2.6 percent of the 1978 national college freshman class were handicapped, and nearly 32 percent of that 2.6 percent counted themselves in the handicapped population on the basis of wearing eyeglasses.

Possibly, the leading issue facing chronically ill youth in higher education happens long before they reach college. The sequential effects of various programs must be considered. Secondary special education lacks precollege programs, and too often, special education students do not have access to qualified counselors. They are rarely involved in college or career days the regular high school offers, and they rarely have access to the school clubs or organizations that help build interest in a college degree and the professions. In short, they are often forgotten in these areas. Chronically ill children and youth and their parents and teachers are often unaware of the employment potential that these students possess. Role models of similarly disabled or chronically ill persons who have achieved their educational and occupational goals are desperately needed.

Physical access to college remains a serious problem. The cost makes removing all architectural barriers impossible. Yet there is a middle ground between inaccessibility and complete accessibility. Efforts are needed to educate educators about barrier-free design principles. Efforts should focus most directly on new construction where costs are neglible. Existing structures should be modified with reasonableness and innovation in mind. There are many ways to accomplish accessibility. Architectural barrier removal is one way; rescheduling, and innovative devices and techniques are but a few alternative ways of achieving accessibility. The most neglected technique is consultation with the disabled person to identify possible adaptive techniques.

Physical-plant access alone is not sufficient. Chronically ill individuals need to process information according to their special needs, and this may require adaptive devices and techniques. Professors and other instructors must be made aware of these needs and be supportive of them.

The area of support services is very sensitive and has been repeatedly contested in the courts. Section 504 of the Rehabilitation Act has been interpreted to mean that support services should be provided by the university or college at its expense. To access the educational program, chronically ill students may require specialized support services including interpreters for the deaf, readers for the blind, and the like. Declining enrollments and increasing costs make it difficult for a college or university to make these expenditures. There may be a subliminal effect as well. Aware that more chronically ill students mean higher costs to the university, avoidance techniques may become more widespread when it comes to recruiting and encouraging special-needs students for college.

Vocational Rehabilitation. The federally funded and state operated vocational rehabilitation program is designed to provide occupational preparation services and independent living skills to chronically ill and handicapped youth and adults. As mentioned earlier, approximately 650,000 special-needs students leave special education and face the transition from school to work or college each year. Of this number, only about 60,000 (or 1 out of every 10 handicapped youths) receive services from vocational rehabilitation. Vocational rehabilitation is not the ubiquitous purveyor of job preparation and independent living skills programs many believe it to be. It is not large enough to meet the needs of such a population.

This means we must conserve vocational rehabilitation resources for the most severely impaired. Conversely, regular programs—that is, regular education, public training programs, public employment programs—must be better organized and implemented so they are able to fulfill their obligation to provide the remaining chronically ill youth and handicapped people with the employment and basic education programs they need but cannot get from rehabilitation. Although vocational rehabilitation needs to concentrate its resources in a particular direction, it also has a leadership role and a responsibility to cooperate with the regular services and with special education.

Sheltered Workshop Programs. Sheltered workshops are independent ventures begun by people in the community who see the need for a sheltered training environment for unserved chronically ill youth and handicapped adults. Nationally, approximately 4,000 sheltered workshops serve more than 100,000 handicapped individuals. Mental retardation represents about 60 pecent of the workshop population.

The placement rate for sheltered workshop clients into competitive employment is relatively low, about 13 percent. This fact, coupled with the average workshop wage of about $1.00 an hour, has precipitated criticism of the workshop movement. To understand the controversies surrounding sheltered workshops, we need to understand what sheltered workshops have been established to do.

There are two types of sheltered workshops. The first provides transitional employment in a sheltered environment. The objective is to train and find outside competitive employment for the client. The other type of sheltered workshop is for severely handicapped people for whom competitive employment is not possible. Rather than institutionalize this segment of the chronically ill population, sheltered workshop programs offer long-term sheltered employment. Here, there is little hope of moving the client into the world of work.

Special legislation allows sheltered workshops exemptions from minimum wage requirements because of the low production levels of their clients. Additionally, they are given preferential treatment when government contracts are awarded for goods and services. The vulnerability of the population, the special exemptions offered sheltered workshops, the lack of uniform accreditation, and the absence of any centralized monitoring authority have tempted a few unscrupulous people to take advantage of the situation and to exploit a source of cheap labor.

Fortunately, unscrupulous and incompetent operators are a minority. If sheltered workshops are to have the public trust, efforts are needed to show the positive work they are doing. Additionally, national accreditation and/or monitoring, either federal or professional, is needed to remedy instances of corruption and incompetency. Accreditation could also help establish professionalism for administrators and trainers and for the untrained parents, volunteers, and other concerned people whose enthusiasm and goodwill do not entirely make up for their lack of skill.

Public Employment and Training Programs. At this writing, the largest public employment and training program is the Job Training Partnership Act (JTPA), which superseded the Comprehensive Employment and Training Act (CETA) in 1982. JTPA is a federally sponsored employment and training program. Blocks of money are apportioned to states and local jurisdictions under the JTPA funding formula. The expenditure of funds is accomplished by prime sponsors, who are guided by JTPA planning councils called Private Industry Councils, which are appointed by the area's political leadership (for example, the office of the mayor, county commissioner, or similar local authority).

Sample studies have indicated a participation rate in CETA and JTPA of about 3 percent for chronically ill and handicapped youth and adults. Only since 1980 have the federal manpower programs begun a major effort to recognize the rights of this population to equal access to their programs. The impetus for this effort can be traced to the preparation of Section 504 regulations for the U.S. Department of Labor, which implements the manpower programs.

The experience with CETA and JTPA prime sponsors demonstrates that local governments fail to recognize that public employment and training programs, like other public programs, should be structured to meet the needs of all the public—including the chronically ill and handicapped. Most prime sponsors have set up planning councils, established outreach efforts, and operated programs without recognition of the rights or needs of the chronically ill. The typical response of a prime sponsor when called on this point has been that they never thought about it.

The implications for national policy are twofold. First, it must be made clear in legislation, regulation, operational directives, and training materials that chronically ill and handicapped youth and adults are to be served by programs that serve the general public. Second, national, state, and local organizations and agencies serving chronically ill and handicapped people must become involved in the mainstream of public activity. These groups tend to deal only with special programs for the handicapped.

Another response often heard from sponsors of manpower programs is that chronically ill and handicapped youth cannot benefit from the training offered and become gainfully employed. Because sponsors have never had a chance to know a chronically ill person who has accomplished training and is employed successfully, they apply the "poster child" image to all chronically ill children and adults. A further concern of local program operators is the expense of training people with chronic illnesses. Apart from legal and humane reasons for their inclusion in public programs, there is a compelling economic argument that should find its way into policy, "Can we afford *not* to train this population for employment?" The alternative is an increase in public assistance rolls. Higher numbers of dependent chronically ill people need institutionalization, Medicare, and Social Security Disability Income when they are not gainfully employed. Nonworking chronically ill people also mean there are fewer taxpayers.

Employment Service. Nearly every local jurisdiction maintains an office of its state employment service. For many years, this federally funded and state operated program has been structured to serve handicapped people. Operational policy and federal law call for each office to maintain a placement specialist who serves chronically ill youth and handicapped people. Over the years, reductions in budget and an increase in collateral duties have tended to limit the placement specialist's availability to fulfill the handicapped placement responsibility.

Federally mandated interagency agreements between the employment service and the area rehabilitation agency have not been effective in a large number of jurisdictions, and competitiveness between the employment service and rehabilitation has festered. Mandated cooperative agreements have occurred mainly in rural areas where cooperation is easier to achieve. In the larger cities, the programs are forced into competition because of accountability needs. For example, rehabilitation is accountable for the number of placements it makes; it tends, therefore, to refer the harder cases to employment services and to save the easier ones for itself. In turn, the employment service reserves its job listings for its own clients. Eventually, cooperation fades as the struggle intensifies.

Affirmative Action. Affirmative action or equal employment opportunity programs operate on two levels for chronically ill youth and handicapped persons. One level is in the legal realm and the other takes shape in voluntary compliance. Both strive to establish a climate supportive of equal employment opportunities for the handicapped population.

The more recent of the two programs comes from Section 503 of the Rehabilitation Act of 1973. This section requires employers who do business with the federal government in the amount of $2,500 or more to employ, and advance in employment, qualified handicapped people. Nearly one half of the nation's employers are covered by Section 503. Consequently, the effect of this affirmative action provision is widespread.

Recent compliance review activities by the Department of Labor have pointed out several problems with this program. The vast majority of covered companies have been found in technical violation of the act for reasons such as affirmative action plans incorrectly written, displayed, or disseminated; failure to establish the correct administrative or staff mechanisms called for in the regulation; and other technical reasons. However, it must be noted that only a handful of companies have shown complete avoidance of the objectives of affirmative action. Once deficiencies have been pointed out or complaints made, compliance is soon achieved. If there is a broad policy issue here, it may be contained in the frequent complaint of employers seeking to achieve good faith compliance. They complain that they cannot find qualified handicapped workers for the jobs offered. They are prepared to meet all the technical obligations set forth in the affirmative action program, but they cannot find members of the protected class to provide with jobs.

The other force in affirmative action is voluntary compliance efforts, which are principally the objectives of the President's Committee on Employment of the Handicapped, state governor's committees on employment of the handicapped, and state divisions of vocational rehabilitation. These long-standing efforts seek to foster, in the United States, a climate of opinion supportive of equal employment opportunities for chronically ill and handicapped youth and adults. Half the nation's employers are covered by Section 503; half are not. The latter group receives its primary motivation to employ handicapped people from public information agencies.

In an era of affirmative action for the handicapped population, some argue that voluntary compliance activities and public information efforts are less germane than mandating complicance by law. But, as we have learned in education and elsewhere, laws can be avoided and even ignored. Reason and understanding come from public relations activities. As a nation, we may be heading away from strict legal affirmative action programs. If so, voluntary compliance may again become the principal tool for advancing the employment situation of chronically ill and handicapped youth and adults.

Union Apprenticeship Training Programs. Most occupations or jobs in trades and industry are covered by trade union agreements. Generally, the agreements mean that, although the employer does the hiring, the union often controls access to jobs by controlling the trade accreditation process. As a consequence, union support and involvement are imperative if chronically ill and handicapped youth and adults aspire to occupations in the trades or industry.

Although no hard data exist to illustrate the actual participation rate of handicapped people in union-related jobs, their involvement can be projected by reviewing data on handicapped involvement in vocational education–related apprenticeship training. The national figure was 0.4 percent. Other less precise measurements, such as field experience with unions, corroborate this implied low participation rate.

Two basic issues face unions on the subject of employing handicapped people. The first results from the seniority system. Seniority dictates that union jobs that require a minimum of physical exertion be saved for union workers who, as a consequence of age or injury, can no longer function in their current position. It is a kind of employment insurance for the union worker and a well-guarded benefit. Even if not currently filled by senior workers, unions prefer not to give the jobs to handicapped people. They feel compelled to save them for the older or injured worker.

The other major issue relates to the strict apprenticeship requirements of many union occupations. These occupations envision a career ladder that includes time spent at a particular job, often one not directly related to the learning of the trade. This unrelated step on the career ladder is often very physical and impossible for handicapped populations. So there are chronically ill youth and handicapped adults who could learn the trade and perform the occupation but who cannot perform duties that are a traditional prerequisite to the career. Because trade union agreements and apprenticeship programs vary from place to place, local efforts need to be mounted to involve unions in resolving this problem.

Employment as a Process

Work Preparation. Work preparation is the beginning step in the employment process. It includes everything from career awareness to skill training. It should begin at the earliest stages of life with stimulation about jobs and career ambition. Every subsequent phase of learning and living should contribute to the development of a person prepared for work.

This process is both subtle and straightforward. What is taught about social and living skills is just as important to work preparation as the teaching of a job skill. Nearly every activity can and should be fashioned to contribute to the overall preparedness of the individual for future employment. This need is intensified with chronically ill youth because, in many instances, their ability to accomplish needed skills may take longer and may require repetition.

Families with chronically ill children face tremendous challenges. They must cope and they must adjust. But, in terms of the employment process, the usual expectations and support for future work seem to be missing. As they cope and adjust, the family often dismisses the eventuality of employment for the child. Activities and conversation exclude elements related to work preparation. Shared hopes and fantasies about wanting to be a fireman or policeman or lawyer or doctor are suppressed by the reality of the chronic illness. Social interaction with peers is either avoided or inhibited for health reasons. Relatives avoid discussing their jobs and their feelings about work to avoid hurting a chronically ill child or youth with an uncertain future.

An important effect of all this is to suppress in the chronically ill child ambition and hope for a work future. Without stimulation, motivation and aspiration tend to fade. The prophecy is self-fulfilling. Little or nothing is expected by the family, so the child aspires to little or nothing in career or work.

The formalized aspects of the work preparation process take place in the education setting. Here academic, physical, vocational, and social skills are taught. Unfortunately, as reviewed earlier, special education lacks the ability to train in many of these skill areas. Its instructional strategies reflect the pervasive low expectation syndrome with respect to the work future of chronically ill children and youth.

Finally, doctors, rehabilitation professionals, social agency personnel, and other professionals tend to be narrow in their treatment of the chronically ill child or youth. They deal, naturally enough, with the issues relating to their specialty. Unfortunately, such treatment often fails to support the child's need for work preparation; it fails to meet the broader needs of the child.

Programmatic issues relating to the work preparation process are:

1. Related service agencies fail to reinforce each other's efforts.
2. Professionals are not sufficiently prepared to provide instruction.
3. Legislative support is meager and unenforced in the areas of rehabilitation, special education, career education, vocational education, and public training programs.

4. Public and private agencies do not maintain needed liaison with the employer community.
5. Inaccessibility is an inhibiting factor. More and better emphasis needs to be placed on barrier-free design principles and program accessibility.
6. Regular programs fail to meet the preparation needs of chronically ill children and youth.

Work Development. Work development includes programs that foster career opportunities. In the case of chronically ill children and youth, work development includes the promotion of equal employment opportunities, the exploration of new careers, and the dispelling of career stereotypes. These activities take place at all levels of administration. National campaigns usually attempt to affect widespread public and employer attitudes with respect to equal employment opportunities, and attention is paid to federal legislation and policy as they may affect chronically ill children and youth in employment. Similar tasks can be directed at the state level of authority. Local action is necessary to ensure the actual development of work opportunities for the chronically ill and handicapped through direct contact with local employers.

Few groups are involved in the work development of the chronically ill youth. As a beginning, groups serving this population should learn more about the employment needs and potentials of the chronically ill. They should seek to identify chronically ill persons who are working, with the view of fostering equal employment opportunities for them.

Work Placement. This component of the employment process is concerned with matching qualified individuals with appropriate jobs. Work placement for the chronically ill person involves counseling, selective placement, and arranging necessary job modifications. The counseling process is designed to document the potential worker's interests, abilities, and needs with respect to employment. Selective placement is the art of finding the right work situation for the individual. Job modification is a reasonable alteration of the worksite so that a chronically ill worker can minimize the negative effects of a disabling condition.

In the main, work placement of the chronically ill is accomplished by three agencies: rehabilitation, the employment service, and education. All three have professionals who specialize in placement of chronically ill youth and handicapped people.

Programmatic issues relating to the work placement process are:

1. Generally, persons practicing the placement of chronically ill youths and handicapped adults have no formal training in the specialized art of job placement.
2. An employer may be contacted by three or more job placement people all of whom are concerned with the placement of chronically ill youth and handicapped adults. This multiplicity of effort confuses employers and leads to struggles among the agencies.
3. Job placement professionals in this field need to learn more about the variety of innovative job accommodations that exist.
4. Job placement agencies need to develop closer working agreements so that cooperation can be more readily achieved.

Work Security. Work security includes considerations and programs that help encourage and protect employment. These forces include employer/employee acceptance, affirmative action, and union or other work rules. Affirmative action is the only one of the three components that is relatively uniform nationwide. Affirmative action offers work security to chronically ill youth and handicapped people with about half of our nation's employers. It offers workers from this protected class a channel to formalize complaints and review the hiring and retention practices of a covered employer. This recent advance has afforded a great deal of assurance and security to the handicapped population. The other two dimensions of work security are local in operation. Both employer/employee acceptance and union or other work rules have a tremendous impact on the likelihood of a chronically ill youth or handicapped adult getting and retaining employment.

Programmatic issues relating to the work security of chronically ill and handicapped youth are:

1. Affirmative action programs for the population cover only one half of the nation's employers. Complete coverage is needed.
2. Both private and public employers continue to be unsure about the work potential of chronically ill and handicapped youth. More education and promotion toward this end are needed.
3. Certain union practices restrict work opportunities for the chronically ill and handicapped. Unions need to be targets of involvement and educational efforts.
4. Private and public employer work rules are often restrictive toward the employment or retention of chronically ill and handicapped youth. This is most notable in the area of medical requirements for hiring and retention. Unnecessary medical requirements and other restrictive requirements need to be identified and remedied.

Work Economics. The fifth and last dimension to employment is work economics. Economic forces fall into three categories: incentives, disincentives, and exploitation.

Reliably, the strongest and most effective work incentive is the prospect of making money. This strong motivator should be used as a way of encouraging chronically ill persons to work. There is a balance to be achieved between providing needed support and services for the chronically ill population and stifling the basic economic motivator. The other consideration under work economics is exploitation. Unfortunately, there continue to be unscrupulous persons who see advantages in hiring the chronically ill and handicapped. First, they can elicit public sympathy, which can help to sell a product. And second, they can underpay handicapped workers on the premise that they do not meet production standards. We must guard against all such instances.

Programmatic issues relating to the work economics of chronically ill and handicapped youth are:

1. Public assistance programs fail to recognize the employment potential of the individual and, as a consequence, help perpetuate their unemployment. Administrators of these programs should initiate policy designed to contribute to the eventual employment of every client with employment potential.
2. Welfare and public assistance programs should be targets of informational efforts demonstrating the employment potential of chronically ill and handicapped persons so they will be as well prepared as possible to encourage eventual employment among their clients.
3. The needs of the chronically ill for insurance as they leave the protection of public assistance for employment must be better understood and addressed.
4. Placement professionals should guard against placements where chronically ill and disabled persons are exploited by an employer.

Major Policy Issues

Every issue, barrier, or problem discussed in this chapter can be addressed with four broad policy initiatives. These are commitment, outreach, continuum, and linkages. These areas represent the most critical ingredients for policy improvement.

Commitment. Policy improvement begins at the top. Each program with the potential to contribute to the employment prospects of chronically ill youth must become the subject of top-level commitment to serve this population. In programs in which service to this constituency is not routine, program heads must assure that the needs of this segment of the public are addressed routinely. In programs that serve the handicapped population as a matter of routine, top-level commitment to the principle of employment must be demonstrated. In both instances, the commitment must be clear, precise, intense, well publicized, and reflected in all written regulations and operational directives. Additionally, commitment must be informed, taking into account needs and wishes of the population itself. Certain staff should have the responsibility to ensure that in-service training and communication make this commitment well known and understood. This staff can record how the program has translated this commitment into concrete action.

Outreach. The need for outreach activities relates mainly to agencies and programs that, although they have not traditionally served this population, can do so. With a commitment to serve, the next critical step is to reach out into the community to alert the chronically ill population that services are being offered. Outreach can be accomplished through public relations activities as well as through direct contact with the agencies, groups, and professionals serving the population. Outreach activities should be augmented or reinforced with consumer involvement activities. Chronically ill youth themselves can help all agencies understand better the needs of the population so they can become more responsive and effective.

Continuum. A continuum of program options makes it possible to place and serve the chronically ill youth in the least restrictive environment possible. A continuum need not be present under one single agency. Related programs can be structured so that the continuum is available among a range of agencies. For example, in the area of work preparation, the area sheltered workshop program could offer both a highly specialized training environment and a long-term sheltered employment and training placement. Vocational rehabilitation could offer the next level of unrestricted work preparation. Special education might offer several programs ranging from a work-study program to cooperative education. Vocational education could provide sites for a work preparation placement of the chronically ill. And the area's public training program could have several levels of placements available to the chronically ill youth. Placement decisions would be based on the training or work preparation desired and the functional capacity of the individual.

To achieve a continuum, representatives of each agency must coordinate their activities. Additionally, each individual agency must ensure that it has within its domain a range of program options, or a continuum, so that chronically ill youth who need the particular service they offer can receive it even though they may have special needs. A continuum should be both community-wide and agency specific.

Linkages. The final critical ingredient for policy improvement is linkage or interagency cooperation. The continuum concept depends on interagency cooperation. In a time of diminishing resources, it is even more imperative that duplication and competition among related agencies be eliminated.

Interagency cooperation requires a shift in emphasis. The client becomes the center, and needs of the agency become secondary. Interagency cooperation most readily permits a mixed array of services to reach the client at the most opportune times. For example, a client of rehabilitation services may be discovered to need special education services at a certain point in order to reinforce a certain level of achievement. With cooperation established, this exchange becomes possible. Needed services reach the client when they are needed, not when the client reaches the service agency.

Interagency agreements are most effective when they are negotiated and written out. This helps ensure commitment to the process. With each agency viewed as an equal partner in the negotiations, a higher level of authority should be available and involved so that impasses can be appealed and decisions reached. Interagency agreements are game plans that reduce confusion, duplication, and neglect.

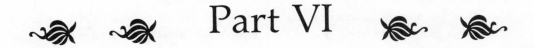

Part VI

Programs and Organizations
Serving Chronically Ill
Children and Their Families

The broad array of organizational approaches to services for chronically ill children and their families is the subject of Part Six.

In Chapter Thirty-five, Arthur J. Lesser provides the reader with a history of child health developments from the late 1800s through the early 1970s. Lesser points out that the legislation establishing the Children's Bureau constituted the first recognition of the federal government's role in public policy promoting the welfare of the nation's children. Studies by the Children's Bureau led to the first public health grants-in-aid program to states, called the Maternity and Infancy Act of 1921 through 1929. Lesser details the variety of forces that led to the enactment of Title V of the Social Security Act in 1935 and then concentrates on Services for Crippled Children, a new program under Title V, and the special projects grants that were provided under its aegis. Lesser discusses the relationship of policy developments in the area of mental retardation to those in the Crippled Children's Services and the Maternal and Child Health Programs as well as the Children and Youth Projects. In the final section he poses some major policy issues for consideration.

Antoinette Parisi Eaton, Kathryn K. Peppe, and Kathleen Bajo, in Chapter Thirty-six, depict developmentally disabled people as a subset of the chronically ill population for the purposes of illustrating the potential for cooperative interagency efforts and policy planning. The authors define elements of interagency coordination and discuss policy factors that indicate the need for it. Presenting common barriers and facilitators to coordination, the authors review three models of successful interagency coordination. Policy considerations and conclusions are stated with an emphasis on the commitment essential for successful interagency cooperation.

Leonard D. Borman reviews recent findings on the nature, development, methods, and effects of self-help/mutual aid groups in Chapter Thirty-seven. He describes in detail several of the groups that exist for chronically ill children and their families, adding the caution that these groups are not a panacea. Self-help must supplement and not supplant existing professional services, Borman states. He reviews some key recommendations to stimulate the development and financing of mutual help groups made by the 1978 President's Commission on Mental Health that are generalizable to all chronic conditions. Finally, he considers policies that could encourage and expand self-help groups and defines roles and skills for professionals and agencies in the support and implementation of such groups.

Carol Milofsky and Julie T. Elworth, in Chapter Thirty-eight, offer a general description of children's health charities and a statement of problems that confront them. Exploring issues of organizational structure, Milofsky and Elworth document differences between the older (and larger) and the newer (and smaller) voluntary health associations with respect to both ideology and politics. Paternalism and corporate central control as opposed to self-reliance and decentralized management are discussed. The authors examine a number of policy issues, including the pros and cons of political activism as well as inequities of fund allocations, reforms in organizational structure, and competition among the charities not only for resources but also for constructive changes in policies and practices.

In Chapter Thirty-nine, Morris Green examines the goals of professional organizations in setting policies that affect chronically ill children and their families. Green notes that most professional health organizations have a generic rather than a categorical interest in policy issues. Using the American Academy of Pediatrics as an example, he describes the structure and methods that are used to translate goals into policy and provides insight into the advocacy process. The importance of professional education, standard setting, coalition building, manpower enlistment, and citizen education are discussed. Green also delineates some of the major deterrents to greater participation of professional organizations in the formulation or direction of public policy. Some of the deterrents include the complexities associated with building consensus among pluralistic memberships, apathy among members, lack of time for involvement, and the belief that their efforts will not make any difference.

35

Public Programs
for Crippled Children

Arthur J. Lesser, M.D.

During the latter part of the nineteenth century, recognition of the distinctive characteristics of children and the effects of early experiences on their development began to emerge slowly, together with growing concern about their particular vulnerability. Leadership was scattered and isolated, but gradually there was documented increasing knowledge about the large numbers of children who were orphans, abandoned, employed in hazardous occupations, homeless, delinquent, and physically and mentally handicapped. It was in the context of a better understanding of childhood as a period of struggle for survival that pediatrics and maternal and child health developed as areas of special interest in medicine and public health. The creation of state and local health departments provided an organizational framework through which preventive health measures could begin to be applied on a large scale.

By 1877, fourteen states had established state health departments, the first being Massachusetts in 1869. During this period were started specialized organizations such as the American Association for the Study of the Feebleminded, the National Association for the Deaf, the Pediatric Section of the American Medical Association, and in 1888, the American Pediatric Society.

The first state hospital for crippled children was established in Minnesota in 1897 for the purpose of providing care and treatment for indigent children "who are crippled or deformed or are suffering from disease through which they are likely to become crippled or deformed" (Bremner, 1970, p. 1032). Additional states developed state hospitals and hospital schools for crippled children and residential schools for the deaf, the blind, the epileptic, and the mentally retarded.

733

This was also a period during which there were many residential institutions for orphans and homeless abandoned children.

The change to a much more dynamic view of child health and prevention of illness for the most part resulted from the remarkable surge of knowledge of bacteriology and communicable diseases toward the end of the nineteenth century. Most of the states began school medical examination programs that basically had the same goals: (1) exclusion of contagious diseases where possible, (2) detection of the most obvious physical defects of school children, and (3) correction of these defects by the municipality (Bremner, 1970, p. 813).

The prevalence of dirty, contaminated milk and the recognition of its relationship to diseases of infancy and childhood and the shockingly high infant mortality provided a dramatic opportunity to demonstrate the possibilities of prevention of communicable diseases and infant deaths. The health officer of Rochester, New York, in a study of the 1896 mortality statistics, concluded that the milk supply was "the great cause for this awful mortality" (p. 871).

Rosenau pointed out that the milk question illustrated better than any single subject many of the fundamental factors in preventive medicine (Schmidt, 1973). In New York City in 1892, Nathan Straus opened the first of nearly three hundred milk stations he was to establish in the United States and abroad to provide clean, wholesome milk for children. In addition to obtaining the milk at these stations, mothers were shown how to prepare feedings and were taught basic principles of infant and child care.

One is impressed by the long delay during this period in using newly acquired medical information for prevention of diseases. The relationship of contaminated milk and water to diseases and mortality was known for decades before effective action began. Similarly, the 1906 report of the New York State Commission on the Blind emphasized that ophthalmia neonatorum was the most common local cause of blindness; yet the use of silver nitrate for prophylaxis for the newborn had been developed in 1881 and would have prevented much sight loss (Bremner, 1970).

The necessity for *social action* was made clear in the report after pointing out the per capita costs of educating a blind child and the savings that resulted from early prophylactic measures. Two points were emphasized: "First, that it is the duty of the State to protect its infant citizen as a minor from the danger of blindness with which he is threatened and second, that it is the duty of the State to protect itself from the burden of caring for the unnecessarily blind" (p. 878). Here was proposed a clearly stated policy that asserted it to be the duty of the state government to adopt available measures to prevent needless blindness in order both to protect children from a dreadful handicap as well as to protect the state from needless expenditures of public funds.

By the end of the nineteenth century, it was well understood that if preventive health services for children were to be effective, they must be accompanied by educational measures to help parents appreciate and adopt fundamental concepts and procedures of child hygiene. Such measures were a major part of the nursing care of children in their own homes. In 1902, at the request of the city health department, a nurse from the staff of the Henry Street Visiting Nurse Association was loaned to the schools. So developed the practice of public health nurses in schools and in the various programs of health departments.

The next significant step was creation of the first Bureau of Child Hygiene in 1908 in New York City, with major innovative program responsibilities for the promotion of the health of mothers and children through the provision of medical, nursing, and health educational services. Interest was also growing in the direction of a more concerted national focus on protection of children against the vicious exploitation of child labor.

The rapid industrialization of the nation following the Civil War led to increased employment of children in a considerable variety of occupations, many of them hazardous. According to the 1870 Census, about one in eight children aged ten to fifteen years was gainfully employed. By 1900, it was one in six, 40 percent of them in industry and 60 percent in agriculture. In the southern mills, one third of the workers were children, many less than ten years old (Bremner, 1970, p. 601). At the same time, the concept of childhood as a period of growth and development was emerging in contrast to the generally prevailing view of children as chattels or little adults. Thus, the voices being raised against child labor and for the protection of children came from several sources including education, psychology, medicine, and public health, as well as labor and social work.

G. Stanley Hall, professor of psychology at Johns Hopkins University, applied the principle of evolution to child development, defining the periods of growth each with its own needs and potentials. Retarding the development of children would arrest also the development of society. The emerging science of psychology emphasized the close relationship of physiology, psychology, and play to normal growth and development. At the same time, the social reform movement opposed child labor because, among other reasons, it deprived children of their natural right to play and to learn.

John Dewey called the realization of a child's potential for development a basic goal of a democratic society. Theodore Roosevelt, speaking for himself and the many citizens concerned with preserving the nation's natural resources, attacked child labor, emphasizing the need for conservation of childhood. The views of many voluntary organizations and individuals led to the formation in 1904 of the National Child Labor Committee, which became a champion for children, opposing child labor and supporting measures to promote child health and welfare.

The Children's Bureau

In 1903, Lillian Wald proposed the idea of a Children's Bureau as an agency of the federal government. Her experience in Henry Street, together with the conviction that interest in the welfare of children was growing, led her to conclude that a federal children's bureau was a necessity. She wrote, "The birth rate, preventable blindness, congenital and preventable diseases, infant mortality, physical degeneracy, orphanage, desertion, juvenile delinquency, dangerous occupations and accidents, crimes against children are questions of enormous national importance, concerning some of which reliable information was almost wholly lacking" (Wald, 1915, p. 164). These concepts were subsequently incorporated into the legislative mandate of the Children's Bureau.

The National Child Labor Committee became the sponsor and principal spokesman for obtaining widespread support for the legislation. The first bill proposing a federal Children's Bureau was introduced in 1906 and finally became law, signed by President Taft on April 9, 1912. The views on the proposed legislation are of particular interest because they presaged the similar debates on the respective powers and responsibilities of the federal and state governments during the New Deal and for subsequent decades. At this writing, we are witnessing once more the advocacy of a greatly reduced federal role in the domestic economy. It is ironic that Senator Borah, who introduced the bill that was finally enacted in 1912, agreed that fifty years earlier the problems of children could be left to the states, but "economic conditions have changed and the responsibilities and duties of government must necessarily change with those changes" (Schmidt, 1973, p. 421).

Considerable impetus for establishing the Children's Bureau was provided by the first White House Conference on the Care of Dependent Children called by President Theodore Roosevelt in 1909. The conference passed a resolution recommending passage of the bill and the president sent a special message to Congress urging enactment.

As passed in 1912, the act directed the bureau "to investigate and report . . . upon all matters pertaining to the welfare of children and child life among all classes of people and . . . especially investigate the questions of infant mortality, the birth rate, orphanage, juvenile courts, desertion, dangerous occupations, accidents and diseases of children, employment, legislation affecting children in the several states and territories" (U.S. House of Representatives, 1911–1912, pp. 79–80). This legislation constitutes the first recognition that the federal government has a responsibility to promote the welfare of the nation's children. For the first time, the federal government's support of studies of agriculture and animal husbandry was extended to children and with it came expression of the belief that a nation's children are its most important resource. A specific public policy that instructed a federal agency to investigate and report on the status of children and on their common as well as special needs was adopted. From the outset, the Children's Bureau studies focused on the child and developed the principle that workers with children and their families concentrate on the child and the child's needs rather than on rules and procedures (Eliot, 1960).

From the very beginning, the program of the Children's Bureau was, in the words of its first chief, Julia Lathrop, "to serve all children, to try to work out the standards of care and protection which shall give to every child his fair chance in the world. It is obvious that the Bureau is to be a center of information useful to all the children of America, to ascertain and to popularize just standards for their life and development" (Bradbury, 1962, p. 6).

A large order? Grace Abbott, speaking to the National Conference of Social Work in 1932, said of Julia Lathrop that with a very broad authority and limited resources

> it was necessary to select carefully those first projects. It would have been the line of least opposition for the Bureau to have concerned itself exclusively with the treatment of symptoms of social disorders as they affected children rather than the discovery of causes; to have sought only methods of providing for the dependent and delinquent, and to have ignored the basic reasons for the suffering of children; to have attacked the problem of the few and the exceptional rather than those which must be solved before one can help to lift the level of life for all children. From the beginning, Miss Lathrop's program of work for the Bureau set up prevention as the goal. She held that, as a democracy, the United States must seek continually new ways of insuring the optimum growth and development of all American children, but the importance of temporary palliatives was never ignored. The slow scientific accumulation of fundamental, basic information about children and child life was begun in no narrow or timid spirit by Julia Lathrop. She was prepared to go wherever the interests of the child might lead her and to accept whatever conclusions flowed from an honest interpretation of facts assembled with meticulous accuracy [Bradbury, 1962, p. 17].

Admirable in its clarity, this statement expresses the policy adopted by the new bureau in carrying out its broad legislative mandate. The first task undertaken by the Children's Bureau was a study of infant mortality, which was carried out by its staff in nine representative cities. The study followed all infants born in these cities for one year or as long as those infants lived during that year. It was the first of a number of studies that related social and economic to medical factors associated with maternal and infant deaths and studies of various patterns of medical care of mothers and children in cities and rural areas. These studies pointed the way to measures that would help prevent illness and reduce mortality. In keeping with the bureau's mandate to investigate and report, the information in these studies was reported to the related professions and to the public in general.

The first annual report states that although it was the bureau's function to serve all children, "this purpose, in the minds of those who drafted the law, by no means overshadowed the needs of those unfortunate and handicapped children. . . . It is a matter of common experience that the greatest service to the health and education of normal children has been gained through efforts to aid those who were abnormal or subnormal or suffering from physical or mental ills. . . . Thus, all service to the handicapped children of the community—an immediate service properly demanded by the popular conscience—also serves to aid in laying the foundations for the best service to all children of the Commonwealth" (Bradbury, 1962, p. 15). Thus, early Children's Bureau studies included such subjects as juvenile delinquency; child labor; daycare; working mothers; institutional care; illegitimacy; mental retardation; mother's aid; nutrition of children; health of preschool children in selected cities; height and weight of children including children with heart disease, rickets, and malnutrition; vocational guidance; maternity benefits in European countries; provisions for the care of crippled children in fourteen states; and numerous other subjects.

The Maternity and Infancy Act of 1921–1929

The legislative history of the act of 1912 establishing the Children's Bureau made it clear that it was the intent of the Congress that the findings of its studies and reports should be used to help state and local groups take appropriate action to improve the care of pregnant women and children (Eliot, 1967). The precedent establishing studies of infant and maternal deaths, showing the relationship of social and economic factors to the medical causes of death, provided the basis for the Children's Bureau to propose a continuing grants-in-aid program to assist state health agencies establish and improve services to promote the health of mothers and infants. The studies of reduction of mortality through better care, instruction of mothers in maternity and baby clinics, popular bulletins, and public health nurses were used as evidence of successful methods of accomplishing the objectives. The authorizing legislation, which expired in 1927, was extended by Congress until June 30, 1929, after which it was not renewed. It was the first public health grants-in-aid program enacted in the United States.

It is not surprising that such precedent-making legislation provoked considerable dissension, and not only within the medical profession. *The Women's Patriot,* a journal of the day, attacked it saying it would make children the best political graft in the country and would give new fat jobs to socialist feminists and childless female bureaucrats. The American Medical Association opposed the original bill and its continuation, causing some of its members to form the American Academy of Pediatrics in 1930. The pediatricians who issued a statement supporting the Sheppard-Towner Act were censured by the AMA in 1922, which led them to create their own forum eight years later. In 1930, the academy stated its purpose: "to improve the health and welfare of our children, to raise the standard of pediatric education and practice, and to encourage research in pediatrics" (American Academy of Pediatrics, 1980, p. 1).

In the eight years of its existence, the Sheppard-Towner Act helped bring about many improvements in health services for mothers and children. Birth registration, one of the Children's Bureau's specific objectives, increased from thirty states in 1920 to forty-six states in 1929, representing 95 percent of the national population. The number of state child hygiene divisions increased from twenty-eight to forty-seven. The number of permanent maternal and child health centers increased greatly, 1,594 being established between 1924 and 1929. There was widespread increase in public health nursing services. And the bureau demonstrated the values of the new partnership of federal and state governments in promoting the health of mothers and children.

Services for Crippled Children

Programs of medical care for crippled children developed more slowly and later than those for pregnant women and babies. Although most of the major cities had hospitals for orthopedically handicapped children by the end of the nineteenth century, the first state to undertake such a service was Minnesota in 1897. Education for the blind and the deaf began between 1850 and 1890. By 1898, there were twenty-four public institutions for the mentally retarded in nineteen states, and by 1920, all but four states were providing some institutional care for the retarded. Various services for the handicapped were a special interest of several voluntary agencies during the early part of the twentieth century, including Rotary International, the American Legion, the International Society for Crippled Children, the Elks, the Lions, and the Shriners.

It was also during the first quarter of the century that the Children's Bureau, in response to inquiries about services for crippled children, carried out a survey of the provisions for their care in rural and urban areas of fourteen states. The findings of these studies later became the basis of recommendations by the Children's Bureau to the Committee on Economic Security in its consideration of the proposals for inclusion in the Social Security Act (Bradbury, 1962).

Considerable impetus to the development of public opinion in support of a comprehensive program of services for crippled children was given by the White House Conference on Child Health and Protection (1933a) whose goals were to study the present status of the health and well-being of the children of the United States and its possessions, to report what was being done, and to recommend what ought to be done and how to do it. The conference was held in November of 1930, and for sixteen months before, some 1,200 people devoted themselves to study, review, and fact-finding.

The Conference Committee on National, State, and Local Organizations for the Handicapped stated in its report, "Grants-in-aid constitute the most effective basis for national and state cooperation in promoting child welfare and in securing the establishment of that national minimum of care and protection which is the hope of every citizen. . . . Maternity and infancy aid is of fundamental importance in the social welfare field as well as in the health field. The benefits of such aid should be made available to the territories and dependencies. Grants-in-aid should be extended to the States to promote the proper care and protection of the dependent, delinquent, and handicapped child" (White House Conference, 1933a, p. 6).

The conference declared that "the solution of the problem of the crippled child will be a program in every state defined by law and given sound financial support" (1933b, p. 166). Such a program must emphasize prevention and be administered in close association with prenatal, infant, and child health, and school health services. It requires the cooperation of all medical, education, social welfare, and vocational rehabilitation agencies. The conference recommended that federal funds be distributed to a properly constituted state service for crippled children in the several states. The programs must include early discovery, diagnosis, and creative and remedial treatment "which will enable the handicapped child to function as normally as possible, this treatment to be available to all handicapped children regardless of financial circumstances and to be a continuing process until a proper adjustment has been effected" (pp. 5–6).

The Social Security Act

A variety of forces led to the enactment of Title V of the Social Security Act with its provisions for three grants-in-aid programs: maternal and child health, crippled children, and child welfare services. As we have seen, some of these forces had been developing gradually since the turn of the century and represented the culmination of federal, state, and local efforts to protect and promote the well-being of the children. Other factors were immediately related to the Depression of the 1930s and the national desire to take the necessary steps to prevent a recurrence. These forces can be grouped into four closely interrelated themes.

First was the growing recognition of the responsibility of the federal government for the promotion and protection of the well-being of children. In the colonial days, the concept of local government responsibility for children began to take shape. During the nineteenth century, state and private agencies assumed responsibility for special groups of children. But the concept of a partnership of the states with the federal government in improving the health of mothers and children did not appear in public debate or federal law until after the beginning of the twentieth century. The establishment of the Children's Bureau meant that the growing concern for children "was translated into a specific public policy to focus attention on the state of well-being of children throughout the country and on their common and special needs" (Eliot, 1960, pp. 135–136).

The Sheppard-Towner Act was the first grants-in-aid program for health services and was based on the principle that federal assistance to state and local health departments would enable them to extend and improve maternity and infant care and help reduce the high mortality rate. The White House Conference of 1930, with its published reports of fact-finding, recommendations, and the strong appeal of its Children's Charter, provided an excellent resource of facts as well as an expression of the climate of opinion that the time had come for action.

The second force was evidence, brought out during the Depression, that far greater needs had existed even in normal times than had generally been realized and that, as a result of the Depression, there had been a decrease in services for children even though the need for these services had increased. The report of the president's U.S. Committee on Economic Security (1935, p. 37) summarized some of this evidence as follows:

> Local services for the protection and care of physically and mentally handicapped children are generally available in large urban centers, but

in less populous areas, they are extremely limited or even non-existent. One-fourth of the states only have made provisions on a statewide basis for county child welfare boards or similar agencies, and in many of these states, the services are still inadequate.

With the further depletion of resources during the Depression, there has been much suffering among many children because the services they need have been curtailed or even stopped. . . .

The fact that the maternal mortality rate in this country is much higher than that of nearly all other progressive countries suggests the great need for Federal participation in a nationwide maternal and child health program. From 1922 to 1929, all but three states participated in the successful operation of such a program. Federal funds were then withdrawn, and, as a consequence, State appropriations were materially reduced. Twenty-three states now either have no special funds for maternal and child health or appropriate for this purpose $10,000 or less. In the meantime, the need has become increasingly acute.

Crippled children and those suffering from chronic diseases such as heart disease and tuberculosis constitute a regiment of whose needs the country became acutely conscious only after the now abandoned child and maternal health program was inaugurated. In more than half the states, some state and local funds are now being devoted to the care of crippled children. This care includes diagnostic clinics, hospitalization, and convalescent treatment. But, in nearly half the states, nothing at all is now being done for these children and in many, the appropriations are so small as to take care of a negligible number of children. Since hundreds of thousands of children need this care, the situation is not only tragic but dangerous.

The third force was the underlying concept that the program of the federal government for recovery from the Depression should include not only ameliorative measures aimed at assurances of adequate income but also preventive measures to safeguard against hazards leading to destitution and dependency of children as well as adults. With respect to the risks to economic security arising from ill health, the committee's report said: "In this situation, there is great need for a nationwide program for the extension of public health services" (p. 37). As was well stated by the committee's medical advisory board in the same report, "At the present time, appropriations for public health work are insufficient in many communities, whereas, a fuller application of modern preventive medicine . . . would not only relieve such suffering but would also prove an actual financial economy. Federal funds, expended through several states in association with their own state and local public health expenditures are in our opinion necessary . . . and we recommend that substantial grants be made" (p. 37). The committee thereupon included grants-in-aid to state and local health departments and funds for an expanded U.S. Public Health Service in its recommendations.

In a special message on January 17, 1935, the president transmitted this report to Congress. His recommendations for legislation that would lead to economic security included federal aid for services for the protection and care of homeless, neglected, dependent, and crippled children, and grants to state and local health agencies.

The fourth force was the widespread conviction that special measures for the protection of children are an essential part of a program for economic security. This conviction permeated the thinking in the development of the provisions that eventually became the Social Security Act. The U.S. Committee on Economic Security stated in its 1935 report to the president that "it must not for a moment be forgotten that the core of any social plan must be the child. Every proposition we make must adhere to this core" (p. 35). In the floor debate on the Social Security Act, Congressman Jenkins of Ohio, discussing the Title V grants, emphasized that the Republican membership unqualifiedly endorsed this Title. "It is not legislation that belongs to any party," he said. "This is legislation that has sprung up out of the desire of the people of this country to have the Federal government participate and help out the States in this great and wonderful work" (*Congressional Record*, 1935, p. 5901).

The provisions of Title V as enacted by Congress followed to a large extent the recommendations of the President's Committee on Economic Security. In 1934, the chairman of the committee, Edwin Witte, asked the acting chief of the Children's Bureau, Katherine Lenroot, for her views on what provisions for children should be included in the proposals for the Social Security Act. Three grants-in-aid programs were proposed: Maternal and Child Health Services, Services for Crippled Children, and Aid to Dependent Children, including social services for children needing special care. Subsequently, the administration of Aid to Dependent Children was transferred to the Social Security Board, but Child Welfare Services was retained in Title V as Part Three and administered by the Children's Bureau. Although the child health and child welfare provisions were closely related through their administration by the Children's Bureau, only the provisions for services for crippled children are discussed in detail here.

Part One. Part One, providing for Maternal and Child Health Services, was an extension of the Sheppard-Towner Act with, however, a most significant new addition. The Children's Bureau had· proposed an appropriation for demonstration programs carried out by staff of the Children's Bureau in cooperation with the states, a concept related to the act of 1912. Congress did not adopt this proposal but instead included appropriations language by which half the grants to the states would be matched dollar for dollar. The other half, called the B funds, would require no matching. The latter fund took into account the per capita income of each state, so the poorer states would receive a larger share of the nonmatching B funds than the richer states. The B fund also provided the basis for subsequent development of special project grants of regional or national significance. The B fund provision was initially included only in the Maternal and Child Health part, but in the 1939 amendments, it was also added to Part Two, Services for Crippled Children. In later years, the use of project grants became widespread throughout the government.

Part Two. Part Two, Services for Crippled Children, was an entirely new program. For the first time, federal funds would be used with state matching funds to provide comprehensive medical care for certain groups of children. The language of the statute is particularly significant in establishing specific requirements for the use of the federal and state matching funds, while at the same time allowing considerable flexibility and recognizing the differences among the states. The purpose clause reads: "Part 2—Services for Crippled Children Appropriation, Sec. 511. For the purpose of enabling each State to extend and improve (especially in rural areas and in areas suffering from severe economic distress) as far as practicable under the conditions in each state, services for locating crippled children, and for providing medical, surgical, corrective, and other services and care, and facilities for diagnosis, hospitalization, and after care for children who are crippled or who are suffering from conditions which lead to crippling, there is hereby authorized. . . ." The statute further states that the state plan must "provide for cooperation with medical, health, nursing and welfare groups, and organizations" and with the state vocational rehabilitation agency (Title V of the Social Security Act, 1935, p. 631).

In contrast to the Sheppard-Towner Act and to most legislation of this type, Congress set no time limit on the Title V authorizing legislation. Congress took the position that Title V is continuing legislation and that the federal government has a responsibility to use its taxing power on a continuing basis to assist the states in their programs to extend and improve the health and welfare of mothers and children (White House Conference, 1933a).

It was clear from the outset that these are state programs with federal funds available to assist the states in carrying out their programs. The statute provided that the chief of the Children's Bureau would approve any state plan meeting the statutory provisions for state plan approval.

With the Social Security Act, the Children's Bureau entered a new era, in which its responsibilities for grants-in-aid administration were quite different from its continuing responsibilities to investigate and report under the Act of 1912. As its staff expanded to administer Title V, the Children's Bureau became increasingly absorbed in grants-in-aid administration. The investigative and study functions decreased, but the reporting functions continued to develop with greater emphasis on Title V programs.

The stated purpose of enabling each state to extend and improve its services meant that a state could not use federal funds simply to pay for what it may have already been doing. Rather, it meant what it said, and emphasis was placed by the Children's Bureau on adopting standards of care and selection of medical personnel that would be consistent with care of good quality.

Title V explicitly requires that state programs must provide services that are comprehensive—for example, including measures for casefinding, diagnosis, treatment including hospitalization, and aftercare. At the beginning, some state agencies, hesitant about going all the way into medical care, proposed doing no more than surveys of crippled children. The Children's Bureau made it clear that such plans could not be approved.

The concept of prevention is of greatest importance in a program concerned with long-term illness or handicaps. Prevention in this context includes not only prevention of onset of illness but also services needed to mitigate crippling and to minimize emotional and social disability.

The statute left the definition of *crippled child* to the states. The predominant crippling conditions during the 1930s and 1940s were orthopedic, accounting for more than 80 percent of the children receiving services. The way was open, however, for broad programs, which did develop subsequently.

There is no mention of a means test for eligibility in Title V, but following recommendations made by the Children's Bureau and its advisory committees, the states have generally adopted procedures for determining eligibility that differ considerably from those adopted for public assistance. Eligibility for treatment services takes into account not only family income and size but also diagnosis; estimated cost of care, including aftercare; and the continuing added costs required by a handicapped child.

An emphasis on rural areas was due to the inadequacy or lack of resources for the care of crippled children in rural areas and the greater availability of such resources in the cities. A notable characteristic of the state plans was the provision for cooperative relationships between the state agencies and the private voluntary organizations. Private groups made significant contributions to the programs by providing related services, such as transportation, and by assisting with organization of clinics, thereby enabling the state agencies to extend their resources (Twenty-Fourth Annual Report, 1936).

Development of Policies. In view of the current concern about the proliferation of detailed federal regulations in recent years, it is of interest that the Children's Bureau issued few regulations in administering Title V. To some extent, this was due to the soundness and clarity of the statute itself, which has needed few modifications since enactment. For the most part, the Children's Bureau relied on consultation with the state agencies, using the policies and recommendations made to the bureau by its advisory committees. Particular attention was given to the quality of medical care, extension of the programs to new diagnostic groups of children, increased employment of multidisciplinary staffs, and focusing state agencies' attention on the child as a person rather than only on that part of the child affected by illness. "This emphasis on quality has been the controlling force within the Bureau" (Eliot, 1960, p. 139).

"As policies were demonstrated with time to be necessary for efficient administration or otherwise in the interests of children, they were formulated into regulations. . . . In 1950, an integrated detailed compilation was promulgated by the Secretary and issued as part of the Bureau's operational manual, a significant compilation of public policy in relation to standards of medical care and the protection of the interests of the patient and the rights of vendors of services. Such regulations, for example, require the states to describe their standards for personnel and facilities in their State Plans; to limit their program's provision of hospital and similar services to individuals receiving medical services under the plan; and to make their diagnostic services . . . available to any child without charge, without restriction or requirement in relation to his family's economic status or legal residence and without requirement that he be referred" (Eliot, 1960, p. 140). The point of the diagnostic services regulation is that, until a diagnosis is made, it is not possible to estimate the kind of treatment required or the cost of care.

A Children's Bureau policy (subsequently issued as a regulation) that became a milestone in medical care administration was the method established to pay for hospital care. Initially adopted for the Crippled Children's program, it reached its most widespread use in the Emergency Maternity and Infant Care Program for wives and dependents of men in the Armed Forces during World War II, as well as by agencies other than the Children's Bureau. Prior to the Children's Bureau regulation, hospital charges varied considerably, there was no standard method of cost accounting in general use, and many hospitals did no cost accounting and did not know what their costs were. Because the hospitals used by the state Crippled Children's agencies were nonprofit hospitals, the Children's Bureau adopted the policy that hospitals be paid on the basis of the average daily cost per patient. The bureau added to its staff a hospital administrator who developed a simplified uniform system of hospital cost accounting that could be used by any hospital and was known as Joint Hospital Form I. With the support of the American Hospital Association, this method of cost accounting was adopted by hospitals providing care under the Maternal and Child Health and Crippled Children's programs, as well as by those that were not. In 1965, with the enactment of Medicare, a different method was included in the statute and the same provision was extended to Title V.

Another issue (of significance for the administration of medical care programs and of concern in the Emergency Maternity and Infant Care (EMIC) program) was whether hospitals and physicians providing care authorized for a patient under the program should be permitted to charge patients more than the amount paid by the state agency. The bureau regulation stated that care authorized by the state Crippled Children's agency be provided at rates or fee schedules established by the state agency. Whether patients would share in the cost and the amount they would pay, including the payment by hospital insurance, would be determined by the state agency; payments to hospitals and physicians were payment in full and additional charges could not be made to the patient.

Special Projects in the Crippled Children's Program

In 1939, Congress increased the appropriation for the Crippled Children's program (at that time largely orthopedic), with the understanding that part of the funds would be used to assist some states to include children with rheumatic fever and heart disease. The Children's Bureau adopted the policy of reserving a portion of the newly appropriated B funds (which did not require matching) and granting them for special projects of regional or national significance to states making applications. As a method of disbursing funds, special projects have the advantage over formula funds of being more flexible and more readily targeted to areas or subjects of particular need. The special project concept was subsequently adopted by other government programs and became the method of grants with widest appeal.

By 1941, nine states had developed demonstration programs for children with rheumatic fever in limited geographic areas, and this was increased subsequently to twenty-eight states. By then, the demonstration phase was over, and children with rheumatic fever and congenital heart disease were included in almost all state Crippled Children's programs.

As appropriations were increased, special project grants were provided for programs for children with such conditions as cerebral palsy, epilepsy, hearing impairment, and congenital heart disease and for graduate training and institutes in specialized subjects. Up to 12.5 percent of the annual appropriation was used for these special projects. Similar provisions were made in the Maternal and Child Health program, and some projects were interrelated. The increased use and diversity of special project grants came about in response to new opportunities to help children with different kinds of handicapping conditions that resulted from the very productive research following World War II. The state agencies also used their appropriations provided by formula to widen the scope of diagnostic problems in their programs.

Significant changes took place in the Crippled Children's programs quantitatively as well as in scope and concepts. The number of children receiving medical care in the program in 1958 was 325,000 or 4.8 per thousand children under twenty-one years of age. This is twice the 1937 rate. The proportion of children in the program who received hospital care decreased from 27 percent in 1937 to 16 percent in 1958, and the average duration of hospitalization decreased by about one half.

In part, the decrease in hospital care is attributable to the changes in the diagnostic composition of the programs. Initially, they were almost entirely orthopedic programs, but in 1958, orthopedic conditions constituted a little less than 50 percent of the reported diagnoses. Changes from 1950 to 1958 include:

> Epilepsy—up 596 percent
> Congenital malformations—up 94 percent
> Congenital heart disease—up 451 percent
> Hearing impairment—up 105 percent
> Mastoiditis—down 43 percent
> Osteomyelitis—down 47 percent
> Acute poliomyelitis—down 89 percent.

These changes are expressions of the response of the Crippled Children's program to the dramatic developments research has produced in medicine. Developments that particularly influenced the Crippled Children's program include:

> Antibiotics for prophylaxis against acute rheumatic fever
> Poliomyelitis vaccine
> Diagnosis and treatment of various types of congenital heart disease
> Development of the science of audiology and the electronic hearing aid
> Drug treatment of tuberculosis

Drugs for the control of epileptic seizures

Increased understanding of the principles of physical and emotional growth and development (Lesser, 1960).

These developments were also among the factors that produced marked changes in pediatrics generally. Better control of acute illnesses meant that, by 1958, a growing proportion of children seen in clinics, hospitals, and private practice had long-term illness and handicapping conditions. In teaching hospitals, children with medical problems congenital in origin constituted between 30 and 50 percent of the inpatients.

The changes in diagnoses mean that the problems change with time but do not go away. Better neonatal survival rates have also meant increased survival of children with cystic fibrosis, neurological deficits, congenital malformations that may or may not be amenable to surgery, and inborn errors of metabolism such as phenylketonuria.

The technology involved in some research developments (for example, in the diagnosis and treatment of congenital heart disease) meant that, for several years, clinical resources available to treat children were limited to some of the teaching hospitals. The success of the Blalock-Taussig operation in 1944 for a common type of congenital heart disease—the tetralogy of Fallot—brought hundreds of children from many states to the Johns Hopkins Hospital for this treatment. A special project grant of B funds was given to the Maryland State Department of Health to pay for the care of children coming to Baltimore from other states for this purpose. Subsequently, similar grants were made to the state agencies in California, Illinois, and Texas for out-of-state children. By this administrative procedure, it became possible for children, living in states that for a time lacked the necessary resources, to obtain promptly what was for many life-saving treatment.

The development of open heart surgery at the University of Minnesota made possible effective treatment of additional kinds of congenital heart disease. The same procedure, providing grants to several state agencies to arrange and pay for care at designated regional congenital heart centers, enabled children, wherever they lived, to obtain care.

Mental Retardation

The considerable progress in the more positive attitudes toward the handicapped, and the development of community programs for them, did not generally include the mentally retarded. It was not until the late 1950s that changes in attitude toward them appeared. In 1957, Congress, with the sponsorship of Congressman John Fogarty of Rhode Island, increased the appropriation for the Maternal and Child Health programs and earmarked $1 million for demonstration clinical programs for mentally retarded children. The states and the voluntary organizations of parents of the retarded responded promptly, and new diagnostic, consultation, and education clinics were established rapidly.

But the major developments on a nationwide scale resulted from the leadership of President John F. Kennedy and the new influence of the National Association for Retarded Children. In 1961, the president appointed a panel on mental retardation "to appraise the adequacies of existing programs and the possibilities for utilization of current knowledge" (President's Panel on Mental Retardation, 1962, p. 201). The recommendations in the Report of the President's Panel relating to Title V of the Social Security Act were included in the President's Message Relative to Mental Illness and Mental Retardation (February 5, 1963) and enacted in P.L. 88-156.

There were three major provisions in P.L. 88-156. First, it increased authorization for Title V, Part One (Maternal and Child Health) from $25 million to $50 million over a period of seven years and did the same for Part Two (Crippled Children). In the Appropriations Committee, Congress earmarked part of the increase for appropriations for special project grants for clinical programs for mentally retarded children. Second, the law authorized a new five-year program of grants to state or local health departments for Maternity and Infant Care Projects. The legislation stated that the program had been authorized "in order to help reduce the incidence of mental retardation caused by complications associated with childbearing. . . . All necessary health care is to be provided for expectant mothers of low income who have or who are likely to have conditions associated with childbearing that increase the hazards to the health of mothers and infants" (Public Law 88-156, p. 274). A separate appropriation was authorized for the Maternity and Infant Care projects for a five-year period (subsequently extended to 1973), rising from $5 million the first year to $30 million for each of the last three years. Federal funds were not to exceed 75 percent of the cost of each project. Third, P.L. 88-156 authorized a new grants program under Title V for research projects that show promise of substantial contribution to improving the Maternal and Child Health and Crippled Children's Services programs.

The provision for a new program of Maternity and Infant Care projects enacted into law one of the major recommendations of the President's Panel on Mental Retardation. In view of the limits of knowledge regarding the prevention of mental retardation, the panel was much impressed by recent published studies of the close association between premature birth and brain damage and between low income, poor or no prenatal care, and premature birth and by the large numbers of women of low income living in major cities who received little or no prenatal care (Lesser, 1963).

In his February 7, 1963, message to Congress, the president had said: "The relationship between improving maternal and child health and preventing mental retardation is clear. But equally clear is the fact that the need for better health services for mothers and children is steadily increasing in general due to the growing child population, the rising costs of medical care, and changes in the practice of medicine and public health" (U.S. House of Representatives, 1963, p. 9). In the president's messages and in his legislative proposals enacted as P.L. 88-156, there are evident not only the specific provisions relating to mental retardation but also the relationship between maternity care and mental retardation, the social and economic factors influencing the health of expectant mothers and infants, and the beginning of an expression of concern for more equitable availability of good medical care for all classes of society.

There was a response to the availability, in early 1964, of funds for the Maternity and Infant Care projects, and by 1969, there were fifty-three projects serving more than 100,000 women and their infants annually in large- and middle-sized cities and rural areas. A major, new, far-reaching policy was the Children's Bureau's express authorization of the use of project funds for family planning services. The 1967 amendments to Title V went further and earmarked 6 percent of the Maternal and Child Health appropriation for family planning services.

The rapid development of clinical programs for mentally retarded children is an indication of the effectiveness of the parents' organization, the National Association for Retarded Children, in bringing to state legislatures and the Congress information about the needs of retarded children and the potentialities for their development. The earmarking of B funds for special projects for the retarded by Congress in 1957 had the result that, by 1962, seventy-seven special clinics were providing diagnostic and treatment services for 20,000 children annually (most of them preschool) in forty-six states. The emphasis was on early diagnosis and help for the parents in childcare and management in their own homes and on interpretation of the problem to the public.

But better recognition and understanding also creates demands; the waiting lists at available clinics were long, and for many families, distances to clinics were too great. Even before the enactment of the 1963 amendments, twenty-four states had asked for additional funds to increase the availability of their services (Lesser, 1964).

With the enormous impact of the president's legislative program, there was rapid acceleration in the growth of that many-faceted program. By 1972, some 250 clinics were in operation with the assistance of Title V funds (both Maternal and Child Health and Crippled Children's appropriations), serving about 60,000 children and their families annually. But major program impact was also evident in areas in addition to direct services.

The clinical teams operating within the Title V framework not only re-emphasized the flexibility of the Maternal and Child Health and Crippled Children's programs to meet special as well as more general needs, "but also clearly demonstrated the unique and specific role which . . . they . . . could play in any health delivery system relating to all mothers and to all children." With the enactment of the 1963 amendments, "the special role and unique contribution of Maternal and Child Health to a total program for the retarded was clearly established and these programs were expected to make a major contribution to state planning efforts for this group of handicapped individuals. The program linkage of MCH and MR played a considerable role in achieving increases in the basic MCH and CC program support on both a State and National level" (Hormuth, 1973, p. 115).

In 1961, Robert Guthrie of the Children's Hospital in Buffalo, New York, published a report of the results of his new inhibition assay screening test, using a few drops of dried blood to detect phenylketonuria (PKU), a metabolic disorder that occurs in about one in 20,000 births and results in severe mental retardation if not treated in the first few months of life. Feeding such infants with a milk substitute low in phenylalanine beginning in the first few weeks of infancy is usually effective in preventing mental retardation. The Guthrie test made it possible to screen newborn infants and to institute the necessary dietary treatment early enough to be effective. In the same year, the Children's Bureau sponsored and financed a mass trial of the screening test to determine its accuracy and usefulness. By 1962, thirty-two state Maternal and Child Health programs participated in the trial, more than 400,000 newborns were tested, and thirty-seven confirmed cases of PKU were diagnosed. Within a few years, forty-three states had enacted legislation pertaining to PKU testing, and mass screening was being done in other countries as well. Since 1970, more than 90 percent of newborns in the United States are tested for this disorder.

As early as 1962, the results were tremendously encouraging, especially to parents of the retarded, with implications for types of retardation other than that caused by PKU. They were also a major stimulus to research in broad areas of inborn errors of metabolism, which became a predominant subject of biochemistry research, especially in pediatrics. The responsiveness to the new interest in the many aspects of mental retardation also had the result that state Crippled Children's programs, which included the phrase *of normal intelligence* (or its equivalent) in their definition of crippled children, discontinued such limitations and there followed an increase in the number of physically handicapped children who are also mentally retarded in the Crippled Children's programs.

There was also considerable support for training of professional personnel. The Public Health Service received funds for construction of university affiliated centers for training, research, and clinical services for retarded and physically handicapped children and adults. The Children's Bureau granted funds for training of multidisciplinary teams. By 1972, with funds authorized by the 1965 amendments, nineteen university affiliated centers in medical institutions were supported with Title V funds and provided training for physicians, psychologists, social workers, dentists, nurses, physical and occupational therapists, nutritionists, geneticists, and others for the health and related care of crippled children, particularly mentally retarded children and children with multiple handicaps.

By the same year, twenty-one projects were in operation supported by Title V funds to provide cytogenetic and biochemical laboratory services as an extension of clinical services in hospitals and medical schools. Projects include chromosome analyses and diagnoses of various medical conditions that may be genetic in origin and may result in physical handicaps or mental retardation. Genetic counseling is provided, and these laboratories also provide continued monitoring of children with metabolic disorders (U.S. Department of Health, Education, and Welfare, 1971).

These developments are indicative of the broad and comprehensive approach afforded by the 1963 amendments in response to the complex problems of handicapped children.

Children and Youth Projects

In response to the same problems that led to the creation of the maternity care programs, a new program of project grants to meet up to 75 percent of the costs of comprehensive health services for children and youth living in areas with concentrations of low-income families was authorized in 1964 as an amendment to Title V of the Social Security Act. In his February 1963 message to Congress on Our Nation's Youth, President Kennedy requested "the Secretary of Health, Education, and Welfare to put a high priority on the Department's studies of school health programs and to make recommendations regarding any action which may be required" (U.S. House of Representatives, 1963b, p. 9).

The secretary's letter, transmitting the report prepared by the Children's Bureau, states, "The material in the enclosed report on 'Health of Children of School Age' emphasizes the gaps in child health supervision in the preschool years with the resultant wide disparity in the readiness of children to begin their education; the great crowding of well-baby clinics and hospital outpatient departments in the cities; the inadequacies in the quantity and quality of medical care received by children in many low-income families; the need for more effective methods of case finding . . . the special problems of adolescents and the handicapped . . . all pointing to the need for new approaches and for concentrating our community resources where they are most needed" (U.S. Department of Health, Education, and Welfare, 1964, p. 1).

The major objective of the legislation was to make possible programs that provide comprehensive health services through the promotion of health as well as medical care, including casefinding, preventive health services, diagnosis, treatment, correction of defects, and aftercare, both medical and dental. This, in fact, is the definition of *comprehensive* in the statute. The emphasis in a project is placed on comprehensiveness and continuity of services; children admitted to the program are to be provided (either directly or through coordination with other local health, education, and welfare programs) with the services they need. In other words, the project takes care of the health problems (personal, as well as environmental) of a given child population. Thus, the projects are involved not only in direct medical services but also in community health activities, such as nutrition education, food demonstrations, working with city authorities to do something about sources of lead poisoning, rat control, and so on.

The Children and Youth Projects were enacted in the same year as the Office of Economic Opportunity Neighborhood Health Centers. This came at a time of great interest on the part of students of the related professions—medicine, social work, nursing, psychology, sociology, and others—in community action on behalf of the underprivileged, which pushed colleges and professional schools to become involved in the world beyond the campus. By 1969, there were fifty-eight Children and Youth Projects, some closely allied with Maternity and Infant

Projects or with Neighborhood Health Centers. In 1968, 335,000 children were registered in the programs. These children were in families in which 37 percent of family heads were women, one third of family heads had less than an eighth-grade education, and 40 percent were unemployed. Early data revealed that about 45 percent of the registered children required immediate care and that the remaining were well and started preventive health services with regular appointments for health supervision (Lesser, 1969).

It was no coincidence that the Children and Youth Projects were authorized in 1965 in the same Social Security amendments that authorized Medicaid. The latter is essentially a means of paying for medical care but does not in itself create clinical resources where they are in short supply. The House Ways and Means Committee in its report on the Social Security Amendments of 1965 pointed out that "communities are finding that they do not have adequate resources to which children can be referred for diagnosis and treatment through school health programs, and their resources for the examination, diagnosis, and treatment of preschool children to help them prepare to enter school are also too few and too crowded" (U.S. House of Representatives, 1965, p. 80).

Thus, for the first time, both the legislative and executive branches of the federal government made clear the important principle that there are two essential elements in any system of medical care: the financing of medical care and the availability of clinical resources from which care can be provided and purchased. This principle has been of particular significance in view of the interest in national health insurance. With the exception of two bills, virtually all of the bills introduced addressed financing but gave little recognition to the need for a more equitable distribution of resources for medical care. This principle was further emphasized by President Nixon in his health message of March 2, 1972, which stated: "One basic shortcoming of a solution to health care problems which depends entirely on spending more money can be seen in the Medicare and Medicaid programs. Medicare and Medicaid did deliver needed dollars to the health care problems of the elderly and the poor. But, at the same time, little was done to alter the existing supply and distribution of doctors, nurses, hospitals, and other health resources. Our health care supply, in short, remained largely the same while massive new demands were loaded onto it. The predictable result was an acute price inflation" (Nixon, 1974, p. 385).

There are few programs that have borne out their stated programmatic objectives as effectively as the Children and Youth Projects. The emphasis is on prevention and increasing the availability of care; it is significant that, if we compare the diagnoses of children at the initial examination with subsequent examinations, we find that the proportion of children with a diagnosis of *well child* is consistently increased by one fourth. At recall examinations for dental services, there is a decrease of more than 50 percent in the number of dental caries. Most important is the fact that since the beginning of the program, there has been a marked decrease in the number of children needing hospitalization—from 7.7 percent of the cases in 1968 to 4.1 percent in 1970. This resulted also in a decrease in the annual average per capita costs.

The language of the Children and Youth Projects amendment is reminiscent of the language of Title V, Part Two, Services for Crippled Children. It is, therefore, of interest to recall that when Grace Abbott, Chief of the Children's Bureau, proposed legislation creating the Crippled Children's program, prior to the passage of the Social Security Act, she saw it as possibly preliminary to legislation for a medical care program for all children. Although limited to projects mostly in large cities with concentrations of low-income families, the Children and Youth Projects fulfill, at least in part, her aspirations for a program of medical care for all children.

The 1967 Amendments

Three new types of medical care project grants were authorized in 1967: Infant Care (neonatal intensive care), Family Planning, and Dental Care. All five types of projects were extended to June 30, 1972, and the authorization was increased to $350 million for all the Title V programs. The amendments specified that 50 percent of the annual appropriation was to be for the formula grants that have a rural emphasis, 40 percent for project grants, and 10 percent for research and training. The amendments further specified that the states were to take over the project grants after June 30, 1972. Each state plan was thereafter to include a program of Maternity and Infant Care Projects, a program of Children and Youth Projects, and so on. To support the new state plan requirement, 90 percent of the annual appropriation would be available for the formula grants (which would also include funds for the projects) and 10 percent for research and training.

The amendments embodied a significant policy decision, in which Congressman Wilbur Mills, Chairman of the House Ways and Means Committee, was the prime mover. It meant that Congress had concluded that the project grants were effective in carrying out their objectives and the legislative intent, that they should be continued, and that all states should be required to have such projects because the need for these programs existed in all states.

To carry out the amendments, each state would have to survey its available resources and requirements—for example, for intensive nursery care for newborn infants. It meant the development in each state of a planned regionalized system of neonatal intensive care nurseries for premature and ill newborns and for infants with congenital anomalies requiring specialized care or surgery. It meant that such resources would be located so as to be available to the population anywhere in each state.

The 1967 amendments had the same significance for all the other project grants. These amendments, together with the 1965 amendment requiring each state to extend Maternal and Child Health and Crippled Children's Services to children in all parts of the state by July 1, 1975, established the *legislative base* for a comprehensive program for handicapped children in each state.

The amendments, delayed one year and modified, were enacted July 1, 1973. Congress recognized that putting 90 percent of the appropriation into the formula with a rural emphasis was in contradiction to programs of project grants that emphasized areas with concentrations of low-income families, such as the major cities. It meant greatly increased funds to rural states (with concomitant matching problems) and greatly decreased funds to states with large cities. At the same time, Congress did not want to drop the rural emphasis. What had happened since 1935 was a polarization of populations with low incomes to rural areas and major central cities.

To solve the problem of grants apportionment and to protect the projects already in existence, Congress enacted amendments that (1) extended the authorization for project grants until June 30, 1974, (2) allocated 90 percent of the appropriation to the states by formula after that date, (3) provided an additional authorization so that no state would be eligible for less funds after June 30, 1974, than the total amount in formula and project grants in fiscal year 1973, and (4) required the states to make appropriate arrangements for continuation of services to the population in areas previously served under the project grants.

It is an indication of the regard with which Congress held the Title V programs, that congressional action took place in connection with H.R. 8410, the 1973 debt limit bill. Each year, this is essential legislation.

Major Policy Issues

Should federal grants-in-aid be categorical or in a bloc? Should there be in the federal government a children's agency whose mission is to improve the conditions in which children live so as to foster their healthy growth and development? Should such an agency not only engage in fact-finding but also administer grants-in-aid in support of child health and welfare? If national health insurance legislation were enacted, would there still be a need for grants-in-aid for Maternal and Child Health and Crippled Children's Services? These interrelated issues are parts of a broader issue: *Should the United States have a national social policy for children that is the basis for the development and continued support of child health services?*

These issues have been discussed ever since the Children's Bureau was established, and they are still being debated. By and large, Congress has been more categorically minded than the executive branch. The latter has tended to be more in favor of organization by function—for example, all health programs in the Public Health Service, social services in another agency, and the Children's Bureau limited to the functions of the act of 1912. Congress generally has been more supportive of Title V and the Children's Bureau and of the categorical approach where there is greater accountability for federal expenditures and readier response to the interests of citizens' organizations.

The Health, Education, and Welfare reorganization of 1967 proposed transferring the Crippled Children's program from the Children's Bureau to the Rehabilitation Services Administration, an agency administering grants for rehabilitation services for handicapped adults. A threat by the Senate Finance Committee to enact legislation keeping the Crippled Children's program in the

Children's Bureau led the Secretary of Health, Education, and Welfare to withdraw his decision. In 1969, the child health grants were transferred from the Children's Bureau to the newly established Maternal and Child Health Service in the Public Health Service.

The relationship of the categorical programs to broad national health care systems has been the subject of considerable study. For example, the Committee for Economic Development stated in its 1973 report, *Building a National Health Care System:* "Basic to the establishment of a national health care system is a determined and adequately supported program to make health services more accessible to people all of whom will be entitled to receive basic benefits. Specifically, this will require a greatly accelerated development of ambulatory and primary care centers particularly in areas of special need; mental health centers; and, especially, organizations that assume responsibility for providing comprehensive and continuous care. . . . Also of vital importance is the continuous financing of such services through a national system and the integration of components into a comprehensive program of health care in each region" (p. 22).

Any health care system financed by insurance needs a service system of clinical resources as an integral part. There is nothing new about this statement—we have only to look at the national health systems in European countries that have had national health insurance for many years.

In 1973, Secretary of Health, Education, and Welfare Elliot Richardson discussed why he favored replacing categorical grants with revenue-sharing grants. However, he recognized the strengths of some categorical programs and used as an example the Maternal and Child Health programs and the close relationship existing among the federal, state, and local Maternal and Child Health and Crippled Children's Services people. The article did not say how such a relationship had developed; undoubtedly, much credit is due the federal Maternal and Child Health staff, but this can be only a minor reason.

What can bring together pediatricians, obstetricians, surgeons, nurses, nurse midwives, social workers, nutritionists, and other professional and nonprofessional people in a productive relationship? Nothing, if not dedication to a common, noble, well-defined purpose—to reduce the inequities in the availability of health services for mothers and children, to enable poor children to have the advantages of continuing health supervision characteristic of that of private patients of pediatricians, to reduce the differences in infant mortality rates between the poor and middle class, to enable crippled children to obtain the benefits of the advances in medical research—in fact, to carry out the provisions of the Children's Charter, a statement of the fundamental rights of the child adopted by President Hoover's White House Conference of 1930.

References

American Academy of Pediatrics. *Fifty Years of Child Advocacy.* Evanston, Ill.: American Academy of Pediatrics, 1980.

Bradbury, D. *Five Decades of Action for Children.* U.S. Department of Health,

Education, and Welfare, Children's Bureau. Washington, D.C.: U.S. Government Printing Office, 1962.

Bremner, R. H. *Children and Youth in America: A Documentary History.* Vol. 2. Cambridge, Mass.: Harvard University Press, 1970.

Committee for Economic Development. *Building a National Health-Care System.* New York: Committee for Economic Development, 1973.

Congressional Record, April 15, 1935, p. 5901.

Eliot, M. M. "The Children's Titles in the Social Security Act." *Children,* 1960, 7 (4), 137–140.

Eliot, M. M. "The United States Children's Bureau." *American Journal of Diseases of Children,* 1967, *114,* 565–573.

Hormuth, R. "Mental Retardation." In H. Wallace (Ed.), *Maternal and Child Health Practices.* Springfield, Ill.: Thomas, 1973.

Lesser, A. J. "Health Services, Accomplishments, and Outlook." *Children,* 1960, 7 (4), 146–151.

Lesser, A. J. *Current Problems of Maternity Care.* U.S. Department of Health, Education, and Welfare, Children's Bureau. Washington, D.C.: U.S. Government Printing Office, 1963.

Lesser, A. J. "Accent on Prevention Through Improved Service." *Children,* 1964, *11* (1), 16–20.

Lesser, A. J. "The Federal Government in Child Health Care." *Pediatric Clinics of North America,* 1969, *16* (4), 891–898.

Nixon, R. "Special Message to the Congress on Health Care." In *Public Papers of the Presidents of the United States: Richard Nixon, 1972.* Washington, D.C.: U.S. Government Printing Office, 1974.

President's Panel on Mental Retardation. *A Proposed Program for National Action to Combat Mental Retardation.* Washington, D.C.: U.S. Government Printing Office, 1962.

Public Law 88-156. "Maternal and Child Health and Mental Retardation Planning Amendments of 1963." *United States Statutes at Large,* Vol. 77. Washington, D.C.: U.S. Government Printing Office, 1964.

Schmidt, W. "The Development of Health Services for Mothers and Children in the United States." *American Journal of Public Health,* 1973, *63* (5), 419–425.

Title V of the Social Security Act of 1935. Chapter 531, *U.S. Statutes at Large,* *XLIX,* Part I, 1935.

Twenty-Fourth Annual Report of the Secretary of Labor, Washington, D.C., 1936.

U.S. Committee on Economic Security. *Report to the President.* Washington, D.C.: U.S Government Printing Office, 1935.

U.S. Department of Health, Education, and Welfare. *Health of Children of School Age.* Children's Bureau, publication no. 427. Washington, D.C.: U.S. Government Printing Office, 1964.

U.S. Department of Health, Education, and Welfare. *Promoting the Health of Mothers and Children.* Washington, D.C.: U.S. Government Printing Office, 1971.

U.S. House of Representatives. 88th Congress, Document No. 60, 1st Session, February 7, 1963a.

U.S. House of Representatives. 88th Congress, Document No. 66, 1st Session, February 14, 1963b.

U.S. House of Representatives. *U.S. Statutes at Large,* 62d Congress, 2d Session, Part 1, Chapter 73, pp. 1911–1912, 79–80.

U.S. House of Representatives, Committee on Ways and Means. "Social Security Amendments of 1965: Report of the Committee on Ways and Means on H.R. 6675." Washington, D.C.: U.S. Government Printing Office, 1965.

White House Conference on Child Health and Protection. *Organization for the Care of Handicapped Children, National, State and Local.* New York: Century, 1933a.

White House Conference on Child Health and Protection. *Section IV. The Handicapped Child.* New York: Century, 1933b.

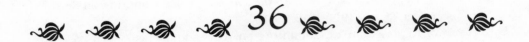

36

Integrating Federal Programs
at the State Level

Antoinette Parisi Eaton, M.D.
Kathryn K. Peppe, R.N., M.S.
Kathleen Bajo, M.S.

Although numerous private and public agencies are committed to the delivery of services for the handicapped, it is well known that the developmental disability service system remains fragmented. Many gaps exist, and rigid eligibility criteria and categories restrict access to certain services. Duplication of services and overlap by governmental agencies with similar target populations are well recognized. It is critical to seek solutions that will meet the needs of clients and, at the same time, be efficient and economical. Therefore, considerable effort across the nation has been directed to the improvement of services through interagency collaboration for children with chronic illness, including those with a developmental disability. For purposes of this chapter, the developmentally disabled are considered a subset of the chronically ill population; our focus is on developmentally disabled children as an example of the potential for interagency cooperation efforts.

Organizations involved in the planning, coordination, and delivery of human services do not function autonomously. They can be influenced by economic, technological, legal, demographic, political, religious, or cultural elements, as well as by the goals of those organizations with which they must share limited resources.

Service delivery systems have occasionally evolved as comprehensive networks, but typically as segmented, divergent, and specialized programs.

Increasing specialization brings increasing reliance on other agencies to meet a wide range of needs for individual persons. The reality facing these diversified agencies is the plethora of systems and networks of "cooperating" organizations; each has a unique focus but provides mutual support to a specific population. The degree of interagency coordination within these systems will often determine the quality, use, availability, and success of the services. However, interdependence is not an easy concept for an agency to accept. Conflict is indigenous to the egocentric nature of agencies as they clarify their roles and develop that part of the system of care they consider their priority and their turf.

Definition and Categories of Interagency Coordination

In its most elementary form, interagency coordination is "the collaboration by two or more agencies or programs in working together to integrate their separate activities for the purpose of improving services to the handicapped" (Elder, 1979, p. 194). Although the literature abounds with details about different ways for agencies to work together, Gans and Horton (1975) describe three general categories of coordination:

1. Voluntary coordination, in which the integrator or lead agency assumes responsibility for provision of selected direct services. Linkages are then developed with autonomous agencies to provide other aspects of care.
2. Mediated coordination, aimed at the development of linkages between autonomous service providers. Utilization of existing resources (rather than creation of new systems) is emphasized to meet the service demands. The lead agency does not assume a significant direct service role.
3. Directed coordination, in which the integrator has the authority to mandate linkages between service providers that are legally subordinate. Directed coordination characterizes the relationship between a state-level department and its local counterparts. The state agency sets all policies and procedures and demands that the local unit carry out the mandated services.

Need for Interagency Cooperation

It has been stated that interagency coordination can reduce cost, maximize limited resources, assure the most appropriate service availability for clients, and improve accountability. Kuzilla (1977) has identified the following factors as indicative of the need for interagency coordination:

1. The need to provide for a continuum of coordinated services
2. The need to provide for the multihandicapped clients who have fallen through the cracks in existing programs and services
3. Larger numbers of developmentally disabled (DD) clients residing in local communities as a result of the depopulation of large state institutions
4. Shrinking resources at a time when health care costs are skyrocketing
5. A need to reduce duplication of effort
6. A need to examine the possibilities of reallocation of resources

7. Service needs of DD clients that cut across agency capabilities
8. A more vocal and active constituency of DD clients and advocates
9. The need for the various professional disciplines to work together for the purpose of providing a safe, secure, and self-actualizing environment for the disabled individual

The need for interagency coordination has increased because of the proliferation of federal programs. Since 1935, a number of programs aimed at the delivery of human services to children and families have sprung from the federal well. The concepts of the programs and the diversity of their bureaucratic authorities have necessitated interagency coordination and cooperation at the state and local levels. Ruth Roemer and her colleagues have stated, in their book appropriately titled *Planning Urban Health Services: From Jungle to System* (1975, p. 4), "The maze of programs in the field of child health . . . each program [with] its own requirements . . . result [in] a patchwork of programs for selected children or selected conditions." Two important federal programs aimed at child health issues are the Maternal and Child Health program (Title V of the Social Security Act) and the Developmental Disabilities program.

"With the passage of the Social Security Act in 1935, an important precedent of federal grants to the states for health services was established, and Title V of that Act became the mainstream of philosophic and financial support in the federal underpinning for child health services" (Silver, 1978, p. 74). The intent of Title V was to "enable each state to extend and improve . . . services for promoting the health of mothers and children" (Department of Health, Education, and Welfare, n.d., p. 3), a broad-based federal policy that gave the interpretation and implementation of this "promotion" to each state and provided a limited appropriation to accomplish it. The Title V program reflected the perspective that public health constitutes care for the masses of people whereas individual care belongs to the private physician and hospital (Silver, 1978). As a result, the Title V legislation gave states the reason to develop general child health services but not the direction or support to ensure strong service programs. The latter task was left to the leadership, skill, and resourcefulness of individual states. Special categorical grants were to channel funds to specific programs.

The primary thrust of the Developmental Disabilities Act was to coordinate the programs that had evolved since 1935, with special focus toward the developmentally disabled population. The goals were to increase cooperation, maximize resources, eliminate service barriers, and increase planning support. Title I of the DD Act recognized the need for these goals in its statement of purpose: to assure that persons with developmental disabilities receive the care, treatment, and other services necessary to enable them to achieve their maximum potential through a system that coordinates and plans services (Title I, 1978). State-level Developmental Disability Planning Councils were established, through legislation, to be the interagency committee charged with implementation.

Thus, the original impetus for cooperation relative to the DD population came from the federal government, which mandated that agencies work together. Many of the resulting agreements were written only to meet regulations and to prevent interruption of the federal cash flow to the agencies rather than to ensure coordination of services. The second impetus was the passage of P.L. 94–142, the Education for All Handicapped Children Act of 1975, which set the principles for delivery systems. These principles necessitated that autonomous agencies regroup to implement the new tenets. A third incentive for coordination is provided by block grants and dwindling resources. In essence, the federal government has shifted from mandating cooperation to encouraging coordination for survival. In the long run, the latter approach can be more effective.

The effective coordination between statewide Maternal and Child Health (MCH) and Developmental Disabilities programs is assumed to have two major outcomes: increased efficiency in the delivery of services to clients who have multiple needs and increased availability, accessibility, and continuity of services (Kuzilla, 1977). Several global factors determine the success of the collaboration:

1. The location and level of authority for the program in the state government unit (MCH programs are located in various departments, such as Health, Welfare, or Human Resources. Their rank varies: they may report directly to department directors or they may constitute small units with limited ability to initiate or implement programs. Similarly, state Developmental Disabilities Councils have a variety of organizational loci, from the governor's office to an insignificant bureaucratic entity with limited clout or support within its parent department)
2. The leadership of the program directors and the qualifications of the staff
3. The level of commitment from the legislature, expressed in both financial support and legislation
4. The effectiveness of state and local advocacy groups
5. Society's attitude and commitment to providing services for DD populations

Barriers to and Facilitators for Interagency Cooperation

There are many barriers to the effectiveness of MCH and DD programs in neutralizing duplicative and competitive agencies and maximizing dollar and human resources. The barriers must be identified and discussed honestly between collaborating agencies. Common barriers are incompatible organizational policies, mandates, or philosophies; poorly defined goals or areas of responsibility; lack of authority to follow through on a defined set of objectives; lack of administrative leadership; desire to remain autonomous in order to retain a competitive edge and maintain control over one's destiny; poor understanding of the overall program goals due to the highly specialized nature of one of the organizations; lack of time and financial resources; past failures of the lead agency, resulting in a low level of confidence in its leadership; and lack of commitment to the goal of program coordination.

Interagency cooperation is facilitated by support from the societal and political environment and by a trusting, cooperative work environment. Facilitators also include good information flow through frequent communication between organizations; participatory management in the negotiations between agencies; excellent leadership; monitoring and evaluation to correct problems; a history of successful programs; commitment to the principles of interagency cooperation, evidenced by the allocation of staff, financial resources, and advocacy directed toward the success of the venture; clear definition of goals, objectives, and anticipated outcomes; solid documentation of need, which continually renews the purpose of the venture and indirectly provides the incentive for progress.

Models of Coordination

Elder and Magrab's (1980) discussion of organization theory raises the question of which comes first, the theory or the practice. They conclude, "In effect, the responders of the concepts and theories, coupled with empirical work, are in the position of trying to codify effectively what is already in existence in the world of organizations" (p. 4). In essence, organizational theory has evolved from observation and documentation of practices that are judged to be effective and successful.

Litwak and his associates view cooperation as one of several types of linkages between agencies (Litwak, 1969; Litwak and Hylton, 1962). They theorize that linkages occur along a continuum where certain conditions exist. Agencies must be interdependent to achieve their individual goals, must be aware of their interdependence, and must possess sufficient resources to provide a basis for negotiation in the chosen linkage areas. The right combination of these elements with the right number and type of agencies can determine the success of the coordination. Linkages run the gamut from sharing staff to sharing processes such as budgeting, to sharing facilities and functions.

An ideal model would include all of the factors mentioned in this chapter. However, the pragmatist recognizes that successful collaboration depends on timing, facile participants, a positive environment that rewards collaboration, and luck. Recognizing that there are numerous successful interagency models, these authors have selected three examples at the state and local levels that illustrate the linkage and collaboration in Ohio between MCH and DD programs.

State Level. An effective mediated interagency coordination model at the state level is illustrated by the regionalized genetic services network in Ohio. Prior to the development of this system, various agencies at the state and local level provided fragmented services. They lacked unified purpose, direction, and coordination to prevent expensive duplication of effort. For example, the Ohio Department of Health provided centralized laboratory services for testing all newborn infants for phenylketonuria (PKU). Later, this service was expanded to include screening for galactosemia and homocystinuria. Another state agency, the Ohio Department of Mental Health and Mental Retardation, provided limited cytogenetic laboratory services. Three medical schools in the state offered clinical, cytogenetic, and biochemical laboratory services to individuals.

The interagency efforts to develop a coordinated genetics system for the state began with an initial meeting in 1972. Individuals were invited to participate on the basis of their potential contribution and relevance to the population to be served. The initial purpose was to discuss the need for an organized approach to delivery of genetic services.

The Ohio Department of Health assumed leadership for development of the planning document, "Ohio Plan for Genetic Services." The plan evolved over two years as the result of meetings with physicians, health professionals, and agency representatives interested in genetics. Prevention and public health were the main thrust of the plan, which called for a regional approach to delivery of comprehensive genetic services. The plan reflected the cooperative efforts of the state departments of Health, Mental Health, and Mental Retardation (now two separate departments); Education; and Public Welfare; as well as the medical school facilities and the March of Dimes Birth Defects Foundation.

During this period, there were discussions of the philosophical approaches, priorities, and mandates on the resources and manpower of all agencies. The establishment of trust among the agencies was a key element in the development of realistic outcomes. The commitment of each participating agency was demonstrated through the allocation of finances, staff support, or advocacy.

The adoption of the written plan by agency directors was, in essence, the "written agreement" between participating agencies. The definition of critical linkages forced the various agencies at state and local levels to follow through because each section of the implementation plan was to be monitored and measured. The commonality of values, goals, and commitment assisted in overcoming barriers, particularly conflicts between mandated authorities. Linkages were defined that were both essential for implementation of the plan and compatible with the mission of each agency. Linkages included staff commitment, funding, programming capacities, referral, outreach, and case management.

The goals of the plan were to reduce the incidence of developmental disability due to genetic disease and to evaluate the impact of a statewide service delivery network. The principal objectives included:

1. Identifying certain genetic and/or metabolic disorders in infants through screening programs. (The Ohio Department of Health continues to screen all newborns for PKU, homocystinuria, and galactosemia. Screening all newborns for hypothyroidism was recently established. When a disorder is suspected, the referring physician is immediately notified. Information regarding the genetic service network for diagnosis, treatment, and follow-up is made available)
2. Identifying mothers and families at high risk for genetic disorders and making the necessary services available
3. Providing public and professional education at the state and regional-center level regarding genetic disorders and services

4.   Developing a centralized information system for data correlation and evalua-
     tion about genetic services, including cost-benefit analysis (Eaton and others,
     1978)

     Since 1976, the Ohio Department of Health, Division of Maternal and
Child Health, has been administratively responsible for the genetic services
network and provides assurance that interagency coordination of efforts continues. Figure 1 illustrates the organization of the genetic network.
     Three advisory groups assist in the implementation and coordination of
the program. The Genetic Services Advisory Committee is composed of twenty-
one members including representatives from other state departments, the genetic
centers, and consumers. Its purpose is to promote cooperation, the exchange of
ideas, public accountability, and a strong service orientation. The Genetic Center
Directors group is composed of the medical geneticists and other key staff
members from each center. Its purposes are to work out details of program
implementation (such as funding allocations), to develop new services, and to
provide information on new approaches to delivery of genetic services. The

Figure 1. Organization Chart for Ohio State Plan for Genetic Services.

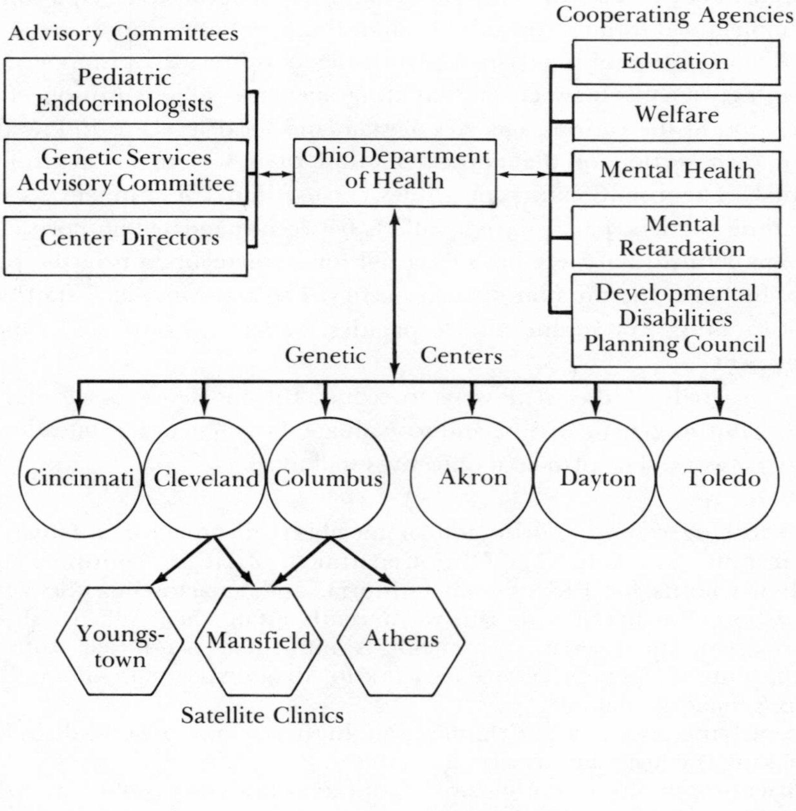

pediatric endocrinologists in the state meet periodically to review and advise on the centralized newborn metabolic and endocrine screening program. They provided valuable consultation for the development of the hypothyroid screening program and continue to monitor the quality and effectiveness of this laboratory service.

The development of statewide hypothyroid screening of all newborns illustrates the extent of interagency coordination in the genetics network. The Ohio Department of Health had the expertise to implement this program but lacked adequate funds to purchase necessary equipment and run a pilot program to determine the most accurate methodology, equipment, and techniques. Because of its focus on prevention of mental retardation, the Ohio Developmental Disabilities Planning Council offered to fund the pilot screening program. Inclusion of hypothyroid screening as a priority in the child development section of the council's state plan provided the clout necessary for the allocation of funds. The Division of Maternal and Child Health of the Ohio Department of Health also provided funds from its state and federal funding resources. One of the medical schools provided a faculty member to assist in the design, proficiency testing, and guidance of the program. The pilot program was expanded carefully for two years, at which time the service was deemed ready to be offered statewide.

Since the inception of the plan, comprehensive genetic services at the local level have grown rapidly from the original three designated regional genetic centers. Currently, six regional genetic centers offer clinical and laboratory services. These centers are all based within medical schools and their affiliate hospitals. In addition, three satellite clinics have been established in rural areas to improve access to services. Medical genetic services from the regional center staff are delivered at the satellite clinics.

Funding of the regionalized genetic services network in Ohio is another example of interagency coordination. The resources used since 1976 (Figure 2) include: federal appropriations through Title V of the Social Security Act, providing formula grant funds for Maternal and Child Health and Crippled Children's Services (changed in 1981 to the Maternal and Child Health Block Grant); state funds for the genetic services network; medical schools and hospital staff and facilities; the Cleveland Foundation's contribution to the Cleveland Regional Genetics Center; the March of Dimes Birth Defects Foundation; the Ohio Developmental Disabilities Planning Council, which contributed funds for the pilot hypothyroid screening program for newborns and funded a public awareness campaign on genetics; and the Ohio Department of Mental Retardation and Developmental Disabilities, which supported a cytogenetics laboratory at a state institution for the mentally retarded.

The coordinated efforts not only benefited clients but also saved funds over the long run through prevention of DD and the achievement of a successful interagency effort. An unexpected reward was the recognition of Ohio as the first state to develop an innovative comprehensive genetics plan. A national model, the plan was used as a resource in the development of federal regulations for the National Genetic Disease Act (Title XI).

Figure 2. Genetics Funding.

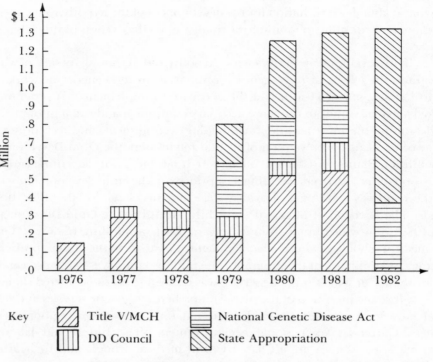

Source: Unpublished data, Ohio Department of Health, 1976–1982.

Local Level. Although there are many examples of interagency coordination at the local level in Ohio, one agency has been particularly committed to this concept. The University Affiliated Cincinnati Center for Developmental Disorders (CCDD) has developed several projects for different target populations in order to improve client services and reduce duplicated efforts (Y. B. Fryberger and J. Rubinstein, personal communication with the authors, 1982). CCDD has successfully obtained both short-term and permanent funding for its interagency efforts.

CCDD is a tertiary care center affiliated with the University of Cincinnati College of Medicine and the Children's Hospital Medical Center. It has a long history of collaborative relationships with United Cerebral Palsy, the Convalescent Hospital for Children, the Children's Dental Care Foundation, local education agencies, and the Adolescent Clinic. The overall goals of CCDD are to provide:

1. Interdisciplinary professional training for delivery of services to persons having developmental disorders
2. Comprehensive interdisciplinary evaluations, reevaluations, and treatment for children having developmental disorders and their families
3. Research and demonstration programs related to the prevention, early

detection, management, and treatment of persons with developmental disorders

4. Outreach continuing education programs for professionals and parents

Two major linkage endeavors of CCDD are examples of effective interagency coordination projects. During 1980, CCDD expanded already existing collaborative relationships with Maternal and Child Health and other Title V–related programs to improve the accessibility and quality of health care for children with developmental disorders and their families. To identify existing needs, establish priority services, and coordinate activities with existing endeavors, an interagency Title V Advisory Committee was established. State and regional representatives from the Maternal and Child Health and Crippled Children's Services (CCS) and representatives from all CCDD disciplines serve on this committee to plan, implement, and monitor CCDD's Title V–related activities. The two major emphases of this interagency endeavor have been the provision of manpower training to Title V–related personnel in the area of developmental disabilities and the implementation of collaborative written agreements between CCDD and Title V agencies.

Accomplishments of this linkage include creation of a satellite Supplemental Security Income–Disabled Children's Program Team at CCDD and the development both of a High-Risk Newborn Early Intervention Team and a comprehensive, interdisciplinary evaluation/management Cerebral Palsy Team at CCDD. Collaborative statewide manpower-training accomplishments have included training of the Ohio Department of Health's nursing consultants in Maternal and Child Health/Perinatal and Child Health, CCS, and Public Health to implement a curriculum on home assessment of handicapped children children for local public health nurses. Some of the statewide training activities were implemented in conjunction with the Ohio Consortium for DD, which included the Case Western Reserve Mental Development Center, the Nisonger Center, and the Ohio University Affiliated Center for Human Development.

Another local interagency collaboration effort occurred when CCDD was awarded a one-year grant by the Ohio Developmental Disabilities Planning Council to address the need for local interagency coordination of services to individuals with developmental disorders. Major goals of this interagency endeavor were (1) to facilitate and/or establish coordination among major agencies involved in providing services to individuals of all ages with developmental disabilities and (2) to facilitate group endeavors among agencies to improve and expand the current local service delivery continuum. In order to accomplish these goals, representatives from seventeen health, education, welfare, mental retardation, mental health, vocational rehabilitation, health, and advocacy agencies were assembled to establish a Local Interagency Consortium. CCDD served as the lead agency and assigned a staff member to work with the consortium. This consortium of agencies has continued to provide a forum for the exchange of information on both a structured and nonstructured level and for the identification of weaknesses and gaps in the local DD service delivery continuum. The success of this local interagency effort was underscored when it was granted permanent local funding by the Community Chest.

Major accomplishments of the Local Interagency Consortium have included: a pilot project that established a centralized case management system among the six major DD adult service programs (Bureau of Vocational Rehabilitation, Hamilton County Board of Mental Retardation, Region I Office of the Department of MR/DD, Hamilton County Board of Mental Health, Living Arrangements for DD, and Ohio Valley Residential Services, Inc.); creation of a comprehensive diagnostic/treatment facility for adults with developmental disorders, head injuries, and strokes; and development of two pilot interagency service coordination projects, one between Head Start and Early Periodic Screening Diagnosis and Treatment (EPSDT) and the other between the Crippled Children's Services and EPSDT.

Summary and Conclusions

Interagency coordination is an evolutionary process that requires time for DD and MCH agencies to develop a working relationship based on mutual trust. It can occur: (1) at various government levels with varying sponsors, settings, and activities, (2) in a variety of organizational models, (3) through provision of a spectrum of health services, (4) with various target groups, target areas, or age groups, and (5) in different environments and influenced by many social and political factors (Gans and Horton, 1975).

The broad goal to be achieved through interagency collaboration between MCH and DD is improvement in the delivery of services to individuals and the efficiency and effectiveness of service delivery systems. Collaboration can be accomplished by strategies ranging from informal communication between agencies to legal documents delineating each agency's responsibility.

Leadership and attitude are important ingredients in successful interagency coordination. Top-level administrative commitment is necessary to negotiate an agreement that may require changes in agency policy or resource allocation. Issues of mutual concern need to be addressed in light of the existing mandates and realistic capabilities of participating agencies in an environment of mutual support and understanding. Channels of communication must be clearly delineated at the decision-making as well as the staff manager level.

Education of agency staff to the scope and types of services provided is an essential element. Sharing of information and resources in a positive manner is vital. There must be wide acceptance of principles and philosophy for successful collaboration in planning, development of mutual agency goals and objectives, determination of personnel and financial resources each can contribute to formulate and implement the plan for action, and agreement on sharing of data for effective evaluation. It is crucial that each agency with potential involvement in the interagency effort be included in this planning and decision-making process.

Certain risks are inherent in the process whenever agencies make decisions or compromises through collaboration. Risks can involve the elimination of targeted population groups or geographical areas that may have been served by the individual agencies. Restrictive or incompatible legislative mandates and limitation on resources force the compromises that may cause the redirection of agencies' goals. The risks should be identified and measured in relationship to the ultimate benefits that can result from the cooperative process.

There is no ideal model of interagency collaboration. There are multiple approaches according to problems identified, age groups, geographical areas or functions, and funding resources. The focus may be narrow or broad for joint planning, programming, or evaluation. The types of organizational structures and advisory committees will vary according to the scope and purpose of each project.

A model is necessary for the development of a coordinated effort because it sets out the basic structure to guide the agencies. The model should clearly identify the facilitators in a successfully functioning process as well as identifying those elements and activities that will be barriers to implementation.

The model developed to make services available in a more efficient manner requires coordination at both the administrative level and the direct service delivery level. Design of a successful model demands that the involved agencies allocate some of their resources—especially time taken by policy makers to attend meetings, determine gaps in services, perform needs assessment, develop strategies to provide quality health services, establish priorities, formulate policies, and make other key decisions. An agency's intent to promote coordination is clearly evident through its level of commitment and attitude to such activities.

The Ohio genetics model is an excellent example of interagency coordination. This type of coordination had a great impact on problem solving and resulted in making services more complementary in content and delivery procedures. It required a commitment of policy makers to work collaboratively to initiate changes through realistic planning efforts that resulted in better integration of service delivery and avoidance of duplication. The State Health Department Maternal and Child Health/Crippled Children's Services Program assumed the lead agency role and responsibility for overall direction. The success of the model was highly dependent on the interagency effort, with the development of linkages as a high priority.

The ultimate reward for agencies and health professionals working jointly is the improvement in services for children with handicaps and their families. Better access to services in an efficient delivery system of the highest quality is the principal benefit, with resultant reduction in frustration as well as in the time and effort that consumers must devote to obtaining effective services. Maximization of resources with avoidance of duplication is achieved through coordinated needs assessment and planning to fill identified gaps. It is assumed that this process will result in the enhancement of interagency communication to the benefit of consumers. However, definitive research is needed to substantiate this assumption.

References

Bonhag, R. C., and others. *A Description of the Health Financing Model: A Tool for Cost Estimation.* Washington, D.C.: Department of Health and Human Services, Office of the Assistant Secretary for Planning and Evaluation, 1981.

Department of Health, Education, and Welfare. "Maternal and Child Health Programs Legislative Base. Title V (Section 501)." Publication no. 77-5221. Washington, D.C.: U.S. Government Printing Office, n.d.

Eaton, A. P., and others. "Genetic Services in Ohio: A Regional Approach." *Ohio State Medical Association Journal,* 1978, *74* (10), 623–626.

Elder, J. O. "Coordination of Service Delivery Systems." In P. R. Magrab and J. O. Elder (Eds.), *Planning for Services to Handicapped Persons.* Baltimore, Md.: Paul H. Brookes, 1979.

Elder, J. O., and Magrab, P. R. *Coordinating Services to Handicapped Children: A Handbook for Interagency Collaboration.* Baltimore, Md.: Paul H. Brookes, 1980.

Gans, S. P., and Horton, G. T. *Integration of Human Services, the State and Municipal Levels.* New York: Praeger, 1975.

Kuzilla, L. A. "Interagency Coordination Model." A paper presented to the Ohio Developmental Disabilities Planning Council—Academy for Contemporary Problems, 1977.

Litwak, E. *Towards the Theory and Practice of Coordination Between Formal Organizations.* The University of Michigan School of Social Work, 1969. (Mimeographed.)

Litwak, E., and Hylton, L. F. "Inter-Organizational Analysis: A Hypothesis on Coordinating Agencies." *Administrative Science Quarterly,* 1962, *6,* 397–421.

Roemer, R., and others. *Planning Urban Health Services: From Jungle to System.* St. Louis, Mo.: Springer, 1975.

Silver, G. A. *Child Health: America's Future.* Germantown, Md.: Aspen Systems, 1978.

Title I (P.L. 95–602), Rehabilitation, Comprehensive Services, and Developmental Disabilities Amendments, 1978.

37

Self-Help and Mutual Aid Groups

Leonard D. Borman, Ph.D.

Since the founding of Alcoholics Anonymous and Recovery, Inc., more than forty years ago, the self-help/mutual aid group movement has grown to address a great variety of conditions and affiliations. A recent directory of such groups identifies nearly 400 different kinds existing in the United States and Canada (Evans, 1979). For the Chicago area alone, 120 different kinds of groups for diverse conditions have been identified (Pasquale, 1981a). Research findings since the 1960s indicate that these groups represent a growing and significant resource for helping vast segments of our society. The early work of Alfred Katz (1961), O. Hobart Mowrer (1964), and Frank Riessman (1965) coupled with recent findings of Lieberman and others (1979) has been recognized by policy making commissions focusing on such critical concerns as mental health, epilepsy, and the crisis in American family life. The President's Commission on Mental Health (1978, p. 24) notes that "Self-help groups . . . have long played a role in helping people cope with their problems. Similar groups composed of individuals with mental and emotional problems are in existence and being formed all over America . . . . These largely untapped community resources contain a great potential for innovation and creative commitments in maintaining health and providing human services. In spite of the recognized importance of community supports, even those that are working well are too often ignored by human service agencies. Moreover, many professionals are not aware of, or comfortable with, certain elements of community support systems. The nation can ill afford to waste such valuable resources. The Commission believes this is one of the most significant frontiers in mental health at all levels of care."

The president's commission as well as other bodies recommending policy have turned attention to self-help/mutual aid groups as ways to reduce costs, to develop community-based alternatives to hospital and other institutional care, and to prevent the far-reaching consequences of countless human afflictions.

This chapter reviews recent findings on the nature of self-help/mutual aid groups, the important mechanisms and processes that seem to help their participants, and some of the recent literature that describes the effects of these groups on their participants. Also reviewed here is some of the major literature (admittedly scant) that focuses on self-help groups for chronically ill children and their families, the kinds of groups addressed, the problems that have received attention, and some of the implications. This includes reports on current studies and findings unpublished to date. Some have been conducted rather systematically with children who have cancer and with families that have been faced with the catastrophic illness of their children followed by death.

Because systematic research has been conducted recently with parents of dwarf children and persons with epilepsy, some of these findings are reported. Although tangential to the major disability concerns of this volume, the research methodologies employed and the findings are generalizable to the chronic conditions addressed. Moreover, the efforts to combine research and extension work (learning with helping) in the epilepsy studies are already finding similar applications with low-incidence chronic conditions.

Finally, this chapter considers some policy implications that address ways in which these important self-help resources might be encouraged and expanded. There are important roles for professionals and agencies to play and new skills and understandings that need to be developed as well as new social agencies that may serve as catalysts and clearinghouses for the developing interest in this phenomenon.

Recent Findings on the Nature of Self-Help/Mutual Aid Groups

Self-help/mutual aid groups are essentially small-scale, voluntary organizations that consist of individuals who face similar problems in health, mental health, or daily living. They are composed of peers who have similar afflictions or those who are related to the afflicted. The groups are a growing phenomenon; recent estimates number approximately 500,000 groups with perhaps 15,000,000 participants. These groups provide social and emotional support for their members, who also acquire information on effective ways to cope with their problems. They often work with other health care providers to stabilize conditions and prevent further disorder or deterioration. Participants, including families of the afflicted, frequently establish long-term friendships that individuals may call upon regularly or in times of special need. Self-help group participants usually have found that conventional sources of help—whether from their own extended families or professionals—have not alone been of sufficient aid.

Recent studies have served to dispel some common misconceptions that have clouded both popular and professional thought about self-help/mutual aid groups (Lieberman, Borman, and Associates, 1979; Borman, 1979b). This is not to suggest that all the issues around self-help groups have been clarified once and for all, but the beginnings of more light than heat on the subject of self-help/ mutual aid groups can be seen. Understanding is being broadened as knowledge on the nature and development of these groups is expanded.

Briefly, there are five dimensions or perspectives around which considerable mythology has prevailed and where our knowledge of self-help groups is being advanced. Self-help groups have an ancient heritage and are not newly emergent phenomena to be regarded as a fashion or a fad. Such groups are found filling existing gaps at the important growing points of our society and do not represent a withdrawal or form of escapism. They provide important help and therapeutic mechanisms for their participants and are not superficial, worthless, or romanticized cults. Self-help groups are varied and evolving, often changing their form of organization rather than remaining firmly fixed in their patterns, programs, and structures.

First, as common interest groups or voluntary associations, self-help/ mutual aid groups indeed have an ancient history. They are small groups based on shared ties, experiences, and common interests rather than on kinship, residence, or territory. As such, they are found in practically all societies of the world and in all stages of humankind's existence. Although some suggest that such voluntary groups emerge when the primary bonds of kinship, neighborhood, the family, and religion are weakened, these groups seem to flourish even when such primary support systems are strong. The ethnographic literature records, worldwide, groups composed of teenagers, bachelors, widows, elderly, warriors, singers, dancers, artists, scientists, and other associations that cut across the bonds of family, clan, and village. Frequently, such groups are dispersed and not geographically based. Often, they are the vanguard, the forerunner, and the gadfly as initiators in every field of human endeavor. In more recent times, they occur in educational, religious, economic, and health arenas.

Second, contrary to much popular and professional opinion, self-help groups are not basically antiprofessional. Contemporary self-help groups have sought professional assistance with most of their endeavors and have encouraged research on the nature of their diverse conditions, and although they provide new and important avenues by means of which the afflicted and their families are able to participate more fully in enterprises, they have often been assisted in their formation by seasoned professionals. A recent review of ten self-help groups disclosed that professionals often played key roles in founding the organizations or giving them a major boost. These include such widely established groups as Recovery, Inc.; Integrity Groups; GROW; Compassionate Friends; Parents Anonymous; and Epilepsy Self-Help Groups (Lieberman, Borman, and Associates, 1979).

Frequently, the professionals involved with self-help groups have been at odds with their conventional colleagues. They have often employed broader definitions for specific afflictions, and they have expanded interest in skills and techniques that would be helpful to the afflicted and their families. They have focused on neglected stages of a condition, such as aftercare for hospitalized patients and the problem of relapse among populations of the addicted. They have frequently advocated new auspices under which helpful programs could be developed to recognize the important role of the afflicted themselves. In general, they have gone beyond the boundary lines of their respective disciplines— whether medicine, psychology, theology, or social work. As a result, they have been ignored or have found it difficult to publish their findings and views. Rarely have their publications been incorporated in training programs and curricula of their fields.

Third, the assertion that self-help groups are an escape or cop-out from the task of making society's services more responsible does not hold up on examination. Although many self-help groups do not deal with confrontation or exposure or take positions on public policies, they do have a long-term and growing impact on the helping systems in our society. They frequently represent new approaches to helping specific populations. Because they represent common communities of fate where survival may be based on coping successfully with the condition, they are more than usually concerned with advanced methods and approaches. For example, parent groups formed for families of children afflicted with autism, Tourette's syndrome, or schizophrenia have prompted research on use of medications, vitamins, allergies, and nutrition in contrast to conventional psychodynamic theories that prevail in treatment. Often, these psychological theories blame the parent for the disturbed conditions of their children.

Alcoholics Anonymous is an example of a group that has developed and promulgated its own view of the nature of alcoholism. Alcoholism has come to be viewed as a disease rather than a weakness of character (the view that prevailed for so long in our society).

Rather than replacing the family, as some assert, self-help groups are serving to strengthen and reconstitute the family in many cases. Note the important spin-off of Alcoholics Anonymous in the development of Al-Anon family groups or the high involvement of couples in Compassionate Friends, the self-help group for bereaved parents. For strengthening, realigning, and understanding family ties, these groups seem to be a valuable resource.

Fourth, the importance of self-help groups in providing helpful therapeutic mechanisms has been grossly underestimated. The fact that most groups are not controlled by conventional agencies and do not exist on professional turf has meant that they have been neglected by researchers concerned with evaluation, assessment, and outcome. We have found, on the other hand, that most groups are willing to cooperate with researchers and, in many cases, seek out researchers for collaborative study. Reported findings indicate that the number of helping mechanisms that exist within such groups are impressive. The importance of universality and acceptance—of being part of a group that shares your condition and understands what you are experiencing—seems to be central. One is not alone, isolated, feeling unique and abandoned. Such universality strengthens elements of cohesion, involvement, and belongingness, which are outside the usual kinds of therapies provided by a conventional therapist or professional. These groups foster communication, provide participants with social support, and respond to their many cognitive and emotional needs. They involve the development of ideologies and belief systems, which appears to be very important in sustaining persons who face a great variety of crises in their lives. Note, however, that these mechanisms are not those commonly described by therapists in terms of insight, feedback, expression of affect, self-disclosure, and so forth. These are additional mechanisms that have been largely ignored by conventional helping service professionals.

Fifth, self-help groups in their development over time do not follow any unilineal theory of development. They represent a zigzag process of groping, trying out new approaches, dropping some and developing new ones. Many changes occur in their organizational size and structure, the number of chapters, and the nature of their leadership. Sometimes, their central focus changes, along with the characteristics of their members. Some groups evolve into professionally run organizations, managed and controlled by trained professionals, and some remain autonomous and firmly in control of their activities. Most support their activities through their own financial efforts, although some seek outside and even public support. The capacity for such groups to sustain themselves and to spread in society reveals a diverse pattern. Social agencies, clinics, hospitals, and universities in recent years are finding ways to articulate with self-help groups and to aid in their development. Because these groups represent creative ideas, forms, and resources that may be so vital for the populations served, such attention on the part of established agencies should be encouraged. Yet, many groups continue to face problems of legitimacy, of being accepted by prestigious decision makers in society. Recent efforts to conduct research with groups as reported here and elsewhere and to understand the ways self-help groups articulate with others of society should accelerate their acceptance considerably.

Review of Literature

The literature on self-help/mutual aid groups, parent groups, and support systems for chronically ill children and their families is limited. A recent review of the social science literature on mental retardation by Rowitz (1974) indicates that a focus on family coping patterns and community network resources is only beginning to receive attention by researchers. Most social research on mental retardation (and other afflictions) has emphasized three other distinct concerns: (1) an epidemiological interest in prevalence of the condition within the larger population, (2) a concern for program planning, evaluation, and studies of professional service delivery systems, and (3) a social system perspective, rather than a medical model, that examines life-style and labeling issues of people with mental retardation in both the community and the institution.

Some conditions have clearly received much more attention than others, although this review does not purport to be exhaustive. Suelzle and Keenan (1980a, 1980b, 1981) have published findings on their survey of parents of developmentally disabled children suffering from mental retardation, cerebral palsy, epilepsy, and autism. Farber (1968) essentially studied mental retardation. Katz's (1961) study of the parents of the handicapped focused on groups formed for coping with four conditions: mental retardation, cerebral palsy, emotional disturbance, and muscular dystrophy. His major study of hemophilia was published more recently (1970) following an earlier paper. McMichael's (1971) study was primarily concerned with the physically handicapped including those with hemophilia, muscular dystrophy, and cerebral palsy. Patten's (1974) discussion of some of the practical aspects of developing parents' groups is addressed to parents of the terminally ill although it is based on information drawn from parent groups formed around a number of conditions including muscular dystrophy, cystic fibrosis, spina bifida, leukemia, multiple sclerosis, and rheumatic diseases. The work of Tizard and Grad (1961) essentially focused on the mentally handicapped, and the work of Birenbaum (1970) addressed findings on the population of the mentally retarded. A number of studies of parents' groups have been published that were conducted in hospitals or outpatient clinics (David and Frankel, 1970; Heffron, Bommelaere, and Masters, 1973; Liebman, Minuchin, and Baker, 1974; Scherzer and Ospa, n.d.). Gorham and others (1975) surveyed parents of the handicapped, covering a variety of conditions from autism to slow learners and pointing out, among other things, the problems of classification and labels.

A number of studies have focused on successful utilization of parents associations and yet, paradoxically, made few recommendations for their expansion or strengthening. Farber (1968) found that parents who participate in such associations are better informed and more involved with communication networks relevant to their particular interest. In this case, the conditions were mental retardation and cerebral palsy.

Involvement with parent associations seems to expose parents to more sources of information than they would otherwise have found. Even in the study conducted by Scherzer and Ospa (n.d.) of professionally directed parent discussion groups of meningomyelocele children, parents indicated that they learned more from other parents than from professionals. The researchers concluded that informal group meetings were particularly helpful "in a supportive way and provided an opportunity of sharing experiences and dealing with feelings in general about having such a handicapped child" (p. 7). Gorham and others (1975, p. 179) noted that "parent organizations are probably the major organized providers of information on the wide assortment of services needed by a child with disabilities as he grows up. The usual estimate is that one-third of the time and energy of such groups goes toward informing fellow patients of the whereabouts of services in the locality." Suelzle and Keenan (1980b) found that parents were willing to participate in groups to a greater extent than opportunities existed. Interest was expressed in such issues as education, group counseling, political advocacy, and participation in governing boards of service agencies. They found that organizational involvement in parent groups seemed to be highest for those with younger children, those whose children had a more severe type of disability, and those whose family incomes were higher.

There appears to be greater interest and involvement in self-help and support groups on the part of the more educated, higher-income, upper-middle socioeconomic families. This was found to be true in our studies of Mended Hearts and Compassionate Friends (Lieberman, Borman, and Associates, 1979), as well as in recent studies of Parents Anonymous (Wheat and Lieber, 1979). Such families may be more highly motivated or knowledgeable about such resources, or more capable of organizing such support networks. Suelzle and Keenan (1980a) found that the better off families were more readily able to overcome such barriers as transportation and obtaining baby-sitters.

Katz (1961) suggests that, as professional staff were acquired by the organizations he studied, there was a reduction of parents' efforts in the work activities. With two of the groups surveyed, the Muscular Dystrophy Association and the League for Emotionally Disturbed Children, parent involvement and participation were de-emphasized, discouraged, and not seen as important in the realization of the group's purposes. The consequences of this for the League for Emotionally Disturbed Children were failure of the organization to grow and lack of enthusiasm among its supporters. For muscular dystrophy, there resulted a difficulty in the development of patient care and community services (pp. 68, 69), although its focus on fund raising through the efforts of a sizable professional staff, along with entertainers and volunteers, has been rather successful.

Katz found, on the other hand, that with a parent-controlled organization such as the New York Association for Help to Retarded Children (AHRC), a strain existed in its relation to the wider community. "Its relative isolation from coordinating groups, its failure to win the support of other community agencies for its legislative program, the overt hostility expressed toward it by some agency professionals—all would seem to derive primarily from the intense degree and quality of parent participation in A.H.R.C." (p. 68).

Why do parents' groups and other self-help/mutual aid groups emerge? Suelzle and Keenan (1980a, p. 18) reaffirm the advocacy function when they note that parent groups are the "single most important factor behind the progress made in recent years in the rights of handicapped children." Katz (1961) explained this social action function in his early study when he noted the methods used by a number of groups to attain more services. These include publicity about needs, pressure on public officials, legislative action, and lobbying. Publicly supported programs for the mentally retarded and cerebral palsied have clearly resulted from these efforts.

There are explanations in addition to their advocacy function for the emergence of self-help groups. In many cases, professional knowledge and skill are simply deficient. For many chronic conditions, as well as addictions, traumas, and life transitions, there is little professional expertise to be evoked. Alcoholics, gamblers, drug addicts, child abusers, widows, and the chronically ill seem to fall between the cracks. Accordingly, those with similar afflictions turn to each other for help (Borman, 1979a). However, not all groups form in response to deficient professional services. Many groups emerge in response to the lack of support once provided by natural support systems, such as the nuclear or extended family, the church, the ethnic group, or neighbors (Lieberman and Borman, 1981a, 1981b).

The therapeutic, beneficial aspects of participating in self-help groups have been a major focus of attention in current research. Katz (1963) recognized this in the study already cited and elaborated on the "great strength" and "less tangible advantages" people with hemophilia derive from self-help groups: "Among these are (1) overcoming the sense of isolation and overwhelming distress, frequently experienced by parents as a first reaction to the diagnosis of hemophilia, (2) provision of accurate information regarding the problems of medical management, child care, blood procurement, and so forth, (3) socialization through contacts and exchange of experience with other families who can contribute to knowledge about developmental phases and problems that can be anticipated, (4) provision of organized or informal opportunities to discuss parents' fear, frustrations, and satisfactions arising from the particular difficulties of caring for a hemophilic child, (5) opportunity to discuss broader and long-range problems that can be anticipated on behalf of the child so that planning can be done, (6) possibility of securing through group action better facilities of a therapeutic and educational nature for their children, and (7) cathartic effects of such personal participation, which helps to relieve anxieties by channeling them into constructive outlets" (p. 98).

Current Studies and Findings

Although research on self-help groups for the chronically ill and their families is in an embryonic stage, a number of studies that have been conducted over the past few years have considerable implication for the utilization and development of self-help group resources. These studies are just beginning to be published, and it may take several years before others will be reported in the literature.

One of the major breakthroughs in our understanding of self-help groups lies in what we are discovering about the helpful mechanisms or processes that operate within the group and about the impact of the group on the participants. Most theories that have developed in small-group therapeutic research have emphasized the role and importance of the professional therapist in the group. "It is axiomatic for a theory of therapy to stress both those conditions that are directly controllable by the therapist and those conditions that do not ordinarily occur in a person's day-to-day life" (Lieberman, Borman, and Associates, 1979, p. 213). Accordingly, theories have focused on insight, feedback, and self-disclosure, including catharsis and other forms of emotional expression. All of these approaches emphasize factors that can be influenced or controlled by a trained professional. "If they are uncontrollable (by a therapist) they usually are not emphasized within the theoretical system" (p. 214).

Examination of the therapeutic mechanisms at work in self-help/mutual aid groups indicates a series of processes that have received little attention as helpful change mechanisms. They include cohesiveness (a sense of belonging in a small face-to-face group); universality (the sense that one's problems are not unique); altruism (the experience of helping others); sharing common values and beliefs, including group teachings, wisdom, and ideology; and information (receiving advice from others). Some examples of these processes or mechanisms in specific groups concerned with chronic and catastrophic illness follow.

Children's Cancer Support Network. In Isenberg's (1981) doctoral dissertation focusing on self-help groups for children with cancer and their families, the role of belief systems is documented as an important mechanism in confronting the dilemmas faced by these families. These ideologies—which represent collective wisdoms, teachings, or beliefs—serve in important ways in helping families and children with cancer in coping with four major dilemmas. First, the medical dilemmas represent difficulties that exist on the part of the child or the family in fully accepting and participating in the often aggressive medical treatment that is required. "The person must resolve dilemmas involving a series of adjustments to health crises, tolerating medical treatments, errors and delays in making medical decisions, doctors' unrealistic expectations for cure, and depleted personal resources when caring for the person with cancer" (p. 155).

A second dilemma occurs around family difficulties that "arise from differences in style and timing of grieving, and the need for family members to also be caregivers while they experience grief and deal with pre-existing problems and developmental issues. Dealing with the needs of various family members during the stress of a life-threatening illness, families experience a sense of helplessness and communication breaks down when members feel over-burdened. The person with cancer is stressed and may feel that the children are a burden and be hostile to family members. The spouse must adjust to new roles, and understand the experiences of the person with cancer. Siblings are often jealous of the attention given their ill brother or sister and lonely during separations. Adolescents struggle with being independent and are pulled back by parents' concern to a state of dependency" (p. 156).

A third dilemma focuses on social issues and involves "isolation as a result of society's irrational fears about cancer. When being honest with others, friends withdraw. Being different in school, losing one's hair or a limb is isolating. Discrimination in one's job blocks career ambitions in the same way. The stigma of cancer erodes self-esteem and daily reminders in irritating incidents make it difficult for the person to separate himself from the disease" (p. 156).

The fourth dilemma focuses around personal issues that "result from emotional responses that are maladaptive. Reactions to losses, as in the loss of the limb or potential future goals or family's anticipated loss of a loved one, are met with anger and blame. Psychological symptoms result. Anxiety increases when looking at the possibility of one's death. An existential dilemma follows from facing death and finding life meaningless. Losing friends to cancer may prevent close relationships from forming with other persons with cancer. After the death of a child, facing life is often devastating" (p. 156).

Isenberg recognized that the ideology of the self-help groups counters these dilemmas through particular teachings and wisdoms that serve, in Antze's (1979) term, as "cognitive antidotes" countering anxious, angry, and destructive attitudes. Focusing on such beliefs as "making today count," or "this instant is the only time there is," helps place the dilemma within a constructive framework.

Such beliefs or teachings, discussed in a supportive context with one's fellows, help the participants "block a response of fear" that could dwell on obsessive ideas of what could happen in the future. These beliefs further emphasize that members rearrange the value they place on relationships and how they spend their time (Isenberg, 1981, p. 157). Additional teachings focus around forgiveness, a determination to see things differently, a rejection of the view of the afflicted as a victim, an effort to resist making judgments about others, rethinking the role of the past and the future, accepting responsibility for one's thoughts, and a value placed on love and peace.

This ideology or belief system developed for children with cancer and their families and promulgated through self-help groups has become the basis for Centers for Attitudinal Healing, which are developing in a number of cities in the United States. Although the ideology is recognized as an important helping mechanism in itself, other reinforcing processes are utilized that serve to provide participants a broad range of continuing and helpful contacts. These include a hospital visitation program, a telephone and pen pal network, school visits for presentations to classes and assemblies, and social outings and other events. Isenberg's study indicated that young people with cancer will provide support for each other when bone marrow tests are required, chemotherapy needs to be administered, or other medical treatments are indicated that require a great deal of time and have the potential of considerable anguish.

Compassionate Friends. Our studies of Compassionate Friends, parents who have faced the death of a child, also reveal the role of ideologies or cognitive antidotes aimed at countering specific problems faced by such parents. Situations around maladaptive responses, family relationships, and reintegrating within the social context are all assisted by belief systems operating within the group (Sherman, 1979).

For Compassionate Friends, these belief systems are fostered through a variety of mechanisms. For example, the tendency to deny that the death occurred is countered by the group setting as a place to remember the deceased child, by developing mementos (such as pictures or trophies), and through the routine group introduction procedure for each meeting when parents give their names and the name of the deceased child along with the date and circumstances of the child's death. Educational materials are used extensively by these parents to understand and facilitate the loss, and most chapters have developed extensive lending libraries of material on death, grief, and personal experiences.

Because the grieving styles of parent-couples are often very different, the group attempts to save marriages and prevent dissolution of the family. Parents are encouraged to attend meetings as couples; modeling is employed in group meetings and workshops where spouses can share their difficulties and discuss workable solutions. The utilization of other parents as third parties is common. The stoic, unemotional role of men is greatly diminished as expression of feelings is encouraged in group discussions.

The group also provides ways and mechanisms for relating to neighbors and friends who have a tendency to withdraw. Bereaved parents and others often find themselves confronting a conspiracy of silence. The group encourages members to initiate social contacts and to take on active roles in teaching the wider community that it is okay to talk about the dead child.

A recent doctoral dissertation by Videka-Sherman (1982) examining the effects of participation in Compassionate Friends found that those parents who became most involved with the self-help group exhibited a greater measure of personal growth and change as compared with those parents who were minimally involved: "Changes in self that parents experienced most frequently included changes in the interpersonal realm, including both empathy for others as well as changes in the nature of one's intimate relations; changes in the parents' belief system, including beliefs about life, death, religion, and what is meaningful and important in life; and changes in the parent's representation of himself in terms of strength and resiliency and in terms of self-betterment and maturation versus deterioration and self-deprecation. These categories corroborate, almost verbatim, the dimensions of change reported by other researchers who have studied existential change as a result of life crises" (p. 10).

Candlelighters. An open and accessible system of communication is made available by Candlelighters, a national self-help network for parents of children with life-threatening illnesses. Candlelighters has more than seventy chapters located throughout the United States and Canada. Field interviews and observations of the groups conducted in Connecticut, St. Louis, and Green Bay, Wisconsin, by the Self-Help Center in 1979 indicated a great reliance on others who are going through similar experiences. A telephone "credit card" (Lifeline) is available for children to talk to each other and for parents to talk with each other as well. Excerpts from the interviews give the flavor of Candlelighters' activities:

> We're a sharing, caring group. We keep in contact with each other; because of the Lifeline, it makes it easy. I can call someone in Stamford and I don't have to worry about my telephone bill. . . . When you know that there is a parent or a child having a difficult time, you let the parents know that you're there; and you'll call them. You'll support them whenever they need to be supported.

Candlelighters, as do other self-help groups, becomes a major repository of information that is shared with participants.

> We have learned a tremendous amount, not only about our own children but about other diseases; you have a very fast course in drugs, and you have to know the side effects. So all this material, which we gather from all over the place, it's always there. Whatever comes in new, everybody can pick up. You end up with a library on your child's disease; you know what everybody thinks all around the country. Another, which is not really advertised that much, not because we're stingy, but we're not a financial aid organization per se. But if we know someone's having a tough time, then we can give them some financial help.

Candlelighters, as with most self-help groups, devotes a considerable amount of time to the educational concerns of participants, as well as emotional support.

Little People of America. An example of another mechanism provided by many self-help groups—that is, a support network often modeled after that of an extended family—is the Parents' Auxiliary of Little People of America. Ablon (1982) describes how this auxiliary, composed largely of normal size parents of dwarf children, meet frequently or are in communication by phone providing help and information to each other.

Little People of America undertakes a variety of activities from regular meetings to national conventions. According to Ablon (1982, p. 35), "Annual national conventions provide both the major forum for the exchange of information and the prime arena for social interaction of families. Daily meetings and workshops for Auxiliary members are scheduled. The topics of discussion deal with varied social, psychological, and medical problems that children are experiencing. The Medical Advisory Board of Little People of America, distinguished clinical specialists who attend conventions and provide free examinations and consultations for LPA members, often present lectures or hold workshops at Auxiliary sessions on such topics as sexuality, nutrition, orthopedic concerns, or the genetic basis of dwarfism."

Role-modeling becomes important for the Parents' Auxiliary, as with most other self-help groups. Ablon (p. 43) writes, "The opportunity to view adult dwarfs who are successful wage earners, parents, and in general, happy and attractive people, relieved many parents' basic anxieties about their child's future. They can project a positive life for their child as they see the successful functioning of these adults, other children of their child's age, and short-statured teenagers, some of whom may actually have more significant physical problems than does their own child. As noted above, most parents have had little or no exposure to profoundly short-statured persons previous to the birth of their own child. Fears and apprehensions bloom most extravagantly with such a void of information."

Epilepsy Self-Help Groups. Studies of epilepsy self-help groups in a number of cities throughout the United States reveal the importance of altruism, of helping others, as an important basis of the self-help group experience (Borman, Davies, and Droge, 1980).

As with the classic twelfth step of Alcoholics Anonymous, "we try to carry this message to alcoholics and to practice these principles in all our affairs," epilepsy groups reach out to others like themselves. In a survey of self-help group participants (Pasquale, 1981b), three kinds of experiences tended to be reported when respondents were asked to describe their single best group experience:

- Being able to help others
- Getting insight into my own problems
- Feeling that a strong sense of commonality existed with one another

An additional process identified by Borman, Davies, and Droge (1980, p. 333) seemed rather universal among the groups visited.

> In our visits with groups in a number of states, we have noted what might be called the restaurant effect. With almost every group we visited, we were invited to a post-meeting session which usually occurred in a restaurant near the meeting site. When the restaurant was not within walking distance of the meeting, arrangements for rides had to be worked out. Many participants reported to us that they would stay in the restaurant until it closed, or until they were ejected. It became clear to us that these post-group sessions were providing help for people with epilepsy in other ways frequently ignored by professionals. For many with epilepsy, the fear of having a seizure in public and either being victimized while helpless, or injured by well-meaning bystanders makes going out of the house a potentially traumatic experience. Indeed, as we visited groups, we continually heard stories of social isolation among group members. Going to a restaurant with someone other than one's parents seems, for many groups members, to be a novel experience. Going with a group of people who understand the embarrassment and discomfort that accompanies a public seizure may be an important part of the member's experience in the group. Furthermore, the informal atmosphere of these post-meeting sessions relieves the necessity to talk about self-help business, and allows members to talk about the weather, baseball or whatever. It frequently allows individuals who may have confronted each other during the course of a tense meeting an opportunity to show some bonds of solidarity and affection. These opportunities for sociability, acquaintance, and friendship may be critical to persons experiencing epilepsy.

Self-Help Groups Are No Panacea. In identifying the profound benefits of self-help groups and their major helping mechanisms, one should entertain the caution that these groups are no panacea. In most cases, they serve to supplement other forms of help. Although we are at the early stages of outcome studies, it is clear that not everyone benefits from self-help group participation, and many choose not to participate at all. Researchers continue to explore the benefits of self-help groups, but studies already conducted indicate that the groups do little harm. In the large surveys we have conducted of Mended Hearts, Compassionate Friends, widows and epilepsy groups, a small percentage (under 10 percent) of the total sample indicate that they receive little help from their group participation. Some find groups boring or uninteresting, and many choose not to return; but no one has yet reported being harmed. And there is no case on record of a self-help group being sued for malpractice. This may be due to the fact that these are voluntary groups for which no fee-for-service is charged and with no professional leader or therapist conducting the meeting.

Although professionally led encounter groups have revealed a relatively high casualty rate, according to Lieberman, Yalom, and Miles (1973), this has not been found among self-help groups. One of the reasons for the casualty rate among encounter groups was the prevalence of confrontation, feedback, self-disclosure, and other mechanisms that often left participants in a high state of anxiety. These professionally led mechanisms are rarely found in self-help groups where the emphasis instead is on providing understanding, assurance of worth, information and advice, and mutual support.

Some Policy Implications

Commissions that have thus far reviewed the work of self-help groups and made recommendations concerning their broader use in society see these groups as supplementing and not supplanting existing professional services. The same can be said for the relationship to natural helping networks as well. At the same time, few self-help groups suggest that the functions of professional services be abnegated or even curtailed. On the contrary, they usually seek more services that are finely honed to specific needs. Many of them advocate shifts in function and emphasis by both human services agencies and individuals rendering professional services. There is an obvious concern for service and research that focuses more on caring and coping in addition to that focused on curing and cause-seeking. This implies that centers for education and training of such professionals need to incorporate findings on self-help and support systems that are gradually accumulating. There are some indications that this is already occurring.

It may be useful here to identify briefly some of the key recommendations made along these lines by the President's Commission on Mental Health (1978, pp. 178–179). These recommendations clearly are applicable beyond mental health settings to hospitals, clinics, and other agencies serving persons with other conditions and afflictions.

1. Mandate that community mental health centers provide directories of mutual health groups and similar peer oriented support systems as part of their resource base and encourage other community organizations, both public and private, to disseminate these directories in order to make such groups more accessible to the public.
2. Develop clearinghouses on mutual help groups and peer oriented support systems in each federal region throughout the country. To integrate information, to publish newsletters and other materials, to provide training and technical assistance, to sponsor periodic regional conferences of self-help, to enable professionals and members of self-help groups to learn from each other.
3. Develop curricula in all undergraduate and graduate programs in the social, behavioral, educational, and medical sciences and professions relating to mental health services delivery on the nature and function of community support systems, and through helping networks, and mutual help groups. The inclusion of such curricula should be considered an essential element in the accreditation process for approval status for graduate professional training programs in medicine, psychology, social work, nursing, pastoral counseling, rehabilitation, psychiatry, and other related disciplines.

4. Experimentation, with program evaluation, to develop new mechanisms for reimbursement of social support services and for community support systems programming as a legitimate part of health and mental health services delivery.
5. Federal money should be made available to state mental health associations, to help catalyze a citizen statewide strategy for the development of locally based, peer-oriented support networks to give technical assistance in the implementation to their local affiliated associations, and to develop information and referral services of mutual help groups.
6. Convene national conferences of voluntary programs in health, mental health, educational, and social welfare programs to identify ways that volunteer programs can be creatively linked to the community's natural support networks in formal caregiving institutions.

Although there has been little federal initiative undertaken to implement these recommendations, considerable effort has been made in various places throughout the country supported primarily from private sources to follow through on these strategies. In a special issue of *Prevention in Human Services,* for example, Borck and Aronowitz (1982) describe the development of self-help clearinghouses as a way of recognizing and strengthening natural networks of self-help groups in various communities. In some cases, these self-help clearinghouses have been developed under the auspices of universities; others are being initiated under the auspices of mental health centers and hospitals. The Self-Help Center in Evanston, Illinois, has spun off from its initial development at Northwestern University and, through private support, has been established as an independent not-for-profit corporation.

In each case, depending on size of staff and budget, these clearinghouses are in fact implementing the recommendations described earlier—from the development of directories of self-help groups in their communities to conducting important research on various aspects of the emergence and impact of self-help groups on various populations. In addition, many are helping develop new groups in their communities and providing practical assistance to new and established groups as they try to reach more persons who may benefit.

The *Plan for Nationwide Action on Epilepsy* prepared by the Commission for the Control of Epilepsy and Its Consequences (1978) also noted that self-help groups often take the lead in opening doors for persons with epilepsy and for others who are seeking new understanding. The commission noted the value of epilepsy self-help groups at three levels: when individuals take responsibility for themselves, when they meet in small groups to help themselves and others, and when they are involved in advocacy efforts. In recommending that local voluntary groups sponsor self-help groups, the commission noted that, "In such a time of strong emphasis on consumer participation, those with epilepsy can be most effective spokesmen for their own cause. They are able to demonstrate most effectively to employers their own capabilities or to describe most accurately for teachers or other groups their problems and difficulties" (Volume One,

p. 102). Clearly, this applies equally to other chronic conditions, suggesting that special efforts, both public and private, could prove productive.

The development of epilepsy self-help groups nationwide since 1976 presents a crucial example of cooperation between the federal government, voluntary agencies, and self-help groups in the establishment of new groups and important collaboration between action researchers and members of groups that followed this development. Through a mixed strategy in which federal funds were provided by the Office of Developmental Disabilities to the Epilepsy Foundation of America, self-help groups in fifteen cities throughout the United States were formed under the auspices of EFA chapters. A critical requirement in the development of these groups was that a service agent, the key person involved in developing and convening the group, be a person with epilepsy. An evaluation of the development of this two-year project revealed that groups have continued in half of the cities where they were developed, and through a radiating effect, others have been formed in other parts of the country (Borman, Pasquale, and Davies, 1982).

Moreover, the follow-up collaboration with researchers and self-help group participants proved equally productive. Through the use of an action learning workshop, such collaboration demonstrated the value of combining research with extension work. Because self-help groups function autonomously and exist primarily in natural community settings rather than under professional control and auspices, researchers need to establish a basis of copartnership. They need to show clearly that such collaboration will benefit the groups as well as the scientific community. This was decidedly the case with the epilepsy self-help workshop. It showed that researchers could assist groups by providing feedback of findings, by holding regular face-to-face sessions with group leaders and participants, and by utilizing newsletters and other reports, written in intelligible language and disseminated widely. Not only do the groups benefit and increase in number and effectiveness, but the researchers become open to dimensions and problems that are not so narrowly defined from an academic perspective. They learn, moreover, that their findings and involvement are most meaningful to the often devastated human communities with which they work. Thus, they are privileged to advance knowledge and human well-being at the same time.

Other voluntary associations focusing on chronically ill children have likewise indicated an interest in forming and sponsoring self-help groups. Ironically, although many of these organizations began as mutual aid groups, they have evolved into more formal organizations concerned with fund raising, research, advocacy, and public education. An increasing number now want to develop their self-help group capacities. The Spina Bifida Association, the American Liver Foundation, and the United Scleroderma Association are examples of such organizations making a major commitment to the facilitation of support networks and self-help/mutual aid groups. As with the Epilepsy Foundation of America, this may require development of specific demonstrations of collaboration with researchers and self-help group participants, both locally and nationally, with potential support derived from both public and private sectors.

Given the increased emphasis on volunteerism, the large numbers of persons that can be reached, and the cost-effectiveness of self-help groups, many more voluntary associations may consider the value of undertaking such programs.

References

Ablon, J. "The Parents' Auxiliary of Little People of America: A Self-Help Model of Social Support for Families of Short-Statured Children." *Prevention in Human Services,* 1982, *1* (3), 31–46.

Antze, P. "Role of Ideologies in Peer Psychotherapy Groups." In M. Lieberman and L. Borman (Eds.), *Self-Help Groups for Coping with Crisis.* San Francisco: Jossey-Bass, 1979.

Birenbaum, A. "On Managing a Courtesy Stigma." *Journal of Health and Social Behavior,* 1970, *11,* 196–206.

Borck, L. A., and Aronowitz, E. "The Role of Self-Help Clearinghouses." *Prevention in Human Services,* 1982, *1* (3), 121–129.

Borman, L. D. "Action Anthropology and the Self-Help/Mutual Aid Movement." In R. Hinshaw (Ed.), *Currents in Anthropology: Essays in Honor of Sol Tax.* The Hague, Netherlands: Mouton, 1979a.

Borman, L. D. "Recent Findings on the Development and Nature of Self-Help Groups." Proceedings of the Fourth International Conference of Therapeutic Communities. New York: Daytop Village, 1979b.

Borman, L. D., Davies, J., and Droge, D. "Self-Help Groups for Persons with Epilepsy." In B. P. Hermann (Ed.), *A Multidisciplinary Handbook of Epilepsy.* Springfield, Ill.: Thomas, 1980.

Borman, L. D., Pasquale, F. L., and Davies, J. "Epilepsy Self-Help Groups: Collaboration with Professionals." *Prevention in Human Services,* 1982, *1* (3), 111–120.

Commission for the Control of Epilepsy and Its Consequences. *Plan for Nationwide Action on Epilepsy.* National Institutes of Health publication no. 78–312. Washington, D.C.: U.S. Government Printing Office, 1978.

David, C., and Frankel, J. "Group Counseling of Parents of Diabetic Children." In Z. Laron (Ed.), *Habilation and Rehabilitation of Juvenile Diabetes.* Baltimore, Md.: Williams & Wilkens, 1970.

Evans, G. *The Family Circle Guide to Self-Help.* New York: Ballantine, 1979.

Farber, B. *Mental Retardation: Its Social Context and Social Consequences.* Boston: Houghton-Mifflin, 1968.

Gorham, K. A., and others. "Effects on Parents." In N. Hobbs (Ed.), *Issues in the Classification of Children.* Vol. 2. San Francisco: Jossey-Bass, 1975.

Heffron, W. A., Bommelaere, K., and Masters, R. "Group Discussions with Parents of Leukemic Children." *Pediatrics,* 1973, *52* (6), 831–840.

Isenberg, D. H. "Coping with Cancer: The Role of Belief Systems and Support in Cancer Self-Help Groups." Doctoral dissertation, Counseling Psychology, Northwestern University, Evanston, Ill., 1981.

Katz, A. H. *Parents of Handicapped Children: Self-Organized Parents' and*

Relatives' Groups for Treatment of Ill and Handicapped Children. Springfield, Ill.: Thomas, 1961.

Katz, A. H. "Social Adaptation in Chronic Illness: A Study of Hemophilia." *American Journal of Public Health,* 1963, *53,* 1666–1675.

Katz, A. H. *Hemophilia: A Study in Hope and Reality.* Springfield, Ill.: Thomas, 1970.

Lieberman, M. A., and Borman, L. D. "The Impact of Self-Help Groups on Widows' Mental Health." *National Reporter,* 1981a, *4* (7), 1–6. (Newsletter of the National Research and Information Center, Evanston, Ill.).

Lieberman, M. A., and Borman, L. D. "Who Helps Widows: The Role of Kith and Kin." *National Reporter,* 1981b, *4* (8), 1–6. (Newsletter of the National Research and Information Center, Evanston, Ill.)

Lieberman, M. A., Borman, L. D., and Associates. *Self-Help Groups for Coping with Crisis.* San Francisco: Jossey-Bass, 1979.

Lieberman, M. A., Yalom, I. D., and Miles, M. B. *Encounter Groups: First Facts.* New York: Basic Books, 1973.

Liebman, R., Minuchin, S., and Baker, L. "The Use of Structural Family Therapy in the Treatment of Intractable Asthma." *American Journal of Psychiatry,* 1974, *131,* 535–540.

McMichael, J. K. *Handicap: A Study of Physically Handicapped Children and Their Families.* Pittsburgh, Pa.: University of Pittsburgh Press, 1971.

Mowrer, O. H. *The New Group Therapy.* New York: D. Van Nostrand, 1964.

Pasquale, F. (Ed.). *Directory of Self-Help/Mutual Aid Groups: Chicago Metropolitan Area, 1981–1982.* Evanston, Ill.: Self-Help Center, 1981a.

Pasquale, F. (Ed.). *Report of the First National Epilepsy Self-Help Workshop.* Evanston, Ill.: Self-Help Center, 1981b.

Patten, M. P. "Parents' Groups and Associations." In L. Burton (Ed.), *Care of the Child Facing Death.* Boston: Routledge & Kegan Paul, 1974.

President's Commission on Mental Health. *Commission Reports.* Vol. 2: Appendix. Washington, D.C.: U.S. Government Printing Office, 1978.

Riessman, F. "The 'Helper' Therapy Principle." *Social Work,* 1965, *10,* 27–32.

Rowitz, L. "Social Factors in Mental Retardation." *Social Science and Medicine,* 1974, *8,* 405–412.

Scherzer, A. L., and Opsa, G. "Effect of a Parent Discussion Group for Meningomyelocele Patients." Manuscript, n.d.

Sherman, B. "Emergence of Ideology in a Bereaved Parents Group." In M. Lieberman and L. Borman (Eds.), *Self-Help Groups for Coping with Crisis.* San Francisco: Jossey-Bass, 1979.

Suelzle, M., and Keenan, V. "Parents as Advocates for Handicapped Children: Untapped Resources for Social Change in the 1980s." Unpublished manuscript, Center for Urban Affairs, Northwestern University, Evanston, Ill., 1980a.

Suelzle, M., and Keenan, V. "Parents' Choice of Services for Developmentally Disabled Children: Final Report." Center for Urban Affairs, Northwestern University, Evanston, Ill., 1980b.

Suelzle, M., and Keenan, V. "Changes in Family Support Networks Over the Life Cycle from Preschool to Young Adulthood." *American Journal of Mental Deficiency,* 1981, *86* (3), 267–274.

Tizard, J., and Grad, J. C. *The Mentally Handicapped and Their Families.* Oxford, England: Oxford University Press, 1961.

Videka-Sherman, L. "Effects of Participation in a Self-Help Group for Bereaved Parents." *Prevention in Human Services,* 1982, *1* (3), 69–77.

Wheat, P., and Lieber, L. L. *Hope for the Children.* Minneapolis, Minn.: Winston, 1979.

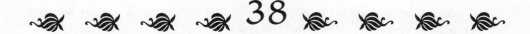

38

Charitable Associations

Carl Milofsky, Ph.D.
Julie T. Elworth, M.A.

Who Are the Voluntary Associations and the Communities They Serve?

The major providers of services to children with chronic diseases include a group of charities that have as their central functions the raising of funds and sponsoring of research and services for victims of particular diseases or groups of related diseases. These children's health charities include such organizations as the Muscular Dystrophy Association, the National Hemophilia Foundation, and the National Foundation–March of Dimes. There are between twenty and thirty national children's health charities affiliated with several thousand chapters at the state and local levels.

Relatively little has been written about these associations either by social science researchers or by policy analysts. The function of this chapter is to provide a description of the associations, a statement of the dilemmas confronting them, and a discussion of policy issues that have most concerned observers of the organizations and the participants in them. This discussion is based on a review of the literature and on interviews with a small number of officials in health charities. Although we try to integrate the material that exists by offering a particular, coherent point of view, what follows should be taken as a starting point for more research rather than an authoritative statement based on extensive data.

There has been harsh criticism of the children's health charities during the past twenty years. Some criticism has been esthetic, challenging the inclination

Note: Partial support for this chapter was provided by the Program on Nonprofit Organizations, Yale University.

of some associations to encourage donations by emphasizing the cuteness of children affected by a disease and the tragedy of their affliction (Katz, 1974; Rosenbaum, 1974; Bakal, 1979). Representatives of the disabled have objected to this portrayal because it suggests that sufferers of chronic diseases are helpless, tragic figures and that help should derive primarily from pity. Other critics have questioned the wisdom of using health charities as a major vehicle for attacking the problem of children's chronic diseases. Health charities have greatly varying success at fund raising. Consequently, the needs of some disease sufferers are better served than those of others, especially as fund raising success does not necessarily coincide with a high incidence of a disease. Because these are nonprofit, tax exempt organizations, our society subsidizes them. We could, in theory, collect as taxes the funds now being donated to the health charities and place them in a single pool for distribution to those serving victims of different diseases—a plan that might make for a more rational service delivery system (Brannon and Strnad, 1977). Such a policy urges dismantling the voluntary health charities in favor of a central governmental allocation system.

We offer a rationale in support of the children's health charities. Although we recognize the variety of administrative and policy problems that plague these associations, the charities play an essential role as interest groups promoting and defending the interests of the chronically ill. One part of their work is lobbying to influence government policy, but their role as interest groups is much more broad. It involves managing the relationship between each disease-oriented community and the society-at-large through fund raising, education, social support, preventive services, and promotion of research and innovation in treatment and sevices.

Taken in strict cost-benefit terms, having many disease associations and investing heavily in the fund-raising process as the associations do may be inefficient. We argue, however, that the decentralization and duplication that characterize this group of organizations are important because many of the diseases have extremely low incidence. If policy making and the allocation of funds were completely centralized (it already has been partly centralized through the collection of federal government services into the National Institutes of Health), those suffering from low-incidence diseases would be in danger of either being cut out of some service programs or facing policies that work against their needs while they serve well those of larger groups of the population. Working as autonomous, self-interested associations, the health charities address the idiosyncratic problems associated with different chronic diseases. In a pluralistic, democratic society like ours, tiny groups with extreme needs are likely to be ignored in favor of larger, more politically important segments of the population unless the members of those small groups form aggressive and well-organized associations to promote their interests. Such an organizational effort is represented by the health charities.

First we offer a demographic description of the health charities as a group. Then we explore issues of organizational structure and a division between the older and newer health charities in terms of their organizational character. Then we discuss the role of health charities in lobbying and in promoting the rights of the chronically ill and disabled. Finally, there is a synopsis of the policy issues raised in this chapter.

Who Are the Children's Health Charities?

There are about twenty national children's health charities, most of which are linked to a network of chapters at the state and local levels. Thus, the organizations are federations with, in most cases, several hundred affiliates. Their national offices are generally responsible for certain large fund-raising programs (such as national telethons), for coordinating training and program design, and for political lobbying. Local chapters sometimes support medical service centers. They carry on local fund raising, the proceeds of which are shared with the national offices. They also provide a variety of information and support services to the families of disease sufferers.

Within these broad outlines, there is considerable variation among the associations. The most important difference is in size. At one extreme are the National Easter Seal Society (income of $133 million in 1979–1980), the March of Dimes Birth Defects Foundation ($71 million), and the Muscular Dystrophy Association ($73 million); these are three of the five largest health charities. At the other extreme are small associations like the Retinitis Pigmentosa Foundation with one- or two-person national offices or no paid staff at all. In most cases, the small associations have national budgets of no more than several hundred thousand dollars.

A large association generally has an elaborately departmentalized national office employing anywhere from 35 to 200 people and supervising a staff of professionals at regional and local levels around the country. According to the National Health Council (1981), the activities of the associations can be divided into the following program service categories: public education, research, patient services, professional education, and community services. In the larger organizations, there is usually a vice-president (with a specialized staff of paid career workers) in charge of each service area. Paid staff and volunteers in the local offices are generally under close control of their national supervisors. Although local programs vary depending on the talents of the staff and histories of different chapters, the administrators in the national offices make strong efforts to oversee local chapters and make them an integrated part of a national program.

In small organizations, there is generally less administrative specialization and less control by the national office. Volunteers and board members do much of the routine work of running the organization. The smaller organizations tend to be dominated and controlled by volunteers, while the larger associations use volunteers mainly to carry out specific functions planned and directed by professionals.

The following descriptions of two health charities, one older and large and one newer and small, convey some sense of what these organizations do and how their organization differs. Statistics are taken from a National Health Council

(1981) report of financial information as well as from interviews with association personnel and the charities' own literature.

A Large Association: Muscular Dystrophy Association of America

The Muscular Dystrophy Association of America (MDA) is one of the largest children's health charities with an annual budget of $77.8 million and a national staff of about 1,000 people. It began in 1950 as a mutual support group of parents and physicians whose primary concern was with the most common of the dystrophies, Duchenne's. In the early years, fund raising was carried out primarily through door-to-door campaigns by volunteers. As the association grew and gained chapters in cities around the country (there are now 230 affiliates), it became more centralized in both its administration and fund-raising methods and more controlled by professional staff.

Today, much fund raising for MDA is conducted through its national telethon, which is hosted by Jerry Lewis. The success of the fund-raising program, coupled with the relatively small number of people who suffer Duchenne's dystrophy or any other of the thirty-four related diseases the association now addresses, has allowed the organization to launch a complex program of research and services that are offered free of charge in 242 clinics across the country. The programs are closely controlled by the professional staff, and most volunteers are allowed only limited service roles in contrast to the substantial policy-making roles thay are given in some of the other health charities. The programs run without government support and there is some pride at MDA that the association can provide sophisticated services to its constituency without relying on government help.

A Small Association: Juvenile Diabetes Foundation

The Juvenile Diabetes Foundation (JDF) was begun in 1970 by a group of parents who objected to what they saw as excessive domination of the older American Diabetes Association (ADA) by medical professionals and paid staff. The parents wanted an association that recognized the competence of families in helping to manage the care of their children. They also wanted an association that would push aggressively for a larger share of government research money and would have as its primary goal seeking a cure for the disease. The founders of JDF felt this plan required more emphasis on the serious consequences of diabetes so the public and politicians would see it as a disease as serious and as in need of research as the other major killers, heart disease and cancer.

Emerging from a reaction against professionals and emphasizing a campaign to build political and popular support for a campaign against diabetes, JDF has had an active national volunteer group. Board members did much of the administrative work of the foundation as well as most of its lobbying. Board administration was seen as necessary partly because funds have been limited (JDF had a total income of $4.7 million in 1980) and because the board wanted to channel as much money as possible to research rather than to administrative overhead.

The antipathy to paid administrators has begun to soften, in large part because, as the association has grown, the informality and lack of specialization in the volunteer organization have become cumbersome. Despite this change, JDF continues to be an organization that sees its role primarily as a catalyst of action to fight juvenile diabetes rather than as the prime provider of services to those who suffer the disease.

Organization of the Health Charities

The dichotomy between the older and newer health charities has both an organizational (or administrative) aspect and a political (or value) dimension. The older associations are best understood if described as formal organizations in the language of administrative theory. The newer organizations are more loosely structured and encourage participation by their clientele. They look more like political movements or interest groups.

Being large and wealthy, the older associations must be concerned with issues of coordination and accountability that newer associations do not face. As a result, volunteers are relatively excluded from decision-making processes in the older groups as compared to the newer ones. A consequence of being relatively closed to grass-roots involvement in decision making is that the older associations are less swayed by changes in the values and politics of their client constituencies.

Political differences between groups of organizations like the old and new health charities can be interpreted in a number of ways. The older associations are more conservative, reflecting perhaps the kinds of people who have become involved in and control them. The politics of the associations also have roots in their administrative structures.

Older Associations: A Charitable Model

The older associations are generally patterned on a protestant, paternalistic model of charity, which has a long history and deep roots in a variety of social welfare institutions in the United States (Milofsky, 1979). This is not intended to suggest that protestants are by nature paternalistic. Rather, the label focuses on a distinctly protestant tradition of helping, which emphasizes that those with wealth, health, and a strong sense of moral responsibility have an obligation to help those less fortunate. Many early helping efforts evolved from basic institutions of the contemporary welfare state, and much good has resulted from the concerned efforts of protestant reformers to carry out their religious and moral obligations (Wilensky and Lebeaux, 1965).

Valuable though these efforts have been, they also have fostered attitudes that have been attacked by some of those being helped and by those wishing to see the government take broader social responsibility. These attitudes—paternalism and corporate control—are built into the programs of the older voluntary welfare associations.

Paternalism. Paternalism is defined as the system, principle, or practice of managing or governing individuals, businesses, nations, and so on, in the manner of a father dealing with his children. There are two manifestations of paternalism in the older health associations. One is in the way resources are acquired and distributed to people with disabilities and diseases. The second is in reliance on the principle that professionals and professional knowledge should be dominant in policy making, program planning, and administration of services. In each case, people receiving assistance or care have little voice in the decision making process.

Paternalism has a negative connotation in our society and, in the case of these health charities, perhaps some of that negativism is deserved. Those who run the associations in the protestant, paternalistic mold tend to depict disease sufferers as helpless victims overwhelmed by a personal tragedy and with limited capacity for personal independence. The emphasis on poster children in fund-raising drives supports this dependence and has raised the hackles of groups, such as the American Coalition of Citizens with Disabilities, that emphasize the self-reliance of the disabled (Varela, 1979). Heart-rending appeals about the tragedies that have befallen helpless children may make it more difficult to raise funds for programs that emphasize and facilitate independence and long-term growth.

Some examples of health association paternalism to which critics most object are probably unintended consequences of important programs. Recipients of services of different associations have complained that they are treated as though they are irresponsible. In their account of raising a child with hemophilia, for example, Massie and Massie (1975) speak of the difficulties of obtaining sufficient blood for the hundreds of transfusions required. As if it were not problem enough that blood plasma was at times unavailable, the Massies complained that the Red Cross and the National Hemophilia Foundation required that they convince friends and community members to give blood to make up for their son's consumption. Although the Massies organized blood drives among family and friends, representatives of the two associations complained that too few people had been attracted and implied that the family was taking unfair advantage of the blood donation system. The Massies argue that families with hemophilia should not be expected to raise the huge quantities of blood required for their care, that this is a responsibility of society in general. Making parents responsible adds stress to what is an already frightening and difficult situation. Luckily, advances in drawing and storage of blood have made this particular horror story for people with hemophilia outmoded. However, the sense of moral reprobation the Massies felt from the Hemophilia Foundation and Red Cross is a common complaint of those receiving services from the health associations.

Paternalism is resented by clients when an attitude of moral superiority seems built into association practices. Viewed from the associaton side, paternalism may be a product of society's failure to support the disabled and chronically ill rather than a failing of the associations. One Muscular Dystrophy Association staff person pointed out that during telethons increasing efforts *have* been made to portray disabled adults and disabled people in independent, mainstream roles. However, people notice and give money because of the poster children.

Professional dominance in the associations may also encourage paternalism. Doctors play an important role in many associations, planning and approving research programs, supervising medical service programs in association-sponsored clinics, evaluating the quality and effectiveness of technological advances, and educating the public. These functions are unavoidably paternalistic when they require that doctors draw on their technical knowledge and experience in treating a disease to make decisions. Expertise is necessarily elitist. However, some critics have complained that medical professionals use their esoteric knowledge to claim an organizational domain they try to protect from competitors whether or not there are technical matters that disqualify laymen from contributing informed opinions (Anderson, 1982).

Distrust of health professionals is partly related to a growing consumerism movement in all areas of health care as people have sought to understand their medical problems and take a more active role in personal decision making and in remediation (Gilbert, 1973; Caplan and Killilea, 1976; Boston Women's Health Collective, 1976; Arms, 1977; Varela, 1979). Those who live with chronic diseases are especially aware of ways medical care could be better and more comfortably organized. They have extensive exposure to a particular disease and, over time, may develop a sophisticated understanding of its medical dimensions. To them, less experienced medical personnel may seem uninformed and ill equipped to make treatment decisions. Furthermore, some needs of the chronically ill require meticulous rather than sophisticated care—for example, turning bedridden patients to avoid bed sores. This care can often be best provided by an attentive family or a private nurse. Finally, hostility toward professionals also grows from institutional insensitivity to the needs of children.

There is an ideological divide among the associations. In some of the new charities, members are suspicious of professional paternalism, and the organization works to help families feel they have more control over the disease they are fighting and the care they receive. In older charities, medical professionals are entrenched. They tend to oppose giving family members and interested volunteers too much control over planning and administering programs.

Corporate Centralism. The older, larger health charities also differ from the newer breed in that policy and services are more centralized and controlled by paid staff and medical professionals. Corporate centralism here refers not to domaination of the charities by business—although some complain that businesses do have an undue influence. Rather, it refers to a style of organization of the nonprofit corporation in which officers and their employees control decision making and in which clients and volunteers are largely excluded from that process. The controlling group is small, and there are sharp barriers between those legitimated to contribute to decision making and those excluded.

Strong corporate control in the older foundations is striking, not only because it creates an atmosphere similar to that of a business but also because it contrasts starkly with the atmosphere that prevails in the newer foundations. The latter are decentralized, democratic, and strongly controlled by local chapters and by volunteers. In the newer associations, roles of paid staff tend to be indistinct. Everyone does everything, including volunteers who work shoulder-to-shoulder with the paid staff.

Tight corporate control has stimulated a number of complaints about the older health charities. One complaint is that too high a proportion of the funds collected supports a large staff and a complex organization rather than helps disease sufferers (Katz, 1974; Bakal, 1979). Families often feel that staff members do not have a proper understanding of the problems that confront the chronically ill and of their priorities in spending to attack the disease.

A different criticism is that, by focusing on building a wealthy, complex institution, those who run the older associations are excessively "patho-centric," focused only on problems caused by their specific disease. Of course, all health charities are primarily concerned with promoting the fortunes of their particular disease. However, it is argued, the older associations try to run the whole show in their areas of interest and pay little attention to coordinating their efforts with the general health policies of the greater society. Some have been active in promoting particular policy positions on issues of immediate interest to their disease—the American Cancer Society's campaign against smoking is an example. But few older associations (the National Cystic Fibrosis Research Foundation is an exception) have paid much attention to general issues of health policy that concern the sufferers of other chronic diseases as well as their own constituents.

Most associations, at least until recently, had few personnel available to monitor legislation and to educate legislators about particular bills important to the disabled and chronically ill (Pollock, 1982). Despite their limited resources, the newer associations have generally been the more active lobbyists during the last two decades. With their visibility and popularity, the older health charities might well have played an important role in shaping public opinion and health policy (Etzioni, 1978), although they avoided this role. The critics suggest that the focus on corporate control has led the older associations to avoid lobbying and coordination efforts that might dilute the control they exercise over their domains.

Paternalism and the Life Cycle of Health Charities

Corporate centralism is partly an unavoidable product of the histories and size of the older associations. The early ones began in the 1950s or before when there were no large-scale or broadly available services for those with chronic diseases and when there was little government funding for medical research. Most associations were begun by families of disease sufferers to raise money for research, provide information for other families, and put professionals familiar with specialized techniques in touch with disease sufferers.

Most associations began with a strongly volunteer force that raised money, sometimes did political lobbying, and helped disease sufferers (Novak, 1973). To raise money, family members who made up the original volunteer force recruited neighbors to help. The rapid progress of research and the improvement in care made possible by systematic efforts of health charities made it clear—at least during the 1950s and 1960s—that fund raising was a vital function for these associations. As fund raising became a more and more central activity and as income increased, relatives of disease sufferers became less able to play a dominant role.

Furthermore, people who know and are respected by people with money must be included in authoritative positions, so the associations drafted community and business leaders to spearhead fund-raising campaigns. These people could gain access to the monied interests, and the associations could play on the career interests and competitive instincts of those in the economic and social elite group of a community (Seeley, Junker, and Jones, 1957).

As association income rose, paid specialists played an increasing role in planning drives, auditing the funds collected, overseeing how money was spent, and training fund raisers (Sills, 1957). Fund-raising techniques, such as telethons and direct mail campaigns, place a premium on tight organization and de-emphasize connections with the informal social networks that are key to fund raising among community elites. Case studies of national charitable organizations again and again report sharp conflict between national central office staff and volunteers in local chapters (Sills, 1957; Zald, 1970). Conflict also concerns coordination: If local chapters control policy, it is difficult to have a national organizational policy or a national program whether in research or patient care.

Administrative reforms are hard to achieve with volunteers. Amateurs tend to participate for idiosyncratic, personal reasons—raising money makes them feel good, they have a sick cousin, they want to impress the boss, they have a strong feeling of Christian responsibility, they want to get out and make social contacts, or they are trying to build a political career (Form and Nosaw, 1958; Wheeldon, 1969; Merton, 1976). Not usually motivated by a desire to make money, they tend to participate for idealistic reasons. Consequently, they may have their own ideas of problems the association should be solving, and they tend to resist supervision. They may want to carry out their own program, gain fulfillment for themselves, and see that they are accomplishing things in concrete, immediate ways (Seeley, Junker, and Jones, 1957; Case and Taylor, 1979).

Not all volunteers suffer these shortcomings. Many health associations—both old and new—rely heavily on volunteers, some of whom take on considerable responsibility. But for large associations like the American Cancer Society or the Muscular Dystrophy Association, this core group is a tiny fraction of all volunteers. There is a national force of thousands in hundreds of communities who do some volunteer work. The problems of coordination and of quality control are immense. The changes in newer associations suggest that corporate centralism in the older health charities is a matter of administrative necessity as well as a consequence of the conservative values critics accuse them of promoting.

Politics and Health Charities

It is tempting to view the contrast between the old and new charities as one between established, conservative, professionally dominated organizations and politically sophisticated, democratic, activist, and consumer-oriented ones. This view is too simple. The dichotomy is partly due to the fact that the two groups of charities are at different stages of administrative development.

Many of the older associations are rapidly becoming more sensitive to state and national policies. They are employing lobbyists and creating new high-ranking corporate positions for the management of political affairs. Some associations are substantially restructuring to give themselves a more activist posture.

There seem to be two distinct social or political movements embodied in health charities. One is primarily service-oriented and committed to making up for the negligence of federal and state programs where care for the disabled and chronically ill are concerned. The other is primarily concerned with moving institutions in society to action.

The service orientation of older charities developed because they were founded prior to 1960 when few government programs provided medical care, counseling, or household help to the chronically ill. They appeal on a symbolic level to sentiments broadly shared among Americans about why it is important to help the needy, sentiments that analysts such as Seeley, Junker, and Jones (1957) and Sills (1957) attribute to the morality of protestantism. Voluntarism is a key to those sentiments. Donating time and money is morally satisfying when the givers feel that denying themselves (even in relatively minor ways by donating a few dollars or several evenings of work) provides a gift the needy cannot obtain elsewhere. Charities are committed to their own causes, not to better health care in general. To the extent charities are successful at fund raising, their leaders also are likely to feel government intervention is not needed.

Government involvement in funding or directly providing services undercuts the effectiveness of this appeal. Once the government is involved, a case can be made that clients have a right to receive care and that society has an obligation to provide it (Janowitz, 1978). A charity that accepts government subsidies for programs it has traditionally supported through voluntary gifts becomes a surrogate government agency—as has happened with many social service nonprofit organizations in the past two decades. Seeley, Junker, and Jones (1957) argue that the moral appeal of the charity is then weakened because donations seem more like taxes than decisions of conscience. This rationale remains strong in a number of the charities today.

The Political Movement in New Health Charities

The newer health charities have a radically different outlook. Emerging in a period of active government involvement in all manner of social and health problem solving, they appeal to different ideologies—those of consumerism and of social action groups. Rather than a need to be organizationally self-sufficient, the newer agencies have grown with the knowledge that federal and state governments would take some responsibility for patient care, with the agencies' major responsibility to be expansion and upgrading of government services. In doing so, two main thrusts characterize the new charities. On one hand, they are pressure groups representing the cause of those who suffer their chronic disease. On the other hand, they are like socially conscious foundations that use their resources to create model programs the government might later take over and expand.

Leaders of new health charities we interviewed were generally aware of several alternative strategies to promote their cause in the political arena. There is a strong sense that for the organizaton to be successful it must influence the political system. The new charities, having a smaller resource base, have a great stake in using their lobbying resources wisely and efficiently. The central question is, how can a small, poorly funded, and obscure pressure group compete most successfully for resources against other pressure groups in the political system?

There are four main modalities by which the new charities stimulate desired social change: leveraging resources, stimulating innovation, lobbying, and mobilizing a public constituency. In each case, the charity tries to act as a catalyst for some broader change rather than to act as a self-sufficient, exclusive service provider to the community concerned with a particular disease.

Leveraging Resources. Leveraging occurs when a foundation provides seed money for a project or creates an administrative presence that helps attract diverse resources to a new project. Presumably, most public service organizations would like to see their programs stimulate increased social and governmental support in their area of concern. Leveraging, however, represents a more self-conscious effort to support projects likely to produce a snowball effect as opposed to projects that simply fulfill immediate service goals.

Since perhaps 1960, a number of foundations, led by Ford, have come to believe they would be more effective if they attacked generic social problems rather than narrowly focused ones. Even large foundations, with meager resources compared with those needed to underwrite the elimination of poverty or comparable broad social problems (Marris and Rein, 1967), have become increasingly concerned with how limited resources could be used to produce maximum returns. Their ideas about what philanthropy can and should do, have changed profoundly.

That new health charities are more interested in leveraging than their older counterparts reflects the more meager resources of the former. Like the pre-1960 general purpose foundations, the older charities are primarily engaged in providing funds for a comprehensive attack on their chosen disease. The new charities focus more on investments in programs likely to affect the entire system of political institutions, health service providers, and research organizations. One can see the leveraging strategy at work in the areas of research and of service provision.

In the research program of a health charity, leveraging is important to the extent that increasing the overall volume of scientific work is important.

Expansion requires attracting scientists and convincing them to commit their careers to working on a disease and its related physical problems. Leveraging is relevant to building public support to the extent that a charity's program of services—as opposed to its self-conscious public relations program—shapes the public perception of how serious a disease is and how urgent the need for research.

An example is provided by the diabetes health charities. A main incentive to founders of the Juvenile Diabetes Foundation (JDF) in 1970 was the perception that the existing diabetes organization, the American Diabetes Association (ADA), had been ineffective at creating a public sense that research was urgently needed. The founders of JDF thought that the low funding level resulted from the ADA's emphasis on patient compliance and the possibilities for a normal life when glucose levels are controlled. Important though compliance may be, emphasizing possibilities for normal living made diabetes seem less serious to the public. The JDF set out to emphasize the seriousness of diabetes, and since the JDF was founded, federal spending on diabetes research has climbed from $10 million to about $130 million (U.S. Office of Management and Budget, 1982).

The Juvenile Diabetes Foundation has also used leveraging to strengthen the community of scientists doing diabetes research. The foundation provides more career development grants than the federal government to stimulate researchers who have a self-conscious identity as diabetes investigators. It has sponsored symposia so that researchers will view each other as colleagues in fighting a particular disease rather than simply orienting themselves to endocrinology or some other broad medical specialty. Finally, the JDF has sought to support speculative and innovative research, which the government tends to avoid. Investment in risky projects has placed foundation researchers at the forefront of scientific advance and has allowed the organization to take credit for important developments in patient care, such as laser surgery of retinal (eye) disease in diabetes. It also gives the foundation special weight as a research advisor when one of its speculative projects leads to a major advance and becomes orthodoxy.

There is a tension in the leveraging between providing support for disease-relevant basic science and providing support for more applied specialized research that might improve care earlier. Especially where low-incidence diseases are concerned, leveraging might do little to advance the narrow purposes of a foundation—that is, improving the lives of disease sufferers and finding a means of reducing the severity of symptoms. The federal government tends to group diseases broadly in terms of the physiological systems involved. Further, physicians and researchers tend to specialize in systems rather than in diseases. Hematologists see relatively little hemophilia (Massie and Massie, 1975). Neurologists see relatively little muscular dystrophy. Spending money to attract federal investments may lead to a broad-gauged focus on basic research rather than investigations to benefit disease sufferers in the short run. Because one or two committed researchers can bring about vast improvements in patient care (as has been true with cystic fibrosis and hemophilia) leveraging might be less effective for small foundations than a more independent approach to supporting research.

Leveraging also can be an effective means for expanding services to clients. Typically, sufferers of childhood chronic diseases confront idiosyncratic problems that run afoul of the policies other health organizations have set to serve the general public in an efficient way. Sometimes investments by a health charity to restructure service provision systems can make services and insurance money more readily available to clients.

Because victims of hemophilia typically require services from many different specialties when they seek health care and often must go to major medical centers, it has been difficult in the past for a child with hemophilia to visit the hematology clinic, a physical therapist, the psychological counselor, and other specialists in one visit. There are administrative duplication and aggravation for the families and children.

The National Hemophilia Foundation attacked this problem by helping to establish special hemophilia clinics with government support. In these clinics, all of the services routinely needed are collected together. Although the government helps fund these clinics, most of their costs are covered through third-party payments so the actual cost to government is low. Without the initial funding and continuing support of the National Hemophilia Foundation, the program would fold, and both the federal and third-party payments would be lost.

Stimulating Innovation. A major contribution nonprofit organizations make to American society is their support for innovative programs. By finding and supporting creative programs and initiatives that have not been tried before, foundation leaders hope they can launch examples of reform or action that will become integrated into and supported by wealthier but more conservative institutions, most notably the federal government.

This strategy has worked best for the health charities in research. Although the federal government funds huge research programs, demands for accountability and the peer review process combine to make their granting programs conservative (Cole, Cole, and Simon, 1981). They conspire to emphasize established lines of inquiry and research likely to advance science in general rather than the interests of particular diseases. Health charities like the Juvenile Diabetes Foundation can help open new lines of inquiry by sponsoring speculative or unusual research.

Health charities also play a role in initiating new treatment modalities by funding unusual programs and supporting their volunteers' or clients' efforts to experiment. The costs and complexity of care for hemophilia were drastically reduced when parents, and eventually patients themselves, began administering transfusions. There was initial resistance to home transfusions by some physicians and by some of the larger state chapters. However, informal volunteer networks and the willingness of some state chapters to train parents from other states gradually forced the change in practice (Massie and Massie, 1975).

A criticism that might be leveled at health charities in general is that they have not played an active role in supporting innovative research programs concerned with the social problems faced by disease sufferers (Anderson, 1982). They might follow the lead of nonhealth foundations in seeking out, supporting, and popularizing innovative social programs for the chronically ill. It is rare, for example, for local chapters of health charities to coordinate their programs to provide respite care or other services needed by people with many different chronic diseases. Experimental coordinating programs could be supported (Varela, 1979) as could programs to help families cope with the death of a child (Brody, 1977; Martinson and others, 1978; McCollum, 1981).

Lobbying. Chronic diseases of children are low-incidence diseases. Legislation and government administrative policy either ignore or sometimes work against their interests. A main incentive for parents to develop voluntary associations has been to create a collective instrument for making their concerns and desires known. Available case studies (Novak, 1973; Massie and Massie, 1975; Schrag and Divoky, 1975) show that when voluntary associations concerned with chronic diseases of childhood have worked as lobbying groups, they have been dramatically successful at convincing legislators and government officials to pass legislation and regulations helpful to their causes. Cheek-by-jowl with successful lobbying programs are examples of diseases for which lobbying did not occur and that were then ignored or cut out of legislative programs. Lobbying matters. Legislators respond to heart-rending stories and hard facts about the needs of the children.

Although lobbying seems essential to promote the interests of the tiny fraction of the population suffering from any particular disease, what the object of lobbying ought to be is more open to dispute. Those active in the health charities focus their energy, for the most part, on initiating, tracing, and educating about legislation or administrative rules that affect their particular disease. Critics of the health charity lobbying effort like Pollock (1982) object to the narrowness of these efforts. He argues that there should be more of a joint effort among health charities to find issues that are of concern across the spectrum of diseases. Perhaps more important, one of the new charity directors suggested that policy makers in government are less likely to seek advice on health issues from a lobbyist who focuses only on narrow, self-interested issues (Etzioni, 1978).

On a broad level, a well-financed, concerted effort by a coalition of health associations might play a significant role in supporting policies that affect the health of the whole population. One area in which such a coalition has been effective has been the campaign for better air quality. Although not concerned with children's diseases, one example of note is the coalition of the American Cancer Society, the American Heart and the American Lung Associations to fight hard for antismoking laws. The March of Dimes and the American Lung Association have lobbied for the Federal Clean Air Act (Pollock, 1982), legislation that does affect children by controlling lead emissions. One can imagine the health charities taking this sort of leadership role in other areas as well—in lobbying for improved national health insurance or improved nutrition or more extensive prevention- and education-oriented public health programs.

Even with full-time lobbyists at work in Washington, however, the health charities might not easily join together to fight for broad changes in health policy. Particularly with federal budget retrenchment, protecting one's interests requires intimate knowledge of the administrative rules that govern relevant government agencies, of the legislative agenda, and of how pending government action might affect spending on a particular disease. The time required to understand the politics of diabetes or hemophilia or cystic fibrosis make it hard for a lobbyist to know the issues for other diseases and between particular disease groups and the general population.

Consider, for example, the struggle to establish a new Arthritis Institute in the National Institutes of Health (Sun, 1982) by breaking off arthritis research and training programs from the present National Institutes of Arthritis, Diabetes, and Digestive and Kidney Diseases (NIADDKD). Such a move has been opposed by the director of NIH, James B. Wyngaarden, who claims that "the start up costs alone for an arthritis institute would total at least $4 million to $5 million. That money would be allocated at the expense of biomedical research, given the budget constraints at NIH in recent years. . . . The formation of a separate institute by disease category runs counter to the trend in biomedical research to study the basic principles underlying the origins of disease. . . . Furthermore . . . the formation of another institute invites the proliferation of others. 'Where does it stop?' " (Sun, 1982, p. 610).

The new institute was also opposed by a variety of biological research and medical groups and was nearly blocked when diabetes groups began lobbying for their own institute. Congress would not establish two institutes. Consequently, when an impasse seemed likely, the Subcommittee on Health and Environment of the House Energy and Commerce Committee proposed a two-year moratorium on new NIH institutes. Faced with this prospect, the arthritis and diabetes interests struck a compromise in which the diabetes interests would be dominant in their present institute, an agreement that might work against the interests of the digestive and kidney diseases that will share the remnants of the NIADDKD.

Lobbying is also important at the state level. A small group of active, articulate parents can have a profound effect on state policy. In Connecticut through the 1950s and 1960s, cystic fibrosis regularly received preferred treatment because it was represented by such a group. Thanks to their work, Connecticut was the first state to provide state support for services to patients with cystic fibrosis. It did so while ignoring nearly every other childhood chronic disease (Novak, 1973).

In addition to staff shortages and conflicts of interest, many health charities avoid lobbying on broad issues that are sometimes associated with sharp value cleavages in society because being associated with a particular position might threaten a charity's ability to raise funds or the willingness of some clients to accept its services.

An example of such an issue is genetic counseling and the attempt to prevent chronic diseases through abortions. Because a number of childhood chronic diseases have genetic origins, preventing them requires an aggressive genetic screening and counseling program. However, doing so runs afoul of the right-to-life movement, which has criticized amniocentesis as a search and destroy process (Henig, 1982). In consideration of this pressure, the Muscular Dystrophy Association (MDA) refuses to take a position on abortion.

A more complex position is taken by the Spina Bifida Association of America, which has lobbied against a national screening program based on the alphafetaprotein test (Cimons, 1979). That test has a sizable false positive rate. The Spina Bifida Association argues that the test should be given only if ultrasound and amniocentesis are available as backup tests to eliminate the false positives and if people have access to medical centers that will perform abortions when the condition is diagnosed. This position clearly accepts abortions. However, the position is also sensitive to right-to-life issues.

It might well be that the Spina Bifida Association can follow this policy only because it is small and speaks mainly to a constituency of families and medical professionals. They represent narrower segments of the population and ones more intensely committed to a single issue—improving treatment for a certain disease. An association like the MDA, with a larger fund-raising program and, consequently, a broader constituency of supporters, would have trouble explaining and legitimating such a complex position.

Constituency Mobilization. Where lobbying refers to efforts by a small number of paid or volunteer staff members to influence legislation or administrative rulings, constituency mobilization refers to efforts by an organization to involve grass-roots constituents in political activity to push for policy changes. Activities may involve demonstrations, letter-writing campaigns to elected officials, or mass visits to state capitols or to Washington, D. C., to visit public officials. Or a constituency may be mobilized to criticize the practices of institutions or local social service agencies.

Among health charities, much activity in recent years has focused on changing the way disease sufferers, their families, and the public think about disease and the disabled. They have become newly aware that their illnesses are partly products of barriers to independence, erected by society, that prevent those with physical limitations from being socially accepted or from caring for themselves. Largely through the efforts or self-help groups and voluntary associations, information has been disseminated to those who suffer from particular diseases or who are limited by physical problems about how to manage relations with professionals and institutions, how to cope with self-care problems, and how to find needed services.

The newer children's health charities have been active participants in the movement to change attitudes. However, activism, political reform, and social change have focused more on the disabled in general. Through constituency mobilization, vast changes have come about in legislation dealing with the disabled including the Handicapped Bill of Rights passed in 1973 and the Education for All Handicapped Children Act passed in 1975. Through these pieces of legislation, disabled people are guaranteed, in theory at least, equal access to public programs and facilities.

The effectiveness of the constituency mobilization approach to political action cannot be measured by looking at a group's effectiveness at changing legislation and launching new social policies. Because constituency mobilization relies heavily on the work of volunteers and the involvement of those who need services, it is a powerful device for educating people, socializing them, and involving them in change efforts at the local level. Despite their small budgets and limited public visibility (compared to the older charities), new health charities have been an important agent of change because they have helped to change the way chronically ill people view themselves and the way that professionals provide them with care.

Conclusion

The political activism of the newer health charities is a phenomenon of our times. We live in an age when classes that have not shared in the wealth, government support, and political processes of American society are forming interest groups to seek these benefits. The new health charities stand alongside civil rights and women's groups as among the most effective lobbyists for their cause (Janowitz, 1978). Vast changes have occurred in a short period of time. Consequently, the organizational style of the new health charities has been championed as *the* model for social services in the 1970s and 1980s by such organizations as the American Enterprise Institute and the National Self-Help Clearinghouse (Sagarin, 1969; Sarason and others, 1977; Levin, Katz, and Holst, 1976; Sarason and Lorentz, 1979; Levin and Idler, 1981; Stokes, 1981).

Contrasted with these organizations, the older health charities seem to some critics to be anachronistic and to pose policy problems that raise questions about their usefulness. For many, the image they present as the servants of the lost and neglected in our society is syrupy and clashes with the fact that they are big businesses whose officers take a utilitarian, market-oriented approach to their work. The metaphors of charity and big business clash to the discomfort of critics (Rosenbaum, 1974), and the fact that some associations (mainly the older ones) win more dollars than others creates vast inequities in the way money is allocated to the attack on chronic diseases. Some have argued that the health charities should not be supported through the tax benefits that are granted them as charitable nonprofit organizations (Brannon and Strnad, 1977).

Childhood chronic diseases are so rare that they are in danger of being ignored by society. Indeed, most of the major associations came into existence precisely because parents felt the needs of their children and of their families were ignored. In large, pluralistic political systems like our federal and state governments, small interests tend to be overlooked unless they have aggressive, visible, and highly legitimate representatives.

Critics of older health charities have not recognized the political role played by these associations. Even though they have not been active as lobbyists or as critics of national health policy, they have been enormously influential as forces for change and investment in new kinds of services—although the newness of those services can be seen only by recalling their lack during the 1950s. The older associations also have created widespread public awareness of their causes and marshalled impressive support. They have not only raised enormous amounts of money but also created an unshakable alliance with the business and cultural leaders of our society. In the absence of reliable government support, the alliance with the private-sector elite provides security, wealth, and recognition of the needs of the chronically ill. It should be no surprise that the older associations see no reason to abandon that fruitful alliance just because for fifteen years the government was prepared to spend money on research and health services.

The inequities among the health charities are disturbing mainly if one views their services as an adjunct to or as a variety of government services. Where government resources are provided, there have been increasingly stringent mandates that all needy groups be treated equally. Thus, the Education for All Handicapped Children Act follows a series of judicial decisions that argues that, if the states require student attendance and claim to provide universal education, the schools have a responsibility to provide the most constructive education for each child regardless of disability (Kirp, 1973; Kirp, Buss, and Kuriloff, 1974; Janowitz, 1978). If the nonprofit, tax-exempt status of the health charities is taken as a reason for viewing those charities as an extension of government (an admittedly controversial position), then inequities in the distribution of services are reason for concern.

If we view the charities as creatures of the political arena rather than of the government service area, however, the inequality across associations, if not less disturbing, is at least natural and predictable. The political arena is a competitive one in which rewards are distributed not through rational planning but through what Lindblom (1977) calls an interactive process. No one runs the political system. Rather, dozens of actors compete for the attention of policy makers, try to mobilize constituency support, and capitalize upon all manner of unexpected events—events like Franklin Roosevelt contracting polio.

Critics such as Brannon and Strnad (1977) who place the health charities in the government arena err in two ways. First, they identify inequalities between charities as a major problem. In the political arena, inequality between competing interests is unavoidable just as inequality between business firms is an unavoidable product of the market. Second, they suggest reforms that replace one style of organizational concentration (the large charities) with another (a centralized government distributional authority). However rational such an authority might be, it would probably allocate its scarce resources to maximize the collective good of the chronically ill. Without a strong lobbying group to represent them, there would be danger that those suffering uncommon diseases would be less well served than those suffering from higher-incidence illnesses.

On balance, we believe it is better for the chronically ill that large charities do exist than for them to be undermined through channeling charitable giving through the government. The health charities raise a lot of money because large numbers of people are attracted to particular causes. Although there is also appeal to collecting money for all health charities simultaneously, as one can see by the growth of combined health appeals around the country, the attraction is different. If particular causes were eliminated, studies, such as those of Sills (1957) and Seeley, Junker, and Jones (1957), suggest less money would be collected, and as a result, the chronically ill would be less well served.

In our view, inequality among the charities is not the main problem. Rather, there are too few organizations representing the interests of disease sufferers. Borrowing terminology from economics, the health charities industry is too concentrated and monopolistic. For each of the major diseases, there need to be a number of organizations that not only compete for resources but also criticize and challenge each other's practices and policies.

Such opposing associations exist in some areas, and their competition and conflict are constructive. When the American Coalition of Citizens with Disabilities attacked the Muscular Dystrophy Foundation for depicting their clients as helpless, that mammoth foundation was encouraged to examine its practices to rebut the accusation. When the Juvenile Diabetes Foundation was formed to challenge the American Diabetes Association, the rapid growth in government research spending that followed helped children with diabetes.

Energy and resources should be invested in making the rest of the sector more competitive with the older charities. This has been happening to some extent as new charities such as the Sickle Cell Disease Foundation emerge and tap major funding sources. However, organizations that compete for big funding money threaten simply to duplicate the large, closed organizational forms assumed by the old associations. A different sort of competition is provided by the more explicitly political new associations. They are outspokenly critical and effective at working within the political arena. As their numbers proliferate, some of them take on as a major function challenging and attacking the older health charities. This sort of competition is important in forcing the older organizations to respond to their constituencies.

One of the major goals of social policy in this area ought to be the strengthening of critical health interest groups that both lobby for government change and attack practices of the older health charities. As federal and foundation money becomes scarcer, however, small gadfly organizations are likely to find it more and more difficult to remain in business. Making resources available to those organizations in the coming years will be a major problem for those concerned with how to improve service provision to children with chronic diseases. Without the small, critical groups, however, it seems likely that power in this sector would become even more concentrated in the large associations.

References

Anderson, J. "Charities Forget Their Purpose." *Washington Post,* January 23, 1982, p. E15.

Arms, S. *Immaculate Deception.* New York: Bantam, 1977.

Bakal, C. *Charity U.S.A.: An Investigation into the Hidden World of the Multi-Billion Dollar Charity Industry.* New York: Times Books, 1979.

Boston Women's Health Collective. *Our Bodies, Ourselves.* New York: Simon & Schuster, 1976.

Brannon, G. M., and Strnad, J. "Alternative Approaches to Encouraging Philanthropic Activities." In Commission on Private Philanthrophy and Public Needs (Filer Commission), *Research Papers,* Vol. 4. Washington, D.C.: U.S. Government, Department of the Treasury, 1977.

Brody, J. "Cancer Project Shows Home Care for Dying Child Helps Families." *New York Times,* April 7, 1977, p. 20.

Caplan, G., and Killilea, M. (Eds.). *Support Systems and Mutual Help.* New York: Grune & Stratton, 1976.

Case, J., and Taylor, R. C. (Eds.). *Co-ops, Communes and Collectives; Experiments in Social Change in the 1960s and 1970s.* New York: Pantheon, 1979.

Cimons, M. "Fears Expressed on Birth-Defect Test." *Los Angeles Times,* August 29, 1979, Sec. 4, p. 1.

Cole, S., Cole, J., and Simon, G. A. "Chance and Consensus in Peer Review." *Science,* 1981, *20* (214), 881–886.

Etzioni, A. "Groups: The Sense of Belonging." *New York Times,* March 29, 1978, p. C1.

Form, W. H., and Nosaw, S. *Community in Disaster.* New York: Harper & Row, 1958.

Gilbert, A. *You Can Do It from a Wheelchair.* New Rochelle, N.Y.: Arlington House, 1973.

Henig, R. M. "Saving Babies Before Birth." *New York Times Magazine,* February 28, 1982, p. 18.

Janowitz, M. *The Last Half Century.* Chicago: The University of Chicago Press, 1978.

Katz, H. *Give!* New York: Doubleday, 1974.

Kirp, D. L. "Schools as Sorters: The Constitutional and Policy Implications of School Classification." *University of Pennsylvania Law Review,* 1973, *121* (4), 705–707.

Kirp, D., Buss, W., and Kuriloff, P. "Legal Reform of Special Education: Empirical Studies and Procedural Proposals." *California Law Review,* 1974, *62* (1), 40–155.

Levin, L., and Idler, E. *The Hidden Health Care System: Mediating Structures and Health.* New York: Ballinger, 1981.

Levin, L., Katz, A., and Holst, E. *Self-Care: Lay Initiatives in Health.* New York: Prodist, 1976.

Lindblom, C. E. *Politics and Markets: The World's Political and Economic Systems.* New York: Basic Books, 1977.

McCollum, A. T. *The Chronically Ill Child: A Guide for Parents and Professionals.* New Haven, Conn.: Yale University Press, 1981.

Marris, P., and Rein, M. *The Dilemmas of Social Reform.* New York: Atherton, 1967.

Martinson, I. M., and others. "Home Care for Children Dying of Cancer." *Pediatrics,* 1978, *62* (1), 106–113.

Massie, R., and Massie, S. *Journey.* New York: Knopf, 1975.

Merton, R. K. "The Ambivalence of Organizational Leaders." In *Sociological Ambivalence and Other Essays.* New York: Free Press, 1976.

Milofsky, C. "Not for Profit Organizations and Community: A Review of the Sociological Literature." New Haven, Conn.: Institution of Social and Policy Studies, Program on Nonprofit Organizations, Yale University, Program on Nonprofit Organizations working paper no. 6, 1979.

National Health Council. *1979/80 Audited Financial Information; Voluntary Health Agency Members of the National Health Council.* New York: National Health Council, 1981.

Novak, B. J. "The Cystic Fibrosis Association of Connecticut, Inc.: Notes on a Special Interest Group in Action." New Haven, Conn.: Yale University School of Medicine Health Policy Project working paper no. 12, August 1973.

Pollock, R. "Making the Grade? CSPI's Report Card on the Health Charities." *Nutrition Action,* 1982, *9* (3), 6.

Rosenbaum, R. "Tales of the Heartbreak Biz." *Esquire,* July 1974, p. 67.

Sagarin, E. *Odd Man In: Societies of Deviants in America.* New York: Quadrangle Books, 1969.

Sarason, S. B., and Lorentz, E. *The Challenge of the Resource Exchange Network: Rationale, Possibilities, and Public Policy.* San Francisco: Jossey-Bass, 1979.

Sarason, S. B., and others. *Human Services and Resource Networks: Rationale, Possibilities, and Public Policy.* San Francisco: Jossey-Bass, 1977.

Schrag, P., and Divoky, D. *The Myth of the Hyperactive Child and Other Means of Child Control.* New York: Pantheon, 1975.

Seeley, J. R., Junker, B. R., and Jones, L. W. *Community Chest.* Toronto: University of Toronto Press, 1957.

Sills, D. *The Volunteers: Means and Ends in a National Organization.* New York: Free Press, 1957.

Stokes, B. *Helping Ourselves: Local Solutions to Global Problems.* New York: Norton, 1981.

Sun, M. "A New Arthritis Institute Nears Approval." *Science,* 1982, *217,* 610–612.

U.S. Office of Management and Budget. *Budget of the United States Government, FY 1983,* Appendix. Washington, D.C.: U.S. Government Printing Office, 1982.

Varela, R. A. *Self-Help Groups in Rehabilitation.* Washington, D.C.: American Coalition of Citizens with Disabilities, 1979.

Wheeldon, P. D. "The Operation of Voluntary Associations and Personal Networks in the Political Processes of an Inter-Ethnic Community." In J. Clyde Mitchell (Ed.), *Social Networks in Urban Situations: Analyses of Personal Relationships in Central African Towns.* Manchester, England: Manchester University Press, 1969.

Wilensky, H. L., and Lebeaux, C. N. *Industrial Society and Social Welfare.* New York: Free Press, 1965.

Zald, M. D. *Organizational Change: The Political Economy of the YMCA.* Chicago: The University of Chicago Press, 1970.

39

Professional Organizations

Morris Green, M.D.

Because a professional organization's role in shaping public policy relevant to chronically ill or handicapped children and their families is determined by its goals, this chapter examines the process by which these goals are established and achieved.

Professional organizations may be concerned with the population-at-large (the American Dental Association, for example) or exclusively with children and adolescents (as is the American Academy of Pediatrics). Although the former type may be committed to the care of persons with chronic illness or handicap, it cannot automatically be assumed that such general advocacy will adequately address the needs of children and adolescents. Therefore, members of generic organizations who have a primary interest in children with chronic illness or handicap must seek an organizational endorsement either of policies chiefly involving children, such as maternal and child health legislation, or support for appropriate attention to the special needs of children in categorical programs, such as programs for diabetes or arthritis. In view of the pluralistic nature of general associations and the competing interests they encompass, intraorganiza-

Note: The author wishes to acknowledge the generous help and support of many individuals, especially Alexandra Calcagno and Jackie Noyes of the American Academy of Pediatrics Washington office and Jean D. Lockhart, Director, Department of Health Services and Governmental Affairs of the American Academy of Pediatrics. I wish to recognize also the contributions of a number of other persons and organizations, identified alphabetically below, who kindly responded to requests for information about the activities of their organizations in relation to chronically ill children: the American Dietetic Association; Virginia E. O'Leary, Ph.D., American Psychological Association; Jeanette Parkin, O.T.R., American Occupational Therapy Association; and Frank T. Rafferty, M.D., American Psychiatric Association. I also wish to thank my secretary, Glenna Clark, for her help in assembling the background information and for typing the manuscript.

tional advocacy for children sometimes succeeds and sometimes fails. In the latter event, the children's advocate may have to pursue other avenues.

In large professional organizations, such as the American Medical Association, one finds examples of both intraorganizational successes and failures. As an example of the former, one may point to the series of American Medical Association Workshops on Child Mental Health that led to publication of a series of handbooks on *The Physician and the Mental Health of the Child*. Much of the content of the handbooks is relevant to advocacy for chronically ill children. The second manual, *Assessing Development and Testing Disorders Within a Family Context* (Grossman and others, 1976), contains information on the emotional concomitants of physical illness along with helpful suggestions and guidelines for treatment. The workshops and the publications were the culmination of an advocacy process that had begun five years before with a presentation by one of its members to the American Medical Association Council on Mental Health. The council endorsed the idea that primary care physicians should be involved with developmental and emotional problems in children. With the support of the National Institute of Mental Health and the American Psychiatric Association, the first workshop was convened in 1976. This accomplishment offers clear evidence that one thoughtful and effective member can achieve the financial support and endorsement of an entire organization for a project benefiting children.

Contrast this to the 1922 censure by the American Medical Association House of Delegates of the Section of Pediatrics following its support of the Sheppard-Towner Act. As a result of that action, the leading pediatricians of the time founded the American Academy of Pediatrics as the national organization to speak on behalf of children.

In the American Academy of Pediatrics, as in other professional organizations concerned exclusively with children and adolescents, no one has to be convinced as to the special needs of chronically ill children. Indeed, one of the academy's ten National Child Goals, adopted in the late 1970s, states, "All children with chronic handicaps should be able to function at their optimal level. . . . Each of America's nine million handicapped children should live in a secure environment where he can reach his potential, partly through his own efforts. For that to be feasible, diagnostic services must be well developed and fully accessible. . . . Special effort should be made to reach children in isolated rural areas, in transient urban populations and in institutions" (American Academy of Pediatrics, 1980, p. 8). Because of the pre-eminence of the Academy of Pediatrics' advocacy of child health and its successes in affecting public policy, frequent reference is made to that organization throughout this chapter. The academy has been the professional organization most prominent in advocating for children with chronic illness; the American Psychiatric Association has held a similar position in relation to chronic mental illness in children.

The record shows, however, that much of the effective advocacy for chronically ill children has come from organizations for categorical chronic illnesses, such as the United Cerebral Palsy Association. Although health professionals have often participated in these organizations, the impetus has come mainly from parents or handicapped persons themselves.

Professional health organizations generally have more a generic than categorical interest; consequently, they usually do not initiate advocacy efforts in relation to a specific illness. Their roles have been more limited to (1) support for efforts initiated by national voluntary organizations, (2) statements defining the specific needs of children, and (3) attention to the role of the specific health professional in the proposed initiative. For example, professional health organizations did not formulate Public Law 94–142, the Education for All Handicapped Children Act of 1975; rather, their efforts have been directed toward participation by specific disciplines in the program.

Translating Organizational Goals into Public Policy

In recent years, many professional organizations have established Washington offices for legislative affairs to facilitate the translation of organizational goals into public policy. In 1970, for example, the American Academy of Pediatrics established an Office of Government Liaison to (1) provide advice to federal agencies responsible for the conduct of child health programs and to congressional committees considering child health issues, (2) keep the members abreast of developing legislative initiatives, (3) help the academy respond effectively to legislation that affects the health of children, and (4) gain recognition for the academy as the professional health organization with a primary interest in children. As is the case with many similar organizations, the academy has a Committee on Government Affairs that works closely with the Washington office.

The Washington legislative affairs offices of national professional organizations have a number of similar duties and responsibilities. Their monitoring role requires reading the *Congressional Record,* the *Federal Register,* legislative newsletters, congressional reports, press releases, and the publications of special interest groups. In their informational capacities, staff prepare commentaries, summaries, comparisons, analyses, and recommendations of various options relevant to proposed or existing federal initiatives. The legislative affairs staff of the American Academy of Pediatrics, for example, maintains background files and prepares commentaries on issues affecting the health and welfare of children, including legislation in which children are part of the target group. Amendments to H.R. 14181, the Arthritis Prevention, Treatment, and Rehabilitation Act of 1974, suggested by the academy were accompanied by the following justifications: (1) children are a major and often overlooked group of victims of arthritis, (2) the problems of the pediatric age group afflicted with arthritis have many specialized characteristics, and (3) medications approved for treatment of rheumatoid arthritis in adults are unavailable for children because of the lack of facilities to carry out the needed clinical trials. Similar statements were drafted in relation to diabetes and other chronic illnesses.

In addition to drafting or editing such communications, a major staff activity involves regular personal communication with congressional staff members, particularly those involved with child health matters, to discuss the organization's policies and concerns relevant to specific issues. For example, in its successful effort to achieve a maternal and child health block grant, key congressional staff members, kept fully informed of all activities, helped the academy staff draft a suitable proposal. In addition to staff contacts, another productive practice is to bring in experts for consultation with the appropriate committee's staff around specific legislation.

The legislative office is also responsible for the coordination, drafting, or editing of testimony to be given in the name of the organization. The stature of the staff of the legislative office must be such that they have ready access to those members of the organization best equipped to make authoritative and influential presentations. If inexperienced in congressional testimony, the member should be briefed on customary procedures and accompanied to the hearing by staff. During the past ten years, members of the Academy of Pediatrics have testified repeatedly in support of funds for maternal and child health and crippled children's programs and numerous other child health initiatives. Indeed, this record of support, established over a decade in hundreds of sessions, provided the credibility for the academy's successful advocacy of a Maternal and Child Health Agency and for the block grant that includes maternal and child health–crippled children's sevices, supplemental security income for disabled children, lead-based paint prevention, and hemophilia and genetic disease research.

To keep its committees and membership informed regarding legislative activities, the Academy of Pediatrics' Washington office sends a monthly Government Activities Report to members who request placement on their mailing list. Such legislative offices also have organized rapid communication systems to advise members to call, write, or wire key legislators on bills and issues to (1) oppose policies not in the best interest of children, (2) seek modification of policies that do not adequately address children's needs, and (3) support those that do. In such a legislative alert, each member is provided a brief background statement, the reason for the organization's position, and the name, address, and correct salutation of the senator and/or representative concerned. On the basis of this information, the member can easily send a personalized message. In addition to the general list, the office should be aware of close friends or acquaintances of congressmen among its membership. These personal contacts are of immense importance when critical votes are needed. All members should be encouraged to know and to communicate regularly with their legislators. The organization's Washington staff may help arrange meetings for members with congressional or agency staff.

In addition to reacting to public policy initiatives, the organization may initiate its own legislation; for example, drafting and lobbying for a separate maternal and child health block grant was beautifully and effectively orchestrated by the Washington office of the American Academy of Pediatrics (AAP). The chronology of that process illustrates how public policy can be constructively shaped by a professional health organization. State chapters were briefed and made contacts with their congressmen; the AAP worked in coalition with other interested groups; testimony was presented in Congress; the AAP leadership met with key members of Congress, congressional staff, and administration officials.

Following Passage of Legislation

It is important not only to communicate with legislators while legislation is pending but also to convey appreciation after its enactment. Recognition awards may be given by the organization to those legislators who render outstanding service to children with chronic illness or handicap. Some organizations have a political action committee, a potent force in policy formation. Others may wish to evaluate legislators periodically on their records of service to children.

Once a law has been enacted, professional organizations can do much to assist its implementation. For example, after the passage of P.L. 94–142, the American Academy of Pediatrics obtained a federal grant to educate pediatricians and other primary care physicians about the legislation and increase their knowledge of the diagnosis and management of developmental disabilities. This major enterprise involved sharing with state chapters information on plans for implementation of the act and suggesting ways in which pediatricians could effectively be involved. In 1979, the academy developed an in-service training curriculum to provide to more than 5,000 primary care physicians advanced training in the care of children with handicaps.

The Members

Although professional staff of an organization play a key role in the area of public policy, in the final analysis it is the commitment of the individual members to the needs of children with chronic illness or handicap that represents its greatest strength. Often, much can be done by a few. A professional who is a close friend of a congressman, a senator, or a staff member may be highly effective in influencing the introduction or support of legislation. The challenge is to tap the membership's tremendous potential to do much more, especially in relation to children with chronic illness or handicap.

In his remarks to a recent graduating class, Harvard president Derek Bok advised the graduates that in their lifetime, there would be no end of opportunities to improve organizations, to brighten the lives of those who work within them, and to do a better job of meeting society's needs. He expressed his conviction that progress is as likely to come from trying to improve individual communities, hospitals, and agencies as it is from a governmental grand design. Leadership in the future, Bok predicted, will pass to those who combine technical competence with an ability to relate their professions and organizations in more satisfying ways to all with whom they come in contact. Those who lead in the effort, he remarked, will have the satisfaction of helping to build more civilized, humane institutions, and those who succeed in building more humane institutions will find themselves in the forefront of building a better world.

This involvement can be fostered in a number of ways. Each member of the organization should have the opportunity, through manuals, workshops, and other means, to become knowledgeable about policy development and legislative action. In addition to education directed toward effective strategies for affecting public policy outside the organization, it would also be helpful to suggest ways in which individual members might advance a personal idea within the organization—for example, how the health of patients with chronic illness could be improved. Some members might be more involved if their participation were assisted and supported by how-to-do-it manuals or workshops.

Another, perhaps visionary, idea would be to have members pledge themselves to volunteer or "tithe" a certain number of hours per week to work on behalf of some aspect of child health, such as chronic illness, including legislative and public policy efforts. A highly successful effort used by the American Academy of Pediatrics to increase participation is an annual forum for state chapter chairmen. In these sessions, the state leaders are briefed about policy matters and asked for their reactions. Such experiences increase capacities of members for regional and national leadership positions.

Working with the Executive Branch

Advocacy in relation to the executive branch includes ongoing liaison with the principal staff in agencies of interest. The Washington office of an organization should maintain a file on those governmental offices concerned with programs affecting children with chronic illness. Each office has its target population, funding, regulations, and operational base. The file should contain information on the organizational structure of those offices, the principal staff members, and copies of the budget. Regular agency visits should be made by staff to discuss matters of mutual concern, especially issues of interest to the organization. Key agency staff should be invited to attend meetings of the professional organization and to serve as consultants to committees and task forces. The organization should also promote appointment of its members to advisory groups for governmental programs and agencies.

Public Image and Effectiveness

The effectiveness of a professional organization with members of Congress, agency staff, and the public is highly dependent on its public image. To be effective, the organization must be perceived as primarily interested in the welfare of children rather than the self-interest of its members. Some members of professional health organizations, however, believe that the primary role of the organization should be to better the status of its members. The only partisan political position suitable is to be for children, not for a specific political party.

The best chance for success of a legislative proposal is the legislators' belief that the action is in the public interest or at least not contrary to the general welfare.

Advocacy at the State Level

Much of the previous discussion is concerned with advocacy of national public policy. Ideally, a professional organization should have the capability to address child health issues on the community and state as well as the national level. Members can enlist support for and publicize the goals of the national organization in their own communities, counties, or states. In addition, state chairmen of organizations can bring to the gestation of national policy on child health problems a special community and regional perspective.

The advocacy of members in their own region may be facilitated by consultation from the organization's legislative office. Some national organizations have assigned full-time staff persons to provide such support to members at the state level. The importance of such consultation has been greatly increased by block grants that shift much of the policy action to the state government. State chapters are more effective in lobbying when their presentations are based on data concerning child health in their state. The national office may offer technical assistance for this purpose in the form of handbooks, workshops, and personal consultations. Some state chapters have found it helpful to have full- or part-time executive directors whose roles include legislative affairs. Training sessions offered by the national office could increase the effectiveness of these staff members.

Committees

Much of the work of an organization is conducted by standing committees and councils. Such groups generally include experts and generalists who have a special interest or investment in the field. If children with chronic illness or handicap have been identified within the organization as an important concern, there likely will be an appropriate standing committee; for example, the American Academy of Pediatrics has had a Committee on Children with Handicaps for many years. In addition to their expertise and interest, the committee members should, if possible, reflect a national geographic distribution. Offering committee positions to a cross-section of the membership is highly effective in increasing individual awareness of policy issues.

A special standing committee to attend to the interests of chronically ill and handicapped children is of great importance in developing a vigorous advocacy for this special population; however, other committees must also be engaged lest, as in much of society, attention to the needs of the handicapped and the chronically ill remain an isolated effort rather than an activity that permeates the organization. In this sense, most of the committees of a large organization like the American Academy of Pediatrics are relevant to the problems of the chronically ill or handicapped child; some pertinent committees are those on Governmental Affairs, Adolescence, Community Health Services, Drugs, the Fetus and Newborn, and Genetic and Environmental Hazards.

Such committees can work jointly toward development of public policy in relation to chronically ill and handicapped children through informal conversations, liaison members, correspondence, and preparation of joint statements. Another method utilized by the American Academy of Pediatrics is to develop a council, comprised of the chairmen of the various standing committees, to identify and pursue issues that have relevance for more than one committee.

Committees have many options for action. They can suggest new policies and programs for consideration by the governing board, such as a recommendation for an action concerning chronically ill and handicapped children. They can draft statements in response to issues posed within or beyond the organization. Committees can also become involved in fostering educational activities such as preparation and publication of manuals, technical bulletins, and films.

To support their work, committees need to be kept advised of relevant legislative and regulatory activities, actions required, and options. Attendance by a member of the Washington staff is especially productive at appropriate committee, council, and board meetings to provide a legislative and regulatory update, answer questions, and comment on agenda items.

Since committee members and chairpersons play a key role in the development of policy, careful attention must be given to their selection. Characteristics of an ideal chairperson include expertise; leadership; willingness to invest the time required; an acquaintance with other leaders in the field; an ability to communicate clearly; understanding of how the organization works; experience in a variety of community, state, and national organizations; the ability to see the large picture; and a record of outstanding achievement. All members should have a true interest in the work of the committee, a willingness to work, and the desire to make a significant contribution to the organization and its goals.

Professional Education

Fundamental to the development of an organizational advocacy position in relation to children with chronic illness or handicap is the informed and active participation of the members. Seminars, courses, conferences, workshops, or self-study packages are the building blocks of an informed constituency. Professionals at all levels should have more training to understand better the needs of children who are chronically ill or handicapped and the importance of the professional's advocacy role in the development of policy.

As mentioned earlier in this chapter, the American Academy of Pediatrics conducted an in-service training project for physicians to improve their understanding and care of handicapped children. The goal of the course was to change physicians' perceptions of handicapped children and their families and to increase their contact with educational and community resources.

Standard-Setting, Prevention, and Manpower

Professional organizations may also provide advocacy for children with chronic illness or handicap through the development and publication of standards and guidelines for care. Such publications, which commonly gain high visibility, may, in part, be incorporated into legislation or regulations. They also provide a measure for the development of quality assurance programs for individuals, agencies, institutions, and communities.

Although much of the advocacy for children with chronic illness or handicap has concentrated appropriately on early diagnosis, intervention, and treatment, prevention is attracting wider interest. Professional organizations can make considerable impact on public policy in relation to chronic illness and handicap by emphasizing the importance of accident prevention, nutrition, prenatal care, control of environmental hazards, early support for family crises, and the dangers of specific health hazards such as alcohol, rotary mowers, and riding in an automobile without safety restraints. The American Academy of Pediatrics has, for example, vigorously pursued a program to ensure the use of child safety restraints, and a large number of state chapters have sponsored or supported state legislation that mandates the use of child restraints. Almost all the other states have initiated comprehensive automobile safety education programs for the public.

Manpower needs represent another important area of public policy. Professional organizations have a major interest in such projections based on what they foresee as the future roles of their membership. The American Academy of Pediatrics, for example, responded to the final report of the Graduate Medical Education National Advisory Committee (GMENAC), appointed to project the national needs for medical manpower over the next decade, by pointing out the inadequacies of the study induced by speculation and compromise on the part of the GMENAC panel.

Liaison and Consortia

Although public policy may be affected by a single professional organization, the impact can be enhanced greatly by the support of other groups. Coalitions, alliances, and consortia in relation to the care of children with chronic illness and handicap are of paramount importance. The American Academy of Pediatrics, for example, recognized early that the influence of that organization on child health policies could be augmented by cooperation with other child health and welfare associations at community, state, and national levels. A policy was established by John L. Morse, the academy's second president: "The policy of the Academy (shall be) to create friendly relations with all professional and lay organizations that are interested in the health and protection of children" (American Academy of Pediatrics, 1980, p. 8). The American Academy of Pediatrics maintains liaison with more than 100 national organizations.

It is also important for key staff members to know each other, especially when their organizations have a mutual interest in specific legislative issues. In this regard, Washington staff members should, on invitation, attend relevant meetings of special interest groups. The Washington office is usually responsible for responding to inquiries from individuals, associations, and agencies regarding activities and policies of the organization or its committees. The staff also maintains contacts with the media, arranges press conferences, and prepares press releases.

Creation of a new Maternal and Child Health Administration in the Department of Health and Human Services to coordinate and strengthen federal Maternal and Child Health programs and reduce fragmentation and duplication of efforts has been a long-time goal of the Academy of Pediatrics. In 1981, the academy's efforts on behalf of this development were greatly helped by other groups interested in child health, including the Maternal and Child Health and Crippled Children's Services directors, the American Academy of Orthopedic Surgeons, the Junior Leagues, the Georgia Council on Maternal and Infant Care, the American College of Cardiology, the American Foundation for the Blind, and the Children's Defense Fund.

In addition to individual liaison members, some associations may develop joint task forces for specific purposes. For example, in the late 1970s, ten pediatric organizations formed a Task Force on Pediatric Education, whose report *The Future of Pediatric Education,* published in 1978, has had an important impact on pediatric education and contributed to advocacy for children with chronic illness. It identified handicapping conditions and chronic illness as important underdeveloped areas in pediatric education. A survey, commissioned by the task force, of 7,000 recent graduates of pediatric residencies revealed that more than half of the respondents believed they had been prepared insufficiently for involvement in child advocacy. The report (p. 24) concluded that pediatric residents "should be knowledgeable regarding community agencies, legislative processes and law which affect the health, education, and welfare of children."

Professional organizations can also advance public policy through collaboration with private foundations that have an interest in chronically ill or handicapped children and their families. For example, the American Dental Association in 1977 began a relationship with the National Foundation of Industry for the Handicapped to assist in providing a broader series of programs for the handicapped. Association and foundation staffs have worked to identify additional funding sources both at the national and state levels. Members of professional organizations may also promote the care of chronically ill and handicapped children through membership on the boards of relevant national, state, and community public and voluntary agencies.

The American Pediatric Society, the Society for Pediatric Research, and the Association of American Medical School Pediatric Department Chairmen have retained a part-time Washington representative to support child health policies that have implications for pediatric education or research.

Actions of academic organizations in relation to child health policy are determined by their councils and by the membership at the annual meetings. In recent years, the resolutions proposed and discussed have not been limited to academic affairs but have included public policy issues affecting children. This broadening of interest and concern has been especially true of the Ambulatory Pediatric Association.

The Ambulatory Pediatric Association has an active Public Policy Committee. Proposals submitted by this committee to the meeting in 1981 opposed the proposed reduction in funds for federal programs relating to the health of mothers, children, and adolescents; supported a maternal and child health block grant in preference to a single block grant; and endorsed the recommendations of the Select Panel for the Promotion of Child Health. Regarding Public Law 94–142, the Public Policy Committee recommended and the membership supported "a continued commitment to the education of all handicapped children as explicitly stated in P. L. 94–142; [and the] active participation of pediatricians at the federal, state, and local levels in the decision process affecting policies and programs for education of handicapped children" (Niederman, 1981, p. 9). In the area of prevention, the Public Policy Committee prepared a proposal on infant seat restraints and lead poisoning.

Passing resolutions at annual meetings probably has little real effectiveness beyond lobbying by individual members. In the president's report in the Newsletter of the Ambulatory Pediatric Association, Dr. Alvin H. Novack (1981) said, "One of the understandings our membership has achieved is that to pass resolutions often has no more effect than to inflate one's own ego. However, for a positive accomplishment of importance to children, it is critical that the APA develop a process which allows it to be effective in this arena. In this regard, I hope to call together an ad hoc group of APA members with 'political' experience at the national and state level to help the membership develop guidelines for organizing itself to pursue health goals for children. It is one thing to have a lobbyist in Washington or at the state level or to pass resolutions as I mentioned above, but it is another to organize oneself to be an effective force in the legislative process."

It is important that residents, especially pediatric house officers, have exposure to and familiarization with the importance of their participation as citizens and child health professionals in public policy and legislative initiatives that affect child health.

Public Education

In addition to development of advocacy among its members, professional organizations may seek to enlist the help of the general public by education directed to parents, children and adolescents, and other citizens through such public media as radio, television, and newspapers and by a speakers bureau. Organizations use different approaches in this effort. In 1978, the Academy of Pediatrics implemented a national child advocacy program entitled "Speak Up for Children!" as an action/awareness campaign "to cause consciousness-raising across the American community concerning the total health and welfare for all children" (American Academy of Pediatrics, 1981, p. 15). In 1979, the first year of the campaign, academy members made more than 500 appearances on radio and television to speak about the program's initiatives. In addition, individual chapters of the organization initiated public education programs, distributing television and radio spot announcements and public information materials and seeking to develop newspaper and magazine articles concerning the objectives of this advocacy effort. It is difficult to be sure about the effectiveness of such campaigns.

Deterrents

Although most of this discussion has been concerned with the promotion of advocacy by professional organizations for children with chronic illness, there are a number of major deterrents. First, the complexity of the problems, arrangements, and processes involved makes it difficult to build consensus with the pluralistic membership of a national organization and within the American community. In any organization, there is a risk that the efforts of a cadre of energetic, committed advocates may be counterbalanced by organizational apathy and the disinterest, passivity, or simple lack of involvement of other members. Some professionals sincerely believe that, in the performance of their daily work with children, they are doing their part or that the demands of academic medicine or practice are such that they have neither the time nor the energy to do more. Physicians often do not adequately appreciate the extent to which their status as professionals with special experience enables them to have influence with legislators and their staffs. Others believe that their individual efforts will not make a difference—a drop in the bucket. Many are uncomfortable because they are outside their area of expertise and lack the requisite background, facts, and sense of proper timing.

Gaining the advocacy of nonparticipators represents a major organizational challenge. The lack of involvement of many physicians with public policy for children with chronic illness or handicap may be due, in part, to the fact that the management of children with long-term problems is usually of a multi- or interdisciplinary character and medical services may not be the major component of care. Although there now seems to be an increased effort by many professional organizations to achieve greater involvement of their members at the community level, there frequently is no tradition for their involvement in formulating public policy. In addition, usually no public recognition is given for such effort. Because positive reinforcement seems to be an effective modifier of behavior, professional organizations must seek ways to provide greater recognition of contributions by individual members to gain their active participation. At the same time, it must be recognized that many physicians may be concerned that their public activities might be construed by their colleagues as self-aggrandizement. Finally, it would seem worthwhile for a study to be made of those members of a health discipline (for example, pediatricians) who have made a contribution to public policy for children to determine what contributed to such behavior, compared with a control group of nonparticipants. The findings of such a study might be useful in enlisting more individual involvement.

References

American Academy of Pediatrics. *An Agenda for America's Children.* Evanston, Ill: American Academy of Pediatrics, 1980.

American Academy of Pediatrics. *50 Years of Child Advocacy: American Academy of Pediatrics, 1930–1980.* Evanston, Ill.: American Academy of Pediatrics, 1981.

Grossman, H. J., and others (Eds.). *The Physician and the Mental Health of the Child.* Vol. 2: *Assessing Development and Treating Disorders Within a Family Context.* Chicago, Ill: American Medical Association, 1976.

Niederman, J. "Public Law 94-142." *Newsletter, Ambulatory Pediatric Association,* 1981, *16* (9).

Novack, A. H. "From the President." *Newsletter, Ambulatory Pediatric Association,* 1981, *16* (3).

Task Force on Pediatric Education. *The Future of Pediatric Education.* Evanston, Ill.: American Academy of Pediatrics, 1978.

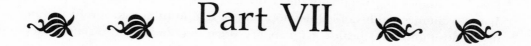

Part VII

Economic Considerations

In America, the system for financing health care for chronically ill children is a complex interaction of federal programs, state programs, and private insurance arrangements. Part Seven discusses the prevalence of disability, the use of services, and the major sources of payment for services.

The first chapter in this part reviews national expenditures for the care of chronically ill children. The authors are John A. Butler, Peter Budetti, Margaret A. McManus, Suzanne Stenmark, and Paul W. Newacheck. They state that there is no national data base to document the amounts and sources of private and public payment for care of children with specific illnesses. Extracting relevant facts from a complex assortment of existing data sources, they report estimates where possible and identify data needs. The chapter discusses the prevalence of disability, the use of services, and the major sources of financial support, both private and public, that help families pay for health care. Two themes recur throughout: (1) there is tremendous variation in both the amount of financial support and the pattern of support for children with differing conditions, for families in differing socioeconomic circumstances, and for similarly situated persons in different states, and (2) there are very serious gaps in private and public insurance coverage and in access to services for many families, especially those who are near-poor or poor but not eligible for Medicaid or Supplementary Security Income (SSI).

David S. Salkever, in Chapter Forty-one, presents selective observations on non-health-sector direct costs of childhood chronic illness. One important component of direct opportunity costs—parental time costs—is emphasized. Salkever reviews the empirical evidence relating to these costs and discusses various methods for computing the economic value of parental opportunity costs. In commenting on and extending the estimates of direct costs, Salkever provides additional data on the distribution of these costs by funding source. Other direct cost components, such as transportation, clothing, and other nonhealth goods and services, are presented. The chapter concludes with comments on future research and policy directions, recognizing a very basic problem—that the financial impact of children's handicaps upon their families is substantial.

In Chapter Forty-two, Karen H. Weeks correlates what is known about health insurance in general with the health care needs of chronically ill children. Weeks examines the historical development of nonprofit and for-profit private health insurance and health maintenance organizations, and the state policy initiatives that contribute to the diversified private health insurance system in the United States. Two critical issues are discussed: who is covered (access) and what services are covered (comprehensiveness). Citing advantages and disadvantages, Weeks explores which funding mechanism—fee-for-service or health maintenance organization—is most likely to meet the needs of chronically ill children. Weeks examines how well the funding of health care through private insurance meets the needs of chronically ill children and describes improvements in the system that merit consideration.

40

Health Care Expenditures for Children with Chronic Illnesses

John A. Butler, Ed.D.
Peter Budetti, M.D., J.D.
Margaret A. McManus, M.H.S.
Suzanne Stenmark, M.S.
Paul W. Newacheck, M.P.P.

For most children in the United States, expenditures on health care are minimal. The bulk of care is either routine and preventive in nature or the medical response to a largely predictable set of acute conditions, most often upper-respiratory infections and gastrointestinal upsets. Because most youngsters do not experience

Note: In preparing this paper, we received indispensable help from a number of federal and state agency personnel and university-based researchers. In particular, we wish to thank Vince Hutchins and Merle McPherson of the U.S. Office of Maternal and Child Health, Mary Grace Kovar of the National Center for Health Statistics, Clyde E. Shorey of the National March of Dimes Birth Defects Foundation, and Stanley Jones of the Blue Cross/Blue Shield Association's Washington office for their many useful comments and the data they provided. Special thanks also go to Suzanne Stoiber and others in the Office of the Assistant Secretary for Planning and Evaluation, U.S. Department of Health and Human Services. Thoughtful reviews of a preliminary draft were offered by Henry T. Ireys, James M. Perrin, and colleagues at the Vanderbilt Institute for Public Policy Studies. Louis Bartoshesky of Tufts University Medical School and Malcolm Holliday of the University of California at San Francisco provided valuable data and information. We also gratefully acknowledge the assistance of Barbara Johnson in typing this chapter.

serious or lasting illness, average yearly health expenditures for children not living in institutions were only $286.07 in 1978, less than half the expense for adults between nineteen and sixty-four years of age and barely one seventh the average expense of the elderly, sixty-five and over (Kovar and Meny, 1981).

These per capita figures can be misleading, however, because the distribution of expenditure across the child population is greatly skewed, with large health care expenditures concentrated on only a small proportion of children. Only 5.3 percent of persons under seventeen were hospitalized one or more times in 1978, a rate approximately one half to one third of that for other age groups, and this resulted in an average of only $102 per capita in hospital expenses (Kovar and Meny, 1981; National Center for Health Statistics, 1979). But those who were hospitalized spent an average of $1,920; the remaining 94.7 percent had no hospital expenditures at all.

Children with serious chronic illnesses or other disabilities are prominent among those with large health care expenditures. The child born with a major congenital anomaly can immediately incur enormous costs for corrective surgery, medical care, and attendant services, sometimes before leaving the maternity unit (Budetti and others, 1981). The child whose illness is prolonged or degenerative can anticipate frequent high-cost health care throughout an indefinite life span (Ireys, 1981a). Although the trajectory of cost and requisite expenditure is largely predictable once a condition has been correctly diagnosed, the financial burden of chronic disease and handicap is seldom adequately anticipated by parents, meaning that financial consequences from the standpoint of the family often are catastrophic.

Many chronic conditions among children conform to what is now understood as the typical profile of high-cost illness in the United States—a longitudinal pattern involving a series of treatments and hospital visits over an extended period of time rather than one medical emergency. Hence, it is not surprising that significant numbers of children are found among the 2 percent of the U.S. population that uses more than 60 percent of all hospital and institutional care resources each year (Zook, Moore, and Zeckhauser, 1981). Although catastrophic illness is less likely to affect children than older age groups, during the past decade, aggregate expenditures for the care of seriously ill children have been rising faster than for the care of adults and the aged; this is largely a result of improved medical care knowledge and technology (Trapnell and McFadden, 1977). In humanistic terms, this trend must be welcomed, but its financial implications remain problematic in a period of straitened family circumstances and fiscal austerity.

Because chronic disability is the high-cost sector of children's health care, one might expect that the financing of services in this realm would have been carefully documented for policy purposes and would have received ample attention in the health services research literature. As it turns out, however, patterns of private and public expenditure on the health care of chronically ill children (how much is paid, who pays, and for what kinds of services) remain poorly documented and understood. In particular, no national data base exists that would permit an understanding of specific child illnesses and family background characteristics as these relate to amounts and sources of private and public payment, either at a single point in time or over the life of the child. Instead, there exists a fragmentary and complex assortment of partial data sources, including elements of national interview surveys, Crippled Children's Services program reports, state Medicaid descriptions, hospital records, disease-oriented studies, and anecdotal materials. Such data enable only a partial analysis, even at the level of simple descriptive statistics.

Mindful that the data are limited, it is with considerable caution that we undertake to review national expenditures for the care of chronically ill children. Our intent is to extract relevant facts from a wide range of existing sources, to report estimates where generalizations can be supported, and to identify areas where information is not yet adequate or remains to be analyzed. This chapter is necessarily incomplete, but we hope it will serve as a starting point for those who would collect and analyze new data in the future. The topic is certain to remain timely for years to come.

To make our task more manageable, we have constrained the chapter's scope in several ways, each of which carries a major caveat. First, although much of what we present encompasses all chronic illness in childhood, special attention is given to the eleven conditions highlighted throughout the work of the Vanderbilt study: juvenile diabetes, the neuromuscular diseases, cystic fibrosis, spina bifida, sickle cell anemia, congenital heart disease, chronic kidney disease, thalassemia and hemophilia, leukemia, craniofacial birth defects, and asthma. These conditions are broadly representative of the full range of chronic illnesses, varying in prevalence, range of severity, cost of treatment, and periodicity of requisite medical care expenditure. As such, they are a valuable set of tracers to be used for financing comparisons. The caveat is simple: Wherever the discussion focuses on the eleven conditions, data are representative rather than comprehensive.

A second caveat concerns the scope of available information on financing. Many of the existing data are oriented to hospital care and physician services rather than health care broadly defined to include routine primary care and health and social support services for the child and family. As a reflection of this fact, more of the chapter is devoted to a review of medical care information than information relating to other elements of care. This should not obscure the fact that, for many families of chronically disabled children, expenses for disease-related medical care are not any more significant than many other forms of necessary expenditures. Moreover, services needed by the chronically disabled children include some that many families simply cannot afford and therefore go without, such as family counseling, mental health services, structural modifications in the home, respite care, and homemaker services. Failure to get these needed services may ultimately increase costs by leading to inappropriate episodic care, hospitalization, and institutionalization. This point is underlined in the recent report of the Select Panel for the Promotion of Child Health (1981). It is also important to remember that being the parent of a chronically disabled child can carry with it very significant indirect and opportunity costs, as pointed out by David Salkever in Chapter Forty-One.

This chapter then principally deals with the multiple sources of financial support that do exist to help families pay for much of the health care of a chronically disabled child. Private assistance comes mainly from various insurance plans, with extra help sometimes available from disease-specific foundations or other nonprofit organizations. A variety of public programs also offer elements of direct service, physician reimbursement, or cash assistance; and eligibility for certain major public programs such as Title XX Social Services or Food Stamps, which are not themselves directly related to the health care of chronically disabled children, can also contribute to child and family well-being. In this chapter, we have decided not to attempt a tour de force summation of all the relevant direct and indirect sources of financial support. Instead, we focus only on those sources offering the largest direct components of payment for health services. In the private sector, these include insurance plans and the major disease-oriented foundations; in the public sector, they include Medicaid, Title V Crippled Children's Services (CCS), and Supplemental Security Income (SSI) programs. The caveat with regard to financing is that these payment sources interact in important and often poorly understood ways with other elements of financial support—both formal and informal—making the true family economics of chronic disability a more complicated matter than program-by-program analysis might suggest. Were better household-based cost and expenditure data available, it would be possible and highly informative to counterbalance program and policy analysis with analysis based on the family's perspective.

An additional limitation is that much of the data is collected only for the noninstitutionalized civilian population. The health care needs of children living in long-term care facilities are not reflected by the national household surveys used in this chapter, particularly the Health Interview Survey. The number of children who are institutionalized because of chronic disabilities is small compared with those who reside in their communities, but the institutionalized ones include many of the most serious, hence most costly, cases. We are unable to compare the costs of institutionalization with costs of community care.

Notwithstanding these limitations in our analysis, we believe existing data enable certain generalizations with potentially significant policy implications. In the second section of this chapter, we review current information on prevalence of disability and use of services by disabled children as those matters relate to the analysis of expenditures. The third section offers an overview of total national expenditure for hospitalization and physician services and of the distribution of private and public insurance coverage for children with disabilities from families above and below poverty income. Following that, each of the major private and public sources of payment and their coverage provisions and limits on eligibility are considered. The chapter ends with a discussion of the policy implications raised by the financing and expenditure data collected in previous portions of the chapter.

Two themes, in particular, underlie much of what we have discovered, and they recur throughout the chapter. These are (1) there is a tremendous variation in both the amount of financial support and the pattern of support for children with differing conditions, for families in differing socioeconomic circumstances, and for similarly situated persons in different states and (2) there are very serious gaps in private and public insurance coverage and service access for many families, especially those who are near-poor or poor but not Medicaid or SSI eligible. Both themes give cause for concern in a period when eligibility and benefits in public programs are causing policy makers to be self-protective regarding the issue of "first-dollar-in." The Omnibus Budget Reconciliation Act of 1981 included a number of provisions designed to reduce federal spending for health care, to consolidate many categorical and formula grant programs, and to increase state authority over health programs. In the first year, reduction in funds for the new Maternal and Child Health Block Grant reflected a 25 percent cut over previous funding levels. In a recent report analyzing the impact of cuts in federal health programs affecting children, Budetti, Butler, and McManus (1982) conclude that the extensive federal funding reductions cannot be accommodated by eliminating excesses and will mean substantially less health care services for low-income children. If current trends continue, the financing of care for chronically ill children may become much more difficult in this decade. Reductions in public coverage and spending are likely to have three effects: increased out-of-pocket expenditures by parents, increased cross-subsidies from private sources to cover expenses of low-income patients, and reduced use of health care services in general.

Prevalence of Chronic Conditions and Use of Services

The prevalence of chronic illness among children and the utilization of services by the disabled are topics discussed in detail elsewhere in this volume. The following section is only a brief review of relevant facts in these two realms as they relate to the financing of care. The definition of chronic illness, scope of conditions included, and estimated numbers of disabled children all constitute important denominators in a discussion of the pattern and adequacy of national expenditure. Similar denominators are provided by relevant facts on use of services and assumptions regarding appropriate use.

Prevalence. Current data sources allow prevalence to be estimated in two ways—according to the epidemiology of specific conditions and according to limitations of activity or functional disability among chronically ill children. Neither is fully satisfactory, but in combination, they enable a fairly good composite picture of the extent and severity of chronic disability nationwide. Epidemiological estimates often suffer from being unreliable, especially with regard to high prevalence/low severity conditions such as mild developmental disabilities, but condition-specific data from numerous sources support the conclusion that only a relatively small portion of all chronically ill children— perhaps one third—have problems likely to require sustained and high-cost health care (Ireys, 1981a). These are the children most severely limited in their ability to perform major activities, such as attending school and playing. In other words, many children may suffer from chronic conditions such as asthma but may not necessarily be limited in their ability to function normally.

Of the total population of children, it is estimated that approximately 12 percent are affected by some physical or mental impairment. Such problems are of widely differing severity and etiology (U.S. Department of Education, 1980; Kakalik and others, 1974). Routinely included in prevalence estimates are physical, sensory, and health impairments along with the additional categories of mental retardation, emotional disturbance, speech impairment, and learning disability. These latter types of disability contribute substantially to the highest prevalence estimates. In contrast, serious physical disabilities involving major health impairment or loss of physical functioning affect approximately 4 percent of all children at any time (Ireys, 1981a; U.S. Department of Education, 1980; Kakalik and others, 1974). In these categories are children with serious chronic or degenerative illnesses, those who suffer from major orthopedic or sensory problems, and those who are multihandicapped. In Chapter Seven of this volume, S. L. Gortmaker estimates that fewer than 2 percent of children under twenty-one experience eleven major childhood chronic diseases including cystic fibrosis, spina bifida, leukemia, congenital heart disease, asthma, sickle cell anemia, chronic kidney disease, juvenile diabetes, muscular dystrophy, hemophilia, and cleft palate. A significant proportion of these children require substantial medical attention over long periods.

Household surveys such as the National Health Interview Survey are the principal source of data on limitations of activity among children. Questions on limitations of activity related to children include:

- Is _____ able to take part at all in ordinary play with other children?
- Is _____ limited in kinds of play because of health?
- Is _____ limited in the amount of play because of health?
- In terms of health, would _____ be able to go to school?
- Is (Would) _____ (be) limited in school attendance because of health?
- Is _____ limited in the kind or amount of other activities because of health?

Limitation of activity (LA) is an important indicator in financial analysis because of its clear relationship to use of medical services. The percentage of chronically ill children who have functional limitations severe enough to restrict their ability to play or to attend school varies among different conditions (Table 1). For example, about 6.4 percent of children with heart conditions are limited in their activities because of those conditions. Children with chronic illnesses such as arthritis, rheumatism, and diabetes report rates of activity limitation on the order of 22 to 25 percent.

Although the numbers remain relatively low, there has been a remarkable increase in the proportion of children with limitations of activity as reported by the National Center for Health Statistics (1979). Between 1967 and 1979, the

Table 1. Selected Chronic Conditions and Limitation of Activity.

Condition	Number of Conditions in Persons Less Than 17 Years of Age (1978)	Persons Limited in Activity Because of Specified Condition as Main Cause, Less Than 17 Years of Age	
		Number	Percentage
Arthritis and rheumatism	114,000	28,000	24.6
Heart conditions	752,000	48,000	6.4
Hypertension	119,000	–	–
Diabetes	88,000	21,000	23.9
Asthma	2,440,000	465,000	19.1
Impairments of back or spine	379,000	59,000	15.6
Impairments of lower extremity or hips	828,000	130,000	15.7
Visual impairments	694,000	49,000	7.1
Hearing impairments	958,000	93,000	9.7

Source: National Center for Health Statistics, 1978.

percentage of children with any degree of limitation nearly doubled, from 2.1 percent to 3.9 percent, and has remained fairly stable since. At the same time, the percentage seriously limited in function also increased proportionately, from 1.1 percent to 2.1 percent. During that twelve-year period, when the total child population of the United States was declining, the number of children with limitations of activity increased from 1.4 million to nearly 2.3 million and the number of children with severe degrees of functional limitation increased from 712,000 to 1.2 million. The reasons for these increases, or even the conditions demonstrating the largest increases, are not entirely clear as yet. Gortmaker (Chapter Seven) argues persuasively, however, that most of the change probably can be attributed to improved cohort survivorship. Incidence of various chronic conditions has been fairly stable during this period. Whatever the cause, as the number of children with activity limitations has increased, so has the cost of necessary services to this group.

Both condition-specific and activity limitation data show a clear and continuing pattern of disproportionate disability among low-income children. Although the estimates from available sources differ in magnitude, the pattern is similar. In 1977, children in families with incomes of less than $6,000 per year showed activity limitation rates approximately 40 percent higher than for other children (Newacheck and others, 1980).

Use of Services. Chronically disabled children require a wide variety of health and social services, ranging from hospital care to transportation. Besides the specialized medical care needed to treat each individual condition, preventive health, dental, psychosocial, and family support services also are needed to assure a child's satisfactory development. Use of services is the basis for the expenditure estimates in this chapter, but patterns and scope of use vary widely by type and severity of condition; hence, generalizations can be misleading. In addition, reliable data with which to analyze disabled children's use of health services are limited to specific medical services, principally hospital care and physician services. Little can be said about use of outpatient and psychosocial services, even though these often impose a substantial financial burden on the family and on various private and public funding sources. Because it focuses on medical care, the following discussion therefore underestimates disabled children's use of more comprehensive health and health-related services. Again, it is important to note that this section only covers use for noninstitutionalized children.

Looking first at short-stay hospital visits, it is apparent that children with chronic conditions, particularly those with limitations of activity, account for a greatly disproportionate share of the inpatient care for their age groups. The National Hospital Discharge Survey (U.S. Department of Health, Education, and Welfare, 1977) reported that in 1977, for all children younger than fifteen years of age, approximately 15.9 million days of hospital care were provided during approximately 3.8 million hospital stays (Table 2). Based upon those diagnoses always considered chronic according to the National Health Interview Survey, 36 percent of the total hospital days were provided to children with chronic condition diagnoses.

The eleven tracer conditions receiving special attention in the Vanderbilt study account for only 6.3 percent of total days of care and 4.6 percent of all admissions (U.S. Department of Health, Education and Welfare, 1977). These data suggest that much of the care for some children with chronic conditions is ambulatory.

By contrast, for children who are chronically ill and limited in activity, the amount of hospitalization required is significantly greater than for those with chronic conditions but no activity limitations and much greater than the average for all children. In 1979, although only 3.9 percent of noninstitutionalized children had limitations of activity, these children accounted for 18.8 percent of

Table 2. Number of Inpatient Discharges and Days in Inpatient Care for Chronically Ill Children Younger Than 15 Years, 1977.

Chronic Conditions	Number of Inpatient Discharges	Days of Inpatient Care
All International Classification of Diseases—A code conditions	3,755,000	15,866,000
All chronic conditions	1,313,000	5,732,000
Eleven specified conditions	172,000	996,000
All chronic conditions as a percent of all conditions	34.8%	36.1%
Eleven specified conditions as a percent of chronic conditions	13.1%	17.4%
Eleven specified conditions as a percent of all conditions	4.6%	6.3%

Source: U.S. Department of Health, Education, and Welfare, 1977.

all hospital discharges (excluding deliveries) and 30.2 percent of child hospital days for the noninstitutionalized population (National Center for Health Statistics, 1981). Average length of stay for children with limitations was twice that of their counterparts without limitations. Each one hundred children with activity limitations averaged 279 days in the hospital compared with only twenty-six days per one hundred children without limitations of activity, a tenfold increase. Even more striking is the amount of hospital care used by those with the most serious limitations, an average of 414 days per 100 such children.

At the extreme of this continuum, there are a few children whose limitations of activity are so severe that they must remain in permanent, long-term, or hospice residential care. Such children do not appear in estimates based on short-stay hospital data, and their precise numbers are hard to estimate. Children in long-term residential care primarily for medical reasons totaled 57,430 in 1976, according to the Survey of Institutionalized Persons (U.S. Bureau of Census, 1978). That figure is an underestimate because long-term residents of acute care hospitals, principally psychiatric ones, were not sampled. The children in nursing homes and other long-term care facilities were not numerous, but they tended to be severely afflicted—38,990 were totally dependent for personal care. Unfortunately, the amount and adequacy of health care received by these children is not well documented, but the amount is likely to be high for those who are severely disabled.

Turning next to ambulatory care for chronically disabled children as compared with others, the distribution of use is similar but not so dramatically skewed. In 1979, the 3.0 percent of children with limitations of activity accounted for 9.0 percent of physician visits. Those with activity limitations had more than twice as many physician visits apiece during the year as other children—9.5 visits per capita compared with 3.9 visits. As with hospitalization, physician visits increase with degree of limitation, and the group with the most severe limitations averaged 13.1 visits.

Although it is known that chronically disabled children use many services provided outside the medical care sector, it is much more difficult to get a clear picture of utilization in those domains. The related services provisions of Public Law 94–142, the Education for All Handicapped Children Act, are an especially significant new element in patterns of care. Public schools are now obligated to offer or assure the provision for various health and health-related services deemed prerequisite to a full and appropriate public education for all handicapped children. At present, approximately 4.03 million chronically disabled children have been identified by the public schools, of whom 169,000, or 4.2 percent, have been judged to need medical services. An additional 355,000, or 8.8 percent, are listed as requiring some other form of related services, including transportation, counseling, psychological services, occupational or physical therapy, social work, audiology, and parent counseling (U.S. Department of Education, 1980; Kakalik and others, 1974). Estimates of child need are based on state compliance data, which may or may not accurately reflect true need and often do not correspond closely to actual receipt of services.

Patterns of Health Care Expenditure

Economists distinguish between direct and indirect costs of illness. Only the first of these are reflected in most estimates of expenditure. As Rice (1967, p. 424) has suggested, direct costs "comprise the expenditures for prevention, detection, treatment, rehabilitation, research, training, and capital investment in medical facilities. In terms of services or types of medical expenditure, direct costs include amounts spent for hospital and nursing home care, physicians' and other medical professional services, drugs, medical supplies, research, training, and other non-personal services." The distribution of payment to meet such costs, by private and public sources and by age, income, region, and other consumer background characteristics, is the traditional focus of expenditure analysis. Expenditures for the treatment of chronically disabled children are the principal topic of this section and those that follow.

Indirect costs are of two kinds; economists term them resource transfer and resource loss (Harris, 1975). The first category includes income and other nonmedical transfers intended to mitigate the burdens of sickness. Income support under the Supplemental Security Income program for families of chronically disabled children or public expenditure necessary for compliance with civil rights legislation for the handicapped are examples of this type of indirect cost. The second category—resource loss—is less easy to define but includes the entire range of opportunity costs to society and the family associated with illness; this includes reductions in labor force participation, productivity, and life expectancy. Indirect costs of this type are analyzed by Salkever in Chapter Forty-one.

Total Expenditures for Care. Personal health care expenditures are for goods and services directly related to patient care. Expenditures in this category are total national health expenditures minus expenditures for research and construction, expenses for administering health insurance programs, and government public health activities. Total personal health care expenditures for children younger than eighteen years of age were approximately 19.875 billion dollars in 1978. Inflationary increases based on the medical care component of the Consumer Price Index would bring this to approximately 24.1 billion in 1980 dollars. Existing data do not enable the total to be partitioned among children with or without chronic disabilities, but some rough estimates can be made on the basis of the data on hospital and physician utilization cited earlier.

Estimated total and per child expenditures in 1980 for physician visits and hospitalization of children with activity limitations are presented in Table 3. Average costs of a visit or hospital day are based on 1977 data from the National Medical Care Expenditure Survey adjusted according to the medical care component of the Consumer Price Index. Estimates of total expenditures are conservative because the average cost of a physician visit or hospital day for a disabled child is very likely to be higher than for all children and highest of all for the most severely disabled.

Table 3. Total and Per-Child Expenditures for Physicians' Visits and Hospitalization of Children with and Without Activity Limitations: 1980.*

	All Children	No Limitation of Activity	With Limitation of Activity	With Severe Limitation of Activity
Physician Visits (average charge per contact with physician = $25.10)**				
Total expenditure (m = millions)	$6,053m	$5,509m	$544m	$407m
Per-child expenditure	$120.46	$98.44	$237.59	$330.00
Hospitalization (average charge per inpatient day for children = $183.20)**				
Total expenditure (m = millions)	$3,868m	$2,698m	$1,170m	$935m
Per-child expenditure	$66.39	$48.21	$510.51	$758.36

* Estimates based on 1979 utilization data from the Health Interview Survey, National Center for Health Statistics.

** Average charge based on 1977 cost estimates adjusted according to the medical care component of the Consumer Price Index for hospital room and board. For 1977 base rates, see Copper, J., and others. "Expenditures for Personal Health Services: Findings from the 1977 National Medical Care Expenditure Survey." Paper presented at the annual meeting of the American Public Health Association, Detroit, Michigan, October 21, 1980.

Estimated total expenditures for physician visits and hospitalization of children with activity limitations were in excess of $1.7 billion in 1980. Hospitalization alone for this group involved a total expenditure of approximately $1.170 billion, which may be compared with total hospital care costs of approximately $3.868 billion in the same year for all children. Per child expenditures for hospitalization show a predictable and strong relationship between levels of expense and severity of disability. Average annual hospital costs for children with activity limitation was $511 compared with only $66 for children without limitations.

Physician visits also represent a significant category of expenditure for disabled children. In 1980, an estimated $544 million was spent on such visits for children with activity limitations. This represents more than 10 percent of all child expenditures for physician visits that year, still disproportionate to the percentage of disabled children in the population but not to the same degree as expenditures for hospitalization. Those with the most severe limitations had the highest per child costs—the range was from $98 for those with no disabilities to $330 for those with the most severe problems.

These figures are rough estimates because they are based only on utilization rates not on actual measured expenditures. Because the Health Interview Survey excludes institutionalized children, no reasonable estimate can be made of the amount of physician and hospital care received by those children. A minimum estimate of the cost of institutionalization for the 38,990 totally dependent children is $413 million annually. Because that is based on average costs for all institutionalized children, not just the handicapped ones, it is clearly an underestimate (U.S. Bureau of the Census, 1978).

Whatever the precise dollar amounts, it is clear that the magnitude of spending for disabled children is substantial and a large share of spending for all children is concentrated on this group. Moreover, although medical expenses among most children are low or nonexistent, they are common and higher for children with disabilities.

Private and Public Insurance Coverage. How well can the families of disabled children meet the high expenses they incur? One way to estimate family impact is by examining variations in private and public insurance coverage. Data of this sort do not satisfy the desire to know how expenditures for individual children are partitioned across various sources—the situation of children with selected disabilities is discussed from this standpoint later. But insurance information does enable important generalizations about the sources of financial help families are able to draw upon because these differ among population subgroups.

Figure 1 shows 1979 patterns of insurance coverage for children according to poverty status and functional limitation. Childhood disability is defined in this model according to functional limitations identified by four relevant questions on the National Survey of Income and Education (SIE). In part because the SIE questions on limitation have slightly different wording, the percent of children in the activity limitation category is somewhat larger in this than the Health Interview Survey—5.5 rather than 3.9 percent.

Figure 1. 1979 Insurance Coverage for Affected Children
Aged Birth Through Eighteen.

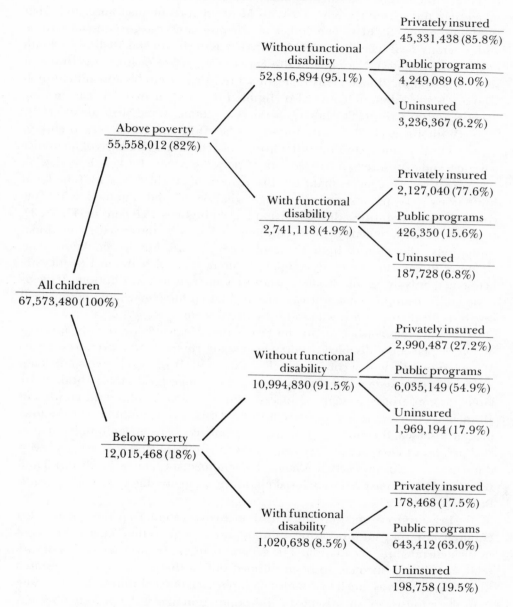

Source: Data derived from U.S. Department of Health and Human Services health financing model. For details, see Bonhag and others, 1981.

On the SIE questionnaire, respondents could indicate multiple sources of coverage. In creating mutually exclusive categories, all Medicaid eligibles were taken first; then, from the remainder, all Medicare, private insurance, and other public program eligibles. The "other public program" category includes those with veterans' health benefits, CHAMPUS (Civilian Health and Medical Program of the United States), National Health Service Corps, free or low-cost clinics, or some other public source. This represents a residual group because all children who are Medicaid eligible and also eligible for Supplemental Security Income benefits and/or Crippled Children's Services are found in the Medicaid category.

With these clarifications in mind, the ASPE model is very useful in showing how disabled children differ from other children in patterns of insurance coverage and exposure to the risk of out-of-pocket payment for health services.

One sobering fact is that fully 10.3 percent of all children with functional limitations have no insurance coverage whatsoever, and among low-income children with disabilities, the proportion is even higher—19.5 percent (Figure 1). It is not known whether these children are among those with functional limitations who require high levels of medical care, but we do know that, whatever the health care needs of these children, they are being met (if they are being met) only by out-of-pocket expenditures and private contributions. It seems reasonable to suppose that at least some of these children generate high medical care bills for their parents, who can least afford them.

Another somewhat surprising fact is that Medicaid covers only approximately 60 percent of disabled children below poverty level. Moreover, for parents of modest income with a chronically ill child, it clearly pays to live in some states and not others. State variations in Medicaid coverage for disabled children are large, ranging from coverage for 10.4 percent of disabled children in families of all incomes in Nevada to 51.2 percent in the District of Columbia. For the low-income disabled, the range is even greater, from 20.5 percent again in Nevada to 86.2 percent in New York. These variations in eligibility and coverage represent the situation prior to the 1981 Medicaid amendments. Changes in Medicaid and state fiscal strain have led to reduced eligibility in many states (National Health Policy Forum, 1981).

Private group and individual insurance covers about 60 percent of disabled children, a significant proportion although not as high as the 75 percent covered in the general child population. The general pattern of a two-tier system of care related to family income, so often pointed out in the health services research literature, applies as much to disabled children as to other children. That is, more than three fourths of the disabled child population above the poverty level has private insurance, with only 15.6 percent relying on public programs and 6.8 percent uninsured. But disabled children below poverty have virtually the opposite situation—nearly two thirds are public program beneficiaries, 17.5 percent have private insurance, and 19.5 percent are uninsured (Figure 1).

The ASPE model reveals patterns of coverage and gaps in eligibility but does not include scope of benefits as part of its matrix or give any sense of how expenditures by the various funding sources are distributed across conditions and types of care. These topics are of obvious importance because even the most generous private and public insurance plans often do not cover needed services or address the full range of disabilities. In the following section, we examine each of the major funding sources to determine in greater detail not only whom they serve but also the adequacy of the services they provide or for which they reimburse.

Sources of Payment

Information on financial support for the health care of chronically disabled children proves much harder to obtain for some funding sources than others. In particular, national data on private insurance payments and the collective activities of various philanthropic organizations are more difficult to come by than data on the Medicaid, Crippled Children's Services (CCS), and Supplemental Security Income (SSI) programs. This is largely because private support varies widely by state and region, and there exists little incentive for national data collection whereas federal programs must fulfill routine national reporting requirements. Furthermore, many states have programs focused on one disease or on a small group of diseases, and these programs are idiosyncratic to that one state. Information from these programs is particularly difficult to aggregate. Where empirical evidence is sparse, we have substituted analysis based on published descriptive materials.

In addition, the organization of this section—which discusses the major sources of support one at a time—tends to obscure the fact that many chronically disabled children receive third-party reimbursement or direct services from several sources at once. At the end of the section, we discuss condition-specific variations in patterns of payment for the care of children with selected disabilities to illustrate that although some children have no coverage, far more common are the complex problems of gaps and limits in service, discontinuities of program eligibility as children grow up or family income changes, and differences in the availability of coverage depending upon the disease.

Private Insurance. As we have seen in the previous section, approximately three-quarters of all American children are covered by some form of private insurance. The vast majority of these—some 68 percent of all children—are eligible for private insurance benefits under group plans, most often as the dependents of employed parents. The rest are covered under a wide range of individual and family plans. Blue Cross/Blue Shield and medical society plans cover approximately half of all families who are privately insured. The rest are covered by commercial insurance, except for a limited number—not more than 5 percent in 1981—who are members of health maintenance organizations (Health Insurance Institute, 1981b).

Private health insurance plans have widely differing scopes of benefits, cost sharing provisions, and premiums. Some cover almost all personal health services; others pay only a limited portion of hospital costs, leaving most expenditures to the family. Because most insurance plans are oriented to high-cost hospital inpatient care, they tend to cover only services that are medical or offered under the direction of a physician. Moreover, with the exception of HMO (Health Maintenance Organization) plans, they seldom contain incentives to use early preventive and primary care. This limitation has serious implications if we stop to consider that one of the major strategies for limiting children's disability is the timely use of family planning, prenatal care, and anticipatory guidance for new parents.

One way to analyze the adequacy of strictly medical coverage under various plans would be to compare claims data to information on child health needs for a national sample of disabled children who are privately insured. Such information is not presently available. In its absence, a next best approach is to review the scope of benefits under various types of plans, and make inferences about what these may imply for disabled children and their families.

In general, scope of benefits is better in large group plans than others because the burden of high-cost care for a few can be distributed across large numbers of subscribers. Survey data on new group health insurance policies written in 1980 reveal the following facts (Health Insurance Institute, 1981a):

> Of 333,212 employees in the 1980 survey, only 8 percent paid their full premium themselves. The rest either had the total cost of their group health insurance paid by an employer (35 percent) or else shared premiums costs with their employer, usually fifty-fifty (57 percent).
> Ninety-four percent had plans that included benefits for dependents.
> Almost half of those surveyed had comprehensive medical expense plans with maximum benefits of $100,000 or more.
> Sixty-five percent of those with major medical plans had out-of-pocket expense limits of $1,000 or less.
> Of the two-thirds of major medical plans with a single deductible, 80 percent had deductibles of less than $150.
> Most had copayment of 20 percent on selected aspects of care.
> Almost 50 percent had nursing home or extended care facility coverage— for 60 days or more in 94 percent of the cases and 120 days or more in 28 percent.
> Seventeen percent had home health coverage. In more than half of these cases, care included physician, nursing, and therapeutic services.

Maximum daily hospital room and board benefits under large group policies improved in the years from 1975 to 1980. In 1975, 38 percent of employees were covered for 120 days or more. By 1980, 58 percent were covered.

Although it is relatively easy to cast the best private plans in a good light, three major problems persist. The first has already been alluded to—inadequate incentives to preventive care. The second is that even the most generous plans usually do not cover custodial care for a disabled child or such essential services as rehabilitative therapy, prostheses, or social services including transportation and family counseling. In the ambiguous realm where custodial or psychosocial services overlap medical or health services, insurance companies are inclined to draw the line conservatively, reimbursing only those activities that are medical or physician-related. This tends to work to the detriment of families whose main expenditures are for long-term health maintenance of a disabled child.

A third major problem is that many families above poverty income with a disabled child do not, or cannot, participate in the more generous group plans. Exclusion may result from inadvertent choice of a less-than-adequate option by the parent, but more commonly, it results from one of several forms of refusal by insurers. Exclusion may take the form of a waiting period for coverage of a pre-existing condition, selective exclusion of reimbursements for services related to a particular condition, or additional high premiums.

The worst case scenarios involve parents who are working but in an occupation that precludes or otherwise fails to provide coverage under a group plan or are unemployed with family income above the Medicaid cutoff but too low to enable them to afford the high premiums for individual or family coverage. If such parents have a child requiring extensive medical services, and perhaps also a significant amount of custodial or psychological care, the financial consequences could be ruinous.

Pooling arrangements for the insurance of high-risk individuals have now been developed by several states. In North Dakota, Indiana, Minnesota, and Wisconsin, commercial and nonprofit insurers share risk for a pool of "uninsurables" up to a maximum cost. In recent years, state legislatures also have passed two types of model legislation that are of major significance for the coverage of disabled children. Forty-four states now have laws requiring that all group coverage policies provide for newborn care. This step was taken to preclude the insurance practice, previously common, of suspending coverage in the first fourteen days of life in order to make an independent determination about whether to insure the infant. This practice confronted the family with a "Catch 22" situation in which they were "fully" insured, yet still vulnerable to potentially catastrophic costs for neonatal intensive care. States still without such a law are Georgia, Iowa, Maryland, Michigan, North Dakota, and Rhode Island. Even in these states, most group policies now provide for neonatal care.

Thirty states also have passed laws stipulating that insurance plans cannot specifically exclude a chronically ill or handicapped child born to parents who are covered by a family plan. The state of Hawaii has gone farther than most other states in attempting to assure adequate health care coverage to all its citizens, although its law presently is being contested in the courts. The Hawaii Prepaid Health Act requires that all employers include specified comprehensive health benefits in their employee plans.

States also can mandate conversion privileges for the insurance of high-risk individuals. Even for those with group insurance coverage, the nature of movements in the labor market and the fact that most private insurance is employer-based make it likely that many Americans will undergo periods when they and their children have no coverage, or move from one plan to another with different benefit structures. If a family loses eligibility for employer-based group coverage, many plans allow individuals to continue coverage without reestablishing eligibility and with no waiting period, although it is often necessary to move to a more costly or restrictive plan.

In recent years, a number of companies have turned to self-insurance for their employees rather than provide standard coverage through Blue Cross, Blue Shield, and commercial carriers. Until recently, self-insurance had been limited to large and well-established firms whose benefit packages tended to be generous. But as computer technology and legal and financial incentives make it more attractive for smaller and less stable companies to self-insure, benefit structures may suffer. In particular, state laws requiring newborn coverage and automatic coverage of disabled children born to insured parents do not apply to the self-insured and increasingly could be circumvented.

The implications for disabled children of legislative proposals for new national health care financing policies based on "pro-competition" approaches are discussed in a staff paper prepared for the Vanderbilt project (Hauck, 1982). Here we only wish to point out that any procompetition model would require some consensus mechanism for establishing a floor on benefits. If the floor is low, this would make it harder than at present for families of disabled children to find adequate group packages or supplemental insurance at reasonable costs. In addition, because marketing strategies will not likely be targeted to families whose children have special health needs, it is not clear how choice among insurance options would be generated.

Another more limited proposal currently being discussed—removal of the provision that health insurance not be counted by employees as taxable income—also could result in more circumscribed employee plans. Both this approach and the other procompetition proposals would have to be designed carefully to avoid isolating families with predictably high medical care costs and making it more difficult and expensive for them to find adequate coverage.

Private Foundations. Associated with each of the major chronic disabilities among children are one or more private foundations or nonprofit voluntary organizations. Generally, these foundations focus on one condition or on a group of related conditions.

The size of the foundations and extent of their resources and influence vary greatly. Each has a different history and different financial base, sometimes originating with one or more major contributors, other times with broad support from a constituency of small contributors. There is no strong relationship between prevalence of a chronic condition and relative magnitude of foundation support. The Muscular Dystrophy Association, for example, spent $56 million on programs in 1979, while the American Kidney Fund expended only $1.5 million in that same year, despite higher prevalence of renal disease (Table 4). Consequently, children with certain disabilities have more resources available to them than others.

As part of the larger picture of health care financing for disabled children, foundation support generally does not constitute a large component of total national expenditure. By and large, the posture of the foundations is to see theirs as a unique role, promoting relevant biomedical research, increasing public awareness, and only assisting families directly as "insurers of the last resort." Although foundations expend a significant amount on direct services, they tend

Table 4. Total Amount and Percentage of Expenses Allocated for Programs of Selected Foundations, 1979 and 1980 (Dollars in Millions; Percentages in Parentheses).

Private Foundation	Total Program Services	Research	Medical Services and Patient Education	Professional Health Education and Training	Public Health Education	Community Services/ Advocacy
Muscular Dystrophy Association, 1979	$56.6 (100)	$18.0 (31.8)	$33.3 (58.8)	$2.0 (3.5)	$ 3.3 (5.8)	--
March of Dimes, 1980	49.9 (100)	10.2 (20.4)	7.6 (15.3)	5.4 (10.8)	13.0 (26.1)	$13.6 (27.3)
Cystic Fibrosis Foundation, 1980	11.1 (100)	1.7 (15.3)	4.2 (37.8)	3.6 (32.4)**	-- **	1.5 (13.5)
American Diabetes Association, 1980	9.7 (100)	1.7 (17.5)	2.7 (27.8)	1.2 (12.3)	2.4 (24.8)	1.7 (17.5)
Arthritis Foundation, 1980	6.0 (100)	2.9 (48.3)	*	1.4 (23.3)	0.9 (15.0)	0.8 (13.3)*
Leukemia Society of America, 1980	3.9 (100)	2.2 (56.4)	1.0 (25.6)	0.2 (5.1)	0.3 (7.7)	0.2 (5.1)
American Kidney Fund, 1979	1.5 (100)	37 k (2.5)	0.9 (60.0)	--	0.2 (13.3)	0.4 (26.6)
Easter Seal Society, 1979***	85.7 (100)	0.5 (0.6)	79.1 (92.3)	1.4 (1.6)	4.7 (5.5)	--

Source: Data collected from individual foundations by telephone interview.
*   The Arthritis Foundation combines patient and community services into one category.
** The Cystic Fibrosis Foundation combines public and professional information and education into one category.
-- No funding category.
*** Easter Seal Society includes the combined expenditures for the national and all state and territorial Easter Seal Societies.

to provide assistance to cover only those services that are not otherwise reimbursable and that place an unreasonable financial strain on families with disabled children. These services include transportation, educational and recreational activities, physical and occupational therapy, special medical equipment, and to a lesser extent, medical care.

Table 4 shows variations in program expenditure for eight of the major foundations, indicating that priorities and amounts expended differ substantially from one organization to the next. On average, these eight foundations devote 45 percent of their expenditures to medical services and patient education, 24 percent to research, and about 14 percent each to community services, public health education, and professional education and training. But the foundations vary greatly in their individual distributions of expenditures across these categories.

Little can be said from existing data about total numbers of children served collectively by private foundations, the extent of their coverage, or the ways in which foundation decisions about coverage interact with those of private insurance companies and public programs. It can be assumed, however, that a complex pattern of advocacy and negotiation takes place continually in most states on behalf of those children whose disability is represented by one of the major organizations. Foundation advocacy is one reason why many state legislatures have been persuaded to support and overmatch the national Crippled Children's Services program under Title V of the Social Security Act.

Medicaid. The main public financing programs for health care of chronically disabled children are Title XIX and Title V of the Social Security Act. Only a limited number of children with chronic conditions, those with end-stage renal disease, are eligible for Medicare. By far the largest public financing program in total dollar expenditures is Title XIX, the Medicaid program.

Medicaid is a joint federal-state program that reimburses providers for medical care benefits to low-income families. The largest group of children receiving Medicaid benefits are those whose families are eligible for cash assistance under the Aid to Families with Dependent Children (AFDC) Program. To qualify for AFDC, a family must include dependent children and one parent must be absent, incapacitated, or unemployed. If the family is in this category, state criteria for family income and financial resources are applied to determine eligibility. In general, these standards are very low and vary from state to state; in 1979, the state income eligibility cutoff for a family of four ranged from $140 per month in Texas to $525 in Oregon and $546 in Hawaii (Rowland and Gaus, 1981).

Disabled children in families that meet AFDC requirements but whose incomes are above the state cutoff may also receive Medicaid if their state has elected to cover the medically needy. In the twenty-eight states with such programs, families meeting the categorical requirements may subtract, or "spend down," their medical expenses from their total income and are eligible for Medicaid once the medical expenses reach a certain level (Table 5). Increasingly, however, states are eliminating or reducing their programs for the medically needy (National Health Policy Forum, 1981).

Table 5. Percent of Handicapped Children (Under 18) Below Poverty Who Are Eligible for or Receive Medicaid, by State: 1979.

20–29	30–39	40–49	50–59	60–69	70–79	80 +
North Dakota*	Nebraska*	Connecticut*	Colorado	Maine	Vermont*	New York*
Kentucky*	Kansas*	Wisconsin*	New Hampshire*	Rhode Island*	Massachusetts*	
Nevada	South Carolina	North Carolina*	Indiana	Pennsylvania*	New Jersey	
	Wyoming	Florida	Missouri	Ohio	Illinois*	
		Arkansas*	South Dakota	Michigan*	Hawaii*	
		Oklahoma*	Washington*	Minnesota*	Delaware	
		Texas	Oregon	Iowa	Washington, DC*	
		Montana*	Alaska	California*	West Virginia*	
		Idaho	Virginia*	Maryland*		
			Tennessee*	Georgia		
			Alabama	Mississippi		
			Louisiana*	New Mexico		
				Utah		

Source: ASPE Health Insurance Model.
* States with programs for the medically needy (28)

Another Medicaid option permits states to provide coverage to children in families that are financially eligible whether or not one parent is absent, disabled, or unemployed. In this case, only the child and not the adults in the family may receive Medicaid. Finally, children who are severely disabled and eligible for benefits under the Supplemental Security Income (SSI) program are frequently eligible for Medicaid. The SSI program is discussed later in this chapter.

Overall, Medicaid eligibility criteria exclude large numbers of poor children from coverage. Nationally, only approximately half of children under eighteen years of age living in families with incomes below federal poverty standards are eligible for Medicaid (Kovar and Meny, 1981). The situation is only somewhat better for disabled children below poverty, 60 percent of whom are eligible (Table 5).

One important ramification of the program's structure, which allows states substantial autonomy in determining eligibility and benefits, is great variation in the coverage of children who have the same economic status but live in different states (Table 5). The proportion of handicapped children below poverty who are covered by Medicaid varies from about 21 percent in Nevada, and 23 percent in Kentucky, to about 80 percent in Hawaii and 86 percent in New York. In thirty-three states and the District of Columbia, more than half of poor handicapped children receive Medicaid. In the remaining states, the majority of such children do not receive Medicaid, and Arizona has no Medicaid program at all.

Benefits under Medicaid are a combination of services required by federal law and those permitted at state option. All states must provide inpatient and outpatient hospital care, other laboratory and x-ray services, physician services, and early and periodic screening, diagnosis, and treatment (EPSDT) services for children up to age twenty-one. States are allowed to restrict the scope and duration of these basic services, however, and some do impose limits—such as Alabama's ceiling of twenty hospital days annually—that may have serious implications for the care of chronically disabled children.

Many of the optional services under Medicaid are also very important for children with chronic disabilities. In 1980, nearly all programs provided institutional services in intermediate care facilities for the mentally retarded (forty-eight states and the District of Columbia) and prescription drugs (forty-eight states), and the vast majority provided skilled nursing facility care for patients under twenty-one (forty-five states) and for prosthetic devices (forty-three states) (U.S. Department of Health and Human Services, 1979 and 1981). A significant number, however, do not provide eyeglasses (no coverage in seventeen states); physical therapy (no coverage in eighteen states); speech, hearing, and language disorder services (no coverage in twenty-two states); occupational therapy (no coverage in twenty-six states); and dental services (no coverage in twenty states). On average, states offer approximately seven out of ten major optional services relevant to chronically disabled children, but state variation is wide. Thus, Medicaid eligibility may mean that a large or small proportion of a disabled child's needs are met, depending on the characteristics of the state program.

In general, the Medicaid program has unquestionably made a very significant contribution to the care of disabled children by financing hospital, long-term care, and outpatient benefits not previously accessible. It has also served to free up CCS monies in most states. As Medicaid budgets face new fiscal limits and constraints, state and local officials will be hard pressed to see that benefits for those most in need do not erode in years to come and that inequities among state programs do not become further exacerbated.

Since the 1972 amendments, Medicare has become the major source of payments for all children and adults with end-stage renal disease, regardless of income. Only a small fraction of the 50,000 patients treated are children. Medicare payments for those less than nineteen years of age were $30 million in 1979 (Fisher, 1980).

Crippled Children's Services. At present, every state and territory operates a Crippled Children's Services (CCS) program supported by federal Title V funds and matching state and local monies. In the past, the CCS component of Title V formula grants to the states has been specified as part of the federal legislation and accompanying regulations, such that a fixed amount of the total Title V appropriation has been awarded to each state based on a formula taking into account a state's per capita income, rural population, and number of children under age twenty-one.

In 1979, $86 million of the total $377 million Title V appropriation was awarded to the states on this basis, with remaining federal Title V monies directed to state maternal and child health programs or used for research and training activities. In that year, the states for their part contributed a total of $194 million for Crippled Children's Services, bringing the total amount available to state CCS programs to $280 million (U.S. Department of Health, Education, and Welfare, 1980). CCS programs served well over a million disabled children in that year, offering a range of clinic, outpatient, and inpatient services through their own facilities as well as through various purchases of service arrangements. The programs plan and promote services and case management as well as reimbursing medical care providers.

Historically, the federal Title V legislation has never specified eligibility requirements for the program, although all states have rationed services in one way or another, usually imposing formal or informal eligibility criteria based on type and severity of condition and on family income. Now as part of the new eligibility standards for the program instituted in 1981, states are required to offer free care to children below poverty.

Considerable variation exists among states in numbers of children served, even when adjustments are made for differences in total size of child populations. For example, the New Jersey program treated 58,930 children in 1979 (2.7 percent of the total child population), California treated 102,827 (1.6 percent), Maine treated 2,096 (0.6 percent), and South Dakota 1,450 (0.7 percent). Differences of this magnitude in percentages served are not likely to be accounted for by variations in the prevalence of handicapping conditions. Rather, they may reflect the relative generosity of state effort—overmatching of federal funds, wider range of conditions eligible for treatment, and greater scope of services. Or, it may be that some states handled certain cases via CCS programs rather than via Medicaid or another funding source. Hence, it is difficult to infer anything about overall state commitment from these data alone.

Using the denominator of all children under twenty-one, state CCS programs in 1979 had average per capita expenditures that ranged from more than $14 in Nevada to a low of twenty-one cents in New York, with a mean of approximately $3.50. Of course, per capita expenditures for disabled children actually served were much higher, averaging approximately $250. Very few states can afford both broad eligibility and broad scope of services. Some states have opted for wider eligibility and more limited benefits; others have constrained eligibility but offer considerable depth of coverage.

Because the CCS program has evolved historically with wide state discretion for selecting conditions to be treated, each state has a unique service profile. The federal legislation mandated that the program serve children who were crippled or with conditions leading to crippling. Each state has discretion for determining the conditions it will serve. Figure 2 shows that states differ significantly in the conditions most commonly treated. For example, refractive errors are most often treated in the District of Columbia, accounting for 12.5 percent of all conditions seen. In Alabama, by contrast, infective and parasitic diseases are the most commonly treated (14.7 percent of all conditions).

Averaging across twenty-two CCS programs, the conditions most often treated in 1979, in rank order, were as follows: congenital malformation of the heart, acquired deformity of the leg, cerebral palsy, otitis media, epilepsy, all other hearing impairments, infective and parasitic disorders, and curvature of the spine (U.S. Department of Health and Human Services, 1979).

Data from the Bureau of Community Health Services (U.S. Department of Health and Human Services, 1979) and Ireys (1981b) show some similarities in the extent of CCS coverage for the eleven tracer conditions. For children with leukemia, diabetes, asthma, and sickle cell anemia, only about half of the states provide coverage. A majority of states, on the other hand, do provide coverage for hemophilia, muscular dystrophy, chronic renal disease, spina bifida, congenital heart disease, cystic fibrosis, and cleft palate.

States also vary in the comprehensiveness of the services they offer, as documented by Ireys (1981b) in a recent comparative national study. Ten conditions (sickle cell anemia is the only tracer condition not included) were investigated and ranked according to scope of coverage (Figure 2).

In 1980, the Cystic Fibrosis Foundation published a survey of state CCS programs that assessed the extent of coverage for this particular disease (Cystic Fibrosis Foundation, 1980). The survey shows that, although children with cystic fibrosis are eligible for CCS benefits in every jurisdiction except the District of Columbia, total and per capita expenditures vary widely, as do specific CCS services provided. Nationally, 2.2 percent of CCS program spending is for cystic fibrosis services, but states range from 0.1 percent to 33 percent. Average expenditure per enrolled child varies from a low of $111 in Colorado to a high

Figure 2. Extent of State CCS Program Coverage of Selected Conditions.

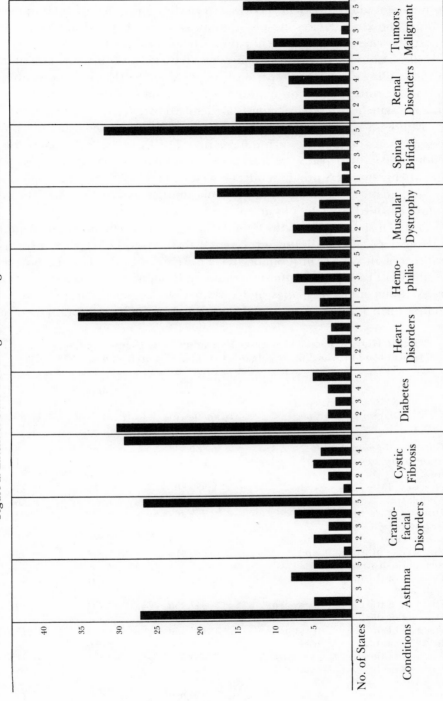

Note: 1 = No Coverage; 2 = Partial Coverage; 3 = Partial Coverage for All Cases; 4 = Full Coverage for Selected Cases; 5 = Full Coverage for All Cases.

Source: Unpublished data, Association of State and Territorial Health Officers, 1979.

of $3,698 in Rhode Island. More than three quarters of all states provided at least some inpatient and outpatient services and medication, inhalation equipment, laboratory and x-ray services, hospitalization, social work, physical therapy, and diagnostic services. Only 35 percent paid for home health services. With increasing fiscal constraints, one in four states has restricted CCS benefits to children with cystic fibrosis during the period from 1977 to 1980. This trend is almost certain to continue and to apply also to other commonly treated conditions as federal and state health service budgets are reduced over the next several years.

Although national CCS data are not available on expenditure by condition, some states do tabulate such information. Michigan, in particular, collects expenditure data that permit at least a rough estimate of per condition expenditure. Michigan's CCS program offers screening and diagnosis, registration for follow-up, financial assistance to low-income families, and care through certified hospitals, enrolled specialty physicians, and specialty clinics.

Table 6 shows that in 1979, more than 63,600 Michigan children under twenty-one registered for follow-up care. Of these cases, 12,541 were treated, at a total cost of almost $17 million, or $1,355 per child served. The data show that by far the most expensive diagnostic groups and conditions to treat are newborn illnesses. Congenital anomalies and certain diseases particular to newborns, including birth injuries, intracranial and spinal problems, cerebral palsy, and

Table 6. Highest Total and Average Expenditures by Diagnostic Groups for Medical Care Provided by Michigan's Crippled Children's Fund, 1978–1979.

Diagnostic Group	Total Expenditure	Average Expenditure Per Child	Rank
1. Congenital anomalies	$6,230,337	1,438	8
2. Certain diseases peculiar to newborn infants	3,010,631	6,811	1
3. Diseases of the nervous system	2,889,507	636	14
4. Neoplasms	1,082,295	1,804	6
5. Diseases of the blood and blood-forming organs	755,802	4,420	3
6. Injuries and adverse affects	714,963	1,765	7
7. Endocrine, nutritional, and metabolic diseases	689,416	1,258	9
8. Diseases of the musculoskeletal system	582,090	791	13
9. Diseases of the circulatory system	347,456	3,994	4
10. Diseases of the genitourinary system	324,190	6,491	2
11. Diseases of the respiratory system	143,580	603	15
12. Infective and parasitic diseases	85,966	1,000	10
13. Diseases of the digestive system	84,738	831	12
14. Diseases of the skin and sub-cutaneous tissue	53,656	2,236	5
15. Symptoms and ill-defined conditions	19,029	951	11

Source: Unpublished data, Michigan Crippled Children's Program.

other diseases, account for more than $9 million (54 percent of total expenditures). This finding is consistent with recent research on high-cost hospitalization (Schroeder, 1979) and with a recent study on the costs of neonatal care (Budetti and others, 1981).

Supplemental Security Income. Supplemental Security Income (SSI), a federal program of income support designed to replace state welfare programs for the aged, blind, and disabled, was passed by Congress in 1972 and implemented in 1974. Low-income handicapped children are eligible for cash assistance under the program, although legislative intent and subsequent enrollment policies in the states have been directed largely toward adults and the elderly (Rymer and others, 1979).

Lack of explicit reference to children in the legislation itself, combined with insufficient incentives for full state participation, may in part explain the low enrollment rates of those under eighteen (Breen, 1980). In February 1979, only 200,488 low-income disabled children were covered by SSI; this represented 5 percent of total program beneficiaries and a small fraction of those children theoretically eligible for the program according to the criteria of income and disability.

As in the case of Medicaid, the percent of potentially eligible children actually enrolled has varied widely across states, ranging from 7.4 percent in Wyoming to 57.8 percent in Illinois. Because the program is administered via the Social Security system, one rather mundane reason for variation has been the difference among states in the numbers of Social Security district offices. Also important as factors explaining state variations have been the availability of state supplementary funds, the relative generosity of Medicaid eligibility criteria, and benefit levels under AFDC. Children eligible for SSI often, although not in every state, are automatically eligible for Medicaid. Unlike AFDC and Medicaid, however, the federal SSI program has a uniform national income standard, and only disabled children themselves—not their families—must meet income eligibility criteria. The child's eligibility is also measured by severity of handicap, usually defined in terms of activity limitation. Section 209b of the SSI law allows states to impose eligibility standards that are more restrictive than those of the federal program if those standards were in effect on January 1, 1972. In a number of so-called 209b states, unless a child meets AFDC as well as SSI eligibility criteria, Medicaid is denied.

SSI children have a wide range of disabilities, only some of them principally health related. Mental retardation is the most often cited handicap (27.4 percent of enrolled children) (Rymer and others, 1979). The percentage of SSI children whose disabilities correspond to the tracer conditions of the Vanderbilt study are as follows:

Congenital anomalies	11.3%
Diseases of the musculoskeletal system and connective tissue	2.5%
Diseases of the blood	1.8%
Diseases of the genitourinary system	1.1%

Neoplasms	0.9%
Diseases of the circulatory system	0.8%
Endocrine, nutritional, and metabolic diseases	0.8%
Diseases of the respiratory system	0.6%

SSI benefits per child have been modest. In 1979, 67 percent of SSI children received a federal grant averaging $158, and 33 percent received both federal and state support, totaling an average of less than $225 per child.

In June 1977, SSI's responsibility for handicapped children was more clearly defined. Title XVI of the Social Security Act was amended to develop the Supplemental Security Income Disabled Children's Program (SSI/DCP), which provides state formula grants. The purpose of this program for blind and disabled children under sixteen is to provide a range of services not available from other programs, especially Medicaid and CCS, including counseling, development of individual service plans, referrals, and for those under seven, medical, social, developmental, and rehabilitative services. The total appropriation for 1980 was $30 million. The majority of SSI/DCP funds are used for equipment (for example, wheelchairs, hearing aids), respite and home care services, physical therapy, and medications. In most states, CCS programs have administered the SSI/DCP program.

This program has been consolidated under the Title V Maternal and Child Health Services Block Grant and no longer retains a separate identity. Some of the same purposes are served by monies under the block grant, although total federal dollars have been significantly reduced.

Condition-Specific Variations in Patterns of Support. Data on eligibility and scope of benefits under the major private and public financing sources do not reveal the patchwork of multiple sources that customarily contribute to payment of services for individual children. Data on selected disabilities are presented in this section to illustrate how complex this pattern can be. These data are exemplary rather than representative because no information base exists to permit national generalizations about how payment sources are partitioned for children with particular conditions.

Table 7 presents information on sources of payment from five major chronic condition centers—the University of Florida Kidney Center, the University of California at San Francisco (UCSF) Renal Center, the National Jewish Hospital Asthma Center, the UCSF Pediatric Malignancy Center, and the University of Oregon Spina Bifida Center. These data illustrate the number of sources that contribute to total payment, the special importance of certain payment sources for particular conditions, the major role played jointly by Medicaid, Medicare, and CCS programs, and the significant amount of out-of-pocket payments parents will incur. Unfortunately, the total number of cases seen at each center is relatively small. Even so, the data are useful in documenting the importance of various sources of payment alone and in combination.

In each of the chronic condition centers, four to six payment sources contribute to total treatment expenditure. These include private insurance, philanthropic support, research funds, Medicaid/Medicare, CCS, self-payment,

Table 7. Percent of Cases Covered by Various Sources at Selected Chronic Disease Centers.

Source of Payment	University of Florida Kidney Center	Condition and Condition-Specific Centers				
		UCSF Renal Center		National Jewish Hospital/Asthma Center	UCSF—Pediatric Malignancies (Radiation Oncology)	University of Oregon Spina Bifida
		dialysis	nondialysis			
Private Insurance	14.5	1.2 {	35.3	71	51.6	22.6
Self Pay	4.5			7	1.3	26.9
Medicaid (or Medi-Cal)	10.5	29.5	18.4	16	15.6	7.2
Medicare	42.4	26.5	14.7		2.6	
Medicare with Medi-Cal		21.2	16.7			
CCS	11.9	21.6	14.9		8.8	21.7
Philanthropy/Research				6		
Kaiser/Champus/Unknown	4.9				19.6	20.1
Other	11.2					1.4

Source: Data collected from individual service programs by telephone interview.

and other sources. For example, at the University of Florida Kidney Center, private insurance accounted for 14 percent of payment, Medicaid 10 percent, Medicare 42 percent, and CCS 12 percent. The UCSF Pediatric Malignancy Center received 51 percent from private insurance, 16 percent from Medicaid, 2 percent from Medicare, and 9 percent from CCS. Comparison of the four conditions according to how payments are partitioned across sources further shows that major payment sources differ by condition. For kidney diseases, the End Stage Renal Disease provisions of the Social Security Act are heavily relied on, making Medicare the largest payer, followed by private insurance and Medicaid. For spina bifida children seen at the University of Oregon, on the other hand, self-payment accounted for 27 percent of expenditure, followed by private insurance expenditure, CCS, and philanthropic contributions.

In comparison with the earlier review of national data from the ASPE model on differences in the distribution of insurance (for example, none, private, and public), the condition-specific examples reveal that differences in payment sources can be found not only according to family income but according to type of disability.

At a further level of detail, the partitioning of payment also differs along at least one additional dimension, the type of service provided. This is exemplified by 1971 to 1974 data from the University of Oregon categorizing cost, utilization, and percent of services paid from public and private sources for 121 cases of myelomeningocele (Table 8). The pattern of support for inpatient care was markedly different from that for outpatient care, allied health services, and social and related services. Another dimension—severity of condition—may also be critical because of variations in insurance payments as individual costs rise (U.S. Congressional Budget Office, 1981).

Both tables support the view that a significant burden of out-of-pocket expenditure remains for parents of chronically disabled children. At the five centers in Table 7, families paid anywhere from 1 to 27 percent of total costs, and that figure does not include supplemental amounts paid for outpatient care, medical equipment, and transportation. In the case of the Oregon children whose costs are documented in Table 8, families paid not only the balance of outpatient and social service costs, but also 10 percent of inpatient care.

The data again make clear the substantial role jointly played by Medicaid, Medicare, and CCS payments. The cumulative effect of simultaneous reductions in these programs over the coming several years could be very serious for children with disabling conditions. If these children are to continue to receive needed services, it seems likely that increased components of expenditures will have to come from self-payment and private philanthropic sources, along with various forms of cross-subsidy. One cross-subsidy at present for children with particular conditions, such as cancer, comes from biomedical research budgets. But such budgets are not likely to provide any meaningful substitute for reduced service dollars, and cross-subsidies from children with private insurance and resources may well increase.

Table 8. Cost and Percent of Services Covered by Various Sources, 1971-1974. Totals for Children with Myelomeningoceles (N = 121).

Payor	Inpatient		Outpatient Medical		Outpatient Allied Health		Social and Related		Total	
	Percent of Total	Dollars	Percent of Total	Dollars	Percent of Total	Dollars	Percent of Total	Dollars	Percent of Total	Dollars
CCS	21.2	191,612	21.9	86,541	10.0	39,520	4.6	9,287	21.8	326,960
Insurance	30.4	274,820	14.6	57,886	2.0	7,711	0.1	135	22.7	340,552
Public welfare	3.1	27,734	0.6	2,429	0.4	1,562	38.6	77,395	7.3	109,120
Kaiser (HMO)	1.6	14,915	1.6	6,371	0	0	0	0	1.4	21,286
Family and other	10.7	96,493	16.0	63,101	32.1	126,915	56.7	113,744	26.7	400,253
Charity*	33.0	298,908	0.8	3,171	0	13	0	0	20.1	302,092
Total		904,483		219,499		175,721		200,561		1,500,263
				Total = 395,220						

Source: David MacFarlane, M.D., Health Sciences Center, University of Oregon, 1976.
* Predominantly Shriner's Hospital for Crippled Children.

Policy Significance

Summary. Health care expenditures for children with chronic conditions have two major characteristics. First, the amount and pattern of financial support vary extensively with differing diseases, with socioeconomic status, and among states. Second, serious gaps and limits in private and public insurance coverage and service access affect the majority of families with chronically ill children, especially low-income families. In particular:

Approximately 12 percent of all children are affected by some physical or mental impairment. A small percent of chronically ill children have functional limitations severe enough to restrict their ability to attend school or to play.

Although the proportion of children limited in activity is relatively low, their numbers have nearly doubled in the last decade—from 1.4 million in 1967 to 2.3 million in 1979.

Data on the prevalence and severity of chronic conditions show that low-income children are disproportionately affected.

Children with chronic conditions, particularly those with functional disabilities, require much greater than average use of hospital and ambulatory care. In 1977, chronic conditions accounted for 36 percent of total hospital days for all children less than fifteen years of age in the United States. Similarly, children limited in activity had greatly increased use of hospitals and visited the doctor more than twice as much as other chronically ill children.

Reliable data on the use of outpatient services, mental health care, and other social services are unavailable, thus limiting any comprehensive analysis of health care expenditures.

In 1980, expenditures for physician visits and hospitalization of children with activity limitation totaled over $1.7 billion; 65 percent of these costs were for hospitalization. Children with the most severe limitations have the highest per-child costs—three times the national average for all children.

Some 10 percent of all children with functional limitations have *no* insurance coverage and almost 20 percent of low-income children with disabilities have no insurance.

The Medicaid program has made a significant contribution to the care of chronically ill children—financing hospitalization, long-term care, and outpatient benefits not previously available. However, Medicaid covers only 25 percent of the disabled child population and only about 60 percent of disabled children below poverty.

State variations in Medicaid eligibility and scope of coverage for disabled children are tremendous. Among low-income disabled children, the percent varies from 20.5 in Nevada to 86.2 in New York.

In thirty-seven states, the majority of poor handicapped children do not receive Medicaid, and Arizona has no Medicaid program at all. Private group and individual insurance covers about 60 percent of disabled children versus 75 percent covered in the general child population. A sharp contrast exists again for poor children: 86 percent of children above poverty and without functional limitations are privately insured versus 27 percent below poverty; 78 percent of those above poverty and with functional limitations are privately insured versus 17.5 percent below poverty.

The role of private foundations in financing care for disabled children is limited to serving as "insurers of last resort." Foundations vary not only in their size but also in their distributions of expenditures for research, medical services, professional education and training, public health education, and community services and advocacy.

On average, states offer approximately seven out of ten major optional services under Medicaid relevant to chronically ill children. Again, state variation is wide.

Crippled Children's Services programs served more than a million handicapped children in 1979, totalling some $275 million. Large variations exist among CCS programs in numbers of children served, generosity of state programs, and conditions eligible for treatment.

Few states collect data on expenditures by disease. Michigan, which does have such information, spends by far the most per child on the treatment of newborn illnesses.

The Supplemental Security Income (SSI) program has been another important federal program for the disabled population, although only 5 percent of the total program beneficiaries are children and the program has now been merged with the new Title V block grant and overall funding reduced.

The percent of SSI-eligible children enrolled has varied widely from 7.4 percent in Wyoming to 57.8 percent in Illinois. Benefits per child have been modest—67 percent received federal grants averaging $158.

To pay for the set of health and social services needed to care for chronically ill children, multiple sources plus extensive out-of-pocket payments are required. The combined effect of simultaneous reductions over the coming years could cause very significant increases in requirements for private expenditure.

The distribution of payments for care for chronically ill children across private, public, and out-of-pocket sources differs not only by income but also by condition, severity of condition, and type of services.

Conclusions. In the 1980s and 1990s, the profile of chronic illness and handicap will continue to change as will the nation's pattern of support. This evolving pattern is complex, with major legislative and funding reforms occurring as well as changes in the child population and reported increases in the prevalence of chronic illness. Determinants that may affect costs and expenditures include trends in the demography of children and epidemiology of childhood disorders; advances in preventive care (including primary prevention, such as prenatal care and genetic counseling, as well as secondary prevention via new screening activities); improvements in medical care technology, especially related to neonatal care, surgery, and other aspects of tertiary care; shifts in the structure of the delivery system, including changes in the balance of hospital-based to non-hospital-based care; effects of inflation on the costs of health care in general, especially medical care; and changes in the balance of public and private responsibility for care, and in particular, how this is affected by recent and anticipated public program cutbacks and other changes in public policy (for example, block grants, procompetition initiatives). Each of these factors is itself complex, making it difficult to fully predict what is implied for the care of children in the coming decade. It is also difficult to know with any precision how these factors will interact.

Hospital care costs probably will continue to present the most serious inflationary sector for health care for chronically disabled children, just as it will for other age groups. Incentives to take care of chronically disabled children outside the hospital are almost certain to increase, which may change the configuration of the delivery system such that more care is delivererd in marginally less expensive settings such as halfway homes, community facilities, or on an ambulatory basis. Already some children's hospitals would prefer to offer care on this basis for all but those most in need of continued medical supervision. But such efforts may be thwarted to some degree if third-party reimbursement patterns persist in paying principally for inpatient care rather than accepting an intermediate reimbursement rate for part-time hospital care that otherwise leaves the child at home or in another community setting.

In order to document the various trends we have mentioned speculatively here, there is a need for much more adequate national data on the changing profile of disability and the changing patterns in the financing of care. We firmly believe that, without a clearer understanding of costs and expenditures in this, the high-cost realm of children's care, the nation will be poorly served. In particular, household interview data seem essential—family-based data, preferably longitudinal, on a stratified sample of disabled children and their parents, with additional research to develop an adequate and reliable picture of the families' financial support as this is distributed across various private and public sources and as it meets or fails to meet the fully costed care of the disabled child.

Policy Implications. One of the major new influences on health care expenditures for chronically ill children is the Omnibus Budget Reconciliation Act of 1981. Three major components of this act have adversely affected handicapped children.

1.   The new Title V block grant legislation incorporates an across-the-board cutback of at least 25 percent in total federal dollar commitment to the entire national Maternal and Child Health and Crippled Children's programs. It seems unlikely that states will make up the difference in lost revenues and equally unlikely that medical care costs will not increase at a faster rate than federal appropriations over the coming years. This suggests that services may have to be curtailed.
2.   The new legislation also departs from the long-standing stipulation that an established proportion of Title V awards to the states must be earmarked for Crippled Children's Services. Monies now will be fungible across MCH and CCS services and the other programs included in the block. It remains uncertain how well CCS programs at the state level will be able to retain their traditional separate identity or compete successfully for their previous component of Title V funds.
3.   The joint effects of cutbacks in Title XIX and Title V may be interactive for low-income disabled children, who stand to lose both optional service

benefits under Medicaid and Crippled Children's Services benefits. It remains to be seen whether private foundations and other sources will be able to make up the difference in reduced services, or whether out-of-pocket costs for families will increase even further. Increasing discussion of the New Federalism suggests that the role of the states is also likely to grow in the coming several years. The implications for disabled children of such a shift in the locus of governance for public programs remain unanalyzed.

It is particularly important, we believe, to gain a clear understanding as soon as possible of the impact of recently mandated cutbacks in federal program support via Medicaid, Title V, and related programs. In relevant sections of this chapter, we have suggested that the joint impact of various federal cutbacks is likely to have three effects: (1) to reduce eligibility and scope of services for children, (2) to redistribute the balance of expenditures from public to private sources, including insurance, philanthropic contributions, and out-of-pocket payment, and (3) to increase the cross-subsidies that already support a significant component of care for the chronically disabled via group insurance premiums, Medicaid hospital reimbursement rates, research budgets, and so forth. Reduced public expenditure would require at least one of these outcomes, and the real issue is which of them will predominate as private and public expenditure patterns for care re-equilibrate in the coming decade. From the standpoint of the children themselves and their families, absolute reduction in program eligibility and financially accessible services clearly would be the worst outcome.

References

Bonhag, R. C., and others. *A Description of the Health Financing Model: A Tool for Cost Estimation.* Washington, D.C.: Department of Health and Human Services, Office of the Assistant Secretary for Planning and Evaluation, 1981.

Breen, P. "Participation of Disabled Children in the Supplemental Security Income Program." Chapel Hill, N.C.: Bush Institute for Child and Family Policy, 1980.

Budetti, P., Butler, J., and McManus, P. "Federal Health Programs Reforms and Proposals: Implications for Child Health Care." *Milbank Memorial Fund Quarterly,* 1982, *60* (1), 155–181.

Budetti, P., and others. "The Costs and Effectiveness of Neonatal Intensive Care." In *The Implications of Cost Effectiveness Analysis of Medical Technology.* Washington, D.C.: Congress of the United States, Office of Technology Assessment, 1981.

Cystic Fibrosis Foundation. *1980 Survey of State Crippled Children's Services Programs for Children with Cystic Fibrosis.* Rockville, Md.: Cystic Fibrosis Foundation, 1980.

Fisher, C. R. "Differences by Age Groups in Health Care Spending." *Health Care Financing Review,* 1980, *1* (4), 65–90.

Harris, S. E. *The Economics of Health Care: Finance and Delivery.* Berkeley, Calif.: McCutchan, 1975.

Hauck, R. J-P. "The Competitive Model: Problems in Achieving Cost Control and Equity." Paper prepared for Vanderbilt project, Public Policies Affecting Chronically Ill Children and Their Families. Nashville, Tenn.: Vanderbilt University, 1981.

Health Insurance Institute. *New Group Health Insurance.* Washington, D.C.: Health Insurance Association of America, 1981a.

Health Insurance Institute. *1980–81 Source Book of Health Insurance Data.* Washington, D.C.: Health Insurance Association of America, 1981b.

Ireys, H. T. "Health Care for Chronically Disabled Children and Their Families." In Select Panel for the Promotion of Child Health, *Better Health for Our Children: A National Strategy.* Vol. 4: *Background Papers.* Department of Health and Human Services publication no. 79-55071. Washington, D.C.: U.S. Government Printing Office, 1981a.

Ireys, H. T. Unpublished data on coverage of selected chronic conditions. Vanderbilt University, Nashville, Tenn., 1981b.

Kakalik, J. S., and others. *Improving Services to Handicapped Children.* Santa Monica, Calif.: Rand Corporation, 1974.

Kovar, M. G., and Meny, D. *Better Health for Our Children: A National Strategy.* Vol. 3: *A Statistical Profile.* Washington, D.C.: U.S. Government Printing Office, 1981.

National Center for Health Statistics. *Current Estimates from the Health Interview Survey, 1978.* Series no. 130. Hyattsville, Md.: National Center for Health Statistics, 1979.

National Center for Health Statistics. "Selected Chronic Conditions and Limitations of Activity." Special Tabulations (unpublished data), 1978 Health Interview Survey.

National Center for Health Statistics. Unpublished data from the National Health Interview Survey. Washington, D.C., 1981.

National Health Policy Forum. "Intergovernmental Health Policy Project." *Recent and Proposed Changes in State Medicaid Programs: A Fifty-State Survey.* Washington, D.C.: National Health Policy Forum, 1981.

Newacheck, P., and others. "Income and Illness." *Medical Care,* 1980, *18* (12), 1165–1176.

Rice, D. "Estimating the Cost of Illness." *American Journal of Public Health,* 1967, *57* (3), 424–440.

Rowland, D., and Gaus, C. "Medicaid Eligibility and Benefits: Current Policies and Future Choices." Paper presented at the 1981 Commonwealth Fund Forum, Lake Bluff, Ill. Washington, D.C.: Center for Health Policy Studies, Georgetown University.

Rymer, M., and others. *Survey of Blind and Disabled Children Receiving Supplemental Security Income Benefits.* Cambridge, Mass.: Urban Systems Research and Engineering, 1979.

Schroeder, S. A., and others. "Frequency and Clinical Descriptions of High Cost Patients in 17 Acute Care Hospitals." *New England Journal of Medicine,* 1979, *300* (23), 1306–1309.

Select Panel for the Promotion of Child Health. *Better Health for Our Children: A National Strategy.* Department of Health and Human Services publication no. 79-55071. Washington, D.C.: U.S. Government Printing Office, 1981.

Trapnell, G., and McFadden, F. "The Rising Cost of Catastrophic Illness." Falls Church, Va.: Actuarial Research Corporation, 1977.

U.S. Bureau of the Census. "1976 Survey of Institutionalized Persons: A Study of Persons Receiving Long-Term Care." *Current Population Reports—Special Studies,* No. 69. Series P-23. Washington, D.C.: U.S. Government Printing Office, 1978.

U.S. Congressional Budget Office. "Protection from Catastrophic Medical Expenses: The Effects of Limiting Family Liability Under Existing Employee Insurance Programs." Staff working paper. Washington, D.C.: U.S. Congressional Budget Office, 1981.

U.S. Department of Education. *Second Annual Report to Congress on the Implementation of Public Law 94–142: The Education for All Handicapped Children Act.* Washington, D.C.: U.S. Office of Special Education and Rehabilitative Services, 1980.

U.S. Department of Health, Education, and Welfare. *Detailed Surgical Procedures for Patients Discharged from Short-Stay Hospitals, United States, 1977.* Washington, D.C.: U.S. Government Printing Office, 1977.

U.S. Department of Health and Human Services, Bureau of Community Health Services. Unpublished data on Crippled Children's Services, 1979.

U.S. Department of Health and Human Services. "Comprehensive NPHPRS Report: Services, Expenditures and Programs of State and Territorial Health Agencies, FY 1979." Washington, D.C.: U.S. Department of Health and Human Services, 1980.

U.S. Department of Health and Human Services. *Data on the Medicaid Program: Eligibility/Services/Expenditures.* Baltimore, Md.: Health Care Financing Administration, 1979 and 1981. Unpublished updated figures.

Zook, C., Moore, F., and Zeckhauser, R. " 'Catastrophic' Health Insurance: A Misguided Prescription?" *The Public Interest,* 1981, No. 62, pp. 66–81.

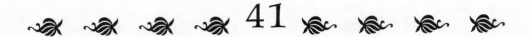

41

Parental Opportunity Costs
and Other Economic Costs
of Children's Disabling Conditions

David S. Salkever, Ph.D.

With the growing prominence of economic concerns in health policy discussions, costs of health problems are receiving more attention. Estimates of economic costs may guide policy formulation (Rice, Feldman, and White, 1976), and expert assessments of policies for confronting major health problems now routinely include consideration of cost estimates (Commission for the Control of Epilepsy and Its Consequences, n.d.; *Report to the President from the President's Commission on Mental Health*, 1978). The importance of the issue has been highlighted by the work of the U.S. Public Health Service (USPHS) Task Force on the Cost of Illness, which is specifically concerned with the use of cost estimates in policy and program evaluation (Hodgson and Meiners, 1982), and by federal funding of several new efforts to synthesize and refine cost estimation methods (Salkever, 1984; Policy Analysis, 1981).

Several different interpretations of cost estimates for policy making have been suggested in the literature. In an early and major work by Weisbrod (1961), these estimates are used as measures of the benefits from preventing the occurrence of health problems. These benefits can be compared with the expected costs of implementing a prevention program, as well as with the costs of the research required to develop more effective prevention methods (such as new vaccines). These benefit-cost calculations can also be used retrospectively to quantify the rate of return on past investments in prevention (Weisbrod, 1971; Mushkin, 1979). Alternatively, economic cost estimates may be viewed not as precise quantitative measures of benefits from specific programs but rather as broad indicators of the economic importance of particular health problems. From this view, economic costs are useful in making decisions about the allocation, across classes of health problems, of funds for basic research, for testing new treatment or prevention techniques, and for developing new modes of organizing medical and support services (Hartunian, Smart, and Thompson, 1980).

Although economic cost estimates have, in fact, been invoked in many discussions of health policy and funding priorities, the systematic use of estimates has been hindered by wide variations in the methods employed in cost studies. The most fundamental variation concerns the definition of costs. Typically, two categories of cost are identified: direct and indirect. Direct costs measure the value of resources used for diagnosis, treatment, rehabilitation, and continuing care. Some researchers have defined the scope of these costs narrowly, including only hospital and physician care or only the costs occurring within the health sector as defined in the official federal estimates of health expenditures (Gibson, 1980). As Scitovsky (1982) has noted, these definitions exclude such non-health-sector items as "cost of transportation to and from providers, special diets, extra household help to care for sick family members, retraining and reeducation, alterations to housing to accommodate invalids . . . and counseling services to both the sick and their families" (p. 473). The relative importance of these exclusions can be gauged with data recently prepared by Mushkin (1979) and her associates. Their estimate of $29.2 to $37.8 billion in non-health-sector costs of illness for the United States in 1975 included $3.9 to $4.3 billion in consumer outlays (for example, for transportation and for property damage due to alcohol and drug abuse), $8.0 to $14.5 billion in government costs of many types ("ranging from extra school costs to added cost of waste disposal processes to anti-trust and insurance commission enforcement" [p. 385]), $4.5 to $6.2 billion in time costs for obtaining health care, and $12.8 billion in costs borne by industry (not specified). Comparing these figures with the $118.5 billion in direct health sector expenses, we see that omission of non-health-sector direct costs from most studies is a potentially serious limitation. Furthermore, differing valuation or estimation procedures can produce highly disparate cost figures within each category of direct cost included in the analyses.

Indirect costs measure the losses in the productivity of individuals due to health problems. These losses relate to (1) the permanent inability of illness victims to work because of premature death or long-term disability, (2) temporary inability to work because of short-term disability and absenteeism, and (3) the reduced productivity of persons who continue to work because of short-term or long-term disability. (The last item is sometimes referred to as debility costs.) Although there is not as much variability in the literature in methods of measuring these costs as is true for direct costs, significant problems remain. For example, debility costs are almost always excluded from cost estimates. The first two types of costs have also been overlooked for all forms of nonmarket work except housekeeping (or "housewife") services. The latter item has been valued in various ways (because earnings or wage figures are obviously not available for nonmarket work) and here again differing methods produce different results (Brody, 1975; Hawrylyshyn, 1976).

Besides employing differing definitions and valuation methods for direct and indirect costs, economic cost studies display other methodological variations (Hu and Sandifer, 1981). Examples are the use of differing discount rates for combining present and future costs and the use of prevalence- versus incidence-based approaches to computing costs. (The incidence approach estimates costs for all cases of an illness beginning within a specified time period; the prevalence approach estimates all costs occurring within a given time period plus the discounted future indirect costs of deaths occurring during this time period [Hartunian, Smart, and Thompson, 1980].) A principal objective of the USPHS Task Force was to avoid further confusion and noncomparability between studies by promulgating guidelines concerning the minimal ("core") elements of cost to be included in all studies, the valuation procedures to be employed, and the range of discount rates to be considered (Hodgson and Meiners, 1982).

Several methodological issues are particularly important for any assessment of the economic costs of children's health problems or, more specifically, of children's handicapping conditions. First, non-health-sector direct costs may be large in both absolute and relative terms. For instance, especially since the passage of Public Law 94–142, a large segment of costs, more than $10 billion in fiscal year 1981, is incurred in the educational sector (Kakalik and others, 1981). Costs borne by parents in the form of additional time spent in childcare, home therapy, and visits to a variety of medical and nonmedical service providers may also be substantial. Second, the demands of caring for a seriously disabled child may also contribute to the occurrence of physical or mental health problems among other family members (Breslau, Staruch, and Gortmaker, 1980). One could reasonably argue that the economic costs generated by these problems should also be included in the cost estimates. Third, the time stream of direct costs generated by these health problems may extend over a long period of time (that is, into adulthood), and much of these costs may relate directly to other health problems that are in fact the result (or partially the result) of the original handicapping condition. Finally, it should be noted that research to date on the economic aspects of children's handicapping conditions has been limited. Thus, an overall assessment of costs must be preliminary, speculative, and incomplete.

Rather than attempt a comprehensive and detailed review, this chapter offers a wide range of selective observations with particular emphasis on one important component of direct opportunity costs, namely parental time costs. We begin with a review of empirical evidence relating to these costs, which is drawn from most of the major studies. We then comment on and extend the estimates of direct health sector costs and report additional data on the distribution of these costs by funding source. A brief review of information on other direct cost components follows, and we conclude with comments on future research and policy directions.

The reader should note that virtually all the empirical data we review pertain to children with reported disabilities due to chronic conditions. As is explained in more detail in Chapter Forty of this volume, many children with chronic conditions that entail substantial economic costs are *not* included in the data because they do not report disabilities (that is, limitations in ability to engage in play and/or school activities).

Parental Opportunity Cost as a Component of Direct Costs

Daily care for a child with a handicapping condition is clearly more demanding and time consuming than care for a child who is free of handicaps. If care is provided by a paid health professional or institutional provider, it will (one hopes) be included in any estimate of direct health costs. If provided by family members, however, it falls outside the scope of direct health costs; instead, it is paid for through reduced time spent by family members in other activities.

Two strategies are conceivable for estimating the costs of this additional care. If detailed data on the time spent by other family members in care-related activities (such as home therapy, visits to health professionals, and assistance with activities of daily living) were available, and if benchmark data on time spent by other families in caring for children without handicaps were also available, we could compare the total childcare time with this benchmark to measure the extra care time required as a result of the child's handicap. For employed family members, the dollar value of this additional time could be computed based on the family members' wage rates. For nonemployed family members, a "shadow price" per time unit would have to be estimated and multiplied by their additional care time to obtain a dollar value. (*Shadow price* is economists' jargon for a per-unit monetary value figure that is not empirically observable and therefore has to be estimated.)

Alternatively, if data were available on time spent by family members in other activities, such as market and nonmarket work, and if similar information for families without handicapped children were available as a benchmark, we could compute the reduction in time spent by family members in other activities as a result of the child's handicap. Dollar values could then be obtained by applying the relevant wage rate or shadow price of time.

Either of these procedures assumes that the family members' wage rates or shadow prices are unaffected by the presence of a handicapped child in the family. This assumption may be questioned for several reasons. Time spent in work provides experience that increases the productivity of the individual in the future. Moreover, wage rates of employed persons may depend upon the intensity of their jobs. If parents of handicapped children spend less time acquiring experience or take jobs that involve less intensive effort, their wage rates or shadow prices will be lower than one would expect if none of their children had handicaps. In principle, of course, one could estimate the magnitude of this reduction.

There have as yet been no comprehensive estimates of opportunity costs based on either of these strategies. A principal obstacle to such research is the difficulty of collecting detailed data on family members' nonmarket time allocations. Although some information has been collected on time spent by parents in broad categories of nonmarket activities, such as housework or childcare (*A*

Panel Study . . . , 1976), data providing more detailed breakdowns of these categories by type of activity, and data allocating time spent in childcare activities to individual children within the family are not available. (It may be possible, however, to use other sorts of data to estimate time spent in some nonmarket activities. For example, data on physician use could be combined with estimates of average traveling, waiting, and visit times to generate rough estimates of parental time spent in obtaining physician care for handicapped and nonhandicapped children.) Another difficulty concerns the estimation of the shadow price of time for nonworking family members. Available statistical procedures for estimating this price have yielded unstable results (Cogan, 1975); however, collection of interview data on "reservation wages" (that is, the wage at which a nonworking family member would take a job) could alleviate this problem.

At present, most of the available empirical evidence on parental opportunity costs relates to reductions in time spent in market work. Although descriptive data from a variety of small-scale studies appeared sporadically during the 1960s and 1970s, statistical analyses measuring the impact of children's handicaps on parental work hours and controlling for a variety of other economic and noneconomic factors did not appear until the last several years. One of the first of these studies, based on data from the 1972 Health Interview Survey (HIS), looked at the work status of mothers of children with reported activity limitations caused by chronic conditions compared with the work status of other mothers (Salkever, 1982a). Results indicated a significantly lower probability (0.353) that mothers in white, two-parent families with a disabled child worked at all during the two weeks preceding the interview in comparison with mothers in similar families without a disabled child (0.396). The estimated reduction in the probability that mothers of disabled children reported working as their usual activity was larger (from 0.289 to 0.230) and also statistically significant.

In other cases (in white, single-parent families and all nonwhite families), the estimated impact of children's disabilities on maternal work probabilities was often negative but never statistically significant in comparison with families of the same group but without a disabled child. Further analysis of the data indicated that overall, the negative impact of the child with a disability on maternal work probabilities was significantly greater for mothers in low-income, white, two-parent families than for mothers in middle or upper income families.

The influence of children's disabilities on parental hours of work has also been studied with data from the 1976 Survey of Income and Education (SIE) (Salkever, 1982b, 1982c). This survey is a rich source of information on the economic status of families with disabled children because of its national scope and huge sample size (151,170 households). As in the HIS, disability is defined with reference to chronic conditions that limit activities; however, the higher prevalence rates in the SIE suggest that more relatively minor activity limitations were recorded (Stewart and Robey, 1978). (Note also that the SIE did not record any disability data for children under the age of three.)

Analysis of SIE data on mothers in white, two-parent families revealed that the overall impact of children's disabilities on maternal work probability was negative but slightly smaller in magnitude than the corresponding estimate with 1972 HIS data. However, maternal work probabilities were significantly reduced when their disabled child's handicap interfered with school work or attendance or when the child's mobility was limited. Conversely, maternal work probabilities were significantly higher when the disabled child was older (aged fourteen to seventeen). Among working mothers in white, two-parent families, annual hours of work were significantly reduced (by about 8 percent or 100 hours) by the presence of a disabled child. Once again, this negative impact was even greater for children with schoolwork, school attendance, or mobility limitations, and annual hours of work increased for these mothers when their disabled children were aged fourteen to seventeen. Similar analyses for fathers of disabled children failed to show any significantly negative effects on hours of work except when the mother was working and when the child's handicap interfered with school attendance.

Even with a data base as large as the SIE, analysis of the impact of child disability on nonwhite, two-parent families was hindered by the fact that only several hundred families with disabled children were contained in the study. The number of such families with severely disabled children was much smaller. Analyses of maternal labor-force status and parental hours of work based on these data failed to show any consistent pattern of significant child-disability effects. However, because of the small number of families, the results cannot be regarded as conclusive.

Data problems were less severe for female-headed, one-parent families. Analyses of data on roughly 700 (white and nonwhite) families with disabled children and roughly 500 comparison-group families showed significant reductions in the probability of working for mothers of disabled children. By contrast, estimated effects of the presence of a disabled child on hours worked by working mothers were uniformly small and insignificant.

A more recent study of maternal work status and hours of work by Breslau and her colleagues was based on household survey data from the Cleveland metropolitan area (Breslau, Salkever, and Staruch, 1982). The data base for the study was a household survey, conducted in 1978 and 1979, of a sample of 369 households with chronically ill children served by pediatric specialty clinics in two teaching hospitals and a random sample of 456 households representative of all households with children three to eighteen years old in the Cleveland area. Although the number of households with chronically ill children was not large in comparison to previous studies, a higher proportion of these children had seriously disabling illnesses and the data gathered on severity was much more detailed.

The results for the two-parent families confirmed the previous finding of a greater negative impact of a child disability on work probability for low-income mothers in comparison to other income groups. The additional finding that child disability had a more negative impact on nonwhite families was contrary to earlier results but was not significant when an indicator of disability severity was included in the model. Negative effects on maternal hours of work were also significant when this severity indicator was used. Work probability and work hours regressions for one-parent families showed no significant child disability effects, though this may be partly due to small sample size ($n = 186$). Although this study does not permit extensive generalization, its conclusions support the notion that a chronically ill child can have a substantially negative impact on the mother's earning power and that this impact appears to be most severe for low-income groups.

To compute the economic value of these parental opportunity costs, it is necessary to translate the reduced time spent working because of the presence of a disabled child into reductions in parental earnings. The analyses of SIE data showed that in two-parent, white families, earnings of working mothers were estimated to be 20 percent lower on average as a result of children's disabilities; earnings per hour were estimated to be about 10 percent lower on average. Negative impacts on earnings were especially large for mothers whose children had disabilities relating to schoolwork, school attendance, or mobility. These reductions increased in size with the age of the disabled child, suggesting that children's disabilities tend to impede the human-capital accumulation process of mothers. Analogous estimates for fathers' earnings and earnings per hour showed no clear evidence of negative effects because of children's disabilities. Results for nonwhite, two-parent families and female-headed, one-parent families also failed to show any clear evidence of decreased earnings. It is interesting to note that the general pattern of findings for white, two-parent families reviewed here is similar to the results from a recent British study of two-parent families (Baldwin, 1981).

Although data on time spent in activities other than market work are limited, some preliminary evidence on nonmarket time allocations has been developed from the 1976 surveys of the Panel Study of Income Dynamics. Analyses of these data for two-parent families (Salkever, 1982c) suggest that the presence of a disabled child increases the time spent in housework by the father by 60 to 100 hours annually. A less significant increase was observed for working mothers but there was no discernible effect for nonworking mothers. No significant effects on maternal or paternal time spent in childcare were observed except for husbands of working wives with moderately or severely disabled children, whose childcare times were increased by about 200 hours per year because of their children's disabilities. The preliminary nature of these findings must be stressed, however, because of the small number of households with disabled children in the Panel Study.

Similar analyses of maternal housework and childcare time have also been carried out on the Cleveland data (Breslau, 1983). Results of these analyses indicate an increase in maternal housework time of about three hours per week in two-parent families because of the presence of a disabled child. No significant effects were found for childcare time of these mothers or for mothers in single-parent families.

Finally, although direct evidence relating to parental time spent in taking handicapped children to providers of health care and related services is not available, it is possible to develop some conservative estimates of this important component of direct opportunity costs for ambulatory services. Butler and colleagues reported in Chapter Forty that the 1979 HIS data show an excess of nearly 6 physician visits per year for children with activity limitations due to chronic conditions relative to their nondisabled counterparts (9.5 versus 3.9 visits). Data collected by Breslau and her associates (1983) in the Cleveland surveys confirmed this finding. O'Grady (1982) reports a smaller differential (3.3 visits per year) between physically disabled and nondisabled children. It is important to remember, however, that the distributions of utilization are highly skewed, with a few children accounting for a large percentage of the visits. Thus, for many families with severely ill children, the actual increases in physician visits may be quite large.

To convert these differential use rates into parental time inputs, we can apply Carpenter's (1980) estimate of ninety-five minutes per physician visit (including travel, waiting, and contact times), based on the 1973–1974 HIS data and 1975 data from the National Ambulatory Medical Care Survey. The 1976 data presented by Aday, Andersen, and Fleming (1980) imply a similar per-visit time figure. It is also likely that per-visit time is longer for disabled children because they rely more on specialist care obtained from large medical centers. O'Grady reports mean travel times of forty minutes and fifteen minutes for disabled and nondisabled children respectively but no significant difference in waiting times. Breslau (1983) reports an almost identical travel time differential, but she also finds that disabled children spend more than twice as long at the site of care (in waiting time and contact time). Based on these data, it seems reasonable to assume that the total per-visit time for disabled children is between 1.5 and 2 times that of nondisabled children. Based on this range and the 9.5 versus 3.9 annual visit differential, we estimate that children's disabilities on average increase parental time in taking children for physician care by about seventeen to twenty-five hours annually.

In addition, parental time is used for visits to other health-related practitioners (for example, dentists, occupational therapists, physical therapists, speech therapists, mental health providers). These visits are, in general, much more frequent for parents of disabled children. There is little comparative data available at present, but results from Breslau's Cleveland surveys indicate a differential of 65.4 visits annually (69.9 versus 4.5 visits) (Smyth-Staruch and others, 1984). Some of these visits occur in school and thus do not involve parental escort time. Time spent in home therapy administered by parents may also be considerable; Breslau reports an average time of four hours per week from the Cleveland data.

Differentials in the use of inpatient services also suggest substantial parental time costs. Butler and his colleagues report that discharge rates are about six times as high for children with chronic activity limitations as for other children (approximately 300 per thousand compared to approximately 50 per thousand); average length of inpatient stay is about twice as high (9.0 days compared to 4.8 days). Breslau's data, according to Smyth-Staruch and others (1984), show similar differentials in discharge rates but even larger length-of-stay differences. It is not possible to convert these figures into time input estimates, however, because data for estimating time spent per discharge or visiting per day by parents are not available.

Direct Health Sector Costs

Because the direct health sector costs of children's disabilities are discussed in much greater detail in Chapter Forty, I shall here summarize the available estimates of these costs. Leaving aside the problem of defining the scope of direct costs, either within or outside of the health sector, we can classify them for purposes of discussion into three categories: physician and hospital costs for noninstitutionalized children, other health costs for noninstitutionalized children, and costs of institutional care. Butler and his colleagues estimate that average per capita 1980 expenditures on ambulatory physician and hospital services were $601.45 higher for disabled children than for their nondisabled counterparts (see Chapter Forty). Based on their estimates of 2.29 million disabled children in 1979, this translates into an excess cost of $1,377 million. An even larger estimate is obtained if we add in the costs for in-hospital physician services. Data from Andersen, Lion, and Anderson (1976) for 1970 suggest that these expenditures are approximately equal to one third of expenditures on inpatient hospital charges for children aged birth through seventeen years. If these expenditures are proportional to hospital expenses for disabled and nondisabled children, the per capita cost differential is increased to $755.55 and the total cost differential rises to $1,730 million. Even this figure may be too low, however, because the figures for per-visit physician cost and per-day hospital charge used by Butler and his colleagues (Chapter Forty) are in the process of being revised upward (J. Kasper, personal communication with the author, 1982).

The relative importance of direct costs other than hospital and physician expenses can be roughly gauged from recent survey data. Andersen, Lion, and Anderson (1976) report that these expenditures comprise about one third of the cost of total health spending for children, or roughly half the dollars spent on hospital care and physician care (including hospital outpatient care). About 50 percent of this component consists of dental expenses, and roughly 30 percent is spending for drugs. The residual 20 percent includes spending on therapists and other practitioners, medical equipment (for example, eyeglasses), and supplies.

Comparative utilization data on these various types of services are extremely limited. Smyth-Staruch and others (1984) report little difference between disabled and nondisabled children in numbers of dental visits but, as one might expect, extremely large differences in use of certain types of practitioners (for example, physical therapists, speech therapists). If we make the simplifying assumption that per capita cost of dental services and drugs is the same for disabled and nondisabled children and that only disabled children use other types of services (the residual 20 percent), the implication is that all costs of these other types of services represent differential costs of disability. Using the result of Andersen, Lion, and Anderson (1976) that these services represent about one fifteenth of total per capita cost and using the per capita cost figures from Table

3 in Chapter Forty plus an additional one third of their per capita hospital cost (for inpatient physician services) to represent two thirds of total per capita cost, we obtain a per capita cost for these other types of services of approximately $20. For a population of almost sixty million children this translates into an additional $1.2 billion in differential costs. Combining this figure with the previous calculations, we obtain an estimate of differential health sector costs in 1980 of roughly $2.9 billion.

Admittedly, these calculations are crude and much additional data and analysis will be needed to develop more precise estimates. Our estimate is much higher than the recent estimate by Callahan, Plough, and Wisensale (1981) of $1.7 billion in total health care spending in 1978 on noninstitutionalized disabled children. The latter figure was obtained by multiplying the overall per capita cost figure by the ratio of physician visits for disabled versus nondisabled children. Apart from minor technical problems with this calculation and adjustment for inflation to make it comparable with our 1980 figure, it results in a large underestimate because the ratio of hospital use for disabled versus nodisabled children is much greater than the physician-use ratio.

Information on the total costs of institutional care is even more sparse. As Butler and his colleagues note in Chapter Forty, their estimate of $413 million is quite conservative. This suggests that a more accurate estimate, combined with the calculations described in the previous paragraphs, would yield direct health sector costs due to children's disability well in excess of $3 billion in 1980.

Additional Data on the Distribution of Direct Health Sector Costs by Funding Source

The magnitude of direct health sector costs for disabled children places extraordinary demands on family resources. The differential cost estimate of $3 billion for noninstitutionalized children and the HIS prevalence estimate of 2.3 million imply a per-child differential cost of more than $1,000 in 1980. Although a variety of public and private insurance and service programs have removed much of this large financial burden from the family, Butler and his colleagues (Chapter Forty) document the significant gaps in this patchwork system.

Several additional tabulations are presented here that confirm the existence and significance of these gaps. The first concerns the receipt of subsidized services by disabled children who report no health insurance coverage. Butler and his colleagues indicate that more than 10 percent of disabled children age birth to eighteen years lack insurance coverage. The financial implications of this lack for their families depends on their access to subsidized sources of care or to coverage under "spend-down" provisions of Medicaid programs if their out-of-pocket medical expenses become large. Many uninsured disabled children do not receive subsidized services even if they are living in poverty (U.S. Department of Commerce, 1978). In particular, in 1975 nearly half of uninsured disabled children below the poverty line (48.5 percent) and about two thirds of their nonpoverty counterparts (65.8 percent) received no subsidized services. Although

Neighborhood Health Centers, Crippled Children's Services, and other publicly supported programs do fill in some gaps in insurance coverage among this population, resources devoted to these programs are limited. Consequently, important gaps in coverage remain.

Data on families' out-of-pocket expenses for health care of children during 1975 were collected in the first quarter of 1976 in the Health Interview Survey (U.S. National Center for Health Statistics, 1978). Mean values of annual out-of-pocket expenses are compared for disabled and nondisabled children in Table 1. The overall differential of $109.36 per child ($198.38 – $89.02) in 1975, when inflated by the 1975–1980 increase in the Consumer Price Index for medical care, amounts to an excess out-of-pocket cost of $173.31 per disabled child. Nearly half of this differential is accounted for by excess hospital costs of $48.85 ($59.25 – $10.40) in 1975, with another third resulting from excess physician costs ($35.00). Excess out-of-pocket costs for prescription drugs and other expenditures account for most of the remaining differential. Overall, it appears that between 15 and 20 percent of the very considerable excess costs for health care of noninstitutionalized disabled children are paid for directly by their families.

Other Types of Costs

Expenditures by families on nonhealth goods and services are likely of considerable importance. A detailed source of information on extra expenses by low-income families is the Urban Systems report on blind and disabled children receiving SSI benefits (Urban Systems Research and Engineering, 1980). In this survey, families reported additional costs on a regular basis for transportation (20.8 percent of respondents), clothing (20.7 percent), diet (10.5 percent), laundry (7.1 pecent), and other nonmedical expense categories (including baby-sitting). Dollar figures were only reported for the "other" category and averaged roughly

**Table 1. Mean Annual Out-of-Pocket Health Expenses for
Disabled and Nondisabled Children, 1975.***

Expenses	Children with Activity Limitations	Children with No Activity Limitations
Total expenses	$198.38	$89.02
Hospital care	59.25	10.40
Physician care	65.21	30.21
Dental care	27.95	29.92
Prescription drugs	25.77	11.37
Optical care	10.20	1.09

Source: Tabulated from U.S. National Center for Health Statistics, Health Interview Survey, 1976.

* Components do not add to totals because children with missing data for some components are included in the calculations for other components.

$20 per month in 1978. In addition, more than 10 percent of the families in this study reported nonrecurring major expenses in excess of $100 for nonmedical goods or services in the year preceding the interview.

Other estimates of nonmedical costs are available from smaller-scale studies that focus on particular types of handicaps. Data on families of children with spina bifida, reviewed by Callahan, Plough, and Wisensale (1981) indicate very large costs resulting, in part, from the need for home remodeling and a larger vehicle for transporting the children. A 1978 general population survey of families in the United Kingdom also reported a wide variety of additional nonmedical expenditures for families with handicapped children (Baldwin, 1981).

An additional component of economic costs arises from the impact of children's handicaps on the physical and emotional health of other family members. This impact has been noted in many descriptive studies; an example is the finding by Breslau, Staruch, and Mortimer (1982) from the Cleveland data that mothers of handicapped children showed significantly higher levels of psychological distress than mothers in a comparison group. The emotional and physical strain of caring for a disabled child may eventually result in health problems that involve expenditures on treatment, earnings loss due to disability, and other sorts of economic costs discussed earlier. The magnitude of these costs cannot yet be estimated because we do not yet know the extent to which prevalence and severity of illness among family members is increased by children's handicaps.

Finally, it is important to recognize that children's handicaps often continue into adulthood. Thus, based on 1978 HIS data, we have calculated that roughly 10 percent of all noninstitutionalized adults with chronic activity limitations in the U.S. population report that their limitation began before the age of seventeen. Roughly 4 pecent report an onset of limitation before the age of two. It seems likely that an even high percentage of institutionalized adults with physical or mental handicaps would report onset of their conditions during childhood.

The persistence of these handicaps into adulthood means the continuation of their economic costs. Of course, some cost elements may become less important over time (for example, costs borne by parents or other family members) but others become much more important (for example, earning losses due to handicaps for the handicapped individuals themselves). On the whole, we suspect that incidence-based approaches to cost estimation (which include costs arising at various ages) would show a much larger economic impact for children's handicapping conditions, relative to other health problems, than is suggested by the prevalance-based cost figures discussed in this paper.

Directions for Future Research and Policy

In addition to documenting our general ignorance, this discussion has identified a number of specific questions relating to the economic costs of children's handicaps, questions worthy of further investigation. In the area of our primary concern, parental opportunity costs, we do not as yet understand how income or race can influence the effects of children's handicaps on parental labor-supply and earnings. Moreover, our data on parental time use are, as yet, inadequate for direct assessment of opportunity costs.

Data regarding health expenditures for noninstitutionalized children are only slightly better. General utilization measures (for example, hospital days, physician visits) can be compared for disabled and nondisabled children using the HIS data, but national data on charges or costs are not available. This problem has diminished, with data becoming available from the National Medical Care Expenditure Survey (U.S. Department of Health and Human Services, 1981) and the National Medical Care Utilization and Expenditure Survey (Dobson, Scharff, and Corder, 1981). Data on nonhealth expenditures are extremely limited at present, and we are not aware of any major efforts analogous to the work in the United Kingdom (Baldwin, 1981) to rectify this situation in the immediate future. This is particularly unfortunate because these expenditures can be quite large and because they are almost entirely financed by families rather than third parties. Collection of these data for a large sample of families will be expensive and thus will not occur until public or private funding sources share our judgment that research in this area is an urgent need.

Research on the effects of children's handicaps on the health of other family members has thus far focused primarily on the psychologial and behavioral functioning of mothers and siblings (Breslau, Weitzman, and Messenger, 1981). A more broadly based assessment of these impacts and their costs may well add substantially to our current cost estimates. Although some analyses with national household survey data are now under way, a more intensive analysis of this category of costs is clearly in order.

A final priority for research is the development of incidence-based cost estimates. As Hartunian, Smart, and Thompson (1980) have noted, these estimates are more useful than prevalence-based estimates for assessing the potential worth of prevention programs or programs aimed at ameliorating long-term disabilities due to chronic conditions. Moreover, these estimates would make explicit the costs of the many disabling conditions among adults that have their onset in childhood.

It is clear that the financial impact of children's handicaps upon their families is substantial. Out-of-pocket spending on medical and nonmedical goods and services directly attributable to handicaps has been estimated to average 12.3 percent of income for families of children with spina bifida (Callahan, Plough, and Wisensale, 1981). Even in other cases where out-of-pocket costs may be relatively lower, income reductions due to reduced labor supply will add to the costs. In the case of many services, it is not possible to purchase insurance to cover their costs; however, the reasons that the private insurance market has failed to offer such coverage are not clear. The possibility of rectifying this market failure or of establishing a publicly funded insurance arrangement that would reduce the financial risks to future parents deserves careful consideration.

References

A Panel Study of Income Dynamics: Procedures and Topic Codes, 1976 Interviewing Year. Survey Research Center, University of Michigan, 1976.

Aday, L. A., Andersen, R., and Fleming, G. V. *Health Care in the U.S.: Equitable for Whom?* Beverly Hills, Calif.: Sage, 1980.

Andersen, R., Lion, J., and Anderson, O. *Two Decades of Health Services: Social Survey Trends in Use and Expenditure.* Cambridge, Mass.: Ballinger, 1976.

Baldwin, S. "The Financial Consequences of Disablement in Children." Unpublished manuscript, Department of Social Administration and Social Work, University of York, 1981.

Breslau, N. "Care of Disabled Children and Women's Time Use." *Medical Care,* 1983, *21* (6), 620–629.

Breslau, N., Salkever, D., and Staruch, K. S. "Women's Labor Force Activity and Responsibilities for Disabled Dependents: A Study of Families with Disabled Children." *Journal of Health and Social Behavior,* 1981, *23,* 169–183.

Breslau, N., Staruch, K. S., and Gortmaker, S. L. "The Burden of Caring for a Disabled Child and the Mental Health of the Mother." Paper presented at the American Sociological Association Annual Meeting, New York, 1980.

Breslau, N., Staruch, K. S., and Mortimer, E. "Psychological Distress in Mothers of Disabled Children." *American Journal of Diseases of Children,* 1982, *136,* 682–686.

Breslau, N., Weitzman, M., and Messenger, K. "Psychological Functioning of Siblings of Disabled Children." *Pediatrics,* 1981, *67* (3), 344–353.

Brody, W. M. "Economic Values of a Housewife." Research and Statistics Note 1975-9, Social Security Administration, U.S. Department of Health, Education, and Welfare, 1975.

Callahan, J. J., Jr., Plough, A. L., and Wisensale, S. "Long-Term Care of Children." Background Paper, University Health Policy Consortium, Brandeis University, July 1981.

Carpenter, E. S. "Children's Health Care and the Changing Role of Women." *Medical Care,* 1980, *18,* 1208–1218.

Cogan, J. F. *Labor Supply and the Value of the Housewife's Time.* Santa Monica, Calif.: Rand Corporation, 1975.

Commission for the Control of Epilepsy and Its Consequences. *Plan for Nationwide Action on Epilepsy.* Department of Health, Education, and Welfare publication no. NIH-78-276. Washington, D.C.: U.S. Government Printing Office, n.d.

Dobson, A., Scharff, J., and Corder, L. "Analysis of the First Six Months of Medicaid Data from the National Medical Care Utilization and Expenditure Survey." Paper presented at the Annual Meeting of the American Public Health Association, Los Angeles, November 1981.

Gibson, R. M. "National Health Expenditures, 1979." *Health Care Financing Review,* 1980, *2* (1), 1–36.

Hartunian, N. S., Smart, C. N., and Thompson, M. "The Incidence and Economic Costs of Cancer, Motor Vehicle Injuries, Coronary Heart Disease, and Stroke: A Comparative Analysis." *American Journal of Public Health,* 1980, *70,* 1249–1260.

Hawrylyshyn, O., "The Value of Household Service: A Survey of Empirical Estimates." *Review of Income and Wealth,* 1976, *22* (2), 101–132.

Hodgson, T. A., and Meiners, N. R. "Cost-of-Illness Methodology: A Guide to Current Practices and Procedures." *Milbank Memorial Fund Quarterly,* 1982, *60* (3), 429–462.

Hu, T., and Sandifer, F. H. "Synthesis of Cost of Illness Methodology." Public Services Laboratory, Georgetown University. Report to the National Center for Health Services Research and Development. February 1981.

Kakalik, J. S., and others. *The Cost of Special Education: Summary of Study Findings.* Santa Monica, Calif.: Rand Corporation, 1981.

Mushkin, S. J. *Biomedical Research: Costs and Benefits.* Cambridge, Mass.: Ballinger, 1979.

O'Grady, R. S. "Use of General Pediatric Health Services by Disabled Children." Doctoral thesis, Johns Hopkins University, 1982.

Policy Analysis, Inc. "Evaluation of Cost of Illness Ascertainment Methodology." Final Report, Parts 1 and 2, 1981, National Center for Health Services Research, Department of Health and Human Services (Public Health Service) contract no. 233-77-2048.

Report to the President from the President's Commission on Mental Health. Washington, D.C.: U.S. Government Printing Office, 1978.

Rice, D. P., Feldman, J. J., and White, K. L. *The Current Burden of Illness in the United States.* An Occasional Paper of the Institute of Medicine. Washington, D.C.: National Academy of Sciences, 1976.

Salkever, D. S. "Children's Health Problems and Maternal Work Status." *Journal of Human Resources,* 1982a, *17,* 94–109.

Salkever, D. S. "Children's Health Problems: Implications for Parental Labor Supply and Earnings." In V. Fuchs (Ed.), *Economic Aspects of Health.* Chicago: University of Chicago Press, 1982b.

Salkever, D. S. "Family Economic Impacts of Children's Handicaps." Final Report on Grant MC-R-240426 submitted to the Maternal and Child Health Service, U.S. Department of Health and Human Services. Baltimore, Md.: The Johns Hopkins University, 1982c.

Salkever, D. S. "Morbidity Costs: National Estimates and Economic Determinants." Final report on Grant HS 04369 submitted to the National Center for Health Services Research, U.S. Department of Health and Human Services. Baltimore, Md.: Johns Hopkins University, 1984.

Scitovsky, A. A. "Estimating the Direct Costs of Illness." *Milbank Memorial Fund Quarterly,* 1982, *60* (3), 463–491.

Smyth-Staruch, K., and others. "Use of Health Services by Chronically Ill and Disabled Children." *Medical Care,* 1984, *22* (4), 310–328.

Stewart, W. F., and Robey, J. "Chronic Conditions of Children and Their Disability Status." Paper presented at the American Public Health Association Annual Meeting, Los Angeles, 1978.

U.S. Department of Commerce, Bureau of the Census. *Microdata from the Survey of Income and Education.* Data Access Descriptions, No. 42. Washington, D.C.: U.S. Government Printing Office, 1978.

U.S. Department of Health and Human Services, National Center for Health Services Research. *NMCES Household Interview Instruments.* Department of Health and Human Services publication no. 81-3280. Washington, D.C.: U.S. Government Printing Office, 1981.

U.S. National Center for Health Statistics. "Current Estimates from the Health Interview Survey: United States, 1976." *Vital and Health Statistics,* Series 10, Number 119. Department of Health, Education, and Welfare publication no. 78-1547. Washington, D.C.: U.S. Government Printing Office, 1977.

U.S. National Center for Health Statistics. "Personal Out-of-Pocket Health Expenses: United States, 1975." *Vital and Health Statistics,* Series 10, No. 122. Department of Health, Education, and Welfare publication no. 79-1550. Washington, D.C.: U.S. Government Printing Office, 1978.

Urban Systems Research and Engineering, Inc. *Survey of Blind and Disabled Children Receiving Supplemental Security Income Benefits.* Social Security Administration publication no. 13-11728. Washington, D.C.: U.S. Department of Health, Education, and Welfare, 1980.

Weisbrod, B. *The Economics of Public Health.* Philadelphia: University of Pennsylvania Press, 1961.

Weisbrod, B. "Costs and Benefits of Medical Research: A Case Study of Poliomyelitis." *Journal of Political Economy,* 1971, *79,* 527–544.

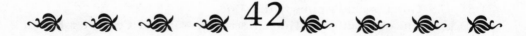

42

Private Health Insurance and Chronically Ill Children

Karen H. Weeks, M.A.

Private health insurance provides a substantial source of financial support—about one third of all expenditures—for health care for children. Families pay out of pocket slightly more than a third of the costs of children's health care so that the total portion paid from private sources is well over two thirds. Moreover, private health insurance and out-of-pocket payments are likely to remain important sources of support, particularly because of current and anticipated reductions in Medicaid and Title V block grant allocations for maternal and child health and crippled children's programs. Yet, despite its importance, private health insurance is poorly understood because of the enormous variation in patterns of coverage and scope of benefits.

Health care needs of chronically disabled children include medical treatment to ameliorate strictly physical conditions as well as the management of care to help children adapt to their conditions and to comply with medical treatment (Ireys, 1981). Some children with chronic disorders require lengthy hospitalizations, and most require regular primary care services. The task here is to investigate how well private health insurance—both fee-for-service and prepaid health plans—serve the needs of chronically ill children. Because health expenditure data for children with these illnesses are at best fragmentary, this chapter attempts to correlate what is known about health insurance in general with the health care needs of chronically ill children. In the discussion, *private health insurance* refers to insurance written by nonprofit voluntary associations such as Blue Cross and Blue Shield; private insurance companies such as Aetna, Connecticut General, and Prudential; and prepaid health plans (health maintenance organizations), which combine the functions of insurance and health care delivery.

During the last fifteen years, expenditures for health care have increased enormously, both in terms of real per capita spending and as a portion of the Gross National Product. Additionally, sources of funds for personal health have changed. While the portion of costs paid directly by patients and their families fell from 52 to 32 percent, the portion paid by third parties increased, with the greatest increase evident in the public insurance (Medicare and Medicaid) share (Gibson, 1980). But there are differences in the patterns of expenditures for children and adults. Private insurance pays a somewhat smaller portion of health care costs for children under age nineteen than for the rest of the population under age sixty-five (33 percent, as compared with 37 percent), public expenditures cover about the same proportion of expenses for both groups (29 percent), and families pay out of pocket a larger portion of children's health care costs than the rest of the population under sixty-five (38 percent as compared with 32 percent) (Fisher, 1980). Significantly, third-party payments concentrate on hospital care and physician services. Third-party reimbursement is important because of its alleged effect upon costs, demand for care, and allocation of resources among various health care services. The current policy emphasis on cost containment has important implications for financing health care of chronically ill children.

In this chapter we examine the historical development of private insurance and the federal and state policy initiatives that encouraged the expansion of a very diverse private health insurance system. We look then at two critical issues: (1) who is covered (access) and (2) what services are covered (comprehensiveness). We then explore the very interesting question of which funding mechanism—fee-for-service or health maintenance organization—is most likely to meet the needs of chronically ill children. In the final section, we look at policy issues and ways of improving the system for children with chronic illnesses.

History

Three themes stand out in the historical development of private health insurance: the parallel and competitive emergence of Blue Cross and Blue Shield and private insurance companies; federal policy initiatives strengthening private health insurance, both fee-for-service and health maintenance organizations; and devolution of regulatory authority to state governments. The complex and simultaneous interaction of the three themes has produced health care plans of enormous variety, having important consequences for the financing of health care for chronically ill children. Therefore it is important to understand the historical antecedents of the current system.

Contemporary health insurance derives from the casualty insurance model. In brief, the purpose of health insurance is protection against the risk of unexpected medical and financial demands, not provision of comprehensive health care. Individuals and families purchase health insurance in order to protect themselves from large health care expenditures that are unpredictable. Critics such as Enthoven (1980) suggest that the casualty insurance model is inappropriate for financing medical care for many reasons, including the difficulty of fixing a value for the loss incurred and the difficulty of determining whether medical care is necessary or unnecessary.

The Blues and Insurance Companies. Private health insurance derives from two separate historical streams: voluntary prepayment plans developed in the early twentieth century and individually underwritten accident insurance begun in the nineteenth century. The first became what we now know as insurance written by nonprofit voluntary associations, such as Blue Cross and Blue Shield, and the second evolved into the plans written by private insurance companies (sometimes referred to as "commercials"), such as Aetna, Connecticut General, Metropolitan, and Prudential.

Blue Cross had its roots in the voluntary, community-sponsored, fee-for-service hospital and medical care system that had been stabilized shortly after the turn of the century. The forerunner of the Blue Cross plans developed in 1929 when teachers in the Dallas area contracted with Baylor University Hospital to provide up to twenty-one days of semiprivate room and board and certain ancillary services in return for payment of a monthly premium. The local nonprofit prepayment prototype, which protected people from the trauma of large medical expenses and provided hospitals a steady income, expanded to include entire communities and then complete states. The American Hospital Association actively promoted Blue Cross plans and in 1937 established a clearinghouse for the plans in Chicago; the new Blue Cross Commission accumulated cost and utilization data and established standards for member plans (Anderson, 1968; Hedinger, 1968).

The Blue Cross plans took on certain characteristics in order to accommodate themselves to the traditions of voluntary hospitals and to differentiate themselves from private insurance companies. Blue Cross plans incorporated as nonprofit organizations; had governing boards representing hospitals, physicians, and the public; emphasized hospital benefits in the form of service rather than cash indemnities; and placed all employees including salesmen on salaries rather than commission (Anderson, 1968).

Within several years of the formation of hospital plans by Blue Cross and private companies, physicians developed plans to offer predetermined payment levels for surgical procedures, laboratory tests, and other services. Historically, Blue Shield plans evolved in close connection with Blue Cross plans and identified closely with state medical societies. In 1978, the national organizations of Blue Cross and Blue Shield merged, although individual plans are still administered locally. At the end of 1979, there were sixty-eight Blue Cross plans and sixty-seven Blue Shield plans.

Private insurance companies also began to market group hospital insurance, typically offering reimbursement in accordance with a fixed fee schedule. And, paralleling the development of Blue Shield plans, private insurance companies introduced group surgical and medical (physicians' visit) benefit plans in the late 1930s and 1940s. Although in the early years Blue Cross enrolled more persons than did private insurance companies, by 1951 the competitive position reversed (Law, 1976). For the last decade, the distribution of enrollees has been 55 percent private insurance company, 40 percent Blue Cross, and the remainder independent plans (principally prepaid group practices) (Smith, 1978).

Blue Cross plans evolved in the context of national debate about the appropriate role of government in assuring adequate health care for its citizens. The possibility of government-sponsored health insurance was a stimulus to their development. Because Blue Cross plans were to be nonprofit community service organizations that substantially covered the costs of hospitalization, the hospital and medical associations successfully sought special enabling legislation that permitted the plans to be classified as nonprofit insurance agencies, supervised by state departments of insurance, relieved of the requirement to maintain substantial cash reserves (because they were offering a service rather than cash indemnity), and exempt from taxes. In later years, several states challenged tax exemption successfully, with courts finding that Blue Cross is essentially engaged in writing insurance in direct competition with private insurers, who have no such favored status (Law, 1976).

During World War II, when wages were frozen, group health insurance became an increasingly important component in collective bargaining agreements. Group health insurance continued to expand following the war, and by the early 1950s the present health insurance structure was in place. The basic policy issue of whether health insurance should be sponsored by government or by private agencies had been settled in favor of a private system (Anderson, 1968).

Federal Initiatives. Over the years, the federal government has taken various initiatives giving impetus to the expansion of private health insurance. These include providing health insurance with favored treatment in the tax code of the early 1940s, providing health benefits to federal employees through private insurance in 1960, allowing participation of insurance carriers in the administration of Medicare and Medicaid in 1965, and stimulating alternative forms of insurance through the Health Maintenance Act of 1973 (and amendments of 1976). But for the most part, as we shall see, the federal government has allocated to the states primary responsibility for regulating health insurance.

Since 1942, the federal tax code has allowed a deduction from income of certain medical expenditures, including expenditures for health insurance premiums. Of greater significance has been the exclusion from an employee's taxable income of employer contributions to health insurance, accomplished first by an Internal Revenue Service ruling in 1943 and later by statute in 1953. Having only a modest impact in early years, the exclusion from income for purposes of income taxation and social security taxes has become increasingly significant to the insured employee as tax rates have increased over the years. By 1981, the annual subsidies for health care resulting from federal tax revenue losses were $25 billion. This represents a tremendous national investment, approximately one fifth of total federal expenditures for health care.

The federal government utilized private insurance to extend health benefits to its own employees when it put into effect in 1960 the Federal Employees Health Benefits Program. The legislation, a compromise among all the principals—the American Medical Association, Blue Cross–Blue Shield, insurance companies, prepayment plans, employee unions, and the federal government as employer—authorized the Civil Service Commission to contract for a service benefit plan (Blue Cross–Blue Shield), an indemnity benefit plan, employee organization plans, and comprehensive medical plans. The federal investment is substantial today, both in terms of number of persons covered and the amount of contribution by the government as employer.

Currently, there are more than ten million employees, retirees, and their dependents covered by governmentwide high- and low-option service benefit plans (Blue Cross–Blue Shield), governmentwide high- and low-option indemnity plans (Aetna), twelve employees' organization plans, and more than seventy comprehensive plans, which are mostly prepaid group practices. The government, as employer, contributes a fixed amount monthly on behalf of each employee (but not more than 75 percent of the premium), which in 1982 was $34.22 for an individual policy and $80.19 for a family policy. Monthly employee contributions to governmentwide plans for family enrollment range from $16.06 to $68.67, depending on the plan. The Blue Shield high-option plan has almost half of all enrollees.

In the early 1970s, health maintenance organizations (HMOs) became the object of federal policy, principally as a means of bringing about changes in the health system and holding down costs by offering an alternative to the predominant fee-for-service system. The term *health maintenance organization,* coined to help win political support, encompassed a range of health plans broader than prepaid group practices (which dated from the late 1920s). The Health Maintenance Organization Act of 1973 (Public Law 93–222), overrode state laws hindering health maintenance organizations and provided for loan and grant assistance to HMOs meeting certain requirements. Few plans qualified, however, and the HMO amendments of 1976 (Public Law 94–460) relaxed requirements regarding services and enrollment. Although membership in HMOs rose from three million in 1970 to eleven million in 1981 (Pear, 1982b), the impact of federal financial assistance has been modest. Since 1973, the federal government has invested only $340 million in grants and loans to HMOs, and in 1985, federal assistance ended. The rise in membership is due to many other factors, one of which is interest shown during the last few years by insurers such as Blue Cross and Blue Shield, Prudential, and John Hancock, which have either started or acquired HMOs.

Currently, federal policy regarding private health insurance is unsettled. The early 1980s saw a flurry of interest in competitive approaches that, by changing the tax structure, would encourage employees to choose less expensive insurance plans (and promote choice among fee-for-service and health maintenance plans). However, legislative proposals encountered stiff opposition from the insurance industry, business groups, and organized labor, and no consensus has yet emerged.

State Initiatives. Since the nineteenth century, responsibility for regulating insurance had been reserved to the states. The Supreme Court ruled in 1868 that insurance was not an act of commerce and was therefore beyond the scope of federal laws that might be enacted under the interstate commerce clause of the Constitution (*Paul* v. *Virginia,* 1868). Regulation of health insurance by the states was grafted onto the existing mechanisms for regulating life, property, and casualty insurance (MacKay, 1980). The arrangement terminated temporarily in 1944 when the Supreme Court held that insurance was a form of interstate commerce subject to federal regulations and that price-fixing arrangements were in violation of federal antitrust laws (*United States* v. *South-Eastern Underwriters Association,* 1944). In response, Congress passed in 1945 the McCarran-Ferguson Act, which expressly reserved to the states authority for regulation of insurance and declared that federal antitrust laws would be applicable only to the extent that the industry was not regulated by the states. Thus, the 1868 decision in *Paul* and the McCarran-Ferguson Act eighty years later assured that oversight of insurance was not in the federal domain and contributed to the very diverse system which later evolved.

Having been granted regulatory authority, the states have been concerned primarily with solvency and with rate setting. In most states, legislation has provided for the prior approval of premium rates by state insurance departments and has sanctioned rate fixing in connection with rate bureaus. In the view of some critics, the health insurance industry has captured health insurance regulation. Since the mid sixties, however, many insurance commissioners have denied premium increases in an effort to curb hospital rate increases (Jacobs, Bauerschmidt, and Furst, 1978). Gradually the states have directed attention to other regulatory areas such as fair practices in marketing, minimum standards, and access to coverage (Jones, 1981).

In the view of many critics, a conspicuous failure of the health insurance regulatory system has been its inability to deal with questions of health care cost control and provider reimbursement. While Congress has assured the growth and expansion of voluntary health insurance by enacting tax subsidies, programs for federal employees, Medicare and Medicaid, and HMO legislation, at the same time it has reserved to the states the function of regulation of health insurance. Gradually, some states (and some insurers) have instituted various mechanisms to control the amount and the method of reimbursement. But the response remains uneven.

Access to Health Insurance

Federal stimuli to private sector health insurance, devolution of regulatory authority to the states, and the parallel emergence of three distinctive types of health insurance—the Blues, private companies, and health maintenance organizations—have each contributed to a system that is diverse by geography, by socioeconomic status, and by employment status. It is thus difficult to generalize about such issues as access and comprehensiveness. But it is possible to present the array of patterns of coverage and to discuss the special problems confronting families seeking adequate protection for their children with chronic illnesses.

Children with chronic illnesses require higher than average use of medical services. Although data for this population are incomplete, the survey of inpatient discharges in Chapter Forty shows that in 1977, children with the eleven chronic conditions specified in the Vanderbilt project accounted for 6.3 percent of days of inpatient hospitalization although they represent only 1 percent of the population of children. There are no comparable data for utilization of physician services by children with one or more of the eleven diseases or for other health care services, but it is reasonable to assume that utilization is considerable, especially because the preferred method of treatment for many of the chronic diseases is on an outpatient basis.

Because the costs associated with utilization of health care services are considerable, it is important to look at patterns of health insurance coverage. In this endeavor we are constrained by the fact that data are most often presented for the population under sixty-five, infrequently for children, and almost never for children with the eleven tracer illnesses. Nonetheless, we can learn a considerable amount from the data for the population under sixty-five because children typically are covered by virtue of their relationship to an adult parent. Parents, in turn, have access to health insurance principally by virtue of their employment status. We examine first access to health insurance and then turn to comprehensiveness of coverage.

Estimates of coverage by private health insurance for the population under age sixty-five vary from 78 percent (National Center for Health Statistics, Health Interview Survey, 1977) to 85 percent (Health Insurance Institute, 1976). Equally important is estimating the proportion of the population that is *not* covered by any kind of insurance, public or private. Surveys generally underreport coverage because respondents are sometimes unaware of their eligibility for benefits. On the other hand, estimates based on program coverage, such as insurance company and public program enrollment figures, tend to overreport because of multiple coverage (for example, both spouses covered under plans provided by separate employers; persons covered under both public and private programs). The U.S. Congressional Budget Office (1979) estimates that the percentage of population under age sixty-five without insurance protection is 5 to 8 percent.

What is significant is the fact that those not covered fall disproportionately into certain segments of the population. In general, they are young and they are in low-income families. Those less likely to be covered include the unemployed, employees of small firms, part-time and seasonal workers, the self-employed, the near poor who are not eligible for Medicaid, persons who are just beginning to seek employment or who are between jobs, and dependent children not included in the coverage of family heads.

Young people are more likely to be without protection than other groups. Fourteen percent of the population under age six are uninsured, as are 20 percent of the population aged six to eighteen and fully 20 percent of the group aged nineteen to twenty-four ("Survey of Income and Education data, 1976," reported in U.S. Congressional Budget Office, 1979). The number of young adults without coverage is disproportionately high for several reasons: many insurance policies do not cover family members over age eighteen unless they are in school; young adults are more likely to be unemployed or in jobs that do not provide insurance; they are not covered by Medicaid unless they have dependent children; and they are among the healthiest of the population and therefore less motivated to purchase health insurance.

Persons in families with incomes below $10,000 are more than twice as likely to be unprotected as those whose incomes exceed $10,000 (U.S. Congressional Budget Office, 1979). Moreover, persons with low incomes are less likely to have access to group insurance, which provides greater coverage and, consequently, lower out-of-pocket costs for health care.

Access to group health insurance is largely determined by employment status and by other factors such as length of employment and type of industry. In 1979, 54 percent of workers over age fifteen were covered by group health insurance plans paid for in part or entirely by an employer or union (U.S. Department of Commerce, 1981). Additional employees are covered by group policies for which they pay the total premium. A surprising 8 percent of employed persons are without health coverage, with part-time workers and self-employed persons being twice as likely to be uncovered as full-time wage earners (U.S. Congressional Budget Office, 1979). Even among the full-time employed, many are not covered because they are subject to waiting periods before they become covered (27 percent of workers are subject to waiting periods of three months or longer) or because they are employed in industries that have a high proportion of intermittent or seasonal workers. A source of growing concern is the numbers of persons who lose health insurance coverage as the result of job layoffs. One estimate in 1982 by federal officials indicates that of the 11.3 million unemployed, 8 million had lost their health insurance coverage, in addition to an unknown number of their spouses and dependents (Pear, 1982a). Under most plans, benefits end within a month or so after a person loses a job.

In addition to the unemployed and marginally employed, dependents of employed persons also often lack coverage. Sometimes family heads are covered but their dependents are not because the heads have waived or were not offered the opportunity to insure them (U.S. Congressional Budget Office, 1979). Typically, when the cost of premiums is shared by both employer and employee, the employee must pay a larger premium for family coverage. The U.S. Congressional Budget Office (1979) estimates that extending coverage of family heads to dependents would lower the number of uncovered by 20 percent; the change would obviously be important for expanded coverage of children.

Access to *group* insurance is particularly important to families with chronically ill children because of its lower price and better coverage. A family has access to group insurance primarily through employment, and this factor is important to a family considering job changes. The price of group plans is less than for individual policies because of economies of scale in administering them and because of reduction in risk through minimizing adverse selection by individuals. Moreover, group policies pay a higher portion of medical expenses when compared to nongroup policies; individuals with group insurance thus have lower out-of-pocket medical expenditures than those with individual insurance (Phelps, 1974).

There has been no systematic evaluation of the provisions of *individual* insurance policies, but a casual examination of individual policies reveals that the policyholder receives less comprehensive coverage requiring higher out-of-pocket payments. In addition, individuals often face age-limit restrictions, waiting periods, and exclusions from coverage because of pre-existing conditions. (It should be noted that such restrictions sometimes apply to group policies).

A pre-existing condition is one that requires medical treatment during a specified period prior to the effective date of the insurance policy. There has been no systematic analysis of pre-existing condition provisions for either individual policies or group policies. Many but not all individual policies exclude coverage of a pre-existing condition altogether. Sometimes in both individual and group policies coverage of a pre-existing condition is subject to a waiting period. For example, if a child has a chronic disease such as hemophilia, which requires treatment during a specified period (such as three months or a year) prior to the effective date of the insurance policy, the child must wait for a specified period, such as one year, before the policy covers the hemophilia.

Another critical problem for children with chronic illness relates to their coverage when they reach the age (typically eighteen or twenty-four) at which their parents' policies no longer cover them. Sometimes the policy provides for coverage of dependents over the specified age if they are disabled or incapable of supporting themselves. However, many children with chronic illness may not be disabled, and because of their chronic condition, they may have difficulty in securing an individual insurance policy. Their best hope is to obtain employment in a firm with a large group policy that does not exclude their illness.

Efforts to expand coverage to the uninsured through the workplace will contribute a great deal, but will not reach all the uninsured. And, indeed, employers participating in a conference sponsored by the Government Research Corporation indicated a willingness to consider extending coverage when there is an employee-employer relationship, such as in the case of over-age dependent children, but less willingness to extend coverage when the employee-employer relationship terminates, as in the case of permanent layoffs or voluntary terminations (Caulfield and Haynes, 1980). The difficulty in extending benefits to part-time, seasonal, or low-wage employees is an economic one. Employer plans cost an average of $808 per employee in 1980; employers express reluctance to extend benefits to employees when the ratio of benefits to direct compensation is too high.

Although only 30 percent of the uninsured are employed by others, certain changes in employer policies could improve the extent of coverage. As noted previously, the U.S. Congressional Budget Office (1979) estimates that if coverage of family heads were extended to dependents regardless of age, the number of uninsured would be reduced by 20 percent. Standardized layoff protection and shortened waiting periods for commencement of employer-provided health insurance would help. The National Association of Insurance Commissioners (NAIC) recommends coverage for at least a month after termination and has proposed model state legislation entitling employees to conversion privileges, which give the terminated employee the option of enrolling in an individual policy of the same insurer. As of January 1979, five states had adopted the NAIC model act and seven others had adopted similar policies (National Association of Insurance Commissioners, 1979). Although conversion privileges would help families with children with chronic illness in that the families would not be subject to waiting periods for pre-existing conditions, premium costs for individual policies are high—typically greater than $100 per month—and coverage is minimal.

Another critical area is lack of access by self-employed individuals to comprehensive health insurance at reasonable rates. Group policies available to self-employed individuals are usually not as comprehensive as those provided to employees of large firms and may not meet adequately the needs of a family with a chronically ill child who presents an unacceptably high risk to a potential insurer. The NAIC Comprehensive Health Insurance and Health Care Cost Containment Act proposes the creation by states of residual market mechanisms (high-risk pools), to assure the availability of comprehensive health insurance to all persons who were previously uninsurable or substandard risks. Insurance carriers would be required to participate in the pool (National Association of Insurance Commissioners, 1979). Six states, Connecticut, Indiana, Minnesota, North Dakota, Rhode Island, and Wisconsin, have established pools for uninsurables. In some states, persons must qualify for the pool by demonstrating that they have been turned down by regular insurers. The insurance industry supports the concept of state pools, but only for bona fide uninsurables (not for standard health risks) who are potential purchasers of individual insurance. Another approach—favored by the insurance industry—is the automatic eligibility of individuals with certain enumerated conditions.

Comprehensiveness: Breadth and Depth of Coverage

Comprehensiveness of coverage is similarly linked to employment status, for, although most group policies cover hospital services, considerable variation by types of employment exists with regard to other health services. Two elements of comprehensiveness are important in this discussion: breadth, which refers to the range of services covered, and depth, which refers to the amount of protection for very costly illnesses. Increasingly, the trend has been for group policies to provide richer packages that cover more services and in greater depth, but there are important exceptions.

To assure optimal functioning, chronically ill children and their families require the following range of medical services: hospital care for the child from the moment of birth, surgical care, outpatient care in physicians' offices or specialty clinics, drugs, medical equipment and applicances, home health care, and well-child care. The task here is to correlate the list of medical services needed by chronically ill children and what is known about health insurance coverage. If the child has a medical condition that requires medical treatment, insurance is likely to provide some coverage. However, health insurance is really medical insurance; it does not and was never intended to cover nonmedical health needs such as transportation, home renovations, compensation for lost work time for parents, and childcare.

Enrollment data are available for numbers of persons covered by the various types of health insurance policies—hospital, surgical, and major medical. In addition, survey data are available regarding persons covered by broad categories of medical services (particularly the employed population) (Price, 1977). However, the data are of limited usefulness for this chapter because they are rarely broken down by age group or disease. Moreover, simply knowing that a certain percentage of children are covered by a policy does not tell very much in the absence of analysis of various features of the specific policy. It is important to understand when and how the various insurance policy components— hospital, surgical, and major medical—come into play and to understand why deductibles, coinsurance features, and partial payments according to fee schedules or prevailing usual, customary, and reasonable reimbursement rates can leave even a covered family with substantial uncovered expenses.

Blue Cross and Blue Shield historically have offered their locally con- trolled plans as prepayment plans that typically combine the following features: service benefits, contracts with providers (hospitals and physicians), and provi- sion of first-dollar coverage. In contrast, private insurance companies serving a national constituency offer insurance against risk through indemnity benefits that are paid directly to subscribers to cover unpredictable and definable events in return for payments based on the experience of the insured group. In practice, the distinctions between the two are not so clear-cut. During the last several decades, and especially during the 1970s, the distinctions have become blurred as both types have competed vigorously in marketing policies.

Basic medical health insurance includes the following three types: hospital (which pays for room and board and certain ancillary services such as use of the operating room and laboratory services), surgical (which pays for surgeons and anesthesia), and regular medical (which pays for nonsurgical doctor fees in hospitals and for physician care outside the hospital). Because these three types of coverage usually have specified limitations, major medical insurance fre- quently supplements their coverage by paying for a wider range of services after satisfaction of a deductible and usually with a coinsurance feature. Sometimes a comprehensive plan combines the features of all four types of insurance.

Basic hospital benefits may be either service benefits or cash indemnity benefits. Plans providing for service benefits cover the full cost of specified room and board accommodations and ancillary services for a specified period. Blue Cross plans provide reimbursement for services under contract with hospitals located in an area served by a plan and pay the provider directly. Typically, Blue Cross plans pay in full for covered services in member hospitals (but pay 80 percent of charges in nonmember hospitals). The Blue Cross contract with the hospital usually specifies what the hospital is allowed to charge the patients covered by Blue Cross. Plans providing indemnity benefits reimburse the cost of room and board up to a fixed amount per day for a specified period. Such plans are more common with private insurance companies than Blue Cross. However, Skolnik (1976) notes a shift on the part of private insurance companies to provide service benefits, in part because of the difficulties encountered by many plans in keeping cash benefits up to date.

In a similar vein, *basic surgical and regular medical benefits* may be provided on a service basis or a cash indemnity basis. When first established, Blue Shield plans covered specified procedures on a fee-schedule basis; however, in the 1950s the plans began to offer coverage based on usual, customary, and reasonable charges (UCR), and this type of plan has been more widely used since the enactment of Medicare. The *usual fee* is the fee that an individual physician usually charges for a service or has charged for a period of time; the *customary fee* reflects the aggregate of fees charged in the community. The concept of *reasonable* allows Blue Shield to adjust a physician's fee to account for a procedure that has unusual complications. When the plan updates the usual and customary allowances, fees increase to reflect the individual (usual) and community (customary) charges of the past accounting period. One way that plans have attempted to hold down costs is to update allowable fees less frequently. If a physician charges in excess of the allowable UCR fee, the patient must pay the excess. An increasing number of private insurance companies, which traditionally have paid in accordance with a fee schedule, now offer contracts that provide for reimbursement on a UCR basis.

Major medical expense insurance, sometimes referred to by the Blues as extended benefits, helps pay the costs of illness not covered by basic coverage and includes such items as home health care, medical appliances and equipment, physician office visits, drugs, and psychiatric treatment. Major medical insurance protects against large expenditures and has experienced the most rapid growth rate in the last decade. Such policies usually feature a deductible and coinsurance. Typically the deductible is $100 per individual per year (although this amount has been increased to $150 in the federal government Blue Cross plans). After the deductible is satisfied, the insurance may cover all or a percentage of costs incurred up to a specified maximum dollar amount, which may be $100,000 or $250,000 or may be unlimited. The typical coinsurance feature requires the insured person to pay a percentage—typically 20 percent—of medical expenses after satisfying the deductible. Sometimes major medical plans include catastrophic protection, which reimburses 100 percent of covered expenses after the subscriber has paid coinsurance of a specified threshold amount, say $1,000 or $5,000.

The important point here is that even though a policy may cover a given health care service, the family is frequently at risk for a portion of the cost of that service. And, typically, private health insurance is more likely to cover certain kinds of services than others. It is more likely to cover hospital costs than office visits and home physician visits. Table 1 shows in the column labeled "Direct Payments" that either private health insurance or public sources pay for all but 3.7 percent of children's hospital care. However, families can expect to pay more than one third of the costs for their children's care by physicians and more than two thirds of the costs of other health care.

It is difficult to analyze adequacy of benefits because of the lack of agreement on what health insurance should protect. One study used an interdisciplinary panel of six persons to develop a consensus of a minimum level of adequate coverage and then used available data regarding benefits provided by employer plans and other data to estimate the number of persons with adequate coverage (Sudovar and Feinstein, 1979). The consensus of the advisory panel established the following minimum adequate standard:

> 80 percent of the costs of medically necessary hospital care, physician services, laboratory and X-ray services, prenatal care, outpatient services and nursing home care should be borne by the third-party program(s);
>
> some of the costs of medically necessary inpatient psychiatric care should be borne by the third-party program(s);
>
> 100 percent of the costs of medically necessary health care in excess of 10 to 30 percent of individual income should be borne by the third-party program(s) (with a stronger preference for a ten percent limit) (p. 1).

It is important to note what services—many of which are important for chronically ill children—were *not* included in the minimum adequate standard. Excluded were certain medically necessary services such as visiting nurses' services, vision care, prescribed drugs, appliances and equipment, outpatient psychiatric care, home care, family planning, dental care, and multiphasic screening because the panel assumed insurance claims would not be justified by the expected benefit and these lower-cost services could be met effectively within the average family budget. The latter assumption, although valid for healthy families, ignores the cumulative nature of such expenses for families with chronically ill children. Also excluded from the minimum adequate standard were intermediate care services performed by providers such as social workers, psychologists, and nurse practitioners (Sudovar and Feinstein, 1979). Despite these limitations, the results of the study are important because they demonstrate dramatically the link between employment and adequacy of insurance coverage.

The standards were applied to public programs and to four categories of private sector insurance: government workers, workers in firms of twenty-five or more workers, workers in firms of fewer than twenty-five workers, and self-employed workers. In the private insurance sector, Sudovar and Feinstein found a tremendous variation in adequacy of coverage by *type of group*. About 90

Table 1. Percentage Distribution of Health Care Expenditures for Persons Under Age 19 by Channels of Payment, Calendar Year 1977.

	Private				*Public*			
	Total Private	*Direct Payments*	*Private Health Insurance*	*Other*	*Total Public*	*Medicare*	*Medicaid*	*Other*
All personal health care	71.5	38.1	32.7	.7	28.5	.1	15.6	12.8
Hospital care	54.6	3.7	50.7	.2	45.4	--	25.0	20.4
Physician care	84.4	38.7	45.7	--	15.6	.4	12.1	3.1
All other care	78.5	70.2	6.9	1.5	21.5	--	9.2	12.3

Source: Adapted from Fisher, 1980.

percent of persons in all groups had adequate coverage for *inpatient acute care,* and more than 90 percent were covered for *inpatient psychiatric care.* In contrast, coverage for *physician office and home services* was significantly less adequate. Although government workers were well protected, only 22 percent of large-group employees and two percent of small-group employees had adequate protection for office visits, and protection for home visits was almost nonexistent; small group and individual policies had almost no protection for office and home visits.

Among the population covered by private health insurance *or* public programs, 61.7 percent had *catastrophic* protection equal to or greater than the panel's unlimited expense protection standard of $250,000. But the adequacy of protection varied significantly by group. Almost all federal government workers and small-group and individual plans reported in this study had an adequate maximum benefit, whereas only about 40 percent of the other groups did. With respect to the second element of catstrophic protection, maximum out-of-pocket limit, almost all federal employees had such a limit, but only about 20 percent of nongovernment workers had such a limit (Sudovar and Feinstein, 1979). The latter element of catastrophic protection is important for families of chronically ill children; for example, if a child incurred repeated hospitalizations and the family was subject to a 20 percent coinsurance payment, a potentially large liability could arise if there were no limitations on out-of-pocket expenses. The findings were consistent with overall data indicating that small groups and individuals tended to insure against high costs and unpredictable events, and to self-insure for lower-cost events.

This study tends to confirm what is known intuitively. Private sector insurance offers reasonably good protection for inpatient acute care, some protection for inpatient psychiatric care, limited protection for physician office and home visits, and protection of widely varying degrees for other services. Government workers, especially federal workers, have the most adequate protection, followed by large-group employees. Small-group employees and individuals tend to insure for high-cost events but to insure less adequately for other benefits. A substantial majority of all groups, except federal employees, do not have an out-of-pocket limitation on expenditures and thus are at risk for at least 20 percent of services, which for chronically ill children could be substantial.

HMO Versus FFS: Does It Make a Difference?

To this point we have discussed primarily private insurance that reimburses subscribers for medical services rendered on a fee-for-service (FFS) basis. A small but growing segment of privately insured persons have chosen health maintenance organizations (HMOs). They represent about 5 percent of the insured population, and their numbers have been increasing in recent years at about 12 percent a year. Expanding opportunities for coverage of chronically ill children by health maintenance organizations deserves consideration because of the breadth of services covered and because of the potential for limiting a family's risk for out-of-pocket payments. There is a growing body of literature comparing the two systems, but there are few data related specifically to chronically ill children. Nonetheless, some studies direct attention to chronically ill persons (adults and children), and it is possible to make reasonable inferences regarding chronically ill children.

In general, health maintenance organizations function both as insurer and health service provider by providing on a contractual basis comprehensive health care services in exchange for regular fixed prepayments to a voluntarily enrolled group. HMOs include both prepaid group practices (PGPs), which typically provide hospital and physician services using salaried staff members, and individual practice associations (IPAs), which typically are sponsored by local medical societies and contract with physicians for the delivery of services to enrollees.

Access and Enrollment. Families are likely to have access to HMOs (especially to prepaid group practices) only if they are members of an employee group. Thus, unless the head of a family with a chronically ill member is employed by an organization that offers an HMO option, the family is not likely to have access to an HMO. Part of the reason for HMO opposition to the federal government mandating open enrollment was their concern that persons with large anticipated health care needs would gravitate to the prepaid plans.

Among the employees who have choices, the literature suggests that on balance there are remarkable similarities among enrollees in both systems. There is little evidence that HMO enrollees are sicker or healthier than persons who receive health care in fee-for-service settings (Berki and Ashcraft, 1980; Marcus, 1981).

One way to examine whether chronically ill persons have access to HMOs is to compare their enrollment patterns with the rest of the population. Several studies (Tessler and Mechanic, 1975; Hetherington, Hopkins, and Roemer, 1975; Juba, Lave, and Shaddy, 1980; Blumberg, 1980; Berki and Ashcraft, 1980) have shown a slight propensity for prepaid plans among families with reported chronic illness. It is equally important to understand why families choose the funding mechanisms they do. Perceived advantages of HMOs reported for the general population in numerous studies include breadth of services covered, lower or predictable costs, and assured access to care. Disadvantages include limitations on the choice of provider, inconvenience of a centralized delivery setting, and the need to terminate an established relationship with a provider. One can speculate that breadth of services and predictable costs would be advantageous to persons with chronic illnesses, while the need to disrupt an established relationship with a provider would be particularly disadvantageous to someone with an illness requiring ongoing care. In an IPA, however, a person could maintain an established relationship.

Comprehensiveness: Utilization and Costs. Discussion of comprehensiveness of care in an earlier section pointed to a number of areas for which private insurance under the fee-for-service system provided poorly. The family is at risk for services that are typically covered by HMOs. One way of looking at the question of comprehensiveness is to go beyond simply enumerating whether or not services are covered services, to look at the extent to which patients actually use them.

Many studies have found that health care financing can have a substantial influence on the kinds and amounts of medical care people receive and, specifically, that health insurance has a direct effect on such things as hospitalization and number of physician visits. As we have seen, insurance coverage on a fee-for-service basis covers rather extensively hospital and acute care but less extensively outpatient and home-based care. Because physicians' fees in HMOs do not depend on the number of treatments they prescribe or the number of hospitalizations they order, one of the theoretical advantages of health maintenance organizations is that they discourage unnecessary utilization and reduce the costs of medical care, especially the costs of hospitalization. One assumption is that HMO physicians encourage more preventive health care than fee-for-service physicians. A contrary assumption is that HMO physicians have a financial incentive to undertreat patients. Thus, caution must be used in interpreting the data: one cannot be certain if a finding of less treatment represents the avoidance of unnecessary treatment or undertreatment.

The evidence regarding utilization of *ambulatory visits* is complex. In general, persons enrolled in HMOs receive at least as many ambulatory visits as persons in fee-for-service plans. Luft's review of recent studies (1978a) indicates that in eighteen of twenty-six pairs of plans, HMO enrolless had more visits than persons in the comparison group. He and others have pointed out that it is important to distinguish among types of ambulatory physician visits. Dutton (1979), for example, distinguishes between patient-controlled use (such as preventive care and other care initiated by the patient) and physician-controlled use (such as follow-up visits). In a study of five different ambulatory-care settings in Washington, D.C., she found that patient-initiated care was highest among enrollees in prepaid group practices, whereas the volume of follow-up care was highest among fee-for-service subscribers.

Several studies suggest that the level of illness, including the presence of chronic or acute conditions, is a predictor of illness-related ambulatory visits. Moreover, there is some evidence that not having a usual source of care, whether HMO or FFS, is a predictor associated with fewer ambulatory visits (Berki and Ashcraft, 1979; Hennelly and Boxerman, 1979; Andersen and Aday, 1978). Hennelly and Boxerman's study is particularly interesting because of the overrepresentation of patients with chronic illness (for example, hypertension and diabetes). The authors found an inverse relationship between the number of visits and the extent to which a patient had to pay expenses out of pocket.

The provision and utilization of *preventive care* is important to persons with chronic illnesses. It is often stated that early identification and ongoing routine care can help stabilize a chronic condition thereby reducing the need for acute care treatment in emergency rooms or in hospital inpatient settings. Luft (1978b) reviews the data related to use of preventive services and finds that one group of studies supports the hypothesis that enrollees in HMOs use more preventive services whereas another group of studies demonstrates that HMO enrollees and FFS subscribers receive about the same number of preventive services. But, he argues, the findings are not inconsistent because the crucial distinction is not HMO versus FFS but whether or not the preventive services are covered by insurance. In the few studies in which conventional insurance covers preventive visits there appears to be no difference in utilization among HMO and FFS enrollees. He concludes that "the greater use of preventive services by HMO enrollees appears to be attributable to their better financial coverage, not the preventive care ideology" (p. 163). A recent study by Marcus (1981) found that HMO members (all of whom had insurance covering health maintenance examinations) reported more recent physical examinations than FFS subscribers. Luft (1980) cautions that it is not clear that having more preventive services is necessarily better and notes the current skepticism regarding the efficacy of many preventive services, such as tests, screenings, and checkups.

An important issue for families with chronically ill children is that an HMO is not likely to include among its staff a physician with specialty training in relatively rare childhood diseases. At various times during the course of a chronic illness, the HMO will need to refer a child to a physician outside the plan. Because the HMO pays for all such referrals, there is an obvious incentive for the organization to handle as much medical care as possible within its own organization. This is an issue about which we know very little and that future research must address.

Studies of *hospital* utilization have yielded fairly consistent results. Summarizing the research findings in a review of studies published since 1950, Luft (1978a) notes that hospitalization among HMO enrollees is about 30 percent lower than it is among the conventionally insured populations. Lower rates of hospitalization are attributable to lower admission rates rather than to differences in average length of stay. HMOs tend to reduce admissions equally in the surgical and nonsurgical categories. The data neither support nor disprove the expectation that HMOs reduce discretionary admissions or procedures. In a later article, Luft (1980, P. 294) suggests two possible explanations for lower hospitalizations among HMOs: "(1) HMO physicians have different practice patterns, so new enrollees immediately experience less hospitalizations; or (2) people joining HMOs are less likely to use hospital services." However, some analysts speculate that Luft's first explanation is correct—that HMOs provide an appropriate level of hospitalization and that fee-for-service physicians, with economic incentives to hospitalize, provide too much (Blumberg, 1980).

Even more important are the findings regarding repeated hospitalizations for the same disease. In a study of six different types of hospitals, Zook, Savickis, and Moore (1980) found that repeated hospitalizations for the same disease represented more than half of the hospitalizations and about 60 percent of total hospital charges. The authors (p. 456) do not differentiate by method of funding but do suggest that, in any changes in major-risk health insurance, attention should be paid "to the use of premium design and co-insurance to channel recidivist patients down the most cost-effective, long-term track of care," and that "financial incentives in health insurance should be structured to discourage costly hospital readmissions when preventive programs and low-cost alternatives are available." Thus, although HMOs have lower hospital admission rates for the general population, we do not know whether this holds true for the chronically ill or whether HMO or FFS systems are more like to devise alternatives to readmissions. However, Luft (1981) notes that HMOs are more likely to emphasize use of outpatient facilities and are more likely to have home-care departments, both of which are important for the management of chronic illness.

In sum, we can say that when compared with FFS patients, HMO enrollees are likely to have fewer hospitalizations (but about the same average length of stay) for both surgical and nonsurgical categories, about the same number of illness-related ambulatory visits, and a slightly greater number of preventive care visits. Because the utilization data comparing the two systems do not disaggregate for persons with chronic illness, we do not know whether these findings hold for them. We do know, however, that persons with chronic illnesses are more likely to be represented in HMOs than in FFS systems.

What, then, are the implications of the data for costs to families? Again, we can only talk about the costs to families in general because there are no separate data for families with chronically ill children. Luft (1981) concludes that average out-of-pocket costs per person and per family are lower in PGPs and to a lesser extent in IPAs than costs for Blue Cross–Blue Shield subscribers, and that HMO enrollees have substantially lower risk of large expenses. Moreover, although there is substantial variation among various plans, prepaid group practices have the lowest total (premium plus out-of-pocket) costs. The mix of services is more heavily weighted toward ambulatory care in prepaid group practices, and the lower total costs are attributed, as we have seen, to lower hospitalization rates. Overall costs in HMOs are 10 to 40 percent lower than in comparable FFS systems. The cost savings are attributable to lower utilization rates rather than lower costs per unit of service. This should not be surprising because HMOs operate within the environment of the larger medical care system and must pay the same for laboratory tests and so on.

Quality of Care. It appears that the cost savings achieved by HMOs have come from reductions in number of services. What is unclear, however, is whether there is an effect, either positive or negative, on quality of care or on health status.

One problem in establishing such a linkage is that many studies that compare HMOs and FFS systems examine health status—such as restricted activity days or the presence of chronic or acute conditions—as a function of *who joins* what kind of health care system. However, health status is rarely a measure of *outcome* of HMO or FFS systems, both because of the wide variation in the definition of health status and lack of agreement about efficacy of services. S. Katz and J. Papsidero (personal communication to the author, 1982) suggest that for persons with chronic conditions, health status should be defined in functional terms because the goals of care are restoration and maintenance of function, in contrast to cure. Functional status includes the dimensions of diagnosis, disability, and activities of daily living. Theoretically, functional assessment could provide information about the effectiveness of care over time.

If we assume, for the purpose of this discussion, that health status is related to quality of care, then Luft's (1981) review of studies assessing quality of care is helpful. The evidence suggests that HMOs are at least as good as FFS providers. HMO physicians tend to have better qualifications than the average FFS physician. Some potential advantages of group practice, such as informal consultations, seem to be utilized about the same in HMOs as in other settings.

Process measures are useful in assessing recorded procedures (such as appropriateness of laboratory tests and prescriptions) but omit interpersonal processes (such as physician-patient interactions). Luft notes that HMOs tend to get higher scores on process measures, but when all patients have the same financial coverage, the difference disappears. Moreover, large-group FFS practices seem to score equally well.

Another outcome Luft reviews is consumer satisfaction. Although HMOs do score lower on such measures as information transfer, humaneness, and continuity of provider, he interprets these findings with caution. Says Luft, "Members like the short waits but are dissatisfied with the amount of time it takes to get an appointment, not seeing their usual physician for urgent visits, and feeling that there is not enough doctor-patient communication and warmth" (p. 298). He notes that despite these reservations, HMOs have tended to increase their market share, only a small proportion of those who disenroll do so because they are dissatisfied (most disenroll because of job changes), and consumers' behavior suggests that many have found HMOs to be the best option for them.

Particularly relevant for this project is continuity of care, a component of medical care that is especially important for chronically ill persons who require repeated visits to one or more providers. The findings are difficult to interpret because of the ambiguity of the concept: does continuity mean obtaining care from one place or one physician? Luft suggests that "it appears that there is less continuity of care among PGP members, particularly if this is measured by the identification of a single physician. However, a group may provide better continuity in terms of record transfer when specialists are required or urgent treatment is needed" (p. 270).

To this point, we have focused on the differences between prepayment and fee-for-service funding mechanisms. It is obviously difficult to separate the effects of funding mechanisms from other organizational characteristics. Certain behaviors, such as informal consultation among physicians and referrals to appropriate specialists, may be more a function of group practice than prepayment. When we do isolate the effects of funding mechanisms, we find in prepaid systems reduced hospitalizations and somewhat increased ambulatory and preventive care services, although unit costs are the same. But increased use of ambulatory and preventive care services is very much dependent on their being covered by insurance; when they are covered for fee-for-service patients, the differential disappears. One tentative conclusion is that in many areas, utilization is less a function of prepayment than whether the service is reimbursable. This conclusion has interesting implications for third-party funding of optimal health care services for chronically ill children.

Policy Issues

The Larger Context. The critical policy issues are how well funding of health care through private insurance meets the needs of chronically ill children and how the system might be improved. We can address these issues more appropriately if we consider first some of the larger issues involving the health care system as a whole. The dramatic increase in the cost of health care in the last ten years has stimulated close examination by economists and policy makers of the relationship between third-party reimbursement and costs. Although many factors, such as inflation, new technology, and an aging population, contribute to increased spending for health care, observers increasingly suggest that the most important cause of the increase is a complex of incentives inherent in our system for financing health care. Enthoven (1980, pp. xvii, xviii) summarizes the incentives of doctors and hospitals in this way:

> The "fee-for-service," or piecework, system by which we pay doctors rewards the doctor with more revenue for providing more, and more costly, services, whether or not more is necessary or beneficial to the patient. Physician gross incomes account for only about 18 percent of total health care spending (16 percent if the laboratory tests they order are excluded), but physicians control or influence most of the rest. They admit people to the hospital, order tests, and recommend surgery and other costly procedures. Yet our system assigns them very little responsibility for the economic consequences of their decisions. Most physicians have no idea of the costs of the things they order—and no reason to care.
>
> Hospitals are paid on the basis of either their costs or charges based on costs. The net effect is that more costs means more revenue. Those who make the decision concerning the use of hospital services, doctors and insured patients, have no reason to be cost-conscious. Most medical bills are paid for by "third-party payors," insurance companies and government agenies that pay the bills after the care has been given and the costs incurred. And they are powerless to control costs. Most consumers' insurance gives them free choice of doctor and hospital and little or no incentive to seek out a less costly doctor or style of care. Their personal insurance premium will be the same whether they go to the most economical or the most extravagant doctor. This system embodies many cost increasing incentives and virtually no rewards for economy.

The argument is, very simply, that the present system creates incentives for overdoing things and that it creates incentives for over-use of high techology.

A frequently cited reason for lack of incentives to control costs is the practice of retrospective reimbursement whereby insurers reimburse hospitals and physicians on the basis of costs incurred. One response has been prospective reimbursement, which, when applied to hospitals, means that insurers negotiate daily rates for the coming year. Today approximately thirty prospective reimbursement programs run by state agencies, Blue Cross plans, or state hospital associations are in operation. The evidence suggests that when prospective reimbursement is mandatory and when programs have been in place for sufficient time to become institutionalized, prospective reimbursement can reduce hospital expenditures by as much as 3 to 6 percent (Steinwald and Sloan, 1980; Biles, Schramm, and Atkinson, 1980; Coelen and Sullivan, 1981). In order to curb the inflationary effects of retrospective reimbursement of physicians, some have suggested disclosure of communitywide and individual fees (that establish the usual, customary, and reasonable charges awarded physicians) (Delbanco, Meyers, and Segal, 1979). Prepaid plans that compensate physicians on a capitation or salary basis more clearly represent prospective reimbursement and have achieved cost savings primarily because of lower hospital admissions.

The difficult policy question is what is the appropriate amount of care? Although many have addressed the issue of incentives that allegedly lead fee-for-service physicians to direct higher levels of physician and hospital utilization than physicians who are reimbursed on a capitation or salary basis, most agree it is difficult to determine whether there are too many operations, tests, and procedures under fee-for-service systems or whether there are too few in prepaid plans.

Nonetheless, as we have seen, the trend is for expanded insurance coverage, particularly in group policies. Several factors have contributed to the growth of insurance coverage. Tax subsidies—both the itemized deduction and the employer exclusion—have encouraged insurance coverage by effectively lowering the price of health insurance to the consumer (Feldstein and Friedman, 1977; Greenspan and Vogel, 1980). This is an important policy issue because the federal subsidy of health insurance through the tax system represents an enormous public investment, which for the period 1975 to 1979 grew at a more rapid rate than either Medicare or Medicaid (Wilensky, 1982).

A growing body of literature relates health insurance to the demand for health care. The concept of moral hazard comes into play here; the idea is that when a risk is insured, the likelihood of the event occurring increases. With respect to health insurance, if the health risk is insured, there is greater likelihood that the patient or physician will seek to treat the condition. The net effect of health insurance is to reduce the cost of covered services to the insured consumer. It is generally agreed that increased health insurance coverage leads to increases in demands for health services and an increase in the total amount of care consumed (Phelps, 1977; Greenspan and Vogel, 1980). Similarly, Newhouse (1978) concludes that the demand for medical services increases as out-of-pocket payments for the service fall.

In addition, insurance coverage of specified medical procedures leads to incentives to choose more costly hospital-based forms of care, which are covered, and possibly reduced incentives to seek preventive care, which is not covered (Phelps, 1977). Thus, insurance coverage may have the unintended effect of skewing health care resources toward more costly procedures. As we have seen, insurers have begun to address this problem by inclusion of less costly outpatient care and ambulatory surgery in benefit plans and a few have included coverage of preventive care. Although some believe that insurance coverage of ambulatory services decreases hospitalization and thus decreases overall costs, the evidence does not confirm this (Newhouse, 1978) and the issue remains unsettled. Similarly, the effectiveness of deductibles and coinsurance in containing costs and restraining unnecessary utilization of health care is a matter of some debate. Deductibles serve to hold down the cost of processing claims by removing from the insurance system routine or minor expenditures. Once the deductible is satisfied, however, there is no incentive not to use a health service. Enthoven (1980) and others have suggested that coinsurance does not work very well in suppressing demand for a service. If the insurance pays 80 percent of the bill above the deductible, the consumer is likely to treat a $50 medical procedure as if it really costs only $10. An out-of-pocket payment of 20 percent will suppress demand somewhat and will probably do so more for people with low incomes than with high incomes.

Some employers have undertaken cost containment initiatives within their insurance benefit programs to inculcate cost consciousness and to change the incentives that had previously caused overutilization of the more expensive facilities. According to the Washington Business Group on Health (1977), employers are increasingly including second surgical opinions, preadmission testing, home health care, ambulatory care, and surgical center care as covered benefits. Many of these changes could work to the advantage of chronically ill children, particularly if the changes redressed the imbalance between hospital procedures and outpatient procedures. Families with chronically ill children might welcome the shift in emphasis from hospital-based care to outpatient or home care—which may be the preferred method for many children having chronic illnesses.

In recent times, policy makers have evidenced considerable interest in cost containment and, following the regulatory approaches of the 1970s, legislative attention has turned in the early 1980s to market strategies (often called competitive approaches) to reduce costs. Policy makers have advocated two competitive approaches, the first calling for an increase in cost sharing by the medical consumer (accomplished by providing insurance packages that are less rich or that require coinsurance) and the second calling for greater use of prepaid health plans (Ginsburg, 1981). The important question for chronically ill children in the implementation of a competitive approach is what the minimum level of benefits should be in a federally qualified plan (a plan that qualifies for federal tax exemption). The question of minimum benefits is enormously important. Omission of needed services from the minimum would place families of chronically ill children at a considerbale disadvantage if healthy families chose low-cost plans with only minimal coverage and unhealthy families were left in high-cost comprehensive benefit plans.

Improving the System for Chronically Ill Children. The discussion of broad issues affecting health care funding through private insurance provides the context for considering improvements to make the system more responsive to the needs of chronically ill children. There are several major problems in financing medical care under the current private health insurance system.

The first is that access to private health insurance is extremely uneven and depends largely on the employment status of the children's parents. Although marginally employed persons and young people are less likely to have insurance coverage of any type, an additional impediment to HMO enrollment is their general limitation to employee groups.

The second relates to comprehensiveness or adequacy of coverage. As currently structured, traditional private health insurance covers rather extensively hospital and acute care but less extensively outpatient and home-based care required for the management of the disease and the prevention of hospitalizations for medical crises. HMOs appear to cover a broader range of services. Moreover, insurance does not cover—and was never intended to cover—many nonmedical expenditures that effective management of care requires. Policy makers are understandably reluctant to expand benefits to the range of services needed by chronically ill children because of possible effects on costs. An unresolved empirical question is whether reimbursement of medical services in other settings might result in decreased hospitalization for this population and in lowered costs in the long run. HMOs appear to have reduced the rates of hospital admissions for their enrollees despite the fact that families with chronically ill members are slightly more likely to enroll in HMOs than in FFS systems, although substitution of one type of care for the other has not yet been demonstrated empirically.

A third problem relates to costs the family must bear in caring for a chronically ill child. Many fee-for-service insurance policies that cover a broad range of medical services are subject to various copayment features that are not well suited for long-term chronic illness. The result is that a family's out-of-pocket expenditures can be substantial. An unresolved policy issue is whether and to what extent families and/or society should bear such costs.

Finally, private health insurance does little to promote the coordination of care for children. Accomplishing this objective by restructuring fee-for-service health insurance is problematic.

However, private health insurance can address the first three problem areas if there is consensus: (1) that society should meet the needs of these children and (2) that private health insurance is the appropriate vehicle. Restructuring the health insurance system to meet the needs of chronically ill children will result in spreading the risk and the cost among the other health insurance consumers. Extending access to persons not now covered and increasing comprehensiveness of coverage means in effect that all insurance policyholders will bear the additional costs. Moreover, any such changes will likely include extension of benefits to the whole population, not just to chronically ill children.

Nonetheless, either federal or state regulation could accomplish the changes. The principal federal levers are provisions in the Internal Revenue Code that define a qualified plan for purposes of (1) deductibility by employers of health insurance premiums as a business expense and (2) exclusion of employer contributions to health insurance from employees' taxable income. The NAIC has suggested direction for state action with respect to access and comprehensiveness in a series of model statutes and regulations.

The organization's Model Health Insurance Act, for example, would require all health insurance carriers in a state to make available to all residents— either through employer or individual policies—a broad range of services including inpatient acute care; care for mental illness (at least twenty professional visits); drugs; services of a home health agency; services of a physical therapist or speech therapist; and other services subject to adequate cost and quality controls. The act would provide for mandatory deductibles (to contain costs) and also for limitations on out-of-pocket expenditures (to insure against catastrophic expense) not to exceed 10 percent of adjusted gross income. It limits the applicability of pre-existing condition clauses and provides for mandatory conversion privileges from group to individual policies. Group plans would be required to make coverage available for spouses and dependents if they are incapable of self-sustaining employment because of mental retardation or physical handicap. Newborn children would be eligible for coverage from the moment of birth. Complications of pregnancy would be covered. A state association would assure coverage to every individual applying for insurance, and a residual market mechanism would be established for high-risk persons. Insurance commissioners would be authorized to review rates. Some states have already enacted legislation mandating changes.

What specific structural changes will correct current deficiencies? The problem of extending *access* to persons not now covered is probably the most difficult, primarily because insurance coverage is linked so closely to employment. One approach already taken by a number of states is to mandate that group policies provide conversion privileges (to individual policies) to employees whose employment has terminated, to spouses of divorced or deceased employees, and to employees' dependent children who marry or reach the age limit under group policies. The latter provision would be especially helpful for chronically ill children who reach the age at which they are no longer covered under their parents' policies. Although purchase of individual policies is likely to be expensive and the coverage inadequate, at least the purchaser would not be subject to waiting periods or exclusion for reasons of a pre-existing condition. Another approach is to expand coverage through the workplace by mandating coverage for seasonal, part-time, and other low-wage employees—an unlikely event because from the employer's perspective the benefit-wage ratio would be unacceptably high. Employers are likely to resist such efforts. Increasing access by mandating coverage of dependents in family policies appears to be more acceptable to employers.

A different approach that is not related to the workplace involves establishment of residual market mechanisms (high-risk pools) in which all insurers doing business in a state share risks for uninsurable persons. Although there is considerable variation among such plans in the six states that have them, participating families or individuals still bear substantial costs; a typical family of four with one chronically ill child might be at risk for $2,500 or more annually in out-of-pocket expenses when premium costs, deductibles, and coinsurance requirements are considered. An interesting question—but beyond the scope of this discussion—is who bears the costs of insuring participating families and individuals? In essence, this method results in spreading the risk of insuring high health risks among all insurance purchasers in the state. To the extent that premiums are paid by employers, the cost is likely passed on to consumers. To the extent that providers are unable to collect on charges, the costs are spread among other health care consumers.

Additionally, to meet the needs of chronically ill children, changes are required to improve the *comprehensiveness* of policies. We have noted that children who are covered by conventional health insurance are likely to be reasonably well protected for high-cost inpatient acute care. Thus, one can infer that the surgical procedures required by children with congenital heart disease, cleft palate, or spina bifida are likely to be covered.

Much more problematic, however, is coverage by conventional (fee-for-service) insurance of blood products required by the boy with hemophilia, drugs and physician visits required by the child with severe asthma, and specialty clinic outpatient services required by children with various chronic illnesses. Office-based or home-based care is, on the whole, much less likely to be covered than inpatient care, and these are precisely the settings in which many chronically ill children receive ongoing care. The rationales for excluding coverage of physician office visits, home care, out-patient drugs, and care provided by nonphysicians (such as nurse practitioners and speech therapists) are that for most of the population such costs are nominal and can be met from within the family budget; the costs of processing small claims (for a physician office visit, for example) are high; and it is allegedly difficult to predict usage of such services. For the typical child, who sees a physician four or five times a year, these rationales make sense. However, chronically ill children require frequent and ongoing visits to pediatricians and multiple specialists, drug therapy, and counseling. Moreover, a family's avoidance of preventive care because of cost may result in more serious and costly episodes of illness. What is needed for these families is a benefit structure that takes long-term needs into account. In some respects, HMOs appear to offer a promising alternative for children with chronic illnesses because such things as physician office visits and care by nonphysicians are usually part of the package (although drugs sometimes are not).

Neither fee-for-service systems nor prepaid plans provide adequately for nonmedical services. Families of chronically ill children repeatedly incur many expenses for which insurance is not intended to provide; these include transportation to tertiary care facilities, home renovations, special equipment needed to manage the illness, childcare, social services, and more. Historically, insurers, employers, and individuals purchasing insurance have been reluctant to include peripheral services for which utilization is not predictable. Coverage of these services is problematic in a competitive market in which there is pressure to keep down premiums (Jones, 1981).

Related to the issue of comprehensiveness is the very important issue of *costs*. Two interrelated aspects of the problem are protecting families against very high or catastrophic expenses and changing the mix of services for improved care and potential cost savings.

In general, *catastrophic* expenses are those that are high absolutely or large relative to income. The traditional definition used in private insurance programs measures catastrophic expense in terms of large absolute expenditures incurred over a specified period of time—typically one year. According to a second definition, catastrophic medical expenditures are those that exceed a threshhold percentage of income. The U.S. Congressional Budget Office (1977) estimated that in 1978, 9 percent of all families would have out-of-pocket expenses for medical care that exceeded 15 pecent of their gross income. The causes of catastrophic expenses include long-term care (the most frequent cause), high dollar expenditures for relatively infrequent care, and high expenditures relative to family income.

The last decade has seen a great deal of interest in protection for catastrophic health expenses as evidenced by the growth in number of persons with major medical policies, the trend in major medical policies toward increased maximum benefits and limits on out-of-pocket expenditures, and consideration by Congress of providing catastrophic protection for those who do not now have it (U.S. Congressional Budget Office, 1981). Four states (Connecticut, Maine, Minnesota, and Rhode Island) have enacted catastrophic insurance requirements for insurers doing business in their states.

Criticism of the catastrophic approach has come from many quarters. Most frequent is the criticism that insuring for high-cost illness or procedures causes a reallocation of health care resources to categories of care that are already receiving a disproportionate share to the detriment of primary care services (Enthoven, 1980; Harvard Child Health Project Task Force, 1977). On the other hand, the Harvard group (p. 81) suggests, "It should be noted that catastrophic insurance could have a very significant effect in one area, namely, in its impact on the new medical technology and the treatment of severe illnesses that affect a small number of children. Hemophilia treatment and bone marrow transplants are illustrations of such highly specialized and expensive procedures. The catastrophic coverage approach, for example, provides an alternative source of funds beyond the current categorical and research support for tertiary care affecting small numbers of children. In this sense, such plans could make a valuable contribution to children's health care." Zook, Moore, and Zeckhauser (1981) note that most proposals for catastrophic health insurance are based on misconceptions about the nature of catastrophic illness. They found that, contrary to popular understanding, high-cost illness "is more often long-term and repetitive than short-term and acute" (p. 67), and that few proposals "contain incentives for providers to develop long-term care programs to reduce readmissions" (p. 73). Moreover, they argue, a benefit structure based on a one-year deductible is inequitable. Persons with chronic illness require a longer-term benefit structure; for example, a child with certain congenital abnormalities or ongoing disease might never qualify in a single year, but might require a series of treatments and hospital visits over an extended period of time. The authors suggest that if Congress considers adoption of catastrophic insurance as a means for filling an identified gap, it should incorporate incentives to providers to develop preventive and long-term management services. Clearly, families with chronically ill children require a benefit structure that limits out-of-pocket expenditures over a period longer than a single year.

In addition to limiting out-of-pocket expenditures, *changing the mix of services* offers possible improvement of care and the potential for cost savings. We know, for example, that for the general population, prepaid group practices have lower hospital admissions. But we do not know to what extent ambulatory services replace hospital services. Nor do we know if HMOs reduce the hospital recidivism rate for chronically ill persons (an important policy issue because the majority of hospital costs are associated with repetitive hospitalizations for the same illness). An interesting hypothesis to test would be whether coverage of ambulatory services or home care results in substitution of ambulatory for hospital care—a desirable result for children, both for reasons of cost containment and for reasons of humaneness. The hypothesis is reasonable in view of the fact that utilization of ambulatory and preventive care is a function of insurance coverage, irrespective of funding mechanism. It appears that HMOs are more likely to cover the services needed by chronically ill chldren than are fee-for-service systems. Moreover, as the payment mechanisms are currently structured, families are less likely to be at risk for large or unpredictable expenses in an HMO. Although substantial variations among plans exist, prepaid group practices have the lowest total (premium plus out-of-pocket) costs.

One policy option is making available prepaid plans to all families with chronically ill members regardless of the employment status of parents. An alternative is encouraging fee-for-service systems to provide coverage for a different mix of services as some are now doing. For example, some Blue Cross–Blue Shield plans are experimenting with coverage of home care as an alternative to hospitalization under certain conditions. Two foundations and twenty-one insurance companies recently announced a study of reimbursement of preventive care services. In addition, coverage by traditional insurance plans of other ambulatory services, rehabilitation, and health education (the latter typically provided by an HMO) would greatly improve care for chronically ill children. Perhaps a solution to the mix-of-services issue would be coverage of specified medical conditions rather than coverage of specified procedures.

Current trends are encouraging, at least with respect to both policies offered federal employees and some other large group plans. Increasingly, there is flexibility with respect to type of care and care provider. Some states have taken initiatives to assure that certain standards are met by policies offered for sale in their states. Although as of 1979 only two states (Connecticut and Nevada) had adopted proposals similar to the NAIC Model Comprehensive Health Insurance Act, various elements of the act have been adopted by other states.

Changing the mix of services would have some interesting implications for the final area of concern, organization of services. It is not at all clear from the evidence whether HMOs or fee-for-service systems are more likely to assure coordination of care. What is clear, at least from the family's perspective, is that there is a need for someone—physician or other provider—to perform the coordination function, which should be adequately compensated. Most chronically ill children receive at least some of their care in a specialty clinic setting, with widely varying services. We need to know more about case management under fee-for-service systems and in prepaid plans. We know very little about what happens in a prepaid group plan if the child needs the services of a specialist outside the group. Most HMOs contract with physicians outside the plan for needed services. But we need to know a great deal more about the interaction between the primary care physician at the HMO and the specialist outside the plan.

In theory, it is possible to change the configuration of private health insurance coverage to better meet the needs of chronically ill children. Indeed, the natural experiments already under way in several states can provide data and experience useful in formulating recommendations for further state action or for federal initiatives. There are two prominent advantages in relying on incremental changes in the private health insurance system. First, since the private sector assumes primary responsibility, this solution is politically acceptable to health providers and insurers and is in tune with the current mood of Congress and the administration. Second, the costs of providing benefits through the private sector are largely hidden and therefore are less susceptible to federal and state budget cuts. A disadvantage is the length of time required to implement an approach that necessitates state-by-state action. More impotant is the problem that expanding the scope of benefits to chronically ill children would entail expanding benefits to the general population—an outcome contrary to the current policy interest in developing incentives for lower cost insurance options.

Achieving improvements in access and comprehensiveness, limitations on out-of-pocket costs, and coordination of care will be a long and slow process. Some children will remain without access to adequate protection. Thus it would seem that discussion about changes in private health insurance should not preclude consideraton simultaneously of financing mechanisms and means of providing service directly targeted to chronically ill children.

References

Andersen, R., and Aday, L. A. "Access to Medical Care in the U.S.: Realized and Potential." *Medical Care*, 1978, *16*, 533–546.

Anderson, O. W. *The Uneasy Equilibrium: Private and Public Financing of Health Services in the United States, 1875–1965*. New Haven, Conn.: College & University Press, 1968.

Berki, S. E., and Ashcraft, M.L.F. "HMO Enrollment: Who Joins What and Why: A Review of Literature." *Milbank Memorial Fund Quarterly*, 1980, *58*, 588–632.

Biles, B., Schramm, C. J., and Atkinson, J. C. "Hospital Cost Inflation Under State Rate-Setting Programs." *New England Journal of Medicine*, 1980, *303*, 664–668.

Blumberg, M. S. "Health Status and Health Care Use by Type of Private Health Coverage." *Milbank Memorial Fund Quarterly,* 1980, *58,* 633-655.

Carroll, M. S. "Private Health Insurance Plans in 1976: An Evaluation." *Social Security Bulletin,* September 1978.

Caulfield, S. C., and Haynes, P. L. *The Gaps in Health Insurance Coverage: An Employers' Symposium.* Washington, D.C.: National Journal, 1980.

Coelen, C., and Sullivan, D. "An Analysis of the Effects of Prospective Reimbursement Programs on Hospital Expenditures." *Health Care Financing Review,* 1981, *2,* 1-40.

Delbanco, T. L., Meyers, K. C., and Segal, E. A. "Paying the Physician's Fee: Blue Shield and the Reasonable Charge." *New England Journal of Medicine,* 1979, *301,* 1314-1320.

Dutton, D. B. "Patterns of Ambulatory Care in Five Different Delivery Systems." *Medical Care,* 1979, *17,* 221-241.

Dutton, D. B., and Silber, R. S. "Children's Health Outcomes in Six Different Ambulatory Care Delivery Systems." *Medical Care,* 1980, *18,* 693-713.

Enthoven, A. C. *Health Plan: The Only Practical Solution to the Soaring Cost of Medical Care.* Reading, Mass: Addison-Wesley, 1980.

Feldstein, M. S., and Friedman, B. "Tax Subsidies: The National Demand for Insurance and the Health Care Crisis." *Journal of Public Economics,* 1977, 7 (2), 155-178.

Fisher, C. R. "Differences by Age Groups in Health Care Spending." *Health Care Financing Review,* 1980, *1,* 65-90.

Gaus, C., Cooper, B. S., and Hirschman, C. G. "Contrasts in HMO and Fee-for-Service Performance." *Social Security Bulletin,* 1976, *39* (5), 3-14.

Gibson, R. M. "National Health Expenditures, 1979." *Health Care Financing Review,* 1980, *2,* 1-86.

Ginsburg, P. B. "Altering the Tax Treatment of Employment-Based Health Plans." *Milbank Memorial Fund Quarterly,* 1981, *59,* 224-255.

Greenspan, N. T., and Vogel, R. J. 'Taxation and Its Effect upon Public and Private Health Insurance and Medical Demand." *Health Care Financing Review,* 1980, *1* (4), 39-46.

Harvard Child Health Project Task Force. *Toward a Primary Medical Care System Responsive to Children's Needs.* Cambridge, Mass.: Ballinger, 1977.

Health Insurance Institute. *Source Book of Health Insurance Data, 1975-76.* Washington, D.C.: Health Insurance Association of America, 1976.

Hedinger, F. R. "The Social Role of Blue Cross: Progress and Problems." *Inquiry,* 1968, *5,* 3-12.

Hennelly, V. D., and Boxerman, S. B. "Continuity of Medical Care." *Medical Care,* 1979, *17,* 1012-1018.

Hetherington, R. W., Hopkins, C. E., and Roemer, M. I. *Health Insurance Plans: Promise and Performance.* New York: Wiley, 1975.

Ireys, H. T. "Health Care for Chronically Disabled Children and Their Families." In Select Panel for the Promotion of Child Health, *Better Health for Our Children: A National Strategy.* Vol. 4. *Background Papers.* Department of

Health and Human Services publication no. 79-55071. Washington, D.C.: U.S. Government Printing Office, 1981.

Jacobs, D. P., Bauerschmidt, A. D., and Furst, R. W. "Hospital Cost Inflation and Health Insurance: A Complex Market Model." *Inquiry*, 1978, *15*, 217–224.

Jones, S.B. "Improving the Financing of Health Care for Children and Pregnant Women." In Select Panel for the Promotion of Child Health, *Better Health for Our Children: A National Strategy*. Vol. 4. *Background Papers*. U.S. Department of Health and Human Services publication no. 79-55071. Washington, D.C.: U.S. Government Printing Office, 1981.

Juba, D. A., Lave, J. R., and Shaddy, J. "An Analysis of Choice of Health Benefit Plans." *Inquiry*, 1980, *17*, 62–71.

Law, S. A. *Blue Cross: What Went Wrong?* (2d ed.) New Haven, Conn.: Yale University Press, 1976.

Luft, H. S. "How Do Health-Maintenance Organizations Achieve Their 'Savings'?: Rhetoric and Evidence." *New England Journal of Medicine*, 1978a, *298*, 1336–1342.

Luft, H. S. "Why Do HMOs Seem to Provide More Health Maintenance Services?" *Milbank Memorial Fund Quarterly*, 1978b, *56*, 140–168.

Luft, H. S. "Health Maintenance Organizations, Competition, Cost Containment, and National Health Insurance." In M. V. Pauly (Ed.), *National Health Insurance: What Now, What Later, What Never?* Washington, D.C.: American Enterprise Institute for Public Policy Research, 1980.

Luft, H. S. *Health Maintenance Organizations: Dimensions of Performance*. New York: Wiley, 1981.

MacKay, M. "The Regulation of Health Insurance." In A. Levin (Ed.), *Regulating Health Care: The Struggle for Control*. New York: Academy of Political Science, 1980.

Marcus, A. C. "Mode of Payment as a Predictor of Health Status, Use of Health Services, and Preventive Health Behavior: A Report from the Los Angeles Health Survey." *Medical Care*, 1981, *19*, 995–1010.

National Association of Insurance Commissioners. *Model Insurance Laws, Regulations and Guidelines*. Kansas City, Mo.: National Association of Insurance Commissioners, 1979.

National Center for Health Statistics. Health Interview Survey. *Hospital and Surgical Coverage—1974*. U.S. Department of Health, Education, and Welfare publication 77-1545. Washington, D.C.: U.S. Government Printing Office, 1977.

Newhouse, J. P. *Insurance Benefits, Out-of-Pocket Payments, and the Demand for Medical Care: A Review of the Literature*. Santa Monica, Calif.: Rand Corporation, 1978.

Paul v. *Virginia*, 75 U.S. 168 (1868).

Pear, R. "Job Cuts Cause Loss of Health Coverage for Over 16 Million." *New York Times*, October 31, 1982a, p. 1.

Pear, R. "Reagan Officials to Halt Aid to Prepaid Health Programs." *New York Times*, April 18, 1982b, p. 17.

Phelps, C. E. Statement Before the Subcommittee on Public Health and the Environment. In *National Health Insurance—Implications,* Hearings before the Subcommittee on Public Health and Environment, House Committee on Interstate and Foreign Commerce. Washington, D.C.: U.S. Government Printing Office, 1974.

Phelps, C. E. *Insurance Benefits and Their Impact on Health Care Costs.* Santa Monica, Calif.: Rand Corporation, 1977.

Price, D. N. "Private Industry Health Insurance Plans: Type of Administration and Insurer in 1974." *Social Security Bulletin,* 1977, *40,* 13-27.

Skolnik, A. M. "Twenty-five Years of Employee Benefits Plans." *Social Security Bulletin,* 1976, *39,* 3-21.

Steinwald, B., and Sloan, F. A. "Regulatory Approaches to Hospital Cost Containment: A Synthesis of the Empirical Evidence." Paper presented at American Enterprise Institute Conference, Washington, D.C., September 25-26, 1980.

Sudovar, S. B., and Feinstein, P. H. *National Health Insurance Issues: The Adequacy of Coverage.* Nutley, N.J.: Roche Laboratories, 1979.

Tessler, R., and Mechanic, D. "Factors Affecting the Choice Between Prepaid Group Practice and Alternative Insurance Programs." *Milbank Memorial Fund Quarterly,* 1975, *53,* 149-172.

U.S. Congressional Budget Office. *Catastrophic Health Insurance.* Washington, D.C.: U.S. Government Printing Office, 1977.

U.S. Congressional Budget Office. *Profile of Health Care Coverage: The Haves and Have-Nots.* Washington, D.C.: U.S. Government Printing Office, 1979.

U.S. Congressional Budget Office. "Protection from Catastrophic Medical Expenses: The Effects of Limiting Family Liability Under Existing Employee Insurance Programs." Staff Working paper. Washington, D.C.: Congressional Budget Office, August 1981.

U.S. Department of Commerce, Bureau of the Census. *Characteristics of Households and Persons Receiving Noncash Benefits: 1979.* Current Population Reports, Series P-23, No. 110. Washington, D.C.: U.S. Government Printing Office, 1981.

United States v. *South-Eastern Underwriters Association,* 323 U.S. 811 (1944).

Washington Business Group on Health. *A Private Sector Perspective on the Problem of Health Care Costs.* Washington, D.C.: Washington Business Group on Health, 1977.

Wilensky, G. R. "Government and the Financing of Health Care." *American Economic Review,* 1982, *72,* 202-207.

Zook, C., Moore, F., and Zeckhauser, R. "Catastrophic Health Insurance: A Misguided Prescription?" *The Public Interest,* Winter 1981, pp. 66-81.

Zook, C. J., Savickis, S. F., and Moore, F. D. "Repeated Hospitalization for the Same Disease: A Multiplier of National Health Costs." *Milbank Memorial Fund Quarterly,* 1980, *58,* 454-471.

Epilogue

James M. Perrin, M.D.
Henry T. Ireys, Ph.D.
Nicholas Hobbs, Ph.D.
May W. Shayne, A.C.S.W.
Linda C. Moynihan

This volume has examined some of the many issues raised by childhood chronic illness in America. The problems have been defined and reviewed from a wide variety of viewpoints: those of parents and children afflicted with chronic conditions, of concerned clinicians who devote their professional lives to the treatment of chronic illnesses, of educators and service personnel, of advocacy groups, and of people who have been involved in the formulation and implementation of policy at many levels. Our own review of the chapters in this volume and of the experience that underlies them has led us to develop certain principles to guide the formulation of new policies concerning childhood chronic illness in America. These principles, which are discussed in more detail in Chapter Eleven of *Chronically Ill Children and Their Families* (Hobbs, Perrin, and Ireys, 1985), should underlie policy, regardless of the specific characteristics of organizations and programs developed to improve the lives of families with chronically ill children. We conclude with a summary of recommendations for policies, the need for which becomes clear on consideration of the principles presented both in *Chronically Ill Children and Their Families* and in this volume.

Principles

First, policy should recognize the central role of families in caring for their own members. Policy should help the family of a child with a chronic illness become competent in meeting the demands of the illness. The burdens borne by families whose children have chronic illnesses will be made lighter through programs and efforts that build on the many strengths of parents and other family members and that strengthen the family's capabilities to nurture their own growing child.

Second, policy should encourage members of the larger community to contribute to the well-being of children with chronic illnesses. The commitment and responsibility of communities involve the sharing of burdens and provision of the generous support needed by the family with a chronically ill child. A community-based policy will assure that attention and resources be applied to development of services at the community level. Many families who face severe illness in their child find themselves socially isolated. A goal of public policy is to strengthen the integration of children with chronic illnesses and their families into the community and into community institutions.

Third, policy should recognize that children with chronic illnesses and their families have special needs that require attention. With few exceptions, these needs are common to all children with chronic health impairments. A review of the chapters on specific diseases in this volume indicates the sorts of specialized medical and surgical care needed by families with rare diseases and also clarifies the persistent needs of families that are repeated in each chapter. Improvements in the financing and organization of general health services for all children carry great promise for those children afflicted with a severe chronic illness. Yet these improvements alone will be insufficient to meet the special needs brought about by chronic illness. For the purposes of policy and for program development, chronically ill children should be considered as a class rather than on a disease-by-disease basis.

Fourth, policy should encourage chronically ill children to stay on task in school to the greatest degree possible. Plans developed for them should diminish the interference of the condition or its treatment with their time in school. And where illness and its treatments do interfere with school attendance, appropriate services should be available to foster the child's educational development.

Fifth, policies should ensure that a suitable array of preventive and treatment services of high quality is available to families with chronically ill children. The types of services needed by these families are broad. Society has provided best for medical and surgical treatments, although even here there are important gaps. Focusing primarily on medical and surgical services leaves unattended many of the needs of the child and family and often diminishes the benefits of the medical or surgical treatments as well. Families require access to quality general and specialty medical services, basic preventive services, and often to nutrition services, homemaker services, education about illness, respite care, and financial counseling, among many others. Policy can help families by ensuring a full range of necessary services.

Sixth, policy should ensure that services are distributed in an equitable and just fashion. Resources for the care of childhood chronic illness should be made available without regard to such nonfunctional criteria as race, sex, religion, social status, or place of residence. Especially in the case of rare disorders that need complex and often expensive treatments and care programs, development of separate programs based on the source of payment may lead to unnecessary and costly duplication of services.

Seventh, policy should encourage professional services of a highly ethical nature. Truth-telling, confidentiality, maintenance of dignity, respect for family preferences, the recognition of limits of effectiveness, and an emphasis on collaboration are key elements of the ethical provision of services. Age-appropriate involvement of children in decision making around their care is also essential. Many daily decisions in the areas of both health and education may have important, long-term effects on the child and the family. Teachers, social workers, nurses, physicians, and others must strive to recognize the ethical nature of many decisions.

Eighth, that many of the tremendous advances in the health of chronically ill children in America have resulted from a commitment to sound basic research should be recognized in public policy by continued and expanded investment in basic research. Along with continued commitment to biomedical research, attention to other areas of promise is needed; these include strengthening understanding of multiple causes of illness or handicap, exploring the processes of coping and adjustment, and defining the mechanisms by which families best receive services. A firm commitment to research requires commitment as well to training of excellent research scientists.

Proposals

The chapters in this volume suggest a number of possible reforms of policies affecting chronically ill children and their families. These incremental reforms are consonant with the principles for policy just set forth. Opportunities for improved policies exist in the organization and financing of services, in the relationship of chronically ill children with their schools, in the training of professionals, and in the stimulation of research of high quality. We provide here a summary of some of the elements of reform available to those who wish to improve the ways that families manage in the face of a child's chronic illness. These elements of reform are delineated in greater detail in Chapter Twelve of Hobbs, Perrin, and Ireys (1985), which examines carefully a series of options to improve policies affecting chronically ill children and their families. Proposed reforms are grouped into the five areas just noted. Each carries some opportunity for improving the lives of children with chronic illness and their families.

Planning and Delivering Services. The following recommendations, many of which have been implemented in part in several areas of the country, contain elements designed to improve access to needed services by children with severe illness and to strengthen the organization of services. Implementation of the recommendations could occur through a targeted project grant program to agencies. Improved efforts to regionalize care could develop through any of a number of present structures including Crippled Children's agencies, the

University Affiliated Facilities (for children with developmental disabilities), academic health centers, or the disease-specific comprehensive care programs (such as those for children with hemophilia).

Regional data systems could be developed that broadly incorporate information on (1) populations and children in need of services, (2) services provided, and (3) regional resources for chronically ill children. Data would reflect both medical and surgical care as well as educational, genetic, psychological, and nutritional services. Such data could lead to the development of areawide plans for chronically ill children, permit identification of major gaps in services, and allow monitoring of the effects of program changes.

The scope of services for each agency should be explicitly defined, and when taken together, available services should be broad enough to meet the large variety of family needs resulting from chronic illness in a child. Family service plans could be developed and monitored periodically for each family with a chronically ill child. Plans would attend to the main realms affected by chronic illness or otherwise important to the progress of the child including medical and surgical, developmental, educational, and family. Although all services will rarely be carried out by one provider, the plan would carefully allocate responsibility for each service to a specific provider. This allocation would prevent omission of a needed service because each of several providers believes another is responsible for that service (Kanthor and others, 1974).

To assure quality technological services, maintenance of the strengths of specialized care centers is essential. These centers, usually in academic health centers, need protection from the potentially negative impact of new, competitive financing proposals. Additionally, greater responsibilities for primary providers could be encouraged (McInerny, 1984). Primary providers are usually closer to families than specialists both geographically and in the sense of knowing the families, and although some are reluctant to assume the added responsibilities of working with families with chronically ill children, many provide excellent treatment, care coordination, and family support. The role of primary providers could be enhanced by (1) more equitable reimbursement for time invested in dealing with complex family and illness problems, (2) effective continuing education, and (3) improved regional communication systems that emphasize the easy transfer of information among different providers.

Case coordination is critical to improving services for chronically ill children and their families. Coordination is a function that can be carried out by any of a number of people including nurses, social workers, pediatricians, and lay counselors. That the function be carried out is far more important than who does it. Effective care coordination could improve the functional outcome for the child and family and reduce unnecessary utilization of expensive medical services. Reasonable reimbursement for care coordination would recognize and affirm the central importance of this service.

Financing of Services. In recent years, policy makers have considered a number of new approaches to the financing of health care. The approaches attempt to meet varying and sometimes competing policy goals: assuring that citizens have access to basic health care, assuring that ruinous cost is avoided, and at the same time, controlling the costs and expenditures in the health care sector. For families with chronically ill children, it is important that policy recognize that chronicity means a financial outlay year after year (not just for the acute episodes that typify most childhood illnesses) and that the high cumulative expenses can ruin families financially. Furthermore, regardless of the parent's employment or economic status, all families with severely chronically ill children require access to financing for a broad range of services. Following are observations on both current and proposed approaches to financing health care as they affect chronically ill children and their families.

Private, fee-for-service health insurance programs could benefit more children with chronic illnesses (see Chapter Forty-Two). Access to the relatively broad coverage of group policies is linked to employment, mainly in large firms. Some of the remedies for exclusion from group insurance policies that could benefit many chronically ill children and their families include extension of coverage to low-wage or seasonal employees, conversion privileges from group to individual policies, and mandatory coverage of dependents in family policies. Conversion privileges for dependent children would be especially helpful to chronically ill children who reach the age at which they are no longer covered by their parents' policies. Several states have mandated high-risk pools in which all insurers in a state share the risks for uninsurable persons; these pools can provide protection to chronically ill children and their families although they entail high annual out-of-pocket expenditures for premiums, deductibles, and co-insurance.

Because most insurance plans are oriented to high-cost hospital inpatient care, they tend to cover only medical services or services offered under the direction of a physician. They seldom contain incentives for preventive and primary care; nor do they cover the broad range of special services and materials, such as outpatient drugs, tests, and home equipment, that are essential for chronically ill children. Fee-for-service insurance systems need encouragement to provide coverage for an expanded mix of services, as some are now doing (for example, recent experimentation with coverage of home care as an alternative to hospitalization). Coverage of ambulatory services, rehabilitation, and health education would improve the care of chronically ill children and might prevent costly hospitalizations. Insurance through prepaid group practices rather than fee-for-service plans might provide a broader mix of services, contain aggregate health care costs, and protect families financially. Access to the highly specialized care required by many chronically ill children needs to be assured in capitation programs.

Catastrophic health insurance, which during recent years has been proposed in a number of forms as one type of national health insurance, could be modified to improve the lives of chronically ill children in several ways (Chapter Forty-Two). Criticism of catastrophic health insurance centers on the likelihood that it will cause reallocation of health resources away from preventive care to higher-cost care, hospitalization, and other services that already receive disproportionate coverage. However, if properly structured, catastrophic insurance could provide valuable protection to chronically ill children and their families. Catastrophic plans have tended to address the costs of a catastrophic event rather than solving the equally serious problem of expensive chronic illnesses. For example, most plans provide reimbursement only after sixty days of hospitalization during a year, a benefit that excludes the large number of chronically ill children whose days in the hospital may be fewer per year, but whose hospitalizations recur year after year. In addition, most of the proposed plans exclude reimbursement for outpatient drugs, often necessary in large and costly quantities for chronically ill children. An alternative provision would be to apply all medical expenses toward a single deductible amount.

The enormous financial burden on families of children with chronic illnesses is not reflected in calculating a single year's expenses. Their large expenses persist year after year. Most catastrophic insurance proposals are directed to cushioning a family against having savings wiped out by a single event. An alternative policy would be longer deductible periods, of perhaps several years. An income-based deductible that limits expenditures on medical care to between 10 and 15 percent of income would be especially important for young adults with severe chronic illnesses. These young people are frequently unable to obtain full-time employment, yet they do not qualify for Medicaid. Income-related insurance protection would make a great difference in access to care and financial independence for them.

Recent proposals to introduce a greater element of competition into the financing of health care as a means of containing the costs are likely to have a negative effect on families with chronically ill children. Most competition proposals would tend to cluster users of many services, and therefore of high-cost care, in the higher-priced plans (Chapter Forty-Two). Adverse selection could price the type of plan needed by chronically ill children out of their reach. Therefore, if competitive approaches are to serve well the families of chronically ill children, they should include methods to share the risk very broadly. Furthermore, although competition plans place limits on the percent of income or the flat dollar amount that individual enrollees must pay out of pocket for health care before the insurance plan pays for care, the narrow definition of eligible services and their definition as related to a spell of illness mean that many services used by chronically ill children are not counted in the deductible. To meet the needs of chronically ill children, the deductible should take into account both all out-of-pocket medical expenses and the price paid for insurance premiums and might be based on a reasonable percentage of income rather than a flat dollar amount. In addition, competition approaches or the removal of tax exemptions for insurance premiums could result in more circumscribed insurance plans. In sum, these approaches must be designed very carefully in order to prevent the isolation of families with predictably high medical care costs, making it more difficult for them to find adequate coverage.

Among directly funded government programs, Medicaid has unquestionably made a significant contribution to the care of chronically ill children by financing hospital and outpatient benefits previously unavailable (see Chapter Forty). However, the uneven pattern of eligibility and benefits among the states has been exacerbated by the reduction of funding during recent years. Additional reductions will only further harm poor chronically ill children and their families. Containing the costs of Medicaid through capitation plans, use of home-based care to substitute for hospitalization, and other administrative rearrangements is vastly preferable to reductions of eligibility and benefits.

Crippled Children's Services (CCS) finance a wide range of inpatient and outpatient services through various arrangements (Ireys, Hauck, and Perrin, 1985). Each state CCS program has a unique service profile and wide discretion in selecting the conditions to be treated. In light of the special services the CCS provides for chronically ill children, maintaining the funding level of the CCS program within the Maternal and Child Health Block Grant is of great importance. Modification of CCS in the direction of developing areawide comprehensive services for chronically ill children and their families would distribute CCS benefits more effectively and equitably.

Schools. The chronically ill child whose condition only mildly or infrequently affects schooling (the child who occasionally requires medications or who needs modified gym classes, for example) is most appropriately served by the regular education system, utilizing counseling and school health services (see Chapters Thirty and Thirty-One). To ensure that the chronically ill child with a mild impairment receives the necessary services within each shool district, each state could adopt explicit school health codes for chronically ill children and mandate their adoption by local school systems. Codes would include policies and procedures in at least the following areas: medication procedures, case registry, emergencies, in-service training, and case coordination.

Special education, as defined in Public Law 94–142, should not be extended or stretched for the purpose of including nonhandicapped children who are in need of related services. However, the related services portion of that law could be revised (or separated in law) to require the provision of related services to all children, handicapped or not, if the services are essential for them to participate effectively in an appropriate education program in the least restrictive environment.

More flexible policies regarding the use of homebound and hospital instruction could be adopted. The consecutive absence period currently necessary to qualify for homebound services results in many chronically ill children going without important instructional services. Schools could adopt internal policies for coordinating regular education and special education. These educational entities should not remain separate service delivery systems with different technologies and goals. In the event that related services are made available to children based upon need, the three sections (regular education, special education, and related services) must interact on a regular basis.

Within the school, training regarding chronically ill children and efforts to educate and sensitize could be directed at both school personnel and other students. Under the direction of a school nurse or physician, school personnel could receive training related to a child's specific condition. Specific curricula or techniques could be developed to explore and modify student and teacher attitudes about chronically ill children. Supportive personal counseling may be necessary for school personnel involved with the education of children with terminal or progressive illness. For proper placement and programming to occur, schools must have health-related information about chronically ill children. Appropriate functions for the physician are the transfer of information to the schools and the fostering of two-way communication between schools and physicians. In general, the physician's role as a consultant rather than an educational decision maker needs clarification.

Research. Support for the training of scientists, especially from the clinical disciplines, to develop strong quantitative and data management skills and incorporate the rapidly growing knowledge in the field of clinical epidemiology needs expansion. Much basic research in child development has come recently from the area of developmental disabilities, often with support from the National Institute of Child Health and Human Development. The skills and developmental knowledge arising from this research have major implications for chronic illnesses in childhood as well and could be applied creatively to this area.

Recent efforts to clarify the ethical considerations in research on children are commendable and outline an area of fruitful future investigation. Although the balance between ethical pursuits of new knowledge and preservation of the rights of children may be difficult to achieve, lack of attention to this problem may lead to haphazard application of potentially dangerous and unproven therapies to children.

The benefits of research should find timely application in service programs for children and families. The development of areawide, integrated programs for chronically ill children will improve the daily interaction between those doing basic research and those providing varied levels of services.

Support for basic biomedical research through the mechanism of the National Institutes of Health should remain a high priority. The investment in basic biomedical research should be balanced with an equally vigorous commitment to basic research in other critical areas including behavioral sciences and health services research (Pless and Zvagulis, 1981). A number of areas appear especially promising—for example, primary prevention of handicapping conditions and improving the process of childhood coping with chronic illness. Support for basic research in genetics; in the development of certain new technologies, such as the insulin pump for diabetes; in epidemiology; and in family coping and adjustment merit special attention.

Several arguments militate against the study of illness only among patients who appear in teaching centers or tertiary care hospitals (see Chapter Six). Population-based studies of childhood chronic illness are essential to understanding the diseases and their onset, ramifications, and treatment. Given the relative infrequency of many childhood chronic illnesses, adequate numbers of children with a specific disease may not be found in a single center. Interinstitutional research should be fostered and supported. Successful collaboration among different biomedical disciplines could be expanded to stimulate joint research ventures among such disciplines as psychology and medicine, physiology and nutritional sciences, and nursing and pediatrics.

Training of Providers. Increased attention to the problems of childhood chronic illness is needed in all health professional schools. Training should emphasize (1) longitudinal experience with the families of chronically ill children during both acute and quiescent phases, (2) collaboration among disciplines working with families, and (3) a broad definition and approach to child and family needs (see Chapter Twenty-Six). Concepts employed in the care of children with chronic handicaps are applicable to several other realms, such as geriatrics and substance abuse. Professional schools need to place special emphasis on concepts from clinical epidemiology, patterns of human adaptation, ethical decision making in long-term care, and principles of patient management as distinguished from disease cure.

Training in the family and developmental impact of childhood chronic illness is important for specialists and generalists alike. Trainees need both skill in diagnosis and treatment of disease processes and a firm understanding of the influences of genetic, familial, environmental, and social factors on chronic illness in children. To enable health professionals to promote healthier behavior and to work effectively with schools, their training must include basic understanding of nutritional concepts, psychological precepts, and educational issues.

A few exemplary training programs in childhood chronic illness could be developed. These would be interdisciplinary in faculty and trainees and would have the goals of producing new researchers in the broad area of childhood chronic illness and other graduates able to provide leadership to public programs for children with handicaps. Unlike most present programs housed in schools of public health, the new training programs could be based within academic health centers, probably in the context of organized areawide programs for families with chronically ill children.

Faculties of nursing, medicine, and related fields could expand attention to the generic problems of chronically ill children by adding new members expert in these problems, who are likely to be graduates of the new training programs. Training for research careers, both in disease-specific areas and in chronic illness in general, remains a high priority. There is increasing need for researchers well grounded in quantitative skills and methodological principles and with good backgrounds in theory applicable to the problems of sick children. Yet outside of specialty fellowships for pediatricians, opportunities for research training in chronic illnesses of childhood (especially in the areas of nursing and psychology) are limited. New interdisciplinary training programs could fill an important gap.

Continuing education for child health providers could address issues in early identification and referral of chronically ill children, new developments in management of chronic illnesses, aspects of care coordination, and advances in understanding of family coping and adaptation.

Summary

Robert Massie documents in Chapter One the strength that he and his family brought to coping with his severe chronic illness and that allowed them to meet the burdens of illness effectively. Although such strength abounds in many families, special trials faced by families with children with chronic illness are well documented in this volume. And the recommendations that flow from the descriptions offer a basis on which to improve the lives of the many chldren shadowed by chronic illness in our communities.

References

Hobbs, N., Perrin, J. M., and Ireys, H.T. *Chronically Ill Children and Their Families: Problems, Prospects, and Proposals from the Vanderbilt Study.* San Francisco: Jossey-Bass, 1985.

Ireys, H. T., Hauck, R.J.-P., and Perrin, J. M. "Variability Among State Crippled Children's Services Programs: Pluralism Thrives." *American Journal of Public Health*, 1985, *75* (4), 375–381.

Kanthor, H., and others. "Areas of Responsibility in the Health Care of Multiply Handicapped Children." *Pediatrics*, 1974, *54*, 779–785.

McInerny, T. "The Role of the General Pediatrician in Coordinating the Care of Children with Chronic Illness." *Pediatric Clinics of North America*, 1984, *31*, 199–209.

Pless, I. B., and Zvagulis, I. "The Health of Children with Special Needs." In L. V. Klerman (Ed.), *Research Priorities in Maternal and Child Health.* Washington, D.C.: U.S. Government Printing Office, 1981.

Name Index

Subject Index